9780387557793
AF788871

This book is dedicated to my wife Frieda
who renounced to innumerable hours of companionship
that I may carry out the forelying work

Arnold Soren

Arnold Soren

Arthritis and Related Affections

Clinic, Pathology, and Treatment

With 572 Figures

Springer-Verlag Berlin Heidelberg New York London
Paris Tokyo Hong Kong Barcelona Budapest

Arnold Soren, M. D., Ph. D., D. O. S.
Professor of Orthopaedic Surgery, New York University Medical Center, New York, N.Y.
University Docent of Orthopaedic Surgery, Medical Faculty of University in Vienna
Consultant in Orthopaedic Surgery, Manhattan Veterans Administration Medical Center
Adjunct Attending in Orthopaedic Surgery, Bellevue Hospital, New York, N.Y.
Former Orthopaedic Surgeon of Rheumatic Diseases Study Group, N. Y. U. Medical Center

ISBN 3-540-55 779-2 Springer-Verlag Berlin Heidelberg New York
ISBN 0-387-55 779-2 Springer-Verlag New York Berlin Heidelberg

This work is subject to copyright. All rights are reserved, whether the whole or part of the material is concerned, specifically the rights of translation, reprinting, reuse of illustrations, recitation, broadcasting, reproduction on microfilms or in other ways, and storage in data banks. Duplication of this publication or parts thereof is only permitted under the provisions of the German Copyright Law of September 9, 1965, in its current version, and a copyright fee must always be paid. Violations fall under the prosecution act of the German Copyright Law.

© Springer Verlag, Berlin Heidelberg 1993
Printed in Germany

Product Liability: The publisher can give no guarantee for information about drug dosage and application thereof contained in this book. In every individual case the respective user must check its accuracy by consulting other pharmaceutical literature.
The use of registered names, trademarks, etc. in this publication does not imply, even in the absence of a specific statement, that such names are exempt from the relevant protective laws and regulations and therefore free for general use.

Typesetting: Ernst Kieser GmbH, 8902 Neusäss
Printing and binding: Appl, 8853 Wemding
2127/3145-543210 – Printed on acid-free paper

Preface

The records of the National Health Examination Survey in 1984 indicate that about 32% of adults in the United States suffered from musculoskeletal affections. The National Arthritis Data Workshop reported in 1985 that about 35 millions of Americans had arthritis or related conditions. Wagenhaeuser [1700] similarly reported in 1969 that 30% of the central European adult population presented changes of the peripheral joints and vertebral spine. Arthritic symptoms causing incapacity in a significant percentage of the population were reported in the United Kingdom and Sweden in 1984.

All relevant statistics emphasize the high incidence and disabling effects of arthritis of various types in all countries. In view of the socioeconomic impact of the joint diseases, intensive research, experimental studies, and the use of diverse therapeutic modalities have been undertaken by the medical profession.

A treatise dedicated to the understanding of articular affections must proceed from the knowledge of the normal organic condition and of the concomitant physiology of joints. Awareness of these properties is the basis for understanding the anatomical changes and the pathological reactions elicited by internal and external factors. Correspondingly, this work, containing very instructive illustrations, endeavors to present the essential features of all known joint diseases, thus providing a basis for the effective treatment of those afflicted by arthritis.

As introduction I like to acknowledge the substantial help provided by others in preparing my text. This book was made possible by the continuous support of Theodore R. Waugh, M. D., Professor and Chairman of the Department of Orthopedic Surgery, New York University Medical Center. For the last 25 years I have had the privilege of working with Norman S. Cooper, M. D., Professor of Pathology at New York University School of Medicine and Director of Laboratories at Manhattan Veterans Administration Medical Center; in weekly conferences we discussed the histopathological features of specimens of articular tissues, and these findings have been incorporated into the present work. I am also very grateful to Prof. Dr. Waldemar Hort, Director Emeritus at the Institute of Pathology at the University of Düsseldorf, and to Prof. Dr. Joseph Thurner, Director of the Institute of Pathology at the Landeskrankenanstalten in Salzburg, both of whom provided me with instructive illustrations and histopathological tissue sections. A number of the histopathological illustrations were published previously in my volume entitled *Histodiagnosis and Clinical Correlation of Rheumatoid and Other Synovitis* (Thieme, Stuttgart, and Lippincott, Philadelphia, 1978). Figures 9 and 206 were published previously by F. Huth, A. Soren, and W. Klein in Current Topics in Pathology (56; 55, 1972) and *Archives of Pathological Anatomy* (359; 201, 1973). Figures 6 and 258 were contributed by Dr. R. Mallinger, Institute of Micromorphology at the University of Vienna. Figure 132 was contributed by Dr. A. B. Ackerman, Professor of Dermatology at New York University Medical Center, and was published by Dr. B. W. Berger et al. in *American Journal of Dermatopathology* (5; 111, 1983); tissue sections for Figures 380 and 381 were also contributed by Dr. A. B. Ackerman. Figures 207 and 208 were contributed by Dr. C. Melone. Associate Professor of Orthopedic Surgery, New York University Medical Center. Figure 267 presents the treatment of Dr. H. C. Amstutz, Professor and Director of the Department of Orthopedic Surgery, University of California in Los Angeles.

Finally, I wish to thank Mrs. D. C. Guyett (Dynamic Business Services) who by outstanding dedication and competence transformed my complicated manuscript into a clear text. The broadmindedness and support of Springer-Verlag have enabled my text and illustrations to appear in an excellent edition.

New York, NY, 1992 Arnold Soren

Contents

Anatomy and Histology of Joints

Human joints have developed along those of other vertebrates and have two main forms. The amphiarthroses are connections between two bones and are filled by dense connective tissue or fibrocartilage; examples of such connections are the intervertebral discs and the symphysis pubis. The diarthroses are contiguous, cartilage-covered bony ends, separated from each other by a capillary joint space and surrounded by a joint capsule; examples include the joints of the extremities and the temporomandibular, costovertebral and apophyseal vertebral joints.

Among the amphiarthroses those of the vertebral column require special description because of their particular structure and frequent degenerative changes. Between each two vertebrae is interposed an intervertebral disc (Fig. 1) attached by its fibers to the cartilage of the vertebral plates. These fibers penetrate into the osseous vertebral end plates and anchor the intervertebral disc firmly onto the two adjacent vertebral bodies. At its circumference, the disc merges with the anterior and posterior longitudinal ligaments and with the oblique intervertebral ligaments (Fig. 2). Structurally the disc is composed mainly of dense fibrous and fibrocartilaginous tissue (Fig. 3), the annulus fibrosus, whose plump fibrocytes and chondrocytes lie in a matrix of short fine filaments. The interstitial matrix is rich in polysaccharides and contains longer and thicker collagen fibers which run interstitially. The central fibers of the annulus course around the nucleus pulposus. The latter is a soft tissue, composed of large vesicular cells and a few collagen fibers interspersed in a mucinous ground substance. Mankin [1019] emphasized the importance of the high water content (up to 65%–70%) of the annulus fibrosus in comparison with other fibrous structures. Besides its collagen content of 50% of dry weight, glycosaminoglycans, chondroitin sulfate, and keratan sulfate are present in high proportions. The nucleus pulposus has a higher water content (up to 88%) and a higher glycosaminoglycan content but a lower collagen content (20%–30% of the dry weight). By virtue of its rich content and the arrangement of the fibers of its annulus, the intervertebral disc holds the vertebrae together. On the other hand, because of its water content and the great elasticity of its nucleus pulposus, the disc also keeps the vertebrae apart. The disc bears the pressure exerted on the vertebral column by the weight of the body and serves as an impact absorber of the mechanical stresses imposed on the vertebral column during its functioning [192].

The diarthrodial joints, by contrast, are characterized essentially by the presence of a patent joint space which separates the epiphyseal ends from each other (Fig. 4). These bones have acquired the property to function as articular ends by virtue of their convex or concave configurations, which enable them to fit more or less congruently with each other (Fig. 4).

The articular ends are further suited to this reciprocal adaptation by an ontogenetically persisting cover or cap of hyaline cartilage (Fig. 4), which varies in thickness both within each joint from joint to joint, and from site to site. The cartilage cover of the acetabulum and femoral head is 3–4 mm thick, that of the patella is 2–4 mm thick, on the tibial condyles it is 1.1–1.4 mm thick, and in the interphalangeal joints of the fingers it is 0.08–0.15 mm thick.

The articular hyaline cartilage has a smooth, shiny, white or bluish-white surface. However, on histological examination [567, 1284] the articular cartilage pre sents furrows and ridges, which have been interpreted [604] as the results of shrinking during histochemical processing, aging or pathological alterations. Histological examinations [603, 604, 1589] further disclose that the articular cartilage has a relatively small proportion of chondrocytes (Fig. 5). The cytoplasm of these cells contains fine granules, a few vacuoles, and a few lipoid globules. Their centrally located nucleus is oval or elongated and has an indented outline; it contains a nucleolus and granular nucleoplasm. On the basis of the typical arrangement and shapes of the chondrocytes, four zones may be discerned in the articular cartilage (Fig. 5). (a) In the tangential zone adjacent to the joint cavity, the chondrocytes and their nuclei are elongated, lying close to each other and with their long axes parallel to the surface. (b) Directly beneath follows the transitional zone, whose chondrocytes are roundish or ovoid, have similarly shaped nuclei, and

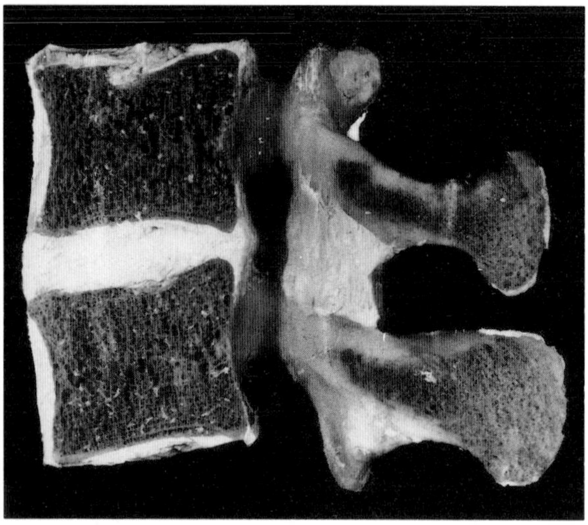

Fig. 1. The bodies of the vertebrae articulate and are held together by the intervertebral discs and by the ligaments. Their apophyseal processes also articulate with each other

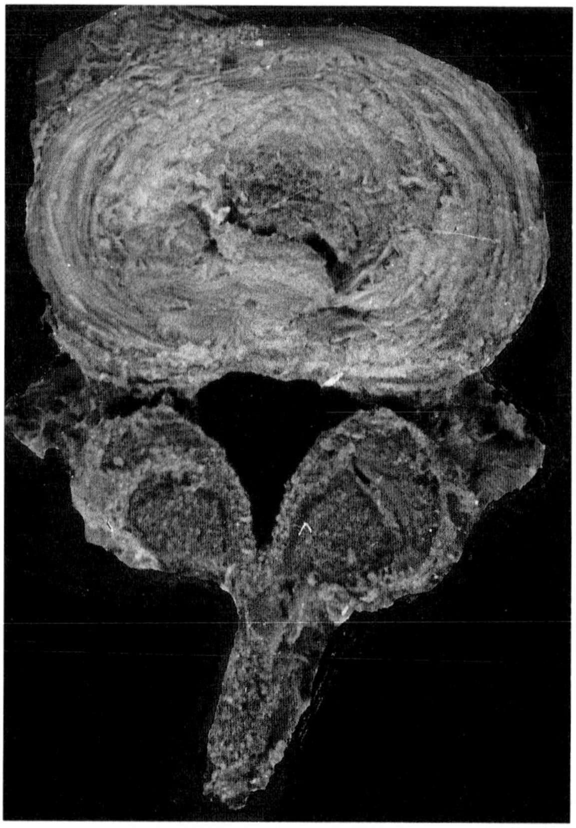

Fig. 2. The intervertebral disc (from a 45-year-old man) fully covers the vertebral body but is disrupted by an extensive central dehiscence and two shorter clefts. The apophyseal joints are well maintained

are irregularly and loosely distributed. (c) In the subjacent radial zone, the chondrocytes are round and generally arranged in vertical columns of six to ten cells. In cartilage covers of greater thickness, the columnar zone contains at its base one to three layers of irregularly positioned chondrocytes, the subzone of resting or mother cells. (d) The deepest zone is that of calcified cartilage, discernible by its darker hue; its chondrocytes, fewer in number and irregularly shaped, are scattered, and many of them have deeply wrinkled, dense, clumpy, fragmented, or no nuclei – an indication of local disintegration processes. This zone is demarcated from the radial zone by the tidemark or provisional calcification line (Fig. 5), an intensely stained, slightly wavy line which can be distinguished from the subchondral cortical bone by its lamellar structure and different staining. While degenerative alterations may also be observed occasionally in the nuclei of the chondrocytes of the upper three zones, other changes are regularly observed in most chondrocytes of all four zones, especially those of the transitional and columnar zones. These chondrocytes individually often present a broad indentation in their outline which partly separates them from the immediately pericellular matrix. The empty space or "lacuna" is formed by shrinking and retraction of the cell membrane caused by the chemical processing for light-microscopic examination and is thus an artifact [604, 1589]. No lacunae are observed with glutaraldehyde fixation.

Electron-microscopic examination [603, 604, 1012, 1079, 1080, 1589] discloses chondrocytes with jagged outlines caused by small processes of the cell membrane, mostly in the chondrocytes of the middle rows (Figs. 258). Their cytoplasm contains a rough endoplasmic reticulum which encloses spaces termed cisternae; some of these are filled with granules. Additionally, several larger vacuoles and small vesicles are found, especially close to the parallel lamellae composing the Golgi apparatus (Fig. 6). Fine filaments and a small number of mitochondria are scattered throughout. The material of the round or ovoid nucleus may sometimes present densification or fragmentation, with its particles scattered in the cytoplasm and in the matrix. These degenerative changes are much more frequent in the calcified zone, which is impregnated with pericellularly and interstitially deposited calcium salts.

With their characteristic distribution in the articular cartilage, the chondrocytes lie in a preponderantly intercellular matrix (Figs. 5, 6). This appears homogeneous under normal conditions [1639]; it stains slightly basophilic with hematoxylin-eosin-phloxin-safran and also stains metachromatically with toluidine blue, Alcian blue, and other polychromatic stains. Rosenberg

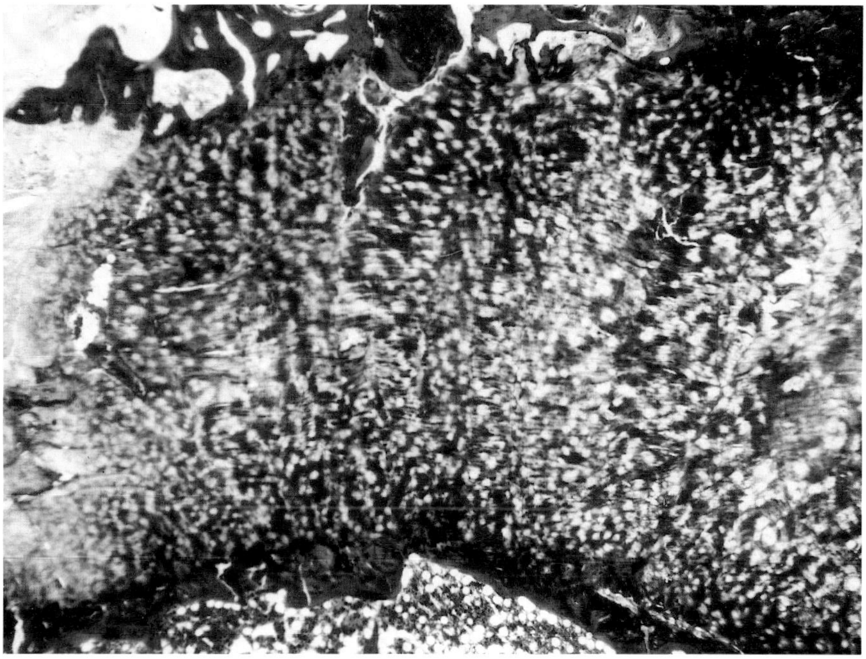

Fig. 3. The annulus fibrosus of the intervertebral disc consists of large chondrocytes which lie in an abundant matrix with pericellular collagen fibers. The ground substance is rich in mucopolysaccharides. The nucleus pulposus is not exposed

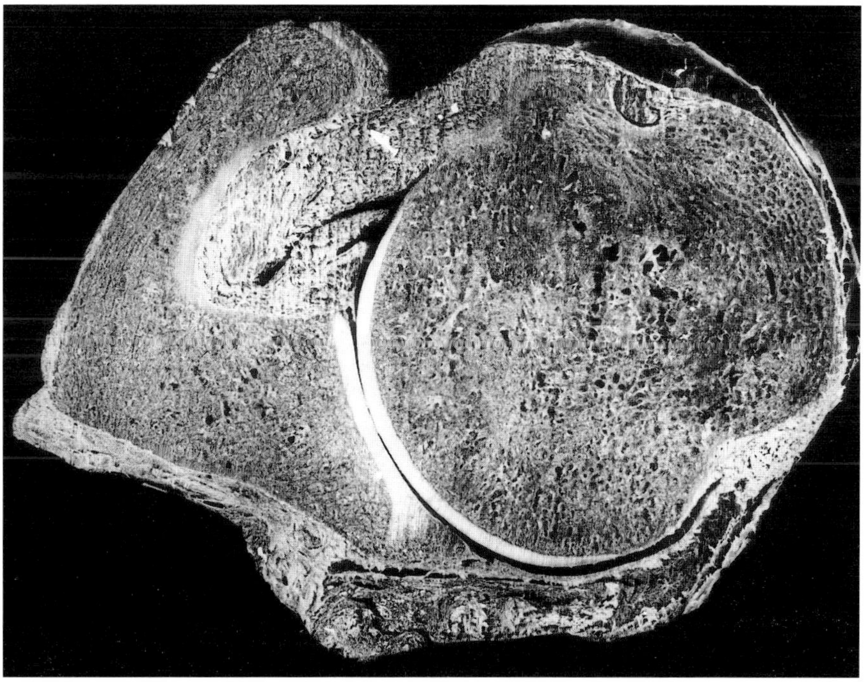

Fig. 4. Horizontal section through a shoulder joint. The epiphyses of the scapula and humerus merge on their contact surfaces with a thick layer of articular cartilage, becoming articular ends. These are surrounded and held together by the joint capsule

[1351, 1353] recommended staining with safranin, a cationic dye, which binds to the anionic groups of mucopolysaccharides. The interstitial matrix consists of 35%–40% ground substance and collagen in almost equal parts of the organic material and of 60%–65% freely exchangeable water [157, 178, 1019]. The material essentially responsible for the staining and for the physical properties of the ground substance and partly also for the properties of the articular cartilage are the proteoglycans [878, 1680]. These consist of a protein core to which are linked polysaccharides, termed glycosaminoglycans, which represent 18%–20% of the dry weight of the articular cartilage. The glycosaminoglycans are composed of a small proportion of hyaluronic acid, consisting of glucuronic acid and acetylglucosamine, and of a larger proportion of both chondroitin sulfates, consisting of hexosamine and glucuronic acid, and keratan sulfate, consisting of hex-

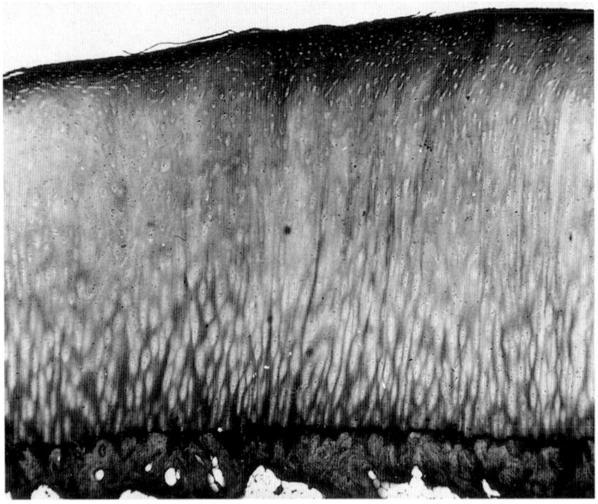

Fig. 5. Normal articular cartilage. The cells have different arrangements and shapes in the superficial, transitional, columnar and calcified zones. Collagen fibers ascend from the calcified zone and wind between the cartilage cells

osamine and galactose [23, 157, 596, 1019, 1350, 1395, 1689, 1778]. Mallinger et al. [1012] used staining and histochemistry to study the distribution of glycosaminoglycans in normal hyaline cartilage; chondroitin sulfate was the most widely distributed glycosaminoglycan, and keratan sulfate was observed intracellularly and in the inner territorial matrix. The important feature in the chemical structure of these glycosaminoglycans is that their repeating units carry closely spaced and negatively charged groups [1352]. In individuals of advanced age or with traumatic defects of the cartilage, the proteoglycans are substituted by dermatan sulfate proteoglycans [1639]. These are formed of smaller aggregates of proteoglycans and are less effectively enmeshed by the surrounding network of collagen fibers [1352].

Special stains [1350, 1352] and electron-microscopic examinations [603, 1035, 1036, 1082] of normal articular cartilage disclose that the intercellular matrix, in addition to the ground substance, consists of a similar proportion of collagen fibers, with their characteristic length and transverse bands. Most of these fibers are thick and run intercellularly in various directions [1036]. In contrast, the directly pericellular fibers are very thin and form a loose meshwork [1082]. The latter structure permits pericellular accumulation of a slight amount of ground substance under physiological conditions and of a greater amount under pathological conditions. This produces the picture of a pericellular halo (Figs. 250, 465) in some tissue sections. On the other hand, the dense and thick intercellular collagen fibers, while crossing each other in various directions, also manifest a distinct course (Fig. 5) within the articular cartilage [1156]. Benninghoff [118] pointed out that the intercellular fibers follow a specific, function-

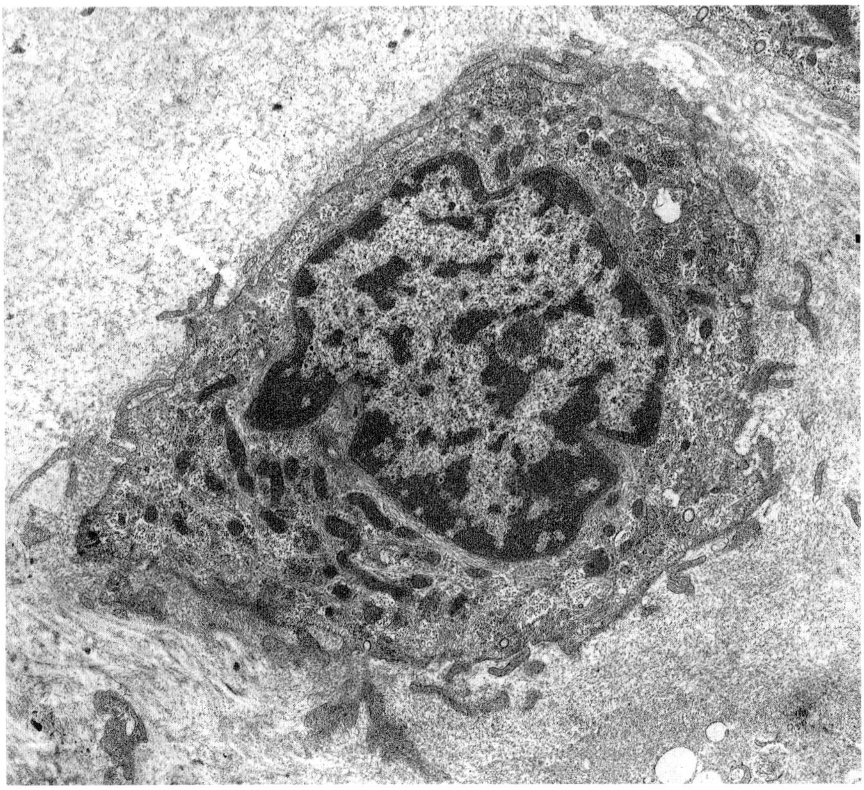

Fig. 6. Chondrocyte from normal tibial condyle contains mitochondria, rough endoplasmic reticulum, and glycogen in the cell body. Its nucleus presents moderate chromatin condensation and secretory vacuoles

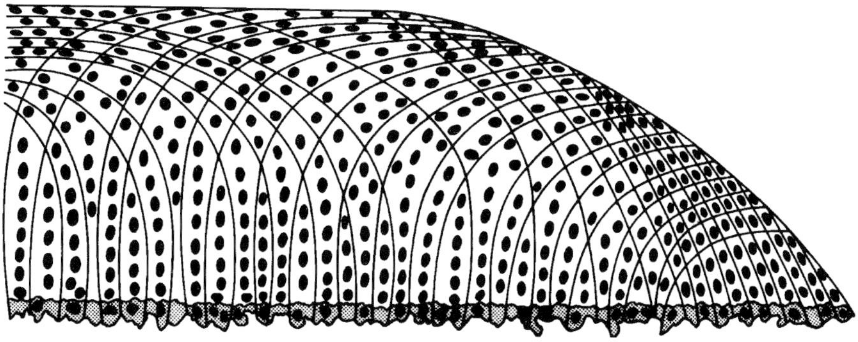

Fig. 7. Modification of the construction scheme by Benninghoff. The differences in arrangements and shapes of the cartilage cells are presented as well as the arcading course of the interstitial fibers

ally purposeful course (Fig. 7). This course can be seen in the interstitial matrix with routine light microscopy generally under circumstances associated with decomposition of the overall ground substance (Figs. 241, 242, 397, 416). Anchored in the calcified cartilage and subchondral bone, the intercellular fibers rise vertically toward the surface. There they run for a short stretch along the surface and then curve backward vertically toward the calcified cartilage and subchondral bone (Fig. 7). Pursuing such a course in all planes of the articular cartilage, these fibers have the spatial arrangement of an inverted U shape and cross each other a number of times. This leads to an overall surrounding network which stabilizes each single chondrocyte on pressure from all sides and accounts for a significant proportion of the mechanical properties of the articular cartilage [118].

The articular cartilage thus attains a differentiated and characteristic structure by the intimate fusion of these three structural elements: (a) cartilage cells shaped differently according to their position, (b) an encompassing network of fibers, and (c) the interposed ground substance. This makes the articular cartilage fit of coping with the mechanical stresses of pressure, shear, and friction. The complex composition of the articular cartilage explains both its physical valency and its lack of capacity for repair. Like other highly specialized tissues, the articular cartilage lacks the ability to regenerate, especially under conditions of excessive wear, unequally distributed mechanical forces, and toxically or enzymatically inflicted damage. Thus physical and chemical alterations of the joint fluid also have here an influence [1428].

The joint fluid, also termed synovial fluid, is normally clear, slightly yellowish, and viscous [306]. Depending on the extent of the joint cavity, it amounts to 0.2–4.5 ml. The synovial fluid has a rather constant composition and contains about 94.8% water and 5.1%–5.2% solid substances. These include salts and albumin in the same concentrations as in the blood, globulin (owing to its larger molecules) in a smaller concentration than in the blood, and 0.9%–1.0% mucin. The latter is the characteristic constituent of the synovial fluid [1498] and consists of protein and mucopolysaccharides, among which hyaluronic acid, composed of glucosamine and glucuronates, is the essential substance. After precipitation of the mucopolysaccharides by an inorganic acid the synovial fluid loses its viscosity and assumes the consistency of blood plasma. Physiologically, the mucopolysaccharides thus convey the average viscosity from 90 to 140 units as determined by the Ostwald viscometer to the synovial fluid and enable it to adhere to the articular surfaces and to serve as a lubricant between them. Because of their high molecular weight the mucin particles cannot diffuse out from the joint cavity and remain within the joint fluid, securing its viscosity. A decrease in viscosity is liable to impair the lubricating function of the synovial fluid and to permit attritional friction of the cartilaginous surfaces. Histochemical and electron-microscopic studies [418, 914, 1443, 1497, 1498] indicate that the liquid part, the crystalloids, and most of the organic compounds of the synovial fluid derive from the blood by transudation through the interstices of the blood vessels and synovial membrane. However, the specific component of the synovial fluid, the mucin, is produced by the synovial membrane.

The innermost layer of the joint capsule – termed synovial membrane, synovialis, or synovium – represents the lining of the joint cavity [1430, 1543]. This membrane is flat in most areas of any joint but has folds in areas characteristic for some joints. The thickness of the synovial membrane thus varies both according to the site within the joint and from joint to joint. Light-microscopic examination [603, 1543] discloses that the most superficial tissue of the synovial membrane consists of a single row of cells, the synoviocytes (Fig. 8). These are aligned with their longitudinal diameters parallel to the surface; they appear ovoid and lie close to each other, with the subjacent tissue being of the areolar type; they appear flatter and with wider interspaces where they overlie adipose or dense fibrous tissue. The synoviocytes have a smaller diameter of 5–9 μm as well as a larger one of 9–14 μm and cytoplasmic

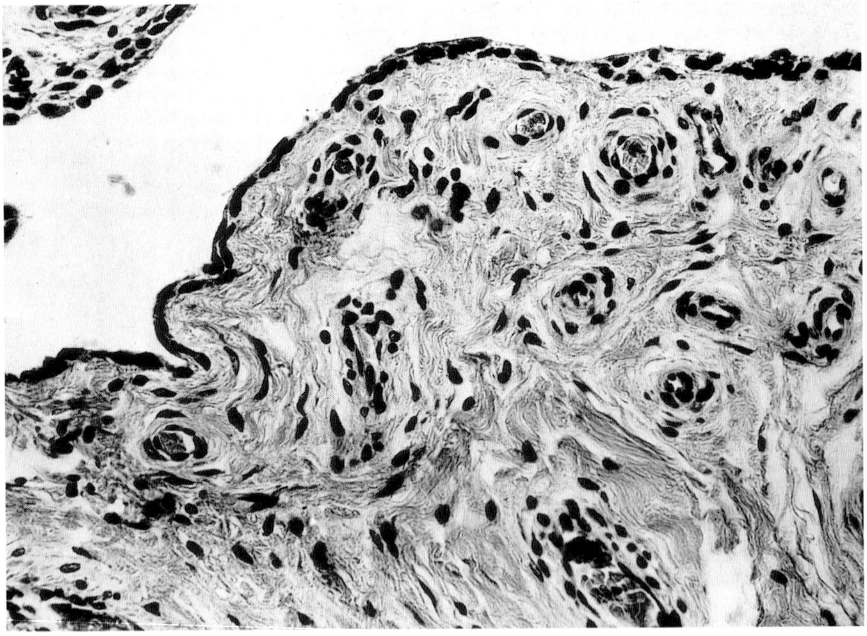

Fig. 8. The synovial membrane bears on its surface a single and continuous row of flat synoviocytes. The subsynoviocytic loose connective tissue comprises fibrocytes, capillaries, arterioles, and venules, and a small number of histiocytes. Between these elements, collagen bundles run in various directions

processes, some of which mesh with the subjacent collagen fibers. Some cytoplasmic processes intertwine laterally with the cytoplasmic processes of the adjacent synoviocytes. They thus connect to form a continuous cover (Fig. 8) which separates the articular cavity from the subsynoviocytic tissue. No cytoplasmic processes are observed extending from normal synoviocytes toward the joint cavity. In the center of the synoviocytes lie their nuclei (Fig. 8), which are fusiform or ovoid and have distinct membranes; their chromatin is dense and evenly distributed. Histochemical examination by Maibach [1004] disclosed the presence of hyaluronic acid and enzymes (peroxidase, phosphatase, diastase, and lipase) in the synoviocytes.

Directly beneath lies the subsynoviocytic tissue (Fig. 8). Depending on the individual joints and the location within the joint, this varies greatly in thickness, degree of vascularity, and amount of interspersed adipose tissue. The zone of immediate subsynoviocytic tissue is composed of a meshwork of thin collagen fibers which contrast with the coarser and more compact collagen bundles constituting the bulk of the deeper subsynoviocytic tissue. The collagen fibers have a wavy shape, are 2–10 µm thick, run in various directions, and are composed of thinner fibers of 0.1–0.4 µm thickness. On the basis of biochemical investigations, Gay et al. [583] differentiated the collagen fibrils according to their varied molecular composition into four types of physicochemical properties and biological functions. The substances composing the collagen fibers are polypeptides – glycine, hydroxyproline, and hydroxylysine. The specific stains for the collagen fibers are van Gieson's solution of trinitrophenol and acid fuchsin and Mallory's aniline blue. Electron-microscopic examination [583] reveals the basic unit of the collagen fibers to be fibrils with the characteristic transverse bands of 640 A periodicity. Other fibers of substantially less quantity in the subsynoviocytic intercellular tissue are very thin, branched reticulin fibers and long, homogeneous elastic fibers which form a loose network.

Between the collagen fibers and in the ground substance are scattered fibrocytes (Fig. 8), which have slender, long or stellate bodies, and extend a few cytoplasmic processes. Generally their cytoplasm is pale and their cell body thin, with the nucleus appearing almost naked. The latter is spindle shaped, oval, or round, depending on the plane in which it was cut. A small proportion of the subsynoviocytic cells is made up of histiocytes, also termed macrophages [494, 495] or wandering cells. These are almost one and a half times larger than the fibrocytes, and their bodies are irregularly shaped by the protrusion of a few broader cytoplasmic processes (Fig. 8). Their nuclei are round, ovoid, or most often kidney-shaped and larger than those of the fibrocytes; they have thick, often indented membranes and contain a few irregularly distributed, clumpy chromatin particles. At the periphery of their cytoplasm lie vacuoles and inclusions of particulate material. All elements of the inner part of the joint capsule are embedded in and bound together by the ground substance, which is rather scant and difficult to stain. Castor [255] explained that much potentially stainable material is leached out during routine fixation; he observed prominent intercellular metachromasia in freeze-dried sections. Meyer [1097]

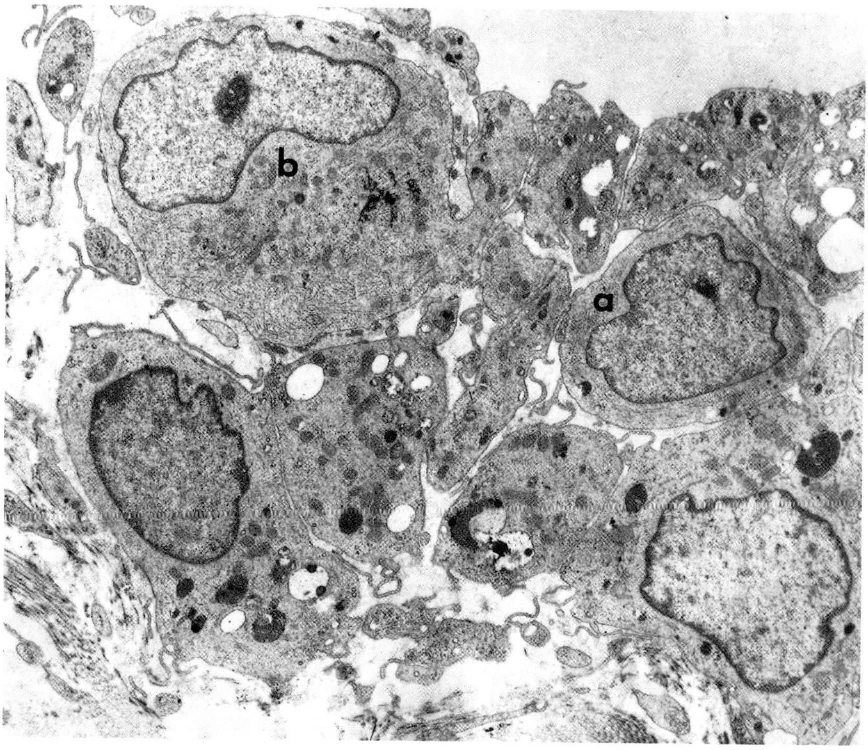

Fig. 9. Two types of synoviocytes can be discerned by electron microscopy: *a*, containing numerous cytoplasmic vacuoles and vesicles; *b*, containing abundant ergastoplasmic material

ascertained that the major component of the ground substance are acid mucopolysaccharides combined with proteins to proteoglycans, which can be demonstrated specifically by toluidine blue and other polychromatic dyes.

The structure of the synovial membrane explains some of its functions and its contributions to the biology of joints. According to histochemical investigations [717, 1434, 1498], the synoviocytes produce the mucin, while the subsynoviocytic blood vessels secure the flow of fluids, crystalloids, and organic substances from the blood stream to the synovial fluid and vice versa. Due to its contiguous cells, the synoviocyte cover seems to represent a continuous delimitation between the articular cavity and the subjacent layers of the joint capsule. Nevertheless, a regular exchange of fluid and solid substances occurs partly by the synoviocytes but particularly through preexistent small interspaces between the aligned synoviocytes. These separations permit the exit of fluids and substances from the blood vessels via the subsynoviocytic tissue into the joint cavity [914]. Equally, these substances can return into the subsynoviocytic lymph spaces and lymph vessels which merge with the blood vessels; this secures the backflow of excessive liquid and solid substances into the blood stream. Under physiological conditions the synovial membrane accordingly regulates the amount and the chemical composition of the synovial fluid. Despite the communicative openings, the synovial membrane represents a well-defined separation between the subsynoviocytic tissue and the joint cavity and converts this cavity into an almost occluded space. Therefore, the exchange of liquid, dissolved and solid substances would occur very slowly if the synovial membrane did not form folds and small protrusions which increase its surface. Hereby both the diffusion and the resorption of substances from the blood stream into the joint cavity and vice versa are materially enhanced.

The synoviocytes, such as the subjacent cells, are connective tissue cells. However, by their position on the surface of the membrane they also display other capacities not observed to this degree in the subjacent cells. The capacities are a special sensitivity and reactivity to all physical, chemical, toxic, and bacteriotoxic forms of damage inflicted upon a joint. These properties of the synoviocytes are also the reason for the easy irritability of the synovial membrane, which is manifested by inflammatory changes of a wide variety. With its rapid reaction to noxious substances, the synovial tissue has largely the same biological function as the reticuloendothelial system with its strong immunobiological defenses.

Electron-microscopic examinations [71, 327, 603, 964] disclose that the synoviocytes are delimited by a membrane with a number of filopodia (Figs. 9, 206). Inside their bodies lies a rough endoplasmic reticulum which comprises cisternae with a proteinaceous materi-

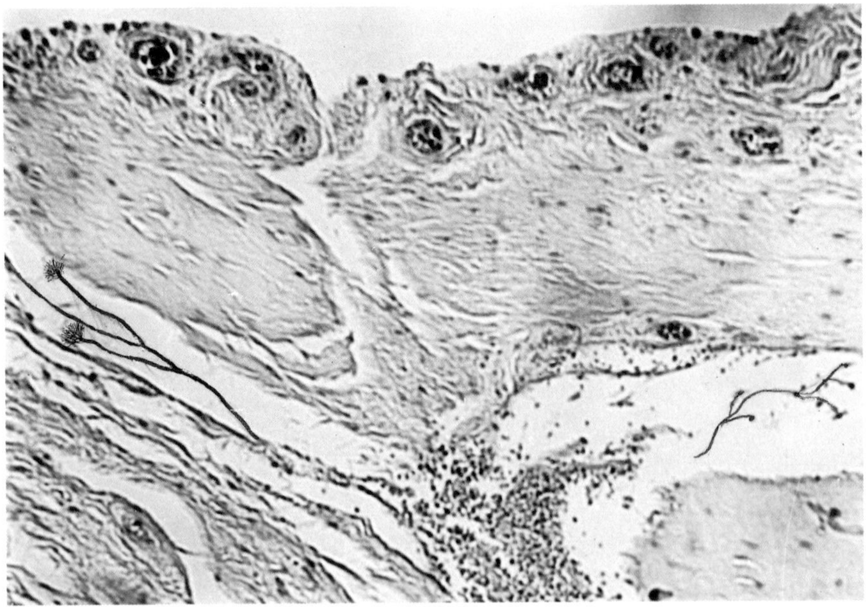

Fig. 10. A nonmyelinated nerve fiber, ending in beadlike terminals, rises close to a blood vessel in the synovial membrane. A myelinated nerve fiber, ending in spray-like terminals, runs between collagen fibers

al. Another prominent intracellular structure is the Golgi complex (Fig. 9), consisting of stacks of parallel membranes and vesicles in which hyaluronic acid has been demonstrated [603]. Other intrasynoviocytic elements are the electron-dense lysosomes, which contain histochemically demonstrable acid enzymes able to digest endogenous and exogenous material [71]. The ovoid, sometimes indented nucleus contains a distinct nucleolus lying in homogeneous chromatin. Barland et [71] classified the synoviocytes into two types, A and B (Fig. 9). Type A contains abundant cytoplasm, a prominent Golgi complex, many lysosomes, and vacuoles (Fig. 9), but a small amount of endoplasmic reticulum; it extends filopodia which surround particles and thus resembles macrophages. Type B contains a few vacuoles and a scant Golgi complex but a larger amount of endoplasmic reticulum, and cisternae filled with homogeneous material (Fig. 9); it is thought to produce protein and hyaluronate. Ghadially et al. [605] also identified a type C which has intermediate features between the two former types. Lever et al. [603] described the surface of the synovial cells as wavy and

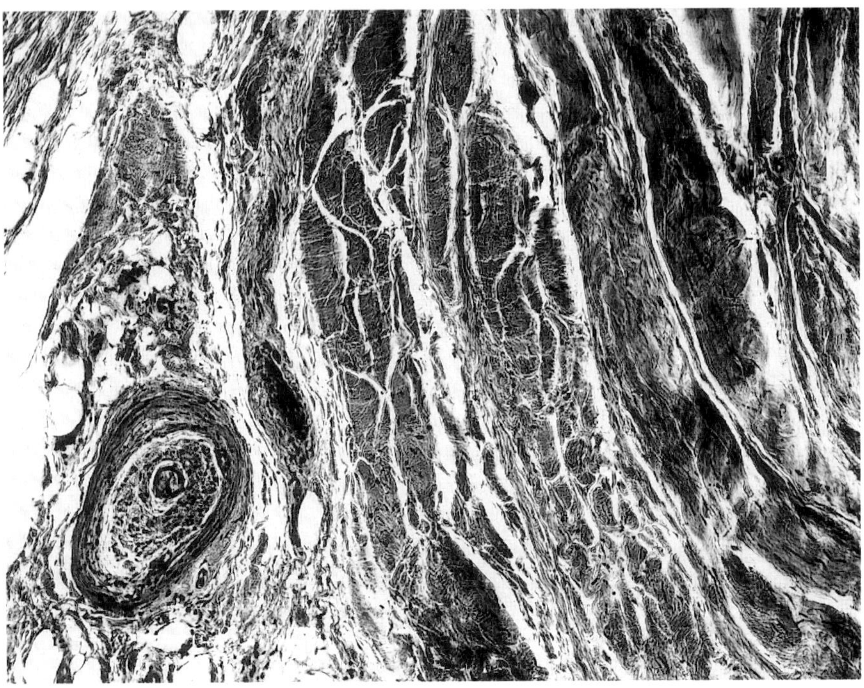

Fig. 11. The dense connective tissue of a collateral ligament contains a transversally cut Vater-Pacini corpuscle with its central axon. A longitudinally cut thick nerve runs in proximity

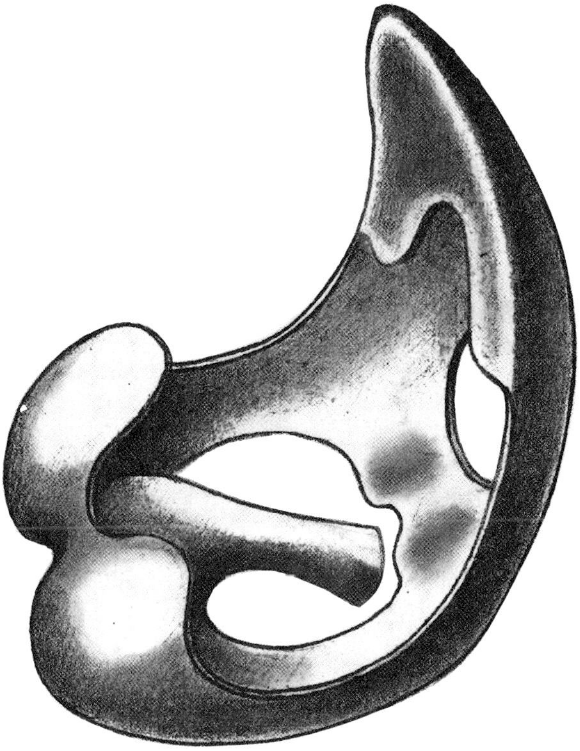

Fig. 12. Differently from all other joints, the synovial membrane of the knee joint is separated to a large extent from the fibrous capsule and has its own course of attachment onto the tibial condyles

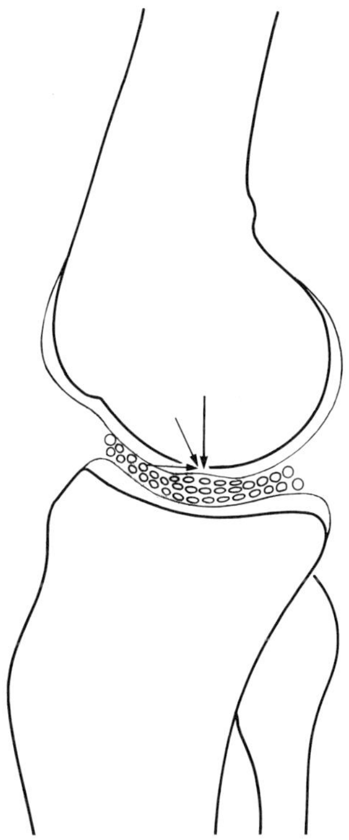

Fig. 13. The oblique gliding force in a joint results from vertical pressure and horizontal friction. The articular cartilage is indented in the area under pressure, and the interposed globules of synovial fluid are compressed and flattened

occupied by many blebs containing large granules. These are discharged into the joint cavity and are thought to be the precursors of hyaluronic acid.

Another sign of the reactivity and vitality of the synovial membrane is its capacity for regeneration after a large part of the synovial membrane has been surgically removed. Small areas of remaining synovial membrane and probably also the denuded subsynoviocytic tissue supplement outgrowing synoviocytes, so that after about 6 months the inner surface of the joint capsule is again endowed with a complete synoviocytic cover [689, 882, 1614] (Figs. 54, 218).

The subsynoviocytic tissue also contains numerous blood vessels (Fig. 8) which derive from the larger blood vessels penetrating the fibrous capsule and continue into the subsynoviocytic tissue. During their course they branch into arterioles and finally into capillaries, which appear more numerous directly beneath the synoviocytes. Here they run for a short distance along the synoviocyte cover, then make a loop, turn back to the periphery, and merge into venules. Each arteriole and small artery is accompanied individually by a pair of venules and small veins, respectively.

In addition, the joint capsule is well supplied in its superficial and deeper zones with nerve endings [61, 386, 571, 871, 1267, 1299, 1794] which partly terminate as myelinated free endings of the spray type, the loop type, or a type with a number of thickenings (Fig. 10). Horten et al. [1782] advised special stains, such as that of the fast blue periodic acid–Schiff reaction for identification of the myelin sheath and that of Bielschowski's silver impregnation for identification of the axon. Another part of the myelinated nerves enter lamellated capsules, in which they become unmyelinated, and terminate in very thin branches or a few buttonlike thickenings. These encapsulated corpuscles of the Vater-Pacini (Fig. 11) and Golgi-Mazzoni types are located chiefly in the ligaments of the joints, an indication of their special sensory function. Additionally, richly distributed nonmyelinated nerve endings form networks principally (Fig. 10) around middle-sized blood vessels and apparently have vasomotor function. All these nerve endings are connected by intermediate neurons to the central nervous system (Fig. 429); their participation in the physiology of the body becomes obvious when their function has been lost. The function of these nerve endings is discussed in "Neuropathic Arthropathies"

In contrast to the strong biological capacities of the superficial layer of the synovial membrane, the deeper subsynoviocytic zone has chiefly mechanical functions. Within the latter, the connective tissue forms regional densities, the ligaments, located differently in each individual joint according to its specific mechanical requirements. The ligaments represent reinforcements to secure the articular ends at certain directions of intense stress movements. Correspondingly, the ligaments consist of parallel bundles of very thick fibers composed basically of collagen and elastin. Another tissue of apparent mechanical purpose is the adipose tissue, which is interspersed scantily in the immediate subsynoviocytic zone and increases toward the periphery. In a way which is regionally characteristic for a few joints, it forms there substantial thickenings which cause bulging of the synovial membrane into the joint cavity. These bulgings are compressible pads which protect the articular ends at certain predisposed areas from shock, pressure, and friction. The overall interposition of the subsynoviocytic adipose layer between the innermost and outermost layers of the joint capsule also has another function – to permit easy gliding of the synovial membrane versus the outer fibrous capsule. This function is essential since the synovial membrane, being inserted along the border of the articular cartilage, invests and accompanies the articular ends and like a muff envelops them at any movement. On the other hand, the fibrous capsule stabilizes the joint by its firmness, residing in its composition of dense connective tissue (Fig. 4) and reinforcement with ligaments and aponeuroses. These hold the articular ends together and prevent their separation even at the extreme ranges of physiological motion.

In this sense the inner synovial membrane, the intermediate subsynoviocytic tissue, and the retentive outer fibrous capsule follow a similar, almost parallel course of insertion and envelope the articular ends like a muff (Fig. 4). However, the joint capsule of the knee differs. While the fibrous capsule here also has the shape of a muff, the synovial membrane deviates from the fibrous capsule and resembles short pants. Its beltlike part surrounds both femoral condyles; a flap expanding from this anteriorly and proximally covers the suprapatellar recessus, but its distal parts are attached separately and individually around each tibial condyle (Fig. 12). The intervening space occupied here by the cruciate ligaments is extrasynovial but still intracapsular. The anterior middle part of this synovial and fibrous capsule has a large opening for incorporation of the patella.

While most joints differ from each other by the configuration of their articular ends and by the mechanical function which they fulfill in their region of the body, certain basic constituents are common to all of them. These are mutually fitting, convex- or concave-shaped articular ends, which merge on their articulating surfaces with caps of hyaline cartilage and are surrounded by an attached joint capsule. The latter has an inner layer which provides the nutrient and the gliding solutions for the biology and mobility of the joint; the outer layer ensures the stability of the joint in any movement and thus makes the joint a reliable effector in the mechanics of the body. In this way the joints manifest the correlation between form and function as well as that between structure and biology [587].

Physiology of Joints

The articular ends are the solid supports and the effectors of joint motion. They are able to serve as such by having mutually complementary osseous configurations and by merging on their surface with a caplike layer of hyaline cartilage. The latter owes its functional capacity partly to its ground substance, whose main constituents are proteoglycans. The characteristic part of the proteoglycans are the glycosaminoglycans [1350, 1352] onto whose negatively charged anions a large proportion of water is attracted [1034, 1035]. The other essential constituent of the articular cartilage is a firmly anchored collagenous fibrillar network (Figs. 5, 7) which enmeshes the ground substance. Due to these components the articular cartilage possesses a high intrinsic pressure and is able to resist the external pressure which arises when two opposing articular surfaces are moved along one another.

The characteristic functional stress of the cartilage caps develops when at the start of motion the opposing articular ends approach each other under pressure and compress one another. The compression of the articular cartilage is thus not one-sided, and the articular motion proceeds under mutual indentation of the articular ends (Fig. 13). This causes a deforming flattening in the opposing areas of maximum load bearing (Fig. 13). The decrease in height of directly opposing zones of the articular cartilage occurs by water contained in their proteoglycanic ground substance beeing squeezed out. This water becomes displaced into directly adjacent areas of the articular cartilage, where the glycosaminoglycans absorb the excess of water [313, 1252]. Concurrently, the local mesh of the collagen fibers, attached in the zone of calcified cartilage (Figs. 5, 7, 13), becomes tilted from its arcading course in the upper zones of the articular cartilage and is overstretched. On discontinuation of the load pressure the fiber network returns by virtue of intrinsic elasticity from the lateral deviation to its original orientation. With this the entrapped globules of glycoproteins in the articular cartilage also return to their original sites and carry along with them the squeezed out fluid. The indented areas of the articular cartilage then resume their previous height.

The compression force of the load causes a tangential shift chiefly of the superficial zones of cartilage cells along their deeper zones. On cessation of the vertical pressure the superficial zones of cartilage cells return to their original position, being pulled back by the tension of the restraining intercellular fibers [1011]. On forward motion of the articular ends, other areas of the articular surfaces come into contact and undergo identical histophysiological changes as the areas previously under pressure. The newly compressed areas also reattain normal structure, when the localized pressure is moved forward. In this way, the compression and elastic reexpansion of the articular cartilage are repeated in a stepwise manner, until the articular excursion has completed its course [1011]. The continued weight bearing capacity of the articular cartilage is made possible by its high content of water, which represents a substantial part of the ground substance. This phenomenon of gliding has thus been designated as hydrodynamic or load lubrication [1019, 1057, 1612].

Although the stepwise deformation of the articular cartilage is transient, it would lead to precipitous wearing off the articular cartilage if the deforming forces were not diverted onto another material. The stresses on the articular cartilage, produced by the gliding of one articular end along the other, are composed mechanically of two forces: vertical pressure and horizontal friction (Fig. 13). The transient deformation of the articular cartilage by vertical pressure was discussed above. The force from horizontal friction is borne primarily by the synovial fluid between the articular surfaces. The droplets of the viscous synovial fluid are composed chiefly of large molecules of hyaluronate and constitute a protective layer, squeeze film [1295], on the articular cartilage. At movements, one droplet is shifted horizontally versus another. In addition, flattening of the synovial fluid globules occurs at the site of the momentarily maximal pressure (Fig. 13), where the deforming forces are largely diverted from the articular cartilage due to the inherent viscosity of these globules. The frictional component of the articular motion is transformed by the fluid film into a lubricated motion [724, 1454, 1609, 1791]. Thus the gliding of the articular surfaces along one other is associated with boundary lubrication. The greater the adhesion of the lubricant synovial fluid and the surface tension of its individual droplets [1019, 1057, 1609], the more vertical pressure and tangential friction is absorbed in the deformation of the synovial fluid layer and is diverted from the articular cartilage.

This consideration also applies to situations in which the viscosity of the synovial fluid has diminished substantially due to altered function of the synovial membrane, the producer of the hyaluronic acid. Such dysfunction occurs in various inflammatory conditions of joints, chiefly in rheumatoid arthritis, in which the viscosity of the joint fluid, normally amounting to 100–140 units as determined by the Ostwald viscometer, is decreased to 45–70. On the other hand, even at its normal viscosity, the synovial fluid cannot fully exert its protective lubricating effect once the cartilaginous cap has become uneven following disruption by injuries or pannus or has disintegrated as in osteoarthritis [427].

In addition to its mechanical function, the synovial fluid provides nutrient material consisting of proteins and glucosaminoglycans to the articular cartilage. These nutrients, produced partly by the synoviocytes and partly derived by diffusion from the subsynoviocytic blood vessels, are conveyed from the synovial fluid by diffusion into the upper zones of the articular cartilage. The nutrition of the cartilage at its junction with the subchondral bone is secured by diffusion from blood vessels which extend from the epiphyseal medullary space toward the subchondral osseous zone. From there, nutrient substances diffuse into the calcified cartilage and the lower zone of the hyaline cartilage [673, 1115]. This establishes a communication with the canaliculi in the deeper zone of the articular cartilage. The overall canaliculi in the articular cartilage provide permeability to the nutrient material in proportion to the size and concentration of its composing globules [1035, 1252].

Since equal distribution of the synovial fluid throughout the joint cavity is accomplished by the movements of the joint [914], these movements are essential for the maintenance of the biology of a joint and for the patency of its cavity. On complete immobilization of a joint for a longer period of time, trophic disturbances set in due to sluggish nutrition of the hyaline cartilage by the lack of adequate diffusion of the regional fluids. A healthy joint may be immobilized in infants up to 3 months without fear of adverse effects. However, thereafter atrophy starts in the regional musculature, as does shrinking in the joint capsule. The joint space eventually becomes limited: this occurs earlier in adults. Where inflammatory changes of the synovial membrane [914] and profound alterations of the articular cartilage preexist, fibrosis of the inner part of the joint capsule and replacement of the articular cartilage by pannus lead more rapidly and more extensively to obliteration of the joint cavity. Yet, independently of the pathological-anatomical factors, the normal joint with fully pervious joint cavity is a merely passive organ which is maintained in its function by the normal regional musculature. Thus a reciprocal relationship exists between the anatomical condition of these cofunctioning organs; only an intact musculature is able to implement the full active motion of a joint, and only a joint with a completely patent cavity permits the regional musculature to contract and relax fully.

The close coordination between the various parts of a joint, on the one hand, and the surrounding musculature and its tendons, on the other, as well as the communications with the body concerning the conditions of the joints is established through nerve fibers by the way of reflexes and long pathways (Fig. 429). The correlated special receptor organs are the sensory nerve endings [61, 386, 571, 871, 1267, 1299, 1794] scattered in the synovial membrane (Fig. 10) and in the ligaments (Fig. 11); they are described in "Anatomy and Histology of Joints", and provide instant information inside the body on the functional status and the position of a joint [571, 572]. By their connections, the sensory nerve fibers establish reciprocal relationships and interactions with the muscles effecting the movements of a joint. In this way all organs and tissues, participating in the function of a joint and contributing to its motion and nutrition represent links of a closed "kinetic chain", and effect the physiology and biology of the joint [724]. On the loss of one link, the operation of this chain and the proper movements of the joint are disrupted. The varying possibilities of disconnection and their untoward effects on the joints are described in "Neuropathic Arthropathies".

Examinations in Arthritis and Related Affections

1. Patient's History

Before examining a diseased joint, it is indispensable to obtain information on all prior diseases of the patient as well as on the course of the present joint disease. The history of past diseases and details concerning the onset and progression of the present disease offer important clues to the etiology and nature of this joint disease. Taking the history also represents the first contact with the patient and provides a useful insight into his psychological reactions, his attitude toward the disease, and his probable cooperation in managing the disease.

Beyond this, the history indicates the necessary tests for corroboration of the tentative diagnosis. In some joint diseases, incidence in the family may be mentioned, implicating a hereditary predisposition. This is often the case in rheumatic diseases and in joint diseases associated with systemic disorders. Hormonal disorders associated with joint ailments may also be observed in the patient's parents or other relatives. Some metabolic disorders such as diabetes, gout, hyperlipoproteinemia, and ochronosis or skin disease such as psoriasis are often preceded in either parent. Hemophilia complicated by joint disease is invariably transmitted by a parent. Similarly, a specific constitutional type with predisposition for certain joint diseases may be transmitted from the parents, such as the pyknic habitus associated with degenerative joint diseases.

Other profound effects on the joints may be caused by the patient himself. Often incriminated as causes of rheumatic diseases are living under conditions of great humidity, or working in a cold wet environment such as in laundries or sewers or chemical factories. Improper nutrition may lead to overweight, with disuse of joints, or to metabolic disorders, among which gout and diabetes may cause considerable joint alterations. Certain occupations, such as those of farmers, veterinarians, and butchers, are associated with joint inflammations from specific microorganisms such as Brucellae or fungi through contact with diseased cattle or material contaminated in certain environments. A large group of patients consist of drivers of vehicles, miners, metallurgical workers, and heavy laborers who are often subjected to injuries of joints. Another ever-increasing group comprise those who sustein manifold injuries to the joints in professional athletics, competitive sports, or recreational physical exercises.

Harm may also be inflicted to joints by infections which primarily affect other organs or the joints by themselves. Various microorganisms invade the body through different portals, and by themselves or by their toxins affect joints. Certain primary organs are usually infected by a specific strain of microorganisms which secondarily infect joints. Streptococci and staphylococci spread from the throat, tonsils, or lymph nodes; pneumococci, tubercle bacilli, and fungi from the lungs; tubercle, typhoid, paratyphoid, and dysentery bacilli and Brucellae from the intestine; gonococci and spirochetes from the urogenital tract; and streptococci and staphylococci, spirochetes, and fungi may be propagated from the skin by the blood or lymph vessels to the joints. The period between infection of any of these organs and inflammation of joints may be so brief that a direct causal relationship between the two conditions cannot be doubted. In other instances, the joint inflammation may develop months or even years after the infection of a distant organ, and it is uncertain whether an etiological relationship exists between the two disease processes. Even more difficulty is presented by a situation in which two or more diseases are active and may elicit a similar clinical picture of arthritis, for example psoriasis and rheumatoid arthritis, gonorrhea and gout, septic tonsillitis and deep skin infection, or ulcerative colitis and idiopathic ankylosing spondylitis. Many of these uncertainties can be resolved by a thorough history, even before the relevant examinations are carried out. At the least, this indicates the proper diagnostic tests and laboratory studies to be considered.

2. Inspection and Palpation of Joints

Information obtained from the patient's history may indicate connections between other diseases of the body and the disease of the joints and therefore requires examination of the entire body prior to that of the affected joints. This examination should be carried out on the undressed patient.

The general development and the body type permit some inference on possible reactions of the organism, and the effects of these on the joints. The asthenic type is often afflicted by rheumatoid arthritis, whereas the pyknic type more often presents degenerative changes or joint diseases related to metabolic or endocrine disorders. The athletic type suffers most from injuries, degenerative alterations, and formations of free bodies in joints. Advanced changes in joints, in conjunction with the primary etiological disease or infection, have a reciprocal effect on the general condition. These joint diseases often lead to psychological and physical impairment due to the associated pain and to the decrease in locomotion and other vital activities. In some infectious processes toxemia survenes; in malignant tumors cachexia is often apparent.

Changes in the skin may provide clues regarding general diseases which also affect joints. For instance, there may be an alteration in the local coloring of the skin. Smoke-gray or blackish pigmentation chiefly in the face suggests ochronosis, whereas bronze pigmentation of the face and/or trunk suggests Gaucher's disease. Yellowish white nodules in the skin over the ear lobes (Fig. 348) or over joints (Fig. 349) are likely urate tophi. Protruding intracutaneous whitish yellow or reddish yellow nodules in the face, ears, hands or trunk (Fig. 377) suggest lipoid dermatoarthritis. Petechiae and small hemorrhages in the skin of the trunk appear in abdominal typhoid fever, and larger hemorrhagic suffusions appear in hemophilia. A multiform erythema may appear in rheumatoid arthritis. Small scaling efflorescences on the body suggest regressing scarlet fever, while larger and inflamed scaling alterations mostly on the back, dorsal aspects of the elbows, frontal aspects of the knees, and in the palms and soles occur in advanced cases of psoriasis (Figs. 324, 325, 326) and Reiter's disease (Fig. 108). Subcutaneous nodes protrude in rheumatoid arthritis, tuberculosis of joints, Gaucher's disease, and malignant tumors of joints. In inflammations of joints the skin color is reddish to red in severe acute inflammation, pale in chronic inflammation, and livid in congestion by a tumor. A draining sinus over a joint with undermined edges and greenish secretion indicates tuberculosis of the joint (Figs. 533, 534). A draining sinus surrounded by inflamed margins of the skin and discharging thick yellowish pus from a joint indicates a coccal infection (Fig. 77), whereas such sinus or sinuses discharging very malodorous pus and crumbs of necrotic tissue occurs in coccidioidomycotic or blastomycotic infection. Fistulae with drainage of fluid containing yellow crumbs occur in actinomycosis. Sharply delimited kidney-shaped ulcers with ham-colored ground are characteristic for tertiary syphilis, and trophic ulcers of the skin with conspicuous thickening of the underlying joint are indicative of neuropathic arthropathy (Fig. 454).

Inspection of an affected joint suggests similar changes in other joints. Extensive blunt contusion by injury may also involve other joints, and recurrent hemorrhagic effusion in one joint (Fig. 403) suggests similar occurrences in other joints due to hemophilia. Conspicuous atrophy of the muscles of an extremity indicates lack of use or paralysis of the regional musculature and/or long-lasting dysfunction of a joint (Figs. 135, 143). Multiple contractures with malalignment often occur in juvenile or adult rheumatoid arthritis (Figs. 178, 186). Owing to its position close beneath the skin and the surrounding, normally thin adipose tissue, each joint, with the exception of the hip joint and the joints of the spine, has its own relief; this permits one to discern the soft structures surrounding a joint and their gross alterations. Small plum- or apple-sized protrusions above or between tendons suggest enlarged bursae (Fig. 163), tenosynovial cysts (Figs. 539, 556), or extraarticular soft tissue tumors. Similar protrusions at the joint may correspond to intracapsular soft tissue or hard tissue tumor (Figs. 507, 522). Blurring of the outlines (Figs. 7, 83, 102, 262, 403) is most frequently caused by swelling of the joint capsule, whereas a blown-up or globular enlargement of the entire joint (Fig. 68) is caused by an increase in the joint fluid. The inspection may also reveal axial deviation within the joint (Figs. 277, 281), caused by deformity of the articular ends or one-sided contracture of the muscles and tendons (Figs. 178, 186).

Palpation, as the next step, is more conclusive because it provides information concerning depth and thereby also changes in volume and consistency of the periarticular and intraarticular constituents. Upon palpating the regional muscles, one may note whether these are atrophied or spastically contracted. The latter condition occurs in acute injuries, contractures of recent onset, and neurological disorders. The palpation should be carried out at relaxed musculature because only then can the examining fingers advance deeply. There the joint capsule is accessible; its areas of tenderness can be detected, its possible doughy swelling or thickening (Figs. 72, 102, 108, 403), and its distension by increase in the joint fluid (Fig. 68). In the latter situation the fluctuation in the joint can be perceived by palpation; ballotement of the patella can be elicited in the knee joint (Fig. 14) by squeezing out the fluid from the suprapatellar recessus and by pressing the patella against the accumulated fluid level. In acute inflammations the joint capsule is boggy and soft all over, but is thicker and denser in chronic inflammations (Figs. 108,

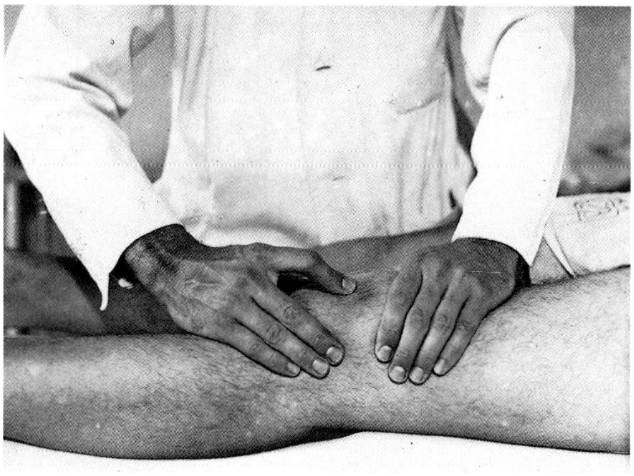

Fig. 14. Substantially increased fluid in the knee joint can be ascertained by ballotement of the patella

262, 403). Spongy enlargement of the joint capsule is caused by acute edematous processes (Fig. 68), whereas fibrous shrinking of the joint capsule is the usual outcome of intensive chronic inflammations (Figs. 186, 324). Recurrent inflammations of the joint capsule cause an unequal consistency, with dense scarified portions alternating with swollen soft portions (Figs. 403). Formation of hard nodes of circumscribed outline may be produced by benign tumors (Fig. 507), and extensive nodes of unsharp irregular delimitation are produced mostly by malignant tumors (Fig. 522). Circumscribed widening of the joint capsule may occur by outpouching of a bursa or a synovial cyst, chiefly at the areas of tendinous attachments (Fig. 539). Within the fibrous capsule of most joints lie ligaments which may be tender either along their course or at their attachments secondary to injury. The joint cleft and articular margins can also be palpated through the joint capsule. The former may be widened by increase of the joint fluid (Fig. 68) or by interposition of loose bodies, detached fragments of cartilage and bone. The latter may be irregularly shaped particularly by osteophytic outgrowths (Figs. 262, 446).

With the presence or persistence of active inflammatory processes within the joint, the local temperature is moderately elevated. The more intensive the inflammatory process, the more pronounced is the rise in local temperature. The palpation also enables one to localize precisely the inflamed areas by testing the tenderness. However, the more intensive the irritation and the more extensive the infiltration, the more tender is the entire joint capsule. With regression of the inflammation and decrease in swelling, the tenderness diminishes and remains localized to some areas from which the inflammation emerged. At normal temperature, the localized tenderness of the joint capsule suggests injury to the ligaments. When confined to the joint cleft and articular margin this suggests either protruding intraarticular bodies or irritated edges of deformed articular epiphyses.

Palpation should be continued with the joint in motion because only then can displacement of loose intraarticular bodies be perceived. Furthermore, the palpating hand on the joint in motion may perceive the fine friction by a fibrosed joint capsule or the coarse crepitation by cartilage-bone friction at uneven articular surfaces.

Finally, the circumference of the joint is measured at various levels and is compared with that of the contralateral intact joint in order to determine precisely the change in volume of a joint either by atrophy of the neighboring musculature or by swelling of the joint capsule.

3. Testing Active and Passive Movements of Joints

The excursion of the articular ends from the resting or midposition to the extreme ranges of motion is an elementary and essential function of the joints, anchored in their construction. Thus the examination for motion is able to provide exact information on the anatomical and functional states of a joint [1454, 1764, 1788]. These states are based on the structural conditions of the individual articular constituents and on the mechanical effectiveness of the organs functioning in and acting on joints. All diarthrodial joints provide active movements carried out by the function of their regional musculature and permit passive movements carried out by the hands. Changes in the execution of a movement of a joint can be determined by comparison with that movement of the contralateral joint or by keeping in mind the average of that movement of such normal joint.

The active movement of a joint is primarily an indicator of the function of the musculature. Since the normal musculature works with optimum effectiveness, an increase in the range of active movement can be obtained only by impairment of the structural barriers of a joint. Thus changes of articular constituents may permit an increase in motion beyond the physiological ranges or concomitant with a new faulty axis. The incongruity of the articular ends secondary to congenital dysplasia, malunited fracture, or partial destruction by a suppurative process, chiefly in childhood, may be associated with an increase in the active movements in one or all possible directions. However, insufficiency of the ligamentous apparatus more often yields an increase in the range of motion. Congenital laxity of the ligaments may permit excessive movements, with deviation of the joints sometimes up to grotesque degrees. Laxity of ligaments during the phases of growth, and sometimes constitutional laxity in women, causes moderate degrees of lasting joint instability. Insufficiency of ligaments often remains as a sequela of nontreated or inadequately healed tears in ligaments. The most conspicuous increase in active movements is seen in tabetic arthropathy, in which the wearing off of ligamentous attachments disrupts the articular connections; in addition, the loss of deep sensation permits the musculature to pull the articular ends without control beyond the normal ranges. A sudden acceleration of the final degrees of motion occurs as a snapping phenomenon (Fig. 478) after the musculature succeeds by forceful contraction in overcoming an obstacle within or around a joint, but the resulting motion does not extend beyond the normal range.

However, if the changes are more advanced and affect larger parts of the articular constituents or their coordinated organs, the active movements of a joint become decreased. The most important factor here are the muscular lesions, which may be of functional or organic nature; the former occur more often, but leave the joints intact. The flaccid paralysis of the regional musculature secondary to neuritis, poliomyelitis, inflammatory or neoplastic processes of the meninges and the spastic paralyses in cerebral palsy, after transverse myelitis, apoplexy, or encephalitis are associated with marked impairment or even complete loss of active movement. The weakening of the musculature by posttraumatic atrophy and the flaccid paralysis in progressive muscular dystrophy or congenital myatonia are also associated with loss of or decrease in the range of active movement of the joint. Similarly, the muscles, which are spastically tense and cannot be relaxed, account for a concentric decrease in the active movement of a joint. If by weakness or paralysis the musculature on only one side of a joint is affected, but the joint capsule does not shrink, the group of functioning antagonist muscles maintains the active movement, albeit in one direction only. When single individual muscles are paralyzed or inflamed, the result is also a one-sided loss of or decrease in active movement. An irritation at one of the muscle insertions caused by bursitis, peritendinitis, or periostitis, may have a similar effect.

Beyond this, even an intact musculature is not able to carry out the active motion without limitation if the resulting effector organ, the joint, underwent significant alterations. Any acute inflammation of the joint capsule with effusion limits the mobility simply by the tenseness of the capsule. The effect of chronic thickening of the joint capsule is similar or even more pronounced. On subsidence of an inflammation, unequal shrinking of the joint capsule may limit the movement to one side only. A complete loss of active movement to any side occurs in fibrous or osseous ankylosis because the entire joint space is obliterated in these situations. Since total inefficiency of the regional musculature entails the same loss of active movement as an ankylosis, it is necessary to differentiate between the limitations of the regional musculature and those of the joint itself.

Examining for passive movement fulfills this need, because it permits discrimination between dysfunction of the joint and that of the muscle. The passive joint movement is carried out by the muscle action of the examiner. One articular end is steadied by the left hand of the examiner, and the other articular end is grasped by the right hand and is passively moved in all possible directions. If the examined joint is in normal structural condition, the action by the examiner succeeds in moving the joint in the physiological directions even if the musculature completely lacks function. As with the active movements, the range of passive movements is measured by a protractor [1388]. Comparison between the ranges of active and passive movements of the examined joints permits an inference whether a decrease in movements is caused by decrease in muscle function or is due to a defect within the joint itself. A decrease in active movement, while the passive movement is fully maintained indicates an impairment of the musculature.

Beyond this, a decrease in concurrent passive movement may also be caused by changes in the musculature itself. A spastic contraction of the regional musculature in neurological disorders cannot be overcome by external force; thus, the passive movement is limited. Idiopathic inflammations of the musculature and all nearby damages extending into the musculature lead to scars of the latter and its adhesions with the neighboring area. This limits any movement. However, changes within a joint account for the limitation in passive movement more often and to a greater degree. A joint capsule thickened by chronic inflammation as well as its shrinking and adhesions onto the articular ends limits the motion of the joint in all directions despite normal musculature. Similarly, articular ends deformed by inflammatory or degenerative processes or by conspicuous marginal protrusions present regional hindrances from which significant limitation of active movement and passive movement may ensue. With fusion of the contiguous articular ends to a block, any type of motion in a joint is completely obviated.

On the other hand, the passive movements of joints may be abnormally increased. The most frequent cause of this is the insufficiency of ligaments. It may occur constitutionally or during the growth of bones with a shift in the points of ligamentous attachments, but it occurs more often as a sequela of nontreated tears in ligaments or of inadequately consolidated fractures of the articular ends. Similarly, growth disturbances or

Table 1. Changes in movements of joints

Active movements

- Increased
  - Normal musculature with changes in ligaments
    - Congenital laxity of ligaments
    - Constitutional looseness of ligaments
    - Insufficiency of ligaments during periods of growth
    - Posttraumatic insufficiency of ligaments
    - Overstretching of ligaments on distension of the joint capsule
  - Normal musculature with irregularities of the gliding structures
    - Snapping at deformities of intraarticular structures, e. g., meniscus
    - Snapping at nodular thickening of the joint capsule
    - Snapping at irregular thickening of articular ligaments or periarticular tendons
  - Normal musculature with deformed articular ends
    - Hypoplasia of articular ends
    - Deformities of articular ends secondary to rickets
    - Deformities of articular ends secondary to osteochondritis
    - Deformities of articular ends secondary to osteomyelitis
    - Malunited fractures of articular ends
- Decreased
  - Normal joint with alterations in the musculature
    - Reflex regional spasm in painful inflammations of joint
    - Persistent spasticity in central neurological affections
    - Flaccid paralysis in peripheral nerve affections
    - Adhesions of the musculature secondary to inflammations
    - Scarified shrinking of muscles secondary to injuries
  - Normal musculature with affections of the gliding apparatus
    - Inflammation of a bursa or tendon sheath
  - Normal musculature with changes of the joint capsule
    - Acute or chronic inflammation of the joint capsule
    - Distension of the joint capsule by large effusion
    - Swelling of the joint capsule in proliferative inflammation
    - Irregular thickening of the joint capsule by tumor
    - Shrinking of the joint capsule with obliteration of the joint space
  - Normal musculature at changes of the articular ends
    - Congenital deformities of the articular ends
    - Deformities of the articular ends secondary to malunited fractures
    - Deformities of the articular ends by inflammatory destructions
    - Deformities of the articular ends in primary or secondary osteoarthritis
  - Changes in the musculature with changes of the articular ends
    - Shortened musculature and malformed epiphyses in congenital deformities
    - Adhesions of muscles secondary to extensive fractures of epiphyses
    - Shrunken musculature and partly destroyed articular ends secondary to healed suppuration

Passive movements

- Increased
  - Normal musculature with changes in ligaments
    - Congenital laxity of ligaments
    - Constitutional laxity of ligaments
    - Temporary laxity of ligaments during periods of growth
    - Overstretching of ligaments in chronic effusions
    - Recent tears of ligaments
    - Inadequate healing of tears of ligaments
  - Relative insufficiency of ligaments with changes in articular ends
    - Congenital dysplasia or hypoplasia of articular ends
    - Deformity of articular ends secondary to osteochondritis
    - Deformity of articular ends secondary to growth disturbance
    - Recent or malunited fracture of articular ends
    - Partial destruction of articular ends in inflammatory conditions
    - Fragmentation of articular ends in neuropathic arthropathy
  - Changes in ligaments with changes in the musculature
    - Flaccid paralysis with secondary overstretching of ligaments
- Decreased
  - Changes in the musculature with normal joints
    - Spasm of the musculature in painful conditions
    - Spastic contracture of the musculature in affections of the central nerve system
    - Shrinking of the regional musculature secondary to injuries
    - Adhesion of the musculature secondary to regional inflammation
  - Normal musculature with changes in the joint capsule
    - Thickening of the joint capsule due to inflammation
    - Posttraumatic or postinflammatory fibrosis of the joint capsule
    - Adhesion of the joint capsule with partial obliteration of the joint cavity
    - Irregular thickening of the joint capsule by tumor
  - Normal musculature with changes in the articular ends
    - Congenital deformity of the articular epiphyses
    - Deformity of the articular epiphyses secondary to malunited fracture
    - Deformity of the articular epiphyses secondary to joint inflammation
    - Deformity of the articular epiphyses secondary to bone inflammation
  - Normal musculature with narrowing of the joint cleft
    - By loose joint bodies
    - By intraarticular granulation tissue
    - By protruding tumor of the joint capsule or articular epiphysis
    - By unevenness of articular ends secondary to fracture or suppuration
    - By unevenness of articular ends in osteoarthritis
  - Changes in the musculature and joint
    - Shortness of all soft structures at congenital deformities of the articular ends

inflammatory destructions of the articular epiphyses are often followed by diminished sizes and by relative overlength of ligaments. A significant insufficiency of ligaments may also be caused by a long-lasting effusion of a joint which forces the articular ends apart and overstretches all ligaments. When the muscle tonus decreases, and the stability of a joint rests solely upon the ligaments, increasing distension of all ligaments of this joint invariably ensues. All flaccid paralyses – especially those in poliomyelitis, temporary insufficiencies of muscles during the growth period, and permanent insufficiencies of muscles due to their adhesions – are followed by overstretching of ligaments. The physiological restraint of motion is thereby lost, and the passive movement of the joint is either abnormally increased in normal directions or is carried out in new, unphysiological directions, or both. Such insufficiency of ligaments and lack of congruity of articular ends is conspicuous in tabetic arthropathy.

Table 1 summarizes the possible changes in active and passive movements of joints.

4. Auscultation of Joints

Under normal circumstances the movement of a joint occurs without sound or noise because the articular ends glide along each other without friction by virtue of their smooth cartilage caps, the interjacent synovial fluid, and the surrounding soft pliable joint capsule. Nevertheless, brusque motions such as in gymnastics, sports, or heavy labor may be associated at the extremes of ranges with a smacking noise followed by a short aftervibration when the articular ends impact against one other. The site of this noise could be extraarticular in the muscles, tendons, bursae, but it is more often intraarticular between the articular ends and joint capsule. In most of these situations the closed joint cavity provides the resonance space in which the noises are intensified and become audible.

One examines the articular sounds with a stethoscope placed alternately on two aspects of the joint while moving the joint actively or passively. Various qualities can be distinguished in the perceived sounds: pitch, timbre, intensity, continuity, and rhythm. These acoustic manifestations have a specific character in the various joint disturbances.

The greatest influence on the sounds, especially on those produced in the joint cavity, is that exerted by the qualities of the joint cavity and its content. The wider this cavity, the more resonance is conferred to the sounds. If the joint cavity is narrowed by pannus, the sounds become muffled, dull, and mat. Substantial increase in the joint fluid spreads the articular ends apart and the joint capsule away; the production of sounds is essentially diminished. However, if the joint fluid is increased to no more than 30–40 ml, it streams at motions from one recessus of the cavity to the other, and a dabble or splashing becomes audible. After resorption of the fluid and with regression, but not complete subsidence of the swelling of the joint capsule, a fine silky crepitation becomes perceivable. This sensation is intensified to raglike friction if the joint capsule becomes thickened and uneven. Finally, if the inflammation healed with fibrosis of the joint capsule, the latter is rubbed at each motion, and a continuous sandlike gnashing becomes audible. The more sclerosed the joint capsule, the louder and coarser is the grating noise.

If alterations in the articular cartilage supervene, the articular surfaces become rough and move along one another with a scratching or rasping noise. More of this is audible when the articular surfaces become very uneven secondary to intraarticular fractures; then the motion produces intermittent cracking noises. In osteoarthritis, the motion of worn-off articular surfaces is associated with a continuous scratching and crepitation, which changes into loud cracking noises when the articular edges and osteophytes rub one another like cogwheels. Intraarticular fragments are pushed under rattling and clashing within the articular cavity. Movement of a loose joint body between the articular ends causes a coarse grinding noise; if catapulted out from the joint cleft, it produces a smacking or popping noise. A torn and displaced meniscus manifests itself similarly. If uncoordinated motion such as in neuropathies is added to these changes, the articular ends crush thunderingly upon each other.

One is thus able to distinguish sounds and noises of different qualities in a joint cavity and may infer from them certain pathological anatomical alterations of a joint. The other value of joint auscultation lies in the fact that joint alterations may be perceived early enough by this simple and innocuous procedure, often before they can be detected by other modalities of examination.

5. Laboratory Studies of the Blood

A reciprocal relationship exists between systemic or local diseases of the body and the joints, as well as between diseases of the joints and the body. These influence each other. The entire organism responds to the pathology of joints by participating in their reactions and defense mechanisms. This mutual communication is carried out by the blood, and thus the interactions within the entire organism are manifested by a series of changes in the blood. Each of these phenomena characterizes the reaction of the body in one way or another; in their entirety they permit conclusions as to the nature and course of the joint affections and their impact on the body [91, 715, 1424]. Accordingly, study of the blood in joint diseases includes: (a) erythrocyte sedimentation rate (ESR), (b) concentration of C-reactive protein, (c) complete blood cell count and differential count, (d) chemical examination for abnormal or abnormally increased metabolites, (e) bacteriological examination, (f) immunobiological tests of the serum, and (g) determination of the histocompatibility complex.

a. If joints undergo damage from extensive injury, intensive inflammation, or neoplastic destruction, protein and proteinaceous substances are released into the blood stream. These substances derive partly from tissue decomposition and partly from general metabolic responses. The increase in proteins in the plasma has, among others, an effect on erythrocytes suspended in plasma by expediting their aggregation. This phenomenon can be measured by the erythrocyte sedimentation rate ESR. The Westergren method enjoys general application for this because it can easily be carried out. The length of the sedimented column of erythrocytes may be read after 1–2 h. More informative is the mean value, obtained by adding one-half the first hour value to one-half of the second hour value.

The normal mean value is 10–15 mm in men and 15–25 mm in women. The Wintrobe method, using a smaller amount of blood, is not as sensitive and may fail in cases in which the Westergren method discloses a distinct increase in ESR.

Most afflictions of joints affect the ESR in proportion to their intensity; the more acute and extensive the inflammation, the more accelerated is the ESR. The type and character of the joint inflammation also have a bearing; exudative and destructive (necrotizing) forms cause a marked acceleration while slowly aggravating granulations affect the ESR only slightly. After resorption of an intraarticular effusion, after regression of inflammatory infiltrates in the joint capsule, or on commencing fibrosis, the ESR gradually declines to normalcy, but it rises immediately in cases of recurrence of infiltrates. Posttraumatic shrinkage of the joint capsule and degenerative changes of the articular cartilage do not have significant affect on the ESR.

Extensive injuries to the joint capsule and articular epiphyses cause an acceleration of the ESR from the 3rd days to a mean to 25–30 mm. In arthritis of rheumatic fever, the ESR promptly rises to 40–50 mm and falls with initiation of successful salicylate treatment; however, recurrences of the fever are accompanied by new rises in the ESR. Chronic rheumatoid arthritis causes an acceleration in the ESR up to 50 mm and even 90 mm but with oscillations for many years and eventually normalizes after all organic changes in inflammation have subsided. Acute joint inflammations with serous or purulent effusion cause a prompt increase in ESR, in joint empyema with extensive tissue disintegration up to 70–100 mm. Gonococcal or pneumococcal arthritis or arthritis in abdominal typhoid fever may cause an increased ESR of up to 60 mm. Arthritis in viral influenza and nonspecific bacteriantigenic arthritis cause sedimentation rates between 25 and 40 mm. In tuberculosis of joints, ESR detects minor changes which are not revealed by roentgenographs; beginning synovial granulations cause less increase in ESR (30–40 mm) than the exudative form with persistent effusion, but disintegrating caseous granulations cause the greatest increases in ESR up to 70–100 mm or more. Mycotic infections maintain a high ESR of 55–95 mm over a long period of time, especially when draining sinuses persist. On the other hand, chronic posttraumatic arthritis has slight to moderate affect on the ESR. Degenerative joint conditions, such as osteoarthritis, neuropathic arthropathies, and endocrine arthropathies, cause a moderately elevated ESR of up to 25–35 mm, unless marked inflammatory changes participate in the response of the joint capsule. Such changes are observed in women aged between 50 and 70 years with pronounced endocrine insufficiencies. In gouty arthritis, the acute attack may be associated with rapid increase in ESR to 40–45 mm, followed by a gradual return to normalcy with the regression in the clinical symptoms. Excessive increases in ESR between 70 and much above 100 mm are observed in the late stage of malignant tumors with extensive disintegration of the articular tissues.

The value of determining the ESR is thus undisputed. While this rate represents a nonspecific reaction of the blood, it permits an evaluation of the severity of a joint disease, provided that no other part of the body has been affected. It is also useful for differential diagnosis between purely degenerative arthritic forms and intensely inflammatory ones. However, the greatest value of the ESR lies in the prognosis for any individual joint disease because comparison of several ESR values obtained after longer intervals indicates the progression or regression of the joint disease, the effectiveness of treatment, and the presence of foci of active inflammation after regional clinical signs have subsided.

b. The onset of inflammation in a joint is also associated shortly thereafter with increased concentration of other proteins in the plasma than those accounting for the elevated ESR. These are the C-reactive components of the complement proteins and the serum amyloid A. Because of the rapid and significant increase in these during the early phase of inflammation these substances have been designated as acute-phase reactants [249, 922, 1240]. C-reactive protein, which is normally present in concentrations of 0.2–0.5 mg/dl in healthy individuals, rises promptly in traumatic and inflammatory conditions of the joints to a concentration of 10 mg/dl. In severe inflammations or infections it may even increase to 30 mg/dl. Measurement of C-reactive protein is thus an informative test which often parallels the ESR; it is even more sensitive because it increases substantially in some cases, before a significant rise in ESR [336]. Furthermore, it decreases earlier than ESR when remission of the inflammation has been obtained by salicylates, gold injections, or corticosteroids and thus provides earlier information on the therapeutic effect. As with ESR, the essential value of determination of C-reactive protein lies in its serial application, which indicates the course of the joint disease and its response to treatment [91, 430, 602, 922]. These tests prove very informative especially in the management of gonorrheal arthritis, arthritis in Reiter's syndrome, enteropathic arthritides, and ankylosing spondylitis.

c. Joint diseases are also expressed in the cytological composition of the blood. Damage to the joints and defense mechanisms of the body lead to qualitative and quantitative changes in the blood picture; increase or decrease in its elements occur as well as episodic shifts in their participation in the blood picture. In most inflammatory joint diseases erythrocytes decrease to 4 times $\times$ 10^6 and even below 3 times $\times$ 10^6/ml. The more toxic the clinical picture, the more pronounced is the anemia; the concentration of hemoglobin decreases concurrently to below 12 mg/dl. Serum iron is also decreased, as is the serum iron binding capacity. The cause of this normocytic normochromic anemia lies in concurrent toxic harm to the blood-forming tissue, the bone marrow. This is noted especially in purulent arthritis and advanced rheumatoid arthritis by the decrease in hemoglobin concentration. If suppuration of a joint has not been adequately drained, a septic condition follows, with concomitant severe anemia. Syphilitic arthritis is usually associated with anemia characteristic for its tertiary phase. In tuberculosis of joints with caseation and cold abscesses, the long-lasting suppuration affects the blood-forming tissues and causes marked anemia.

The count of white blood cells is subject to more characteristic changes [475]; their total number shows an increase to 25000–30000 and even up to 70000/ml or more on aggravation of the inflammatory changes in joints. This reaction sets in earlier than any other response of the blood, often within 2–3 days. On the other hand, a decrease in the normal leukocyte count may set in primarily or may follow an increase in leukocytes if the sites for formation of leukocytes have been profoundly harmed. Since the various blood-forming organs differ in sensitivity, the various groups of white blood cells respond differently according to the type of toxic harm. Thus the differential count of white blood cells is an instructive and essential addition to the total count. This indicates the intensity of inflammation, the selective site of harm and/or response, and the defense reaction of the organism. The basic evaluation of the various cellular elements of the blood can be carried out on slides thinly smeared with blood. The stain according to Wright or May-Grünwald-Giemsa is used for differentiating the cells as to variations in their cytoplasm and nuclei.

Polymorphonuclear neutrophilic leukocytes are very responsive cells and represent the first defense troops against any inflammatory irritation. The greater the number of neutrophilic leukocytes, the more effective is the protection of the body. Here the bone marrow also releases immature forms: myelocytes, unsegmented metamyelocytes, and large promyelocytes. Thereby a considerable increase in the number of neutrophils up to 75%–80% results versus the other types of leukocytes – a left shift. This is observed to a small extent in the acute stage of rheumatoid arthritis and is very pronounced in acute specific arthritides provoked by pneumococci, gonococci, or enteritis bacilli. Neutrophilic leukocytes may also be increased briefly by 50% in an acute attack of gout. The most conspicuous increase in polymorphonuclear neutrophilic leukocytes is caused by empyema of a joint; this pattern may lead to a considerable decrease in granulocytes, agranulocytosis, due to harm to the bone marrow in cases of long-lasting, severe suppuration.

Eosinophilic leukocytes are indicators of a special state of disease. Their number is increased in all allergic reactions of joints, such as seroanaphylactic arthritis and intermittent hydrarthrosis. Cases of seropositive rheumatoid arthritis with pronounced extraarticular manifestations are also associated with increased eosinophils, suggesting in addition to other findings that rheumatoid arthritis may represent an allergic reaction to noxious factors. In other chronic processes, such as tuberculosis of joints, eosinophils decrease with expansion of the caseinating process and increase at the start of healing. An overwhelming toxicity with breakdown of the defense mechanism causes a disappearance of eosinophils from the blood stream; such a reaction is regarded as an ominous sign in suppurative arthritis and arthritis in abdominal typhoid fever. Changes in the number of basophilic leukocytes are not observed in joint diseases. Segmented (staff-nuclear) leukocytes and monocytes are increased when the inflammation of joints has passed its peak and is in the phase of regression and healing. Thus the increase in monocytes signals a favorable change and is observed at the completion of rheumatoid arthritis, cessation of joint suppuration, the healing of nonsuppurative bacterial arthritides, and the scarification of tuberculous granulations in joints. On the other hand, a decrease in monocytes occurs in the absence of healing of a protracted articular process, in the recurrence of rheumatoid arthritis or metastatic bacterial arthritides, and in tuberculosis of joints after miliary spread and affection of other organs, such as the meninges.

Lymphocytes [1380, 1405, 1624, 1765] represent the immunobiological reaction of the body and joint, and they also participate in the metabolizing of tissue remnants. Lymphocytes thus prepare for the restructuration of harmed tissue. An increase in lymphocytes to more than 65 % of the white cell count may be regarded as a sign of regressing joint inflammation or of the beginning of healing. Rheumatoid inflammations, specific bacterial joint infections, and articular tuberculosis are associated with lymphocytosis when they enter the phase of healing. However, if an aggravation occurs, and the toxicity of the articular process increases, lymphocytes decrease to 18 %–22 %. Lymphopenia is therefore an alarming sign in the course of a rheumatoid articular process with marked exacerbation or in tuberculosis of joints with mixed infection of a draining sinus. Arthritis in abdominal typhoid fever is associated throughout its course with lymphopenia; lymphocytosis sets in at the onset of healing. A relative lymphopenia below 15 %–18 % may be observed due to an increase in polymorphonuclear neutrophilic leukocytes in an intensive joint inflammation.

Since the various inflammations of joints are caused by different etiological factors and are associated with the particular course of the disease, a characteristic predominance of one or an other type of white blood cells may be noted in certain joint diseases. In the acute phase of rheumatoid arthritis a general leukocytosis appears without significant left shift. However, septic or metastatic arthritis is associated with neutrophilic leukocytosis and a left shift. In empyema of a joint, a strong neutrophilic leukocytosis starts and is followed by lymphopenia; leukopenia with relatively increased proportion of neutrophils versus lymphocytes may set in on aggravation of the suppuration. In gonorrheal arthritis the blood contains degenerative forms of leukocytes and monocytes. In arthritis following abdominal typhoid fever, the blood initially shows a brief leukocytosis and then leukopenia and lymphopenia; on general improvement a relative lymphocytosis follows, then an eosinophilia and finally an absolute lymphocytosis; an incidental absolute lymphopenia carries a dismal prognosis. In paratyphoid fever with arthritis a tendency to neutrophilic leukocytosis is noticed, which may revert to leukopenia in longer lasting abdominal conditions. The arthritis in dysentery is initially associated with leukocytosis and a strong left shift; remission of the disease complex is manifested by monocytosis. Arthritis in brucellosis displays a leukopenia with a specific decrease in eosinophilic leukocytes; lymphocytes and monocytes increase rather early during recovery. Arthritis in secondary and especially tertiary syphilis is usually associated with persistent monocytosis and lymphocytosis. The more intensive the inflammatory changes are in the course of tuberculosis of joints, the more pronounced the leukocytosis is too; a distinct left shift is regarded as serious because it indicates caseous decomposition or a mixed infection. Although monocytosis suggests a decrease in the inflammation, it can be observed for a longer period of time; but it is the lymphocytosis and the appearance of eosinophilic leukocytes which herald the phase of healing. Osteoarthritis does not cause any change in blood values, which is relevant diagnostically in distinguishing it from primarily inflammatory arthritides; however, at more pronounced inflammation of the joint capsule, lymphocytosis, but not leukocytosis is noticed.

Depending on the character of the joint affection, the changes in the blood picture display phases regarding the prominence of some types of blood cells and regression of other types; these correspond to the biological leukocyte curve observed in general inflammatory processes. The conflict between the noxious agent and the organism begins with the neutrophilic battle phase. In the fluctuations of progression and regression of the inflammation, the participation of neutrophilic leukocytes changes until this phase is resolved. The monocytic phase follows, and then the lymphocytic phase.

Due to its rapid and nonfailing changes, the blood picture offers instructive insights into the reaction of the body to the noxious agent, most often spread by the blood stream, and to the damage in joints. Although no specific diagnostic value may be attributed to the differential leukocyte count, this test is very informative by indicating the phase and/or nature of inflammation of a joint. The value of the differential leukocyte count corresponds to that of a specific serological reaction but lies in a different realm; it mirrors the reaction of the body and allows prognosis on the basis of results obtained at intervals. Of these findings, a decrease in neutrophilic leukocytes below 30 %–35 % is of major importance because it indicates a breakdown in the defense mechanism of the body and carries a very ominous prognosis.

d. Differential diagnosis is often possible on the basis of qualitative and quantitative identification of organic and anorganic substances, which as final products of normal metabolism or as intermediate products of a faulty breakdown appear in the blood during the course of a joint disease. In this chemical determination, attention is usually paid first to uric acid because joint inflammations are often of a gouty nature. The normal levels of uric acid are 6.5–7.2 mg% in men and 6.0–6.5 mg% in women, but the difference diminishes in elderly persons. Uric acid is usually increased following nutrition with food rich in purins and occasionally in pneumonia. Only in the absence of such conditions and in the presence of a joint affection does an elevated concentration of uric acid suggest the diagnosis of gouty arthritis. The levels of uric acid may then be increased up to 17–20 mg%. The causes of this may be: (a) primary metabolic abnormality with increased activity of phosphoribosyl-pyrophosphate synthetase and decreased activity of glucose-6-phosphatase [868, 869, 870]; (b) increased cell breakdown in hematological disorders such as leukemia, plasmacytoma, polycythemia vera, and secondary polycythemia; or (c) impaired kidney function with diminished glomerular filtration and decreased urate clearance. Thus the presence of hyperuricemia does not necessarily indicate that the articular symptoms under investigation are of gouty nature, and other possible causes of the articular symptoms should therefore be considered. Clinical situations associated with increased concentrations of urates (intake of diuretics, azotemia, cardiovascular conditions) but without eliciting articular symptoms must also not be disregarded [664, 1449].

The determination of other organic substances – such as total lipids and cholesterol in their concentrations [543, 1633] (normal: total lipids 450–1000 mg/dl, phospholipids 125–300 mg/dl, lipoprotein 260–400 mg/dl, fatty acids 220–370 mg/dl, cholesterol 140–250 mg/dl, triglycerides 30–150 mg/dl) – is essential in hyperlipoproteinemia. In this inherited disorder of lipoproprotein metabolism, chiefly the phospholipids and cholesterol are substantially increased and are deposited in articular tissues and especially in paraarticular tissues. Similarly, in lipoid dermatoarthritis (multicentric reticulohistiocytosis) most of the lipids are moderately or substantially increased due to a nonfamilial disorder of fat metabolism and are deposited, in addition to the skin, in articular structures, especially in articular epiphyses. An extensive deposition of a substantially increased lipid, glucocerebroside, in articular epiphyses and metaphyses occurs in Gaucher's disease.

The normal phosphorus concentration in blood is 3–4 mg%. In inflammations of joints associated with extensive osteoporosis of articular ends phosphates are released, and the concentration of phosphorus in the blood rises. Similarly in therapeutic administration of calcium preparations, increased phosphoric acid is released into the blood to buffer the calcium ions. The determination of calcium in the blood parallels the above test. Furthermore, the calcium level is symptomatically increased in the blood above the normal values of 9–12 mg% in joint diseases such as tuberculosis, in neuropathic arthropathies such as syringomyelia, and in malignant tumors causing destruction of articular epiphyses. Even more informative is the increase in calcium to 12.4–14.1 mg% in hyperparathyroidism, when with articular and paraarticular calcinosis and at concurrent increase in alkaline phosphatase to more than 100 IU, phosphate is decreased to 3.0–3.2 mg%. By the opposite hormonal influence, hypoparathyroidism, serum calcium is decreased to 7.3–8.2 mg%, and the phosphate level may reach 4.2–5.0 mg%. Decrease in calcium salts may occasionally be noted in secondary degenerative changes of several joints which are associated with sclerosis of the articular ends and paraarticular calcinosis.

e. Since inflammations of joints are occasionally caused by localization of microorganisms, demonstration of the latter in the blood is essential for ascertaining the etiology. The probability of success here is especially great when the blood specimens are withdrawn in the early phase of joint inflammation or in an episode of hematogenous spread manifested by elevation in temperature and/or chills. The microorganisms can then be demonstrated primarily in the blood smear stained with methylene blue or according to May-Grünwald-Giemsa, Wright, or Gram. The latter is preferable because it permits differentiation of the microorganisms, of which several have similar shapes, spread, stain, or arrangements. Gram-positive microorganisms pathogenic in joint infections, include staphylococci, streptococci, pneumococci, mycobacterium tuberculosis, actinomyces, and other mycotic fungi. Pathogenic gram-negative microorganisms include gonococci, meningococci, Shigella, Salmonella, Brucella, and influenza bacilli. A special stain for mycobacterium tuberculosis is the Ziehl-Neelsen stain which is used for blood specimens treated primarily with antiformin solution. Spirochetes are detected especially by contrast in dark-field illumination. Fungi are stained especially with periodic acid–Schiff or methenamine–silver nitrate Gomori stain. However, microscopic demonstration of microorganisms in the blood does not always succeed, especially because inflammation of the joints occurs mostly when the dissemination of microorganisms by the blood has been concluded with the localization in joints. Therefore, the presumably small number of microorganisms in the blood is increased by culture, which also helps to differentiate them by use of various culture media, such as plain agar, blood agar, chocolate agar, peptone agar, bouillon agar, or Sabouraud's glucose agar. Even then the demonstration of microorganisms is not always successful, and a negative outcome of a blood culture must not be interpreted as unequivocal proof of the absence of bacterial infection. On the other hand, the demonstration of microorganisms in the blood is proof of infection of a joint, unless other infected areas are also present in the body.

f. Nevertheless, the search for causative microorganisms in the blood in situations of many arthritides is often unsuccessful except in instances of septic arthritis in which staphylococci or less often streptococci, meningococci, or pneumococci can be detected in the blood by culture or occasionally by stained smear. Therefore, the search for harmful bacteriogenic effects also focuses on identifying antigenic substances emitted by these microorganisms and/or on identifying products of the human body which counter these harmful substances present in the serum and joint fluid. The antigens affecting joints are: proteins, lipoproteins, polysaccharide proteins, nucleoproteins, nucleic acids, and other chemicals [1021]. These antigens derive from: (a) exogenous sources (food, drugs), (b) microbial sources (bacteria, viruses, parasites) [26, 29, 1271], and (c) endogenous sources (autoantigens, tumor antigens). The identification of a specific antigen eliciting an immunological reaction, manifested by inflammatory response in a joint, may prove necessary for the diagnosis of a specific infectious disease. This can be performed by hemagglutination inhibition [1732], radioimmunoassay [986], and counter immunoelectrophoresis [1385].

Since the search for the emitted antigenic substances does not always yield positive results, the search for specific antibodies produced to combat an infection often provides a useful diagnostic modality. These antibodies are present in the serum and can be ascertained by exposing the serum to known specific antigens in the presence of sheep erythrocytes. The relevant serological tests are for agglutination, precipitation, and flocculation; these are used individually or to control each other and are often also controlled by the complement fixation test (discussed below). Agglutinins in the serum of patients can be identified by exposing the serum to a suspension of killed microorganisms considered to be pathogenic antigen for the disease in question. Agglutination at a high titer (above 1:128) can be taken as proof of an infection by the suspected pathogenic microorganism. Agglutination by the patient's serum of erythrocytes coated with meningococcal polysaccharide is tested, in addition to other infectious agents, in clinical conditions suggestive of meningococcal infection, but without isolation of meningococci. The agglutination test is similarly applied against the somatic antigen and the flagellar antigen in Salmonella infection. Agglutination is also tested in suspected Brucella infection. In this way an infection caused by a microorganism can be ascertained. Another, less often investigated antibody is antilysin, which is formed in response to the lysin produced by hemolytic streptococcus, the causative agent of upper throat inflammation and subsequent rheumatic fever. The above types of tests, which ascertain the presence of specific antibodies against presumed microorganisms or their antigens, show their positive outcomes by the concomitant participation of specific protein substances, the complements. This indicates the major importance of complements in a great number of immunobiological tests, as discussed below.

Chemical and electrophoretic examinations of the serum, as reviewed by Frangione and Buxbaum [538], reveal the peculiarity that, besides fibrinogen and other proteins, the gammaglobulins are particularly significantly increased in numerous types of joint inflammations. This increase is considered to be elicited by antigens of various natures. The globulins manifesting the immunological response to antigens are antibodies and are termed immunoglobulins. According to their different structural composition – length and polymerization of their amino acid chains, number of combined polysaccharides, antigenic properties – the immunoglobulins are subdivided into five main classes: IgA, IgD, IgE, IgG, and IgM [536, 537, 538, 539]. IgA participates chiefly in the defense against acute inflammations of infectious etiology. IgD is a minor immunoglobulin which together with IgM serves as a surface receptor on B lymphocytes. IgE contains reagins which interact with the cells causing the release of histamine and other substances responsible for the clinical manifestation of allergic states. IgG is the major immunoglobulin which provides the bulk of antibody in active and chronic inflammations. IgM predominates in many immune responses active for longer periods of inflammation [539].

Various immunological complexes result from the interaction of the antibodies, produced by polyclonal B lymphocytes [1021], with antigens, in varying concentration of each of these components [381, 711, 754, 837, 1348, 1818]. These are deposited especially in histiocytes, fixed macrophages, reticuloendothelial cells, and synoviocytes [934]. By interaction with the receptors of these cells, the immune complexes, especially those containing IgG and IgM antibodies, activate a complement system. This consists of nine distinct, enzymatically interacting proteins which are designated by the letter C and a sequential number. The first component is C1, which consists of three subunits: C1q, C1r, and C1s [1444]. The initial step in complement activation occurs by binding of C1q to the immune complexes. The complement proteins regulate the antigen-antibody complexes and thereby participate in the inflammatory response by the synovial tissue, among other tissues. They also participate in the elimination through lysis of microorganisms and irreversibly harmed tissue such as synovial tissue and articular cartilage [126, 381, 468, 518, 586, 588, 595, 743, 1021, 1158, 1187, 1372, 1444, 1649, 1818]. The levels of complement components are measured by immunodiffusion and by immunochemical assays using antisera specific for a given complement protein. These levels are higher in the serum of patients with rheumatoid arthritis, juvenile rheumatoid arthritis, gonococcal arthritis, and Reiter's syndrome [535, 1444, 1654] but are lower in those with very destructive rheumatoid arthritis and pronounced extraarticular manifestations, clinically similar juvenile rheumatoid arthritis, extensive psoriatic arthritis, and gouty arthritis [595, 1774].

Determination of complement levels in the serum is used clinically to evaluate the intensity of an active inflammatory process or the therapeutic response in this process. Participation of the complement proteins in the immunobiological process was suggested by Bordet et al. [162, 163]. Wassermann et al. [1717] demonstrated that when extracts of treponema pallidum are exposed to the serum of syphilitic patients, an interaction follows with concurrent binding of the complement proteins in the serum of the patient. Upon this reaction the complement fixation test is used not only for the etiological diagnosis of syphilitic arthritis, but also for identification of antibodies present in gonorrhoic arthritis and in arthritis caused by Shigella, Salmonella, Brucella, viruses [1255], actinomyces, or coccidioides. The formation and local deposition of antigen-antibody complexes in joints is associated with harm to the synovial membrane and articular cartilage and is followed by inflammation of the former. Identification and quantitative determination of immunoglobulins provide significant information as to the implication of an immunological complex in the reaction of an articular affection; thus they are of diagnostic value. Furthermore, their serial quantitative determination provides additional information, because increasing or decreasing titers of immunoglobulins indicate persistence or regression of the impact on joints. These determinations are of importance in evaluating the course in gonorrheal arthritis, Reiter's disease, Lyme's disease, and rheumatoid arthritis, among others.

In addition to the routine serological tests, immunofluorescence has received increasing acceptance for identifying specific antigens. Serum specimens containing a presumed antibody are mixed with a specific fluorescein-labeled (conjugated) antigen and then examined under a fluorescent microscope. In a positive combination, the resulting antigen-antibody complex emits a brilliant green-yellow light [321]. Thus, this technique is used in chronic gonorrheal arthritis with negative bacterial findings; the serum of the patient is exposed to fluorescein-conjugated gonococci. Similarly, in suspected meningococcal infection, the diagnosis can be corroborated by immunofluorescence of the relevant antibodies. In the late stages of syphilis, when the results of routine laboratory tests are often negative, the immunofluorescence method is also very useful because it detects the adsorption of antibodies onto fluorescein-conjugated treponemas [479].

In addition to the antibodies to antigens introduced into the body by external factors, secondary antibodies are formed against the initial immunoglobulins. These secondary antibodies are termed autoantibodies and are produced by activated polyclonal B lymphocytes [1536, 1812] mostly against IgG and IgM. They are detected chiefly in progressing rheumatoid arthritis (rheumatoid factor) and in some types of infectious arthritis. The autoantibodies are identified, for example, by the sheep cell agglutination and latex fixation tests [15, 456, 910, 1176, 1177, 1505, 1699]; their presence in at least 1:80 dilution accounts for the positive outcome of these tests.

g. The individually varying response of the body to identified antigen-antibody complexes has been explained in the past two decades by the varying histocompatibility complex located in the genes, termed the human leukocyte antigen (HLA) [909]. Three major categories of it HLA-A, HLA-B and HLA-C, have been identified by typing. The significance of this complex has been indicated by the clinical experience that carriers of the specific HLA-B27 gene manifest a conspicuous susceptibility for ankylosing changes of the spine. About 80% of patients with idiopathic ankylosing spondylitis, 60%–70% with Reiter's syndrome, 40% with psoriatic arthritis, and 10% with rheumatoid arthritis, all of them carriers of the HLA complex, develop ankylosing changes of the vertebral spine [415, 489, 1058]. Similarly, 15%–20% of individuals with positive findings of the HLA-B27 histocompatibility complex have an affection of the vertebral spine in any general disease. It appears that the HLA antigens, encoded in genes, are not by themselves responsible for the occurrence of inflammation of the spine. However, they influence the mode of general reaction of the body in the presence of an intensive disease and facilitate the establishment of a profound affection of the spine.

6. Urinalysis

In some joint diseases the pathogenetic microorganisms or abnormal metabolic products pass through the barriers of the blood stream and are eliminated through the kidneys. Examination of the urine constitutes a useful supplement to that of the blood since diseases and conditions affecting joints may also be reflected in the urine. Detection and identification of harmful agents in the urine is a simple and essential part of the investigations relevant to the etiology of articular affections.

The color of the urine may change to dark yellow or brown if urobilinogen in larger amounts is converted into urobilin; this occurs regularly when a large blood effusion in traumatic hemarthrosis or hemophilic arthritis is being absorbed. A more intensive discoloration to dark brown or black develops when the urine contains homogentisic acid; the latter, an intermediate product in the catabolism of tyrosin and phenylalanin, appears in the blood and accounts for the changes in ochronotic arthritis.

Of the substances normally contained in the urine, phosphorus and calcium may be increased in rheumatoid arthritis due to extensive osteoporosis of the articular ends. A decrease in excreted phosphorus occurs in gouty arthritis due to retention of phosphonucleotides in the body. Of greater significance in gout is the determination of urate concentration in the urine, which decreases from normal values of 0.5–0.7 g/l to 0.2–0.3 g/l. A decrease below this level characterizes the acute attack of gout and may last 2–3 days until the urate level in the urine rises with elimination of the increased purin amounts in the blood. Increased levels of uric acid in the urine also occur in secondary gout, in which substantially increased amounts of uric acid in the blood derive from excessive disintegration of nucleic acid in leukemia, erythroblastosis, multiple myeloma, and other conditions associated with an abnormal increase in red or white blood cells.

The amino acids tyrosine, leucine, and histidine do not normally occur in the urine but may do so in abdominal typhoid and paratyphoid fever. A wider range of protein substances is detected in the urine in chronic suppuration of joints, advanced rheumatoid arthritis, fungal mycotic arthritis with draining sinuses, disintegrating tumors of joints, and particularly in caseous tuberculosis of joints. An abnormal protein substance is the amyloid, which consists of light-chain immunoglobulins and is identified in the urine by the Bence-Jones test. A positive outcome of this test is considered characteristic for plasmacytoma (Fig. 422), but it is also occasionally positive in rheumatoid arthritis and psoriatic arthritis, which in extensive plasmacyte infiltrations are sometimes associated with amyloid deposition in the joint capsule (Fig. 426). In other conditions, intermediary metabolites such as phenylalanin and homogentisic acid are present in the blood and urine because of incomplete catabolism of protein and account for the joint changes in ochronosis (Figs. 359, 362). These can be identified in the urine by their chemically reducing property of solutions containing mercury, silver, or copper salts, whereby the urine becomes discolored black. Copper salt is routinely used in the Benedict's test for identifying abnormally increased glucose levels in the urine, as occurs in diabetes. Copper salt in solution is also reduced by metabolites from penicillin and other antibiotics. This diversity can be clarified by testing the urine for glucose with the more sensitive Fehling's reagent or Nylander's reagent. The corroborated increase in glucose in the urine, also checked with the glucose concentration in the serum, confirms the presence of diabetes, which may be an important factor in the etiology of arthropathy.

Thus the demonstration of abnormal substances or normal substances in abnormal concentrations in the urine is of diagnostic significance because it indicates disintegration of articular tissues by such substances.

The urine may also be examined for the presence of microorganisms by staining its sediment and by inoculating its specimens into culture media on which sensitivity tests are also carried out. In this way microorganisms may be detected which are either growing primarily in the urogenital tract, such as gonococci or tubercle bacilli, or have been transmitted by the blood stream into the urine. Other generalized infection may have been caused by streptococci, staphylococci, Escherichia coli, Brucella, Shigella, or Salmonella. Their identification in the urine confirms a specific metastatic inflammation of joints.

7. Radiological Examination of Joints

Radiological examination is very informative by providing insight into the conditions of joints, information not obtainable by other routine examinations. Therefore, radiological (especially roentgenographic) examination must not be excluded from any complete examination of joints. Although very instructive, radiological examination has its limits for diagnostic uses. Regardless of the etiology of the pathological process, only the physical densities of the various tissues are represented in different shades. Changes in soft tissues and cartilage are perceived only to a small degree, and only those changes of the soft tissues, cartilage, and bones are perceived which have macroscopically detectable size and thickness. The attempt to read the etiology and diagnosis primarily or solely from the roentgenographs and/or other radiographs must be regarded as speculative. By not taking the complete history of the patient, not performing the physical examination, or obtaining the indicated laboratory tests, one deprives oneself of certain etiological considerations and pathological-anatomical concepts. However, the corroboration of the diagnosis is provided by the radiological examination, which should be carried out as one of the final and concluding steps of the examinations.

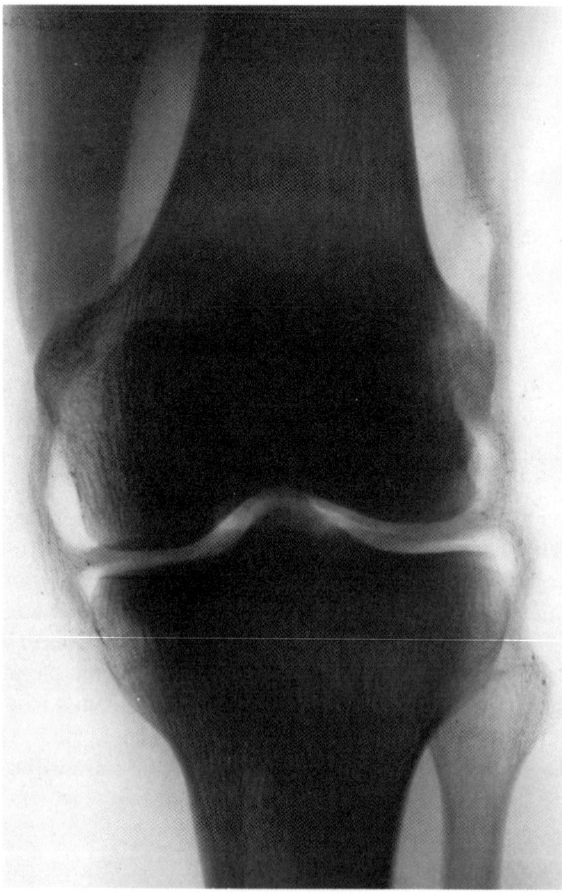

Fig. 15. In the AP view of the air-filled knee joint, the wedge-shaped filling defects in the joint cleft correspond to the menisci. The suprapatellar recessus expands far proximally

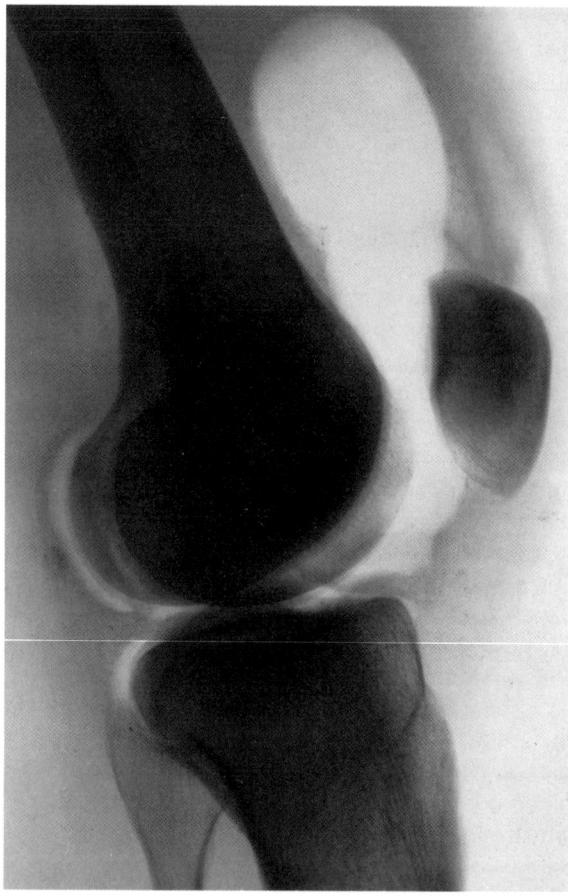

Fig. 16. In the lateral, view of the air-filled knee joint, the extent of the suprapatellar recessus and the infrapatellar fat pad, the wedges of the anterior and posterior horns of the menisci, and the extent of the posterior joint cavity are evidenced

Roentgenographic examination of the joints is performed in at least two planes, anteroposterior and lateral (Figs. 15, 16). Two additional oblique views should also be taken. The part of the articular epiphyses placed nearest to the cassette becomes most sharply focused. Physical details of roentgenographic exposure such as voltage and amperage should also be considered. Low voltage is used when evaluation of soft tissues is desired [425, 592]. The resulting structure-rich roentgenograph provides advantageous survey of the soft tissues and substantially assists in detecting changes within the joint cleft and regional variations in the calcium content of the articular epiphyses. A complete survey includes changes of the articular epiphyses, joint cavity, and articular soft tissues [315, 528, 592, 1276, 1471] for evaluation of the condition of a joint. In this examination, a basic knowledge of the normal structure of a joint and its variations within physiological limits, as revealed by routine roentgenographs, is indispensable.

When viewing the articular epiphyses, also termed articular ends, their shapes and configurations should be surveyed. Congenital malformations, injuries to bones with displacement, and subsequent callus formation, advanced osteoarthritis, and neuropathic arthropathies generally result in deformities of the articular epiphyses (Figs. 138, 432, 433, 447, 448, 455, 461). Their smooth outline may also be changed by destructive and/or proliferative processes within the bone or at the cortex (Figs. 115, 121, 136, 144, 146, 440, 447, 461). The contours of the paraarticular metaphyses become uneven (Figs. 115, 136, 181, 182, 447) secondary to traumatic or inflammatory periosteal apposition. Inside the articular epiphyses, areas of radiolucency or radiodensity may be perceived as sequelae of resorption, substitution, suppurative destruction, or necrosis which originated within the epiphyses and secondarily perforated into the joint or emanated from the joint cavity and secondarily invaded the articular epiphyses (Figs. 80, 81, 98, 115, 116, 147, 165, 166, 265). Recent infectious destructions are characterized by poorly delimited foci of radiolucency with loss of the bone structure and osteoporosis in the vicinity (Figs. 80, 81, 98, 105, 170). After healing of the inflammatory processes the margins of the foci become smoother, and the calcium content returns (Figs. 121, 122, 144, 146). On the other hand, irregular but sharply delineated densifications in the soft tissue or osseous tissue may occur secondary to local deposition of calcium salts or to benign new bone formations (Figs. 285, 389). A frequent change following regional hyperemia is decalcification of the osseous parts with rarefaction of the trabecular structure. The osteoporosis may homogeneously involve the entire epiphysis but is more often manifested by poorly delimited radiolucent areas (Figs. 234, 235, 264). Metabolic and blood disorders as well as tumors are also able to produce changes in the structure of the articular epiphyses (Figs. 351, 399, 405, 406, 407, 420). These conditions cause lentil-sized or more extensive areas of partial or more profound radiolucency, which in most cases are irregularly outlined (Figs. 63, 291, 351, 366, 378, 379, 419, 424) but rather sharply delineated. However, in malignant tumors the radiolucencies are intense and are invariably of blurred outlines (Figs. 523, 524). As the late sequelae of inflammatory processes and of all degenerative processes, marginal osteophytes develop which distort the roundness of the articular epiphyses and are very deforming components (Figs. 110, 111, 238, 263, 265, 438).

The joint space, or more appropriately the cartilage space, is formed by the end-to-end apposition of the epiphyses, which by merging on their articulating surfaces with a cover or cap of hyaline cartilage have become the articular ends. The clarity of this space is determined by the radiolucency of the contiguous cartilage covers, and the width of the joint space corresponds to the thickness of the cartilage covers plus the width of the interposed articular cleft and synovial fluid. The actual articular cleft is only a little wider than a hair line (Fig. 4). The width of the cartilage space averages about 4 mm but shows physiological variations depending on the thickness of the contiguous cartilage covers in correlation with the size of the joint. This space is narrower in the interphalangeal joints (Fig. 378) and wider in the shoulder (Fig. 554), hip (Fig. 223), and knee (Fig. 234) joints. The exact thickness measurements of the articular cartilage are presented in "Anatomy and Histology of Joints". In children the cartilage space is broader due to the greater thickness of the cartilage cover of the incompletely ossified articular epiphyses (Fig. 147). In the elderly the cartilage space becomes narrower due to attritional thinning of the cartilage cover (Figs. 263, 264). In evaluating the cartilage space, the following criteria are used: congruency, width, delimitation, and transparency. Congruent articular contact is determined by the normal alignment and physiological configuration of the articular ends. In congenital or posttraumatic malformation or traumatic displacement of the articular ends, this congruency is diminished (Figs. 432, 433, 439, 447, 448, 449). Axial deviations in acquired deformities lead to one-sided widening and/or one-sided narrowing of the cartilage space (Figs. 45, 121, 145, 150, 234, 430, 438, 440, 461). Unequal or one-sided widening of the cartilage space may also be caused by the interposition of radiolucent solid structures, such as malformed menisci, cartilaginous loose joint bodies, or nodular protrusions of the joint capsule. In a similar way, interposed loose bodies of bone density stemming from osteochondritis dissecans, osteocartilaginous metaplasia in the joint capsule, or separation of marginal osteophytes may account for one-sided widening of the cartilage space. A uniform widening of the joint space is caused by interposition of increased joint fluid in fresh or recurrent traumatic or inflammatory effusions (Fig. 147).

On the other hand, narrowing of the cartilage space is caused by decrease of the thickness of the articular cartilage, occurring most often in degenerative attrition (Figs. 264, 285, 330, 357). The remaining cartilage space is usually evenly delimited, and the subchondral cortical borders of the articular epiphyses are rather sclerosed (Figs. 144, 146, 192, 285, 430). Suppurative destruction or enzymatic disintegration of the articular cartilage, erosion by granulation tissue, or wearing off of portions of the articular cartilage account for one-sided or overall narrowing of the cartilage space (Figs. 81, 95, 98, 105, 116, 149, 150, 170, 219). In any of these events, uneven delineation of the joint space may be associated with irregular spots of osteoporosis expanding into the subchondral bone (Fig. 291). When both adjacent cartilage covers are completely worn off, the subchondral cortical margins of the apposed articular ends are contiguous with each other, and the joint space is partly or totally absent (Figs. 88, 189, 192, 492, 500). Nevertheless, the outline of the denuded articular epiphyses is sharp and anatomically normal (Figs. 263, 264) if the subchondral bone has remained intact. Irregular, sharply delimited indentations may develop (Figs. 110, 219, 432, 446) secondary to localized grinding of sclerosed margins. The ossification line of the articular epiphyses may also be disrupted by eroding granulations of the synovial membrane which advance deeply or by proliferations from the subcortical marrow; the delineation of the articular epiphyses becomes irregular or indistinct (Fig. 81). In advanced osteoarthritic changes cartilage portions may become dislodged into the subcortical bone marrow and produce cystic areas of radiolucency there (Fig. 291).

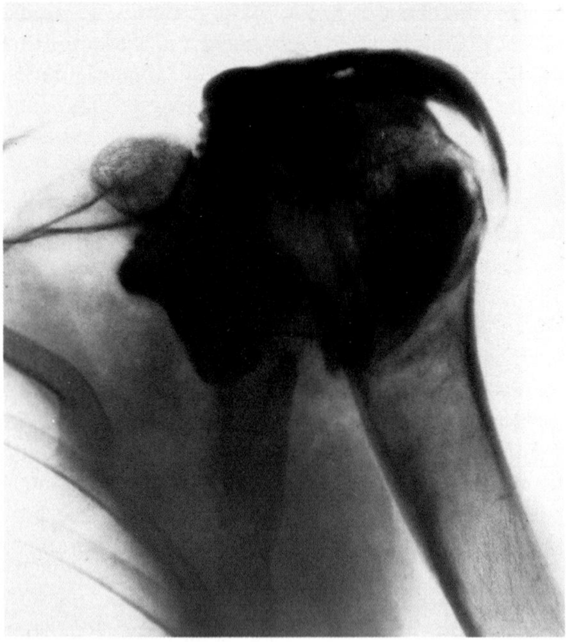

Fig. 17. Contrast filling of the shoulder joint outlines the subacromial bursa and indicates a large tear of the rotator cuff

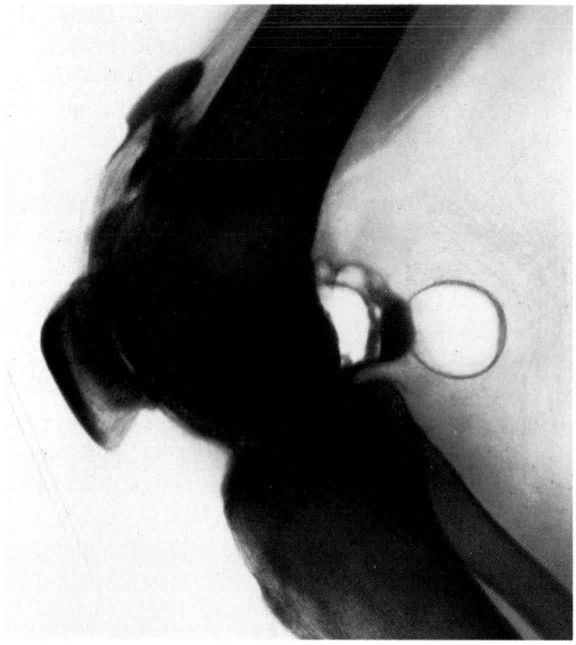

Fig. 18. Contrast filling of the knee joint discloses accumulation of air and positive contrast material in a posterior outpouching, indicative of a popliteal cyst

On the other hand, when enchondral ossifications appear at the edges of the articular surface, they form marginal small protrusions or beaklike osteophytes (Fig. 291).

In order to perceive the cartilage space, its radiolucency and width must have been preserved. However, overlying soft tissue formations of increased density may produce interfering shadows. An essential effect is exerted here by the joint capsule which, when densified by extensive inflammatory infiltrates or by fibrosis, overlaps the cartilaginous and osseous portions of the articular ends as an indistinct curtain. The joint capsule partly interferes here with the penetration by X-rays; the cartilage space is shadowed. The more intensive the density of the joint capsule, the more blurred is the structure of the articular epiphyses (Figs. 105, 136, 523, 524). The normally faint perceptibility of the joint capsule is substantially enhanced by intracapsular new formations of dense tissue as in fibromata or chondroosteomata (Figs. 56, 514) or by intracapsular deposition of osteocartilaginous fragments in neuropathic arthropathies (Figs. 446, 454). One can also distinguish whether this or an increase in joint fluid causes the enlargment of a joint. If the cartilage space is filled with very dense fibrous or osseous tissue, its radiolucency is diminished or lost (Fig. 357).

Roentgenographs thus noninvasively provide reliable information on the condition of the articular components and permit an interpretation of the pathological-anatomical changes in a joint. Serial roentgenographs ascertain progression or regression of any articular changes, as well as the response to therapeutic measures.

The routine roentgenograph, as informative as it may be, is not able to provide information on the capillary joint cleft or on the extent of the joint cavity or its delineation by the joint capsule. For the visualization of this, the joint cavity is filled with contrast medium having a different penetrability to X-rays than the articular tissues.

As negative contrast material, plain air, oxygen, carbon dioxide, or nitrogen is used. As in all interventions in joints, aseptic precautions must be observed. After administering local anesthesia, a long needle, connected to a manometer and a cylinder containing the gas of choice, is introduced into the joint cavity. Repeated perforations of the joint capsule must be avoided, so that no air escapes into the paraarticular spaces which could lead to misinterpretation of the findings. If the joint fluid is increased, it is aspirated. Air or gas is permitted to flow in, until the manometer indicates a rise in the intraarticular pressure from 8 to 100 mm. Roentgenographs in a few planes reveal the configuration of the joint cavity, inner outline of the joint capsule, shape of intraarticular structures, and extent of all recesses (Figs. 15, 16). These roentgenographs are used chiefly for demonstration of abnormal outpouchings of the joint capsule (Fig. 18), of the presence of free bodies, or of tears of menisci.

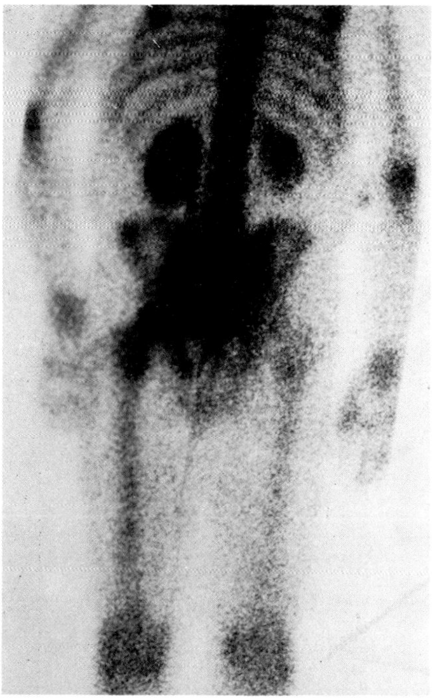

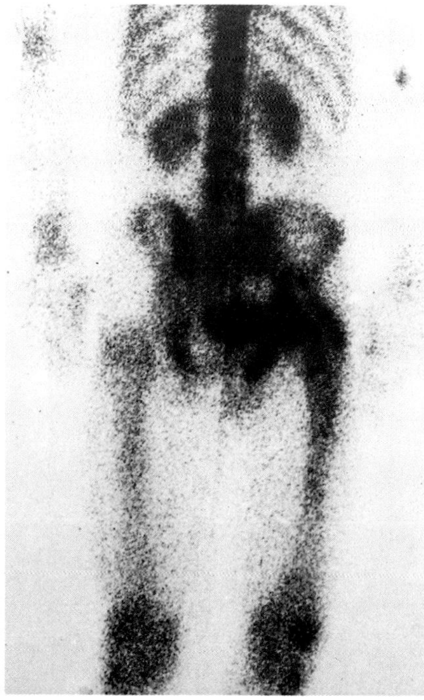

Fig. 19. Scintigram discloses a distinct decrease in uptake of radionuclides in the left femoral head, neck, and entire shaft, suggestive of avascular necrosis

Fig. 20. Scintigram discloses a distinct increase in uptake of radionuclides in the left femoral head and neck secondary to arthrodesis

For positive demonstration of the joint cavity, 3–4 ml water-soluble contrast material is injected into the joint and distributed as a thin film by movements of the joint over its entire inner surface. The contrast layer provides a view of the inner outline of the joint capsule and the configuration of the joint cavity, articular epiphyses, intraarticular structures, and suspected outpouchings of the joint capsule (Figs. 17, 18). Inflammatory changes of the joint capsule cause an irregular wavy, serrated or bumpy outline. The contrast filling was formerly also used in the intravertebral canal for visualization of the spinal cord, but this has been widely replaced by computed tomography (CT) in view of the meningeal irritation sometimes following myelography. Furthermore, the intraarticular contrast solution is usually injected in combination with a gas or room air for better and overall even distribution. Although applicable to any joint and any type of joint pathology, the combined positive-negative (double) contrast roentgenography is used mostly in the shoulder, elbow, or knee joint for demonstrating lesions of the meniscus, marked proliferations of the synovial membrane, changes or outpouching of joint capsule, or the presence and location of free bodies [358, 745, 1186, 1276, 1664]. However, misinterpretation may occur because of the possibility of irregular distribution of the contrast material. Therefore, only unequivocally positive or negative contrast roentgenographic findings may be used for corroboration of a clinical diagnosis.

In addition to the routine and the contrast techniques, other modalities of radiological technique have proven of diagnostic benefit in special conditions of the skeleton and for elucidation of specific questions of osteoarticular conditions.

The tomogram is a roentgenographic image of a specific layer, obtained by moving the roentgen tube and the film cassette. Thereby one layer of tissue is sharply demonstrated while the structures of the areas above and below are blurred. Precise information is provided on the extent and delineation of a lesion as well as on the level of its maximal manifestation.

Radionuclide imaging is based on the fact that injected radioactive substances arrive through the blood stream into the skeleton in concentrations commensurate with the local blood supply. The radionuclides are then localized by chemoabsorption into the hydroxyapatite crystals of the bony substance depending on the regional vitality of the examined tissues [361, 418, 592, 593, 677, 908, 1173, 1664, 1816]. Being well tolerated and promptly absorbed, the radioactive substance technetium-99m [17] has received general application. By its decreased or increased uptake in bone, technetium provides very instructive information on the changes developing in bone [17]. These changes occur either by obliteration of the blood supply and concomitantly decreased uptake (Fig. 19) or by restored blood supply and by restructuring of the osseous tissue with increased uptake (Fig. 20). Therefore, the scintigram is used for verification of necrosis of the femoral head

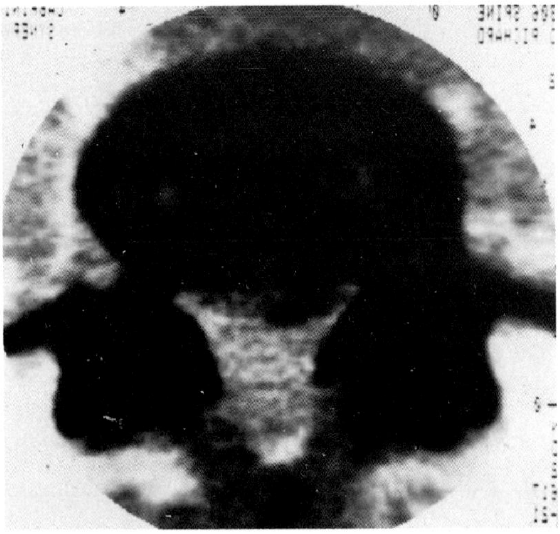

Fig. 21. CT scan discloses a herniated disc at L4–5, and an extrusion totally effacing the left nerve root of S1

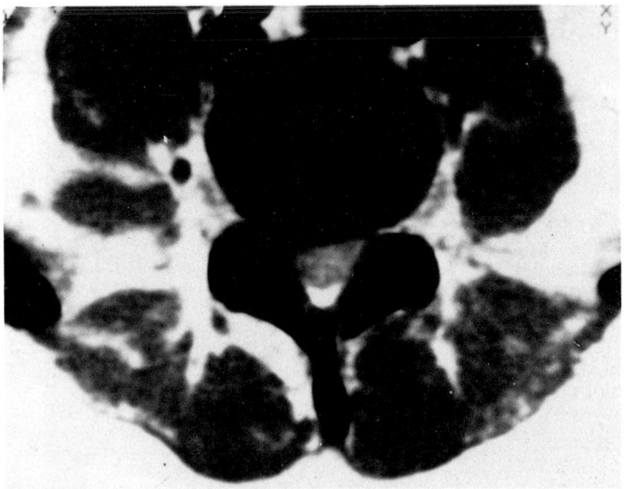

Fig. 22. CT scan through the L4–5 interspace shows a posterior protrusion of the intervertebral disc. The right nerve root of S1 is displaced by the herniated disc

and its stages arising from prolonged intake of corticosteroids, chronic alcoholism, hemoglobin abnormalities, fat embolism, and other conditions associated with substantial decrease in the local blood supply. The scintigram is also useful for ascertaining increased or decreased uptake of radionuclides in stress fractures, infections, and metastases in which the destructive or reconstructive phase can be evaluated.

High-resolution radiography obtains images directly magnified up to four times by the use of small focal spot tubes and fine grain films. It thus provides enhanced visualization of fine structural changes and is of value especially for clarifying articular and trabecular alterations of small bones [425, 592, 1280].

A higher resolution can be obtained by the computerized tomography CT which clarifies the spatial relationship of neighboring organs by distinctly delineating soft tissue from osseous tissue. The image is obtained by measuring the density of rays emanated from a roentgen tube moving above the patient and differently absorbed by various tissues of the body. The resulting information is fed into a computer which produces a roentgenographic-like image on a cathode ray tube. By the identification of organs of different structural density, the CT scan [250, 512, 514, 740] provides circumspective information on the outlines of all organs present at one level. The CT scan is thus able to detect soft tissue tumors in areas physiologically free of such densities [539]. CT can also be used at any level of the axial and peripheral skeleton affected by intra- and periarticular disorders [512, 514]. It is used mostly for otherwise unclarified conditions of the vertebral spine, sacroiliac joints, pelvis, and extremities. The special value of the CT scan is in questions regarding the relationship of the vertebral spine to the spinal cord, chiefly in compression of the spinal cord assumed to be caused by a herniated intervertebral disc. CT enables the visualization of this disc and its relationship to the neighboring spinal cord and the ascertainment of a possible compression of the latter and its nerve roots (Figs. 21). CT has widely complemented or substituted myelography in situations of neurological symptoms presumably resulting from compression by a herniated intervertebral disc (Fig. 22). CT is also helpful in outlining invasive tissue of a malignant tumor in a joint [639].

Magnetic resonance imaging (MRI) has recently found increasing application. This modality obtains images by nuclear magnetic resonance [1138, 1673] owing to the fact that the protons in the hydrogen nuclei emit signals when subjected to a magnetic field. The strength of these signals is proportional to the local and characteristic density of hydrogen protons present in any type of organic tissue. The emitted signals are encoded with spatial arrangement, producing a magnetic resonance image. This has the advantage over a CT scan of improved contrast sensitivity, and that it can be obtained with sagittal, frontal, axial, and oblique views. It is also used in articular disorders [1134, 1504] in which abnormities of the synovial membrane, articular cartilage, and intraarticular fibrocartilage can be visualized distinctly (Figs. 23, 24). Firooznia [513] emphasized the diagnostic value of MRI in detection of traumatic, inflammatory, and neoplastic disorders of ligaments, tendons, and muscles. Firooznia [512], Chafet et al. [267], and Modic et al. [1122] indicated the usefulness of MRI in diagnosing lesions of the spinal cord, spinal nerves, and intervertebral discs.

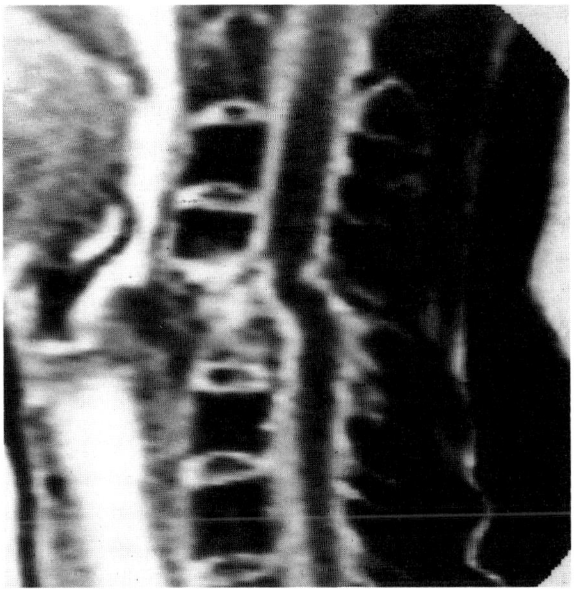

Fig. 23. MRI of the cervical spine discloses extensive destructive changes at C5–C6 and distortion of the spinal cord

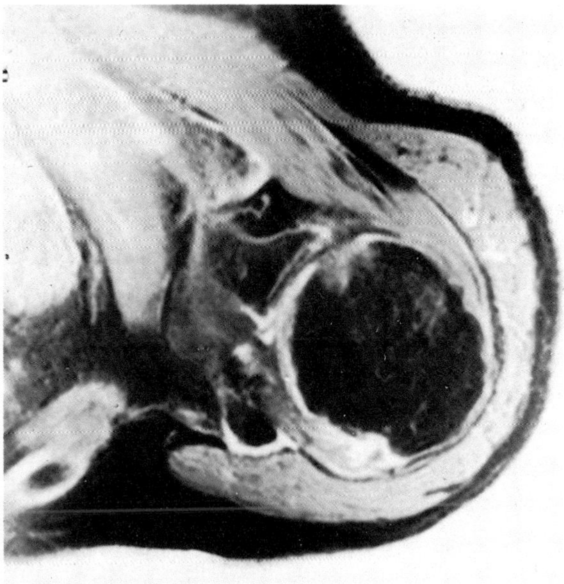

Fig. 24. MRI of the shoulder joint discloses erosive changes of the glenoid cavity and humeral head

8. Arthrocentesis and Examination of the Synovial Fluid

Increased joint fluid is removed primarily for therapeutic considerations in all situations in which the joint fluid does not absorb within 2–3 days despite conservative treatment, and secondarily for diagnostic purposes. Since the potential complications of this procedure resemble those of a surgical intervention, it must be performed with aseptic precautions. The skin of the region must be cleansed thoroughly with pHisohex and then with alcohol, and it should be covered with sterile towels. All necessary utensils and instruments are arranged on a table covered with a sterile sheet: sterile sponges, a sterile anatomical forceps for directing the injection needle, injection needles of gauges 22, 20, and 19 and 1.5–2.0 in. long (4 in. for the hip joint), disposable syringes, a vial with 1% anesthetic solution, sterile test tubes, heparin-filled tubes, and glass slides.

The insertion site for the aspirating needle should be chosen for the shortest route from the skin to the joint cavity. The decision as to site also takes into the consideration the area where the increased joint fluid causes the most prominent or palpable bulging and the anatomical route which avoids vulnerable tissues (blood vessels and nerves) and overlying thick structures, such as tendons. The following routes are generally used for the major joints. The shoulder joint is entered at its anteroinferior aspect between the convexity of the humeral head and the more deeply located anterior rim of the glenoid cavity. The elbow joint is entered superoposteriorly between the lateral humeral condyle and the olecranon. The hip joint can be entered either anteroposteriorly at a point lying laterally from the femoral blood vessels and on a line connecting the tip of the greater trochanter with the ilioinguinal ligament or anterofrontally along the anterior aspect of the femoral neck and on a line connecting the tip of the greater trochanter with the center of the femoral head. The knee joint can best be entered superolaterally to the base of the patella (Fig. 25); the needle enters the suprapatellar recessus and from there the cavity between the patella and the patellar groove of the femur. In an effusion of smaller quantity in the knee joint and depending on the predominant site, the needle is inserted medially or laterally to the apex patellae directly into the medial or lateral compartment. For the ankle joint,

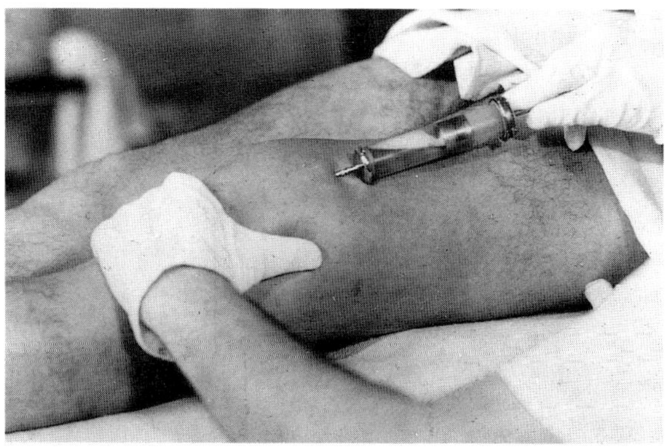

Fig. 25. Arthrocentesis of the knee joint by the aspirating needle inserted into the suprapatellar recessus

the anterior approach laterally to the dorsalis pedis artery and the tendon of extensor hallucis longus represents the most direct route.

The injection needle is attached to a syringe filled with anesthetic. After anesthetizing the skin, the needle is advanced toward the joint cavity, while simultaneously infiltrating the tissue in its pathway. One senses the penetration of the joint capsule by the sudden plunging of the needle into a space without resistance; prompt aspiration of joint fluid confirms that the needle is in proper site. When a larger amount of joint fluid is noticeable by the extent of fluctuation, it is advisable to intercalate a three-way stopcock between the needle and the syringe in order not to detach repeatedly the syringe from the needle for repeated emptying of the syringe. After most of the joint fluid has been withdrawn, the needle with the syringe is gently moved forward and to the sides to aspirate any remnants of fluid accumulated in side pockets or outpouchings of the joint capsule. On the sensation that the entire joint fluid has been removed, the syringe with the needle is withdrawn under continuous aspiration. However, sometimes in the presence of a remaining palpable quantity of joint fluid, the syringe, even by force, does not succeed in aspirating further fluid. This indicates that the needle has been plugged by clots of fibrin or fragments of synovial tissue. Therefore, the needle must be cleared by pressing air or physiological saline solution with the syringe through the needle. If this does not succeed, a 19- or 20-G needle attached to another syringe should be inserted along a new, although similar route.

Since arthrocentesis is an intraarticular procedure which may aggravate an existing irritation of the joint capsule, the latter should afterward be either compressed with a firm strapping or immobilized with a splint for 1 week. Administration of antibiotics for the following 3 days is indicated. In the case of posttraumatic, rheumatoid, or nonseptic joint inflammations, ampicillin 0.5 g orally six times daily suffices. However, in cases of suspected septic inflammation, ampicillin 1.0 g orally, six times daily or penicillin 10×10^6 U daily in divided doses should be administered intramuscularly until the culture and sensitivity test of the synovial fluid have clarified whether microorganisms are present and whether antibiotics are further indicated.

Examination of the synovial fluid provides information on the biology and pathology of a joint [195, 354, 465, 616, 774] and partly on participation by the body. The synovial fluid is by its hyaluronate a genuine product of the synoviocytes, and by the admixture of proteins, diffused from the subsynoviocytic blood vessels through synoviocytic stomata, a contribution from the plasma. Under normal conditions no joint fluid can be removed because it amounts even in major joints (hip and knee joints) to no more than about 4–5 ml. This amount is spread in a thin layer over the inner surface of the entire joint and is slightly more accumulated in outpouchings of the joint capsule. An increase in synovial fluid may occur in any traumatic, allergic, chemical, or toxic irritation or in bacterial infection of the inner part of the joint capsule; it may range from 15 to 450 ml in volume. A greater quantity of increased fluid occurs mostly in the knee joint (Figs. 68, 77) which has the widest articular cavity.

To obtain as complete an evaluation as possible, the increased synovial fluid is analyzed by the following methods [717, 1051, 1266, 1439]: (a) macroscopic and physical examination, (b) microscopic examination, (c) microbiological examination, (d) chemical examination, and (e) immunobiological examination.

a. The color of the aspirated fluid varies from pale yellow to brown due to admixture of bilirubin resulting from hemoglobin of extravasated erythrocytes; the synovial blood vessels are hyperemic in all situations of irritation. The synovial fluid is uncolored only in intermittent hydrarthrosis and in allergic serum effusion. However, its appearance may resemble nonclotted blood in fresh traumatic effusions and in effusions in hemophilia. Hemorrhagic admixtures in clouds or stripes to yellow effusions are mostly caused by perforation of blood vessels at the time of arthrocentesis. On the other hand, gray or whitish yellow creamy appearance of the synovial fluid is caused by increased admixture of white blood cells. The effusion in rheumatoid arthritis is light to dark yellow, that in gonococcal and pneumococcal arthritis greenish yellow, and that in abdominal typhoid arthritis yellowish gray. Fresh nonhemorrhagic and nonpurulent effusions are clear. However, when colloidal substances and elements formed from the blood and inner joint capsule are admixed to the joint fluid, the effusion becomes turbid. Accordingly, one distinguishes serous, serofibrinous, hemorrhagic, and purulent effusions. The increase in globulins in rheumatoid and tuberculous arthritis and the shedding of minute cartilage or synovial fragments in osteoarthritis cause a cloudy turbidity. The increase of fibrinogen in gonococcal arthritis causes a flaky to spider-web turbidity, and the increase of mucin in abdominal typhoid fever and syphilis causes an opalescence of the synovial fluid. In effusions of longer duration, the fibrinogen precipitates in yellowish white flakes. In gout, long white needlelike crystals or amorphous crumbs precipitate; in actinomycosis sulfur-yellow granules, and in ochronosis blackish granules occur almost invariably in the synovial fluid. With the admixture of proteins [1497, 1498], especially fibrinogen and prothrombin from the blood, and in proportion to their increase, the normally non-

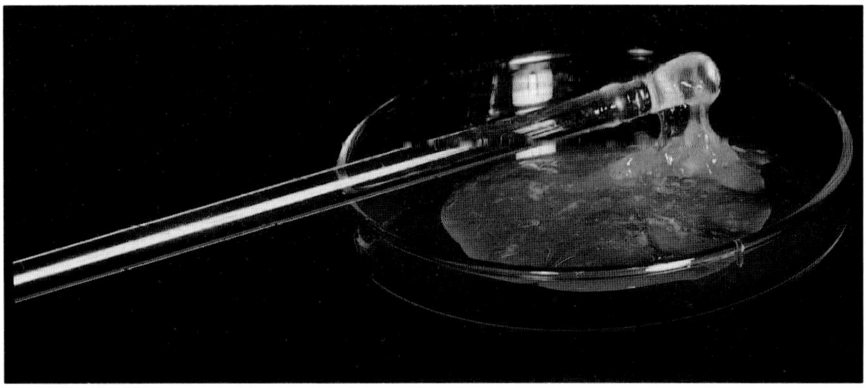

Fig. 26. This synovial fluid, aspirated from a knee joint with myxoma (Fig. 509), has a viscosity of 410, as manifested by its dense string formation

clotting synovial fluid coagulates rather fast. Therefore, addition of heparin to the test tubes is necessary to prevent clotting of the synovial fluid and to permit numerical and morphological determination of its cellular admixtures. Concurrently also the specific gravity of clear fresh effusions measuring 1018–1022 increases to 1025–1045 in longer lasting and very turbid effusions and rises even more in purulent effusions.

Beyond these, a very fundamental examination is that for viscosity, a property determined by the reciprocal friction of the component organic particles. This test evaluates the presence, concentration, and polymerization of the hyaluronate serving in the lubrication of joints. The viscosity can be estimated roughly by its property of string formation when slowly ejected from the aspirating syringe, or when pulled between two fingers. By these tests, the viscosity is found to be normal or may be increased in degenerative joint conditions [374], is substantially increased in benign joint tumors, but is essentially decreased in chronic joint inflammations [1335] due to enzymatic degradation of the hyaluronate [41, 1196]. Another simple, yet sufficiently practical evaluation of the degree of hyaluronate polymerization is rendered by the test for mucin clot formation [1341, 1342]. In this test, 10% acetic acid is added to the synovial fluid; a firm ropy clot is formed at normal or degenerative conditions of the joint, but a loose, flocculent clot results from chronic inflammation of the joint [772]. Precise determination of the viscosity of the synovial fluid, as measured in units against the flow time of water, can be obtained by the viscometer of Ostwald [75, 153, 827]. This examination of the synovial fluid yields an intrinsic viscosity of 90–150 units in normal joints, normal or increased viscosity of 165–280 units in degenerative joint conditions, and increased viscosity of 300–

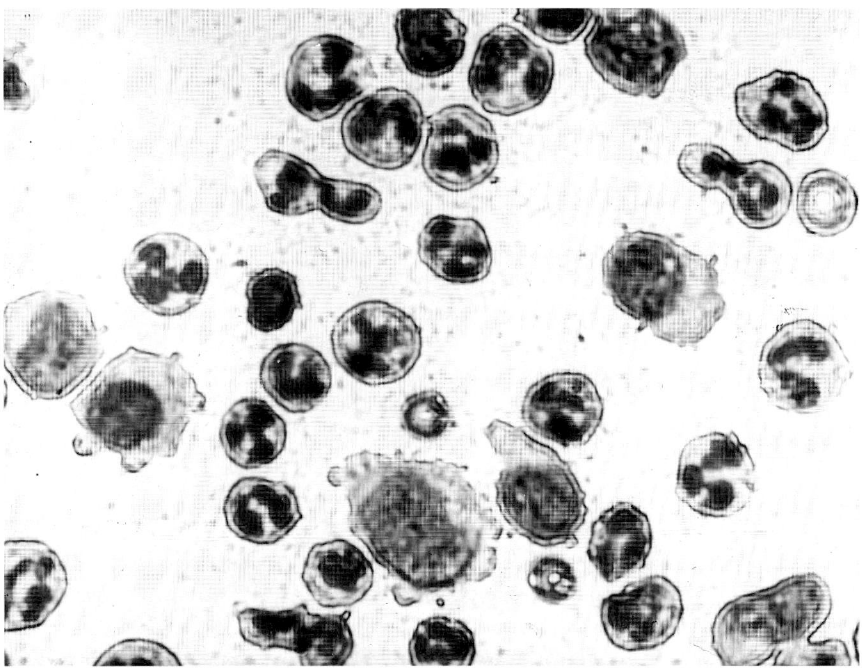

Fig. 27. The synovial fluid from rheumatoid arthritis in an acute phase presents a larger proportion of polymorphonuclear leukocytes and a smaller proportion of plasmacytes, lymphocytes, histiocytes, and synoviocytes

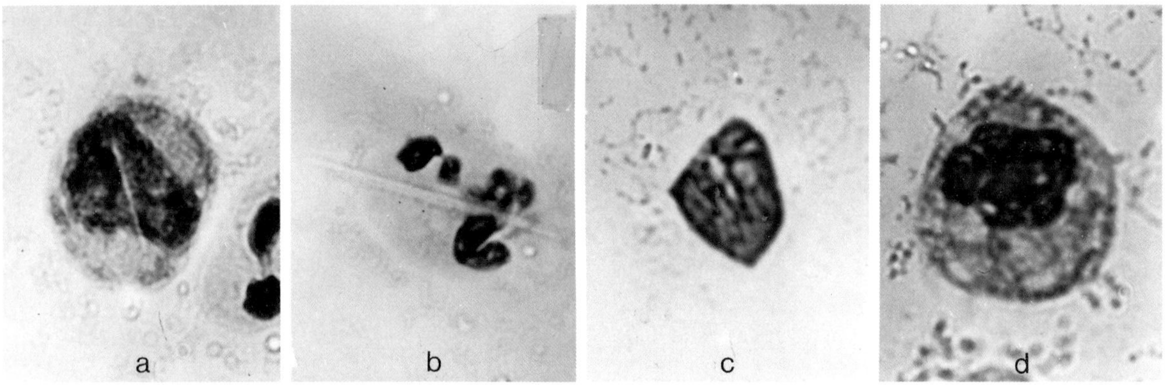

Fig. 28. The synovial fluid, mostly in degenerative arthritis, sometimes contains: *a* calcium pyrophosphate long thin needle crystals in histiocytes; *b* calcium pyrophosphate long thin needle crystals in leukocytes; *c* apatite plump rod crystals in histiocytes; *d* apatite small clumps in histiocytes

420 units (Fig. 26) in benign joint tumors. On the other hand, secondary to degradation of the hyaluronate by the enzymes originating from the synoviocytes and leukocytes, the viscosity is moderately decreased to 65–90 units in traumatic effusions and to 35–70 units in rheumatoid arthritis and other chronic inflammations of joints.

b. Microscopic examination of the synovial fluid [547], to which 0.3% saline or heparin solution has been added, starts with the total count of white blood cells. The normal synovial fluid contains about 50–100 cells while these are increased to 200–2000 in mild irritations and to 2000–40000 in any distinct inflammation, including rheumatoid arthritis (Fig. 27); they increase above 50000 to 100000 in septic inflammation [958]. Further information by identification and differential counting can be obtained in wet smears, but more instructively on dried smears and stained with methylene blue or according to Wright or May-Grünwald-Giemsa. In normal synovial fluid and that at mild irritation or degenerative alteration of the joint, synoviocytes and monocytes predominate among the cellular elements, but the lymphocytes predominate (Fig. 30) at more pronounced inflammation and chronic course. With intensified inflammation and mainly in its acute phase, polymorphonuclear neutrophilic leukocytes assume an increased proportion up to 90% (Fig. 27). Such proportion, sometimes reaching even 95% (Fig. 29), is highly suggestive of a purulent inflammation [916].

On longer duration of a septic process, neutrophilic leukocytes display degenerative changes with swelling of the cell bodies and vacuolization of the cytoplasm; some of them show loosening of the nuclear structure, and others show shrinking and pyknosis of the nuclei. The proportion of intact to degenerated leukocytes permits an inference on the toxicity and duration of the septic or purulent process. The participation in the cleansing from inflammatory alterations is noticeable in a great number of the leukocytes (ragocytes) by their peripheral inclusion bodies. Some of these inclusions are of irregular outline and probably stem from disintegrated synoviocytes, while other roundish inclusions are immunoglobulins and immune complexes [1819]. On regression of the inflammatory phase, the proportion of polymorphonuclear neutrophilic leukocytes decreases, and that of the lymphocytes increases. Some of the latter have larger nuclei or broader cytoplasmic rims, an indication of their various transformational phases secondary to activation by antigens. They then amount to 40%–50%. Additionally, monocytes and larger macrophages – also containing irregularly shaped inclusion bodies, some of them from the ingestion of cellular debris and disintegrated leukocytes – appear among the cellular elements [193, 874]. Differentiation of the latter cells can be effected by staining with Sudan black since synoviocytes and lymphocytes do not absorb this [1439]. Furthermore, the monocytes stemming from the blood have round dense nuclei, while macrophages have larger, ovoid or slightly indented, reticulum-containing nuclei. The latter cells are present chiefly in the reparative phase of the inflammation, and are also present in chronic inflammations.

Synoviocytes also occur in the synovial fluid (Fig. 27) but mostly in proliferative and degenerative alterations of the joint capsule. They vary in diameter from 15 to 26 μm, are usually of irregular outline, and have a few cytoplasmic processes, but they may be roundish due to swelling. Their cytoplasm is homogeneous; the nucleus is large and ovoid. A moderate increase in synoviocytes suggests a proliferative joint alteration; a marked increase suggests advanced degeneration or intensive harm with disintegration. Other synoviocytes may have a diameter up to 40 μm, and a

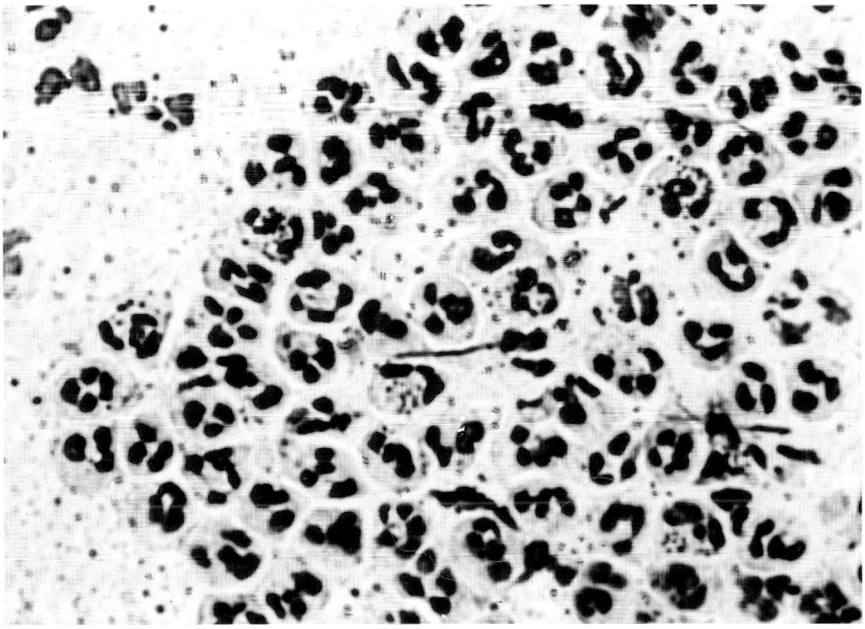

Fig. 29. The synovial fluid in gonorrhoic arthritis contains a great number of polymorphonuclear leukocytes, among which many gonococci are scattered

20 μm large nucleus containing two nucleoli and dense chromatin, often in atypical amitotic division. These are malignant tumor cells which lie together in demarcated clumps.

In addition to the cellular content of the synovial fluid, amorphous materials may be noted stemming from fibrin or globulin deposits, lipid or proteinaceous material emerged from the synovial membrane, or fragments of articular cartilage. Furthermore, microscopic examination of the stained smear and particularly of the wet smear occasionally discloses the presence of crystals of different outline (Fig. 28). Most of these lie intracellularly, being ingested by polymorphonuclear leukocytes and macrophages; others lie extracellularly. Such are the urate crystals 2–14 μm long and shaped like long needles or blunt rods, the calcium pyrophosphate crystals 1–10 μm long and shaped like needles (Fig. 28), rods, or chipped rhomboid platelets, and the hydroxyapatite crystals 6–12 μm long and also occurring like straight or slightly curved sticks, irregular rhomboid crystals, or clumps (Fig. 28). These crystals can be further identified and differentiated by polarized microscopy; the urate crystals are strongly and negatively birefringent, the hydroxyapatite crystals are also strongly but positively birefringent, and the pyrophosphate crystals are weakly and positively birefringent. Of lesser frequency in the synovial fluid cholesterol crystals can be observed; these are also shaped like flat or rhomboid plates or needles and are strongly negatively birefringent. Similarly, crystals of calcium oxalate, square or rhomboid in shape and, positively birefringent plates may occur [1051, 1266, 1439]. To detect calcium compounds in synovial fluid, staining with alizarin red has been recommended [1228].

c. Continuing the differential evaluation, the slides with stained smears are microscopically further reviewed for the presence of microorganisms which are seen at higher magnification when present (Fig. 29). Especially the budding fungal organisms are very obvious by their sizes up to 50–55 μm and their multiple small inclusions or by their mature, sharply delimited yeast form of 7–12 μm belonging to coccidioides (Fig. 30), blastomyces, histoplasma (Fig. 172), or sporothrix (Fig. 174). Periodic acid–Schiff and the methenamine–silver nitrate Gomori stains indicate fungi. However, differentiation of the bacteria and cocci can best be carried out by the Gram stain, which brings the microorganisms into prominence versus other cellular elements originating from the blood or synovial membrane; here the fungal microorganisms are irregularly stained, except for actinomyces which is gram-positive. When considering the possibility of infection by mycobacteria tuberculosis, the Ziehl-Neelsen stain is indicated. Further identification of the suspected microorganisms is possible by inoculating the synovial fluid on culture media of meat broth, plain agar, blood agar, chocolate agar, or peptone agar on which the microorganisms grow in characteristic colonies, when incubated aerobically, anaerobically, or under CO_2 tension. On suspicion of the presence of mycobacteria tuberculosis, Löwenstein-Jensen medium should be used; this provides growth of the microorganism after an incubation of 6 weeks. The fungi grow in typical colonies on blood agar or best on Sabouraud's glucose agar. Coccidioides, blastomyces,

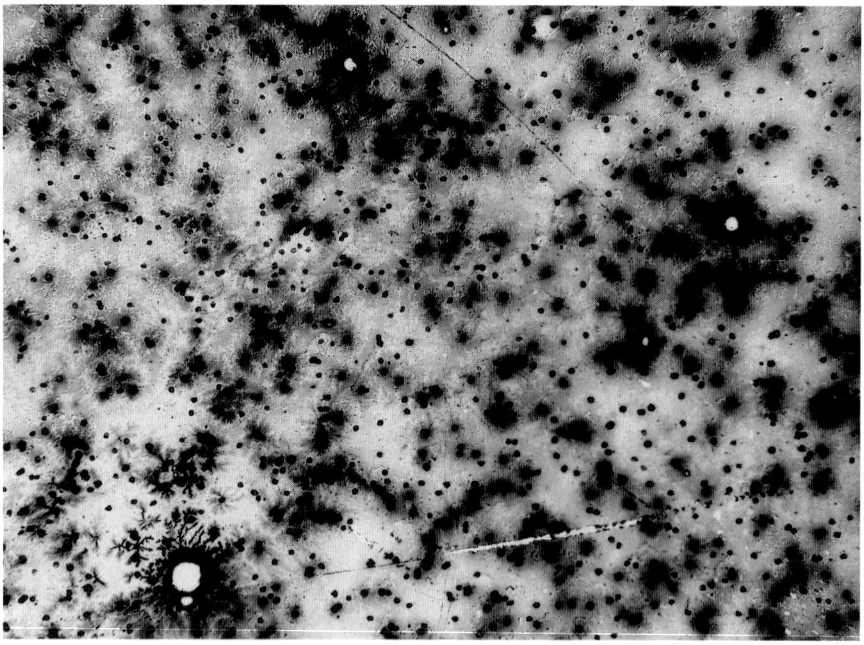

Fig. 30. The synovial fluid in coccidioidomycosis contains a few coccidioides yeasts with their highly refractile capsules

histoplasma, and sporothrix display here the phenomenon of dimorphism [1266] by growing as fluffy mycelium (Fig. 31) at 22° C, while multiplying as small yeast cells at 37° C; candida albicans and cryptococcas grow in yeast form at both temperatures.

d. The synovial fluid in recent effusions has the characteristics more of a transudate to which crystalloids and proteoglycans are admixed from the blood and synoviocytes; the effusions in chronic inflammations of greater intensity contain substantially more proteins. The ion concentration of the synovial fluid also varies, corresponding to the intensity of the inflammatory changes, to the diffusion of crystalloid buffer substances, and to the entry of protein substances [165]. The pH of the normal joint fluid is 7.2–7.4 and is similar in traumatic effusions. The more intensive the inflammation of the synovial membrane, the stronger is the acid reaction and the lower the pH. The more chronic and milder the inflammation, the more frequent and/or more pronounced is the alkaline reaction. The effusions in rheumatoid arthritis, osteoarthritis, tuberculosis, and syphilis have a pH of 7.3–7.8;

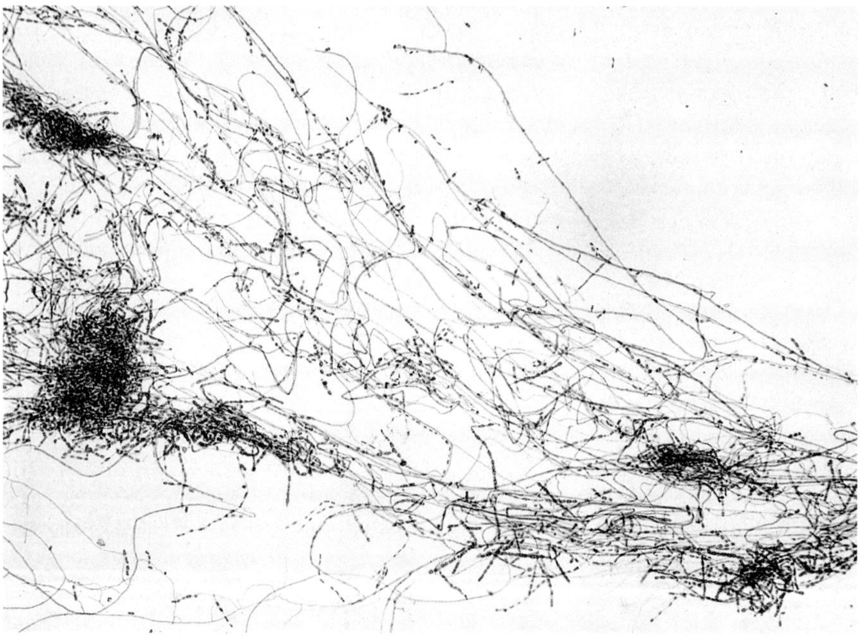

Fig. 31. Coccidioidomyces grows as a fluffy mycelium on Sabouraud's agar at lower temperature

the effusions in metastatic infectious arthritides and in empyema have a pH of 6.8–7.0. Low pH at repeated aspirations indicates the tendency to recurrences; the change of acid reaction to alkaline heralds a good prognosis. The glucose concentration in synovial fluid is 60–80 mg%; bacterial inflammations cause its decrease due to its greater use; chronic mild inflammations leave it relatively unchanged or only slightly decreased. In conjunction with this, the level of lactic acid in the synovial fluid can be determined by gas chromatography, which shows that lactic acid is distinctly increased in inflammation by gram-positive and gram-negative cocci [195, 1266]. The total concentration of protein is 1.5–2.5 g% in normal synovial fluid and contains albumin to 60%–65%, while the percentages of globulins and lipoprotein are less than in plasma [1443, 1584]. However, with intense inflammation and commensurate hyperemia of the synovial blood vessels such as in rheumatoid arthritis and Reiter's syndrome, the percentage of globulin [134], especially gammaglobulin, rises substantially in relation to that of albumin. Thereupon the total protein concentration may increase to 4.5–7.2 g%, even to 8.9 g% [717], but not in posttraumatic synovitis, other noninflammatory articular conditions, or osteoarthritis. The concentrations of fibrin and fibrinogen [301] and phospholipids vary similarly [1288, 1289]. Total bilirubin expresses the bilirubin content derived from hemoglobin and amounts to 0.2–0.6 mg/dl. An increase above 0.7 mg/dl indicates traumatic etiology while a decrease below 0.6 mg/dl suggests inflammatory nature, and a decrease below 0.3 mg/dl suggests a degenerative nature of the joint affection. In concurrence with Bombardieri et al. [158], Punzi et al. [1288, 1289] pointed out that prostaglandin is significantly increased in the synovial fluid of inflammatory arthritic conditions. This increase is attributed to enhanced production by the synoviocytes which are stimulated by the interleukin accumulated in inflammations.

e. Antigens being carried into joints [1385] lead to an inflammatory reaction which is associated with diffusion of antibodies from the serum through the dilated synovial blood vessels, as well as with arthrogenic formation of antibodies. Consequently immunoglobulins appear in the synovial fluid in a significant concentration, which is nevertheless lower than that in the serum. The combination of antigens and antibodies results in formation of immune complexes which probably play an essential role in the intensity and duration of the joint inflammation. Todesco et al. [1649, 1650] noted a distinct increase in B_2 microglobulins in rheumatoid arthritis and other active inflammations of joints, in comparison to noninflammatory joint conditions. Similarly, Gambari et al. [564] pointed out that, in proportion to the globulin, the complement fractions C3 and C4 are also increased in the synovial fluid of rheumatoid arthritis but not in other arthritic conditions.

Upon contact with reticuloendothelial cells and lymphocytes in the body and upon contact with synoviocytes and lymphocytes in the joints, the immune complexes elicit the enzymatic formation of a series of proteins, the components of the complement system [735, 1224, 1225, 1371, 1774, 1822]. These can be qualitatively and quantitatively determined by immunochemical diffusion and by radioimmune assay [1818]. The concentration of complement in the synovial fluid is lower than in the serum and is partly correlated with the concentration of proteins in the synovial fluid and partly with the concentration of intrasynovial antibodies [788]. Therefore, determination of protein and antibodies in the serum and synovial fluid is indicated [212]. These procedures disclose the complement to be decreased in seropositive rheumatoid arthritis, juvenile rheumatoid arthritis, septic arthritis, and crystal deposition arthritis [535, 1051, 1372, 1443, 1655]. The level of complement proteins in the synovial fluid is also instructive in evaluating the activity of an inflammatory, particularly infectious process within a joint. In association with the antigen-antibody reaction a significant level of complement proteins initially results, but on intensification of the local inflammatory process the level of complement proteins locally decreases due to increased utilization of these proteins. The synovial fluid in seropositive rheumatoid arthritis is shown by determination of the rheumatoid factor to contain altered immunoglobulins, such as the IgG and IgM, to which the subunit C1q of the complement proteins is bound. As a consequence of this or from blocking of the binding site for C1q by a high concentration of esterase, a significant decrease results in the titer of complement proteins. On the other hand, this titer is increased in Reiter's syndrome, other very active arthritis, and gout. Further information on the concentration of complement is provided by measuring the total hemolytic complement, which includes all protein components of the complement system in the synovial fluid. Antiimmunoglobulin components of the complement complex, among them IgM rheumatoid factor and properdin factor, are also synthesized by the synovial cells [1774]. The complement concentration largely parallels the degree of the inflammation [1233] but is lower in very active rheumatoid arthritis, as is the hemolytic complement activity [1655], probably due to local consumption by the immune complexes [354].

In addition to the quantitative determination of complement proteins as a sign of the intensity of an inflammation, the presence of complement can be used diagnostically in the complement fixation test for ascertaining the presence of an antibody against a specific

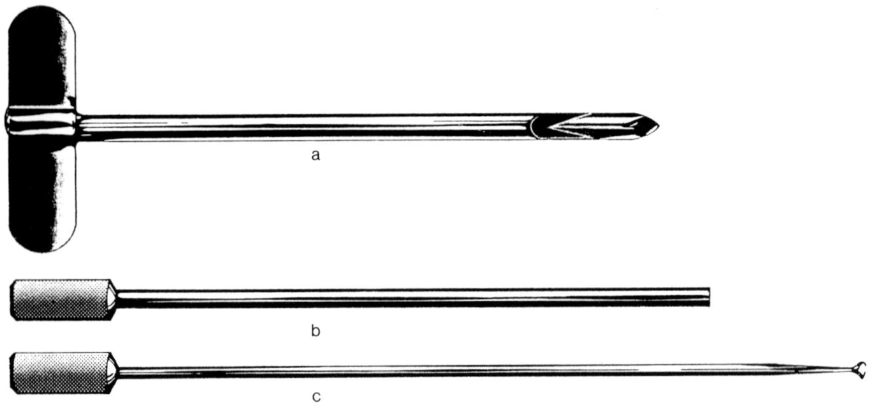

Fig. 32. The Polley-Bickel set is composed chiefly of: *a*, trocar pointed tube with a hooked fenestrum; *b*, tubular knife; *c*, stylet with sharp corkscrew tip

antigen. In this test, known antigens, either killed microorganisms or their component substances, are exposed to the synovial fluid thought to contain antibodies (agglutinin, precipitin, flocculin) directed against specific antigens. Complement is added, followed by sensitized sheep erythrocytes. If an antigen-antibody complex exists, the complement becomes consumed; no lysis of the erythrocytes occurs; the test is positive. Complement fixation can ascertain the etiological diagnosis of a specific joint inflammation even in the absence of causative microorganisms. Thus the outcome of the complement fixation test can be of substantial value in gonorrheal arthritis when no gonococci are detected in the synovial fluid. The test is also informative in viral arthritis. Furthermore, the identification of antibodies such as agglutinins or precipitins in the synovial fluid can be usefully tested in meningococcal arthritis, pneumococcal arthritis, Salmonella arthritis, or Brucella arthritis by exposing erythrocytes coated with a specific antigen to the synovial fluid. The more recent immunofluorescence test exposes synovial fluid containing antigen-antibody complexes to a fluorescein-labeled antibody, and is a diagnostically very informative method. This identifies complexes by fluorescent microscopy [190, 321, 1002].

Examination of the synovial fluid from several points of view thus provides very instructive insights into the biology of joints, their reaction to various noxious factors, the reciprocal relationship between the body on one side and the joint on the other, and the mutual influence in all harmful situations affecting one or the other of these.

9. Punch Biopsy of Joint or Arthroscopy and Examination of Articular Tissue

While the history, clinical examination, and laboratory studies may render sufficient information for the diagnosis of a joint disease, only microscopic examination of the articular tissue enables one to verify the changes relevant to the particular type and phase of the joint disease. This examination therefore provides clarification or confirmation of the diagnosis in a good number of cases.

For obtaining tissue portions at minimal risk a joint cavity can be entered with an injection needle [1239, 1707]. However, the material obtained in this way consists of tissue fragments and permits examination of only single component cells. Thus needle biopsy lends itself chiefly to microscopic examination in the context of suspected tumors.

Adequate portions of synovial tissue to permit informative histopathological examination without exposing the patient to greater intervention can be obtained by punch biopsy; for this the Polley-Bickel set [1269] and the Parker-Pearson needle [1435] are available. Since the histopathological examination is more instructive, the larger the reviewed tissue portions are, the Polley-Bickel set (Fig. 32) is more informative as its trocar has a wider lumen. Being an intraarticular procedure, the punch biopsy should be carried out with aseptic precautions. The site for inserting the biopsy set is selected according to the palpable, most pronounced swelling of the joint capsule. Local anesthesia is administered here from the skin down into the joint cavity. If the joint fluid is increased, it is aspirated through the anesthesia needle and is subjected to examination. The trocar (Fig. 32a) in its surrounding tube (Fig. 32b) is then inserted through the skin along the anesthesia tract until it perforates the inner lining of the joint capsule and enters the joint cavity. The surrounding tube is withdrawn and leaves uncovered the protruding hook of the trocar, which by pressure is hooked onto a portion of the inner joint capsule. Thereupon the surrounding tube is reinserted, and its sharp edge cuts off the grasped portion of the synovial membrane. A third instrument, terminating with thin corkscrew hooks (Fig. 32c) pulls out the separated portion of the synovial membrane. This procedure may be repeated in other areas of the inner part of the joint capsule until a number of adequate portions have been obtained. The trocar is withdrawn, the punch wound is covered with sterile dressing, and the joint is compressed with an elastic bandage. Bedrest and elevated extremity for 1 day is advisable, as are antibiotics (ampicillin or cephalosporin 3.0 g in 24 h) for 2–3 days.

The tissue portions thus obtained are fixed in buffered 10% formol or in Bouin's solution and routinely stained with hematoxylin-eosin-phloxin-saffran; in appropriate instances special stains include Mallory's phosphotungstic acid hematoxylin, Weigert–van Gieson's stain, and Masson's trichrome stain. On suspicion of the presence of crystals, the heat-fixed and methylene blue stained slides are examined microscopically under polarized light. The histopathological features to be examined [322, 1543] for significant alterations in the synovial membrane are:

Hypertrophy of synoviocytes (Figs. 70, 198, 199, 336)
Hyperplasia of synoviocytes (Figs. 54, 57, 337)
Hyperemia of synovial blood vessels (Figs. 53, 70, 71, 113)
Edema of synovial membrane (Figs. 70, 71, 106, 131, 175)
Inflammatory cells in the walls of synovial blood vessels (Figs. 123, 340, 524)
Inflammatory cells in perivascular infiltrates (Figs. 175, 176)
Focal accumulations of polymorphonuclear leukocytes and/or lymphocytes, plasmacytes, histiocytes (Figs. 84, 100, 106, 128, 472)
Diffuse infiltrates of polymorphonuclear leukocytes and/or lymphocytes, plasmacytes, histiocytes (Figs. 67, 85, 96, 118, 427)
Nodules of lymphocytes and/or plasmacytes
Ulcer of synovial membrane
Fresh fibrin on synovial membrane (Fig. 100)
Organized fibrin on synovial membrane (Figs. 96, 97)
Fibrin in synovial membrane
Hemorrhages in synovial membrane (Fig. 40)
Hemosiderin in synovial membrane (Figs. 401, 414, 415)
Fibroblasts in synovial membrane (Figs. 198, 199)
Increased fibrocytes in synovial membrane (Figs. 112, 124, 261)
Giant cells in synovial membrane (Figs. 155, 168, 383, 535)
Villi of synovial membrane (Figs. 54, 55, 65, 67, 76, 140, 183, 200, 343, 347)
Proliferating capillaries in synovial membrane (Fig. 54)
Increased blood vessels in synovial membrane (Fig. 54)
Thick-walled blood vessels in synovial membrane (Figs. 134, 337)
Necrosis and/or inflammation of blood vessels in synovial membrane (Figs. 229, 341)
Degeneration of collagen fibers in synovial membrane (Fig. 394)
Necrosis of synovial membrane (Fig. 394)
Hemigranulomata in synovial membrane (Fig. 124)
Granulomata in synovial membrane (Figs. 140, 155, 157, 159, 171, 354, 538)
Fragments of cartilage and/or bone in synovial membrane (Figs. 314, 363, 445, 459)
Crystals in synovial membrane (Figs. 355, 548)
Deposits of amyloid or lipid in synovial membrane (Fig. 383)
Fibrosis of synovial membrane (Figs. 114, 119, 129, 261, 546)

The results of electron-microscopic examinations of synoviocytes in inflammatory changes have been noted in various joint conditions but most elaborately in rheumatoid arthritis [72, 603, 796, 797, 1194, 1195]. The description of characteristic electron-microscopic findings in inflamed synoviocytes has therefore been incorporated in "Rheumatoid Arthritis" (Fig. 206). Statistical evaluation of the incidence of histopathological changes of the articular cartilage is presented in "Arthrotomy, Excision and Examination of Articular Tissue".

Recording histopathological features of the synovial membrane and other relevant factors such as age of patient, duration of symptoms, physical findings, and laboratory studies permits the study of possible correlations among them. These parameters offer instructive information on the phase, activity, and nature of the joint disease and may provide thereby a clue to the diagnosis [568, 570, 587, 589, 1009, 1543]. No definite diagnosis, however, may be made from the histopathological alterations alone.

Nevertheless, a solitary granuloma or, more particularly, abundant proliferation of large fibroblasts (Fig. 199) are highly suggestive of rheumatoid arthritis, while the absence of polymorphonuclear leukocytes, scantness of infiltrates by other inflammatory cells, and overall increase in fibrocytes (Figs. 260, 261) are highly suggestive of osteoarthritis. Extensive dense infiltration by polymorphonuclear leukocytes (Fig. 85) is a strong indication of acute bacteriogenic inflammation probably associated with suppuration, and extensive dense infiltrates composed predominantly of plasmacytes are often observed in gonococcal arthritis (Fig. 107), syphilitic arthritis (Fig. 139), and psoriatic arthritis (Fig. 336). Dense infiltrates of lymphocytes mixed with a few polymorphonuclear leukocytes are observed in arthritis caused by Brucella or Salmonella (Fig. 121). Formation of numerous granulomata associated with Langhans' giant cells indicates tuberculous etiology (Figs. 155, 157, 538), and extensive granulomata without giant cells but containing large centers of necrosis indicate arthritis in tertiary syphilis (Fig. 140). Extensive granulomata with large giant cells and both of them containing inclusions of fungal spores (Figs. 168, 171) are indicative of mycotic infection. Intracellular and interstitial deposits of hemosiderin as residuals of hemorrhages are sometimes observed in traumatic synovitis, but invariably in hemochromatosis (Fig. 401), hemosiderosis, pigmented villonodular synovitis (Fig. 65), and particularly in hemophilic arthritis (Figs. 414). Crystals of needle shape and lying superficially and deeply (Fig. 355) are of uric acid, whereas crystals of needle or rod shape are of dihydrocalcium phosphate, crystals of rhomboid or irregular shape are of hydroxyapatite, and crystals of rhomboid shape or in rosette arrangement (Figs. 521, 548) are of cholesterol. Finally, a few small fragments of cartilage or of cartilage and bone occur in osteochondritis dissecans (Fig. 314) and osteoarthritis, whereas larger fragments, in greater number, and lying superficially and deeply occur in neuropathic arthritis of diabetes (Fig. 445), tabes, and syringomyelia (Fig. 459). Although some of these features are rather characteristic for one or another entity of joint disease, in view of their multifold and varied occurrence they are not pathognomonic for any specific joint disease.

Similarly, electron-microscopic examination (Fig. 206) does not provide a clue for diagnosis. However, by revealing elementary details in the synoviocytes, such as lysosomes, endoplasmic reticulum, Golgi complex, mitochondria, and micropinocytotic vesicles, this examination is able to provide an explanation of many microbiological and histochemical phenomena observed in the pathologically altered synovial membrane [568, 570, 587, 589, 1009]. Consequently, electron-microscopic examination, similarly to light-microscopic examination, is used in immunopathological studies for detecting the presence of immunoglobulins and their complement proteins in antigenically elicited inflammatory conditions of the synovial membrane [176].

In addition to the identification of various morphological alterations in tissue elements and of abnormal components occurring in the inflammatory changes of the synovial membrane, ascertaining the participation of the synovial membrane in immunological inflammatory events can be highly informative. The immunofluorescence test [321, 863] and the immunoperoxidase test [752, 1171] are used as diagnostic methods.

The immunofluorescence test [190, 1002] can be used as a direct method, in which fixed tissue sections are exposed to antibodies conjugated with fluorescein isothiocyanate and directed against a suspected microorganism or antigen. In the presence of the suspected etiological factor, localized fluorescence is observed by immunofluorescent microscopy. In the indirect immunofluorescence method, homologous antisera conjugated with fluorescein isothiocyanate are used to identify immunoglobulins as the antibodies against a suspected etiological factor (Fig. 130). By the latter method, Geiler [586] identified IgG, IgM, and IgA in intensely inflamed synovial membrane of rheumatoid arthritis. Similarly, Kinsella et al. [890] observed deposition of fluorescent granules in synoviocytes and fluorescent clumps lying interstitially as well as along vascular walls in seropositive rheumatoid arthritis, Sjögren's syndrome, and psoriatic arthritis. Since immunofluorescent studies of the synovial membrane are more sensitive (Fig. 130) than immunological studies of the serum, they can be diagnostically useful. In view of the great variety of suspected or possible etiological microorganisms or antigens, a great number of specific fluorescein-conjugated antisera must be used to obtain a specific diagnosis [1237, 1256].

The direct immunoperoxidase method [752, 1171] uses antibodies conjugated with a stable enzyme, horseradish peroxidase, which in contact with the pertinent antigen releases free oxygen radicals. These cause a concurrently added chromogenic substrate, diaminobenzidine, to polymerize as a brown precipitate at the site of the antigen-antibody reaction. In the indirect method, the primary antibody directed against the relevant antigen is unlabeled. A second antibody, directed against immunoglobulins of the species in question, is conjugated with horseradish peroxidase and is used to detect the primary antibody. The indirect method is more sensitive than the direct method and can detect smaller amounts of antibody, thus also of antigen. Nevertheless, both methods are useful in the immunochemical evaluation of histopathological changes in the synovial membrane. Using the indirect method with class-specified antisera, Fritz et al. [554] realized that the immune response of the synovial membrane in rheumatoid arthritis is much more pronounced than that in osteoarthritis; demonstration of the rheumatoid factor by specific antisera offered the possibility of immunohistochemically differentiating between rheumatoid arthritis and osteoarthritis.

Inflammatory activity in the synovial membrane is also associated with release of oxidase by histiocytes and macrophages, with molecular oxygen being converted into superoxide. The latter leads to formation of hydrogen peroxide, an oxidizing factor of the enzymes on proteins and accounting for some of the ensuing tissue changes in inflammation [58, 834, 1175]. Determination and quantitation of the hydrogen peroxide by precipitation of benzidine hydrochloride into granules permit histochemical evaluation of the presence and intensity of inflammation.

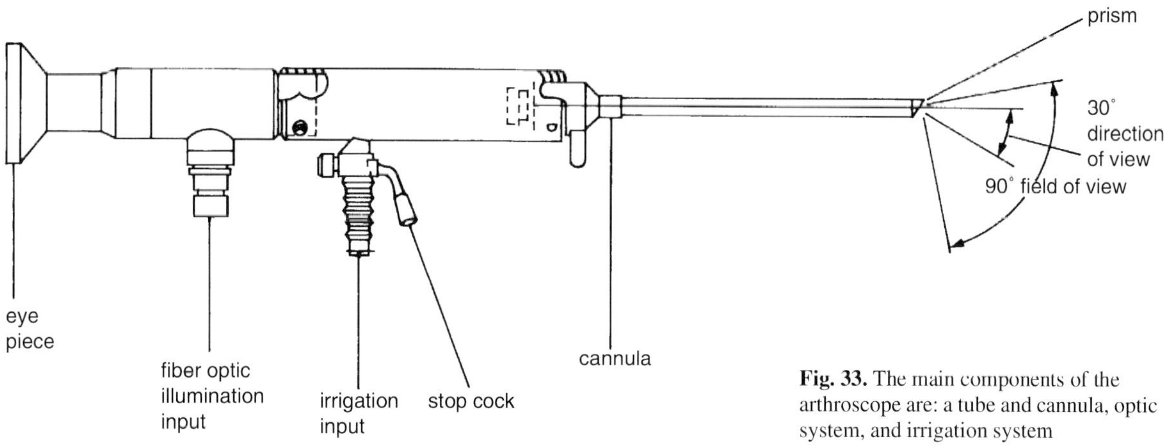

Fig. 33. The main components of the arthroscope are: a tube and cannula, optic system, and irrigation system

While punch biopsy provides portions of synovial tissue from a joint, these tissue specimens are rather small, having been removed from limited areas. Thus one needs to obtain substantially larger tissue portions from areas representative for the existent articular pathology; especially the desire to visualize internal tissue changes led to the use of the arthroscope in numerous situations of articular pathology. This was initially developed by Takagi and subsequently perfected by Watanabe [1718, 1719]. The arthroscopy has been widened into an operative procedure [1049, 1533] by adding new features to the original technical design. The optical instrument (Fig. 33) consists of a 4-mm-wide cylinder, the arthroscopic sheath, through which a tube is inserted, the actual arthroscope. This has both an objective and an ocular lens, surrounded by glass fibers propagating the light from the electric source into the joint cavity. Designing the arthroscope for various angles has provided a scanning effect which allows an optimal field of visualization [1469]. By supplementing the arthroscope sheath with an inflow and an outflow channel (Fig. 33) for continuous irrigation of the joint cavity with physiological saline solution and by adding another channel for inserting surgical instruments, the optical device has been converted into a surgical apparatus. The basic instruments include: a probe, grasping forceps, biopsy forceps, curved basket forceps, straight and curved scissors, bone curette, file, osteotome, and, if needed, motorized instruments.

After visualization [811, 831, 1469] of the forelying pathology, excessively enlarged or other abnormal-appearing portions of the inner part of the joint capsule (Fig. 34), floating fragments of the synovial membrane, fronds of the articular cartilage (Fig. 35), or loose joint bodies can be grasped. Concomitantly, frag-

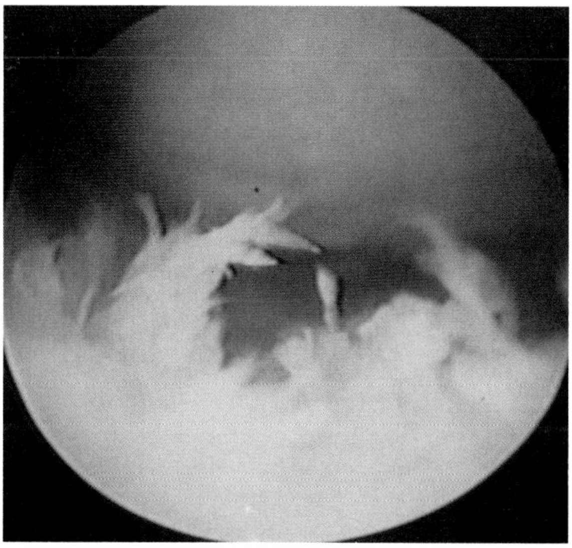

Fig. 34. Arthroscopy discloses that several large and ramified villi rise from the synovial membrane

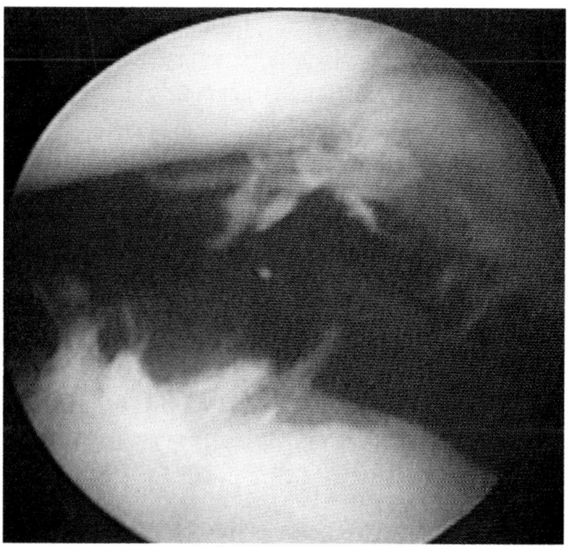

Fig. 35. Arthroscopy discloses that the contiguous articular surfaces of the patella and femoral condyle are very uneven by elevations and indentations

ments in osteochondritis dissecans can be pinned in situ, defects in articular cartilage can be smoothed, and obstructing exostoses can be osteotomized and removed.

Because of its relatively small field of visualization, however, the arthroscope must use various approaches to a joint cavity, and it therefore enters a joint through a number of specific sites of incision, designated as portals. Thus, selecting the most direct route to the site of pathology requires knowledge of the complete case history, thorough physical examination, and study of the roentgenographic views of the affected joint. The most frequent portals for the knee joint [363, 1067] are the anteromedial, anterolateral, suprapatellar, and midpatellar approaches. These permit to perceive and to deal with excessive proliferations of the inner part of the joint capsule or synovial plicae, tears of the menisci or cruciate ligaments, nonseparated osteochondritis dissecans or defects in the cartilaginous surface, incongruent osteocartilaginous protrusions or marginal osteophytes, and loose joint bodies. The other major joints are less often objects of arthroscopy since they are less often affected [478]. The shoulder joint [1756] can be entered through an anterior or posterior portal. Through the former one can also inspect the biceps tendon, rotator cuff, and subscapularis tendon. Through either of these portals the glenoid cavity, labrum glenoidale, and cartilaginous surface of the humeral head can be inspected. Incident pathological changes can be treated, especially a detached labrum glenoidale, osteocartilaginous fragments in the joint cavity, and old tears of the joint capsule followed by its excessive local proliferation. It is of substantial benefit here to have traction applied on the arm by an assistant in order sufficiently to separate the humeral head from the glenoid cavity; adequate inspection of the joint cavity, is thereby obtained. Traction is also of benefit at arthroscopy of the elbow joint; which can be entered through an anterolateral or a posterolateral portal; the joint capsule can be distended by abundant irrigation. Such irrigation is also of benefit for the ankle joint, which can be entered through an anterior, anteromedial, anterolateral, or posterolateral approach. Approaches for inspection and operation have recently also been used for the hip joint.

Arthroscopy thus offers intraarticular visualization which can be extended by turning and tilting the arthroscope or by removal or extraction of obstructing tissue alterations [252]. The limitation in visualization and surgical treatment of tissue alterations can be compensated partly by versatile directing of the arthroscope and partly by entering the joint through more than one portal. Arthroscopy also has the advantage that it can be carried out under local anesthesia in a significant percentage of cases. Consequently, Klein et al. [898] expanded the use of arthroscopy on an outpatient basis by performing it under local anesthesia. Nevertheless, the potential complications from arthroscopy must not be disregarded, and all precautions and care should be taken. The untoward effects [1426, 1475] arise: (a) preoperatively, from incorrect diagnosis, (b) intraoperatively, from misuse of operative equipment, faulty operative equipment, inadvertent major injury of articular cartilage, blood vessels or nerves, or complication during general or epidural anesthesia, and (c) postoperatively, from recurrent intraarticular effusions or hemarthroses, synovial herniation, and deeply seated infections.

10. Arthrotomy, Excision, and Examination of Articular Tissue

Arthroscopy permits visualization of a joint and removal of articular tissue, yet to a limited extent. The wide opening of a joint only is satisfactory in situations requiring extensive inspection of a joint cavity for diagnostic or, more particularly, for therapeutic necessities. These situations present themselves when the alterations affect broadly the synovial membrane, such as in advanced posttraumatic, villonodular, nonspecific, or rheumatoid synovitis, in other proliferating chronic joint inflammations, in benign tumors such as fibroma, hemangioma, chondromatosis, or in malignant tumors such as synovial sarcoma or chondrosarcoma. In all these conditions the possibility of unlimited inspection of the joint cavity is essential for being able to deal adequately with the diagnostically anticipated alterations.

Arthrotomy is further indicated in all situations in which the alterations extensively affect the articular epiphyses. Such are irreducible intraarticular fractures, osteochondritis dissecans, several loose joint bodies, advanced primary or secondary osteoarthritis, congenital or acquired deformities of the articular ends, and benign or malignant tumors of the articular ends. In all these conditions the grossly deformed and often hard osteocartilaginous tissue can be handled only by routine surgical instruments.

Arthrotomy (Figs. 36, 243) offers a substantial view into a joint and of any pathological changes in it. Thus, it allows confirmation of the clinical diagnosis and performance of the indicated therapeutic procedure. This may consist of excision of diseased synovial or osteocartilaginous tissue, repair of damaged structures or deformed epiphyses, or insertion of organic or artificial articular substitutes. Since the opening of a joint is a major and serious precedure, with complications possibly leading to tragic consequences, arthrotomy is indicated upon persistent symptoms only after exhaus-

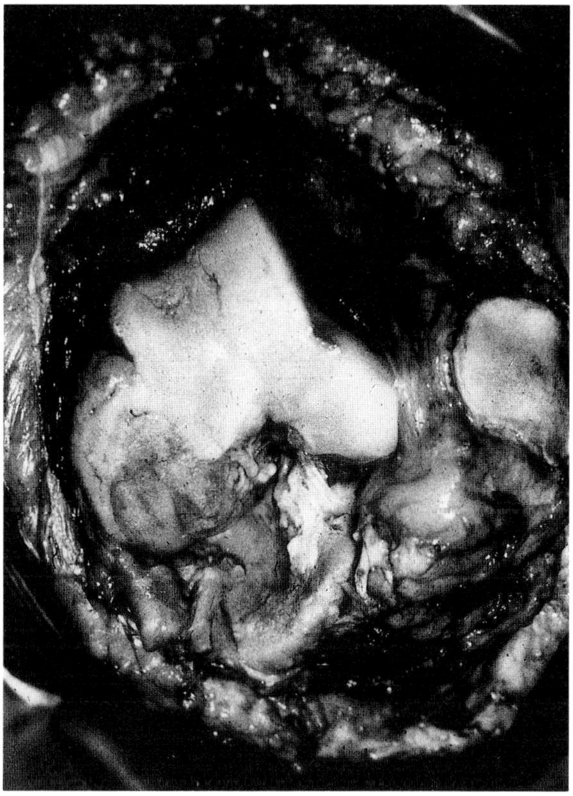

Fig. 36. Wide anterior arthrotomy of the knee joint with lateral retraction of the patella and exposure of the entire articular surfaces. A large part of the medial femoral condyle is deeply worn off, as are the medial and lateral tibial condyles

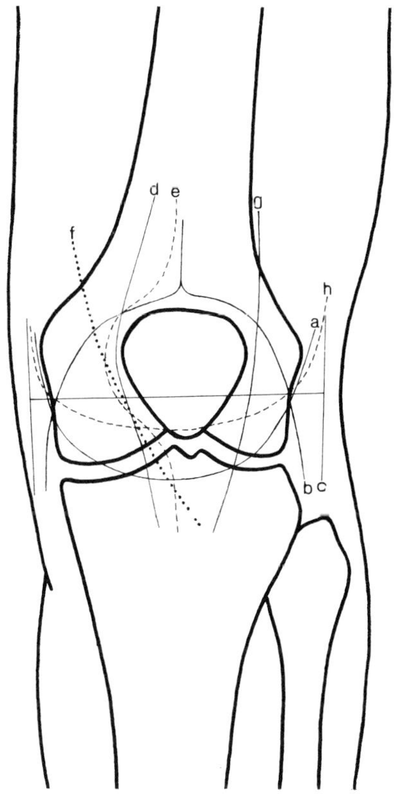

Fig. 37. Anterior arthrotomies of the knee: *a*, distal dome incision, *b*, proximal curvilinear incision, *c*, transpatellar H incision, *d*, medial parapatellar incision, *e*, medial parapatellar curvilinear incision, *f*, medial oblique incision, *g*, lateral parapatellar incision, *h*, transpatellar dome incision

tion of all diagnostic tests and after all attempts at conservative treatment have failed.

Before embarking on such procedure, a complete medical examination is indispensable to ascertain generalized or local infection, organic disease, or a regional skin inflammation – which would represent a contraindication to an elective surgical procedure. The arthrotomy best fulfills its purpose in removing or repairing a markedly altered articular constituent if the direct approach to this constituent is used, and any harm to the other constituents of the joint is avoided.

In the performance of arthrotomy, proper positioning of the patient and the joint is essential to permit adequate survey of the joint cavity. The shaven skin at the area of the joint and proximal and distal to it should be thoroughly scrubbed and thereafter draped with sterile sheets far beyond the area of operation. It is advisable for complete relaxation of the musculature to perform the operation under general anesthesia; in interventions on the arm anesthesia of the brachial plexus may suffice, and in interventions on a lower extremity, including the hip, epidural anesthesia may suffice. Whenever regionally feasible, a pneumatic tourniquet should be applied to provide a blood-free operative field. Where a tourniquet cannot be applied, electrocauterization of the smaller blood vessels and ligation of the larger blood vessels is necessary to ensure unimpeded performance of the surgical procedure. The skin incision follows the most direct route to the area of the joint to be surgically treated [488].

Experience indicates the following approaches for the major joints; the steps in these approaches are described by Crenshaw [343].

Shoulder joint [574, 1105]: anteromedial, anterosuperior, transacromial, anterior transaxillary, or posterior

Elbow joint: medial, lateral, or posterolateral

Wrist joint: dorsal, volar, medial, or lateral

Hip joint [240]: anterior iliofemoral, anterolateral, lateral, posterolateral, or posterior

Knee joint: anteromedial, anterolateral, medial, lateral, posteromedial, or posterolateral

Ankle joint: anterior, anterolateral, posterolateral, or posterior

Besides these basic approaches, various modifications, designed for specific situations, are used especially for the shoulder, hip, and knee joints (Fig. 37). The apophyseal joints of the vertebral spine are exposed through a posterior approach, the sacroiliac joint through a posterior or anterior approach, and the vertebral bodies through an anterior transabdominal approach. In view of the rather long duration of most intraarticular operations, it is a wise precaution intraoperatively to irrigate the field of operation one or two times with an antibiotic solution and postoperatively to administer antibiotics for 2–3 days. The closed wound is covered with a sterile dressing, and a drain is inserted to prevent accumulation of a large hematoma in an extensive operation. Concurrently, the joint is immobilized by a strapping, splint, traction device, or plaster cast for an individually determined period of time. Subsequently, the joint is mobilized by active exercises selected in terms of the purpose of the operation. The indicated types of operative procedure are described in each type of joint affection.

At its opening, the joint should be inspected in the full extent of the incision for anatomic-pathological changes in the joint capsule, articular epiphyses, interepiphyseal space, and joint cavity. Changes in the inner joint capsule may be:

Swelling by edema or hyperemia (Fig. 69)
Thickening at partly maintained evenness (Figs. 52, 248)
Moderate unevenness by shrinking and fibrosis (Fig. 249)
Moderate unevenness by small to moderate-size villi (Figs. 52, 64, 138, 345)
Marked unevenness and thickening by large or plump villi (Figs. 74, 75, 103, 411)
Brown to very dark discoloration by hemosiderin deposits (Figs. 52, 64, 400, 409, 410, 411)
Defects by ulceration
Tumorous outgrowth (Figs. 525, 526).

Changes in the articular epiphyses may be:

Unevenness by attrition of the articular cartilage (Figs. 247, 249, 434, 435, 442, 443, 450, 455)
Unevenness by erosion or ingrowth of granulation tissue (Figs. 82, 83, 99, 137, 138, 169, 196, 197, 245, 335)
Deep defect by injury (Fig. 39)
Deep defect by abscess (Figs. 83, 99, 117, 152, 169)
Cavities filled with blood clots (Figs. 412, 413)
Deposits of urate or calcium (Figs. 352, 353, 391, 392)
Extensive fragmentation (Figs. 152, 334, 449)
Extensive destruction by tumor (Figs. 525, 526).

Changes in the interepiphyseal space or joint cavity may be:

Narrowing by ingrowth of granulation tissue (Fig. 288)
Narrowing by attrition of articular cartilage (Figs. 245, 246)
Widening by excessive attrition of articular surfaces (Fig. 449)
Widening secondary to deep destruction of articular surfaces by abscess (Figs. 117, 151)
Partial obstruction by loose joint bodies (Fig. 332)
Partial or complete obstruction by fibrous tissue (Fig. 494)
Partial or complete obstruction by osseous tissue or malignant tumor (Figs. 495, 525, 526).

After completion of the intraarticular operation, histopathological examination of the surgically obtained tissue portions is indispensable. These tissues are fixed in 10% formaldehyde or Bouin's solution. The synovial tissue portions are stained and examined as described in "Punch Biopsy and Arthroscopy of Joints". The articular cartilage portions are stained with hematoxylin-eosin-phloxin-safran and also with safranin [1350].

Histopathological examination of the articular cartilage – not obtainable by punch biopsy and only insufficiently so by arthroscopy – constitutes an integral diagnostic and highly informative part of the evaluation after arthrotomy. The following tissue changes are quantified at microscopic examination of the articular cartilage and considered statistically as parameters [323]:

Irregular spotty staining of the cartilage ground substance (Figs. 241, 370, 416)
Loss of basophilia of the ground substance (Figs. 323, 356)
Decrease in or loss of the ground substance and unmasking of the interstitial fibers (Figs. 524, 249, 397, 416)
Horizontal cleft formation (Figs. 250, 396)
Vertical cleft formation (Figs. 41, 42, 242, 250)
Fragmentation of articular cartilage and separation of flakes (Figs. 184, 339)
Necrosis of chondrocytes (Figs. 41, 251, 311, 397)
Empty or shadow lacunae (Figs. 41, 251, 437)
Decreased number of chondrocytes without empty lacunae (Figs. 41, 356)
Hypertrophy of chondrocytes (Figs. 250, 273)
Pericellular halos with increased ground substance (Figs. 250, 465)
Hyperplasia of chondrocytes (Figs. 250, 396, 466)
Thinning of articular cartilage down to its complete loss (Figs. 43, 417, 459)
Articular cartilage and subchondral bone plate partly or completely replaced by inflammatory tissue (Figs. 86, 158, 159, 200, 202, 338)
Articular cartilage and subchondral bone plate partly or completely replaced by granulation tissue (Figs. 44, 310, 311)

Articular cartilage and subchondral bone plate partly or completely replaced by connective tissue (Figs. 44, 89, 120, 184, 203, 236, 458)
Fibrocartilage cover on subchondral plate (Fig. 458)
Hyaline cartilage below subchondral bone plate (Figs. 41, 252, 253, 417)
Multiplication of tidemark (Figs. 250, 437)
Vascular tufts in subchondral bone plate (Figs. 41, 42)
Vascular tufts penetrating the tide mark (Figs. 42, 43)
Thinning of subchondral bone plate (Figs. 184, 311)
Thickening of subchondral bone plate (Figs. 204, 252, 254, 255)
Eburnation of subchondral bone plate (Figs. 204, 254)
Necrosis of subchondral bone plate (Figs. 436, 437)
Cyst with myxoid tissue in subchondral bone (Fig. 25)
Cyst with connective tissue in subchondral bone (Figs. 255, 453)
Cyst with hyaline cartilage or fibrocartilage in subchondral bone
Focal inflammation of subarticular marrow (Fig. 437)
Diffuse inflammation of subarticular marrow (Fig. 370)
Necrosis of medullary bone (Fig. 453)
Hypertrophy of medullary bone (Fig. 254)
Atrophy of medullary bone (Figs. 184, 236, 417)
Formation of marginal osteophyte (Fig. 339).

Recording these features on computer sheets permits the study of their correlation with symptoms, physical and radiological findings, laboratory studies, and clinical diagnosis. They also suggest the degree and probability of inflammatory arthritis, primary osteoarthritis, or secondary osteoarthritis. The correlation results from electron-microscopic examination of articular chondrocytes in degenerative joint conditions (Fig. 258) are described in "Osteoarthritis".

Classification of Arthritides

Disorders of the joints present varying clinical pictures which, independently of their etiology, have some features in common. Nevertheless, it is necessary to group the various pictures into entities by certain criteria in order to systematize consideration of the different aspects of joint diseases [1474] and to rationalize treatment. Subdivision according to the clinical course in acute, subacute, and chronic diseases would not be informative because the same etiological factor, commensurate with the degree of its impact and the defense of the individual, may sometimes elicit an acute and other times a chronic disease. Inflammations of joints generally start as nonspecific reactions and are followed by multifaceted immune reactions, especially in those situations in which microorganisms or antigenic substances are or are assumed to be the etiological factors. In addition to these determinants, it is inherent in the anatomical substrate and in the slow reactivity of the articular tissues that acute joint diseases often persist and take a chronic course. This results in transitions between the individual courses in joint disorders. Furthermore, differentiation between atrophic and hypertrophic joint diseases is hardly of use because many diseases of different etiology may present similar pathological-anatomical pictures. On the other hand, the same disease may be associated with varying changes in the articular tissues, depending on its course, phase, and the individual reaction of the body.

In consideration of the therapeutic necessities, a subdivision from the etiological point of view appears most useful. Such a grouping, however, encounters difficulties because the etiology of a large group of rheumatic arthritides and their variants, as well as of a few other entities has not yet been clarified definitely [587, 588]. With this limitation in mind – and taking into account the pathogenesis of degenerative joint diseases and the identified etiology of both the specific joint infections and the joint involvements in systemic diseases [1474] – disorders of the joints may be classified as follows:

I. Traumatic alterations of joints
II. Idiopathic inflammations of joints
III. Specific inflammations of joints by microorganisms
IV. Allergic, rheumatic, and etiologically unclarified inflammations of joints
V. Degenerative changes in joints
VI. Trophic alterations in joints
VII. Joint affections in systemic diseases
VIII. Acquired dysfunctions and deformities of joints
IX. Tumors of joints.

I. Traumatic Alterations of Joints

In daily life, the joints are exposed to injuries which may act either directly on the joints or indirectly through neighboring areas of the body or the extremities. According to the type of impact, its extent, and the injured structures, the injury may cause either a contusion or a sprain or an inflammation.

1. Contusion of Joints

Contusion or bruise to a joint is caused by a direct blunt injury which causes damage to the skin, compression of the subcutaneous tissue, and disruption of the joint capsule as well as of the articular cartilage, but not of ligaments. The injury is greater and causes more profound damage to the articular components when the joint is struck against a hard object, or when a heavy object falls on the joint. The most severe impact, however, occurs by the patient falling from a height on the upper or, more often, the lower extremities. The joints then sustain profound damage by the excessive vertical load, often extending beyond the articular components into the subchondral bone and even more deeply into the articular epiphyses. Severe contusions occur chiefly in sports, work injuries, and traffic accidents.

The general condition of these patients depends on the size of the injured joint, the extent and depth of the impact on the articular tissues, and the number of injured joints; this varies from moderate discomfort to deep shock. Concomitantly, the local changes in the injured joints vary; these can be well perceived in the superficially located joints (Fig. 38) but are not obvious in those surrounded by a thick cloak of soft tissue, such as the hip or vertebral joints.

The skin at the bruised areas is usually discolored, from blue to greenish yellow, by ecchymoses. These areas are also very tender down to the joint, which is often enlarged due to distension of its capsule by an intraarticular hemorrhage (Fig. 38). Here the motion of the joint is mechanically impaired. The active movement is otherwise limited only by pain, while the passive movement retains the full range, as long as the regional musculature is not spastically contracted due to pain.

Roentgenographs reveal no fracture but a widening of the joint cleft when a more substantial intraarticular hemorrhage accumulates. Nevertheless, a fine fissure through the subchondrol bone may be present, and this can be ascertained by an enlarged roentgenograph [425]. Obvious fracture extending into the depth of the subchondral bone, whether with or without displacement, is not the subject of this treatise.

Gross anatomically the contusion is characterized by occasional abrasion of the epithelium, disruption of subcutaneous and capsular tissues, and tear of their blood vessels. The hemorrhage expands in the subcutaneous tissue, which becomes swollen, thus separating the skin from the joint capsule. In addition, intraarticular hemorrhage often also occurs. On injury to larger blood vessels, this hemorrhage may reach a great extent, until it ceases by autotamponade. The intraarticular free blood initially remains liquid due to admixture

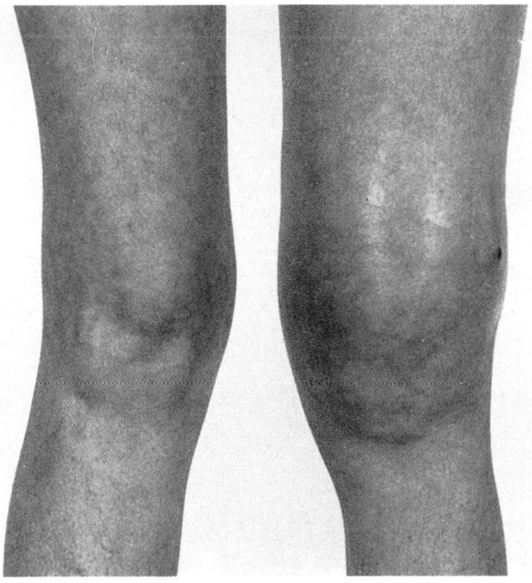

Fig. 38. Marked enlargement of the knee by swelling of soft tissue and increase in joint fluid secondary to direct bruise

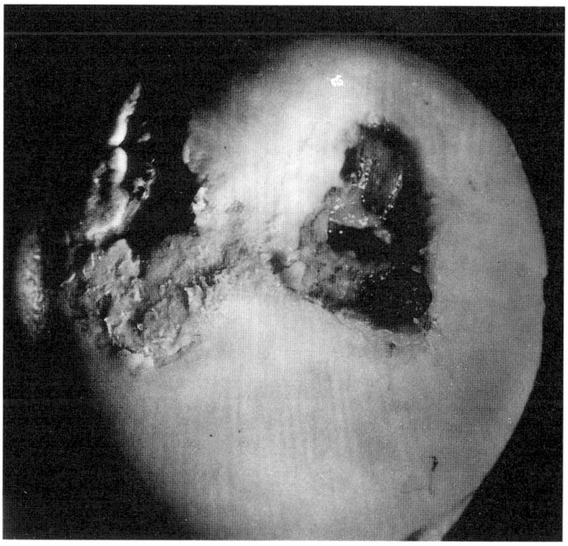

Fig. 39. Extensive defect in the articular cartilage of the femoral head secondary to contusion by a fall from a height

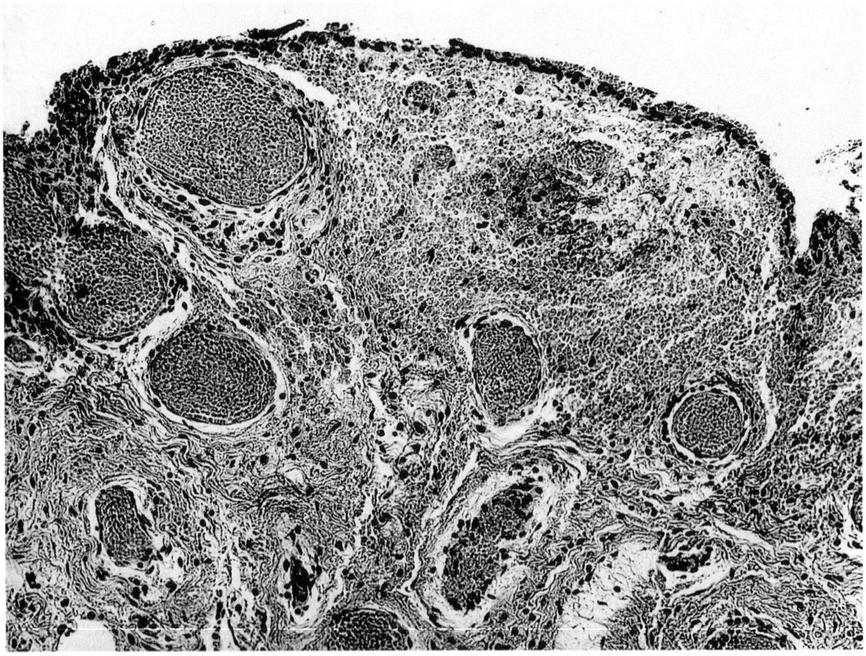

Fig. 40. All blood vessels of the synovial membrane are extremely engorged with blood. Fragments of a disrupted blood vessel lie in the subsynoviocytic tissue and are extensively surrounded by erythrocytes

to the synovial fluid, which lacks fibrinogen and thromboplastin [306]. If the hematoma persists in the joint in smaller quantity, it can be resorbed through the stomata and the lymph vessels of the synovial membrane. However, if accumulated in larger quantity and persisting for a longer period of time, the blood clots lying on the inner surface of the joint capsule elicit a reaction of the synovial membrane. Capillaries, fibroblasts, and fibrocytes intrude into the deposits of the hematogenous fibrin and organize it. Histiocytes also densely infiltrate the subsynoviocytic tissue. By these deposits and the hypercellularity of the synovial membrane, the joint capsule eventually becomes thickened. However, in addition to the immediate traumatic changes, intraarticularly manifested in accumulation of a hematoma and by hemorrhagic suffusion of the inner part of the joint capsule, the surfaces of the articular ends may also present traumatic changes. These are

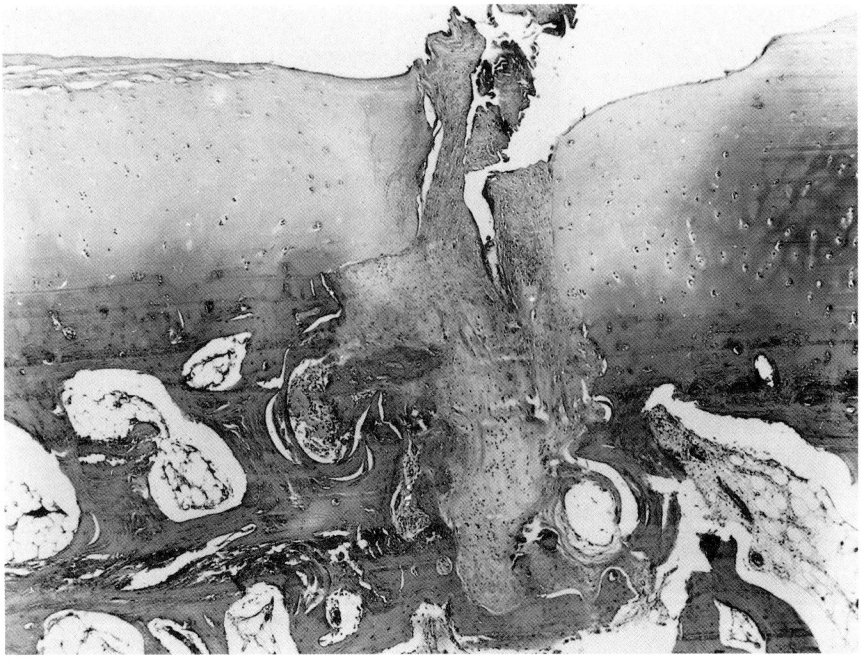

Fig. 41. The articular cartilage is partly disrupted by a few vertical clefts; one of these extends together with articular cartilage into the subchondral bone and is penetrated by capillaries. The superficial clefts are without ingrowth of capillaries

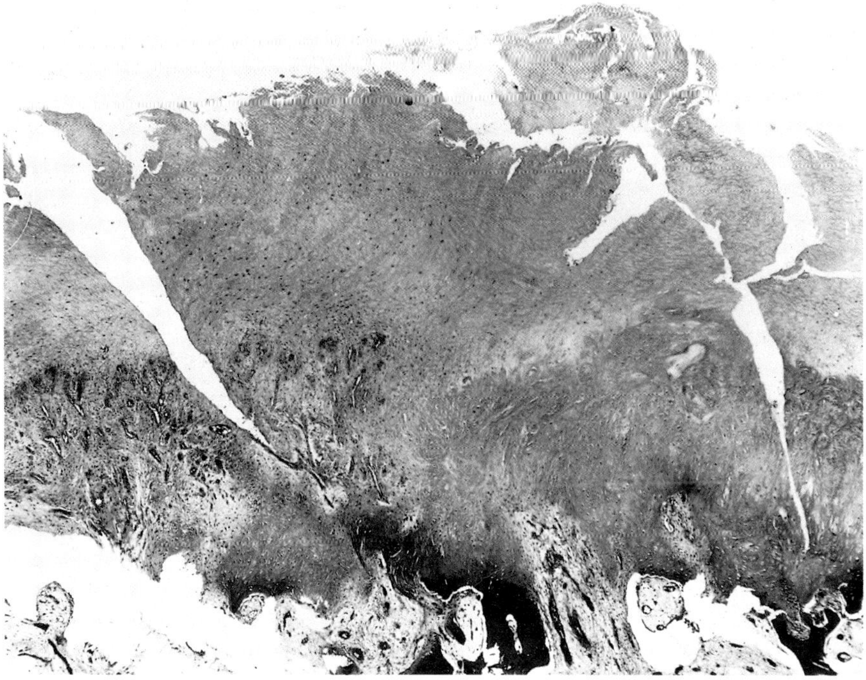

Fig. 42. The articular cartilage is disrupted by oblique and vertical clefts which expand deeply into the subchondral bone. Numerous small blood vessels proliferate here into the articular cartilage

narrow clefts which penetrate the thickness of the articular cartilage or somewhat broader gaps with dehiscences of their margins in the articular cartilage. In rare occasions, cartilage fragments of rather wide extent are completely separated from the articular surface, exposing the subchondral bone in larger areas through the resulting defect (Fig. 39).

Histopathological examination of the synovial membrane discloses disruption in some places of the synoviocyte lining, moderate dilatation of the smaller blood vessels, and extensive, rather dense permeation of the subsynoviocytic and peripheral tissue by extravasated erythrocytes (Fig. 40). This blurs the structure of the tissue, and the inner part of the joint capsule becomes substantially thickened. Disruptions of collagen bundles are noticeable in places. More essential are the occasional disruptions of various extent within the articular cartilage. The shorter disruptions (Fig. 41) extend in oblique or vertical lines from the superficial zone through the thickness of the articular cartilage but not beyond the zone of calcified cartilage. The other disruptions are vertical discontinuities, also not extending beyond the zone of calcified cartilage but combined with horizontal discontinuities within one of the zones. Here small flakes or larger fragments are completely separated from the articular cartilage. Defects of various extent and depth within the articular cartilage are the result of the latter type of disruptions. Furthermore, vertical clefts may extend through the entire thickness of the articular cartilage into the subchondral bone (Figs. 41, 42), where communication with the subchondral marrow spaces becomes established. The eventual outcome varies with the types of discontinuities [938]. In the superficial discontinuities, some of the marginal chondrocytes hypertrophy, and other chondrocytes multiply to small clones, with concomitant increase in ground substance (Fig. 41) but not to the extent of filling the gap between the separated margins. Nor does the occasional ingrowth of small blood vessels (Fig. 42) cause a substantial proliferation of chondrocytes. The more frequent outcome is degeneration and necrosis of chondrocytes (Fig. 43), as manifested by pyknosis of their nuclei, large lacunae in their cell bodies, or empty cell spaces, with concomitant staining changes in the intercellular matrix over a broad zone. These observations have also been made by DiPalma [403], Ghadially [604], and Otte [1213].

In contrast, Dustman [450] and Puhl [1286] observed, in experimentally elicited superficial cartilage defects, regional proliferation of undifferentiated cells, which under the influence of mechanical function differentiated to chondrocytes. Similarly, Thurner [1641] demonstrated that chondrocytes have the ability to regenerate and to close a defect by cartilagelike tissue in superficial defects of the articular cartilage; however, this healing capacity exists only in young individuals. On the other hand, pronounced disintegrational changes are found in the deep and broad cartilage defects remaining after separation of large fragments (Fig. 43). No signs of repair are seen here on

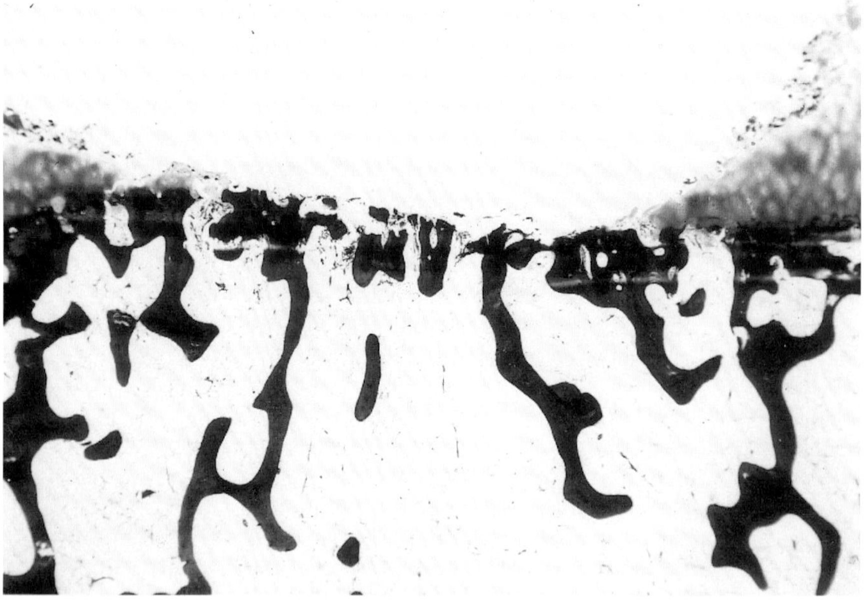

Fig. 43. The subchondral bone, which remains intact beneath torn-away articular cartilage, is without proliferation of blood vessels to the surface and without cover by connective tissue

the part of the chondrocytes, but the marginal zones present necrosis of the chondrocytes and disintegration of the ground substance [1190].

An entirely different reaction is noticeable once the gap in the articular cartilage extends through the subchondral bone into the marrow space. Even at a narrow cleft, fibroblasts accompanied by capillaries advance from the marrow space and fill the gap with gradually maturing connective tissue (Fig. 44). Cotta [329], Ghadially [604], Salter [1390], and Thurner [1641] demonstrated that the fibrocytes occasionally and gradually assume the appearance of chondrocytes, with concurrent disappearance of the capillaries and with occasional degeneration and necrosis of chondrocytes. Nevertheless, despite potential conversion to chondrocytes, the intercellular matrix is inadequate due to lack of formation of sufficient ground substance [1016, 1081].

The hemorrhage in the subcutis and joint indicate the injuries of these organs, while the absence of circumscribed tenderness at the attachment of ligaments and of abnormal passive motion excludes damage to ligaments. Negative findings in roentgenography exclude the presence of an articular fracture.

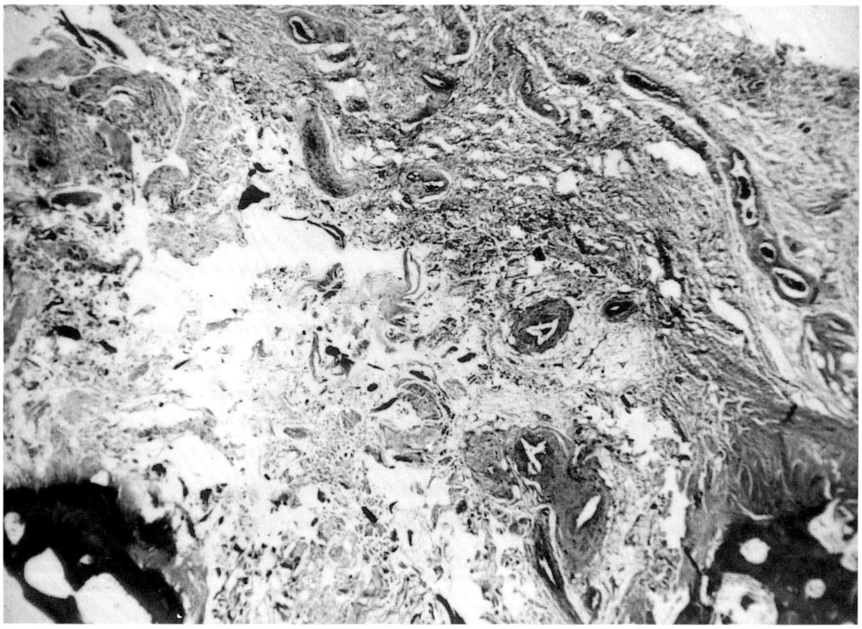

Fig. 44. On deep disruption of the articular surface through the subchondral bone, granulation tissue expands from the marrow spaces and extensively fills the defect with maturing connective tissue

After the diagnosis has been established, complete bedrest with elevation of the injured extremity on two pillows should be instituted. The injured joint should be surrounded with compresses soaked in cold water at least three times a day for 3 h each time or, better, around the clock. An ice pack has a similar vasoconstrictive effect but not the same pain-relieving effect. Enzyme medications (containing streptokinase-streptodornase or papase) are of benefit for expediting the absorption of the swelling. If the hemorrhage is small and chiefly extraarticular, the symptoms regress after 2–3 days. Use of the injured joint may be resumed with an elastic bandage wrapped around the joint during the day for 3–4 weeks. However, if the intraarticular hematoma is large and is not absorbed or at least decreased by the above management within 1 day, it should be removed [329, 1286]. The technique of aspiration is described in "Arthrocentesis". Arthrocentesis immediately after the injury is not advisable because the torn blood vessels have not yet thrombosed, and renewed leaking of blood may start from them. On the other hand, delayed removal of the hematoma may permit the enzymes contained physiologically in the blood to initiate a disintegration of the articular cartilage [329, 1286] and leaves a large amount of fibrin precipitated on the synovial membrane. Permanent thickening of the joint capsule may then ensue. A joint emptied by its blood effusion either by spontaneous resorption or aspiration must be compressed by a firm strapping for 3–4 weeks. Resumption of function without this constant compression may cause recurrence of intraarticular hemorrhage or effusion.

Partial active mobilization should be instituted early since longer immobilization impairs the trophic aspect of the joint [329]. After sufficiently long compression, full mobilization of the joint by active exercises is necessary. While early mobilization of bruised joints appears advisable, it is questionable whether this consideration applies to the joints of the lower extremities involved in a severe injury. In view of the possibility, or even probability, of disruption of the articular cartilage, avoidance or at least minimization of weight bearing for 6–8 weeks is advisable here as a useful reconstructive factor. As aftercare, physical therapy with six to eight sessions of massage and ultrasound (its effects are described in "Contracture of Joint") at low intensity, 2–3 W/cm^2, may be indicated [687, 1541] if soreness of the joint persists.

2. Sprain of Joints

Sprain is the designation of an articular injury which involves principally the articular ligaments and joint capsule but leaves the articular epiphyses intact. The sprain is caused either by a direct trauma or, more often, by an indirect trauma which exceeds the range of passive movement of a joint in one and or possibly further axes. Here the retentive structures of the joint, the ligaments, are overstretched. The inner layer of the joint capsule may also be overstretched but without incurring severe damage by virtue of its folds and pliability.

Depending on the intensity and duration of the trauma, the following three degrees of damage to the articular ligaments may be distinguished, as manifested by the clinical signs.

a. A few fibers of a ligament are elastically overstretched without suffering a rupture. Thus no discontinuity is present, and the clinical symptom of swelling is slight or absent, but a moderate, circumscribed tenderness along the ligament is noticed. The active and passive movements have normal ranges or are slightly limited.

b. Some fibers of a ligament are disrupted, with local swelling and moderate to pronounced tenderness. Since the major portion of the ligament retains continuity, the stability of the joint to any side is not impaired. Nevertheless, the attempt of passive movement in one or another direction elicits severe pain along the course of the injured ligament or at its points of attachment. When the ligament has been overstretched and not treated shortly thereafter, a reflex spasm of the regional muscles often sets in which protectively keeps the joint in contracture for 1–2 weeks. The attempt to correct this deviation elicits pain at the site of the injury.

c. A complete tear is one in which all fibers of a ligament are disrupted. An irregular discontinuity exists either in the course or at the attachment of the ligament. In conjunction, the outer part of the joint capsule is often also torn. If the tear involves the midportion of the ligament, bleeding into the joint cavity occurs, with considerable swelling of the joint. Marked pain and substantial impairment in the function of the joint, due to instability, characterize the situation. Depending on the site of the tear, circumscribed tenderness is present either at the level of the joint cleft or in the area of the ligamentous attachment. The attempt to tilt the joint passively to the opposite side of this ligament elicits pronounced pain at the site of the injury. After release of the passive hold, the tilted articular end returns suddenly and with a snap or click to its normal alignment to the contiguous articular end. The possibility of such abnormal passive tilting exists in a fresh, complete tear of a ligament only in the first 24 h following the injury. Thereafter a reflex-elicited tenseness of the regional musculature sets in, lasting 1–2 weeks, during which the abnormal laxity cannot be ascertained.

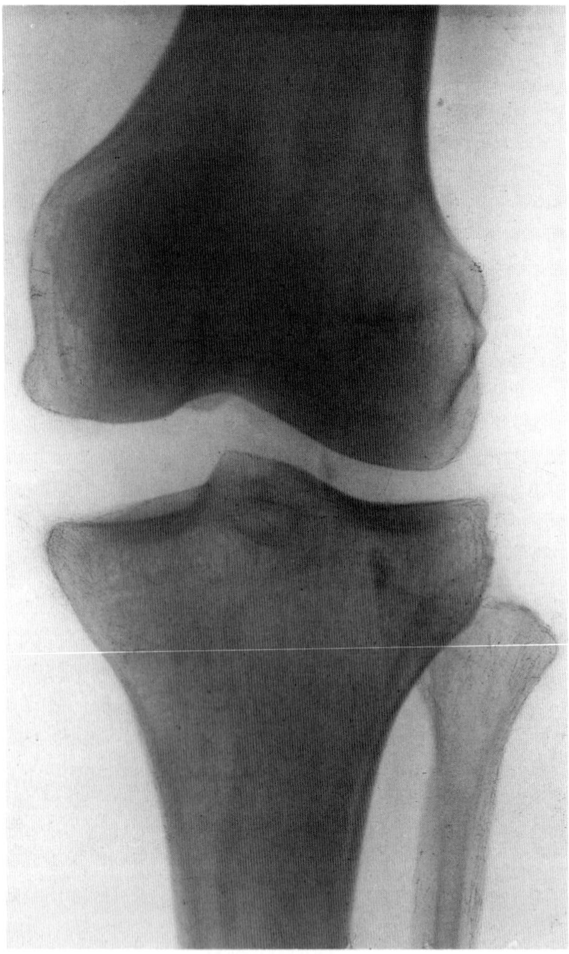

Fig. 45. Passive angulation of the lower leg and widening of the medial joint cleft, due to tear of the medial collateral ligament, is ascertainable after an injury

Roentgenographic examination excludes bone injury and indicates the degree of discontinuity in a ligament by a posttraumatically, abnormally tiltable articular end (Fig. 45). However, such a roentgenograph can be obtained only as long as muscular spasticity has not set in or after it has subsided. Additionally, the directly posttraumatic abnormal passive angulation in a joint can be ascertained by a stress roentgenograph. After infiltrating the area of tenderness with a local anesthetic, one articular end is passively tilted in the direction opposite to the side of the ligament. A distinct angulation of 10°–30° can thus be measured and a one-side widening of the cartilage space is detected (Figs. 46, 47). Nevertheless, a constitutional laxity must also be taken into consideratin upon a directly posttraumatically positive roentgenograph, and this can be ascertained by testing the mobility of the corresponding joint of the other extremity.

The above symptoms and diagnostic evaluations apply chiefly to sprains of the joints of the extremities. Among these, the knee joint deserves special attention because of the variety of structures which either alone or in combination can be injured in a sprain [506]. These are the collateral ligaments, cruciate ligaments, and menisci. Therefore, differential diagnosis here is more complicated and the examination more elaborate. Often, all diagnostic modalities, including contrast roentgenography, magnetic resonance imaging, and arthroscopy, are required to confirm the diagnosis or to make it as precise as possible. Nevertheless, the basic and specific tests on the knee joint are those of abduction stress with medial instability upon tear of the medial collateral ligament, adduction stress with lateral instability upon tear of the lateral collateral ligament (Fig. 46), anterior drawer stress with anterior instability upon tear of the anterior cruciate ligament (Fig. 47), and posterior drawer stress with posterior instability upon tear of the posterior cruciate ligaments. The specific tests in injuries of the menisci and the modalities of their treatment are not discussed here because the menisci are not structures which hold together as the ligaments are.

The ankle joint also frequently suffers sprain, especially in women due to the constitutionally weaker musculature and habitual use of high-heeled shoes. These factors lead to usual and excessive supination of the foot. The ligaments, fibulotalar and fibulocalcaneal, on the lateral aspect are thus overstretched, often also partly disrupted. Intense tenderness and marked swelling (Fig. 48) at the lateral aspect of the ankle are often associated with blue discoloration. The attempt of passive supination in the ankle joint elicits sharp pain on its lateral aspect, and this is countered by contraction of the peroneal muscles.

Treatment of a sprain of any peripheral joint [506] aims in the first 2–3 days to reduce the swelling and pain. Complete bedrest with the extremity elevated on two pillows, and cold wet compresses around the injured joint, applied continuously for 1–2 days, provide great relief and improvement. With intraarticular hemorrhage, arthrocentesis is indicated if no absorption of the effusion is attained within 1–2 days by this treatment. Subsequently, in an overstretching of a ligament, the joint should be compressed by a firm adhesive strapping for 3–4 weeks. However, in a tear of some fibers the joint should be immobilized with a splint or a brace for 4–6 weeks at concurrent avoidance of strenuous activities. Otherwise the inadequately treated overstretching of a ligament and especially the partial tear of a ligament are followed by soreness lasting several weeks or months and by impaired use of the joint due to insufficiency of the ligament. In complete tear of a ligament, as revealed by stress roentgenograph, exposure of the ligament by arthrotomy and approximation of its ruptured ends by sutures, followed by splinting

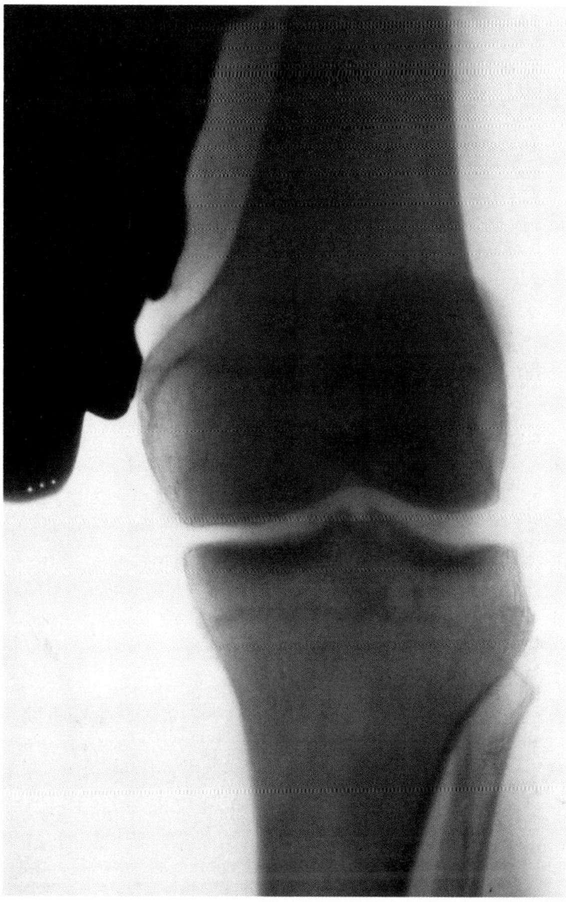

Fig. 46. Stress view of injured knee. The lower leg can be passively tilted into adduction, an indication of injury of the lateral collateral ligament

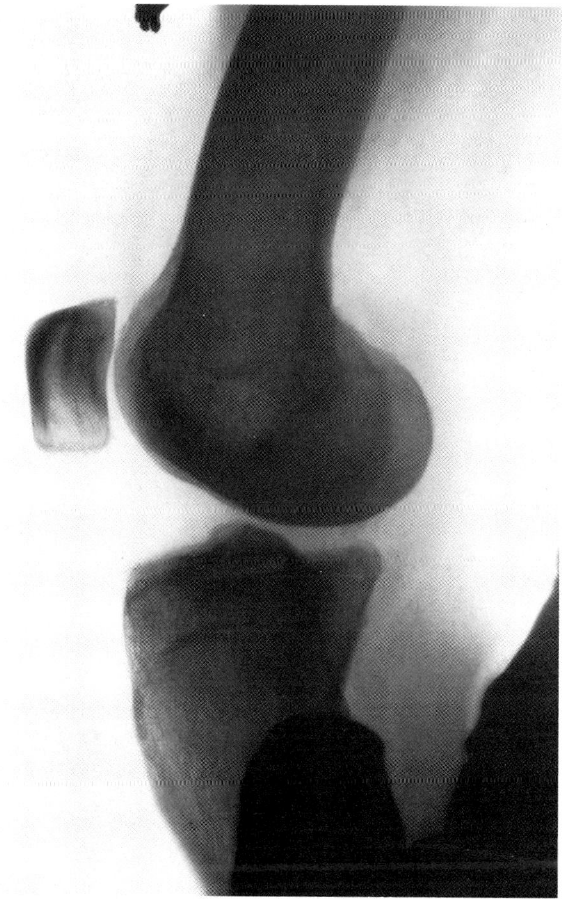

Fig. 47. Stress view of the knee in Fig. 46. The lower leg can be passively subluxated anteriorly, an indication of injury of the anterior cruciate ligament

for 4 weeks, is the method of choice. When open approximation is not feasible for any reason, the joint should at least be immobilized with a splint or a plaster cast for 4–6 weeks; the result may be satisfactory for the knee and other peripheral joints. Some authors [66, 471, 801, 840, 1392] recommend concurrent, immediate immobilization even as the primary treatment for tear of a ligament; parallel follow-up examinations reveal the final outcome of this nonoperative treatment to be not inferior to that of primary surgical repair of the torn ligament [1199].

In old, nontreated injuries of ligaments of peripheral joints causing persistent soreness and swelling (Fig. 48), the pain may be eliminated by massage, eight to ten ultrasound treatments with 3–4 W/cm^2 or two or three topical hydrocortisone injections. However, with persistent mechanical inadequacy of the joint, regular strapping with an elastic bandage or firm splinting is necessary. If these modalities do not suffice, a plastic repair of the ligament by its plication or its reinforcement by transposed tendons from the neighboring area is indicated [805, 1214, 1451]. Additionally, strengthening of the regional musculature by regular isometric exercises, massage, and faradic stimulation over a period of 4–6 months often compensates by an increase in muscle tonus for the diminished stability of the joint. A splint may sometimes also be necessary.

The joints of the vertebral column are also subject to sprain. The joints of the cervical spine are sprained principally in car accidents of head-on or rear collision. Marked circumscribed tenderness, especially at the apophyseal joints and along the interspinal line of the middle and lower parts of the cervical spine, is the clinical finding which indicates an overstretching of the intervertebral and longitudinal ligaments. This situation is most often associated with spasm of the paravertebral musculature and sometimes also of the sternocleidomastoideus musculature. Hereby the active and passive movements of the cervical spine are substantially limited in all directions. However, the concurrent irritations of the nerve roots emerging from C4, C5, C6, and C7 (Figs. 298, 299) lead to greater impair-

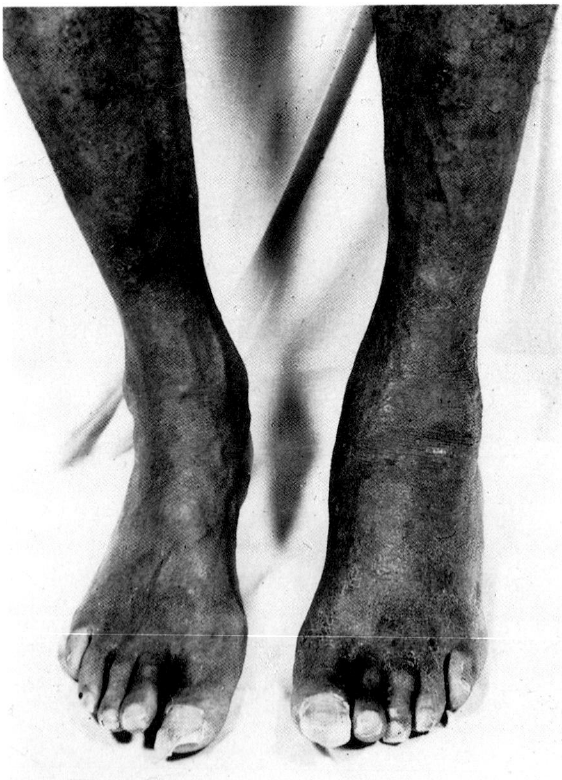

Fig. 48. Old untreated sprain of the left ankle joint with residual marked thickening and instability

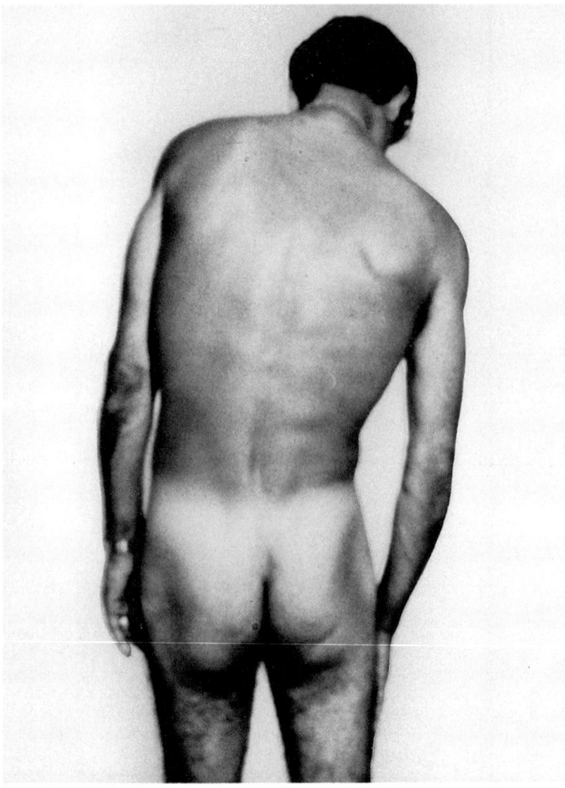

Fig. 49. Recent sprain of the lower thoracic and entire lumbar spine with resulting tenseness of the paravertebral musculature and tilt of the trunk to the right side

ment [341]. These symptoms may appear a few days or even a few weeks after the injury. They are most often caused by compression of the nerves in their bony canals when the intercervical joints are moved to excessive excursions. Other causes of compression of nerve roots are swelling and hemorrhages of the adjacent capsular ligaments or subsequent narrowing of the intervertebral exits by fibrotic thickening of the ligamentous and capsular tissues [809, 810]. Such nerve root symptoms occur bilaterally in 15%–18% of cases and are caused similarly as the unilateral nerve root symptoms [809, 910].

The lumbar spine is subjected even more often to acute sprains, caused not only by car accidents but also, almost as often, by its excessive movement in sports, professional, or routine activities. The symptoms are similar to those in sprains of the cervical spine, manifested [968] by persistent pain in the lower back, pronounced tenderness of the lumbar spine and lumbosacral junction, and marked tenseness of the regional paravertebral musculature. These injuries are associated with substantial limitation of movement in the direction of ventral and lateral flexion. The injuries sometimes involve the articular and paraarticular structures of the lumbar spine only at one side, but with greater intensity. Here the homolateral paravertebral musculature becomes very contracted, causing a tilt of the lumbar spine and trunk to the affected side (Fig. 49). However, sometimes the contralateral musculature is contracted, causing the trunk to be tilted to the opposite side. Most sprains of the lower lumbar spine are associated shortly afterward with nerve root symptoms in the buttocks and thighs. Neurological, examination in the initial phase indicates pressure on the nerve roots most often at L4, L5, and S1 and less often at L2 and L3 [341], expressed in intense, radiating pain into the areas of their distribution (Figs. 300, 301). These symptoms change after longer duration to those of paresthesias, anesthesias, and diminished reflexes. Roentgenographs in a number of views and various inclinations reveal no fracture or subluxation but sometimes osteoarthritic changes with narrowing and irregular delimitation of the intervertebral spaces by sclerosed vertebral plates carrying marginal osteophytes. In some cases, an abnormal tilting of a vertebral body is noticeable whereby the physiological alignment and relationship between vertebral bodies in disturbed, and the intervertebral foramina are narrowed. All these changes are more frequent and more pronounced in the lumbar spine [968] than in the cervical spine.

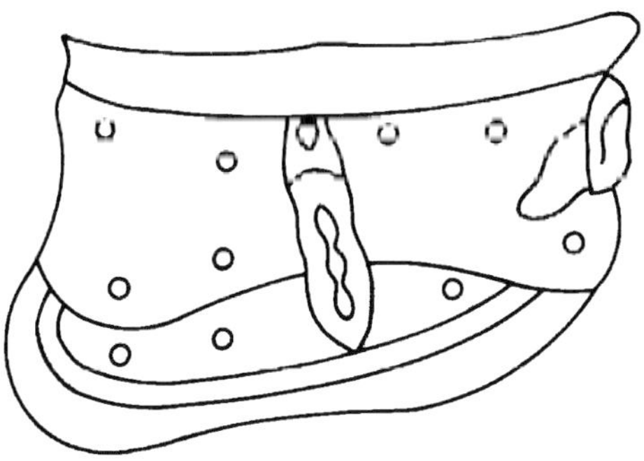

Fig. 50. Cervical collar of plastic material with adjustable metallic supports

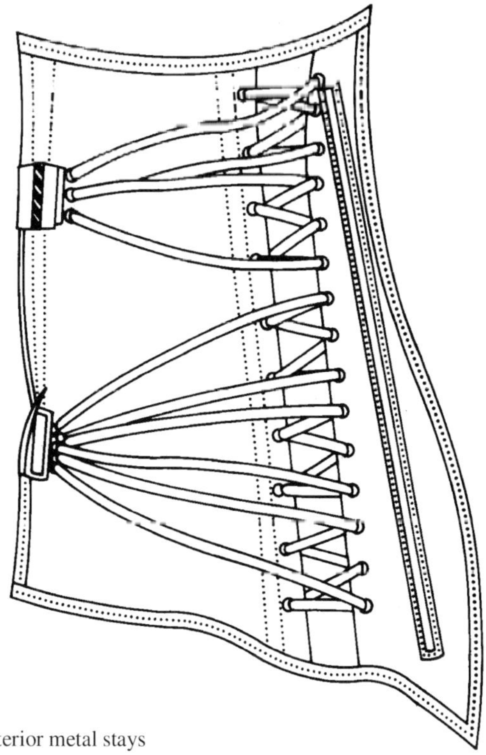

Fig. 51. Thoraco lumbar belt of firm canvas with lateral lacings and posterior metal stays

Initial treatment of a sprain of the vertebral column consists of complete bedrest, lying flat on a firm mattress, if necessary reinforced by a bedboard, and regular application of moist warm compresses to the affected area of the vertebral column. These compresses have a relieving effect on the sensory nerve fibers and thus mitigate the pain. Moderate or strong analgesics, even narcotics, and muscle relaxants are also necessary as long as the reflex muscle tenseness persits. Salicylates are not effective in the initial phase, but in larger doses they may subsequently be sufficient when the acute intense pain regresses. Then the temperature of the moist compresses is changed to very warm, leading to regression of the muscle tenseness. The patient is permitted to resume ambulation, provided that the affected area is protected by a reliable support. A plastic collar with metal stays is necessary for the cervical spine (Fig. 50), and a high lumbosacral corset of firm canvas with metal stays in the back is necessary for the lumbar spine (Fig. 51). In patients who are overweight or who have more extensive and severe symptoms affecting the lower thoracic spine, entire lumbar spine, and lumbosacral junction, a leather-metal spinal brace is indicated. However, if the muscle tenseness does not regress within 4–6 weeks, and the nerve root symptoms persist, continuous cervical and/or lumbar traction is necessary. This can be effectively carried out only in a hospital, and a substantial mitigation in the neurological condition can be obtained. If this modality is not fully effective, intra-paravertebral nerve blocks with lidocaine solution injected at the involved nerve roots provide a distinct relief. When the nerve root symptoms regress and full ambulation has been resumed, protective immobilization of the affected part of the spine by a collar, corset, or brace should be continued for at least 6 months. Physical therapy with muscle-strengthening exercises and massage [1613] and/or ultrasound [687, 1541] in two or three series of six to eight sessions may be very beneficial, as is the abstaining from vigorous activities for a period of about 6–12 months.

3. Traumatic Synovitis and Posttraumatic Synovitis

In addition to specific articular structures such as the ligaments and cartilage, direct and indirect injuries to joints harm primarily the inner part of the joint capsule, the synovial membrane. Even after the immediate effects on some parts of a joint have subsided, its synovial membrane may remain in a state of irritation; this inflammation is termed traumatic synovitis.

The clinical symptoms are moderate swelling and diffuse soreness related to the joint capsule along its entire extent. Local temperature is not elevated. Neither specific points of tenderness nor a protective reflex of the regional musculature is detected. The range of active movement is limited at the extremes of excursions in any direction, and the attempt of increased passive movement elicits pain. The function of the joint is distinctly limited and becomes even more limited when the joint is enlarged by thickening of the joint capsule or increase of the joint fluid. This is tested by fluctuation or by ballotement of the patella (Fig. 14) when the knee joint is affected.

Aspiration in this situation (Fig. 25) yields 60–100 ml pinkish clear or slightly hemorrhagic synovial fluid, which contains 800–5000 erythrocytes and 200–2000 lymphocytes per milliliter, and increased content of albumin at normal viscosity, and fair degree of mucin clotting. Roentgenographs present no abnormal findings. Histopathological examination of the synovial tissue (Fig. 53), obtained by punch biopsy, discloses slight hyperplastic thickening of the synoviocyte cover, moderate rarefaction of the subsynoviocytic tissue by edema at pronounced dilatation of the blood vessels, and slight focal infiltration by lymphocytes. Hemorrhages are rarely noticed.

Absorption of the effusion is expedited by prolonged bedrest, elevation of the extremity, and regular application of cold to mildly warm wet compresses. If this modality does not succeed within 1–2 days, arthrocentesis under local anesthesia is necessary for removal of the joint fluid. Immediately thereafter the joint should be compressed by a soft strapping reinforced with adhesive tape or by an ACE bandage to be worn throughout the day for the following 3–4 weeks. Elevation of the extremity at bedrest during the night is necessary for 1–2 months. Beyond this, the normal use of the affected joint should be resumed gradually and slowly; recurrence of the synovitis and impairment in the function of the joint may follow.

In contrast to traumatic synovitis, posttraumatic synovitis develops not concurrently with but at an interval after an injury. The case histories of these patients reveal the occurrence of a direct or indirect injury in the past at work, traffic, sports, or in everyday activities. Due to minimal disturbance at that time, no medical care was sought. However, after many months the injured joint becomes painful and often swollen. Eventually, pronounced disturbance in the function of the joint ensues, with impaired motion and sometimes instability, while no additional trauma or supervening disease provoked further local lesions. In view of the relatively long interval between the traumatic event and the appearance of symptoms, the designation of posttraumatic synovitis seems appropriate. This term is also justified histopathologically. The examined synovial membrane no longer displays the changes produced by a recent injury but mostly those of the chronic state which developed in the intervening period.

Physical examination discloses that predominantly the knee joint is affected; shoulder, wrist, and ankle joints, are affected less often. The joint is enlarged by the swelling of the joint capsule, which may be more conspicuous when atrophy of the regional musculature set in. A moderate increase in joint fluid often aggravates the enlargement of the joint. The entire joint is diffusely tender. In cases of longer duration, its motion is limited partly due to thickening of the joint capsule and partly due to tenseness or contracture of the regional musculature.

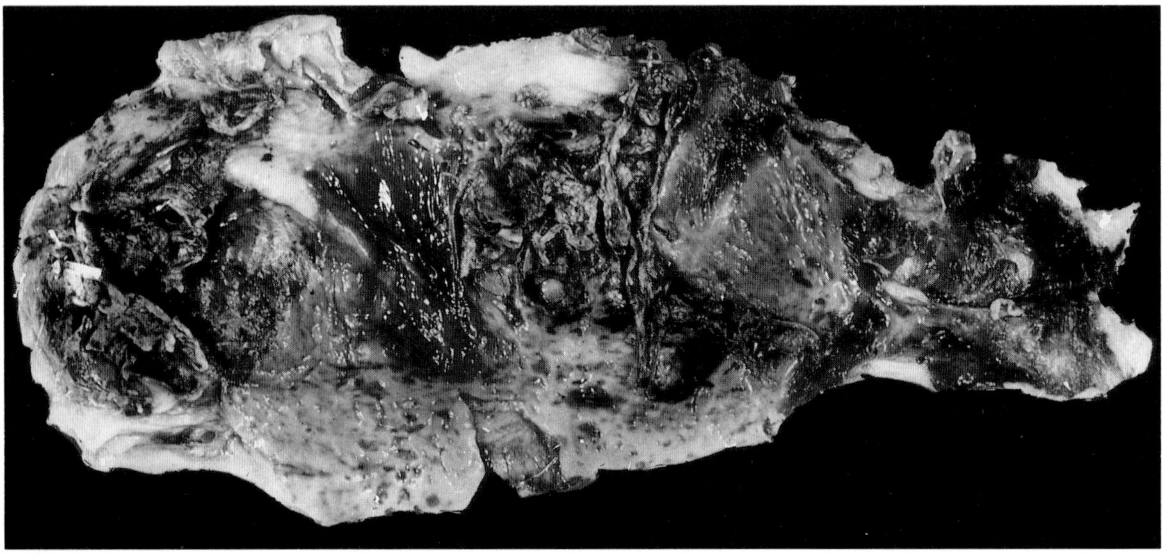

Fig. 52. The inner part of the joint capsule is hyperemic on most of its extent and is uneven by elevation of villi and small polypous outgrowths. In a few other areas the tissue is thickened but rather even and is discolored grayish white

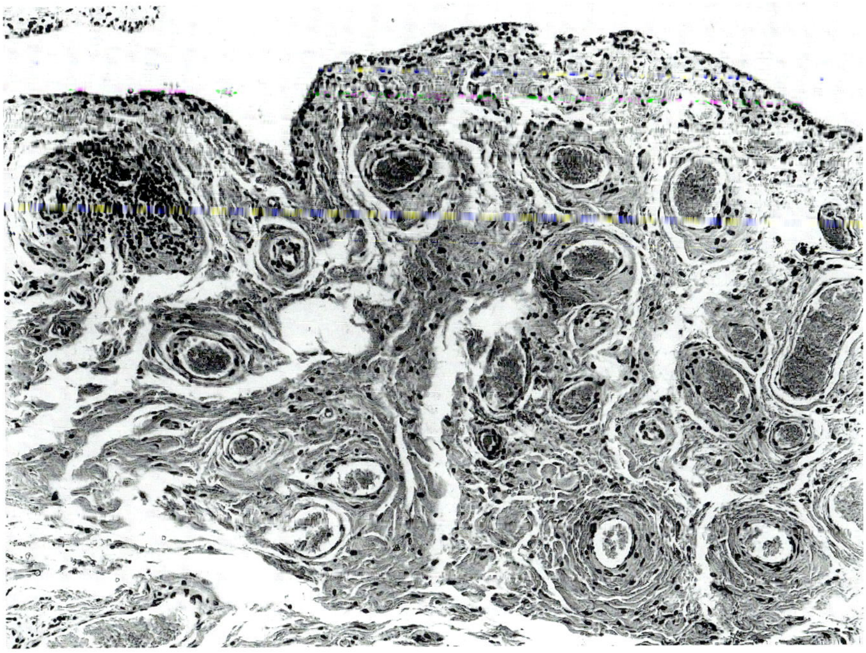

Fig. 53. Below slightly hypertrophic synoviocytes, all blood vessels are dilated and hyperemic. Some blood vessels have thickened walls. The subsynoviocytic tissue is moderately loosened by edema; lymphocytes are perivascularly accumulated in one area

The aspirated joint fluid is clear and straw- to amber-colored. It sometimes contains an increased number of erythrocytes, but its albumin and globulin content is normal. Roentgenographs reveal thickening of the joint capsule or its distension by joint fluid and widening of the cartilage space. Calcified densities occasionally lie in the joint capsule.

On gross-anatomical examination the inner part of the joint capsule is shiny and hyperemic. In some instances, islands of tissue discolored from reddish-hemorrhagic to tan-brown lie amid more extensive areas of grayish white color and firmer consistency. Occasionally the inner surface is uneven and thickened into a few plump folds, but most often it is occupied by numerous thin villi (Fig. 52). A few small loose bodies of cartilage-bone consistency may be attached to the synovial membrane, where it merges with the articular cartilage. The latter is smooth, shiny, and even.

Histopathological examination of the synovial membrane [980c, 1543, 1548] discloses hyperemia in the

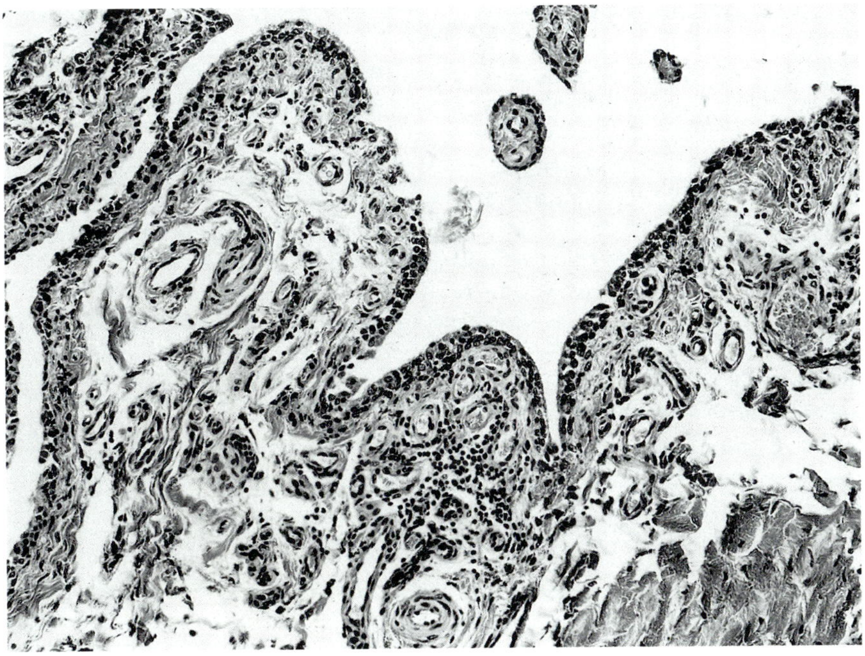

Fig. 54. The synovial membrane is elevated in plump villi which are covered by moderately hypertrophic hyperplastic synoviocytes. The subsynoviocytic tissue is loosened by edema and contains small infiltrates of lymphocytes

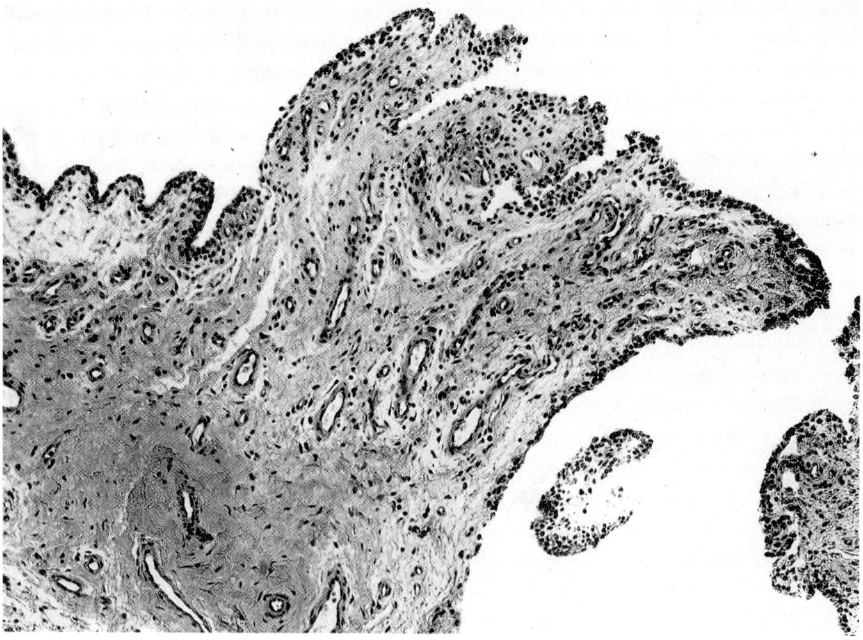

Fig. 55. Synovial membrane, specimen excised 4 years after synovectomy, bears a few small villi covered by single rows of normal-sized synoviocytes. The subsynoviocytic tissue is free of inflammatory infiltrates

early phase (Fig. 53) and hyperplasia of the synoviocytes to two or three rows, which delimit areas of even surface, as well as long villi in the advanced phase (Fig. 54). The subjacent blood vessels are often thickened by increased smooth muscle cells and concentric collagen fibers.

Hemosiderin is sometimes deposited in the subsynoviocytic tissue, but more often small agglomerations of lymphocytes are situated perivascularly and/or loosely scattered. In other instances the fibrocytes are increased and usually associated with fibrosis of the subsynoviocytic and deeper tissue.

In view of the soreness and signs of irritation, the joint should be compressed with an elastic bandage throughout the day. Wet warm compresses applied regularly and eight to ten sessions with shortwave diathermy are very beneficial. When the joint fluid is increased, it should be removed by arthrocentesis, followed immediately by application of a firm compression strapping for 4 weeks. In the rare situations when this modality is not successful, immobilization with a brace or a plaster cast may stop the irritation of the joint capsule. However, if the symptoms, especially the marked thickening of the joint capsule, continue despite the above therapeutic modalities and remain associated with mechanical impairment, arthroscopy or arthrotomy for complete inspection of the joint cavity is indicated. Partial or total synovectomy may be necessary (Fig. 52). This operation should not be deferred, in view of the otherwise frequent fibrosis of the deeper zones of the joint capsule and the concomitant limitation of movement. A further indication for the excision of the thickened inner part of the joint capsule derives from the experience that the chronically inflamed synovial membrane by its concomitant abnormal enzymatic activity may cause degradation of the articular cartilage [330, 1432]. Following the operation, joint mobilization exercises and muscle strengthening are necessary. Long-term follow-up examinations disclose resumption of normal configuration of the joint in the full range of movements [1124]. Histopathological examination of biopsied specimens obtained at a longer interval after the synovectomy disclose restructuration of the synovial membrane, yet with formation in some places of villi which are of distinctly smaller size and less inflammatory changes (Fig. 55) than those at the time of the operation [689, 882, 1614].

4. Infrapatellar Liposynovitis

A specific type of posttraumatic synovitis is manifested by an anatomically and clinically conspicuous enlargement of the inner part of the joint capsule caudal to the patella [416]. This condition was originally described by Hoffa [768].

The cause of the alteration was initially thought to be proliferative growth due to tuberculosis or a tumor. However, upon further evaluation the enlargement is interpreted as an abacterial inflammation, whose etiology lies in frequent indirect injuries or in local mechanical irritations [1101, 1263]. As a sequela of these, an increase in synovial connective and subsynovial adipose tissue elements results in concomitant enlargement of the inner part of the joint capsule in this area [339]. That concentrated injury is the eliciting cause is supported by the fact that this enlargement is often associated with injuries of the medial meniscus or anterior cruciate ligament. This coincidence may be explained by the concurrent effect of the trauma on the meniscus and the infrapatellar synovial pad. The result is a thickening of the pad which due to its protrusion into the joint cavity is constantly exposed to mechanical irritation. Another explanation for such development may be found in the fact that, secondary to internal derangement, abnormal mobility of the meniscus and/or of the tibia may persistently cause mechanical irritation of the infrapatellar synovial tissue leading to its thickening and plumpness. Continued local pressure on the anteroinferior aspect of the knee in certain professional activities (floor or street repair, tile paving) is also able to provoke hypertrophy of the infrapatellar tissue. Occasionally, marked inflammatory processes of the adjacent bursae cause inflammation and thickening of the infrapatellar synovial pad. According to other concepts [416], alterations in the infrapatellar synovial pad represent aspects of a generalized chronic synovitis.

Enlargement of the infrapatellar joint capsule occurs in middle-aged adults, chiefly in men (athletes, craftsmen). Characteristic is their complaint of experiencing, after sitting for more than 1 h, a bothersome tightness in the anterior compartment of the knee. This sensation is produced by the interposition of the enlarged joint capsule into the joint, and it vanishes by retraction of the joint capsule on extension of the knee joint. Other patients report the opposite complaint; they feel that something is "drawn into" the knee joint on extension, while this tissue is being released from the interior of the knee joint on flexion. The differences in complaints may be explained pathomechanically by the frequent connection of the infrapatellar fat pad with a persistent median septum in the latter situation. Accordingly, on standing up from sitting position, the patient feels a snap between the anterior aspects of the femoral and tibial condyles. Caudally to the patella, a noticeable, palpable, and moderately tender thickening protrudes on both sides of the ligamentum patellae. Otherwise the contour of the knee is not changed, unless a moderate effusion is present. Active flexion is not impaired, but active extension may be limited; even a temporary blocking before full extension may occur [1137, 1263]. The diagnosis can be corroborated by palpation of an infrapatellar thickening which glides inward or outward of the joint cavity upon flexion or extension of the knee joint.

Examination of the moderately increased joint fluid discloses the presence of a moderate number of lymphocytes and erythrocytes and numerous cells from the synovial-adipose tissue.

Roentgenograph in the lateral view (Fig. 56) reveals a densification and enlargement of the infrapatellar soft tissue, an alteration seen more distinctly in the air contrast roentgenograph.

Gross-anatomical examination discloses that the anterior inner surface of the joint capsule is reddish and contains a few small hemorrhages. Villi of the inner joint capsule protrude at both sides of the patella, but the plump enlargement of the joint capsule caudally to the patella is more conspicuous. This enlargement protrudes backward into the anterior space of the joint cavity, ingressing as a wedge between the anterior insertion of the medial meniscus and that of the lateral meniscus. The diverging plicae alares of the joint capsule are often also enlarged. The infrapatellar synovial pad has a lobulated configuration and is of sclerosed consistency. Its sagittal section discloses a yellowish surface traversed by grayish white dense strips.

Histopathological examination (Fig. 57) discloses hyperplastic thickening of the synoviocyte cover, proliferation of broad villi, and focal infiltration of the subsynoviocytic tissue by a small number of lymphocytes. The blood vessels are widened and hyperemic, and a few small hemorrhages are scattered. The subsynoviocytic adipose layer is substantially enlarged and is traversed by broad septa composed of fibrocytes and a prevailing proportion of thick bundles of collagen fibers [1101].

Differentiation between generalized posttraumatic synovitis and infrapatellar liposynovitis may be difficult if the infrapatellar thickening is not very pronounced. Similarly, a history of locking episodes without characteristic pain areas makes the differential diagnosis versus an injury to a meniscus rather difficult. The benign lipoma has a coarse lobulated surface, is well delimited, and may be located in any area of the joint cavity. The chronically inflamed and thickened infrapatellar bursa is palpable outside of the joint capsule and in front of the patellar ligament [1101].

If conservative treatment by regular local application of moist heat, physical therapy with shortwave diathermy in eight to ten sessions, elastic compression by an ACE bandage during the day, and antiinflammatory medication does not provide a substantial decrease in the thickening, arthrotomy is indicated. This is indicated especially if a blocking phenomenon in the knee recurs. Arthroscopy does not permit a sufficiently wide removal of the fat pad. The knee joint must be opened by a parapatellar incision which offers a sufficient survey of the joint cavity and permits adequate resection of the infrapatellar joint capsule, preferably under tourniquet ischemia. Excision and diagnosis of the enlarged infrapatellar capsular pad are possible here, preferably

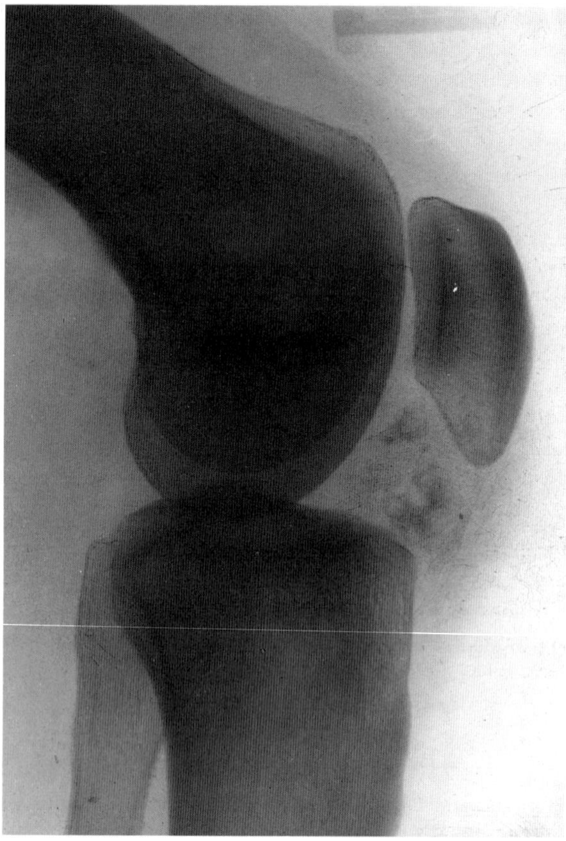

Fig. 56. An osteoma has formed in an enlarged and densified infrapatellar fat pad

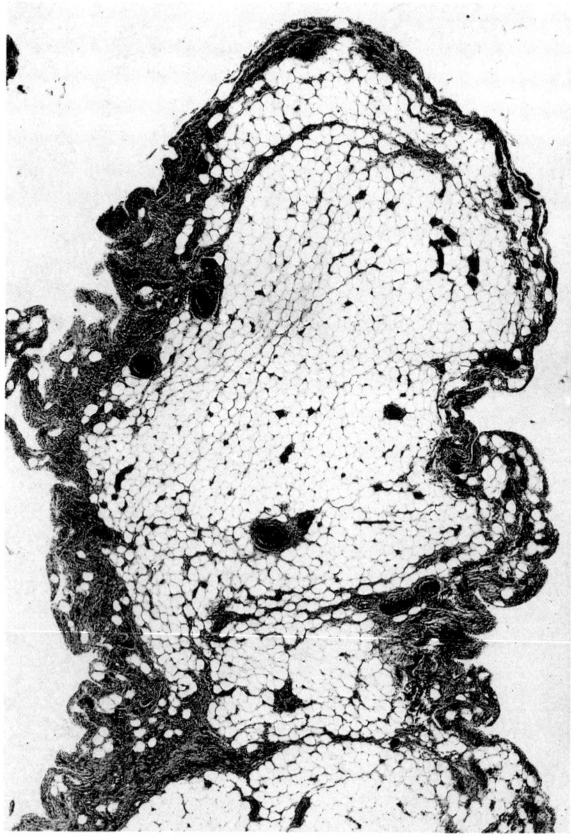

Fig. 57. Marked enlargement of the infrapatellar fat pad by numerous plump villi on the surface and by increase of the intrinsic adipose tissue. The synoviocytes are hyperplastic, and the subsynoviocytic fibrocytes as well as the collagen bundles are substantially increased

by electrocautery. Postoperatively, the knee joint is compressed and immobilized by a firm strapping or a plaster cast for 2 weeks and is subsequently mobilized by active exercises. In addition, continued elastic compression of the knee joint and isometric quadriceps-strengthening exercises are advisable for further 3–4 months. Thereupon the normal configuration and function of the knee joint are restored.

5. Posttraumatic Fibrosis Ossificans of Joints

Injury and/or mechanical irritation of the outer zone of the joint capsule or of the paraarticular structures may lead to fibrosis and subsequent ossification of these tissues [21, 22]. Such ossification was initially described by Pellegrini [1235] and Stieda [1585] at the medial aspect of the knee joint, but it may also be observed in the shoulder, elbow, hip or ankle joint, although at substantially lower incidence [201, 1169].

The cause of this alteration is usually a trauma which either directly bruised the articular ends or indirectly caused an angulation of the articular ends with overstretching of the articular fibrous structures. Periosteal tears occurred in the former situation, and partial discontinuities of ligaments and/or tendons or avulsions of periosteal slips occurred in the latter situation. In all these cases collagen fibers were torn, blood vessels were disrupted, and hemorrhages appeared [1554]. The hematoma is organized by ingrowing granulation tissue which becomes fibrosed and finally becomes transformed into osteoid and osseous tissue. However, in other cases no single unequivocal trauma can be identified in the past history – only repeated and intensive localized stresses imposed by forced activities at sport or professional work. The heterotopic formation of bone may be explained by the fact that fibroblasts and fibrocytes in the vicinity of the articular epiphyses have an ontogenetic penchant for transformation into osteoblasts and osteocytes [21, 22]. Where periosteum has been avulsed, its continuation of bone deposition in the

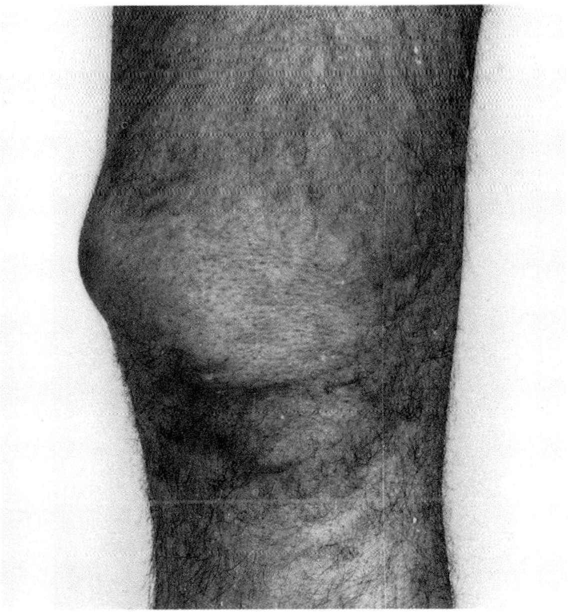

Fig. 58. A circumscribed thickening, hard on palpation, is noticeable close to the medial femoral condyle

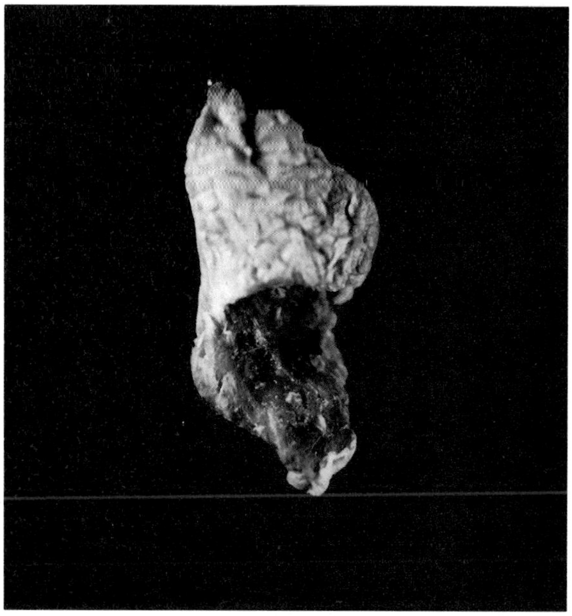

Fig. 59. The excised thickening is firm bone embedded in the dense connective tissue of a collateral ligament

neighborhood is a pathophysiological process. The regional hematoma provides a favorable medium for continued formation of bone. This interpretation and concept of the occurrence of bone in the vicinity of articular ends has been termed *osteome metatraumatique* by Leriche [963].

Posttraumatic ossification appears at the earliest 6–8 weeks after injury but generally later, and chiefly in young individuals. It causes vague symptoms, diffuse pain, impairment in the use of the joint, and moderately circumscribed deformity (Fig. 58). One can palpate in the depth of the area of tenderness, close to the articular epiphysis (Fig. 58), an immovable, uneven resistance which is very tender in the first few months of its formation. With longer duration, the tenderness decreases, but the hardness increases. When attaining larger size, this hard thickening causes substantial fatigue at the joint and may limit the motion of this joint.

Roentgenographs (Figs. 60, 61) reveal an irregular, hazy shadow of ossification extending in close proximity along the convex contour of the femoral condyle. This shadow is generally of curved outline and is separated by a narrow translucent zone from the condyle (Fig. 60). With longer existence the shadow becomes broader, denser, rather sharply demarcated, and also longer by extending proximally above the condyle and distally to the level of the joint cleft (Fig. 61). The beginning changes may be differentiated from an infraction or avulsion by the intact cortical outline of the femoral condyle.

Gross-anatomically (Fig. 59), a long bone spur or a curved brooch is noticed immediately beneath the fibrous joint capsule and within the collateral ligament. It is interconnected throughout with the dense fibers of this ligament and can be separated only by sharp dissection. If it has existed for a longer period of time, it extends proximally beyond the attachment of the joint capsule into the tendinous insertions and is of hard osseous consistency.

Histopathologically (Fig. 62), portions of cancellous bone lie in cellular connective tissue and are delimited by seams of osteoid tissue which contains numerous osteoblasts. The central parts of these bony inclusions resemble membranous bone while the peripheral parts of this bone have the structure of lamellar bone. In some areas the connective tissue is transformed into fibrocartilage [582].

In the differential diagnosis, an avulsion fracture must be considered, but this is noticed in roentgenographs obtained immediately after the injury. On the other hand, a negative roentgenographic result at the time of the injury, with a subsequent ossification about 6 weeks or later after the injury, confirms the nature of the alteration in question as a posttraumatic event.

Treatment aims at suppressing the pain by moist warm compresses applied every evening, and six to eight shortwave diathermy sessions, followed if necessary by ultrasound treatment of 3–4 W/cm^2. Massage is contraindicated because it irritates the tissue mechanically and may stimulate further bone formation. On the other hand, two or three topically administered injections of hydrocortisone may suppress any tendency to further bone formation. However, if these formations are so extensive that they essentially limit the

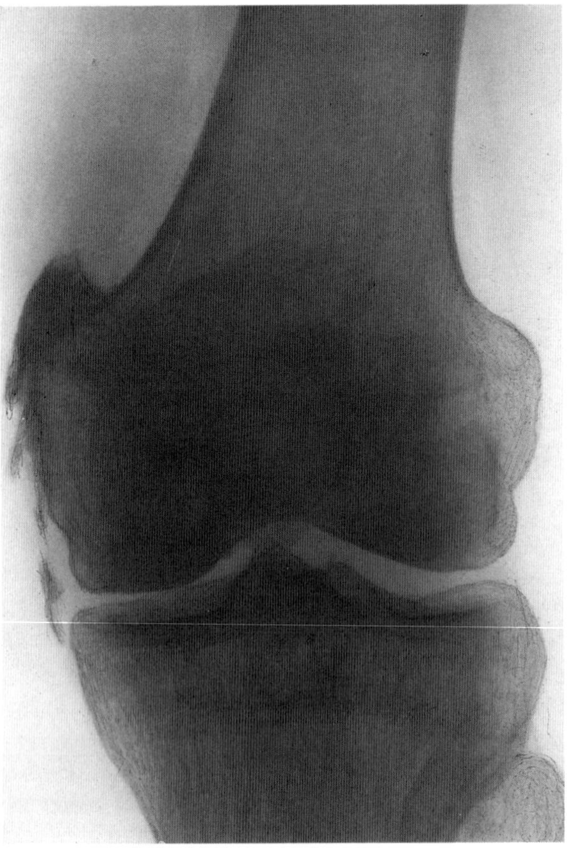

Fig. 60. A delimited ossification starting in the insertional area of the adductor tendons and expanding along the medial collateral ligament to its distal insertion

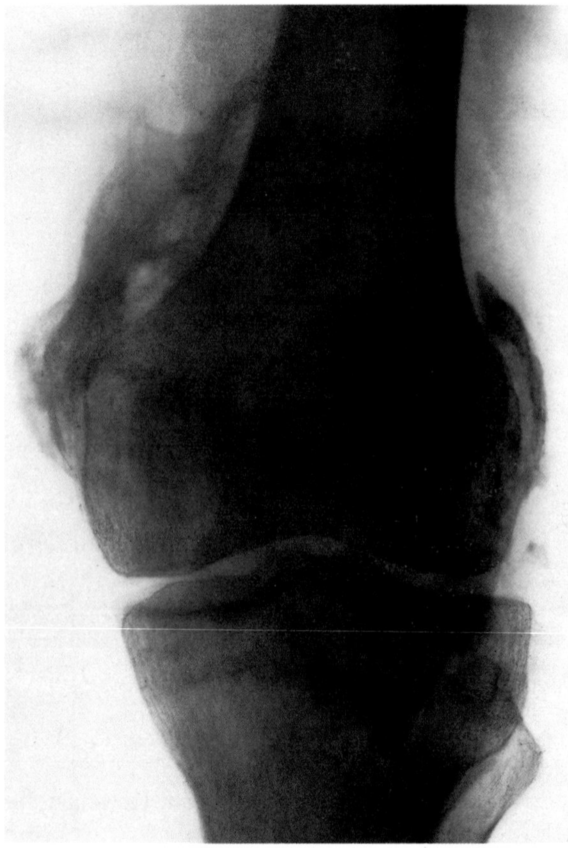

Fig. 61. An extensive and broad ossification occupies the area of the adductor tendons and their insertions into the medial femoral condyle. A curved, separated ossification expands in the lateral collateral ligament

movements of the joint or cause persistent discomfort, they and the neighboring connective tissue are excised. Such excision may be performed at the earliest about 1 year after the injury, when it appears probable that the ossification process has reached its maximum, and no further ossification would occur [582]. Prolonged mobilization exercises should follow.

6. Pigmented Villonodular Synovitis

Pigmented villonodular synovitis is the term used by Jaffe [817] for a condition which was previously referred to as xanthogranuloma, xanthomatous giant cell tumor, fibrohemosiderin sarcoma, or hemorrhagic synovitis. It is characterized histopathologically by conspicuous proliferation of the synovial membrane with an extensive increase in stromal cells, many of them laden with hemosiderin granules and some of them enlarged by deposition of lipids.

On the basis of the clinical signs and histopathological findings, this condition has been regarded as an inflammatory reaction elicited by traumata. The extensive deposition of hemosiderin in the synovial membrane indicates the precedence of hemorrhages into the joint. The experimental work by Young et al. [1802], who produced similar lesions in the joints of dogs by intraarticular injections of blood, strongly supports this concept. Myers et al. [1166] observed that an acute injury or recurrent injuries preceded the development of pigmented villonodular synovitis in more than 50% of their patients; their other patients did not recall an injury to the ailing joint. The incidental histopathological finding of giant cells or lipid-laden foam cells leaves open the possibility of other etiological factors. Therefore, Jaffe [817] considered the changes in pigmented villonodular synovitis to represent a reactive synovitis to a variety of factors. Nevertheless, the invariably present and extensive deposits of hemosiderin indicate strongly that hemorrhages were initial and essential synovial changes. In view of a reported trauma or traumata in the histories of the majority of the patients, pigmented villonodular synovitis is classified among traumatic joint conditions.

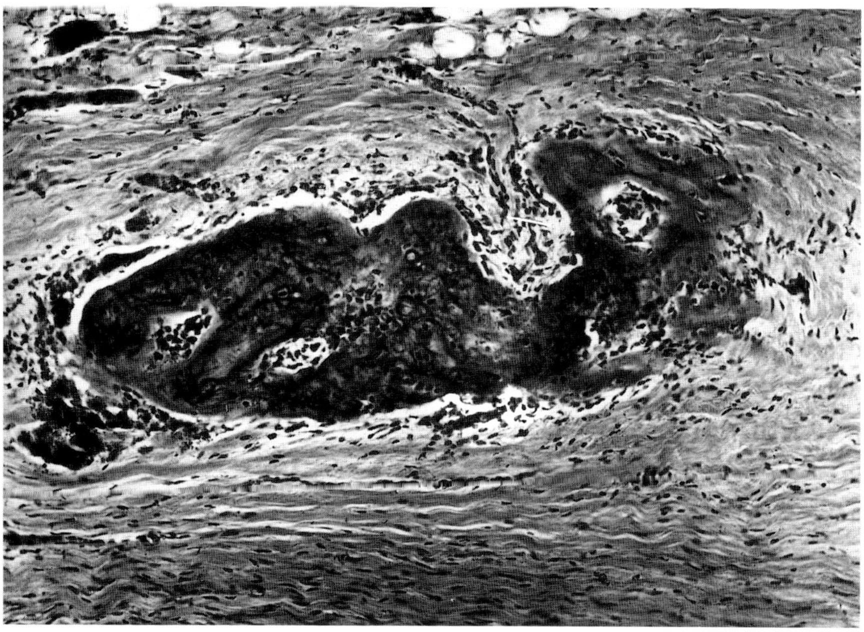

Fig. 62. Intramembranous ossification has developed in a ligament. Numerous osteoblasts lie along the convex outline, while large osteoclasts cause resorption on the concave outline of this ossification

Pigmented villonodular synovitis [431, 945] involves principally young adults of both sexes, but it may occur in patients aged up to 65 years. The most commonly affected joint is the knee; the hip, ankle, shoulder, elbow, and wrist joints follow with lesser frequency. Tendon sheaths at the wrist or ankle and bursae (trochanteric) are rarely affected. The initial symptoms are vague and are expressed as diffuse aching which is aggravated when a swelling of the joint develops. Analogously, the symptoms diminish, when the swelling of the joint partly regresses. However, with time and gradually increasing swelling, pain arises on prolonged use of the joint, especially the joint of lower extremity. The pain may eventually become almost constant. In some patients the pain is localized to specific areas of the joint. Yet more disturbing to the patient are occasional episodes of transient locking or blocking of a joint, which must be shaken out or resolved by manipulations.

Clinical examination [220] generally discloses a circumscribed enlargement of the joint due to regional thickening of the joint capsule, which is sometimes combined with a moderate increase in joint fluid. This area of the joint, usually one joint only, is slightly warmer than the neighboring tissue. Palpation discloses further that the thickening of the joint capsule is not always homogeneous, but it may be confined to a circumscribed area, being an enlargement often of lobulated configuration. Such capsular thickening can be shifted by digital pressure within the joint. This area usually presents a pronounced tenderness. Besides, a moderate, diffuse tenderness is noted along the circumference of the joint. The ranges of active and passive movements are limited depending on the degree, extent, and firmness of the thickening. On longer duration of this condition and continued impairment in the use of the joint, the regional musculature eventually becomes atrophic.

The laboratory studies regarding sedimentation rate, blood count, and lipids in the serum do not disclose abnormal findings. The bleeding, clotting and prothrombin time, and the number of thrombocytes are usually within the normal range. The aspirated joint fluid in the amount of 30–80 ml is serous, invariably tinted reddish brown, and contains 5000–60000 erythrocytes per milliliter.

Roentgenographs at soft tissue exposure reveal enlargement of the joint capsule with increased density in some areas. The cartilage space, irregularly delimited in the late phase by erosion of the cartilage cover, is usually widened by the mass of the interposed thickened joint capsule. In addition, Cohen et al. [308], McMaster [1075], Monghal et al. [1132], and Scott [1450] have described a few cases with erosion beneath the articular surface at the insertion of the joint capsule into the cartilage-bone junction. Such erosion is followed by secondary subchondral cyst formation (Fig. 63). Similar subcortical lytic lesions, delimited by sclerosed borders, arise by ingression of the synovial membrane through vascular channels into adjacent bone. Irregular, sharply delimited defects also occur in the corticalis by direct erosion. Such lytic lesions are observed mostly in the iliac and/or pubic bone (Fig. 63), in the femoral head close to the hip joint, or in the femoral condyles close to the knee joint. Amouroux [34] noted that the vascularization of the

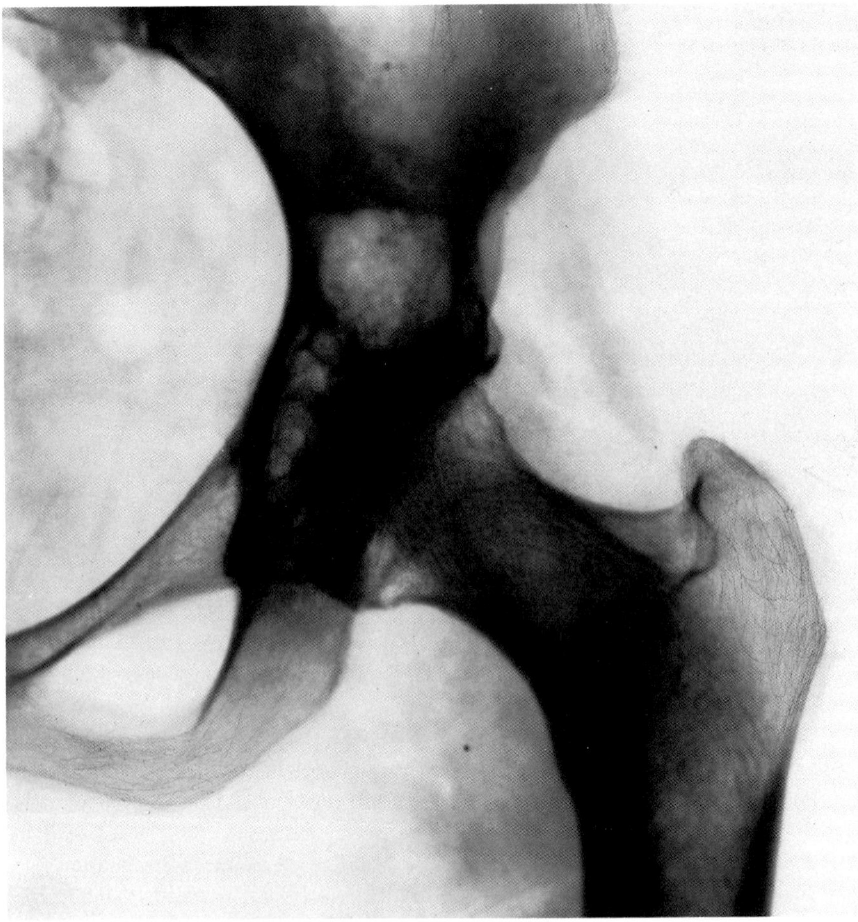

Fig. 63. Rather well-delimited areas of distinct radiolucency are located at the junction of the femoral head with the femoral neck. Similar, even larger areas are located cranially and medially to the acetabulum

intraosseal synovial protrusion depends entirely on the intraarticular synovial membrane and has no connections to the intraosseal blood vessels.

On the basis of gross-anatomical findings (Fig. 64), ascertained by arthroscopy [812] or arthrotomy, the following types of villonodular synovitis may be discerned: (a) the solitary nodule of walnut or larger size, wrinkled surface, orange or yellowish brown color, and connected by a rather long stalk with the uneven joint capsule; (b) the multiple nodular type (Fig. 64) in which the greater part of the inner surface of the joint capsule is occupied by numerous sessile nodules of pea to cherry size with a rather smooth yellowish brown surface; and (c) the mixed villonodular reddish brown type in which the sessile nodules present the smaller elevations while numerous long slender villi, many of them ramified and others merging with each other, occupy the greater part of the inner surface. From its very spongy appearance, the elevated tissue resembles a scraggly beard [817], a piece of worn-out rug, or a dense moss.

Histopathological examination [34, 1441, 1795] discloses that the synovial membrane is arranged in numerous rather long villi which rise high above the surface (Fig. 65). By branching and fusion, these villi enclose numerous cystlike spaces, all of them lined by one to two rows of enlarged synoviocytes. Similarly, all villi and nodules are covered by hypertrophic synoviocytes which surround a stroma (Fig. 65) amply comprising large cells with ovoid nuclei (young fibrocytes), and polyhedral cells with indented nuclei (histiocytes). The latter cells contain golden brown granules of hemosiderin which stain blue with potassium ferrocyanide due to their iron content. Similar granules, although in smaller amount, lie in the fibrocytes and synoviocytes. Furthermore, hemosiderin granules in greater amount lie extracellularly and interstitially. The stroma of the nodules sometimes contains giant cells with 2–12 nuclei, either dispersed between the other cells or clustered in the center, and a small number of lipid-laden foam cells. In some cases, the stroma of the nodules presents a substantial increase in the amount of the collagen fibers and narrowing of the lumina of the blood vessels, indicative of extensive fibrosis. The occasional cystic spaces in the subcortical bone contain synovial tissue with smaller villonodular elevations than those of the synovial membrane in the joint cavity. Apparently, this tissue expanded through

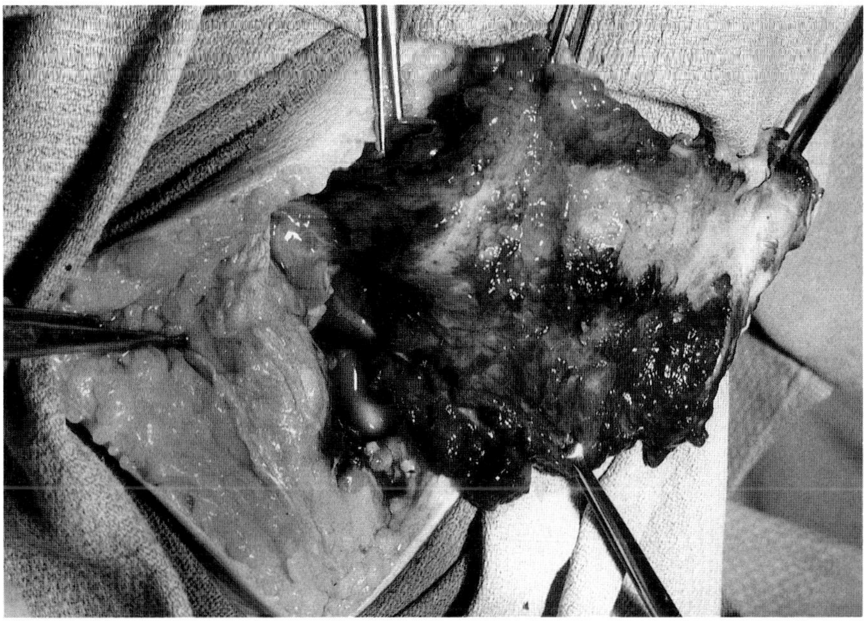

Fig. 64. Arthrotomy of the knee yields tumorlike enlarged tissue composed mostly of dark brown, small and larger nodules. A small part of the nodules have retained whitish yellow color

preexistent bone channels, ligamentous attachments, or bone erosions.

Differential diagnosis must consider: (a) recurrent traumatic hemarthrosis preceded by injuries; (b) arthropathy in hemophilia which starts in childhood and presents extensive deposits of hemosiderin in the synovial membrane (Fig. 415), without the occurrence of giant cells or foam cells, and with the invariably associated abnormal findings of extensive alterations in the articular epiphyses and deficiency of factor VIII in the blood; (c) synovial sarcoma originating from intraarticular or paraarticular synoviocytes and characterized histopathologically by a very varied structure containing cystic spaces lined by large synoviocytes or spindle-shaped cells (Figs. 528, 529), yet none of these cells containing hemosiderin granules. However, the most important, distinctive features of the synovial sarcoma are its invariable tendency diffusely to invade the neighboring bone and to metastasize, neither of which are observed in pigmented villonodular synovitis.

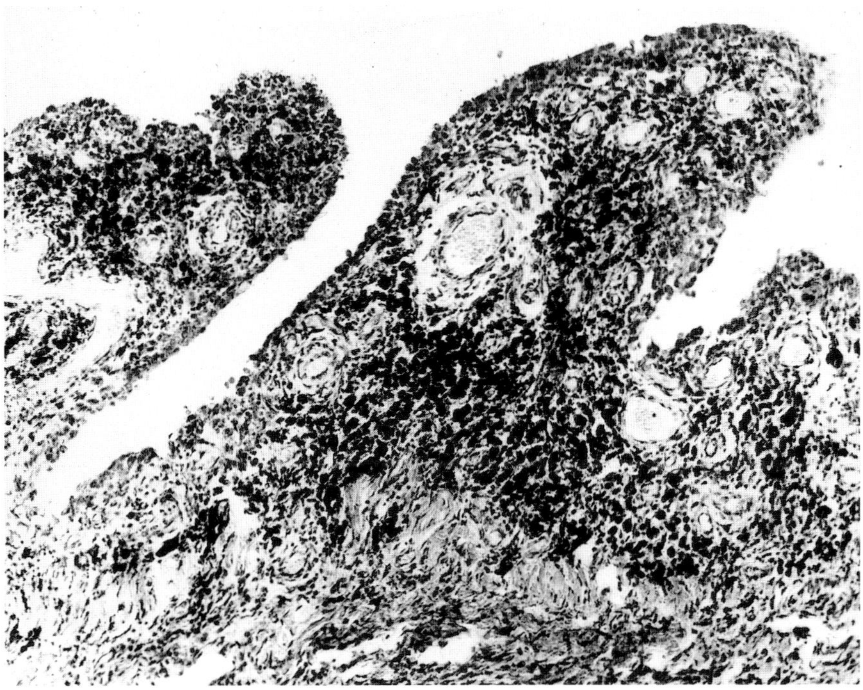

Fig. 65. The synovial membrane is raised in plump, rather long villi delimited by hypertrophic synoviocytes. Most of these cells as well as the subjacent large fibrocytes and histiocytes contain dark brown hemosiderin granules. In addition, many granules lie interstitially

Nevertheless, the treatment of the latter [220, 614] should be initiated early, after the diagnosis has been confirmed by arthroscopy and histopathological examination. The treatment of choice is total synovectomy, which should be carried out as extensively as possible and preferably by electrocautery. Since even under the best of circumstances this operation is a subtotal synovectomy, postoperative radiation treatment (cobalt radiation) of 15–20 Gy is indicated over 3–6 weeks depending on the size of the joint and the severity of the alterations. The rationale for radiation treatment is consistent with the general experience that local recurrences with extensive synovitis follow in 20%–40% of operated patients [662]. The tendency for recurrence raises the question of possibly malignant transformation of pigmented villonodular synovitis [476, 825], but histopathological examination and the absence of metastases do not support this view. Postoperatively, the joint should be protected from undue strain by a brace or a splint. The follow-up examinations largely reveal satisfactory results as to restoration of the joint capsule and function of the joint. However, the results are poor where extensive cystic cavities develop in the articular epiphyses of the lower extremities. In these situations the cysts should be curetted and be filled with grafts of cancellous bone. Weight bearing on these joints should be deferred until adequate restructuration of the articular epiphyses has been attained. Without such build-up, the articular surfaces are prone to collapse or to sustain fractures on stresses or weight bearing. Pronounced osteoarthritic changes eventually ensue.

II. Idiopathic Inflammations of Joints

1. Nonspecific Synovitis

The inner part of the joint capsule, the synovial membrane, plays an essential role in the biology, function, and pathology of the joints. By virtue of its structure, a richly vascularized loose connective tissue delimited on its surface by the very reactive synoviocytes, the synovial membrane is the first of the articular components to participate in any inflammatory condition of a joint. Anatomopathological and histopathological examinations [603, 1436, 1543] show that inflammation of the synovial membrane by itself may occur without affection of the other joint constituents and may remain confined to this tissue. The conclusion drawn from such findings is that synovitis can occur as an entity by itself. While most inflammations of joints primarily affect the synovial membrane and later expand to other constituents of the joints, synovitis – strictspeaking – refers to those conditions in which clinical and roentgenographic examinations on long-term follow-up provide no evidence of extrasynovial involvement. Additional gross-anatomical examinations by arthroscopy or arthrotomy, and histopathological examinations are needed to confirm the confinement of inflammatory changes to the synovial membrane. Only then is the designation synovitis justified.

In these cases of synovitis, the history and physical examination do not establish any causal relationship or give clues to external factors or to systemic diseases which could explain the occurrence of synovitis. The uncharacteristic course and the insignificant laboratory findings at follow-up examinations do not present sufficient features to permit inclusion of this type of joint affection into any of the currently recognized arthritic entities. No evidence exists of a connection to trauma, infection, allergy or autoimmunity. The condition is therefore referred to as nonspecific synovitis especially since its etiology is obscure. It is probable that repeated or chronic mild injury of any nature causes an irritation of the synovial membrane. Besides the extrinsic noxae, a dispositional sensitivity of the synovial membrane is apparently necessary to react with distinct changes to minor irritants. Most cases of nonspecific synovitis affect the knee joint; other involved joints are the wrist, elbow, hip, or ankle joint, rarely the shoulder or sternoclavicular joint.

Inflammation of the joint starts insidiously, and the elicited symptoms are rather slight. The joint is moderately and diffusely tender, but its movements are not impaired. However, on longer persistence the inflammation of the joint capsule becomes manifested by a slowly increasing swelling which is sometimes associated with slight local elevation of temperature. The swelling is not noticeable or palpable in joints surrounded by a considerable cloak of soft tissue, such as the hip and shoulder joints. The affected joint then is moderately sore and becomes painful especially at the start of active movements; eventually it is limited in the extreme ranges of motion. In these situations the regional musculature becomes moderately atrophic. The joints of the lower extremities are also impaired in their weight-bearing capacity and become painful after prolonged standing or walking. On the other hand, with timely regression of the swelling of the joint capsule, before fibrosis sets in, the movements eventually regain the normal ranges.

Blood studies disclose no changes except for a moderate leukocytosis and elevation in the sedimentation rate to 30–40 mm/h in a small percentage of patients. Results of the tests for C-reactive protein are positive in about 20%–25% of cases, and those for rheumatoid factor yield false-positive results in about 3%–5% of cases, not significantly different from those in the age-related population. Smears of blood stained according to Wright or Gram disclose no circulating microorganisms, nor do so the cultures of blood on plain agar, chocolate agar, or peptone agar. Similarly, examinations of the serum by agglutination, precipitin, flocculation, or complement fixation tests provide no indication of the presence of an antigen active in this inflammation. The joint fluid contains an increased number of lymphocytes, 1200–3000/ml, and an increased concentration of globulin to 3.7 g%. Smears of the occasionally and slightly increased joint fluid, stained with methylene blue and according to Gram, show no microorganisms or polymorphonuclear leukocytes but do show lymphocytes and synoviocytes with large ovoid nuclei. A small number of histiocytes with indented, reticulum-containing nuclei are also present. Roentgenographs reveal the maintenance of the normal cartilage space but a blurred structure of the articular ends, when the joint capsule is very thickened. Osteoporosis of the articular ends follows in cases of longer duration.

On gross-anatomical examination [1087, 1808] the synovial membrane initially presents a moderate redness which regresses in longer lasting inflammation. The superficial layer is edematous (Fig. 66). In chronic cases, villi appear on some areas of the surface and enlarge slowly to considerable sizes. Eventually the synovial membrane loses its soft consistency and becomes dense and thickened.

On the basis of histopathological findings [236, 1543], nonspecific synovitis presents itself in three phases. (a) The initial phase is associated with hyperemia of the blood vessels and small perivascular infil-

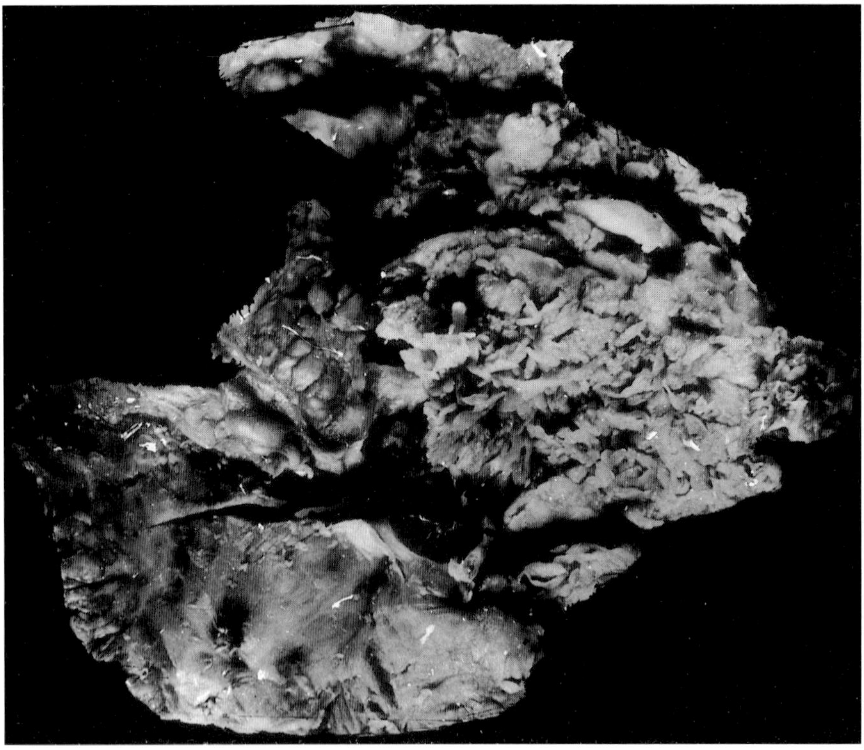

Fig. 66. The inner part of the joint capsule is moderately thickened but rather even in one part; it is elevated in small nodules and long thin villi in the larger part

trates mostly of lymphocytes. The subsynoviocytic tissue is edematous. (b) The subsequent phase is characterized by slight to moderate hypertrophy and hyperplasia of the synoviocytes. The subsynoviocytic tissue contains infiltrates composed chiefly of histiocytes and lymphocytes. Fibrocytes and a few fibroblasts proliferate in the subsynoviocytic tissue. A change by formation of villi is noticed on the surface. Neither the immunofluorescence test nor the immunoperoxidase test applied by the direct method to synovial specimens with advanced inflammatory changes identify antigenic substances in the synovial membrane. (c) In the advanced phase, the inflammatory infiltrates have substantially expanded, and large, broad villi have formed (Fig. 67). Regressive synovitis changes have set in, associated with hyalinization of the superficial layer, and sometimes with loss or desquamation of the synoviocyte cover. In some areas the capillaries and small blood vessels are increased; in others the middle-sized blood vessels are thickened by fibromatosis of the media. Similarly, the subsynoviocytic connective tissue is dense by hypercellularity and/or fibrosis (Fig. 67).

Differential diagnosis must include all types of arthritis, especially rheumatoid arthritis and its variants. However, as the inflammation continues, clarification of the clinical picture, the negative outcome of all laboratory studies of the blood and joint fluid, and negative roentgenograph results militate against the diagnosis of rheumatoid arthritis or any other specific inflammation. The diagnosis of nonspecific synovitis remains as the final solution.

Treatment is directed at the symptoms and depends on the stage of the disease. In the acute phase, the affected joints should rest as much as possible, with the extremity elevated; avoidance of strenuous activities is of primordial necessity. Moist warm packs should be applied around the joint one or two times daily for 30 min, and the joint should be compressed with an elastic bandage when upright and ambulating. Eight to ten sessions of shortwave diathermy are very effective [944, 1613]. When the joint fluid is increased, it should be removed by arthrocentesis, and the joint be compressed with a tight adhesive strapping. Immobilization for 3–4 weeks with a plaster cast or a rigid splint is advisable in all cases of longer duration because limitation of joint movements accelerates the healing by minimizing mechanical irritation of the joint. Medications are additionally indicated; acetylsalicylic acid should be administered regularly in divided doses of 2–3 g daily. If satisfactory regression of the symptoms is not attained, nonsteroidal antiinflammatory drugs are indicated, but their potential adverse effects (especially suppression of the bone marrow) should be borne in mind. If the symptoms persist, an intraarticular injection of hydrocortisone may bring a dramatical regression the inflammatory condition, but the potential detrimental effects of this medication, leading possibly to

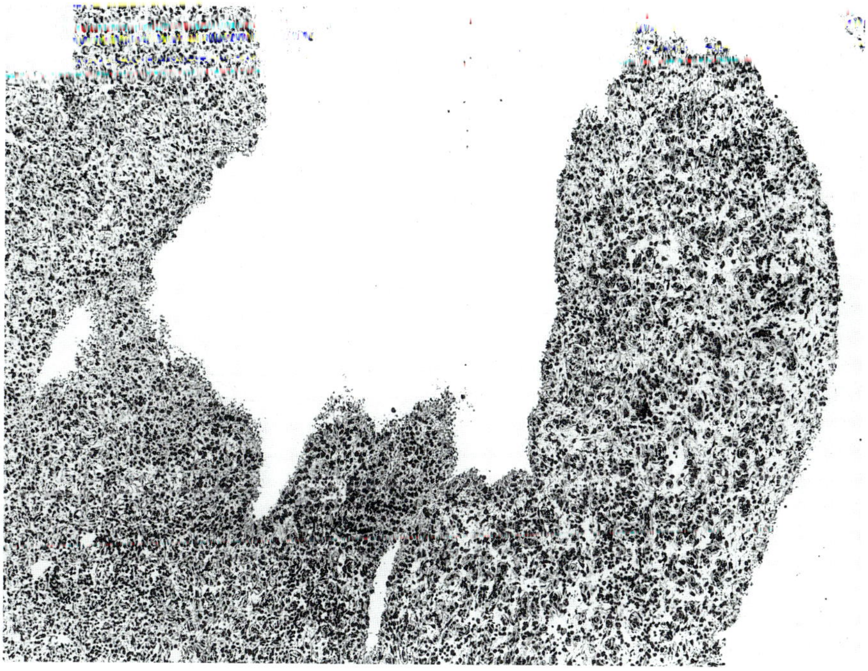

Fig. 67. The synovial membrane is elevated in plump villi and is very hypercellular with fibrocytes, histiocytes, and lymphocytes

disintegration of the articular cartilage [121, 269, 655, 1018, 1126, 1149, 1389, 1572] makes this modality nonadvisable. Less untoward effects may be obtained from oral administration of corticosteroids.

It is therefore sometimes advisable to consider a modality which removes the thickened synovial membrane without endangering the articular cartilage. Chemical synovectomy (synovioorthesis) by intraarticularly injected methotrexate or alkylating agents [685, 1216, 1644] is of brief and/or uncertain effect. A similar result is obtained with osmium tetroxide and radioisotopes [685]. On the other hand, surgical treatment, performed in terms of the particular alterations as a subtotal or a total synovectomy, effectively removes the thickened portions of the joint capsule [689, 1285]. The value of this procedure was confirmed by the findings of Key [882], Swett [1614], and others [1125] that the synovial membrane regenerates to almost normal structure 6–12 months after synovectomy. Mohr [1125] observed that formation of an inner cover of the joint cavity starts 5 weeks after the synovectomy by fibrin and granulation tissue. This fibrous membrane is subsequently covered by a multicellular synovial lining.

Concurrently the follow-up examinations [689, 982, 1124] confirm that not only has the previous thickening of the joint subsided, but also that the soreness or painfulness of the joint arising especially on movements or weight bearing has become essentially mitigated or even completely abolished. Further support for this operation derives from the observation that the chronically inflamed synovial membrane, by its abnormal enzymatic activity, may cause damage to the articular cartilage.

2. Intermittent Hydrarthrosis

Repeated stimuli causing recurrent irritation of the synovial membrane are followed by intermittent production of an increased amount of joint fluid which accumulates in the joint cavity. The knee joint is most often affected; the elbow, wrist, hip, or ankle joint is much less often, even rarely affected. Excluded from this clinical picture are recurrent joint effusions caused by traumata, bacterial infections, rheumatoid arthritis, or identified injuries emanating from systemic diseases, and manifested by distinct alterations.

The etiology of idiopathic intermittent hydrarthrosis has not yet been completely elucidated, but it appears that two factors contribute to or determine the occurrence of effusions [344, 950, 1090]. The first is a hormonal and/or constitutional factor, and the second is an individual predisposition of the synovial membrane [1807]. The latter manifests itself in general hypersensitivity of serous membranes to certain facultatively harmful substances [124] and in increased permeability to serous fluid.

The hormonal influence is seen in the fact that idiopathic intermittent hydrarthrosis occurs in adults, predominantly women. A relationship to the menstrual cycle is observed since the effusions often occur

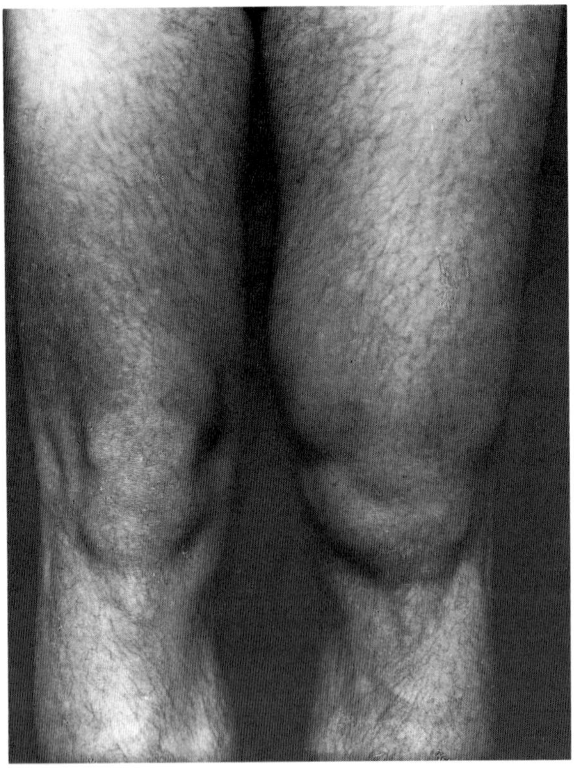

Fig. 68. The left knee is blown up like a balloon at the distal third of the thigh. The regional folds are effaced

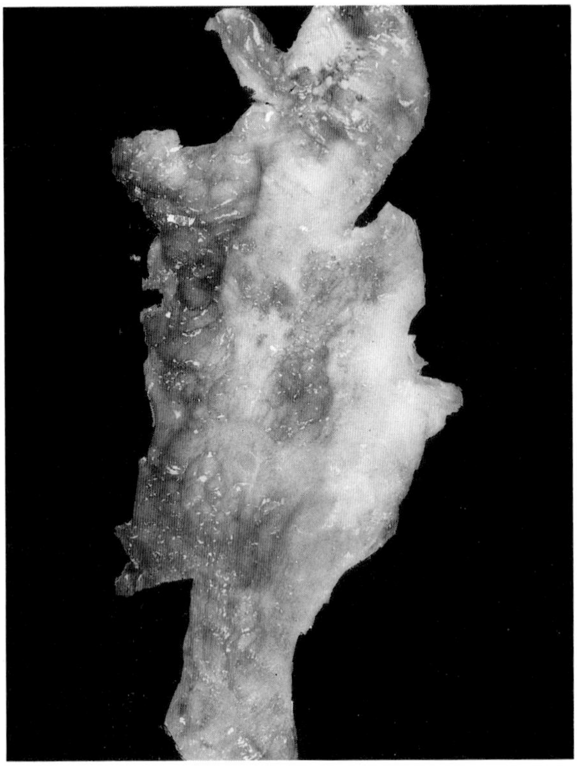

Fig. 69. The inner part of the joint capsule is elevated in a large area, which is rather pale and slightly uneven

5–7 days prior to menstruation and subside with the onset of the menstrual period. The dependence of effusion on follicular activity was verified in two patients. In one woman menstruation was deferred by hormone deferment, and with it the spontaneous resorption of the effusion for 7 days. In another woman, menstruation was brought on 4 days earlier by administering high doses of folliculin, and with it the concurrent absorption of the effusion. In some women, the tendency to develop effusions disappears with pregnancy, while in others this tendency ceases with the menopause.

The central nervous system also seems to play a role because recurrent effusions without ostensible external causes are observed in neurotic men. A disturbance in the automatic vegetative innervation concomitant with increased permeability of the synovial membrane may account for the sudden synovial effusions associated with edemata in other parts of the body. These effusions are the outcome of exudative swellings of the joint capsule, analogous to the Quinke edema, and may be explained by angioneurotic disturbances [1413]. In this category belong also the intermittent effusions of joints which accompany vasomotoric rhinitis or bronchial asthma.

Furthermore, a systemic susceptibility of the joint capsule may account for effusions which recur as manifestations of an anaphylactic process [1113]. Criep [345] reported joint effusions recurring after ingestion of eggs, fish, tomatoes, nuts, or grapes. Similarly, an allergic reaction of the synovial membrane to proteinaceous substances was suggested by the observation of a 28-year-old woman who developed an effusion in both knee joints 1–2 days after sexual intercourse. Since an effusion in the knee joints could experimentally be elicited by intramuscular injection of sterilized sperm, the etiology of this joint effusion was attributed to hypersensitivity to sexual mediators. The occurrence of effusions in this case was averted by desensitization using increasing, parenterally administered doses of sterilized sperm. Thus it appears that proteins, lipoproteins, mucoproteins, and polysaccharides may be antigens which are able to elicit hypersensitivity responses manifested by synovial effusions.

Intermittent hydrarthrosis can be differentiated from other joint effusions by the periodicity of its occurrence, the duration of 3–10 days, and its difficult management by conservative modalities. Occurring mostly in women, it manifests also a certain dependence of the menstrual cycle [461] as well as a spontaneous disappearance in phases of hormonal change such as pregnancy, lactation, or menopause.

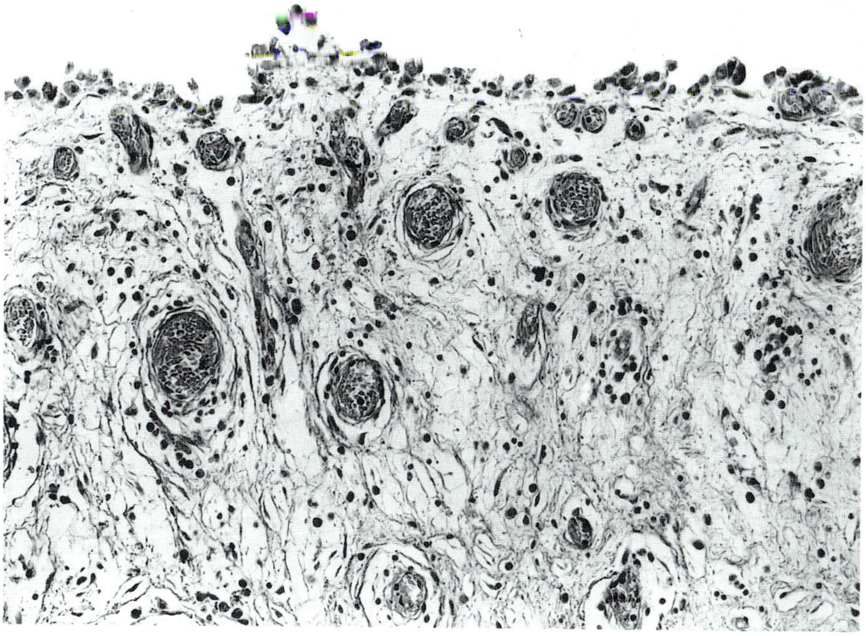

Fig. 70. The synovial membrane bears one flat row of rather hypertrophic synoviocytes. The subsynoviocytic tissue is extensively rarefied by interstitial edema. All blood vessels are markedly hyperemic

On physical examination the ballooning of the joint is sometimes a very conspicuous sign (Fig. 68). The outlines of the joint are blurred; all grooves and indentations characteristic of the configuration of that region are evened out. Fluctuation in the joint is distinctly noticeable on palpation. Acute effusion may be associated with elevation of the local temperature. In the knee joint ballotement of the patella can be tested by manually squeezing out the joint fluid from the suprapatellar recessus and by pressing the patella onto the subjacent fluid level (Fig. 14). The joint is moderately tender but becomes very painful due to tenseness of the joint capsule on excessive increase in the quantity of the joint fluid. In such situations the movements of the joint are limited, but they return to normal ranges after the effusion subsides. However, with longer persistence of the effusion the joint capsule and its ligaments become overstretched, and instability of the joint ensues.

The sedimentation rate is moderately elevated to 30–45 mm, but the leukocyte count is usually within normal limits. The skin test for tuberculosis is often positive in adult patients with intermittent hydrarthrosis; however, this test is positive in many adults with normal joints. Its negative outcome is of greater significance. On the other hand, the serological test for syphilis is negative in the tertiary stage of the acquired form; therefore, only a positive test has diagnostic value.

Thorough examination is given to the joint fluid [1731], which can accumulate up to 450 ml (in the knee joint; Fig. 68) and is clear, serous, and yellowish. Sometimes it is discolored brownish due to hemorrhagic admixture; it becomes slightly turbid with a greater content of formed elements. Its specific density lies between 1025 and 1040; the concentration of protein is usually between 3.0 and 4.5 g% and that of glucose is 85–90 mg%. The pH ranges between 7.20 and 7.40, indicating that the effusion is of noninflammatory nature. As the fluid becomes slightly turbid, its acidity increases. Examination of the formed elements provides information on the intensity of the inflammation. Their number ranges between 200 and 1500/ml and comprises lymphocytes, monocytes, and a fair number (6%–7%) of eosinophils. The more active the exudation, the greater are the numbers of cells in the joint fluid; the more it is a transudate, the fewer are its formed elements. Besides these cells, synoviocytes at a proportion of about 10%–12% of the total cell count are observed in the joint fluid. They have ovoid or polygonal shapes and a pale, rather homogeneous cytoplasm; their nuclei are large and contain fine chromatin particles arranged in a reticulum. An effusion which contains more than 15% synoviocytes indicates proliferative changes of the synovial membrane. Complete examination of the joint fluid also includes complement levels in the complement fixation test for syphilis and their comparison with identical studies of the blood levels. A part of the synovial fluid is centrifuged; the sediment is stained with methylene blue and with special stains according to Gram, May-Grünwald-Giemsa and Ziehl-Neelsen. Concurrently the fluid should be submitted to culture for streptococci, staphylococci, diplococci, and tubercle bacilli.

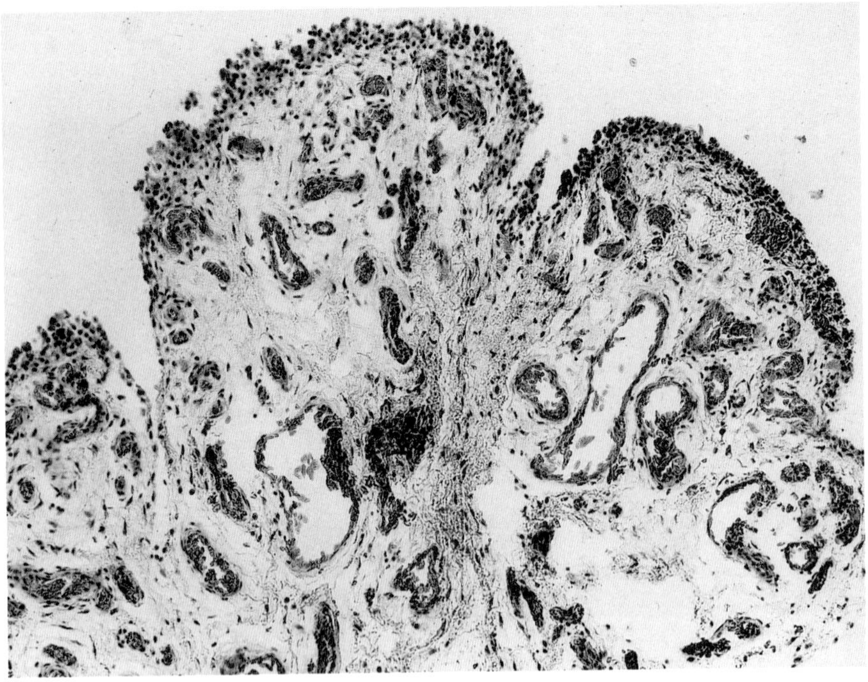

Fig. 71. The synovial membrane is raised in plump villi delimited by moderately hypertrophic hyperplastic synoviocytes. The subsynoviocytic tissue is extensively rarefied by interstitial edema. All blood vessels are markedly dilated

To ascertain an etiologically possible allergy, tests are carried out using extracts from the suspected allergens (aliments or other substances, sex glands) and injecting them intracutaneously in increasing concentrations. A positive skin test result, manifested by a wheal and/or erythema, provides a valuable clue to the etiology.

Roentgenographic examination does not reveal abnormal findings except for a widening of the cartilage space. The articular epiphyses have smooth outlines.

On gross-anatomical examination (Fig. 69), the inner part of the joint capsule is markedly swollen and pale, in places discolored slightly reddish, and of boggy consistency. Small flaky precipitates of mucin or fibrin lie on the surface of the synovial membrane. With more extensive transudation, the edema expands to the outer part of the joint capsule, which also becomes boggy. Histopathological examination (Fig. 70) in the early phase shows loosening of the synovial membrane with wide separation of its formed elements by an increase in interstitial fluid; nevertheless, these elements retain their outline and normal structure. All blood vessels are markedly dilated and hyperemic. A few very small perivascular and focal accumulations of lymphocytes are scattered in the subsynoviocytic tissue. In the chronic and advanced stages, the synovial membrane is raised in broad villi (Fig. 71) which are delimited by moderately hypertrophic hyperplastic synoviocytes. All blood vessels are markedly dilated and hyperemic. The subsynoviocytic tissue is extensively rarefied by edema; a few small infiltrates by lymphocytes are scattered.

Differential diagnosis must consider all specific inflammations of joints and especially palindromic rheumatism, a variant of rheumatoid arthritis. Each may be accompanied by recurrent effusions. Studies of serum, joint fluid, roentgenographs, and biopsy specimens enable one to exclude such conditions. Beyond these eliminations, the periodicity and self-limited duration of the effusions, occurring more often in women and then dependent on hormonal phases, provide a strong clue to the presence of intermittent hydrarthrosis.

Despite all investigations, the etiology of intermittent hydrarthrosis cannot always be elucidated, and therefore no specific treatment can be instituted in these cases. Treatment therefore remains symptomatic and seeks to remove the joint fluid and to prevent its recurrence. In a recent effusion, complete or at least prolonged bedrest, elevation of the extremity, and mildly warm wet compresses often applied around the joint help in the resorption of the effusion within 4–7 days. Antihistamine medications, 50 mg twice daily, are often helpful in relieving or suppressing an incipient case of hydrarthrosis, as are intramuscular injections with increasing amounts (1–4 ml) of sterilized milk. Enzyme tablets (varidase, papase) expedite the absorption of the fluid. After resorption of the swelling the joint should be compressed with a snug strapping to prevent distension of the joint capsule and to minimize movements; thus mechanical irritation of the

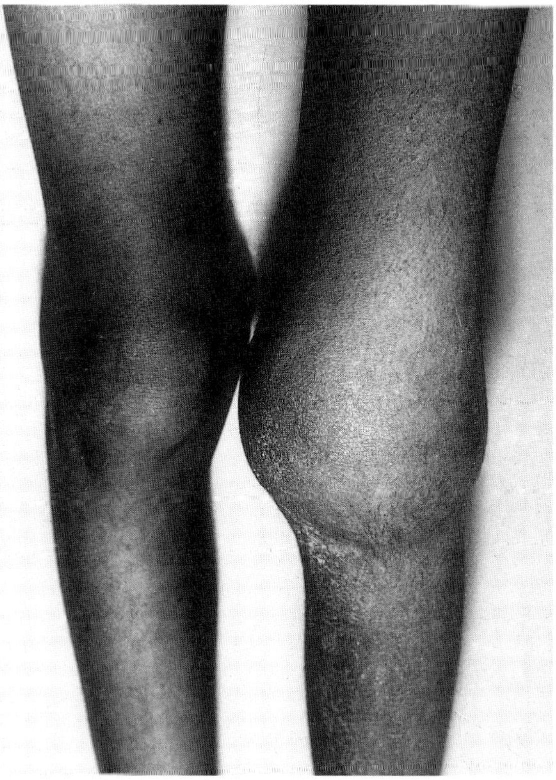

Fig. 72. The left knee is globularly enlarged by extreme thickening of the joint capsule

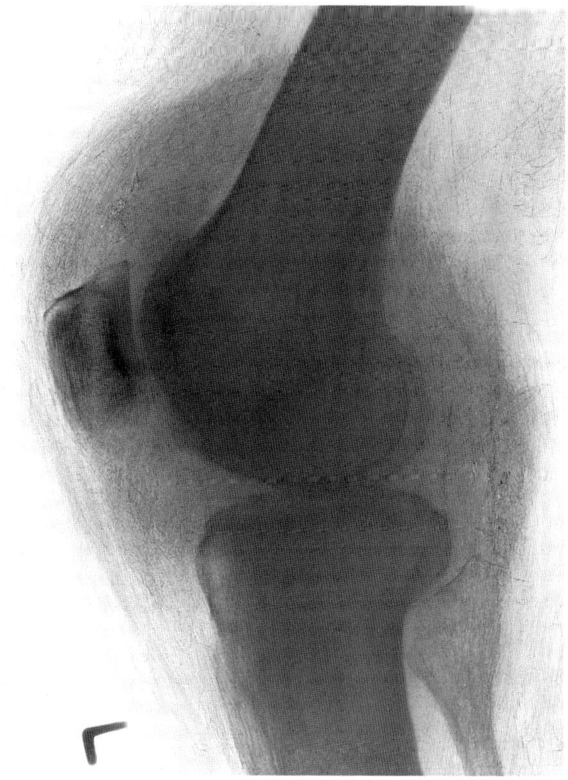

Fig. 73. Roentgenograph discloses marked thickening of the joint capsule at its anterior and posterior aspects

joint, will be prevented. This requirement is indicated especially when the joint effusion recurs a few times; it should be carried out by applying a thinly padded, well molded plaster cast which keeps the joint immobilized for 4 weeks.

However, if the joint effusion does not absorb after the above modalities, it should be removed by arthrocentesis as described in "Arthrocentesis of Joints". Aspiration of the joint effusion should be carried out, as all interventions on joints, with aseptic precautions. By tilting the aspirating needle in various directions any remaining joint fluid can be removed from all outpouchings of the inner joint capsule. It is debatable whether arthrocentesis should be followed by intraarticular injection of corticosteroids. Although the beneficial effect of intraarticular steroids has been demonstrated [663, 773, 1466, 1572, 1600] and thus could be of use in recurrent effusions, their deleterious effect on the articular cartilage is also known [121, 269, 655, 1018, 1125, 1149, 1389, 1577]. Despite proper aftercare the effusions of the joint may recur periodically and should be treated in the same way as the first effusion. In addition, physical therapy with diathermy may be applied regularly in repeated series of six to eight sessions. In women with hormonally elicited recurrence of effusion, folliculin, stilbestrol, or testosterone is also administered on the day prior to the anticipated swelling in intermittent hydrathrosis. If allergy against certain food stuffs has been confirmed, desensitization against protein substances (peptone) and/or polysaccarides should be performed. Such a joint may eventually cease to produce excessive synovial fluid.

If all conservative methods fail to prevent subsequent effusions, a partial synovectomy, termed fenestration, is advisable. The rationale for this operation is the experience that recurrent effusions eventually cause irreversible changes in the inner part of the joint capsule, and that fenestration often succeeds in preventing or minimizing these changes. The technique of fenestration involves a surgical approach at an easily accessible site, in the case of the knee joint at the suprapatellar recessus. There the regional muscles and attached tendons are retracted, and the fibrous capsule is exposed and divided. The subsynoviocytic adipose tissue is separated from the innermost part of the joint capsule, and a flap of 3–5 cm^2, depending on the size of the joint, is excised from the latter part. This defect is left open; the fibrous capsule as well as the subcutaneous tissue and skin are closed by sutures. The joint is compressed and immobilized for 2 weeks. The beneficial effect of this fenestration results from mechanical drainage of the joint fluid into the loose subsynoviocytic tissue [880, 933, 1121, 1614]. A long period of aftercare is necessary, involving regular compression of the joint with an elastic bandage, and by avoidance of vigorous activities of the involved extremity for protection from strain. However, if despite the above listed modalities the effusions recur, irreversible thickening of the inner part of the joint capsule eventually develops by formation of long villi and organization of fibrin deposits (1272). In this situation, a total synovectomy (Fig. 69) succeeds to bring cessation of the effusions.

3. Arborescent Liposynovitis (Lipoma Arborescens)

The synovial membrane reacts to traumata or other types of harm even of slight intensity if their repetition results in cumulative intensity. In addition to the local response of the synovial tissue, one must presume an individual, constitutionally determined excessive reactivity to be able to explain the conspicuous alterations [1087] observed in arborescent liposynovitis. Injury and inflammatory proliferation alternate here, eventually resulting in such pronounced response.

Arborescent liposynovitis should be distinguished clinically and pathologically from the pronounced synovial proliferations noted in traumatic conditions, rheumatoid arthritis of long duration, tuberculosis, syphilis, or fungal infection. Anatomopathologically and histopathologically it is neither a circumscribed benign tumor nor an invasive malignant tumor. Thus the designation as lipoma should be abandoned. This condition is an idiopathic proliferating articular disease, whose etiology has not yet been fully clarified. No definite physical, chemical, bacteriological, antigenic, or other harmful factor has ever been proven to be causal. However, the probability of traumatic etiology has been implicated [1264, 1741].

Arborescent liposynovitis occurs chiefly in middle-aged men, and thus far it has been observed only in the knee joint [84, 215, 416, 746, 1264]. While in some patients (farm workers with frequent mild injuries from agricultural machines) repeated contusions are recorded, others show a tendency to excessive keloid formation. In others the knee joint becomes enlarged without any identifiable cause over the course of 4–6 years until the function of the joint is substantially impaired. The initial symptoms are minor and consist of diffuse soreness and frequent fatigue of the leg. In time, an insecurity in the knee joint is experienced, the range of motion decreases in all directions, and eventually locking episodes in the knee may occur. Most patients seek medical help rather late, alarmed by the progressive enlargement of the joint and fearful of cancer.

The knee is conspicuously, almost globe-like enlarged (Fig. 72), much more than in fungus tuberculosus (Fig. 143) or hemophilic arthritis (Fig. 403), but the regional musculature is only slightly or not atrophic. The net of the veins around the knee is widened, and the lower leg is thickened by chronic edema. The joint capsule is markedly thickened along its entire extent, and it sags caudally on upright standing due to its weight in advanced cases (Fig. 72). Thereby the distal part of the knee appears thicker than the proximal part. Palpation discloses a doughy consistency of the joint

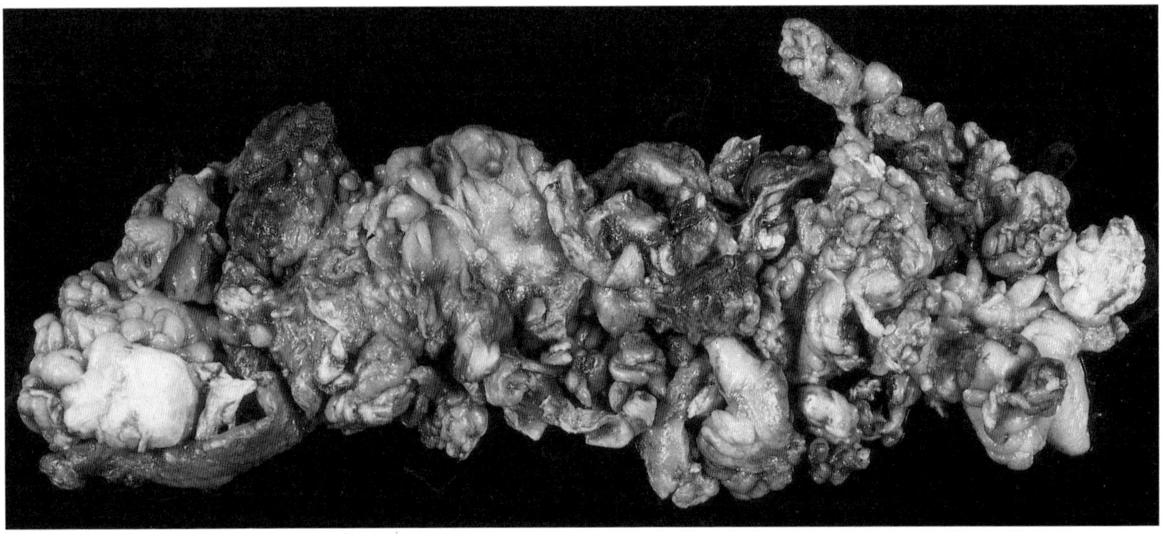

Fig. 74. Synovectomy yields a very thickened inner part of the joint capsule, which bears plump villi, large lobes, and thick folds, all of them of whitish yellow color

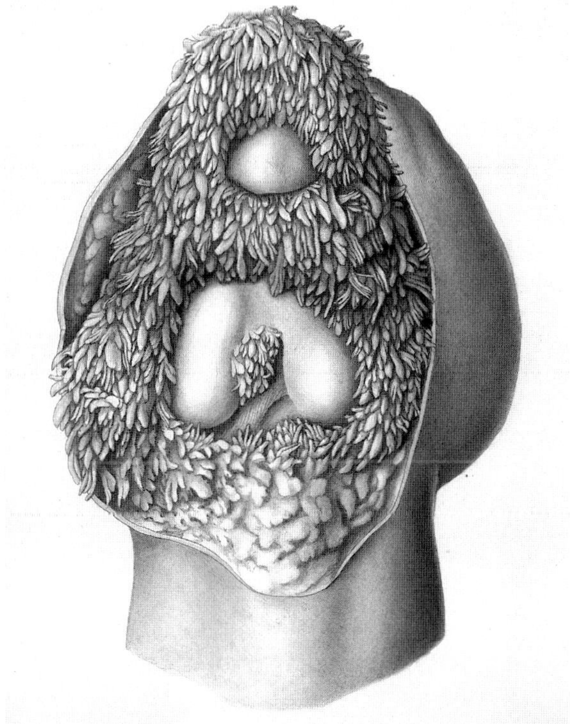

Fig. 75. Arthrotomy in another patient discloses that the entire inner surface of the joint capsule bears many and very long thin villi

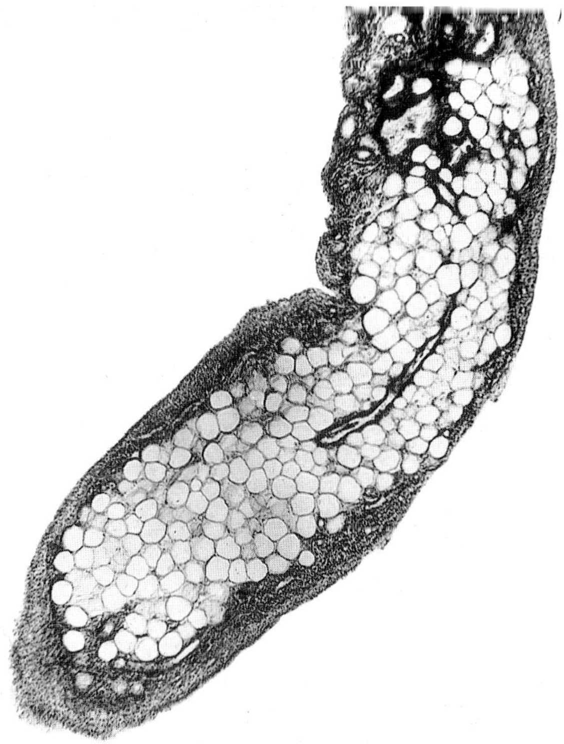

Fig. 76. A fingerlike villus has a hypertrophic hyperplastic synovial cover, beneath which the adipose tissue is much enlarged

capsule, with numerous nodular or lobular densities which can be shifted manually. The thickening is hindering throughout, and the range of movements is diminished. Aspiration yields only a small amount of joint fluid, much less than that suggested by the shifting of the soft masses of the joint capsule.

Laboratory studies disclose no abnormal findings which could provide clues to the etiology. Roentgenographs (Fig. 73) reveal excessive thickening of the tissue around the articular epiphyses, whose structure is slightly blurred by the overlying dense joint capsule [215, 746]. Moderate widening of the cartilage space is sometimes noticed.

On gross-anatomical examination [229, 817, 1087] arborescent liposynovitis presents a very characteristic picture (Figs. 74, 75). The entire inner part of the joint capsule is enormously thickened while its fibrous capsule is minimally changed. The synovial membrane is no longer even but has the appearance of a sheep fleece, with its inner surface elevated in numerous excessively long villi (Fig. 75). Some villi have the size of small fingers, others resemble polypoid outgrowths or apronlike overlapping flaps (Fig. 74), and others float like ramified tree branches in the joint fluid. Many of these villi display inflammatory redness or hemorrhagic infarctions. In its surface the synovial membrane comprises a few areas of dense grayish white tissue. However, the articular cartilage is usually not altered.

Histopathological examination discloses marked thickening of the synoviocyte cover by hyperplasia. Most of the surface is elevated in a great number of villi of unusually large size. Some villi have a stroma of connective tissue with numerous capillaries and small blood vessels and sparse focal lymphocyte agglomerations, but most of them (Fig. 76) have a stroma of adipose tissue traversed by strips of connective tissue. The subsynoviocytic tissue of the areas with uneven surface contains perivascular and small interstitial accumulations composed chiefly of lymphocytes and a few histiocytes and plasmacytes. The tissue here is dense by moderate fibrosis.

Differential diagnosis includes fungus tuberculosus, fungus albus syphiliticus, benign synovial lipoma, and malignant synovial tumor. The presence of a normal cartilage space, negative results on the VDRL test, lack of periosteal apposition, and lack of osteoporosis or extensive bone erosion indicate the absence of an invasive inflammatory process. The overall thickening of the entire joint capsule in arborescens liposynovitis permits differentiation from the circumscribed and moveable thickening which is characteristic of a solitary lipoma. The slow growth of the capsular thickening with soft consistency, the continued general good health of the patient, and the absence of bone destruction and metastases permit differentiation from a malignant tumor.

Conservative treatment with antiinflammatory agents does not effect a regression of the excessive synovial thickening. X-ray radiation, 10 Gy in six to eight sessions, has a limited success. Thus, given disturbing appearance and impaired function, an operation is indicated. Total synovectomy is the procedure of choice. The proliferated inner part of the joint capsule is broadly dissected in its entirety (Fig. 74), as a fleece, along the proper layer of the subsynoviocytic tissue. It is advisable here to use electric cauterization to avoid profuse bleeding. After closure of the wound, the joint should be compressed and immobilized with a firm strapping. Subsequently, the regional musculature needs to be strengthened by regular active exercises, massage, and faradic stimulation in two series of eight sessions. These modalities are indicated to compensate for the overstretching of the ligaments during prolonged distension of the joint capsule. In view of this insufficiency, the patient should wear an elastic knee cap with metal hinges for a period of 6–12 months until adequate strength of the musculature has been attained.

III. Specific Inflammations of Joints by Microorganisms

1. Suppurative Arthritis

Suppurative arthritis, the most feared complication in a joint, has become less frequent in recent decades. It may be caused by any type of microorganism of virulence or toxicity, but it is most often due primarily or secondarily to staphylococci.

The suppuration of a joint may originate in the following ways: (a) contusion to a joint by violent blunt injury with consequent necrosis and infection of the local soft structures; (b) penetrating wound into a joint by a weapon or sharp tool (including surgical instrument) or compound intraarticular fracture with spread of infection from the skin into the joint; (c) propagation by the lymphatic route from suppurating processes of soft tissues in the vicinity, such as a furuncle in the skin, an abscess or a phlegmon in contiguous organs, or fascial necrosis; (d) extension of an active osteomyelitic focus from the epiphysis into the joint; (e) hematogenous metastatic spread from active infectious processes such as tonsillitis, pneumonia, enteritis, abdominal typhoid, or erysipelas. In some of these cases, the primary focus may be insignificant, for example, pyorrhea in the mouth or paronychia of the big toe. A preceding blunt injury to a joint or a preexistent, even inactive arthritis, creates the basis for the localization of a purulent process [680, 682].

Suppurative arthritis [93] may involve individuals of any age group, but it involves chiefly adults whose professional activities expose them to the risks of open wounds. It also involves debilitated persons whose diminished resistance makes them susceptible to infection in any part of the body. In all of the above etiological possibilities, suppurative arthritis affects the knee joint most often among the peripheral joints; in declining frequency of infection follow the hip, elbow, wrist, finger, and ankle joints.

Clinically, three degrees of severity of purulent inflammation of a joint may be distinguished. The mildest and most frequent type ist purulent effusion which causes swelling, increased local warmth, and tenderness but does not involve the deeper portions of the joint capsule. The second type is empyema with extensive infection of the joint capsule (phlegmon) and articular cartilage; this expresses itself in severe pain, marked constitutional symptoms, continuous elevation in temperature to 39.4°–41°C, and acceleration of the pulse to 120–130. On protracted duration of the empyema, the third type, septicemia, develops with general decay, anemia, and irregularity of the easily compressible pulse. In the second and third degrees of severity the joint is swollen and intensely tender along its entire extent; its outlines are completely blurred. The skin is tense, reddened, and much warmer than in the neighboring area. Any movement is anxiously avoided, and the joint soon becomes contracted in midposition. By expansion of the suppurative inflammation into the outer layer of the joint capsule, the joint becomes very swollen (Fig. 77), a tense tumor results. Due to compression of the surrounding blood vessels and lymph vessels, the entire extremity becomes swollen by edema. Finally, the muscle attachments around the joint become sore; radiating pain into all directions characterizes this stage. On liquefaction necrosis of the capsule, the pus penetrates into the surrounding tissues and breaks through the skin (Fig. 77). The pain in the joint decreases due to diminution of the tenseness, but the swelling of the entire extremity increases.

Blood studies reveal a leukocyte count of 35000–100000/ml with predominance of polymorphonuclear neutrophilic leukocytes and their toxicdegenerative forms. Soon thereafter hypochromic anemia follows, with a decrease in erythrocytes to 2.5×10^6. The sedimentation rate may be accelerated to 70 mm/h, but it decreases once the pus has been evacuated, and the swelling of the joint capsule decreases. However, with continued suppuration the serum contains significantly

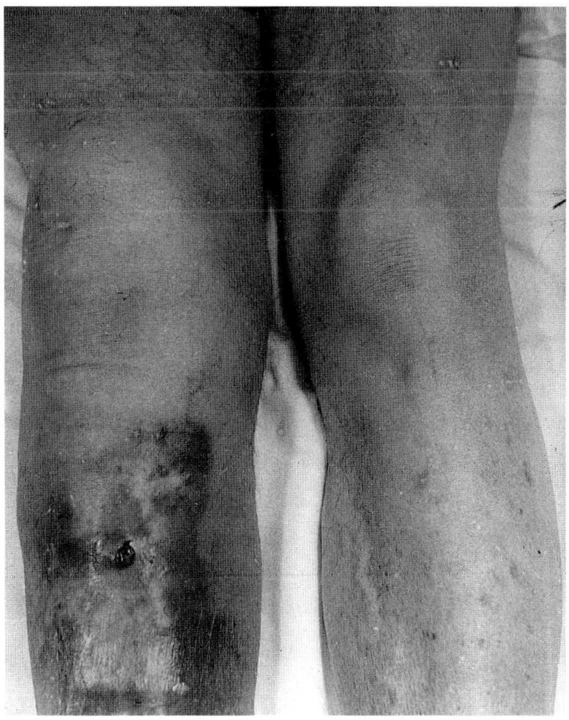

Fig. 77. The right knee is markedly swollen, and its outlines are blurred. A draining sinus is open at the anterior aspect of the lower leg

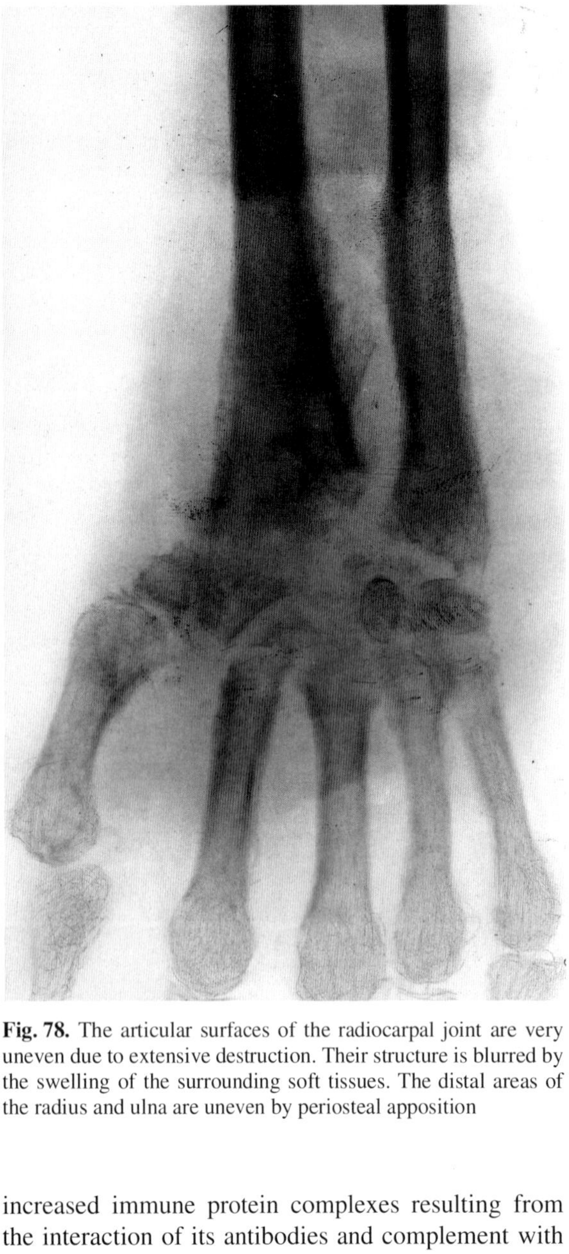

Fig. 78. The articular surfaces of the radiocarpal joint are very uneven due to extensive destruction. Their structure is blurred by the swelling of the surrounding soft tissues. The distal areas of the radius and ulna are uneven by periosteal apposition

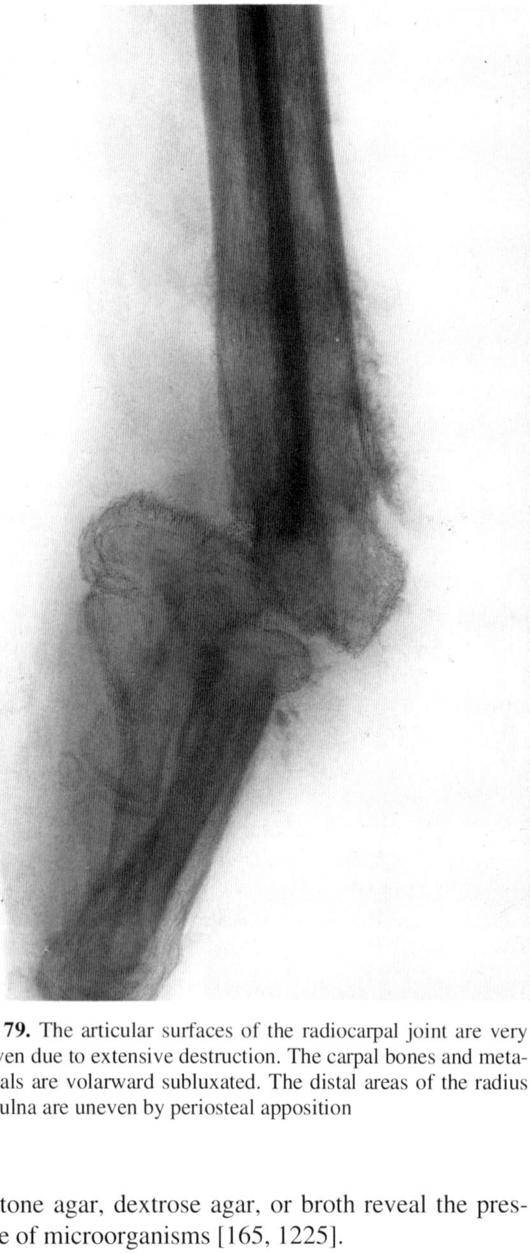

Fig. 79. The articular surfaces of the radiocarpal joint are very uneven due to extensive destruction. The carpal bones and metacarpals are volarward subluxated. The distal areas of the radius and ulna are uneven by periosteal apposition

increased immune protein complexes resulting from the interaction of its antibodies and complement with the microbial antigens. Intermittent high temperature and persisting high sedimentation rates indicate the persistence of foci of pus. Similarly the appearance of urobilinogen in the urine is an unfavorable sign. The purulent joint fluid is greenish, dense, malodorous, and may have a protein content up to 10 g%, correlated with the increased immunoglobulins and complement complexes as in the serum. It contains 50000–100000/ml leukocytes with 90% polymorphonuclear neutrophilic leukocytes, 7% mononuclear leukocytes, 3% lymphocytes, and 50000 erythrocytes. In about 90% of cases numerous bacteria may be seen lying free as well as intracellularly in the smears stained with methylene blue, May-Grünwald-Giemsa or Gram stain. The cultures on agar, blood agar, chocolate agar, peptone agar, dextrose agar, or broth reveal the presence of microorganisms [165, 1225].

Most purulent infections of the joints (64%) are caused by staphylococci. The other purulent infections of joints are caused by diplococci (20%), streptococci (12%), and hemophilus influenzae, Escherichia coli, Salmonella, or pseudomonas aeruginosa (4%) [1165]. The Gram-positive staphylococcus aureus is a round microorganism which lies single or typically in clusters; it produces a yellow-golden pigment on routine culture media and causes hemolysis on blood agar. This staphylococcus consists of peptidiglycan, techoic acid, and protein A [1418]; its peptidiglycan and protein bind the IgG globulin, while the techoic acid induces the formation of antibodies. Thus the prime resort in combating a staphylococcal infection are the antibodies in the host's serum, acting in combi-

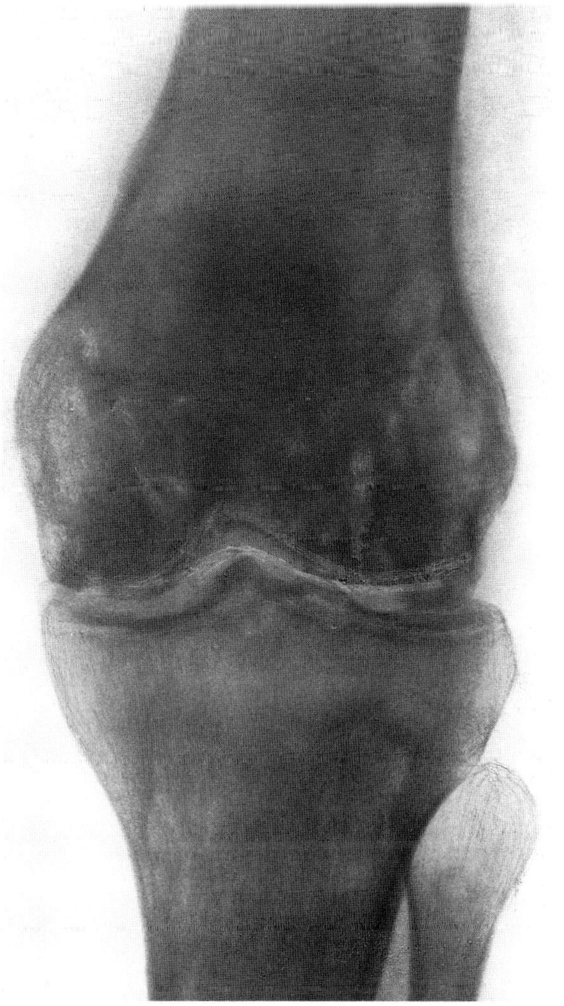

Fig. 80. The femoral condyles present several areas of irregular, intensive radiolucency, which are surrounded by osteosclerosis. The articular surfaces are uneven, and their borders are paralleled by a line of subcortical radiolucency

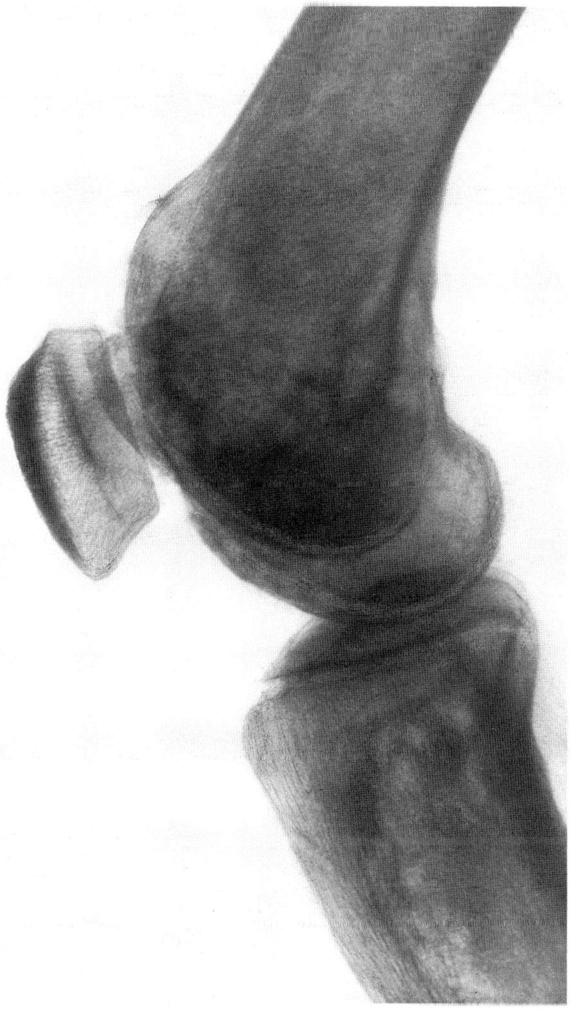

Fig. 81. The metaphyses of the femur and tibia comprise several irregular areas of radiolucency bordered by osteosclerosis. The femoral condyles and, less so the tibial condyles present lines of osteoporosis parallel with their articular contours

nation with complement fixation [1558]. However, this defense is diminished in individuals with anemia, debilitating disease, diabetes, leukemia, or after prolonged steroid medication.

Roentgenographic examination discloses in the early phase a widening of the cartilage space by an increase in joint fluid. Following the damage and erosion of the articular cartilage, the bone marrow proliferates and causes irregular, uneven delimitation of the articular epiphyses. The associated toxic osteoporosis in the subchondral subcortical zone of the articular epiphyses is manifested by a strip about 2–3 mm in width of markedly decreased bone density, resembling a mourning border, beneath and along the cartilage-bone junction (Figs. 80, 81). With the expanding bone destruction, areas of intense radiolucency extend deeply into the bone and are delimited by zones of sclerosis (Figs. 78, 79, 80, 81). Concurrently the cartilage space gradually becomes narrower and irregularly delimited secondary to disintegration of the hyaline cartilage and to erosion of the articular epiphyses by the encroaching synovial pannus (Figs. 78, 79). The adjacent articular ends become connected to each other, and the already narrowed cartilage space is obliterated. The increased density and occasional calcification of the joint capsule cause further obscuring of the structure of the articular epiphyses. Rafii et al. [1297] emphasized the diagnostic advantages of computed tomography versus conventional roentgenography, especially in acute septic arthritis of deepseated axial joints. This permits identification of early swelling of soft tissues, accurate location of the disease process, and early articular erosions.

Gross-anatomical examination [37, 1438] enables one to distinguish empyema (pyarthrosis) with involve-

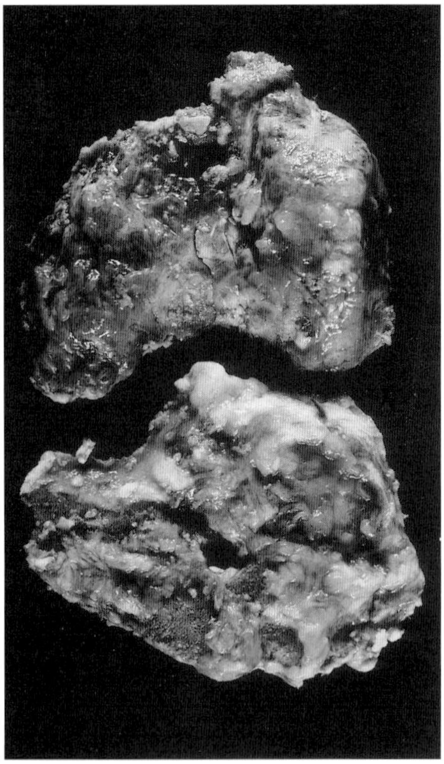

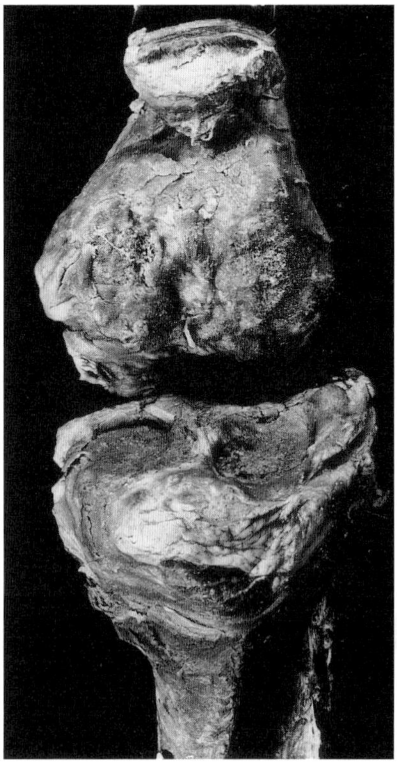

Fig. 82. This defective articular cartilage has been excised in toto from the femoral condyles and tibial condyles. Portions of the articular cartilage have been destroyed due to delayed administration of antibiotics

Fig. 83. The articular surfaces of the femoral condyles and tibial condyles are bare of cartilage and are very uneven. Remnants of the posterior horns of the menisci partly surround the tibial surfaces

ment of the innermost part of the joint capsule, phlegmon with involvement of the entire joint capsule, and purulent panarthritis with additional involvement of the articular cartilage (Fig. 82). The initially serous yellow exudate of the joint cavity becomes progressively more turbid, assumes a yellowish green color and thick-fluid consistency, and sometimes contains admixed blood. The inner part of the joint capsule is very swollen and hyperemic. If the suppuration expands into the fibrous capsule, the periarticular structures also become involved. In this stage, necrosis of the entire joint capsule may occur, perhaps resulting in tubular abscesses which spread along the muscle sheaths and septa. On continuation of the intraarticular suppuration the hyaline cartilage disintegrates. Defects then expand into the depth of the articular surface (Fig. 82), exposing the reddish yellow subchondral bone (Fig. 83). These defects are soon covered by intensely proliferating granulation tissue from the marrow spaces. Concurrently the joint cavity becomes obliterated (Fig. 494) secondary to vigorous reaction of the inner part of the joint capsule. With the subsequent shrinking of the fibrous capsule and due to adhesion of all folds, the entire joint becomes encased in dense, scarified tissue (Fig. 496). On expanding suppuration and destruction, the epiphyses eventually become fused to osseous ankylosis (Fig. 495). However, if the inflammation is of milder course and the suppuration quickly subsides, the alterations are confined chiefly to the joint capsule. The articular cartilage may remain partly intact (Figs. 95, 98), but the motion of the joint is restricted because of the only partly maintained articular cavity.

The infecting microbes in the joint cavity provoke the invasion of polymorphonuclear neutrophilic leukocytes which ingest the microbes and by their proteolytic enzymes, also contribute to the decomposition of the ground substance of the articular cartilage. This harmful effect is initiated by the toxins of the microbes. The synoviocytes, hypertrophic in response to the inflammatory stimuli, also produce protease, cathepsin, and collagenase by their substantially increased lysosomes. In addition to the ground substance, the collagen fibers of the articular cartilage are also dissolved, and the latter becomes extensively disorganized. Similar harm is inflicted on the chondrocytes, of which many become necrotic [355].

Accordingly, histopathological examination [37, 568, 1438] discloses that the superficial zone of the synovial membrane is partly necrotic and is covered with hemorrhages and fresh fibrin in some areas and with leukocytes and microorganisms in others. Free and intracellularly located microorganisms are spread in the superficial and somewhat deeper zones of the synovial membrane (Fig. 84). All blood vessels are markedly hyperemic. On continuation of the inflammation, the synovial membrane becomes diffusely and densely infiltrated predominantly with polymorphonuclear neutrophilic leukocytes (Fig. 85). Portions of ne-

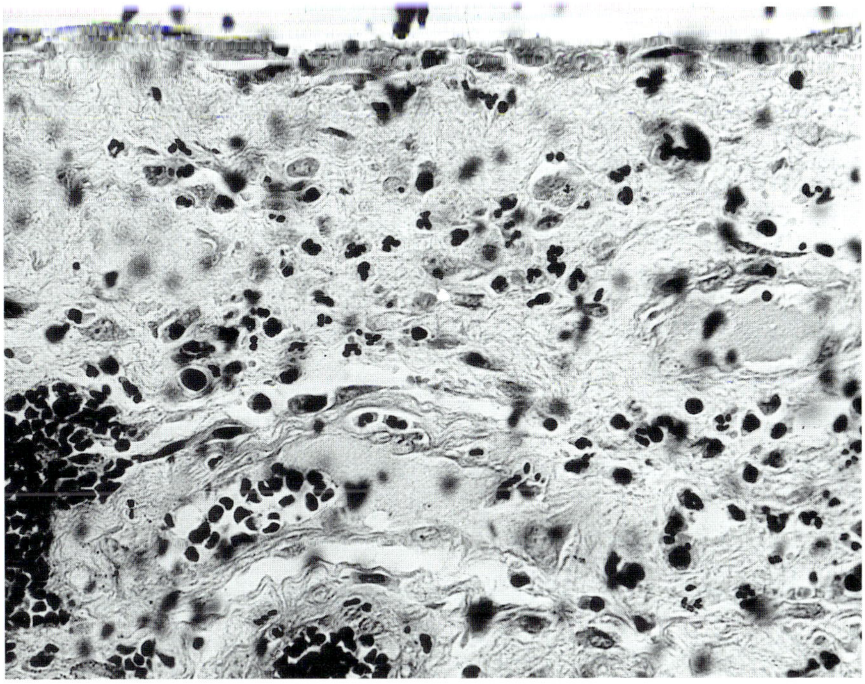

Fig. 84. The synovial membrane is moderately hyperemic and edematous and contains polymorphonuclear leukocytes, fibrocytes, histiocytes, and lymphocytes, among which staphylococci are scattered

crotic tissue are desquamated from the surface, leaving ulcers and deep defects in the synovial membrane. When the dense infiltration by inflammatory cells persists through the subacute phase, it extends into the depth of the subsynoviocytic tissue (Fig. 85) and beyond into the fibrous capsule. In the articular cartilage the chondrocytes are ballooned, and mucinous degeneration as well as decreased staining of the ground substance are observed (Fig. 86). Polymorphonuclear leukocytes, some of them laden with microbes, penetrate the intercellular spaces (Figs. 86, 101), which have lost their ground substance by the enzymatic influence of the bacterial toxins and leukocytes. Those also cause dissolution of the chondrocytes. Similarly by toxic influence, the subchondral bone becomes porotic; it often also undergoes suppurative inflammation and necrosis. Eventually the defects in the articular cartilage (Fig. 87), the ulcers in the synovial mem-

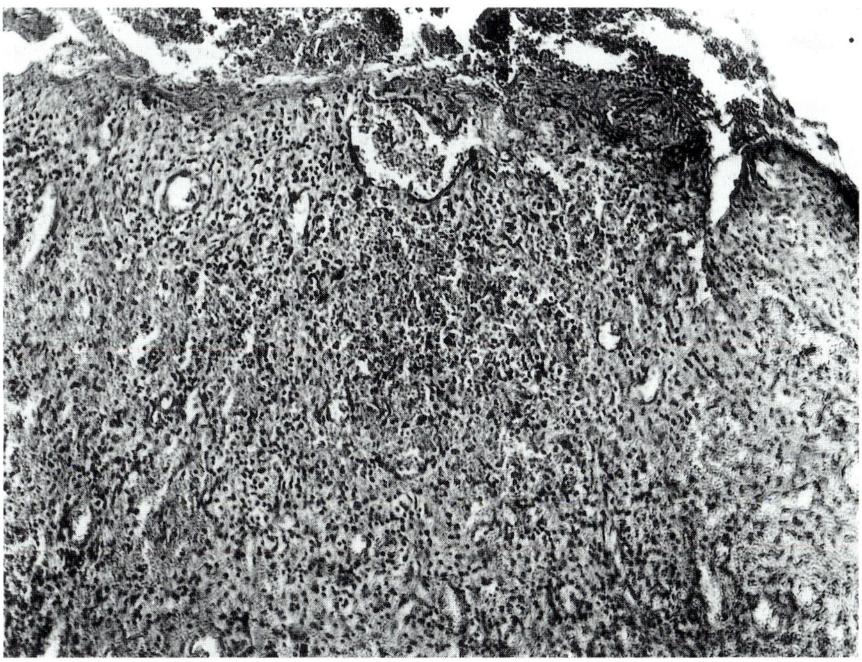

Fig. 85. The synovial membrane bears on its surface dense accumulations of polymorphonuclear leukocytes and is also extensively infiltrated by polymorphonuclear leukocytes. Among the latter, fibrocytes and histiocytes are increased

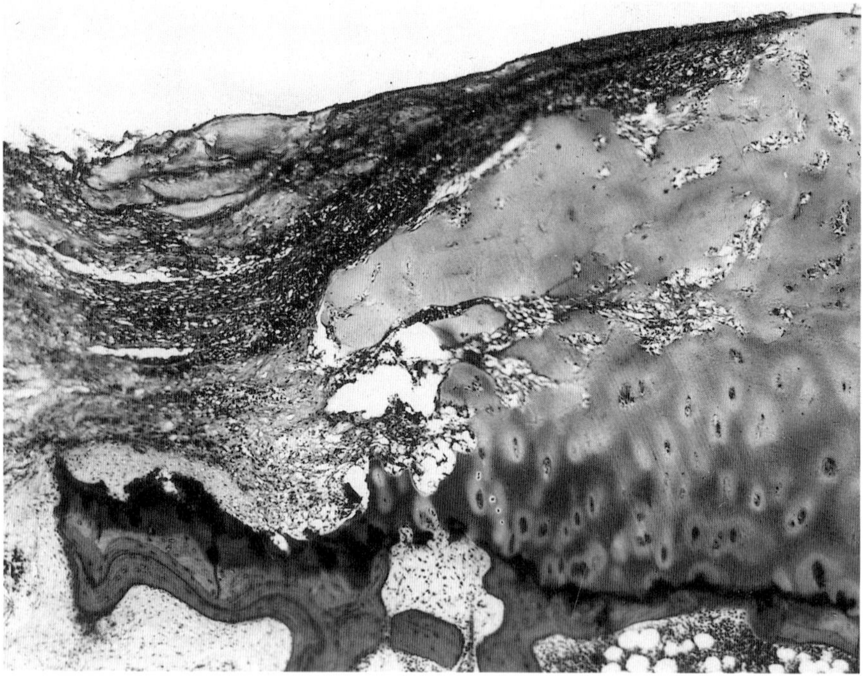

Fig. 86. The articular cartilage is invaded on its surface and at its junction with the subchondral bone by very cellular granulation tissue

brane, and the articular cavity are filled with proliferating granulation tissue which subsequently transforms into dense fibrous tissue. A fibrous ankylosis becomes established there (Figs. 494, 496). Blood vessels and osteoblasts protrude from the marrow spaces and may lead to osseous fusion and ankylosis of the joint by ossification of the interstitial fibrous tissue (Figs. 495, 497).

With incipient suppurative arthritis, differential diagnosis must consider especially the acute arthritis in gonorrhea or in gout, because of the similar clinical picture. However, the generally unequivocal case history, with indication of an infected wound or a suppurative process in the proximity or at a distance, provides a clue to the nature of the underlying process.

The best treatment of purulent arthritis [541, 1355, 1712] is prophylactic because many joint infections can be avoided by proper attention to all internal and external infections. Abscesses of the skin or deeper tissues of the extremities or the trunk should be incised,

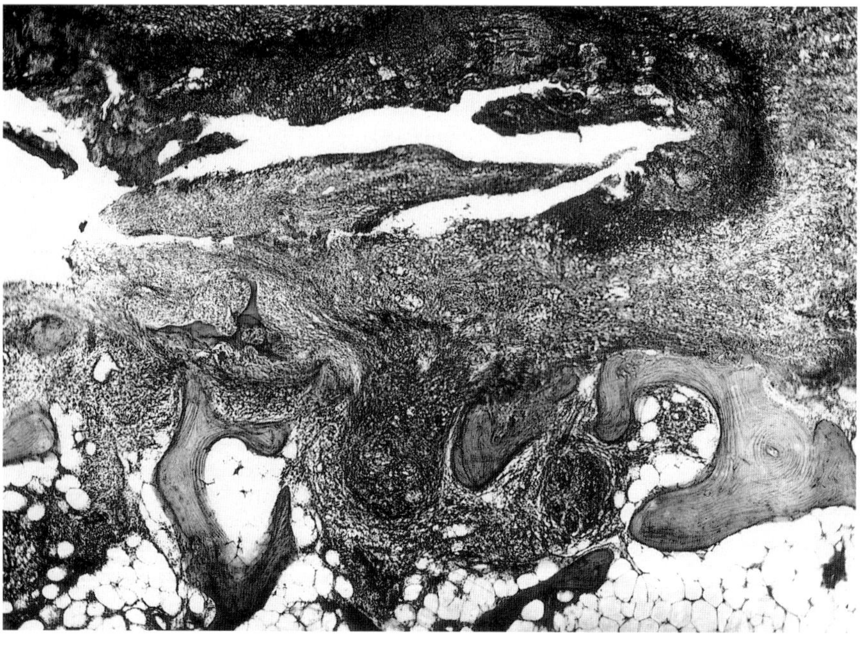

Fig. 87. The cartilage on the articular surface has been extensively replaced by granulation tissue and young connective tissue, which also expands into the subchondral marrow spaces

drained, and treated with the antibiotics indicated by culture and sensitivity test of the pus. Similarly, internal suppurations should be evacuated by draining and should be treated concurrently with the indicated antibiotics. Wounds of the skin which also involve joints should be débrided and thoroughly irrigated with a solution of antibiotic (preferentially penicillin 1×10^6 U in each 10 ml); the joint capsule and the skin are closed loosely with sutures, and the extremity should be immobilized with a splint. Penicillin G is the antibiotic of choice and is effective against most suppuration-causing microorganisms (staphylococcus aureus, streptococcus pyogenes, Escherichia coli, pneumococci, gonococci, Salmonella typhi); this is administered parenterally in daily doses of 10–15×10^6 U divided at 3- to 4-h intervals [1180]. A similarly effective antibiotic is ampicillin, 3.0–4.0 g daily and administered orally in divided doses. However, if the concurrent sensitivity tests disclose resistance of the microorganisms to penicillin (in about 65% of cases) due to their production of penicillinase and coagulase, the antibiotic of choice is cephalosporin 2.5–4.0 g daily and orally or intravenously, tetracycline daily and orally according to the brand from 400 to 2000 mg in divided doses, erythromycin 2.0–4.0 g daily and orally in divided doses, or chloromycetin 2.0–4.0 g daily and orally in divided doses. However, chloromycetin may cause serious blood dyscrasias (aplastic anemia, granulocytopenia, and thrombocytopenia), and all the above antibiotics may cause hypersensitivity reactions of some severity. The cephalosporins have received wide acceptance because of their lower incidence of allergy complications and their effectiveness against penicillinase-producing staphylococci and a range of other microorganisms.

If a noninjured joint becomes swollen, and its fluid is increased, the latter should be aspirated and examined from all points of view, especially as regards the presence of microorganisms and their sensitivities to various antibiotics [1180]. With turbidity of the joint fluid, this joint is irrigated copiously with saline solution through the arthrocentesis needle left intraarticularly, until clear fluid returns. Then, depending on the site and capacity of the joint, 10–30 ml penicillin solution with 300,000 U/ml is injected intraarticularly. Concurrently penicillin G daily is administered parenterally [1222] until the results of culture and sensitivity tests indicate the presence and type of microorganism and the proper antibiotic. The above discussion dealing with wounds of the skin and concurrent wounds of joints – on the effect of penicillin (or cause of its occasional lack of efficacy) and the possible use of other antibiotics – applies as well to noninjured, probably infected joints. Aspiration of the joint fluid, followed by irrigation of the joint cavity and intraarticular instillation of the indicated antibiotic solution, should be repeated daily. Often the swelling of the joint eventually decreases; the joint fluid becomes clear and is resorbed [58, 628, 631]. Experience shows that the antibacterial effect of intraarticularly administered antibiotics is greater than that of generally administered antibiotics, and that the closed joint capsule treated by this modality is well able to fight infection [682].

In infections of joints by microbes other than staphylococcus, the following antibiotics show effect. Streptococcus responds to penicillin G 8000000–10000000 U, erythromycin 3.0–4.0 g, vancomycin 2.0–3.0 g, or cephalosporin 3.0–4.0 g daily in divided doses. Diplococci respond to penicillin G 10000000 U, ampicillin 2.0–4.0 g, erythromycin 3.0–4.0 g, chloramphenicol 2.0–3.0 g, or cephalosporin 3.0–4.0 g daily. Escherichia coli [143] responds to ampicillin 2.0–4.0 g, cephalosporin 3.0–4.0 g, tetracyclin 2.0–3.0 g, or sulfamethoxazole 3.0–4.0. Salmonella [367] responds to ampicillin 2.0–4.0 g or chloromycetin 2.0–3.0 g daily. Enterobacter, Klebsiella, proteus vulgaris, and anaerobic microbes [615] respond to ampicillin 3.0–4.0 g, tetracycline 2.0–3.0 g, or cephalosporin 3.0–4.0 g daily. Pseudomonas aeruginosa responds to tetracycline 2.0–3.0 g, gentamicin 100–300 mg, tobramycin 40 mg intravenously or amikacin 0.5–1.0 g daily. Hemophilus influenzae responds to ampicillin 3.0–4.0 g or chloramphenicol 2.0–3.0 g daily [272, 460, 766, 767]. While the effect to these antibiotics is highly salutary, the potential adverse effects occurring in some patients must not be overlooked. These complications are generally longlasting gastroenteritis and in some patients aplastic anemia, granulocytopenia, and thrombocytopenia. Therefore, blood studies must be carried out in the course of protracted antibiotic administration, and immediate discontinuation is indicated upon manifestation of untoward effects.

However, if despite treatment the joint remains swollen, and the joint fluid becomes thick and purulent, complete and continuous evacuation of the pus by arthrotomy should be performed without delay [1512]. An incision is made at the site of the most prominent swelling, combined with a counterincision to prevent retention of the pus in a pocket of the joint capsule. Through these incisions drains are inserted around the articular ends and are used for twice daily irrigation of the joint with the indicated antibiotic solution. The surgical modality is necessary particularly for the hip joint, which is not easily accessible to aspiration due to its thick cloak of soft tissue. If the first aspiration of the joint fluid and irrigation of the hip joint is technically unsatisfactory or does not provide a satisfactory result, the joint should be opened by an anterior incision, preferentially combined with a lateral incision. The

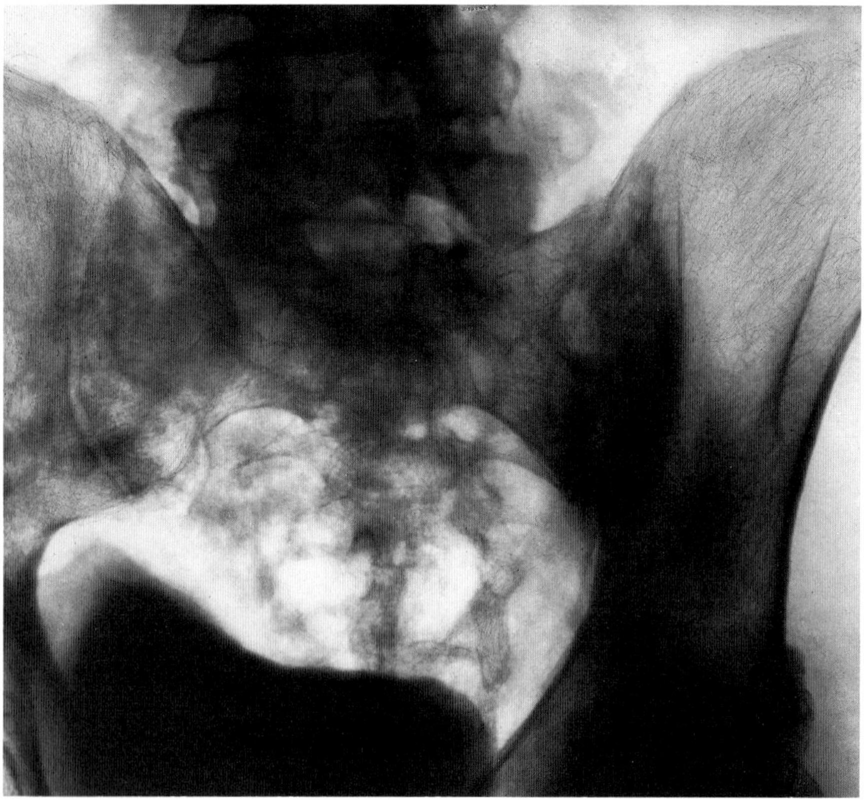

Fig. 88. The left sacroiliac joint is almost obliterated by dense bone formation, which also comprises a few small areas of osteoporosis

wide accesses permit adequate drainage of purulent fluid from the hip joint as well as from other major peripheral joints, especially with the patient kept in prone position. Essential benefit is obtained here by regular and extensive irrigation with the indicated antibiotic solution [1046]. If despite thorough drainage the septic condition persists, and the joint remains swollen and painful, a strong indication exists that one or all contiguous articular epiphyses (Fig. 495) have become involved by the suppurative process [682]. Roentgenographic examination may reveal an osteomyelitic focus in the articular epiphyses. The resection of these articular epiphyses [613] succeeds in eliminating the suppurative process, but a late sequela may be deformity of the joint with axial deviation, instability, and subluxation. To prevent the accumulation of pus in the joint and its expansion into the articular epiphyses, Willems [1761] recommends broad incision of the joint capsule without insertion of drains, but gentle active movements of the joint carried out a few times daily. The purpose of these movements is to separate the adhesions of the capsular folds from the articular epiphyses and to squeeze out pus from the joint cavity. However, if elevated temperature and pain in the joint continue, the active movements are discontinued. Compared with the traditional principles to maintain a suppurating joint at rest, the concept of Willems [1761] appears a controversial method.

When the suppuration of the joint terminates, the temperature normalizes, and the pain subsides; but this joint is most often stiff. Therefore, the joint should be mobilized [65] as soon as the general and local conditions permit, by progressively increasing active exercises. If necessary, passive mobilization exercises should be added. These modalities stretch the shrunken joint capsule and periarticular structures and separate the adhesions as long as the epiphyseal surfaces have not fused with each other. Regular performance of the exercises in a warm bath helps to soften the shortened tissues and to increase the range of motion. However, if the motion of the joint progresses only slowly, and the exercises cause unbearable pain, mobilization of the joint can be carried out by manipulation (Figs. 483, 488, 489) under general anesthesia as discussed in "Contracture of Joint". In the hands of a physician experienced in such technique, the manipulation succeeds in providing a substantial increase in the range of motion without the complication of a fracture through the osteoporotic metaphyses. It is very advisable to administer antibiotics during and several days after this manipulation to prevent the activation of possibly encapsulated foci of suppuration.

With the timely use of general and perhaps local antibiotics, the suppuration of a joint can often be arrested before the articular cartilage becomes damaged. Recovery of full or alt least a functional range of mo-

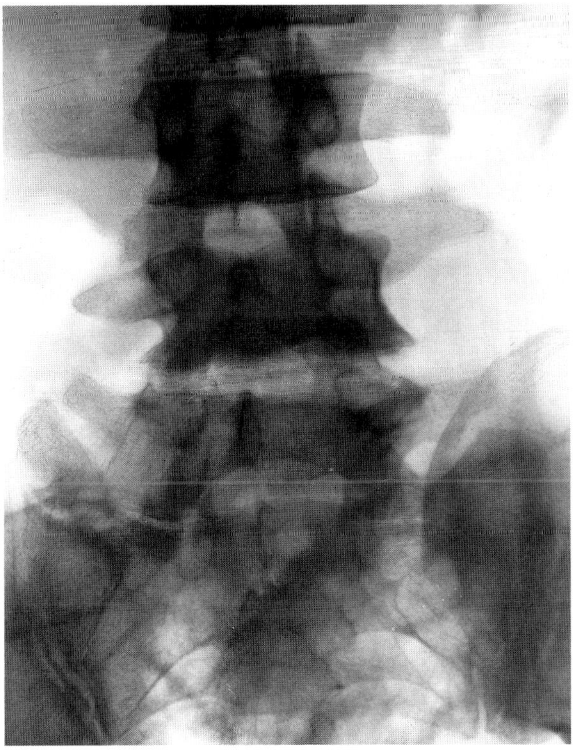

Fig. 89. The adjoining borders of the vertebrae L4 and L5 are uneven, and the vertebral bodies are of irregular structure, mostly sclerosed

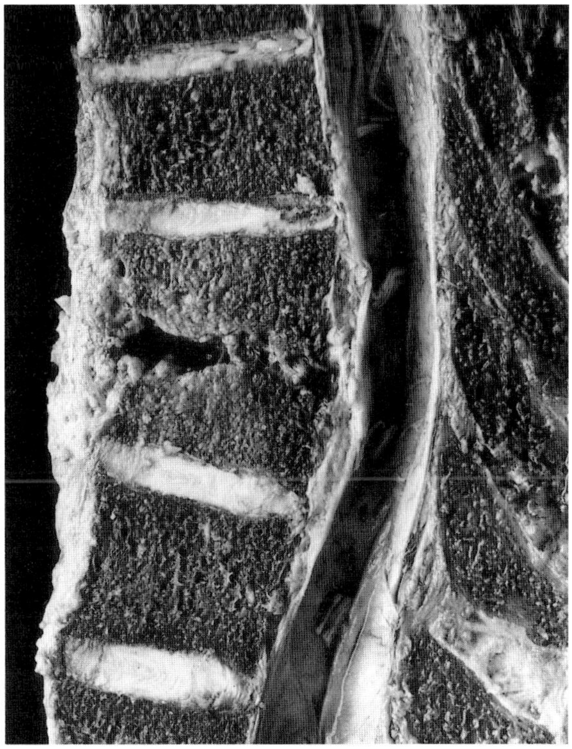

Fig. 90. Two vertebral bodies of the lumbar spine are partly united secondary to destruction of the intervertebral disc. A large gap persists between the other part of the vertebral bodies

tion may be expected in 70 % of patients treated in this way [1103]. However, in about 25 % of these cases the articular surfaces become involved and remain uneven and partly incongruent (Fig. 82). Herefrom a secondary osteoarthritis eventually results which may be associated with impaired motion. In the remaining 5 % of patients, the joint develops a fibrous or osseous ankylosis (Figs. 494, 495) which, lacking any motion in this joint, permits the pain-free use of the limb. For those desiring to regain the motion in the joint, arthroplasty may be undertaken, but only when the sedimentation rate, leukocyte count, and roentgenographs reveal the absence of any active inflammatory process in the articular epiphyses. Additionally, a test by three irradiations with shortwave diathermy is indicated to ascertain whether this modality would cause pain, local increase in temperature, or elevation of the general temperature, suggestive of a dormant bacterial focus. The prinicples in the treatment of such condition are discussed in "Ankylosis of Joints".

Besides the joints of the extremities, those of the axial skeleton may develop septic arthritis; among these the sacroiliac joint is often the seat of such infection [337, 395, 652, 1165]. It is usually propagated from furuncles in the covering skin, rectal abscess, or persistent inflammations of the colon, adnexae, or urogenital tract. The symptoms are increasing pain and pronounced swelling at the posterior aspect of the sacroiliac area, marked circumscribed tenderness at the site of the affected joint, compression pain from both sides, and positive results from straight-leg raising test and Gaenslen's test. Aspiration of the scant, yellow, turbid fluid most often discloses by smear and culture the presence of Escherichia coli or streptococcus pyogenes, less often that of pseudomonas aeruginosa or staphylococcus viridans. Roentgenographs (Fig. 88) reveal uneven delimitation of the affected joint cleft by erosion of the adjacent bones, more often of the iliac bone than the sacrum, and irregular structure by osteoporosis alternating with areas of sclerosis of bone. Besides complete bedrest in supine position, treatment consists of 15 millions U penicillin G daily administered parenterally in four divided doses should begin without delay and be continued for 4–6 weeks. However, if culture reveals resistance of the microorganisms to penicillin, and the symptoms – especially swelling, pain, and fever – continue, tetracycline 1.5–3.0 g, cephalosporin 2.0–4.0 g, or chloramphenicol 1.5–2.5 g should be given daily in divided doses and continued until unequivocal subsidence of the symptoms. This is the usual outcome and avoids the need of surgical intervention. Nevertheless, the lower part of

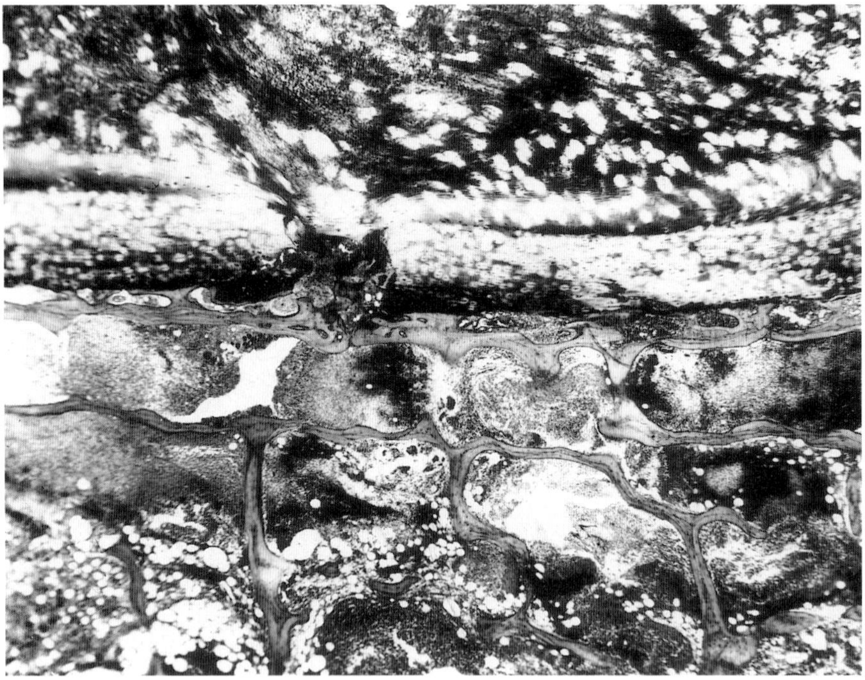

Fig. 91. Chronically and intensely inflamed connective tissue expands from the subchondral marrow spaces through the cartilage endplate into the intervertebral disc.

the vertebral column should be supported by a firm lumbosacral belt with metal stays extending sufficiently far caudally (Fig. 51). Immobilization of this part of the vertebral column is continued for 9–12 months.

Similarly as the sacroiliac joints, the intervertebral joints of the lower thoracic or lumbar spine may become infected (Figs. 89, 90, 91) by the above microorganisms. Other microorganisms which may cause here inflammation and/or suppuration include Salmonella (Fig. 116) and Brucella (Figs. 121, 122). All these microorganisms elicit an affection principally of the intervertebral disc and adjacent vertebral plates. Herewith are associated intense, rather diffuse pain, pronounced spasm of the paravertebral musculature, and substantial limitation of motion. The vertebral bodies are less often affected and respond as well as the intervertebral inflammations to prolonged administration of the antibiotics indicated by culture of the obtained suppurative material. Surgical intervention is therefore generally not indicated. In addition, complete immobilization by a dorsolumbar brace (Fig. 51) for a period of 12–18 months (longer than for the sacroiliac joint) is necessary to obtain healing, often resulting in ankylosis of the affected intervertebral joints. In contrast to tuberculous spondylitis, the healing occurs much faster. In the rare situations of expansion of the suppurative process into the intramedullary space, complicated by compression of the spinal cord and resultant paraplegia [182, 1241], a laminectomy for decompression of the spinal cord is indicated.

Purulent arthritis in infants [1772] differs from that in adults by etiology, the course of the disease, and the generally favorable prognosis [943]. Therefore discussion of this condition is indicated separately. Its etiology may be any bacterial infection of the body: suppuration of the skin as pustule or furuncle after variola or varicellae, suppuration of the umbilicus, otitis media, stomatitis aphthosa, parotitis, bronchitis, pneumonia, various kinds of enteritis, meningitis, or influenza. In summary, any inflammatory process which affects the infantile organism may be the source for dissemination of microorganisms. The causative microbes may thus be streptococci, staphylococci, pneumococci, diplococci, enterococci, hemophilus, Escherichia, or Salmonella. The intraarticular localization of microbes is generally caused by hematogenous spread or lymphatic propagation, and rarely by injuries. It often starts as primary colonization of the microbes in the bone marrow of the metaphysis. The physiologically enhanced tissue activity in the metaphyseal growth zone is accompanied by an increased blood supply which propagates the microbes into the trabecular meshes. Here the microbes provoke an abscess which may remain localized, but the microbes more often transgress the barrier of the cartilage growth plate and penetrate into the epiphysis. By expanding suppuration in the latter, the border of the subchondral bone to articular cartilage is eventually perforated. Masses of pus are then evacuated into the joint cavity, where they infect the inner part of the joint capsule. Thus in addition to the possibility of primary affection of the joint

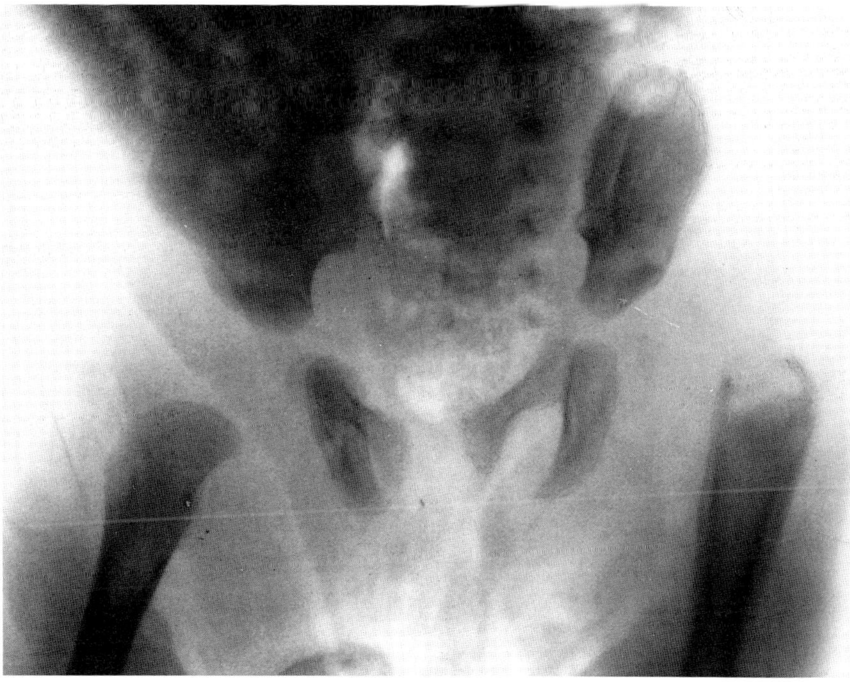

Fig. 92. Superolateral dislocation of the proximal femoral end in a recent suppuration of the left hip joint

capsule, the characteristic type of purulent arthritis in infants starts as osteomyclitis in the metaphysis and affects the joints by expansion.

As in adults, purulent arthritis manifests itself as empyema of the joint cavity, phlegmon of the joint capsule, or totally suppurative arthritis. Due to less tendency to spread the articular empyema is the more frequent occurrence.

The joint inflammation [1140] begins with all symptoms of a virulent infection. The general condition is substantially impaired, the young patients lie moaning and whining, unable to go to sleep or to accept food. The temperature rises rapidly to 40.5°–41°C, and the body weight decreases fast. These symptoms are not as pronounced in the suckling as in the infant; the course of the disease is slower and more sparing in the former. The clinical picture of joint inflammation develops rather rapidly, with swelling, redness, increased joint fluid, and distinctly elevated local warmth. The joint is held in midposition by the distended joint capsule and reflectory muscle tenseness. The most often affected joints are those of the knee, hip, elbow, shoulder, and ankle. The joint fluid contains 35000–80000/ml polymorphonuclear leukocytes and is examined for the presence of microbes by stained smear and by inoculation of various culture media (agar, blood agar, pepton, bouillon). Roentgenographs in the early phase reveal widening of the cartilage space (Fig. 92) by an increase in joint fluid and hazy structure of the epiphyses by the thickened joint capsule. Areas of radiolucency bordered by normally structured cancellous bone appear subsequently, and the outlines of the articular epiphyses are blurred. The past suppuration of a joint is recognizable even after many years in the deformation of the articular epiphyses, partly by destruction but more commonly by growth disturbance (Figs. 93, 94). The articular epiphyses then present a bizarre appearance, and areas of radiolucency alternating with sclerosis, as caused by destruction, necrosis, and incomplete restructuring (Fig. 94). The cartilage space is irregularly but sharply delimited.

Accordingly, the gross-anatomical examination discloses one larger or a few smaller confluent areas of destruction in the cancellous bone of the articular epiphyses. The larger area usually has the outline of a wedge, whose apex is in the subchondral spongiosa; the smaller areas have irregular configurations with openings into the joint cavity. At these sites, the articular cartilage presents rough defects and undermined ulcers. The smaller areas have grayish yellow, softened, necrotic centers containing fragments of osseous trabecula and are surrounded by broad red hyperemic borders. The inner part of the joint capsule is swollen and intensely reddened; an edema occasionally expands into the fibrous capsule. The joint cavity is filled with yellowish green exudate.

Histopathological examination discloses ulcerous defects in the synovial membrane filled with free microbes and with leukocytes containing microbes. The blood vessels of the subsynoviocytic tissue are dilated, engorged with blood, and surrounded by leukocyte agglomerations. Similarly, the entire subsynoviocytic

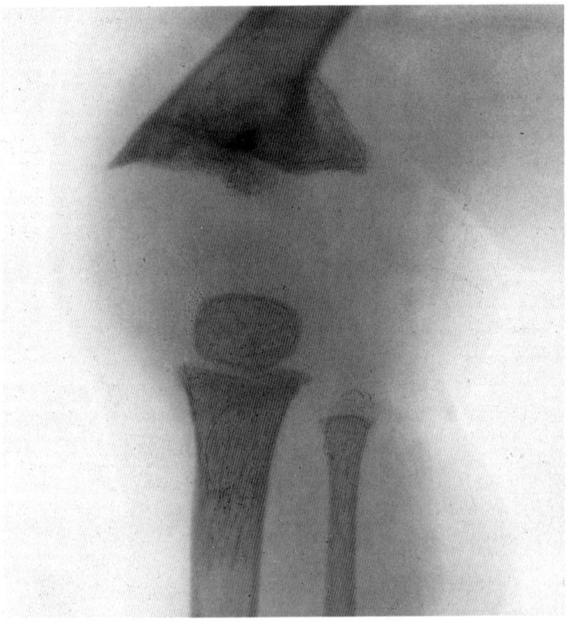

Fig. 93. Destruction of the distal femoral epiphysis at concurrent marked swelling of the joint capsule in suppuration of the knee joint

tissue is diffusely infiltrated, principally by polymorphonuclear neutrophilic leukocytes and less so by lymphocytes.

In the differential diagnosis, primary osseous tuberculosis must be considered, but this affects only children older than 4 years and begins without grave septic symptoms. On the other hand, in primary osseous tuberculosis secondarily invading a joint, areas of the metaphysis and epiphysis may, as in purulent arthritis of infants, present irregularly delimited areas of radiolucency due to destruction.

The local fluctuation indicates the presence of an intensive inflammation with an increase in joint fluid. Arthrocentesis is indicated to examine this fluid from all points of view. If aspiration reveals turbid fluid, the joint is irrigated through the arthrocentesis needle left in situ – at first with physiological saline solution until clearance and subsequently with penicillin G solution containing 100,000 U/ml. Of the latter, 10–25 ml depending on the space of the joint cavity is injected intraarticularly. Concurrently 5,000,000 U penicillin G daily is administered, divided into 3 to 4 h doses either orally with tea or in rectal infusion, provided that the tests disclose sensitivity of the microbe to penicillin. It is advisable to administer penicillin intramuscularly for 1 week to obtain reliably high levels. Thereafter penicillin is orally administered for 3 weeks. The swelling of the joint decreases, and the temperature normalizes. In the presence of penicillin-resistant microbes, the next antibiotic of choice [777, 1091] indicated by the initial sensitivity test is erythromycin 0.6–1.5 g or cephalosporin 1.0–2.0 g given daily in divided doses. The adverse effects of these antibiotics may be gastrointestinal symptoms, anemia, and leukopenia. When smear and culture disclose the presence of microbes other than staphylococci, the same antibiotics are indicated as described above for such infections in adults.

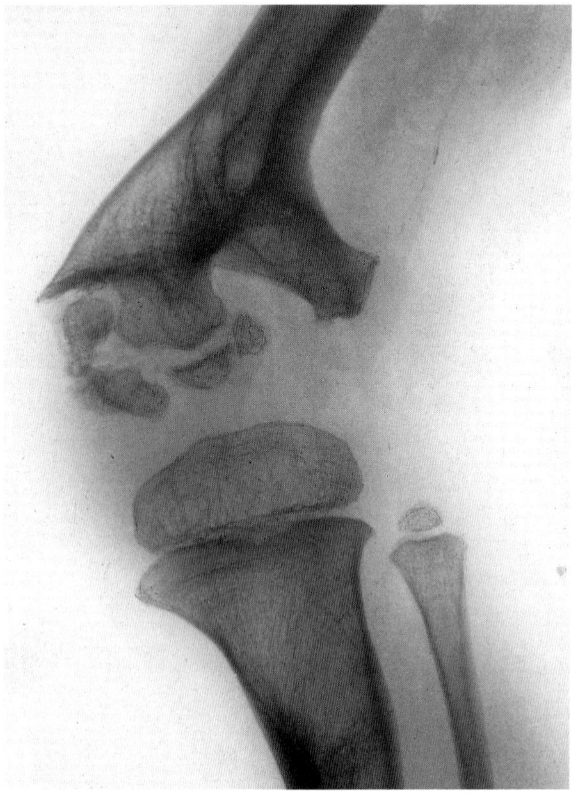

Fig. 94. Pronounced angulation at the distal metaphysis of the femur and malformation of the distal epiphysis secondary to suppuration

However, if general administration of the indicated antibiotics does not provide an improvement in the general and the local condition [272, 1772], and arthrocentesis discloses the presence of frank purulent effusion, the joint capsule should be opened by two counterincisions. Such sites of incision are indicated especially when roentgenographs exclude a primary osteomyelitic focus in the epiphysis or metaphysis. This ensures complete evacuation of the pus, and thorough irrigation of the joint cavity is made feasible – twice daily through drains extending into the joint cavity. The primary irrigation with physiological saline solution is followed by instillation of the indicated antibiotic solution in 10–20 ml. The effects of this treatment are noticeable in an essential change in general and local conditions. The infant sleeps quietly, deeply, and sufficiently long, and its appetite returns; the temperature drops to 37.5°–38.2°C, and the swelling and warmth of the joint regress. The drained fluid from the joint becomes clear, free of microbes, and gradually decreases in amount until complete cessation. In this situation the joint should be passively and gently manipulated in all directions of physiological movements to prevent adhesions and gradually to restore the range of movements. These manipulations are more performed energetically after the incisional wounds have closed. Nevertheless, a contracture caused by fibrotic cicatrization of the joint capsule and shrinking of the periarticular tissue may sometimes follow. Therefore, the energetic manipulations need to be continued for several months until reattainment of the normal range of motion. The regular application of moist warm packs is here of substantial benefit by decreasing the soreness of the joint and by softening the contracted regional tissues, including the musculature.

In the presence of persistent suppuration of a joint despite adequate administration of antibiotics, and when roentgenographs reveal an osteomyelitic focus in the epiphysis or metaphysis, this area must be opened by a drill or a frazier. The necrotic and purulent material is removed by curettement, and a drain is inserted, through which the abscess cavity is irrigated daily with physiological saline solution followed by 10 ml of the indicated antibiotic. The effect of this modality, which must sometimes be carried out for 1–2 months, is noticeable in the gradual clearance and decrease in wound secretion until its complete cessation and closure of the drainage wound. Concurrently, the indicated antibiotic should be administered by any feasible route (oral, rectal, or parenteral) for 2–3 months. The recovery in terms of afebrile state, reattainment of good general condition, and restoration of the function of the joint needs a much longer period of time than when only the joint capsule is infected. Prolonged treatment is indicated especially in view of the potential for profound harm to the articular cartilage and extensive destruction of the articular epiphyses. This may result not only in impairment of the motion of the joint but also in disturbance in epiphyseal growth, with consequently faulty alignment, subluxation, and osteogenically determined deformities. A supportive brace maintaining the articular epiphyses in proper alignment often succeeds in preventing such sequelae and should be worn for several years, usually until puberty or until completion of growth.

Suppuration of joints in children usually regresses under adequate antibiotic administration. Destructive changes in the epiphyses and growth disturbance follow only in a few cases, with resulting angular deformity, yet with a sufficient range of motion. In any of the cases of purulent arthritis in infants, the outcome is determined primarily by the defensive forces of the patient and by the virulence of the microbes. Of these, hemophilus influenzae is the most toxic, while staphylococcus causes severe local harm, and streptococcus and Salmonella are overcome rather quickly. Nevertheless, the expansion of a joint infection can be contained by the timely initiation of antibiotic treatment, thereby safeguarding the proper configuration and mobility of the joint. Therefore, the prognosis of purulent arthritis in infants may be characterized as fair to favorable [943]. In very rare cases of excessively virulent infection with panarthritis and concurrent hematogenous spread into the brain, kidneys, liver, and spleen, generalized sepsis may lead to a fatal outcome.

2. Meningococcal Arthritis

Arthritis caused by meningococci [1159] is a rather frequent complication, occurring in about 5%–8% of meningococcal infections of the meninges, lungs, endocard, or pericard by hematogenous spread. Arthritis sets in on the 5th–11th days after the start of this infection [947, 1763, 1800]. Meningococci may also emanate from the nasopharyngeal cavity in company with other microbes and then cause a mixed infection. In exclusively meningococcal sepsis the joints are affected more virulently, and the infection of the meninges may linger in the background.

Inflammation of the joints begins polyarticularly, but it eventually becomes localized in a single joint: knee, wrist, elbow, or ankle joint [219, 1205, 1258, 1399]. Children are affected more often than adults. The general condition is markedly impaired by the signs of meningeal irritation: fever, nausea and vomiting, general weakness, headache, and malaise or lethargy. If meningitis is the predominant manifestation, the irritation of the sensory and motor nerve roots results in pronounced hyperesthesia and in hypertonicity of the musculature. Characteristic of meningococcal sepsis are widespread small hemorrhages, such as petechiae and suggillations, in the skin of the trunk and extremities. The affected joint displays intense changes of acute inflammation. It is distinctly warmer than the surrounding area, is enlarged by capsule swelling and effusion, but is less tender than in other acute bacterial joint infections. The motion of the joint is limited by reflex contraction of the regional musculature. Regional tendon sheaths and bursae may also be involved.

Three types of joint affection may be distinguished [490] clinically as well as pathological-anatomically. The first is arthralgia with transient hyperemia of the synovial membrane. The second is hydrarthrosis associated with a serous inflammation of the synovial membrane and increase in synovial fluid. This is clear, light green in color, and contains fibrin flakes. Examination of the synovial fluid discloses a moderate number (800–2000) of polymorphonuclear leukocytes and lymphocytes, no microorganisms, but a significant in-

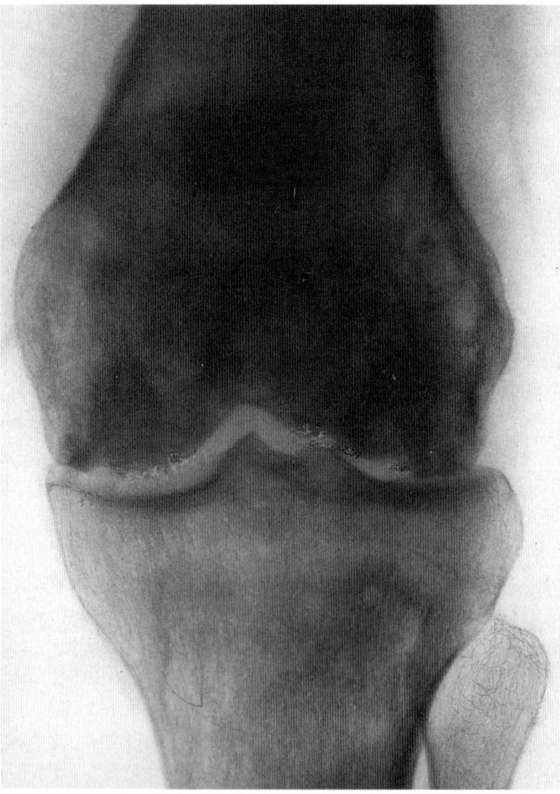

Fig. 95. The articular borders especially of the lateral femoral condyle are uneven and the lateral joint cleft is narrowed. The proximal tibial epiphysis is osteoporotic, and the femoral condyles contain areas of radiolucency

crease in immunoglobulins [674]. The third type is pyarthrosis characterized by marked hyperemia of the synovial membrane, with ulcerations on larger areas and fibrin precipitates in other areas. The inflammation may expand into the fibrous capsule, where it tends to form abscesses. The purulent, yellow synovial fluid contains an abundance of microorganisms, 40000–65000/ml polymorphonuclear leukocytes, mucus, and fibrin; protein is increased to 4.2–6.3 g%, and glucose is decreased to 15–25 mg%.

Infection of the meninges, which in most cases precedes or is concurrent with the joint complication, provides a clue to the etiology of the joint inflammation. However, if no irritation of the nerve roots is manifest, the blood, joint fluid, and if possible cerebrospinal fluid should be examined by smear with Gram stain and culture. Meningococci are Gram-negative, extra- and intracellularly occurring microorganisms which lie in pairs with the along sides flattened, having the shape of a biscuit or bean. They grow readily on chocolate agar and Thayer-Martin agar. On the basis of serological studies identifying their capsular protein and polysaccharides, the meningococci have been classified into several groups, of which the groups A, C, and Y are most commonly observed in joint infections. However, in the majority of nonpurulent joint inflammations, examinations of the joint fluid by smear and culture fail to disclose the presence of microorganisms. In these situations the inflammatory joint alterations must be interpreted as immunocomplex reactions to the antigen emanating from the meningococci, circulating in the blood stream, and arriving in the joint [674]. Laboratory studies for antibodies contained in the immunoglobulins ascertain the agglutinin in the patient's serum against erythrocytes coated with meningococcal capsular polysaccharide. The presumed complement in the serum and joint fluid is identified by the fixation test [1248]. The immunofluorescence method has received increasing application for detecting antibodies, and it is of substantial help in the diagnosis and in explaining the pathogenesis of the meningococcal arthritis [9]. The immunoglobulins are usually within the normal ranges [9].

Roentgenographic examination reveals no changes specific for the meningococcal infection. In the rare cases in which suppuration sets in and becomes aggravated, osteoporosis of the articular epiphyses in associated with narrowing of the cartilage space (Fig. 95). In children the articular involvement may proceed from an osteomyelitic epiphyseal focus which perforates into the joint cavity; deformity of the articular epiphyses may be the outcome.

Histopathological examination of the synovial membrane discloses marked hyperemia, free hemorrhages, and diffuse infiltration by polymorphonuclear leukocytes. In some areas the synoviocyte cover is missing and is generally substituted by fibrin deposits (Fig. 96). The latter and the synoviocyte cover contain intracellularly as well as free lying diplococci which stain Gram-negative. The subsynoviocytic tissue is infiltrated extensively (Figs. 96, 97) by leukocytes, lymphocytes, and histiocytes and is loosened by edema which expands into the fibrous capsule. The articular cartilage contains numerous necrotic chondrocytes and is disintegrating in several areas (Fig. 97); this exposes the zone of calcified cartilage and the subchondral bone.

Differential diagnosis may present difficulties in those cases in which no meningitic symptoms preceded the articular symptoms. Acute rheumatic arthritis and arthritis elicited by pneumococci or gonococci present similar clinical pictures. Therefore, microscopic and culture examinations of the blood and joint fluid should be performed in all equivocal situations; this clarifies the etiology.

Treatment of meningococcal arthritis is prophylactic and should begin immediately with the manifestation of meningeal inflammation or sepsis. Penicillin G is given parenterally in divided doses of 10,000,000–15,000,000 U at 4 h intervals for 14 days until the gen-

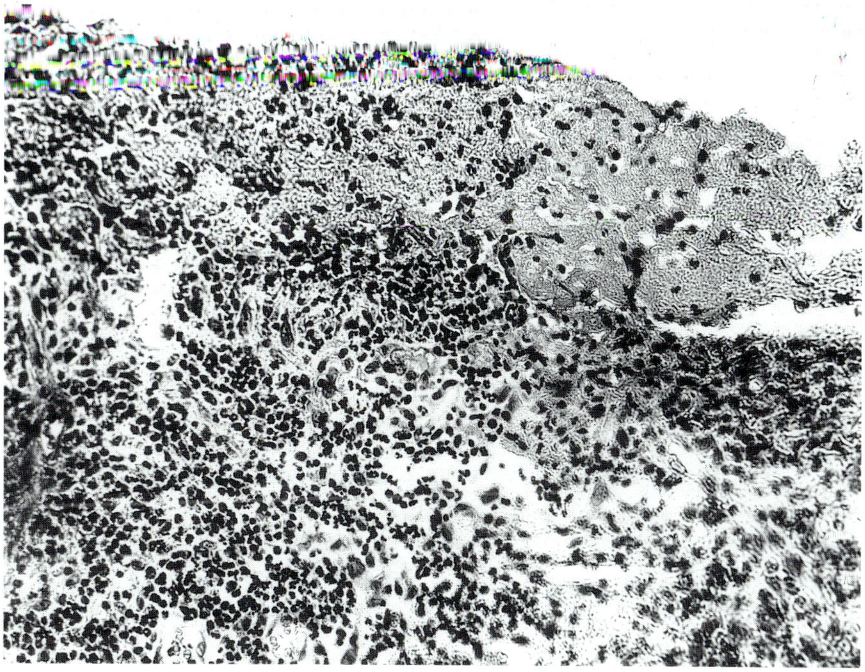

Fig. 96. The synovial membrane is mostly bare of synoviocytes and is covered by fibrin. The latter and especially the synovial membrane are hypercellular with fibrocytes, polymorphonuclear leukocytes, and histiocytes. Meningococci are scattered among them

eral symptoms and especially the fever regress or subside. Thereafter penicillin is continued at the same dose as long as the joint symptoms persist. In cases of microbial resistance to penicillin or of allergy on the part of the patient, chloromycetin 1.5–2.5 g or tetracycline 1.5–3.0 g, given daily in divided doses, is effective. The general and articular symptoms are thus resolved within 2–3 weeks [961]. The involved joint is surrounded by moist warm compresses and is immobilized with a splint. If the joint fluid is increased and does not absorb, it should be removed by arthrocentesis and examined for the presence and type of microorganisms by stained smear, culture on blood agar, and sensitivity tests. The outcome of these findings determines the type of the antibiotics administered both generally and once or twice daily in articular irrigations, which follow the aspiration of the joint fluid.

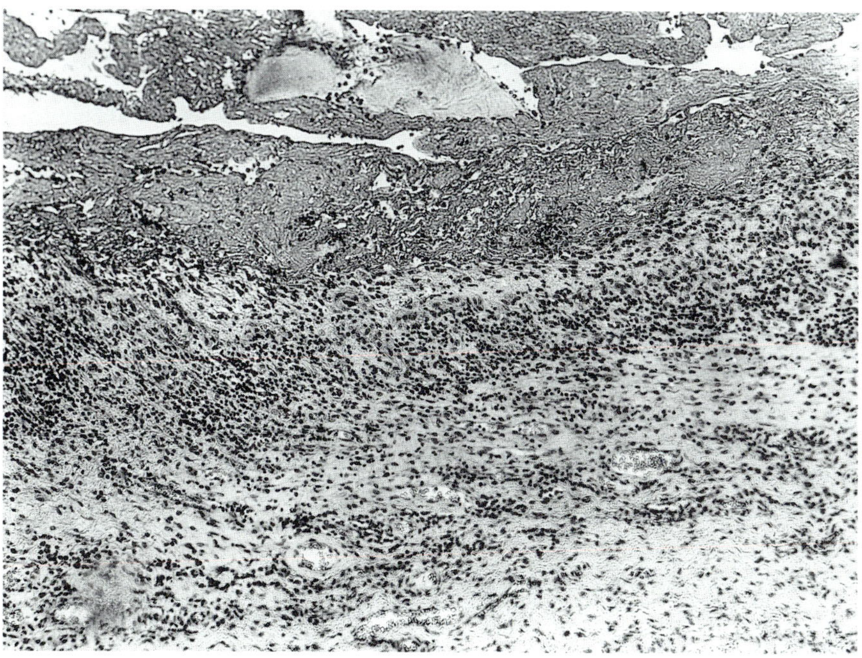

Fig. 97. Fragments of necrotic articular cartilage lie in extensive deposits of fibrin. The synovial membrane is hypercellular with fibrocytes, lymphocytes, polymorphonuclear leukocytes, and histiocytes

If the temperature nevertheless rises or continues to be elevated, and the joint fluid assumes a purulent character, the joint capsule should be opened by two opposite incisions through which drains are inserted into the joint cavity for outflow of the pus. Regular irrigations of the joint cavity are carried out through the drains twice daily with a solution of the antibiotic indicated by culture and sensitivity tests, performed after the first arthrocentesis. With this treatment the suppuration eventually ceases. After the incisional wounds in the joint capsule and skin have closed, the joint should be mobilized by active und passive exercises. If the result is not satisfactory and a substantial deficit in the range of motion persists, the joint should be mobilized by manipulation (Figs. 482, 488, 489) under general anesthesia. In very rare cases the destruction of articular constituents is so extensive that a permanent deformity of the joint results.

Infection by the meningococci, especially when affecting the meninges, may be so virulent as to result in death. However, in most other meningococcal inflammations, the antibiotic treatment is usually able to control the infection of the joint, especially if no indication for incision of the joint capsule arises. The inflammation then usually resolves, with full recovery and normal function of the joint. The good healing tendency in children permits reattainment of a satisfactory range of motion of the joint, even with partial deformation of the articular epiphyses.

3. Pneumococcal Arthritis

Infection by pneumococci (Fraenkel-Weichselbaum [1728]) is the most frequent cause of pneumonia, which in 2%–4% of the cases is complicated by arthritis, also caused by the pneumococci. This arthritis typically develops between the 5th and 14th days of pneumonia, but also often in the second week after the crisis. Any other site of infection (pharynx, endocard, meninges) by pneumococci may also be the source of articular inflammation. In the infant, pneumococcal arthritis may also derive from the middle and inner ear, peritoneum, mucosa of the nose and mouth, and skin. The joint infection [861, 902, 1653] usually develops by hematogenous spread. Prior traumatization of the joint probably favors the localization of the microorganisms. Direct propagation from infection of the skin is rare.

Pneumococcal arthritis may be polyarticular but more commonly occurs monoarticularly, involving the middle-sized or large joints. This arthritis affects infants more often than adults. It sometimes presents as arthralgia with slight symptoms, but it is usually associated with pronounced inflammatory changes. Concomitant disturbances vary with the primary pneumococcal infection. The typical clinical picture is that of a virulent infection. The general condition is markedly impaired. Headache, vomiting, nausea, and confusion may be compounded by conspicuous weakness. The temperature is always elevated and may reach 39.4°–40.2° C. The fever is continuous but may show a septic course in the presence of bacteremia or the formation of pus in the joint. In moderate affection, the joint may be ballooned by an intraarticular effusion. In severe affection, the articular and periarticular tissues are very swollen and tense; the skin is reddened and much warmer, giving the impression of a phlegmon of the joint capsule. The joint is very tender, and its motion is substantially limited.

The number of leukocytes in the blood is increased and may rise in children to 50000/ml. The synovial fluid is turbid, creamy, or frankly purulent. Microscopic and culture examinations disclose the etiology in cases of difficult differential diagnosis. Pneumococci are Gram-positive, oval or lancet-shaped diplococci which in the exudate lie chiefly in pairs or short chains, less often singly. They grow on blood agar in green colonies, similarly to streptococcus viridans. Depending on the composition and antigenicity of their capsular polysaccharides, pneumococci have been classified into many (about 80) types. Their typing is carried out by sera which contain specific antibodies against the individual antigens, and which were also therapeutically used in the preantibiotic era [228]. In view of related antigens in gonococci, cross-reactions by agglutination and complement fixation may occur without gonorrheal complications. Detection and differentiation of the capsular antigens is presently carried out by counter immunoelectrophoresis [437].

Roentgenographic examination of the inflamed joint reveals no specific changes which would point to the presence of a pneumococcal infection. In hydrarthrosis of longer duration, a diffuse osteoporosis develops. In severe infection or empyema, prominence of the trabecular design and areas of osteolysis in the articular epiphyses are prevalent, as well as narrowing with irregular delimitation of the cartilage space (Fig. 98). Regression of the osteoporosis signals the beginning of the healing process.

Depending on the gross-anatomical changes, two types of inflammation may be discerned. One is hydrops (hydrarthrosis), whose inflammatory changes are confined to the innermost part of the joint capsule and are associated with exudation. The articular cavity contains an increased amount of mucinous greenish yellow fluid to which threads of fibrin are admixed. The second type ist empyema (pyarthrosis), in which the articular cavity contains yellowish green pus. The latter may perforate externally or may affect all constituents

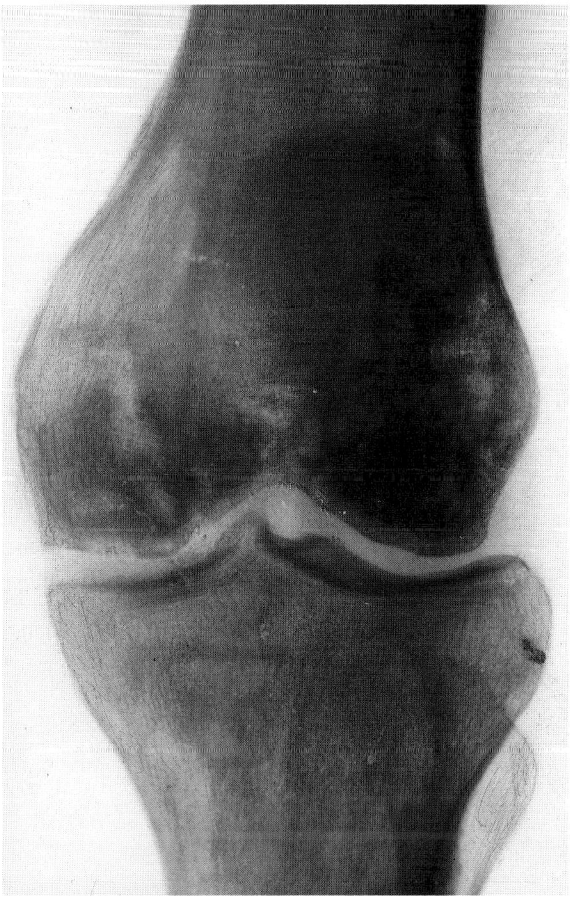

Fig. 98. The femoral condyles present a few areas of circumscribed osteolysis, and the proximal tibial epiphysis presents diffuse osteoporosis. A narrow zone of osteoporosis parallels the articular border of the medial femoral condyle

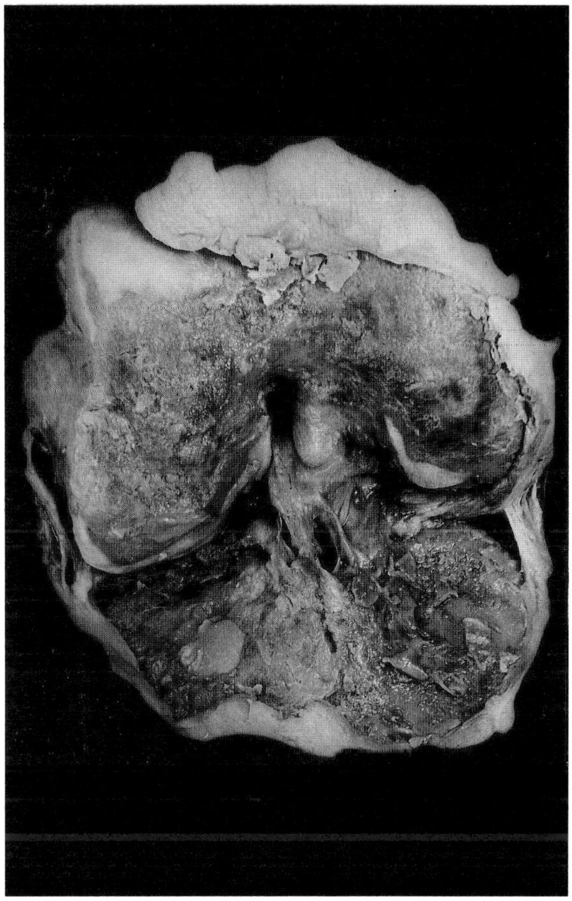

Fig. 99. The articular surfaces of the femoral and tibial condyles are almost entirely bare of their cartilage cover, and these surfaces of the lateral condyles are also deeply eroded

of the joint. Diffuse infiltration of all layers leads to marked thickening of the joint capsule. The periarticular soft tissues also become swollen by edema. The dusky red synovial membrane displays ulcers covered by membranes of fibrin. The hyaline cartilage is disintegrated, denuding the subjacent bone on larger areas (Fig. 99). Ankylosis may subsequently result. However, if the suppuration is stopped at an earlier phase, before the entire articular cartilage is destroyed, secondary osteoarthritic changes gradually develop.

Histopathological examination discloses marked widening and hyperemia of the synovial blood vessels. In some areas, the synoviocyte cover presents defects filled with fibrin precipitates containing leukocytes and diplococci (Fig. 100). The superficial and deeper zones of the synovial membrane are densely infiltrated by polymorphonuclear neutrophilic leukocytes; edema expands into the fibrous capsule. The articular cartilage also displays extensive defects and areas of disintegration of the intercellular matrix. These changes in the articular cartilage are caused by ingression of densely infiltrated synovial tissue (Fig. 101).

Differential diagnosis poses difficulties versus other, etiologically different types of severe joint inflammation, especially when the joint inflammation was not preceded by a pneumonia. In infants and children, several sources of infection and other microorganisms must be considered. In such cases, the etiological agent should be identified by culture of the blood, and by microscopic and culture examination of the joint fluid. Once pneumococcal infection has been confirmed, the type of pneumococcus should be identified. Type III pneumococcus is most often responsible for the joint inflammation.

The treatment of choice is parenteral administration of 10,000,000–20,000,000 U penicillin G daily in divided doses for 10–14 days. The effect is seen in the regression of pain and decrease in the swelling of the joint. In children, ampicillin or other synthetic penicillin 1.5–2.0 g daily is given orally in divided doses. If

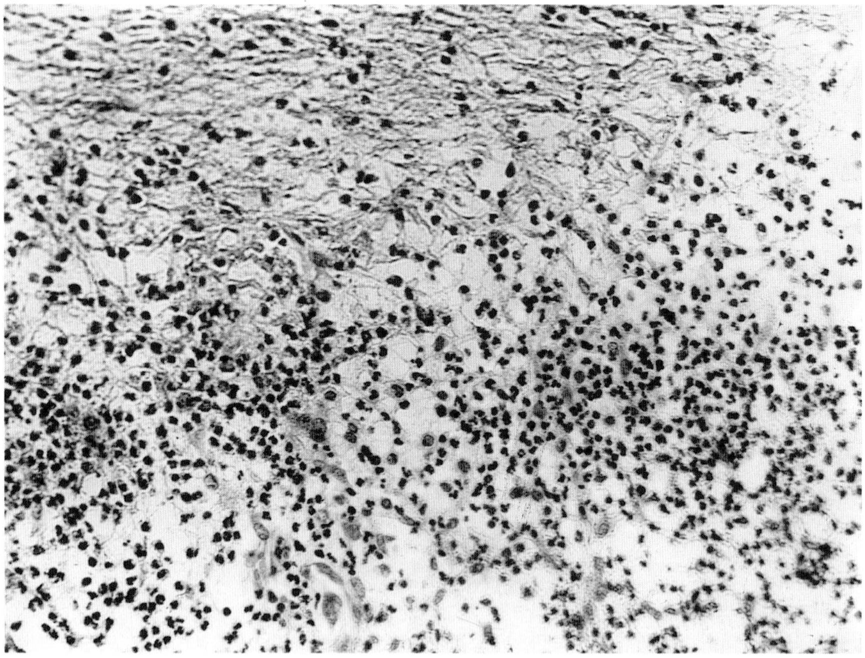

Fig. 100. The synovial membrane, bare of synoviocytes, is covered by a loose fibrin net and is infiltrated by polymorphonuclear leukocytes, histiocytes, and lymphocytes. Among these, diplococci are scattered

penicillin or ampicillin is not effective due to microbial resistance [813] or is not tolerated, erythromycin 2.0–3.0 g, cephalosporin 3.0–4.0 g, tetracycline 2.0–3.0 g, or chloramphenicol 2.0–3.0 g should be given daily in divided doses for 2–3 weeks [813]. The doses of these antibiotics are decreased to one-half in infections of children. Local treatment of the affected joint includes immobilization with a splint or Buck traction and by surrounding it with mildly warm wet compresses.

If suppuration of the joint nevertheless occurs, as evidenced by aspiration of purulent fluid, this fluid should be evacuated at once. The joint is opened by two transcapsular incisions carried out at opposite sites to each other and permitting the insertion of drains. Through the latter, the joint is irrigated twice daily with physiological saline solution followed by penicillin solution containing 10,000 U/ml. The latter, if ineffective, should be substituted by a solution of the antibiot-

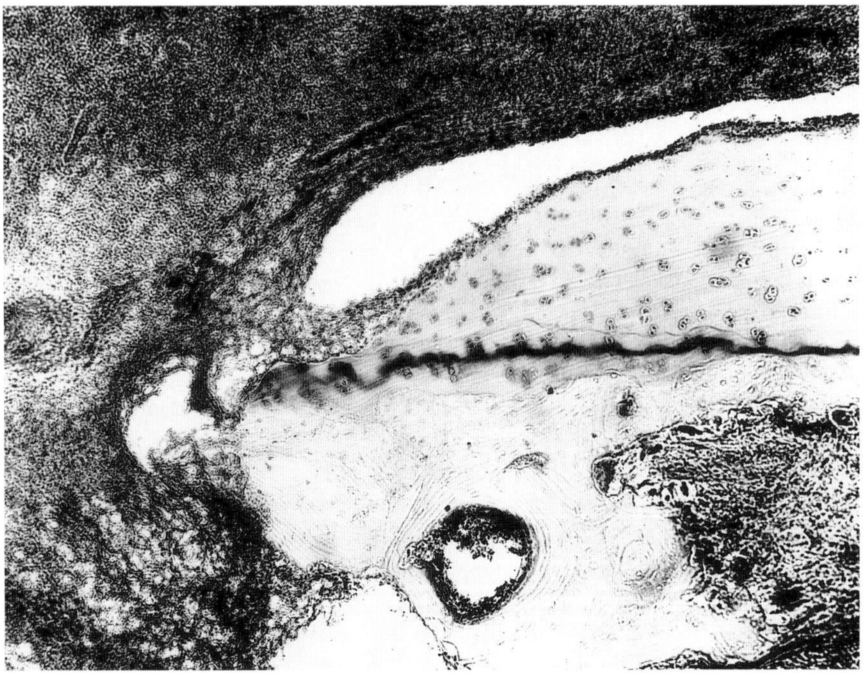

Fig. 101. Loose connective tissue, very densely infiltrated by polymorphonuclear leukocytes and lymphocytes, expands over the articular cartilage and undermines it at the junction with the subchondral bone as well as from the subchondral marrow spaces

is indicated by culture and sensitivity test of the pus. It is important concurrently to observe the general condition of the patient; ample fluid (fruit juices) and vitamin C in high doses are given. Special attention is paid to heart action; digoxin 0.25 mg is administered when irregularity or weakness of the heart supervenes. After drainage from the joint has stopped, and wounds of the joint capsule have closed, mobilization of the joint is started without delay. Active and passive exercises should be instituted. In those rare cases in which the articular cartilage has been extensively destroyed by suppuration, fusion of the articular surfaces and ankylosis of the joint may be the outcome (Fig. 495). In infants the prognosis appears more favorable because even with suppuration the joint heals rather quickly and retains mobility, unless osteomyelitis has set in [290]. However, disturbances in the physiological growth of the articular epiphyses may subsequently appear.

The more serious complications in pneumococcal arthritis include generalized sepsis and heart failure. Timely administration of antibiotics can prevent the transition from the serous to the purulent type of arthritis and thus may essentially improve the prognosis.

4. Gonococcal Arthritis

Arthritis arising as a complication from gonorrhea often confounds by the opinion prevalent among lay persons that this venereal infection is innocuous. Arthritis occurs in 3%–6% of the patients with gonorrhea and represents about 1%–2% of the joint affections in an average population suffering of arthritis. It generally follows in the third week after gonococcal infection, but may sometimes follow closely after the genital inflammation has healed. Penetration of gonococci or their antigens into the blood stream accounts for the associated inflammation of joints, as this inflammation is caused by hematogenous spread. It appears that forceful manipulations in the genital tract, sexual excesses before healing of the gonorrhea, or physical exertions permit such penetration into the blood stream. The ensuing localizations indicate that the gonococci and their toxins have a specific affinity for synovial joints, tendon sheaths, and tendinous insertions into bones. In view of the manifest primary source of infection, the obvious means of propagation, and the clear pathogenesis in the affection of joints, arthritis in gonorrhea may be considered a typical example of specific infectious arthritis.

This arthritis involves principally young adults and usually starts as a very acute, intense inflammation which with regression of intensive symptoms may proceed to the chronic stage. The course is rarely mild or moderate from the very beginning. In this case, several joints are affected in a polyarticular form which shifts from one to another joint until a monoarthritis follows its course. In men the knee joint (Figs. 102, 105), in women the wrist (Fig. 104) and finger joints are predominantly affected. The ankle, elbow, shoulder, and hip joints may also be affected but at a substantially lower frequency [177].

On the basis of the pathological-anatomical changes which determine the clinical picture, three types may be discerned among the manifestations of arthritis in gonorrhea [317, 867, 1042]. The first is arthralgia expressed in subjective soreness without objective changes; probably rapidly subsiding episodes of synovitis account for the symptoms. The pain appears especially on change of weather to cold and may initially be confused with rheumatic pain. However, characteristic for the former condition is the short, stabbing, or lancinating character of *douleur fugitive*, since it alternates between joints or in another region of a joint. The second type is the serous or serofibrinous form [1354], which is manifested by swelling of the joint and intraarticular effusion, persistent pain, and slow progression, but without a tendency to ankylosis. It results ultimately in a chronic thickening of the joint capsule [1354] (Figs. 102, 103). The third type is the densely infiltrative form, which presents a very painful swelling sometimes associated with suppuration. It leads in rapid course to fibrous contracture or to ankylosis of the joint (Fig. 493). A septic, generally toxic state is associated with this type.

The serofibrinous and especially the purulent form of arthritis are very characteristic and pronounced. In a sudden onset, marked swelling and warmth of the joint develop, indicating a virulent inflammation. The pain is severe and continuous and allows the patient neither rest nor sleep. Sometimes steps by another person on the floor of the room or a slight commotion of the bed aggravates the pain to an unbearable degree. The outlines of the joint are blurred by swelling, the doughy edema of the joint capsule is considerable, and the joint fluid is often increased. The surrounding skin is tense, shiny, and sometimes speckled brownish. Any motion is anxiously avoided, and the joint soon assumes a contracture by muscle reflex. Due to the continuous pain and sleepless nights, the general condition of the patient becomes markedly impaired; he sometimes conveys the impression of sepsis. The temperature is elevated to 40°–41° C, but does not have such septic course as in the presence of pyarthrosis. The pulse is accelerated commensurately. Other concomitant extragenital affections in gonorrhea include hemorrhagic petechiae, papules, and ecchymoses in the skin of the chest, abdomen, or extremities (Fig. 102). Tenosynovitis of the extensors of the wrist or of the peronei and extensors of the toes is very frequent [1014]. A rare but

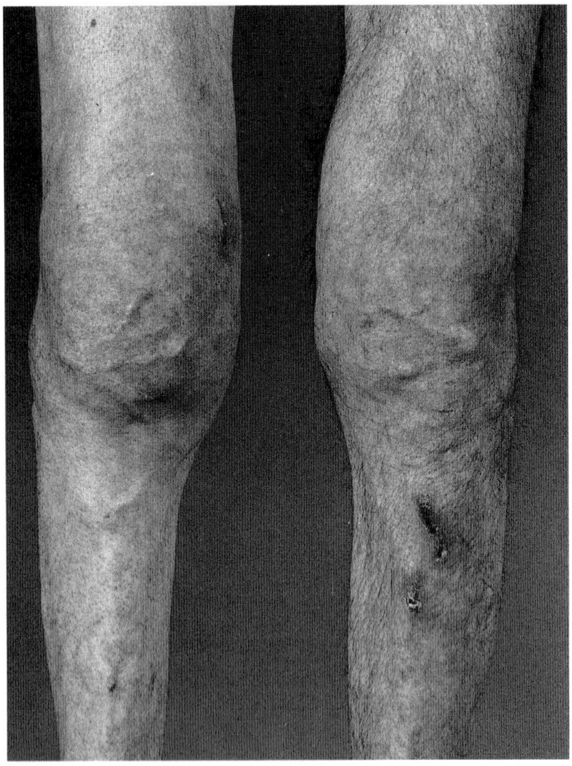

Fig. 102. Chronic thickening of both knee joints secondary to untreated gonorrhea persisting for more than 25 years. Trophic ulcers are present on the anterior aspects of the lower legs

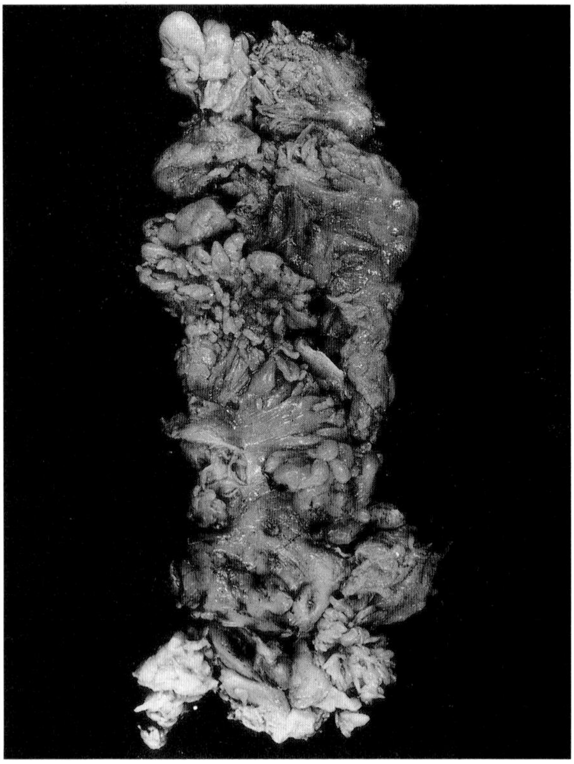

Fig. 103. The inner part of the joint capsule of the patient in Fig. 102 is very thickened and uneven by numerous villous and nodular elevations

rather characteristic affection is inflammation of the plantar fascia and the subsequent formation of a spur on the plantar aspect of the calcaneus in young people. Further dissemination of the gonococci or their toxins may lead to iridocyclitis, pyelonephritis, meningitis, pericarditis, or endocarditis.

Examination of smears of the secretions from urethra, vagina, cervix, prostate, and/or rectum substantially assist in the identification of gonococci and are thus of essential help in ascertaining the etiology of the joint inflammation [392]. This applies chiefly to patients who have had an associated inflammation of the prostate or adnexe [558, 751, 1336]. Gonococci (Fig. 29) are Gram-negative diplococci lying singly or in pairs, with their adjacent sides flattened; their form is that of a kidney or biscuit. Due to their varying shapes gonococci resemble staphylococci, other types of diplococci, or enterococci. The leukocyte count in the blood may be as high as 30000/ml, in which particularly polymorphonuclear leukocytes participate. The sedimentation rate is accelerated to 40–65 mm/h in the acute and subacute phases but declines soon thereafter. The results of blood cultures are positive in only about 10%–14% of cases of mono- or polyarthritis. Neisseria gonorrheae grows only on blood agar under conditions of increased carbon dioxide tension, which ensure optimal pH. In view of the frequently negative outcome of the blood culture, the complement fixation test (Müller-Oppenheim) appears very informative because it is positive in 65%–75% of cases with deep gonococcal infection. The results of the complement fixation reaction are negative in acute genital gonorrhea, become positive within 2–3 weeks after transgression of the gonococci or their toxins into the blood stream, and may be positive even after the inflammatory articular changes have subsided. Serology tests are therefore of use only in cases of longer duration of the infection, which enable the patient to develop the pertinent antibodies. However, deficiencies in the complement system may occur, and these account for the chronicity of the infection [1248] as well as for the occasionally negative outcome of the relevant test. Another possibility for ascertaining active gonococcal infection is the identification of its antigens by polyclonal sera [365]. Diagnostic confirmation can also be obtained by the immunofluorescence technique, which uses heat-treated, strong antigenic and fluorescein-labeled gonococci and exposes them to the presumed antibodies in the patient's serum on a slide. The latter is examined under a fluorescent microscope. Another mo-

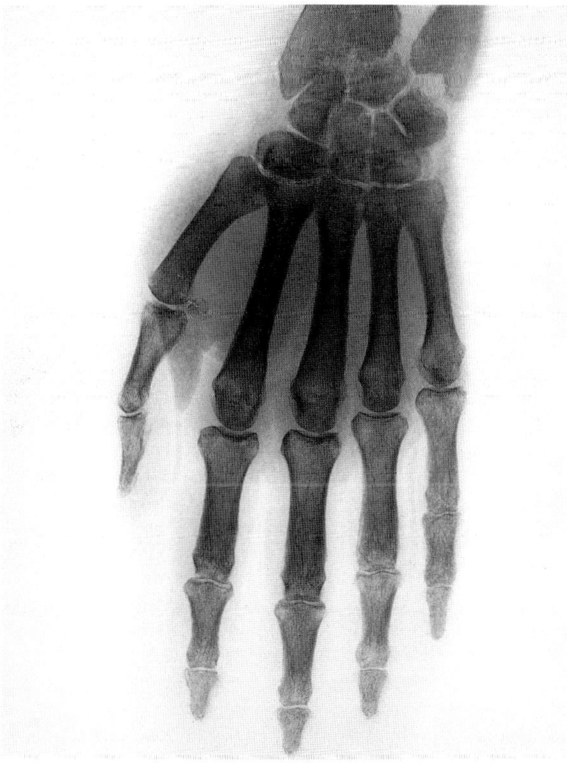

Fig. 104. The articular surfaces of the radiocarpal joint are deeply eroded, and their joint space is widened. The epiphyses are osteoporotic

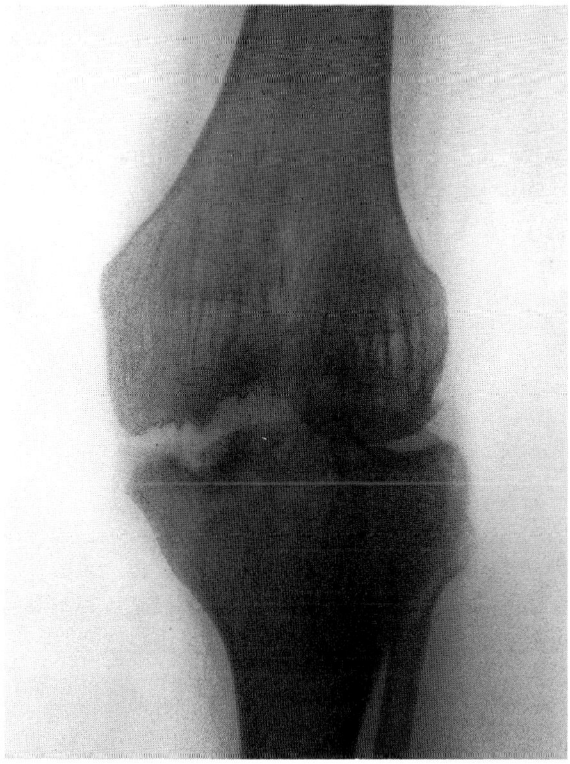

Fig. 105. The articular surfaces of the medial femoral and medial tibial condyle are deeply eroded, and their joint space is widened. The vertical trabecula are very pronounced secondary to extensive osteoporosis

dality endeavors to detect gonococci by treating smears from secretions or from cultures with immune serum labeled with fluorescein isothiocyanate [382].

The synovial fluid is not increased as much as would correspond to the intensity of the inflammatory swelling and amounts only to 30–50 ml. It is yellow, slightly to strongly turbid, contains flaky fibrin admixture, and may sometimes have a purulent character. The number of white blood cells in the synovial fluid is then increased to 20000–90000/ml, with polymorphonuclear neutrophilic leukocytes predominating at 70%–96%, and presenting toxic degenerative forms and vacuolization. Free or intracellular gonococci can only rarely (8%–15%) be identified in the synovial fluid (Fig. 29) by any stain. Ultrastructural examination of the gonococci [627] disclose their cell wall to consist of an outer capsule of protein filaments and a membrane of protein and liposaccharides. Several of these components are of structural and serological differences which may account for the variations of the gonococci in terms of biological behavior, virulence, resistance to the antibodies in normal human sera [466, 1322, 1425], and response to antibiotics. Similarly to that of the blood, examination of the synovial fluid for gonococci by culture rarely yields positive results despite the use of special culture media [177]. On the other hand, results of the complement fixation test with synovial fluid are generally positive (60%–75%). Similarly to serum, the synovial fluid can be tested for the presence of gonococcal antibodies by the immunofluorescence technique.

Roentgenographic examination reveals, in the beginning phase, swelling of the soft tissues and widening of the cartilage space. In the 3rd week of articular affection, a glassy osteoporosis appears which is confined to the articular epiphyses; the extraarticular bone has a normal structure. On aggravation of the articular affection, the cartilage space becomes narrowed, and the subchondral calcification line subsequently becomes irregular and indented (Figs. 104, 105). On advancing fibrous union, the cartilage space becomes abolished. Since the regional osteoporosis has not yet subsided in this phase, the vertical, mechanically stressed trabeculae come more clearly into evidence and simulate the pattern of a rain stream (Fig. 105). When osseous fusion is fully established, the cancellous trabeculae pass in continuity from one to the contiguous articular epiphysis (Fig. 493). However, if neither

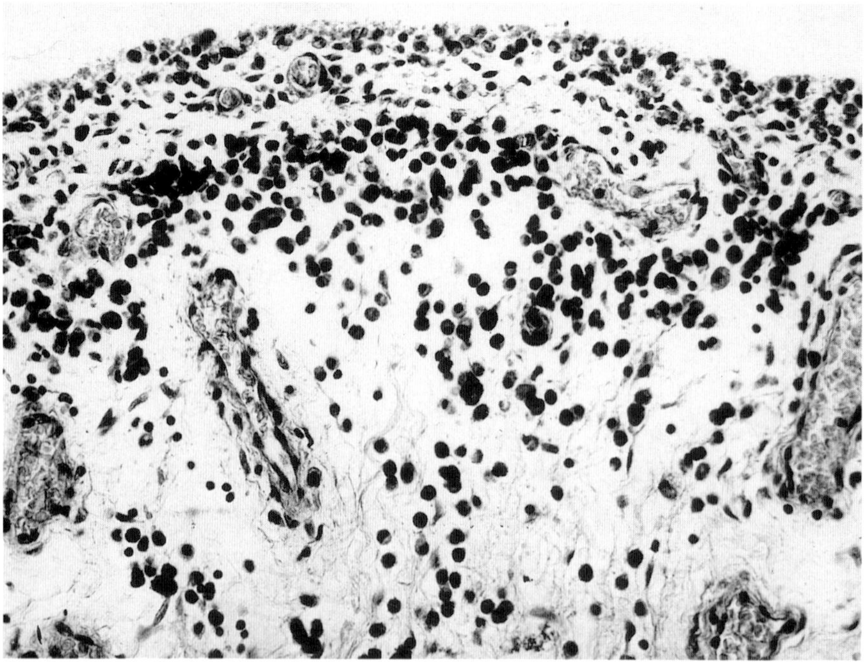

Fig. 106. The synovial membrane in acute gonorrhoic arthritis is extensively rarefied by edema. All blood vessels are hyperemic, and those beneath the surface are surrounded by plasmacytes. Small agglomerations of plasmacytes are also scattered in the deeper subsynoviocytic tissue

type of ankylosis ensues, the eroded articular surfaces eventually develop the uneveness and marginal osteophytes of secondary osteoarthritis.

Gross-anatomical examination discloses intensive redness and gelatinous swelling of the joint capsule, which may extend beyond its inner part to the fibrous part and the periarticular structures. The synovial membrane proliferates and forms numerous moderate-sized villi and small nodules (Fig. 103) which often expand as pannus over the articular cartilage. The latter lacks its smooth, glistening surface and disintegrates, leaving extensive, irregularly delimited defects. When the effusion is purulent, the cartilage rapidly melts away. The proliferating synovial membrane completely fills the joint cavity and connects the contiguous articular epiphyses. Joint inflammation by gonococci or their toxins is characterized by the formation of extensive granulation tissue and rapid dissolution of the articular cartilage. The outer joint capsule becomes densified by fibrosis, and secondary to its shrinking the joint assumes a faulty position. When fibrous ankylosis has affected the greater extent of the joint cavity, osseous ankylosis often follows by metaplasia of the intraarticular syndesmosis.

Histopathological examination discloses marked hyperemia of the synovial membrane with distension of its blood vessels and extensive edema (Fig. 106). In the very early phase focal agglomerations of polymorphonuclear neutrophilic leukocytes predominate; these and the fibrin precipitates on the synovial cover occasionally contain gonococci. Subsequently the agglomerations expand and are composed of a significantly greater proportion of plasmacytes and a small proportion of lymphocytes (Fig. 106). Such changes in the synovial membrane persist on a large extent (Fig. 107) in those chronic cases in which no destruction of the articular cartilage follows. In most other cases, extensive areas in the synovial cover disintegrate by necrosis and are substituted by organized fibrin and granulation tissue, which comprises fibroblasts, capillaries, and plasmacytes. In a few places, proliferations of the synovial membrane encroach upon the articular cartilage. In the latter, probably due to the action of proteolytic enzymes released from the gonococci and hypertrophic synoviocytes, chondrocytes become necrotic, as manifested in fragmentation and dissolution of their nuclei. Their intercellular material vanishes, and portions of the cartilage disintegrate. The decomposition of the cartilage leaves widening areas of expansion to the intruding synovial pannus. Eventually, opposite articular epiphyses become fused, with the occasional interposition of a strip of connective tissue (Fig. 496), in which a few islands of hyaline cartilage persist.

Differential diagnosis may present much difficulty if the soreness of the joint is mild, and if the results of stained smears of the urethral secretion and joint fluid as well as those of the cultures of blood and joint fluid are negative. Arthritis in acute rheumatic fever, a bout of gout, or an acute phase of any septic arthritis may present a similar clinical picture [1159]. In view of the urethral inflammation associated with peripheral arthritis, among others, Reiter's syndrome must not be disregarded. Therefore, a thorough search for gono-

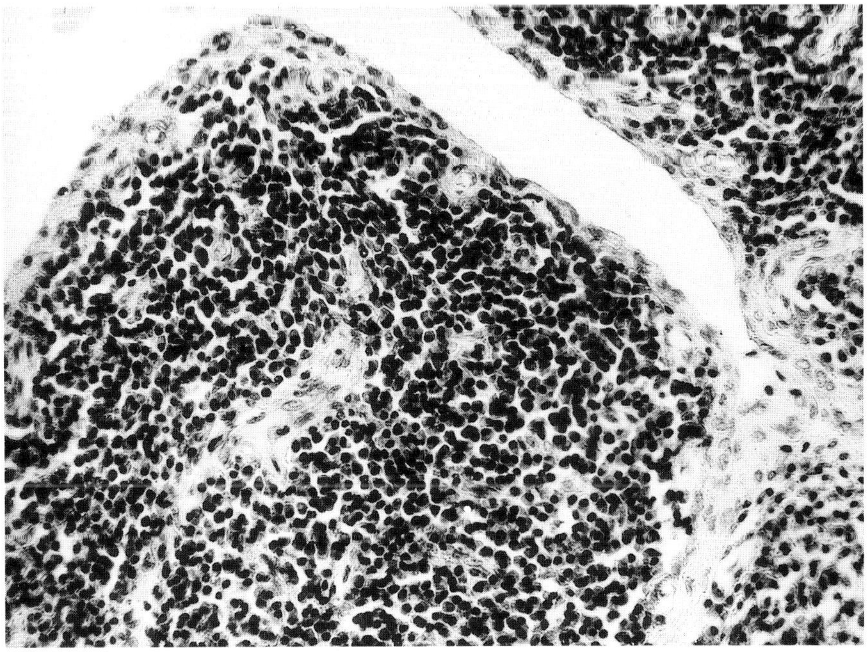

Fig. 107. The synovial membrane in long-lasting gonorrhea (Fig. 102) is elevated in broad villi and is extensively and densely infiltated chiefly by plasmacytes

cocci by repeated examinations of urethral and rectal secretions, of expressed prostrate secretion, or of smears of premenstrual vaginal discharges is necessary. Eventually the outcome of the complement fixation test for gonococcal antibodies succeeds in clarifying the etiology. The clinical picture and the determination of etiology become especially complicated when the gonorrhea is associated with syphilis.

In view of the absence of gonococci from the blood and joint fluid in a significant percentage of the microscopic and culture examinations, even with marked inflammatory articular signs, it appears that the joint inflammations are elicited not directly by the gonococci but by their potent antigenic substances spread by the bloodstream into the joints. The ensuing inflammatory changes in the joints and other organs are the outcome of a reaction determined by the emanating antigen and the available or absent antibodies in the human body. The serological tests presently in use for extragenital complications in gonorrhea attest to this concept [1385].

Once the presence of a gonococcal infection has been ascertained, the source of infection must be eradicated. After obtaining smears from the genital tract and submitting them to culture and sensitivity tests, the treatment should be instituted immediately by giving 1,500,000 U penicillin G regularly and parenterally every 3 h. If parenteral administration is not possible, ampicillin 0.5–1.0 g should be given orally every 3 h. This treatment should be continued for 10–14 days unless sensitivity tests disclose (as is presently increasingly the case) resistance against penicillin [1329]. The medication should then be shifted to an alternative antibiotic, which is continued for 10–14 days further after the clinical signs of active infection of the genital tract and those of inflammation of the joint have completely subsided [721]. Effective antibiotics include tetracycline 250–500 mg, erythromycin 300–600 mg, or cephalosporin 500–750 mg given every 3–4 h. In unreliable patients, hospitalization and parenteral administration of the indicated antibiotic is advisable.

Concurrently with the medicamentous treatment, the involved joints should be surrounded with moist warm packs and be immobilized with a splint of metal or plastic material to eliminate movements. Potent analgesics are necessary at the beginning of treatment. Daily sessions with shortwave diathermy may be beneficial since the gonococci are very sensitive to heat. If the joint nevertheless becomes more swollen, and the joint fluid increases, the latter should be aspirated. Furthermore, if the joint fluid turns purulent, a bilateral incision into this joint is necessary without delay to ensure quick and general evacuation of the pus. This may forestall necrosis of the hyaline cartilage. Through the intraarticularly positioned drains the joint is irrigated two or three times daily with physiological saline solution and thereafter with the indicated antibiotic. These procedures are continued until clearance of the joint fluid and regression of the acute inflammatory signs.

In addition to the general etiological and local symptomatic measures, the management is guided by the attempt to prevent adhesions in the inflamed joint. Immediately after regression of the acute symptoms, mobilization of the joint is instituted by active and passive exercises, carried out preferentially in a warm bath or with moist warm compresses surrounding the joint. The exercises are carried out to the final degrees of excursion despite the arising pain and require analgesics, energy, and will power. If fibrous adhesions develop nevertheless, they can be disrupted by forced manipulation (Figs. 488, 489) under general anesthesia. In extreme cases of osseous ankylosis (Fig. 493), mobility of the joint can be restored by arthroplasty, as described for each joint in "Rheumatoid Arthritis", "Osteoarthritis", and „Ankylosis of Joints". This operation may be undertaken only after all relevant examinations ascertain the complete healing of the inflammatory process; it appears very promising in cases without initial purulent involvement of the bony ends. Regardless of the modality of plastic procedure which is used, the end result also depends here on the determination and cooperation of the patient.

5. Arthritis in Reiter's Syndrome

Reiter [1315] originally described a type of arthritis associated with urethritis and conjunctivitis and preceded by diarrhea. Clarification has since been added to the clinical aspects of this disease [510, 1483] but its etiology has still not been fully elucidated. Since Reiter's syndrome may be preceded by diarrhea, the cases of arthritis following enteritis caused by Shigella, Salmonella or Yersinia should be discussed as separate entities in view of their differing bacteriological findings. The same exclusion applies to arthritis following gonococcal infection, especially in view of its different clinical picture, treatment, and prognosis. Thus, in accordance with Wilkens et al. [1758], the diagnosis of Reiter's syndrome should be confined to arthritis of more than 1 month duration, and following a nonspecific urethritis and/or cervicitis.

The complete picture of the syndrome [213, 351, 1472, 1787] develops 3–4 weeks after inflammation of the primary organ, the urethra, with associated prostatitis or cervicitis and mucopurulent abacterial discharge secondary to sexual contact. The most affected joint is the knee; with less frequency follow the ankle, foot, hip, elbow, shoulder, and wrist joints. Affection of the lumbosacral spine, less frequent than that of the knee joint, may be more frequent than that of the other peripheral joints. A conspicuous feature here is the fact that men are involved substantially more often than women; this proportion has changed in the past two decades. Marked impairment in the general condition with high fever characterizes the onset of arthritis, especially if it starts polyarticularly. Eventually it becomes pauciarticular or monoarticular. The affection of the peripheral joints is usually asymmetrical. It manifests itself either as arthralgia with moderate, diffuse tenderness and a duration of 3–4 weeks or as arthritis with distinct capsular swelling (Fig. 108), increased local warmth, persistent ache or pain, and occasional moderate effusion lasting several months to a few years. Nevertheless, the possibility of full recovery of the joint function exists as long as the articular cartilage does not become affected, and substantial narrowing of the joint space does not ensue. Otherwise, secondary osteoarthritis and painful movements are the outcome. Similar problems result in the peripheral joints if the joint capsule and periarticular structures shrink, and a contracture with limitation of motion develops. Affection of the joints of the vertebral column, usually confined to its lumbosacral segment, causes frequent discomfort, especially at the start of motion. Circumscribed tenderness and gradually increasing stiffness sometimes lead to complete loss of motion in this area, yet without neurological symptoms. Affection of the sacroiliac joints is sometimes more painful than that of the lumbosacral spine [1197]. Other symptoms may be tenderness at the insertion of the paravertebral lumbosacral musculature into the vertebrae and tenderness at the insertion of the Achilles tendon and/or plantar fascia into the calcaneus.

Secondary to the urethritis and its associated discharge, inflammation of the glans penis often follows with small, confluent vesicles of balanitis. Lesions of hyperkeratosis (keratodermia blenorrhagica), resembling the pustular lesions of psoriasis, may develop on the palms and soles. Masses of yellow, waxy hyperkeratotic material may accumulate under the nails and lead to their separation [1730]. The skin of the trunk and extremities sometimes presents extensive areas of inflammatory lesions, with macules and papules which eventually result in hyperkeratosis (Fig. 108). Shallow ulcers surrounded by a hyperemic border may be observed in the mucosa of the lips, tongue, and oral cavity, but these are of short duration. Completing the clinical picture, inflammation of the eyes may occur; the conjunctivitis is usually mild and may be associated with iritis, uveitis, or keratitis [259].

Laboratory examinations disclose a moderate leukocytosis (12000–20000/ml in the blood, and increase in the sedimentation rate to 60 mm/h as long as the joint disease is active. Results of tests for rheumatoid factor are false positive in 8%–12% of patients. The presence of the histocompatibility antigen HLA-B27 is observed in about 60%–70% of patients with Reiter's syndrome [188]. This finding must not necessarily be interpreted as the causative factor for development of arthritis in Reiter's syndrome, especially since it is often observed in healthy members of the patient's family [951, 1804], being transmitted by inheritance. Nevertheless, the presence of the HLA-B27 antigen

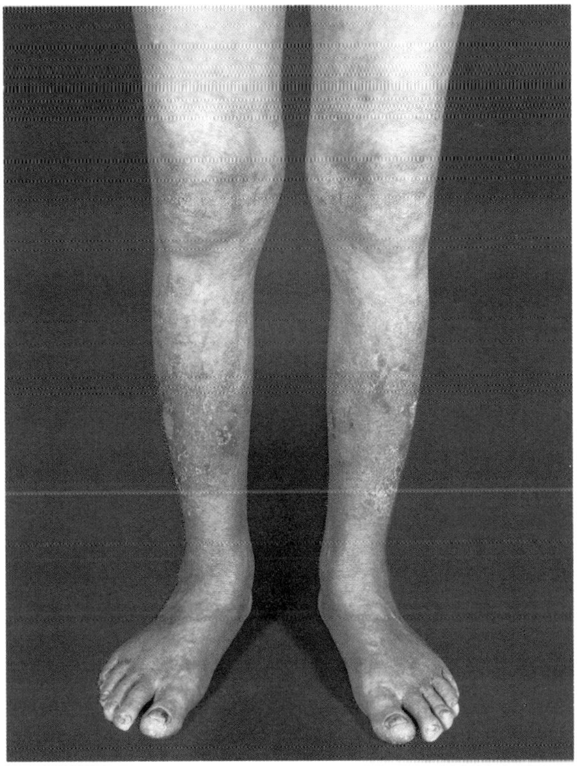

Fig. 108. The knee joints are moderately thickened chiefly in the suprapatellar area. The skin of the lower legs presents extensive areas with macules, papules, and hyperkeratosis. Also ulcers and scars secondary to ulcers are present

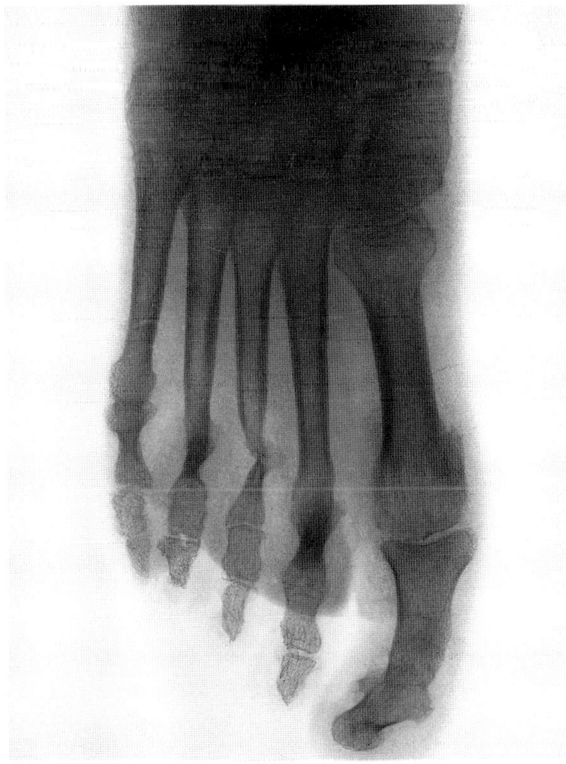

Fig. 109. The third and fourth metatarsal bones are sharpened pencil-like

indicates the influence of a genetic factor, which determines the susceptibility and response of mesodermal tissues to some infectious agents. Herefrom results the manifestation of a disease process. In this way the rather great incidence (30%–40%) of partly ankylosing spondylitis and/or sacroiliac arthritis in patients with Reiter's syndrome may be related to the concurrent findings of HLA-B27 [956, 1347, 1348, 1433]. The synovial fluid is moderately increased to 30–70 ml, slightly turbid, less viscous, and contains 3000–14000/ml white blood cells with 50%–60% polymorphonuclear neutrophilic leukocytes. The smear of the urethral secretion displays abundant polymorphonuclear neutrophilic leukocytes but no microorganisms.

Extensive studies have been undertaken [419, 1483, 1730] to ascertain a possible bacteriological etiology of the arthritis but have failed to provide unequivocal proof. However, two types of inclusion bodies have been observed [83] in the cells of the synovial fluid. One type are large inclusion bodies stemming from leukocytes phagocytosed in macrophages, and the other type are small inclusion bodies most probably corresponding to phagocytosed viruses. The latter have been termed pleuro-pneumonia-like-organisms (PPLO) and were isolated by Amor et al. [33] and Dienes et al. [419] from the synovial fluid of joints affected in Reiter's syndrome. Other authors [1234, 1400, 1472] have confirmed this finding. Schirmer et al. [1409] conclude that these inclusion bodies belong to the group of psyttacosis-lymphogranuloma-trachoma viruses. However, the examinations by Claus et al. [297] disclosed the presence of PPLO in only a small percentage of their specimens of synovial fluid and synovial tissue, but no viruses. Therefore, the participation of these microorganisms in the etiology of Reiter's syndrome appears doubtful. Nevertheless, Pekin et al. [1234] found high levels of hemolytic complements in the synovial fluid of these joints, probably reflecting the intensive inflammation occurring in these joints. Accordingly, the presence of significantly increased immunoglobulins [64] and complement proteins indicates that immunological reactions account for the pathogenesis of Reiter's syndrome [884, 1348, 1799].

Roentgenographs of the peripheral joints reveal [1037, 1045] thickening of the joint capsule, widening of the cartilage space due to effusion, and juxtarticular osteoporosis in the beginning stage. However, on aggravation of the joint disease and involvement of the articular cartilage, this space becomes narrowed, and the articular ends are irregularly delimited (Fig. 110).

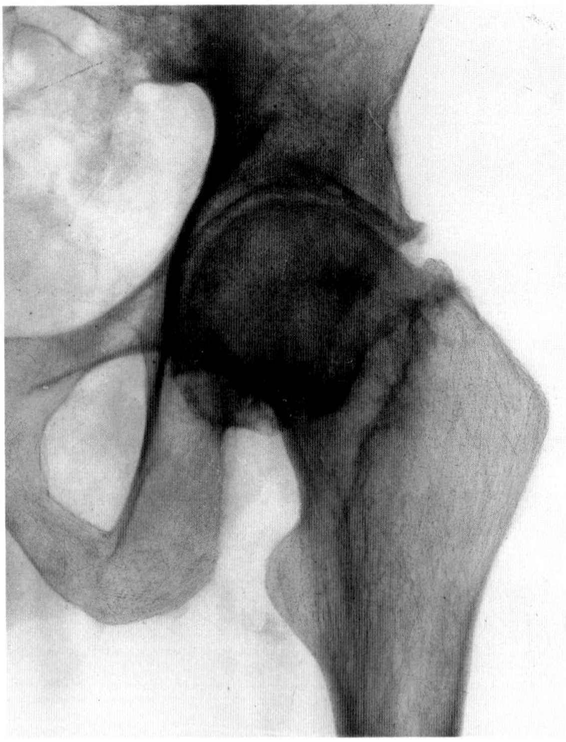

Fig. 110. The cartilage space of the hip joint is narrowed and is irregularly delimited due to erosions chiefly in the outline of the femoral head. Marginal osteophytes have formed

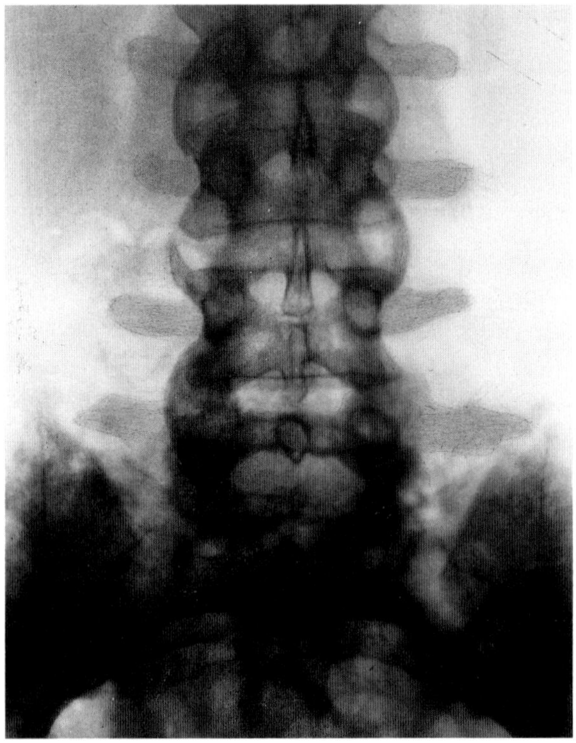

Fig. 111. The sacroiliac joints are very narrowed by the sclerosed iliac bones. The vertebral bodies T12 to S1 are fused by marginal osseous bridges

On further erosion of the latter, faulty alignment in the joints follows. Concurrently, thin periosteal appositions secondary to periostitis may sometimes be noticed in the metaphyseal cortex close to the joint capsule of the knee, elbow, hip, and/or ankle. Similar thin periosteal appositions may occur on the diaphyses of the phalanges, metacarpals, and metatarsals, with the latter sometimes also undergoing a pencillike sharpening (Fig. 109). On the other hand, bone formation is sometimes observed in the insertional portions of the Achilles tendon and the plantar fascia onto the calcaneus. In a great number of patients, the sacroiliac joints are irregularly delineated, being partly narrowed and partly widened. The structure of the adjacent epiphyses, chiefly in the iliac bone, is very uneven by large areas of density (Fig. 111). The lumbar vertebrae are connected in some places by ossified longitudinal ligaments which bridge the intervertebral spaces. In other cases, large marginal osteophytes expand from the vertebral plates to the adjacent vertebrae and thereby form almost complete connections [302] (Fig. 111).

Histopathological examination [322, 1194, 1543] of the synovial membrane discloses marked hyperemia with distension of all blood vessels and extensive edema. Some of the hypertrophic synoviocytes and subsynoviocytic histiocytes contain granular inclusions. Numerous focal agglomerations – initially composed predominantly of polymorphonuclear neutrophilic leukocytes and subsequently of plasmacytes, lymphocytes, and histiocytes – are dispersed in the subsynoviocytic tissue. These infiltrates decrease in the chronic stage, when fibrocytes increase substantially and occupy the subsynoviocytic zone (Fig. 112). While in some places of the latter granulation tissue has developed by the proliferation of fibroblasts and the advancing of small blood vessels, in numerous other places dense fibrosis accounts for the thickening of the joint capsule. Examinations for immunoprotein deposition [43] indicate that an immunobiological process has taken here place. Secondary to hypertrophy and hyperplasia of the synoviocytes, villi of moderate size form (Fig. 112) and encroach from the margin on the articular cartilage. The latter then undergoes dissolution in large areas, where the subchondral bone becomes covered by granulation tissue. In other areas, the articular surface becomes partly denuded. On the following sclerosis and uneveness of the articular surfaces, marginal osteophytes of moderate size are formed.

Differential diagnosis must include rheumatoid arthritis, arthritis in gonorrhea, arthritis in psoriasis, as well as arthritis in specific or nonspecific inflamma-

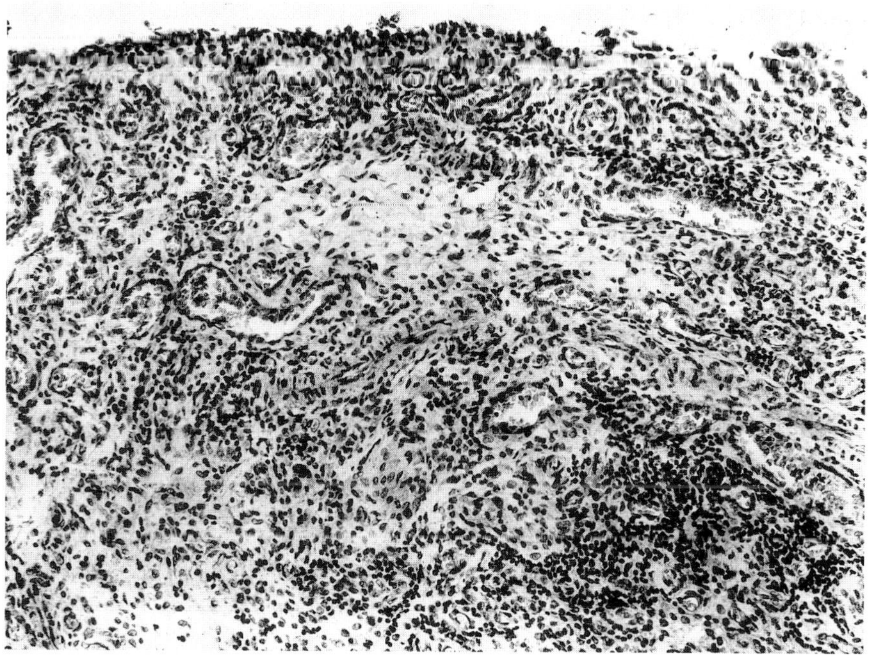

Fig. 112. Moderately hypertrophic synoviocytes form small villi. The subsynoviocytic tissue is moderately hypercellular with fibrocytes and fibroblasts and comprises small perivascular and focal agglomerations of lymphocytes

tions of the intestine, such as in dysentery, abdominal typhoid, and ulcerative colitis. Metaphyseal periosteal appositions on the long bones of the extremities are also observed very often in syphilitic arthritis.

Since no specific etiological agent has yet been identified, no specific treatment can be administered. However, tetracycline 1.0–2.0 g or erythromycin 2.0–4.0 g daily given in divided doses over the course of 4–6 weeks appears to be an effective medication, especially in the acute phase. This benefits the affected joints as well as the urethral and/or intestinal inflammation. Subsequently, salicylates 2.0–3.0 g daily are given, leading to moderate symptomatic relief. Similar results are provided by nonsteroidal antiinflammatory medications. Phenylbutazone 100 mg two or three times daily given for 2–3 weeks decreases the swelling and improves the mobility of the joints. However, periodic blood studies with leukocyte count are necessary here in view of the potential depression of the bone marrow. Even greater precaution must be given to the cytotoxic drugs (methotrexate 4–6 mg daily for 5 days and repeated after 4 weeks; cyclophosphamide 50–100 mg daily for 1 week and repeated after 3–4 weeks). Their results are not superior to the above medications, but the potential complications (pernicious anemia, granulocytopenia, thrombocytopenia) are much more serious [493]. Concurrently, moist hot packs should be applied regularly to the affected joints of the extremities and axial skeleton. Similarly, physical therapy with shortwave diathermy in two series of eight sessions is of benefit in the subacute phase [944, 1613], whereas ultrasound at 2.5–3 W/cm^2 in one or two series is indicated for the chronic phase [687, 1541]. Splinting of the peripheral joints is very beneficial for prevention of deformities. Support for the lumbosacral spine by a firm, high lumbosacral belt with metal stays (Fig. 51); is indispensable especially in the stage of early painful inflammation. In the case of established deformity of a peripheral joint with contracture, a correction can be obtained by synovectomy, possibly combined with tenotomies, and followed by a protective splint. Total arthroplasty with insertion of arthroplastic components, as discussed in "Osteoarthritis", may be indicated in advanced secondary osteoarthritis of the hip or knee joints. Arthrodesis appears indicated more in secondary osteoarthritis of the ankle joint. Nevertheless, the general prognosis is guarded in the situation of multiple joint affections [218, 533, 1387].

6. Arthritis in Bacillary Dysentery

Arthritis concomitant with bacillary dysentery was first reported by Sydenham in 1672 [657]. The causative Shigella is a Gram-negative, nonmotile plump rod, from whose large family the Shiga-Kruse and the Flexner-Noguchi strains generally account for the intestinal and articular infections. The general condition of the patient is poor. especially in infection with the Shiga-Kruse strain; the pulse is rapid and easily compressible. Stupor alternates with confusion. The intestinal disease may present itself under a moderate clinical picture with gastrointestinal discomfort and a few diarrheic stools. However, more often it begins directly as a severe condition with intense abdominal pain, prostration, marked weakness, and numerous bloody stools sometimes mixed with pus. The temperature is elevated to 40°–41.2° C and is of irregular but not septic course. The spleen is not enlarged. The strength decreases, and septic shock may lead to death.

Inflammation of joints occurs in 4%–6% of cases with bacillary dysentery. Various forms of arthritis may be observed, especially during periods of epidemics. Schittenhelm et al. [1411] emphasized that the frequency of joint affections is in inverse proportion to the seriousness of the intestinal infection. Bacterial toxins, resorbed through the intestinal wall, are spread with the bloodstream and affect serous membranes and joints. This ellcits a reaction of the synovial membrane. The dysenteric joint complication develops as so-called dysenteric rheumatoid 1–2 weeks after onset of the intestinal infection, but it may also appear during convalescence between the 6th and 12th weeks. Concurrently, conjunctivitis, iridocyclitis, urethritis, pleuresy, and very painful neuritis may develop.

The usually monoarticular or pauciarticular manifestation [647, 975, 1500] ranges from arthralgia without clinical findings to serous arthritic inflammation. In the latter condition, the outlines of the joint are blurred by swelling of the soft tissues and by intraarticular effusion. In very rare situations septic arthritis may set in due to direct invasion of the joint by the bacilli, facilitated by concurrent chronic illness such as diabetes, anemia, leukemia, or liver disease. The local temperature is then elevated, and the entire joint is diffusely very tender. With increasing enlargement and soreness of the joint, the regional musculature becomes contracted, and the motion of the joint is concentrically limited.

Examination of the blood discloses an increase of the hematocrit resulting from chronic dehydration. The sedimentation rate is invariably elevated to 60–85 mm/h. Results of the agglutination test for Shiga-Kruse or Flexner-Noguchi strain become positive toward the end of the 1st week, but are considered to confirm infection only at a dilution above 1:128. The concentration of serum complement is increased. The pinkish colored joint fluid is clear and mucinous and has a high titer of agglutinins but does not contain bacilli in smear or culture unless septic arthritis sets in. It then also contains a significantly high number (30000–50000/ml) of polymorphonuclear neutrophilic leukocytes. The diagnosis may be confirmed by the presence of the microorganisms in mucus flakes from the intestine and in the feces. The Shiga-Kruse and Flexner-Noguchi strains can be distinguished from each other by their different ability of fermentation and acidification on lactose agar culture media.

Roentgenographic examination reveals no pathological findings since the inflammation of the joint capsule usually subsides before bony changes would set in.

Gross-anatomical examination discloses accumulation of serous-hemorrhagic fluid in the joint cavity. The inner part of the joint capsule is very reddened and swollen in a jellylike way; these changes may extend

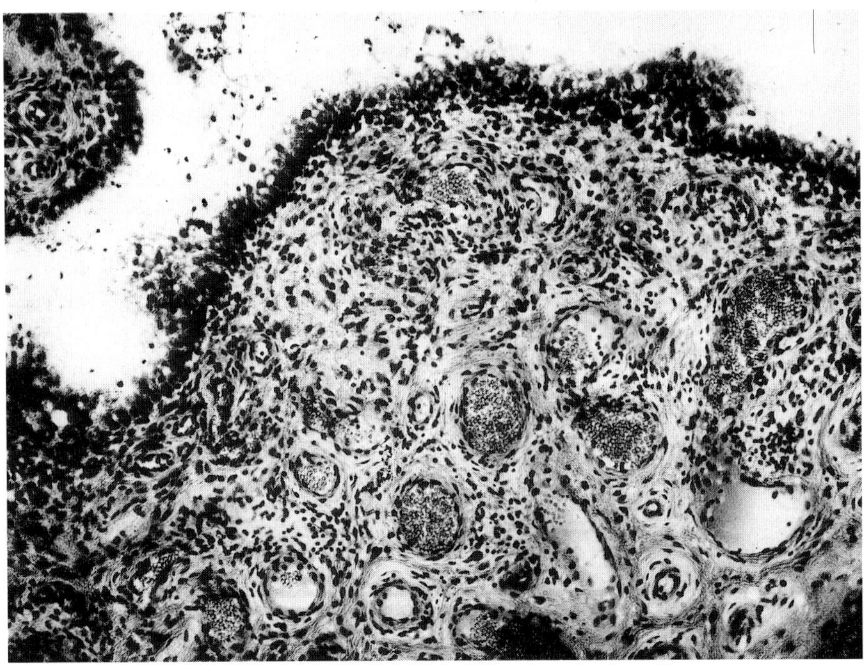

Fig. 113. The synoviocytes are moderately hypertrophic and markedly hyperplastic. The subsynoviocytic tissue is also hypercellular with fibrocytes, fibroblasts, and histiocytes and contains small agglomerations of lymphocytes. All blood vessels are dilated and hyperemic

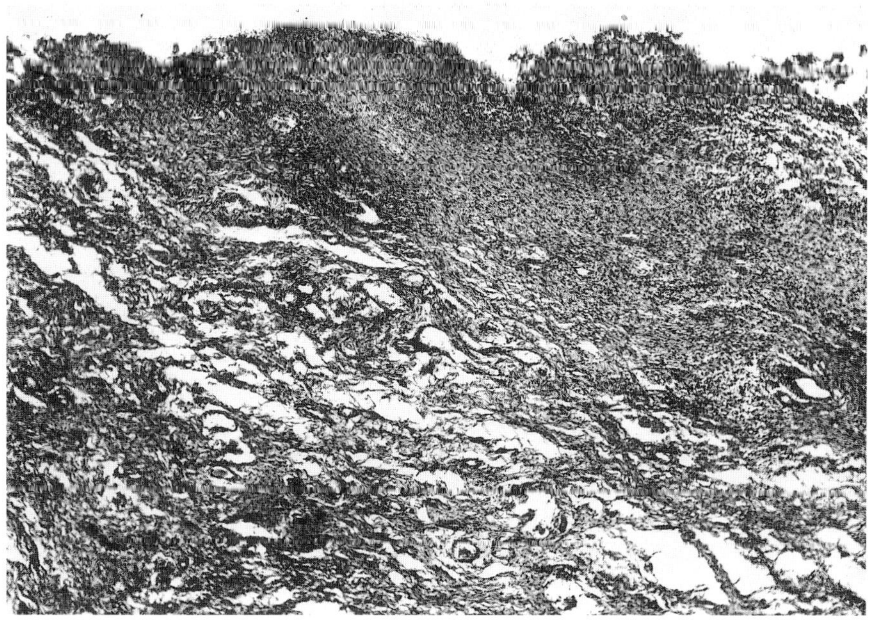

Fig. 114. The synovial membrane is very densified by hyperplasia of the synoviocytes, a marked increase in subsynoviocytic fibrocytes, and a substantial increase in the collagen fibers

into the periarticular tissues. Neither suppuration of the joint capsule nor destruction of the articular cartilage are observed.

Microscopic examination discloses edema of the synovial membrane which is diffusely but moderately infiltrated by lymphocytes. All blood vessels are engorged (Fig. 113). Numerous erythrocytes and leukocytes have emerged on the surface of the synovial membrane. With longer duration of the inflammation the edema and the infiltrates regress; the fibrocytes increase substantially. Fibrosis of the joint capsule results (Fig. 114).

Differential diagnosis must consider acute arthritis in rheumatic fever, gonococcal arthritis, typhoid arthritis, and arthritis of Reiter's syndrome. The absence of changes of the heart, refractory attitude to salicylate medication, absence of a genital infection or enlargement of the spleen, positive outcome of specific agglutination tests in the blood and joint fluid and bacteriological examination of the stool in view of the pronounced intestinal symptoms help to clarify the etiology of the arthritis in bacillary dysentry.

In the general treatment, prophylactic measures are very necessary during epidemic periods. The consumption of boiled water and carefully cleansed food contributes to the prevention of infection. Of similar benefit are the identification and treatment of the microbe carriers. In fully developed dysentery, sulfaguanidin or sulfanilamide 4.0–6.0 g daily in divided doses is administered until subsidence of the intestinal symptoms. Among antibiotics, ampicillin 3.0–4.0 g or tetracycline 1.5–2.0 g daily given in divided doses is indicated for 2–3 weeks. However, their efficacy is not always secure in view of the spread of Shigella resistant strains to antibiotics [289]. In such situations sulfamethoxazole 4.0–6.0 g daily for 2 weeks provides healing. Supportive measures by ample supply of fluids and vitamin C are a prime necessity. In severe dehydration, the parenteral supply of fluids and electrolytes is urgently needed. The food is bland and rich in protein and carbohydrates. Spasmolytics and charcoal are very helpful against the intestinal spasms.

Local treatment consists of moist warm compresses applied regularly around the affected joint, which is also immobilized with a splint or compressed with a strapping. When the acute soreness regresses, shortwave diathermy is administered in eight to ten sessions. On restoration of function, an elastic bandage is applied around the joint throughout the day. If sensitivity of the joint persists after subsidence of its inflammation, the application of hot mud packs or treatment in a balneo-therapeutic station prove very helpful for suppression of the symptoms.

Since dysenteric affection of the joints does not generally show a tendency for suppuration or destruction, subsidence of the inflammatory articular changes is the usual outcome upon application of all modalities of treatment, provided that no general, life-endangering complication supervenes.

7. Arthritis in Abdominal Typhoid Fever and Abdominal Paratyphoid Fever

Abdominal typhoid fever is a widespread disease caused by ingestion of water, milk, or food contami-

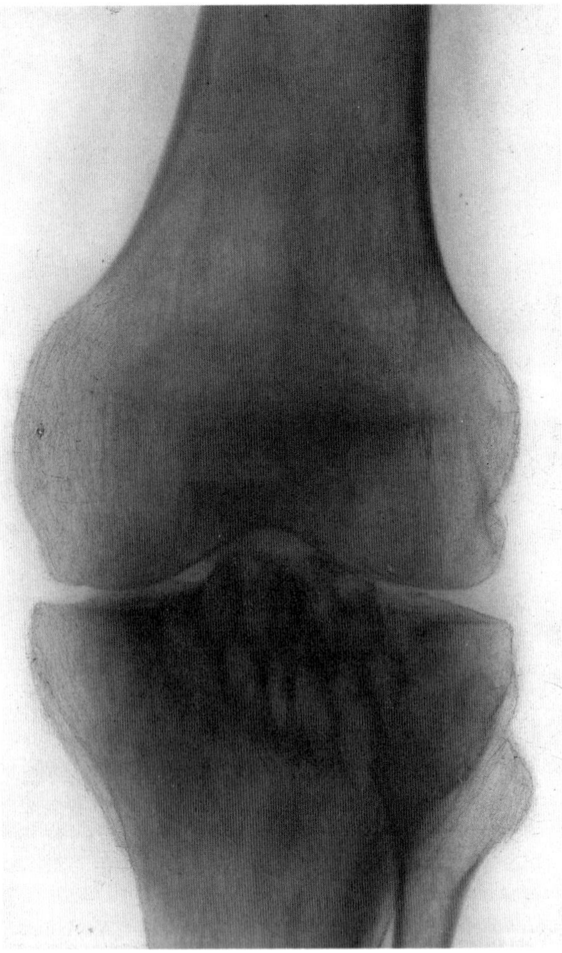

Fig. 115. The tibial epiphysis presents several areas of osteoporosis surrounded by marked densification of the bone. Some of these areas expand into the joint space, which is hereby irregularly delimited and narrowed. This epiphysis also presents periosteal apposition

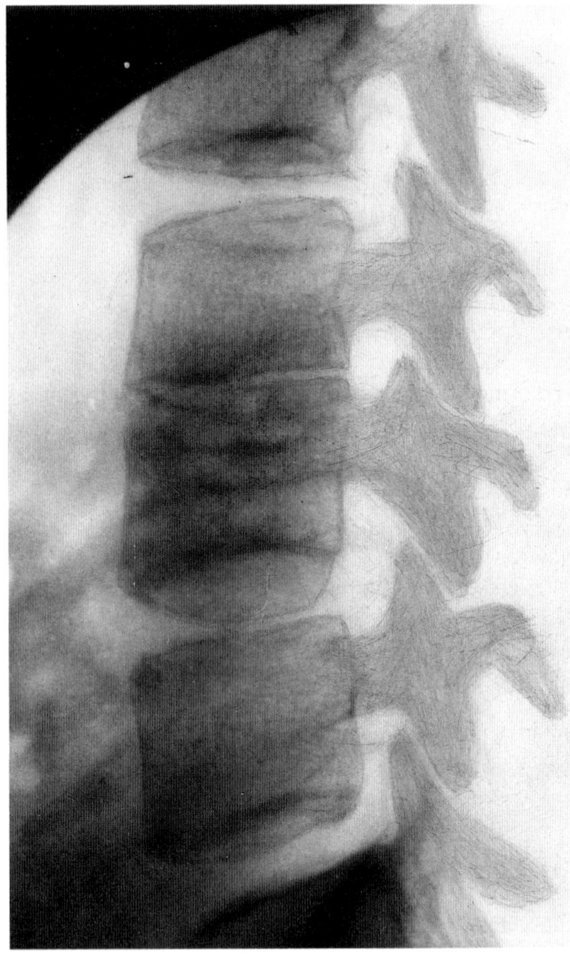

Fig. 116. The vertebra L4 presents an irregular area of radiolucency which is bordered by osteosclerosis and expands into the intervertebral space. The latter is markedly narrowed, and the contiguous vertebral endplates are uneven

nated with Salmonella. Gastrointestinal symptoms set in, with frequent stools and concomitant fever up to 39.5°–40° C. In the course of abdominal typhoid fever, the 3rd week represents the critical period in which complications usually develop. By the beginning desquamation of the necrotic Peyer's plaques from the intestine, bacteria and their toxins are spread throughout the body. Typhoid inflammations of bones and joints occur as concomitant complications in about 5%–8% of cases.

In the period when inflammation affects the joints, the characteristic symptoms of abdominal typhoid fever usually begin to regress. The general condition improves, appetite returns, intestinal complaints lessen, the tumor of the spleen decreases, and the petechial hemorrhages in the skin of the trunk diminish. However, on occurrence of joint complications between the third and sixth weeks after eruption of the abdominal typhoid fever, the temperature rises again. Headache and pain in the joints characterize this stage.

Joint inflammation in abdominal typhoid fever chiefly occurs in adults, but may also appear, albeit more rarely, in children and adolescents. It manifests as arthralgia, serous inflammation, or purulent inflammation. The former two types are often multiarticular while the latter type is monoarticular. Whereas the arthralgia is fleeting and does not elicit any noticeable alterations, the serous exudative inflammation provokes an enlargement of the joint, which is caused less by swelling of the joint capsule than by an increase in joint fluid. When empyema develops, the joint is enlarged principally by dense swelling of the joint capsule; it is reddened, much warmer than the neighboring area, and very tender. Movement is not substantially limited as long as no regional muscular spasm or epiphyseal osteomyelitis supervenes in septic arthritis. The latter complication occurs by hematogenous spread, particularly in individuals with diminished defense capacity, and may also affect the metaphyses of the long bones as well as the lumbosacral vertebral bodies [1324, 1477].

The most frequently affected joints are those of the lower extremity, the knee and ankle joints; the shoulder and wrist joints are rarely affected. However, the joints of the lumbar spine are also rather often affected [367, 1679, 1716]. Depending on the initial localization of the inflammatory focus, a primary synovial and a primary osseous joint inflammation may be distinguished. The primary synovial inflammation occurs as a serous synovitis associated with hydrops or as suppurative arthritis associated with an empyema. The primary osseous form expands from an osteomyelitic focus in the epiphysis or metaphysis; here the joint fluid has a high content of bacilli. It invariably is of the suppurative type, which prevails in children and adolescents. Occasionally a typhoid focus close to a joint (Fig. 115) elicits a "sympathetic" serous inflammation.

Blood studies disclose elevation in the sedimentation rate to 70–80 mm/h and absolute lymphopenia, which turns into leukopenia and relative lymphocytosis on aggravation of the condition. In the latter situation, the urine presents a positive diazo-reaction. Culture of the stool, blood, and urine discloses plump, Gram-negative rods with numerous flagellae; these are stained well with methylene blue. The various types and subtypes of Salmonella (S. typhi, S. typhimurium, and S. enteritidis) can be differentiated from each other by the antigens both in their cell bodies and in their flagellae. The patient's serum agglutinates typhoid bacilli at a dilution over 1:128. The Widal reaction, testing the presence of antibodies O and H in the serum of the patient against the somatic antigen and flagellar antigen of Salmonella, is significantly elevated in the 3rd–4th weeks of infection. However, the results often become negative after regression of the abdominal typhoid fever. In these situations, immunofluorescence helps to establish the diagnosis. The typhoid bacilli may be distinguished from the paratyphoid and coli bacilli by their different ability of fermentation and acidification on lactose agar. The appearance of eosinophilic leukocytes in the blood is a good prognostic sign, whereas the intensification of the diazo-reaction indicates a poor prognosis. Examination of the serous joint fluid yields negative results for bacilli, but that of the purulent joint fluid shows it to be rich in typhoid bacilli.

Roentgenographic examination [112, 173] on longer peristence of the inflammation reveals a spotty osteoporosis of the articular ends. Characteristic for typhoid osteomyelitic changes are a smooth thickening of the juxtarticular cortical bone by periosteal apposition and ovoid foci of radiolucency delimited by homogeneous sclerosis inside the epiphysis (Fig. 115). On more extensive destruction beyond the subchondral bone, the cartilage space becomes narrowed and irregularly delimited. The lumbar spine presents narrowing but maintenance of intervertebral spaces, with erosion and irregular delimitation of the adjacent vertebral plates.

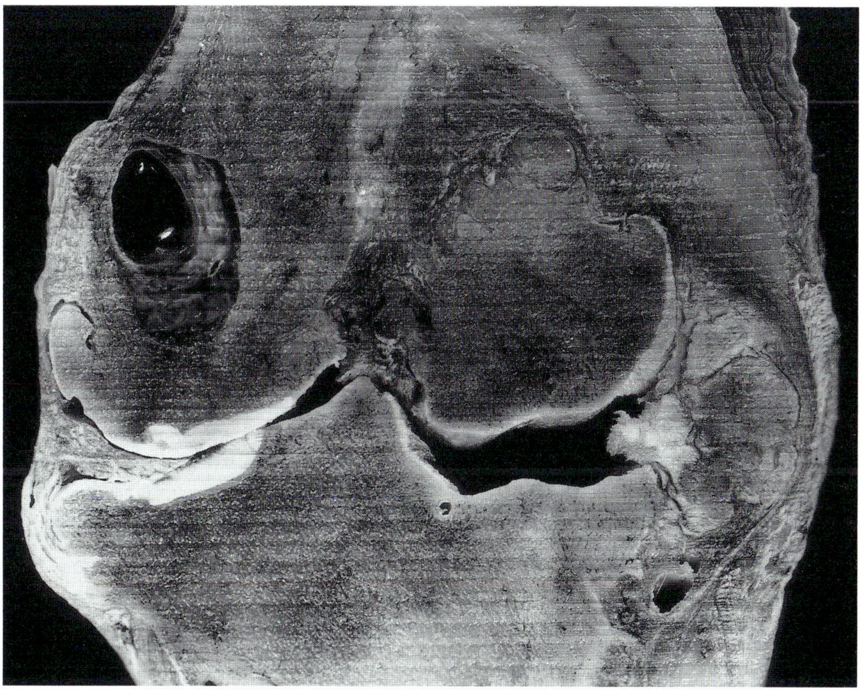

Fig. 117. One femoral condyle contains an abscess cavity, and the other femoral condyle is almost completely bare of its articular cartilage – as is the adjacent tibial condyle. The interjacent joint cavity is thus markedly widened

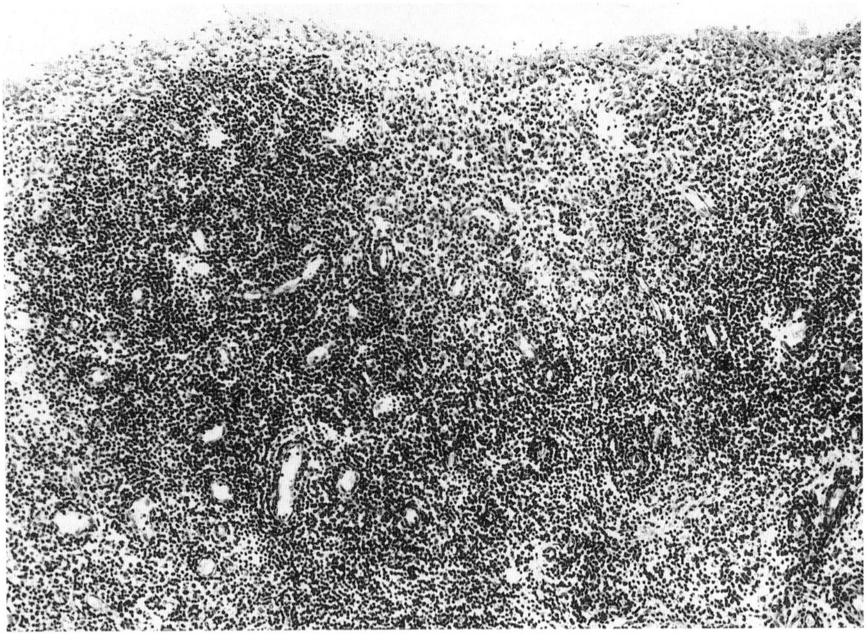

Fig. 118. The synovial membrane has a synoviocyte cover loosened by edema and is extensively and densely infiltrated by lymphocytes

Areas of bone destruction as well as those of bone densification are noticed in the affected vertebral bodies (Fig. 116).

Gross-anatomical examination of serous synovitis discloses active inflammatory changes such as redness and swelling confined to the synovial membrane but without involvement of the articular cartilage. The joint capsule is distended by accumulation of abundant seromucinous, opalescent yellowish-gray fluid. However, on penetration of an osteomyelitic abscess (Fig. 117), the joint fluid becomes frankly purulent and greenish yellow, and the local articular cartilage becomes destroyed. The purulent joint effusion may be discharged spontaneously through a fistula.

Histopathological examination discloses hyperemia and edema of the synovial membrane with perivascular and focal accumulations of lymphocytes. The suppurative inflammation is associated with a diffuse and dense infiltration in which the polymorphonuclear neutrophilic leukocytes predominate over the lymphocytes in the very early phase. Subsequently, lymphocytes and plasmacytes expand in the synovial mem-

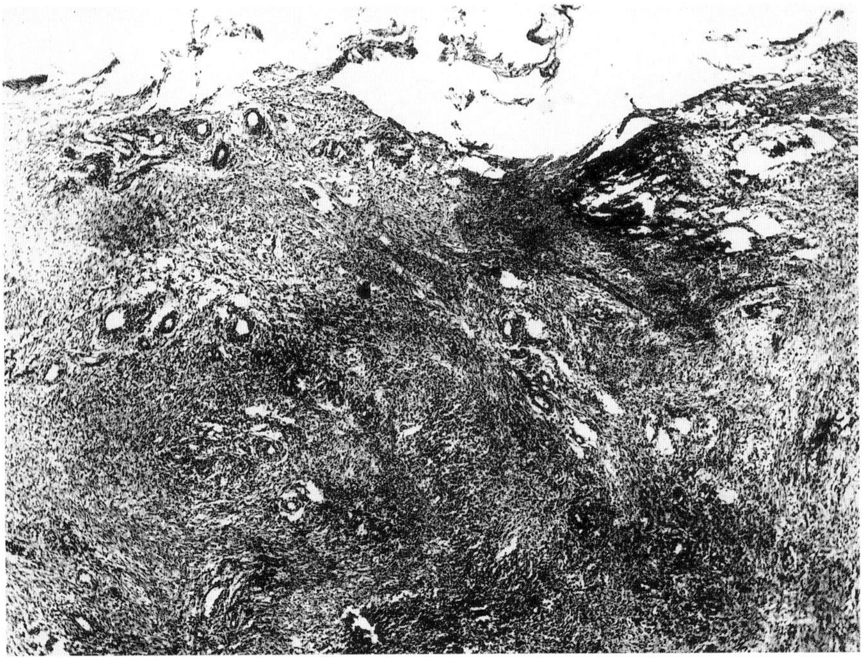

Fig. 119. The synovial membrane is very cellular throughout with lymphocytes and fibrocytes and is also densely fibrosed in a few areas. Its surface is disrupted

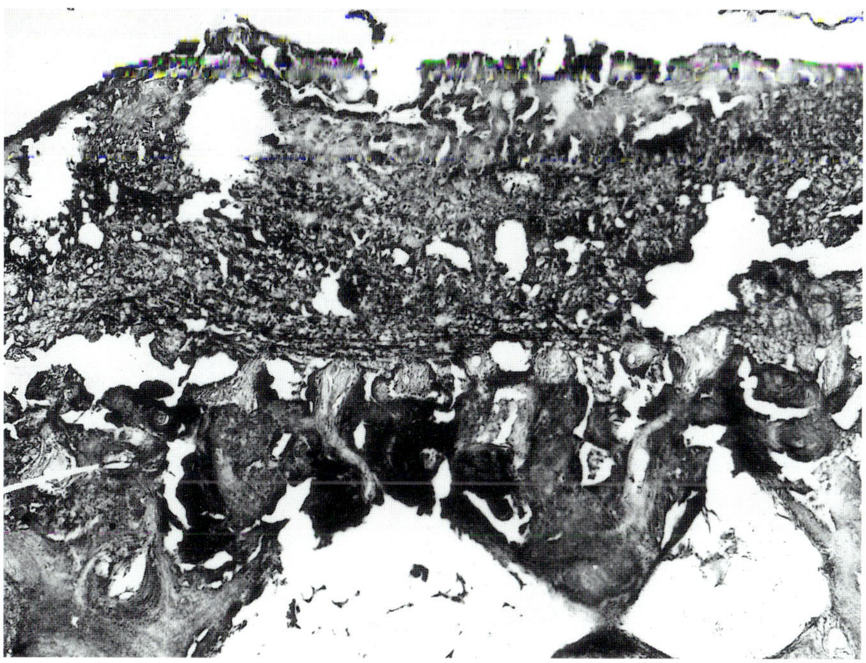

Fig. 120. The articular cartilage is almost entirely fibrosed and has retained hyaline structure only in superficial areas. It is also disrupted by several large, sharply delimited cavities. Similar cavities of larger extent disrupt the subchondral bone

brane (Fig. 118). No special histopathological feature is observed which would suggest the diagnosis of typhoid arthritis. On regression of the acute inflammatory changes, the fibrocytes increase in number and are eventually associated with fibrosis of the superficial and deeper zones of the synovial membrane (Fig. 119). The articular surface is devoid of its cartilage cover on several larger areas (Fig. 120). One of these undermined erosions often leads through a defect in the subchondral bone into a cavity, which represents an osteomyelitic abscess filled with purulent material and fragments of osseous trabeculae.

Differential diagnosis includes staphylococcal or streptococcal osteomyelitis, primary tuberculosis of the articular ends, purulent arthritis, paratyphoid arthritis, and arthritis in Brucellosis. The diazo-reaction of the urine, agglutination tests of the blood, typical blood picture, bacteriological examination of the synovial fluid and stool, and roentgenographs help to establish the diagnosis of arthritis in abdominal typhoid fever.

The infection can be prevented in periods of endemics by prophylaxis. Once such infection occurs, ampicillin 2.0–3.0 g or chloromycetin 1.5–2.0 g daily are administered in divided doses until normalization of temperature and beyond that for another 14 days. These antibiotics succeed in turning negative the results of cultures from urine, blood, and stool and in preventing complications [161]. Nevertheless, these antibiotics may elicit allergy reactions, and chloromycetin may also cause serious complications such as aplastic anemia, granulocytopenia, and thrombocytopenia. In situations of resistance to these antibiotics, sulfamethoxazole 4.0–6.0 daily given in divided doses for 2 weeks is very effective. Much attention is paid to general strengthening of the body and increasing the host defenses. The bland food is rich in protein and carbohydrate and should be supplemented with vitamin C 500 mg three times daily. Regular warm baths provide an invigorating feeling.

Local treatment includes the application of mild warm compresses to the affected joints and immobilization with traction or splinting of the elevated extremity. This relieves the pain and expedites absorption of the effusion. If the increased joint fluid is not absorbed completely, it should be removed by arthrocentesis and be examined; the joint should be compressed with a tight adhesive strapping. Subsequently, application of an elastic bandage is necessary for a longer period of time to minimize the tendency to swelling of the joint capsule. By these modalities, the serous joint inflammation may heal completely, thus leaving the joint intact. However, in persistent or recurrent joint effusions the joint capsule becomes chronically thickened and widened. In these cases regular compression of the joint by an elastic bandage, physical therapy with shortwave diathermy in two series of eight to ten sessions, and application of moist warm packs are indicated. Similarly, in affection of the vertebral column application of moist warm packs and shortwave diathermy in two series of eight to ten sessions are of substantial benefit. These are followed by prolonged immobilization with a lumbosacral belt of firm canvas reinforced by metal stays (Fig. 51).

If empyema of a joint develops, and repeated aspirations of the joint fluid followed by irrigation with normal saline solution and thereafter with ampicillin or chloromycetin solution of 1.0 g in 50 ml distilled water does not succeed in clearing the infection, the joint should be opened by two opposite incisions. Through drains left in situ, the joint is irrigated two to three times daily with normal saline solution and thereafter with ampicillin or chloromycetin solution. The infection then subsides, and the healing of the wound progresses quickly. In primary osseous suppuration with persistent inflammation of the joint, the extraarticular focus must be evacuated by a direct surgical approach, which also permits local irrigation with ampicillin or chloromycetin solution until subsidence of the drainage. In prolonged suppuration of a joint due to delayed evacuation of the pus, a secondary osteoarthritis with impaired motion or an ankylosis may develop.

Paratyphoid fever affects in its complications usually a few joints and causes a more virulent type of joint inflammation than typhoid fever. It leads either to a persistent serous or to a more destructive suppurative inflammation.

The paratyphoid bacilli cultivated from the blood, stool, and joint fluid can be distinguished from typhoid bacilli by their inability to ferment tartrate in culture media. The temperature curve is less characteristic and shows more remissions. A tumor of the spleen is usually not present, and the urine manifests a negative diazo-reaction. Leukopenia is rare and less pronounced.

Treatment is the same as that in abdominal typhoid fever. However, in infection with virulent strains of paratyphoid bacilli, the prognosis regarding life and function of the joint is very serious.

8. Arthritis in Brucellosis

Brucellosis, or Malta fever, so named because of its principal occurrence on islands and shores of the Mediterranean sea, is associated [654, 723] with affection of joints, tendon sheaths, and bursae. Two hundred ninteen cases of Brucellosis were reported in the United States in 1979 [1015]. Comroe [314] and Buchanan [202] emphasized a high frequency of complications in Brucellosis in the United States and explained this incidence by the greater toxicity of the regional microbe strains. The causative agent is Brucella Melitensis, a Gram-negative, nonmotile, small aerobic bacillus which can be differentiated from other Brucella strains by its inability to ferment sugar on lactose agar or to produce hydrogen sulfide on blood agar.

Brucella penetrates the human body through the mucosa of the intestine or through the skin. Brucellosis therefore appears primarily in individuals employed as livestock breeders, butchers, meatpackers or in related professions and who thus come into close contact with infected cattle, sheep, goats, or swine. The infection also commonly occurs by ingestion of cheese, raw milk, or meat from infected animals. The disease begins suddenly with weakness, characteristic loss of appetite, headache, sleeplessness, and decrease in body weight. Another characteristic sign is the course of fever: steep increase in the evening, profuse night sweat, and remission in the morning. Unless the pronounced anorexia and nocturnal fever prevail in the clinical picture, the diagnosis may be rather difficult. The periods of fever may last 3 weeks to 4 months in untreated cases and are interspersed with episodes of feeling well. However, the sensation of malaise generally prevails, and this is aggravated in 7%–10% of patients by pain in a number of joints.

Brucella Melitensis affects joints by way of the bloodstream. The affection occurs between the second and third weeks after the start of fever. It may manifest as arthralgia or pronounced arthritis [1357, 1561]; the former is associated with intense pain but no other symptoms, and the latter appears in the major peripheral joints and in the vertebral column. The most commonly affected peripheral joint is the knee, which is distinctly warmer and is enlarged by an increase in joint fluid. Consequently, the joint is held reflectorily in slight contracture; the joint capsule is swollen and diffusely tender. The frequent affection of the lumbar spine is very painful, especially when complicated by irritation of the nerve roots; this is associated with impairment in general condition and with high fever. Other regular signs include marked localized tenderness, pronounced defense of the regional musculature, and significant limitation of movements. With progressing destruction of the vertebral plates, the lumbar spine loses its lordosis and becomes flattened, but it is not convexed into a gibbus as in tuberculosis. Affection of the sacroiliac joint is less frequent [1467] and presents fewer symptoms than does the lumbar spine. The liver is slightly enlarged, and the spleen is markedly enlarged.

Blood studies disclose moderate leukopenia with relative lymphocytosis; eosinophilic leukocytes are sometimes completely absent. Results of the Brucella agglutination test are positive at dilutions of 1:160–1:1280 during the active phase, and those of the complement fixation test are positive at titers of 1:128–1:256. Both tests give evidence that the immunoglobulins, especially IgG and IgM, are significantly increased [879, 1363]. Further confirmation of the infection can be obtained by exposing heat-treated Brucella to fluo-

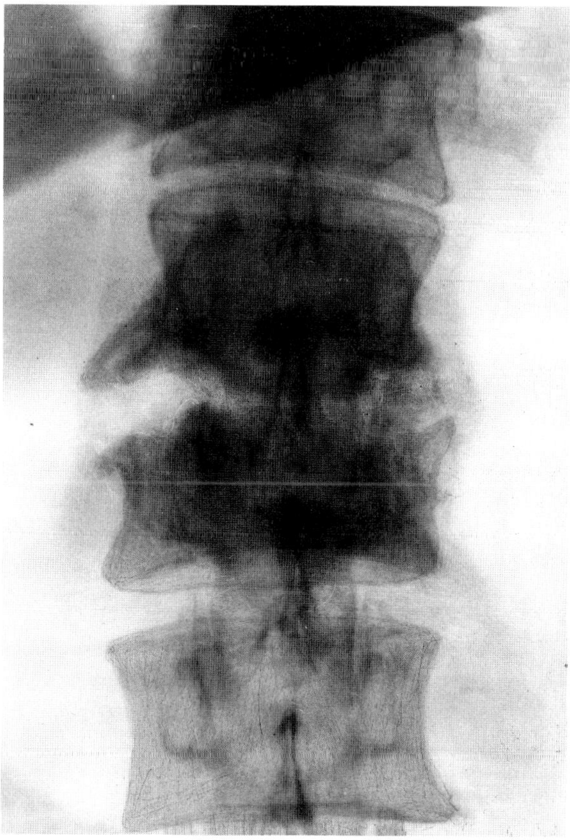

Fig. 121. The intervertebral space L1-2 is narrowed and unevenly delimited secondary to erosion of the bordering vertebral plates. The bodies of L1 and L2 are partly densified and of irregular structure

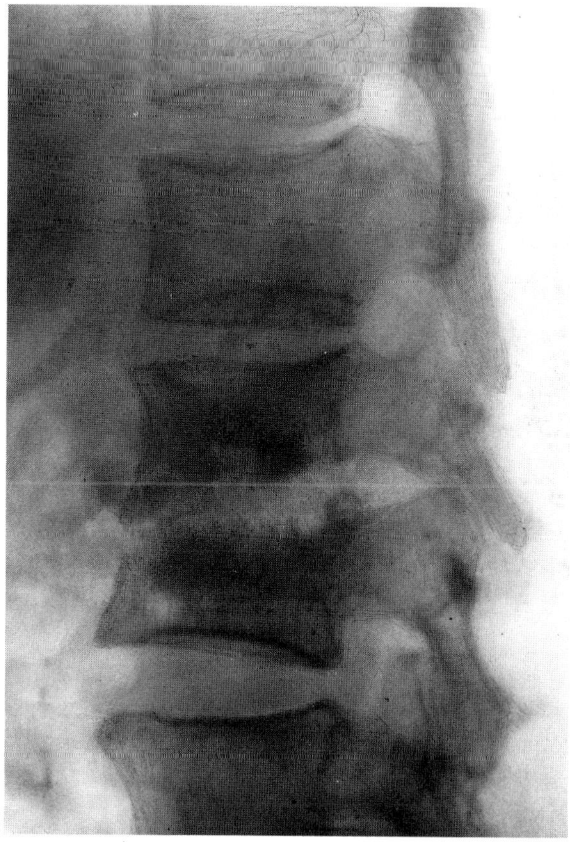

Fig. 122. The bodies of L2 and L3, including their articular processes, are extensively eroded, partly sclerosed, and unevenly delimited. Concomitantly, the intervertebral space is irregularly widened

rescein-conjugated serum of the patient and examining this mixture under a fluorescence microscope. Tissue typing is also used for the diagnosis of Brucellosis [376]. HLA-B27 is present in the majority of patients with affections of the spine. The diazo-reaction in the urine is often positive. Brucella Melitensis can be demonstrated by smear and culture (especially on agar containing soybean-casein digest) of blood and urine during the fever episodes as well as in the joint fluid. The joint effusion is yellowish, dense, and contains abundant fibrin flakes. In the chronic stage of Brucellosis, the intracutaneous injection of a filtrate of Brucella Melitensis culture may be very informative [1467]. Weed et al. [1725] identified Brucella in articular tissue removed at surgery.

Roentgenographic examination discloses no specific or characteristic changes in the peripheral joints. The articular ends are osteoporotic and sometimes irregularly delimited [959]; the cartilage space is slightly narrowed or fully maintained. However, the vertebral column (Figs. 121, 122), chiefly in the lumbar region [1391, 1467] and rarely in the cervical region, presents typical narrowing of one or two intervertebral spaces with irregular but sharp delimitation. The adjacent vertebral endplates undergo erosion extending deeply and/or destruction. The residual vertebral bodies have diminished heights, but their structure is very dense in the healing phase [111, 615, 865, 978, 1391]; rather bizarre osteophytes extend from the lateral margins (Fig. 121). The neighboring vertebrae are osteoporotic (Fig. 121) and in distinct contrast to the affected and sclerosed vertebrae.

Gross-anatomical examination of the joints of the extremities discloses intensive redness of the inner part of the joint capsule, which is covered in a few areas by precipitates of fibrin. No involvement of the peripheral part of the joint capsule or of articular cartilage is noted. Suppuration of the joints is very rare; the turbid joint fluid does not have the thick consistence as in other, especially coccal, infections.

Histopathological examination in the initial phase discloses marked hyperemia and edema of the synovial membrane, which contains focal agglomerations of lymphocytes and plasmacytes (Fig. 123). In the subacute and chronic phases larger infiltrates composed of lymphocytes, plasmacytes, and a smaller number of

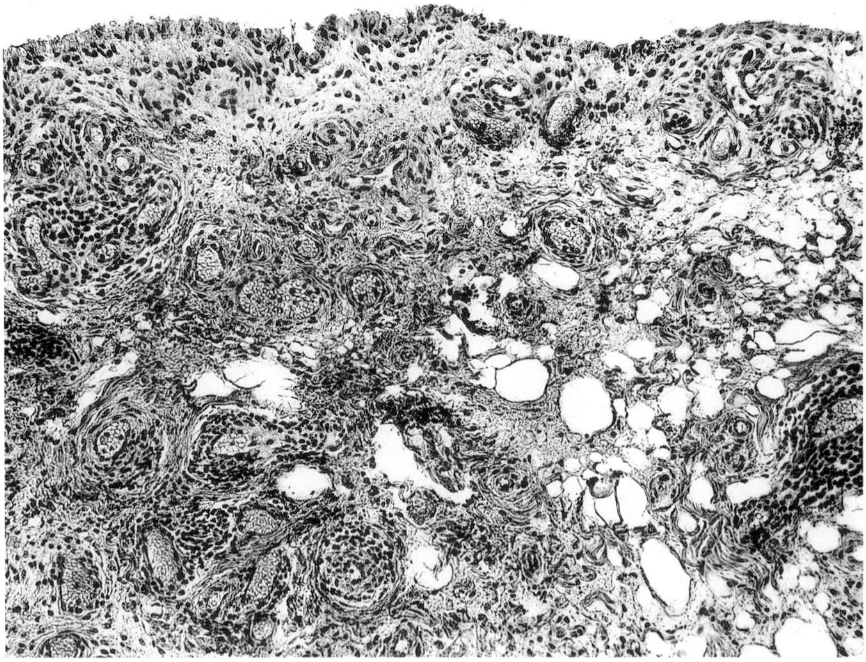

Fig. 123. The synoviocyte cover is moderately hypertrophic. The subsynoviocytic tissue is moderately hypercellular with plasmacytes and histiocytes. The blood vessels are very hyperemic and are surrounded by inflammatory infiltrates

histiocytes expand in the subsynoviocytic tissue. Similarly fibroblasts appear in a small number, eventually leading to a general increase of fibrocytes. By the concurrent increase in synoviocytes small villi are formed, which in granulomalike structure surround and organize deposits of fibrin on the surface (Fig. 124). This formation is considered very instructive [684] as it indicates the high reactivity of the synovial membrane in seropositive cases.

Diagnosis is based in the active phase on the characteristic wave of the fever curve and on the demonstration of microbes in the blood, urine, and joint fluid; it is based in the later phase on the reaction of serum. The negative outcome of the sheep cell agglutination test and the negative response to salicylates speak against the diagnosis of rheumatoid inflammation, but the decrease in leukocytes suggests the possibility of typhoid inflammation. Roentgenographs reveal the main-

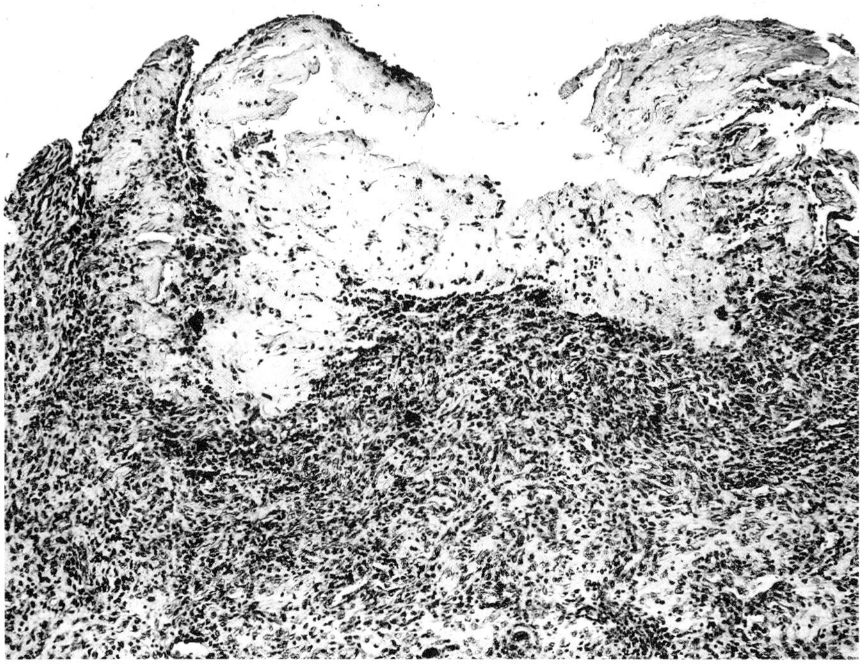

Fig. 124. The synovial membrane is markedly hypercellular with fibrocytes, lymphocytes, and histiocytes. On the surface lies a deposit of fibrin which is very sparingly organized and, like a hemigranuloma, is bordered by the synovial membrane

tenance of the intervertebral space and the absence of a paravertebral abscess, excluding the possibility of tuberculosis of the spine.

Treatment is primarily prophylactic by treating all skin lesions of persons occupied in growing and meat processing of cattle, sheep, goats, and swine, and by thoroughly boiling the milk and cooking the meat from endemic regions suspected of having diseased animals. However, when the disease has already been acquired and is active, as manifested by the characteristic fever curve, tetracycline or chloromycetin 0.5 g is administered four to six times daily for at least 4 weeks. The effect of these medications is substantially enhanced, and the potentiality of recurrence minimized by combination with streptomycin 1.0 g given daily for 2 weeks. The temperature then normalizes, and general symptoms regress [750, 875, 1208]. The administration of antibiotics should be continued beyond this, if blood and urine studies reveal the presence of microorganisms – which may be for 3–4 more months. Otherwise, patients will remain carriers of the microorganisms, and their joint symptoms are likely to recur. In such situations, sulfathiazole 4.0–6.0 g daily for 4 weeks or other sulfadrugs or rifampin 600 mg daily for 3 weeks provides the expected benefit. Fever treatments with parenteral protein injections or physical hyperthermy may provide recovery from the infection. The articular symptoms are concurrently treated with regularly applied moist hot packs until regression of the swelling. Subsequently, shortwave diathermy in two series of eight to ten sessions and firm compression with elastic bandages are very beneficial. In affections of the lower spine prolonged support by a high, firm lumbosacral belt with metal stays (Fig. 51) or a lumbosacral brace is indicated. An operative fusion of the spine is not necessary, but decompression may be necessary in the rare cases of compression of the spinal cord [978].

A less virulent strain, Brucella abortus (Bang's bacillus), is propagated by diseased cattle to persons in contact with them; this occurs particularly in southern Europe. Chiefly affected are veterinarians and butchers. It is a small, ovoid, Gram-negative microorganism which can be differentiated from Brucella Melitensis by monospecific sera. Entry portals for this microorganism are the skin and the gastrointestinal tract by raw milk and meat. Infection with Brucella abortus also causes joint affections, but these are of lighter degree than those with Brucella Melitensis. The joints display moderately painful swelling of the joint capsule but no effusion or limitation of motion. With the start of antibiotic administration, tetracycline 2.0–3.0 g daily in divided doses and then orally or intravenously for 4–6 weeks combined with shortwave diathermy in two series of eight sessions, the changes of the joints soon regress. However, in lack of response to tetracycline, chloromycetin 1.5–2.5 g is administered daily for 4 weeks. One must bear in mind, however, it potentially serious adverse effects: aplastic anemia, granulocytopenia, and thrombocytopenia. In cases with protracted thickening of the joints, regular application of hot mud packs and antiinflammatory medications (as listed in "Rheumatoid Arthritis") are beneficial.

Prolonged administration of antibiotics and regular application of local modalities normally lead to subsidence of the inflammatory affection and reattainment of normal function in cases of Brucella infection. Surgical intervention is generally not needed [959, 1467].

9. Arthritis in Scarlet Fever

Inflammation of joints is a rather frequent complication during the course of scarlet fever. In 10%–15% of these children, the fingers, wrists, elbows, hips, and knees become affected. The toxins in scarlet fever are transported by the bloodstream to the joints and cause an abacterial synovitis. In the rare cases with gangrenous abscesses of the tonsils, hemolytic streptococci may enter the bloodstream and upon arriving in joints elicit a bacterial inflammation. Suppurative arthritis is the potential outcome here. However, it appears that with the decreasing severity of scarlet fever over the past three to four decades [106, 786, 1029] the articular complications have also decreased in frequency and intensity. This phenomenon is explained by the lower virulence of the causative microbial strains (streptococcus B hemolyticus or streptococcus A pyogenes) and/or by the timely administration of antibiotics.

Inflammation of joints [786, 1374] appears as the so-called early scarlet rheumatoid arthritis between the 5th and 14th days after the onset of scarlet fever. In this phase the characteristic fine-papular, erythematous skin rash is regressing. The joint inflammation represents a reaction to bacterial toxins and is characterized by rapid and complete subsidence of all signs. As the scarlet fever is healing or shortly afterward, usually 6 weeks after its onset, late scarlet rheumatoid arthritis may occur. Clinically this resembles the early rheumatoid form but is of much longer duration. During the course of 1 day, all symptoms of scarlet rheumatoid arthritis are manifested, associated with pain radiating into the regional musculature. Multiarticular asymmetric arthralgias are present, or a monoarticular synovitis with slight effusion may have settled. Whereas the arthralgias are characterized by fleeting soreness without objective findings, the synovitis is expressed in a diffuse and soft swelling of the joint capsule. In the latter condition the entire tissue is moderately sensitive, but no area of marked tenderness is noticed. The motion of the joint is not limited, and no contracture ever develops. In the overwhelming majority of affected joints, no further alterations ensue. The inflammation is usually of mild degree and remains confined to the inner layer of the joint capsule. The regional musculature, although often very sensitive, does not become swollen.

When the articular complication appears, the main signs of scarlet fever are in regression. The temperature is normalizing, and the exanthem is blanching. However, the pharynx is still red, and the tonsils are swollen and comprise deep clefts. The retromandibular and submandibular lymph nodes are enlarged. Heart action is not impaired. The spleen is sometimes enlarged.

The smear from the throat confirms the diagnosis by presenting streptococci which grow on blood agar with transparent hemolytic halos. Blood studies disclose a persistent leukocytosis, and in generalized sepsis a lymphopenia; polymorphonuclear eosinophilic leukocytes appear in the healing phase. The blood has an elevated antistreptolysin-O titer and sometimes contains streptococci. The joint fluid of serous inflammation is sterile and contains 600–1000 white blood cells, chiefly lymphocytes. Roentgenographs of the joints present normal findings.

Histopathological examination of punch biopsy specimens discloses thin deposits of fibrin on the synovial surface and sparse agglomerations of lymphocytes in the subsynoviocytic tissue. Occasionally, deep focal agglomerations of lymphocytes and histiocytes are noted which are considered [880] as formations similar to Aschoff's nodules.

Differential diagnosis must take into consideration acute rheumatic inflammation and allergic arthritis after serum injection. The etiology is indicated by the history, initial symptoms and exanthem, absence of heart symptoms, changes in the blood picture, and results of the culture for streptococci as well as the search for streptococcal antibodies.

Treatment primarily consists in immediate administration of ampicillin 2 g daily in divided doses for 14 days; penicillin-resistant children are given erythromycin 1–2 g or cephalosporin 1–2 g daily for 14 days. Moist warm compresses are applied around the joint two or three times daily for 1 h, and the joint is immobilized with a splint or by a traction device. With regression of the symptoms the joint may benefit from eight sessions of shortwave diathermy and should be protected with an elastic bandage during the day. In the rare and serious situations of beginning joint suppuration, presenting a complication of bacteremia, all therapeutic modalities must be used in addition to high doses of the indicated antibiotic. These modalities are discussed in "Suppurative Arthritis".

Some patients experience fleeting, rather disturbing pain in a previously affected joint for a longer period of time, even for several years afterward. The application of moist hot mud packs or a sojourn on a beach with warm sand helps to eliminate this pain.

10. Bacteriantigenic Arthritis

A great number of arthritides are elicited by various microorganisms which can be identified in the blood, joint fluid, and/or an organ representing a portal to the bloodstream. In contrast, in nonspecific bacteriantigenic arthritis no causative microorganism can be identified either in the blood or in the joint fluid [314]. Such microorganisms can only occasionally be identified in a primary organ presenting a chronic or a regressing inflammation. The etiology of this type of arthritis can reasonably be explained by the presence of a remote inflammatory focus [60, 1683] as a center which spreads noxious substances, bacterial debris [704], or components of cocci [359, 568, 775] with antigenic properties into the body. This results in an immunologically reactive joint inflammation [523]. Thus the term bacteriantigenic arthritis appears appropriate and descriptive.

Proof that antigens may cause inflammation in joints was provided by Dumonde et al. [444] who injected antigens into the joints of sensitized rabbits and provoked a very active inflammation replete with characteristic changes in the synovial membrane. These findings were corroborated by Brackerts [171], Cromartie [347], Greenblatt [670], and White [1749].

It is of significance to note in bacteriantigenic arthritis that the search for a primary focus is sometimes unsuccessful, because the changes in this focus either are inconspicuous or are already healed, and thus escape detection. Thus, the bacteriantigenic arthritis is a cryptogenetic inflammation in many cases. To identify the rather active inflammation in a joint, as opposed to the mild reaction in the primary focus, one must assume a change in the character of the bacterial antigen to organotropic toxicity [1326]. Recalling that, for example, in the case of Reiter's syndrome, nonspecific urethritis can be the source of joint inflammation, it is easy to accept that toxins or antigens emitted from microbes may settle in any organ of the body and elicit arthritic conditions there. Ford [523] demonstrated that inflammatory arthritis can arise from the host's response to microbial substances by mechanisms which are probably similar to those operating in Reiter's syndrome [951]. Meak [1083] and Proell [1283]

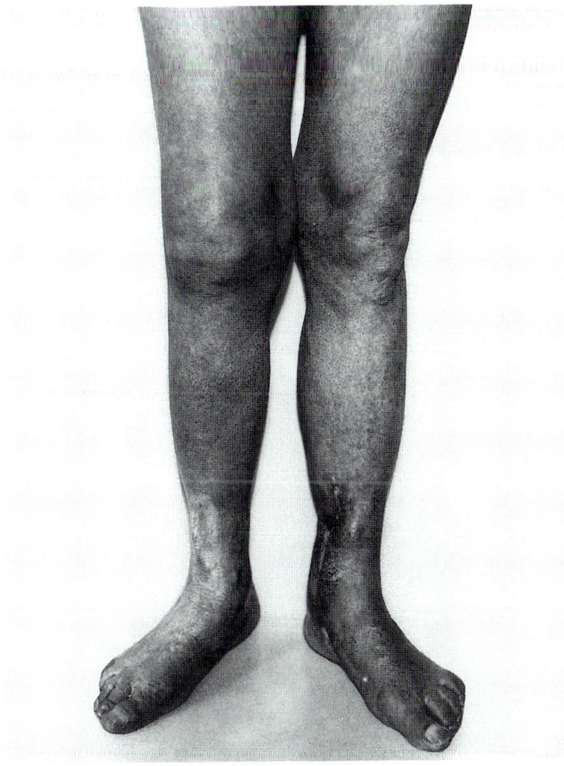

Fig. 125. This patient with chronic osteomyelitis of both tibiae has recurrent effusions in the right knee joint. Repeated examinations of the joint fluid disclosed the absence of microorganisms

considered here a selective ability of localization, terming it organ affinity.

Three stages in bacteriantigenic arthritis may be distinguished [364]: (a) invasion and localization of microorganisms in a primary focus, (b) transformation of microorganisms, or rather mutation of their antigens, and (c) metastatic affections as arthritis or nephritis by these antigens. Metastatic antigenic arthritis presumes an individual constitutional propensity of the mesoderm. If this did not play a role, it would be impossible to explain the differing reactions from patient to patient in terms of the clinical picture which results from the same type of microorganism or its antigen.

The causative agents are generally streptococci, rarely staphylococci, and sometimes other microorganisms (hemophilus, enterobacter, Escherichia coli), acting by their antigens at a distance. The disseminating focus may be any organ of the body which presents an active or a regressing inflammation caused by bacteria, and which emits their toxins and antigens [1283]. The most frequently incriminated source are the tonsils; the large ones are not at fault but rather the small indented ones, from whose clefts ample secretion can be squeezed out. Controversy exists as to the view [1683] that inflammatory alterations in the teeth and alveolar pyorrhea, periodontitis, caries, granulomata, and root abscesses may serve as originating foci of joint inflammation. The view has led to the coining of the term oral sepsis. Inflammations of the paranasal and maxillary sinuses are often responsible for joint affections, as are inflammations of the bronchi. Chronic inflammation of the gallbladder, appendix, or their surrounding tissues may be the source of antigens; this is also true particularly of chronic inflammations of the intestine caused by a mixed flora of bacteria. Catarrhal inflammation of the urinary bladder, chronic adnexitis, or persistent prostatitis often elicit an inflammation of joints. Also panaritia, carbuncles, or abscesses may be the sources of antigenic arthritis.

Bacteriantigenic arthritis [1230] shows a brief stage of acute, often rather painful inflammation which changes into a chronic and milder, but occasionally exacerbated, aggravated form. Accordingly, the temperature rises for briefly to 38.3°–38.9° C and then fluctuates persistently between 36.8° and 37.8° C. The general condition is not impaired unless the inflammation of the primary focus (sinus, tonsils, teeth, gallbladder, appendix, or urogenital tract) causes marked disturbance. The changes in the larger and smaller joints (shoulder, elbow, knee, ankle) of the extremities are not very pronounced. These joints are slightly enlarged by swelling of the joint capsule, and they become larger when their synovial fluid is occasionally increased (Fig. 125). The local temperature may be slightly elevated, but no redness is ever observed. The entire joint is moderately and diffusely tender. The regional bursae and insertions of tendons are also tender. Nevertheless, the motion of the joint is not limited unless occasional episodes of more pronounced pain temporarily impair the use of the joint. In addition, the clinical picture varies from joint to joint. In the shoulder, the joint capsule is moderately tender while the acromial and subcoracoid bursae are very tender, thus limiting the active movements of the shoulder joint. On longer duration an adduction contracture may result. The wrist and finger joints present a moderate thickening of the joint capsule, yet without residual deformity. In the hip joint, the affection may be followed by sensitivity to a change in weather or secondary to strain. In the knee joint, the chronic thickening of the joint capsule may sometimes be associated with a moderate, slowly resorbing effusion (Fig. 125) following strain or overactivity. In the ankle joint, the tenderness of the joint capsule may expand into the adjacent tendon sheaths. The lower part of the thoracic spine and the entire lumbar spine are tender at the apophyseal joints, with the paravertebral musculature becoming moderately tense. The movements of this segment of the spine are diminished. Occasionally, nerve root hyperesthesias occur here, and these are more impairing than are affections of the apophyseal joints.

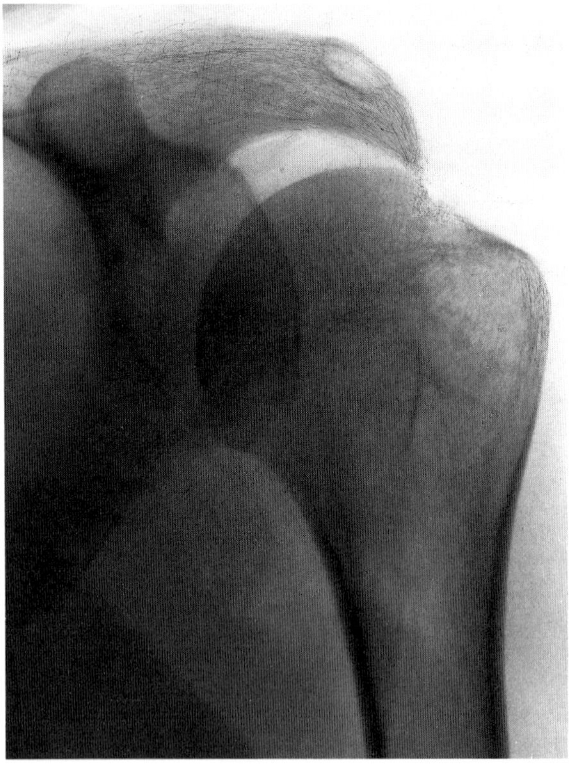

Fig. 126. The shoulder joint, with arthritis secondary to prostatitis, presents small areas to osteoporosis at the attachment of the joint capsule to the scapula and humerus

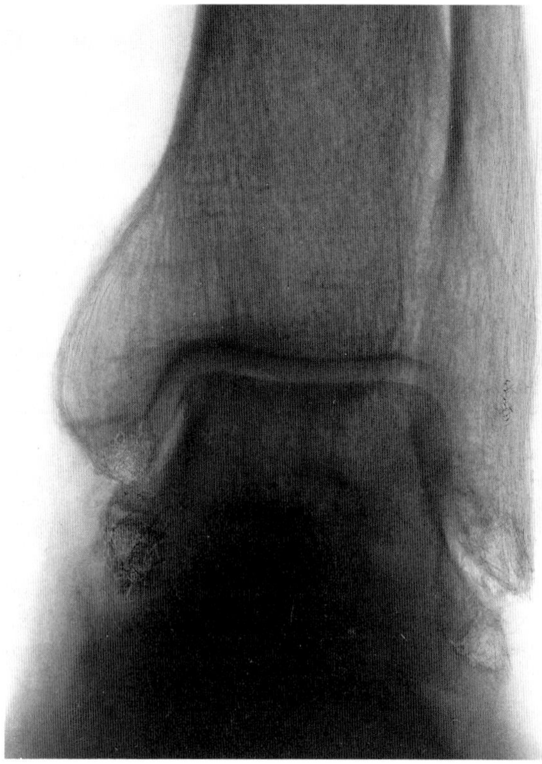

Fig. 127. The ankle joint, with arthritis in chronic adnexitis, presents small areas of osteoporosis at the attachment of the joint capsule to the malleoli and calcaneus

The sedimentation rate is accelerated and remains so for a longer period of time without reaching excessive values; average findings fluctuate between 25 and 50 mm/h. Blood studies disclose a moderate leukocytosis. Serum proteins are increased to 6.0–7.3 g% and globulin to 3.3–4.0 g%. The antistreptolysin titer is positive at a dilution of 1:80–1:320 in 35%–40% of patients, indicating streptococcus as the initial agent in a number of these articular affections.

Blood cultures are usually sterile, as are those of joint fluid. The urine of patients with primary urogenital inflammation contains increased proteins and cellular elements. The clear to slightly turbid joint fluid contains 800–5000/ml polymorphonuclear neutrophilic leukocytes, lymphocytes, and plasmacytes. Examination by smear or culture of the blood, secretions or discharges from internal organs, and joint fluid rarely discloses the presence of microorganisms; however, their circulating antigenic components in the blood can be detected by immunochemical analysis and immunoelectrophoresis [1385]. In immunochemical analysis, individual proteins and other substances are exposed to specific antisera whose antibodies bind to the appropriate antigen and permit quantification of the resulting precipitate by staining. Immunoelectrophoresis analyzes the various components of a protein complex after having exposed it to a heterospecific antiserum directed against various classes of immunoglobulins. The antiserum produces precipitation bands whose reactants are analyzed and quantified by staining and electrophoresis. Furthermore, by the use of antibodies labeled with fluorescent thiocyanate [321], the corresponding microorganismal antigens and/or their proteins can be identified in the blood, as well as their antigen-antibody complexes. Available antibodies labeled with fluorescent compounds can be used for detection and identification of antigenic substances in the synovial membrane (Fig. 128) and synovial fluid [190, 321, 863, 1237, 1256]. They can be visualized under the fluorescence microscope and are identified in the majority of patients as deriving generally from hemolytic streptococci and less often from nonsuppurative staphylococci, pneumococci, or mixed gonococci and staphylococci. These direct methods permit one to ascertain the presence of bound antibodies and microorganismal antigens which elicit nonspecific articular inflammations [318, 1739]. The indirect immunofluorescence test as described in "Arthrocentesis and Examination of Joint Fluid" can here very informatively be applied too.

Serial roentgenographs (Figs. 126, 127) obtained after a longer duration of the joint inflammation reveal

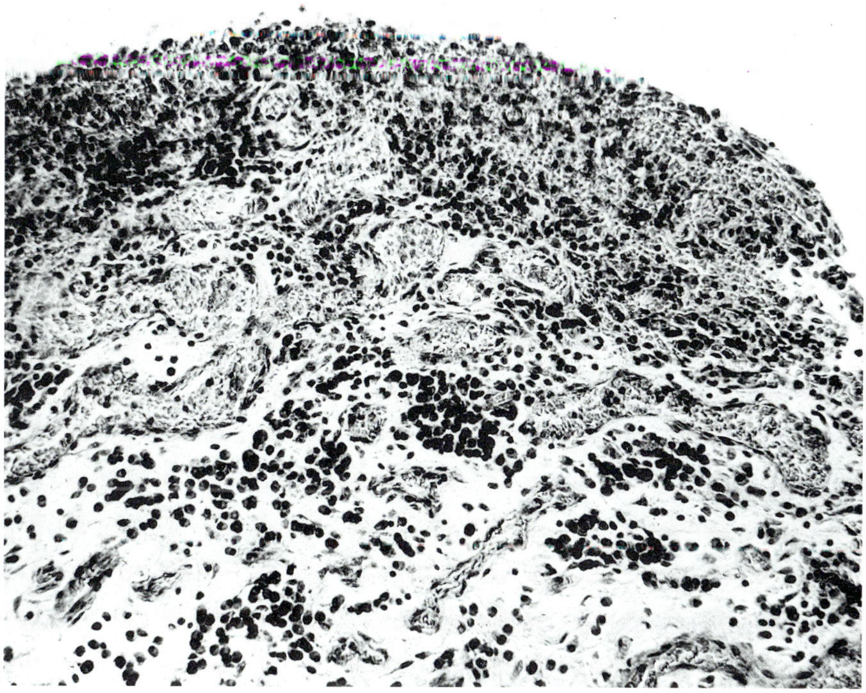

Fig. 128. The synovial membrane presents a marked increase in histiocytes in the subsynoviocytic zone, hyperemia of the blood vessels, and rather large focal accumulations of plasmacytes

a spotty, subchondral osteoporosis in the articular epiphyses, without surrounding sclerosis. Particularly the knee, shoulder (Fig. 126), and ankle (Fig. 127) are affected in this way at the areas of attachment of the joint capsule and/or ligaments. The cartilage space has normal width and even delimitation. In rare cases, the structure of the articular epiphyses is blurred by a densified joint capsule.

Gross-anatomical examination discloses swelling and redness of the inner part of the joint capsule, which on longer duration of the condition becomes thicker and protrudes into the joint cavity. However, the articular cartilage is not altered. Histopathological examination (Fig. 128) discloses a few areas of the synovial surface covered by necrotic detritus, while the subjacent tissue presents a few small hemorrhages and focal

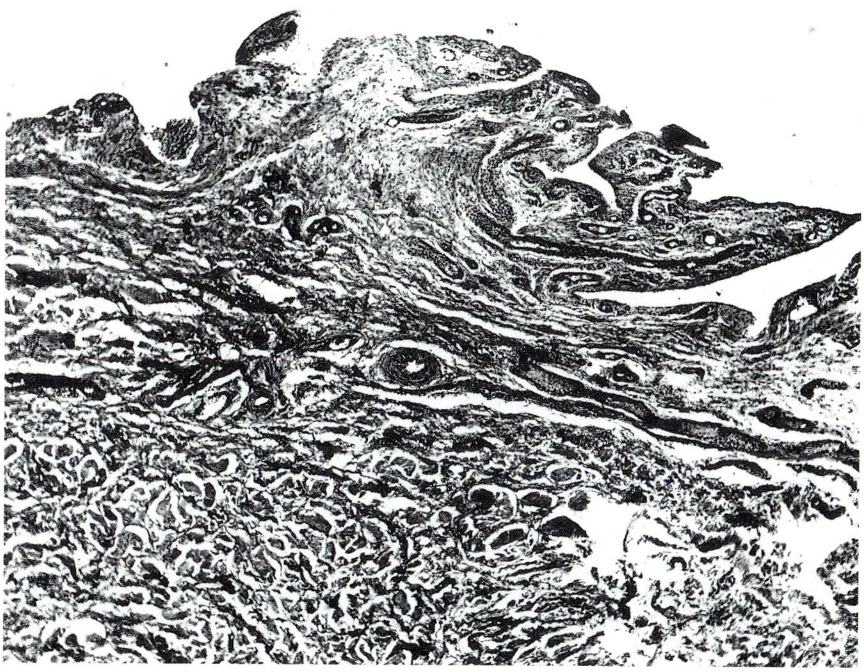

Fig. 129. The synovial membrane presents in the chronic phase moderate formation of villi and moderate hypercellularity of the subsynoviocytic tissue with fibrocytes and histiocytes. The collagen fibers are increased in the deeper zone

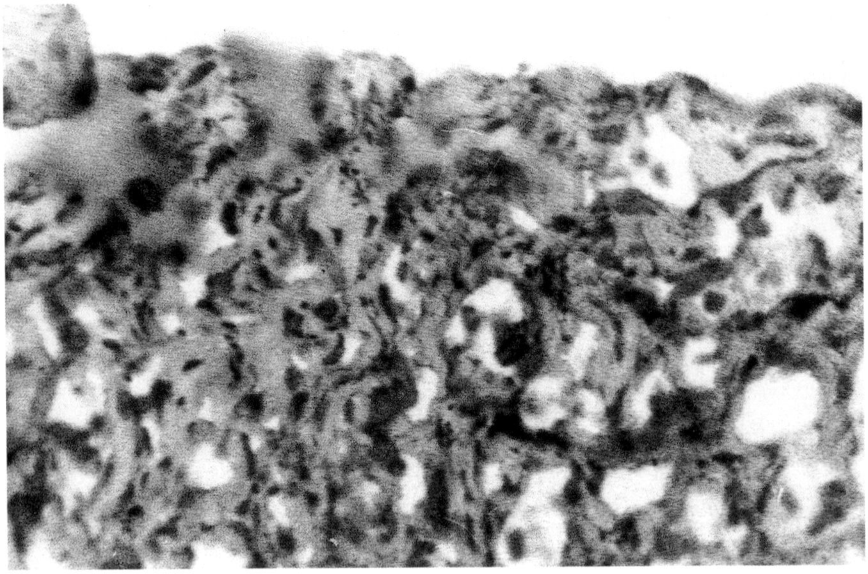

Fig. 130. The synovial membrane, from a patient with chronic adnexitis and chronic arthritis of the knee, presents spotty immunofluorescence on exposure to fluorescein-conjugated antiserum against streptolysin

agglomerations of lymphocytes and plasmacytes. These infiltrates gradually regress and are followed by a moderate increase in fibrocytes and by hyperplasia of synoviocytes. Formation of small villi on the surface and fibrosis in the deeper zone (Fig. 129) eventually results. Specimens of synovial tissue, fixed with ethanol ether, were exposed to fluoresceinconjugated rabbit antisera against human IgG, IgM, IgE, C3, and C4. Subsequent examination under the fluorescence microscope disclosed that immunoproteins containing IgG, IgM, less IgE, C3, and C4 were deposited chiefly in synoviocytes and perivascular tissue (Fig. 130) and less in lymphocytes and histiocytes. These findings indicate that immune complexes absorbed in the synovial membrane mediate its inflammatory reaction [670]. The demonstration of antigen-antibody complexes in the synovial membrane by the direct method and/or by the indirect method provides a clear proof for the causation of joint inflammation by antigens originating from microorganisms.

The milder the primary focal infection, the less pronounced is the clinical picture in the affected joint. Of great importance for the differential diagnosis is the complete case history and the thorough search for inflammatory foci in the body. The fulfillment of these requirements, the pauciarticular involvement, and the absence of articular deformities help to avoid confusion with chronic rheumatoid arthritis [1729]. The inflammation in specific infectious arthritis caused directly by invasion of bacteria is much more painful, presents a distinct clinical picture, and yields specific reactions of the blood as well as positive results in the culture of blood and synovial fluid.

Treatment of the nonspecific bacteriantigenic arthritis should be etiologic; therefore it aims at identifying and healing or eliminating the disseminating focus. The tonsils are inspected and should be removed if enlarged and discharging secretion. Inflammation of the sinuses is treated with local application of moist heat, warm inhalations, and oral administration of antibiotics and vitamin C. Granulomata, cysts of the teeth, and purulent root canals are treated surgically. Diseased teeth should be extracted, if an inflammatory focus has developed around them despite the administration of antibiotics and has caused roentgenographically detectable changes. These extractions should be carried out in intervals so that the opening of the infectious foci would provide a vaccinating effect. An inflamed gallbladder or appendix should be removed. A catarrh of the intestine should be treated by diet and high doses of antibiotics. Inflammation of the renal pelvis is treated with ample fluid and high doses of antibiotics, sulfonamides, or furacin. Inflammation of the prostate or adnexa is treated with rectally applied shortwave diathermy in two series of ten sessions, parenterally administered penicillin G 5,000,000 U daily, or orally administered cephalosporin 3.0 g or chloramphenicol 3.0 g daily for 2–3 weeks, and hormones. A generally underestimated or neglected cause of nonspecific bacteriantigenic arthritis is the common cold. The concomitant activation of ubiquitous microorganisms, especially in the upper respiratory tract, probably accounts for the dissemination of bacterial toxins or antigens and the frequent inflammation of joints. Complete bedrest, regular intake of antibiotics (ampicillin 3.0 g, erythromycin 3.0 g, or cephalosporin 3.0 g daily), followed by salicylates 2.4 g daily, warm fluids, and vitamin C 1.0 g daily succeed in improving the general condition and expediting regression of the joint affections.

At the acute inflammation of a joint, moist warm packs should be applied regularly around the joint and supplemented with shortwave diathermy in one series of eight to ten sessions. With increased and nonabsorbing joint fluid, an arthrocentesis is indicated; this should be accompanied by a firm strapping for compression and immobilization. The aspirated synovial fluid is examined from all points of view as outlined in "Arthrocentesis and Examination of Joint Fluid". On transition to the chronic phase, moist hot packs or hot mud packs and intensified shortwave diathermy radiations are applied in two or three series of eight sessions. When a chronic joint inflammation with thickening persists, nonspecific protein or autogenous blood may be injected intramuscularly [1534] if a longer series of nonsteroidal antiinflammatory medications does not provide substantial benefit. The joint is mobilized by gentle active and passive exercises. Combination of the above therapeutic modalities, applied according to the phase, succeeds in influencing both causally and symptomatically nonspecific bacteriantigenic joint disease and bringing the subsidence of this affection.

Since the inflammation of the synovial membrane usually subsides without involvement of the articular cartilage, the designation of synovitis in the majority of these cases appears more indicated than that of arthritis.

11. Arthritis in Influenza

Influenza is an acute infection of the respiratory tract and is characterized by contagiousness and rapid spread. Its causative agent was originally considered to be the small Gram-negative coccobacillus hemophilus influenzae, which grows in colonies on blood containing culture media, and which resemble transparent dew drops. However, since this bacillus cannot always be demonstrated even in pronounced cases of influenza, its role as the etiological agent in influenza has been doubted; its secondary role seems probable. On the other hand, the studies of Andrews [44] and others revealed that the causative agent of influenza is a filtrable virus belonging to the group A myxoviruses. This can be cultivated by continued animal transferences and thereby gains in toxicity. On the basis of the different nucleoprotein antigens in its composition and the differences in the elicited clinical picture, the influenza virus is distinguished into types A, B, and C [1423]. Type A causes the wider epidemics and serious complications. Nevertheless, the occurrence of hemophilus influenzae does not appear to be an incidental finding because it is noted at least as coexistent in a significant number of toxic cases with severe pneumonia and lethal outcome. The pneumococcus is much less often observed in these pneumonias. Thus the viral pneumonia in influenza is superimposed by a bacterial pneumonia. Some authors [695] consider hemophilus influenzae as a sensitizing agent which prepares the terrain for the localization of the influenza virus. This infection occurs characteristically during cold, moist seasons and in epidemical outbreaks of varying extent [1423].

The symptoms of influenza are well pronounced. Characteristic is the acute and marked impairment in general condition associated with headache, fever, chills, and anorexia. This is followed by pain in the respiratory, gastrointestinal and/or urinary tract. Children are much more afflicted by laryngobronchitis with croup and by gastrointestinal upset [79]. The temperature rises abruptly to 39.5°–40.5°C and declines after 3–5 days, when most major symptoms regress. However, in a smaller percentage of these patients the pain in the chest is followed by a longer lasting pneumonia of serious character. Death follows in most of these patients due to extensive and dense infiltration of the lungs, causing an incorrectible hypoxia [79]. On the other hand, many of those who recover experience a few days later a dragging sensation in the muscles of the back and limbs, especially in those of the lower limbs [1084, 1102]. These symptoms last 4–6 weeks and are often aggravated by myositis with increased production of muscle enzymes. Lancinating pain in the joints and aching of the entire body are associated.

The joints are affected [25, 1150, 1162, 1459, 1678, 1810] usually 3–5 days after the onset of influenza. The ensuing arthritis is believed to result either from direct viral infection of the synovial tissue or from the immunological response of the host to the virus, with formation of antibody complexes in the synovial tissue [1422]. Arthritis in influenza usually presents itself as fleeting arthralgia or as hydrops (hydrarthrosis) and affects the knees, ankles, shoulders, and/or elbows and sometimes the hands. It usually regresses within 7–10 days, but may persist a few weeks with increased local warmth and swelling in some patients. These varying symptoms may be explained by the varying intensity of changes in the synovial membrane. The joints present moderate diffuse swelling of the soft tissues with mild blurring of their contours. The joint capsule is tender along its attachment onto the epiphyses, but the motion of the joints is not limited. The joint fluid is slightly increased. The lymph nodes and the spleen are sometimes enlarged. Purulent arthritis rarely occurs; it affects mainly small children and is caused by hemophilus influenzae, pneumococcus, or staphylococcus. This is discussed in "Suppurative Arthritis".

Laboratory studies in the acute phase disclose the presence of influenza virus type A or B inclusion bod-

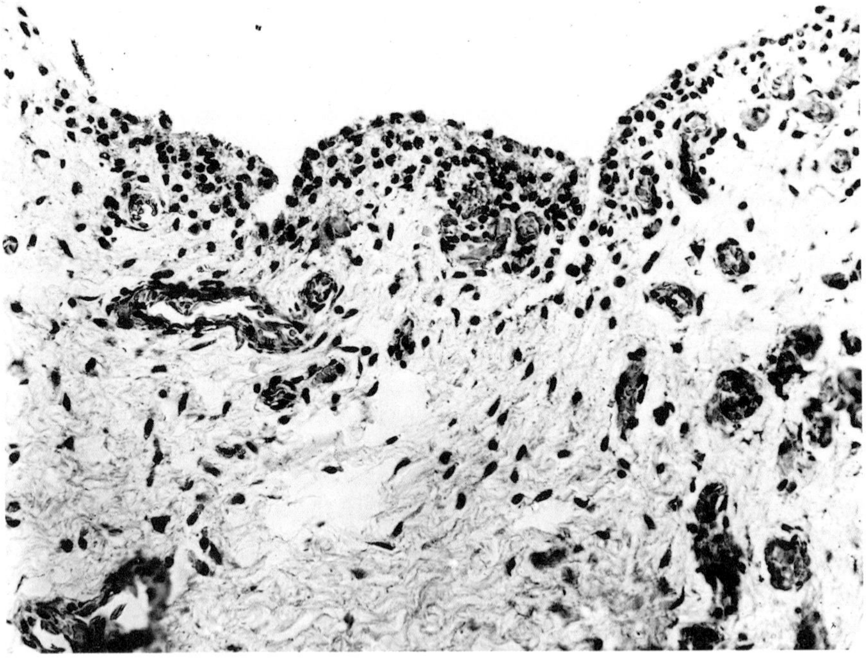

Fig. 131. Beneath slightly hypertrophic synoviocytes, histiocytes are increased, and a few lymphocytes are interspersed. All blood vessels are hyperemic, and the subsynoviocytic tissue is extensively rarefied by edema

ies [423, 565, 1422] in the cultures of blood and of smears from nose and throat secretion. The spherical virus particles consist of nucleoprotein, lipoprotein, and glycoprotein. The response to their presence can be ascertained [1154] by serological studies for identifying immunoglobulins, complement fixation, and hemagglutination inhibition, as well as the neutralization assay [1202]. All these disclose the presence of antibodies in a significant titer. Viral antigens can also be detected by immunofluorescence in the synoviocytes [1422]. A moderate leukocytosis without characteristic changes may be present. Leukopenia occurs in the very toxic forms of this disease. Urine studies show decreased output of keto- and oxysteroids, indicative of corticotropic hypofunction. The moderately increased joint fluid is very thin, clear, and pale greenish and contains abundant admixtures of mucin and 800–1400/ml white cells, mostly lymphocytes; no virus particles are observed.

Roentgenographic examination seldom reveals any changes except for moderate swelling of the joint capsule. However, in beginning but rare suppuration, intensive thickening of the joint capsule blurs the structure of the articular epiphyses, which progressively become more osteoporotic until partial dissolution.

The histopathological picture of the tissue obtained by punch biopsy corresponds to that of acute synovitis with hyperemia of all blood vessels and extensive edema of the subsynoviocytic tissue (Fig. 131). The latter contains scattered, moderate agglomerations of lymphocytes and plasmacytes but no feature suggestive of a specific etiology. The synovial membrane is swollen but not enlarged by villi.

Differential diagnosis of this arthritis is aided by the history of an initial influenza and by negative bacteriological findings in the blood and/or synovial fluid.

Treatment of arthritis in influenza focuses primarily on general measures such as complete bedrest and ample intake of warm fluids. Antiviral agents as amantadine 100–200 mg, adamantanamine 800 mg, or ribavirin aerosol or acyclovir 800–1000 mg daily are administered in divided doses until complete subsidence of the fever. However, if not effective within 2 days, and because of the frequent copresence of hemophilus influenzae or other microbes in concurrent inflammations of the lower respiratory tract, ampicillin 2.0–3.0 g, tetracycline 1.0–1.5 g, cephalosporin 2.0–4.0 g, or chloromycetin 2.0–3.0 g should be given daily in divided doses for 10–14 days. Afterward, salicylates (3.0 g daily) are indicated for the myalgias and circumscribed arthralgias. Additionally, moist warm compresses are applied around the joints as well as splints for immobilization. If a joint effusion develops and is not absorbed, it should be removed by arthrocentesis; the joint should be afterward compressed with an adhesive strapping. On persistence of swelling of the joint capsule much beyond the acute phase, one to two series with eight sessions of shortwave diathermy in addition to moist warm compresses and the application of an elastic bandage during the day are necessary for a period of 2–3 months.

Since conservative treatment is able to restore the function of the affected joint within a relatively short period of time, joint inflammation in influenza usually has a favorable prognosis. This experience applies chiefly to adults, due in part to their acquired immunity; however, it may not be so in children with hemophilus influenzae in their blood and joint fluid. With them the prognosis is incomparably more guarded [1710], and treatment of the joint inflammation as discussed in "Suppurative Arthritis" may be indicated.

12. Arthritis in Lyme Disease

Lyme disease owes its name to the town of Old Lyme, Connecticut, USA, where it was originally identified as an arthritic condition of undetermined etiology. Similar arthritic conditions were previously observed in other areas of Connecticut and elsewhere in the United States. Because of the larger number of affected children, it was initially considered a form of juvenile rheumatoid arthritis. The efforts of Steere et al. [1568, 1569, 1571] succeeded in elucidating the etiology of this arthritic condition as being initiated by a skin lesion caused by the bite of the tick, ixodes Dammini. The occurrence of an annular erythematous skin lesion was already described by Afzelius [8]. Subsequently, Lenhoff [960] reported that he found spirochetes in lesions of erythema chronicum migrans. Burgdorfer et al. [216] isolated a treponemalike spirochete in the ixodes ticks and thus established an etiological relationship between the implanting of spirochetes and the following skin alterations and systemic diseases. The spirochete (Fig. 132), Borrelia Burgdorferi [216] resembles the treponema in syphilis by its flagellae. It is either injected into the skin of the patient by the bite of the tick or is deposited on the skin by the discharge of the tick. The hosts of the ticks are mice, dogs, squirrels, and deer. This disease, observed in a significant proportion (444) of the 12000 inhabitants of Old Lyme, was subsequently confirmed also to occur in other northeastern and western states of the United States [1571]. Other reports were published in France [277, 800], Germany [4], Switzerland [600], and Australia [1580].

Following its penetration into the skin of the thigh, groin, or axilla, the spirochete provokes an initial red macule or papule [1568, 1569] after an incubation of 3–30 days. This skin affection gradually enlarges to erythema chronicum migrans, measuring 15 cm or more in diameter. Its center is intensely red and indurated and may become necrotic or vesicular. At its periphery several annular lesions follow after a few days by the spirochetal spread within the skin (Fig. 132). These are much smaller and less red and regress within 1–2 weeks. Similar annular lesions follow. The skin manifestations are associated with regional lymphadenopathy, general malaise, headache, fatigue, fever, and chills [1568].

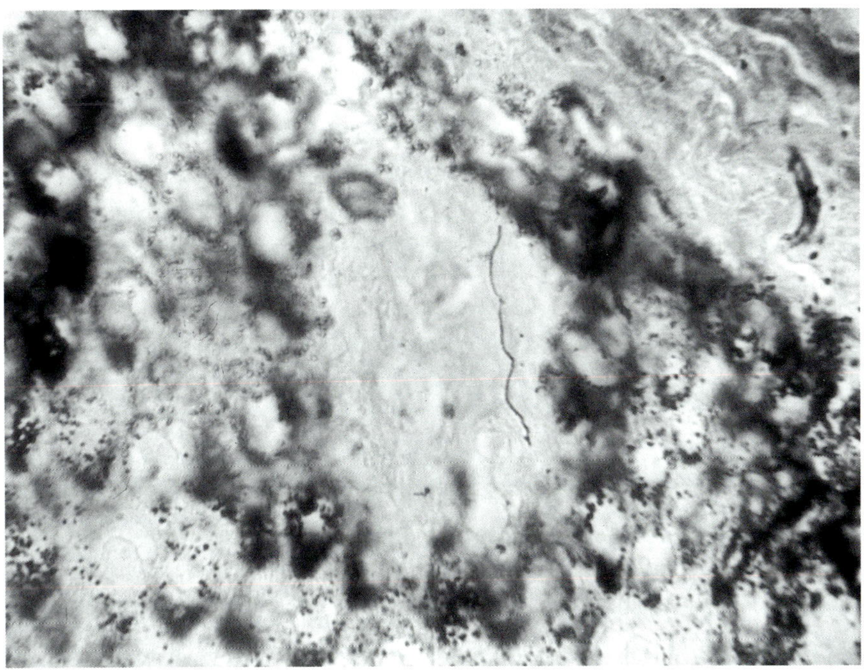

Fig. 132. A spirochete is located in a dermal papilla at the periphery of an erythema chronicum migrans

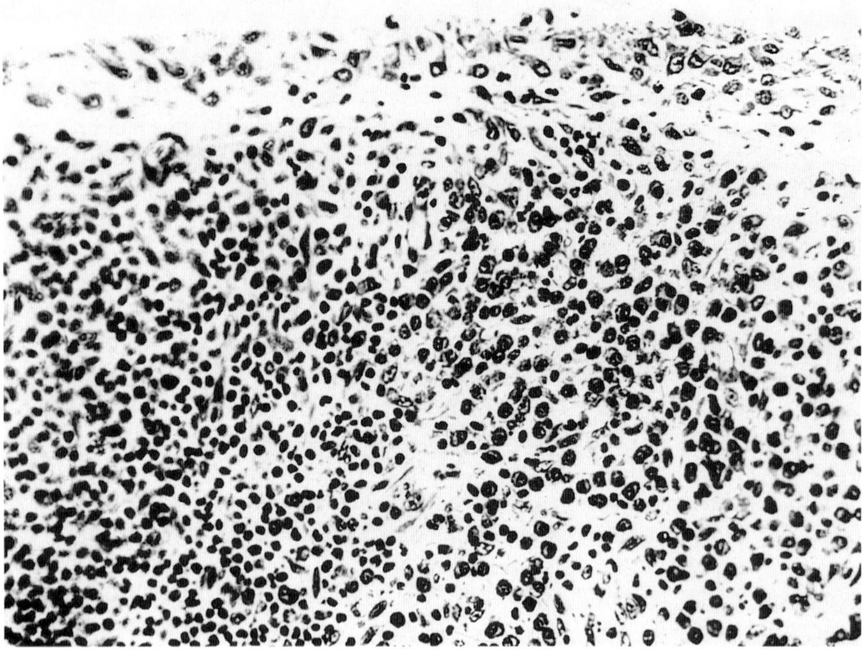

Fig. 133. The synoviocytes are moderately hypertrophic-hyperplastic. The subsynoviocytic tissue is extensively infiltrated; lymphocytes are agglomerated at one side, and plasmacytes are agglomerated at the other. Cells in the intermediate zone represent transitional elements

Secondary to intrusion and spread of the spirochete in the blood stream, the central nervous system [1313] and/or the heart become affected a few weeks to months later in 15% of these patients [1568]. The initial headache becomes more pronounced and is associated with pain and stiffness in the neck. Symptoms of encephalitis and meningitis with chorea, cranial neuritis, and/or myelitis with sensory and motor radiculoneuritis follow. After a period of 3–6 weeks the neurological symptoms usually regress completely. Regression is also seen of the cardiac symptoms, which are manifested in changes in the electrocardiogram with atrioventricular block, suggestive of acute myocarditis and pericarditis [1568].

A few weeks or as long as 2 years after onset of the skin condition, arthritic symptoms develop [1568] in about 60% of the patients. These symptoms are migrating pains in joints and their regional tendons or frank arthritis. The large joints, among them principally the knee and ankle joints, are affected by marked swelling of the joint capsule, intense pain, increased local warmth, and increased synovial fluid. The arthritic episodes may last a few weeks to a few months, may recur after years, and eventually subside, except in 10% of patients in whom they lead to residual arthritis [640].

Laboratory studies [69, 1568, 1571] disclose elevated serum IgM and IgG levels as specific antibodies 3–6 weeks after onset of the skin condition. These antibody titers rise when an affection of the central nervous system or of the major joints sets in. In the presence of relevant clinical findings an antibody titer of 1:256 or above (against Borrelia antigen) is strongly suggestive of Lyme disease [340], but cross-reaction with antigens in syphilis or leptospirosis must be considered. Serial determinations of IgM levels are very informative on the course and extent of this disease [340]. The indirect immunofluorescence assay for antibodies is diagnostically useful in the cases of Lyme disease with involvement of the central nervous system and/or cardiovascular system [1041]. A further and recently more frequently used serological test is the enzyme-linked immunosorbent assay, which is highly specific above the titer of 0.90 in complicated Lyme disease but is relatively insensitive in patients with erythema chronicum migrans [69, 1378]. Nonspecific findings include the high elevation in sedimentation rate (up to 70 mm/h) and increased levels to serum glutamic oxalacetic transaminase. Since the serological tests are not absolutely specific due to cross-reaction with syphilis and other infectious diseases, direct demonstration of the etiological spirochete has received increasing attention. The cultures for spirochete from the blood or skin exudate yield positive results on a modified medium [876] in a small percentage of these cases. Positive results provide unequivocal confirmation of the etiology [216]. Berger et al. [123] identified spirochetes of the same type as those isolated from ixodes dammini by silver stain in tissue sections of erythema chronicum migrans (Fig. 132). In addition, the spirochete has been demonstrated [216] in the synovial tissue in cases of capsule swelling. The yellowish, slightly turbid joint fluid contains substantially increased white blood cells, on average 25000/ml, most of them polymorphonuclear neutrophilic leukocytes.

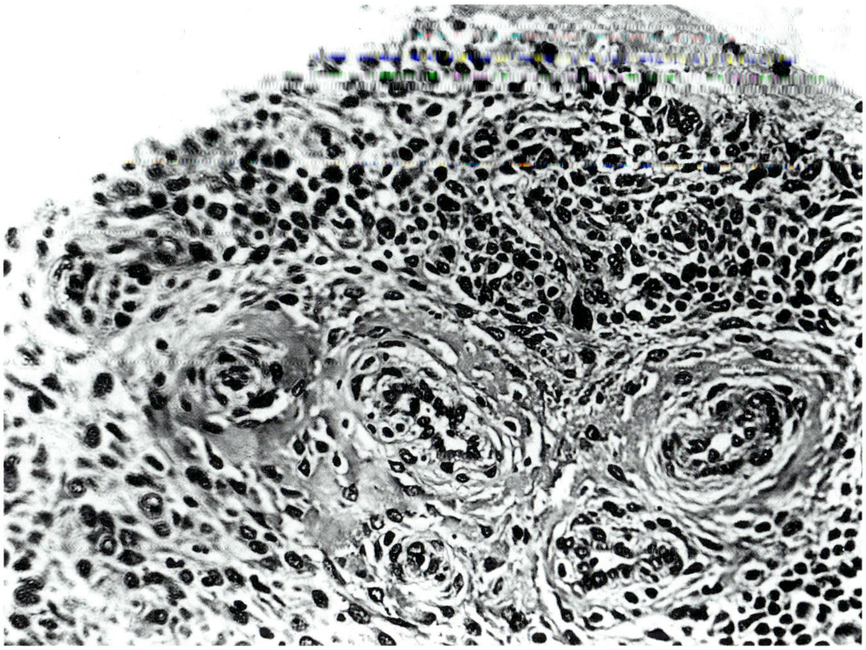

Fig. 134. Arterioles and venules in the subsynoviocytic tissue have thickened walls by enlargement of the cells in their media and by an increase in the cells in their adventitia

Synovial biopsies [1571] disclose surface deposits of fibrin, villous hypertrophy, vascular proliferation, and heavy infiltration by mononuclear cells including plasma cells (Fig. 133). These cell agglomerations resemble those observed in the synovial membrane in early syphilitic arthritis [841]. Some arterioles and venules in the subsynoviocytic tissue have markedly thickened walls by enlargement of the cells in their media and by increase of the cells in their adventitia (Fig. 134). Johnston et al. [835] detected spirochetes in microangiopathic lesions in the synovial membrane. In about 10% of cases of persistent or recurrent inflammation of large joints erosion of the articular cartilage and subchondral bone follows [640].

The diagnosis cannot be missed in those cases in which an expanding erythema chronicum migrans is followed by affection of the central nervous system and/or heart and eventual arthritis. An insect bite can be ascertained in only 60% of these patients. However, the diagnosis becomes difficult when the primary skin affection is only a papule which does not expand or merely resembles a local urticarial rash. In these situations, serum arthritis, Reiter's syndrome, or rheumatoid arthritis must be considered [1571]. Laboratory tests (especially the enzyme-linked immunosorbent assay ELISA) and the search for spirochetes in skin lesions help to ascertain the diagnosis.

Once the diagnosis has been established on the basis of the primary and typical skin manifestation and/or subsequent laboratory studies, routine treatment consists of tetracycline 250 mg six to eight times daily and orally given for 2 weeks, followed by ampicillin 500 mg six times daily for 2–3 more weeks [1041, 1571]. If tetracycline is not tolerated, erythromycin 500 mg four to six times daily is given for 3 weeks. However, in view of the experience [1041, 1571] that the skin lesions are followed in 15%–20% of cases by affections of the central nervous system, meninges, and/or heart and are followed in 60% of cases by arthritis, it appears a wise precaution to begin treatment with the most effective medication. Thus 10–20,000,000 U penicillin G daily should be administered intravenously for 3 weeks. If indicated by clinical signs and laboratory studies, the above oral antibiotics should follow, or the series of penicillin injections may be repeated for longer periods of time. This policy derives from the experience that arthritic episodes may recur even after several years.

13. Syphilitic Arthritis

Syphilitic arthritis occurs in 2%–3% of those infected with acquired syphilis and in an even higher proportion of those with inherited syphilis. Among all joint inflammations, that of syphilitic etiology represents 0.1% in frequency [1238]. The causative microorganism is the 8- to 18-μm-long treponema pallidum of the spirochete family; its body has an axial filament, is wound up in a few spirales, and is in continuous motion when examined in body fluids.

The joint affection appears in the second stage of acquired syphilis [1448]. This begins with an exanthem

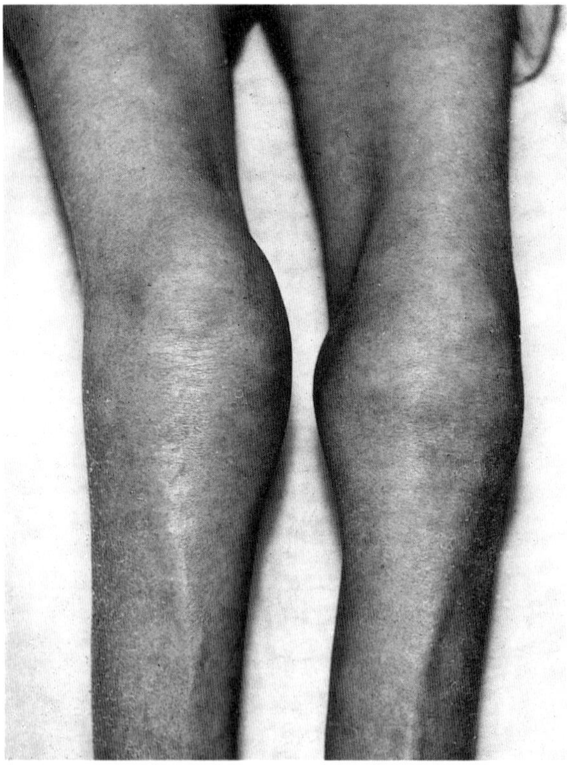

Fig. 135. Both knee joints are extensively thickened, and the contours of the knees are distorted. The knees are held in slight flexion contracture

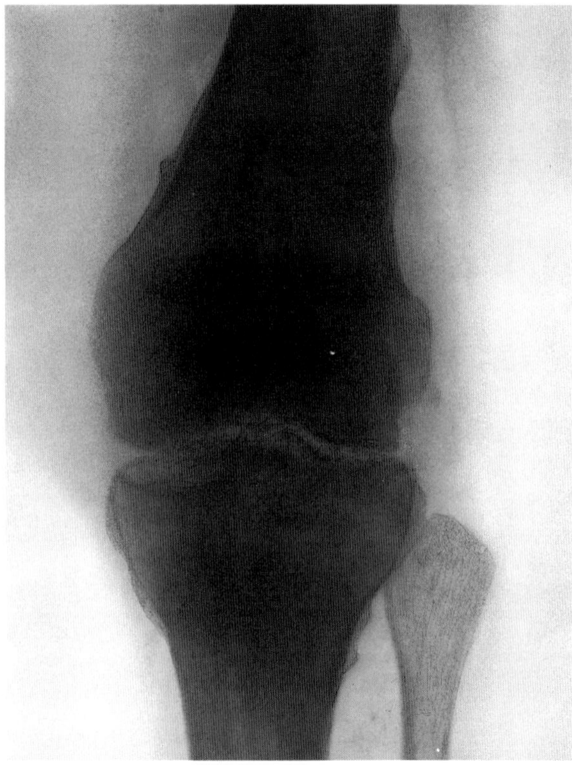

Fig. 136. The articular contours of the femoral condyles and tibial condyles are uneven and unsharp. The medial joint space is widened secondary to deeper erosion of the medial tibial condyle. The femur and tibia are sclerosed, and their cortices are uneven by periosteal apposition. The periarticular soft tissues are densified

showing very red, oozing and/or dry macules, and crusty papules which disintegrate into pustules and ulcers extending over the trunk and/or extremities. Similar aphthes are observed on the mucous membranes, but a moth-eaten-like alopecia develops in the scalp. Of the internal organs, the liver and spleen are enlarged; frequent icterus points to the parenchymatous damage of the liver. The harm to the kidneys is associated with persistent albuminuria. Affection of the eyes is manifested in iritis and/or retinitis and that of the central nervous system is associated with cerebral meningitis involving chiefly the optic, facial, and acoustic nerves [103].

The treponema entering and being spread by the bloodstream can settle in the joint capsule or the articular epiphysis. It elicits in these tissues inflammatory and disintegrating changes and thereby causes in them a susceptibility to subsequent other harmful influences. Syphilitic arthritis imitates joint inflammations of various etiologies and can appear in the following diagnostic types: (a) pseudogonococcal arthralgia, (b) pseudorheumatoid arthritis with effusion, and (c) pseudotuberculous fungus with occasional draining sinuses.

Accordingly, the clinical picture is very varied and changing. Pain often occurs especially in the night, and is localized chiefly in bones and/or joints (dolores osteocupi nocturni). These sensations have a drilling or cutting character and sometimes a certain steadfastness in a single bone or joint. In other patients, the painful sensations shift from the knee to the ankle, hip, shoulder, wrist, or finger joint. When a joint effusion representing a syphilitic enanthema develops, the symptoms are those of rheumatoid arthritis; the general condition is impaired, and the temperature is elevated at times. Patients have a pale appearance, and their internal examination, especially in the tertiary stage, may reveal changes in the cardiovascular system (endocarditis, mesaortitis, aneurysm). The most commonly affected joint is the knee, less frequently the sternoclavicular junction or ankle joint. The joint is enlarged but not warmer. Characteristic for the syphilitic etiology is the relative freedom from pain despite the obvious swelling (Fig. 135), the scantness of local inflammatory changes despite effusion, and the pauciarticularity, as well as the frequent symmetricality of the joint affection (Figs. 135, 137). While the effusion

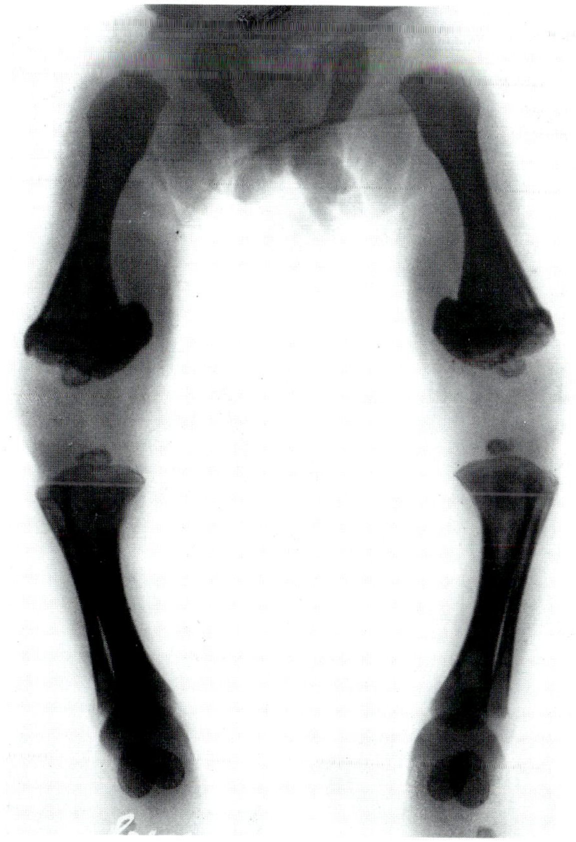

Fig. 137. The distal femoral metaphysis is very deformed and enlarged in congenital syphilis. The proximal tibial metaphysis is less deformed, and the joint capsule is densified

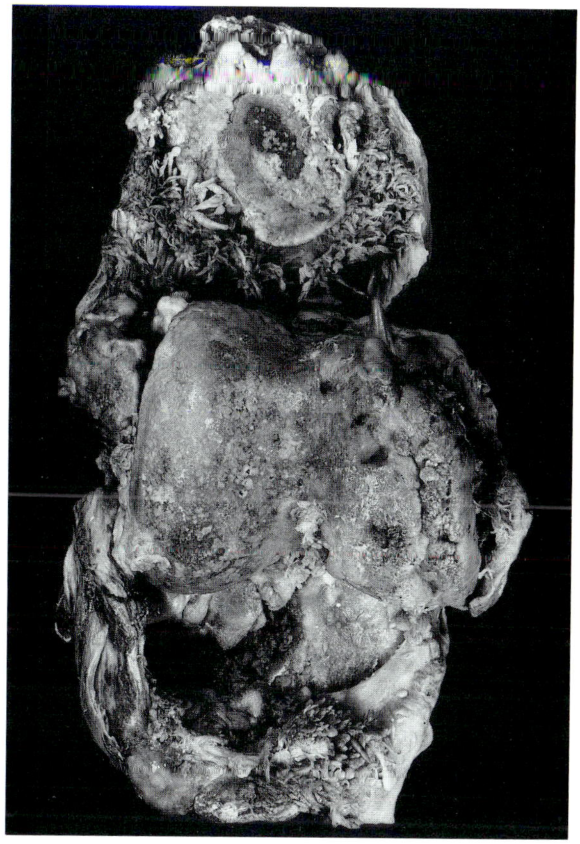

Fig. 138. The articular surfaces of the patella, femoral condyles, and tibial condyles are uneven secondary to estensive erosion of their cartilage. The medial tibial condyle is deeply defective. The inner joint capsule is raised in many slender villi

regresses, the joint capsule becomes diffusely infiltrated. It presents on palpation the sensation of being padded with cotton. On very progressive thickening of the joint capsule, the joint becomes enlarged and globe-like. The surrounding skin is overstretched, anemic-pale, and shiny; therefore it is termed tumor albus syphiliticus. With longer duration of the joint affection, the regional musculature becomes atrophic (Fig. 135) and the movements of the joint are limited.

In the laboratory studies, the sedimentation rate is only moderately elevated. Following invasion of the human body by the treponema pallidum antibodies are formed which are ascertained serologically in the diagnosis of syphilis. The test, inaugurated by Wassermann [1717], uses an extract from human syphilitic tissue (liver) as antigen in complement fixation for demonstration of the antibodies in the patient's serum. The Kolmer test [1670] directly employs treponemal antigen, but from another strain of treponema than pallidum, also in a complement fixation test. On the other hand, the Venereal Diseases Research Laboratory (VDRL) uses nontreponemal antigen (an alcoholic extract from cardiolipin [842], lecithin, and cholesterol) in a slide flocculation test with the patient's serum [1670]. However, a positive result of the VDRL test is not always proof of the syphilitic etiology of a joint affection; rheumatoid arthritis is associated in 2%–3% of cases with false-positive VDRL test outcomes. This test as well as that of Wassermann have a specificity of 76%–90% particularly in the primary and secondary stages of syphilis, but they are deficient in a great percentage of cases in the tertiary stage [818, 1273]. In these situations, immunofluorescence study is regularly employed; this uses treponema pallidum which is exposed to the patient's serum and thereafter to a fluorescein-labeled anti-human globulin. The latter identifies the presence of the patient's immunoglobulin on the surface of the treponemal body [479]. Arthrocentesis yields a greenish yellow opalescent fluid containing 3%–5% protein and 4000–20000 cells/ml, most of them lymphocytes and plasmacytes. The sediment contains abundant fibrin flakes, lymphocytes, and plasmacytes. In tumor albus, spirochetes may be demonstrated in the joint fluid and/or in the synovial tissue by dark-field examination and immunofluorescence [1310]. The VDRL test on joint fluid has often been the

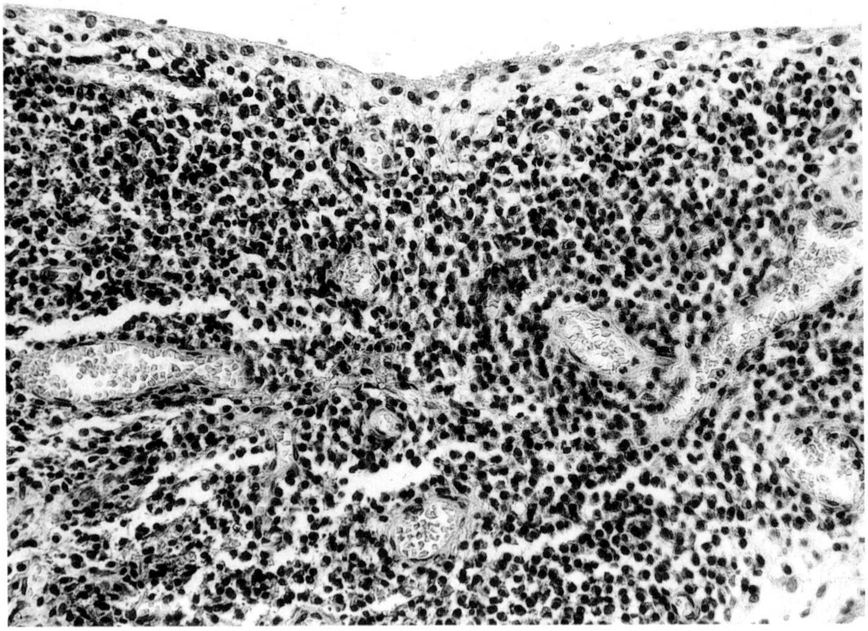

Fig. 139. The synovial membrane is extensively and densely infiltrated chiefly by plasmacytes. The blood vessels are hyperemic

subject of research because a reliable indicator is sought in view of the inconsistency of the serum reaction. Schlesinger [1415] reported a positive reaction to the Wassermann test on joint fluid in 30% of cases of syphilitic arthritis, but he also emphasized that the joint fluid yielded a negative result in 70% of cases. Therefore, the immunofluorescence study for treponemal antibodies in the joint fluid represents a very conclusive test [842, 1647].

Roentgenographic examination reveals no changes at the onset of the joint affection. With densification of the joint capsule the joint space becomes overshadowed. Secondary to inflammation of the periosteum, cortical apposition and irregular delimitation of the metaphysis (Fig. 136) follows close to the epiphysis. The metaphysis then becomes sclerosed and thickened due to cufflike apposition. By disintegration of gummatous foci at the attachment of the synovial capsule and in the subchondral area, lentil- to pea-sized defects delimited by sclerotic borders develop in the articular epiphysis.

Gross-anatomical examination in the initial phase discloses that the synovial membrane is reddened and edematous. Subsequently, the inflammation spreads into the fibrous capsule and from there into the periarticular organs such as tendons and/or bursae. When the joint capsule is directly affected by spirochetes, the synovial membrane is covered in places with masses of fibrin and becomes substantially thickened by numerous large and ramified villi (Fig. 138); here it resembles a shaggy cover. All layers of the joint capsule are diffusely thickened and contain dense nodules which consist of reddish gray gelatinous tissue with occasional central caseation. Their sites of predilection are the synovial folds and the inner layer of the fibrous capsule at the margin of the articular cartilage. On longer duration of the joint affection, serrated, sharply delimited defects as if punched out by a instrument develop in the hyaline cartilage (Fig. 138). This loss is subsequently compensated by connective tissue which fills the ground of the indentations. The resulting scars represent a characteristic alteration of syphilitic etiology (Fig. 138). Following further expansion of the cartilage defects and their substitution by peripheral granulation tissue, the articular cavity may become obliterated. On the other hand, necrotic nodules within the joint capsule may perforate externally, leading to draining sinuses with mixed infection.

Histopathologically [107, 841, 1310, 1659] the synovial membrane displays marked dilatation of the blood vessels (Fig. 139) and focal agglomerations of lymphocytes and particularly plasmacytes which expand progressively to infiltrates. In some places the lymphocytes are aggregated in nodules. In the chronic phase, numerous large villi covered by hyperplastic synoviocytes rise above the surface into the joint cavity (Fig. 140). The lymphocyte infiltrates expand through the subsynoviocytic tissue into the fibrous capsule. In a few areas of the subsynoviocytic tissue, gummata are scattered (Fig. 140), and resemble tuberculous granulomata since they also contain centers of necrotic tissue. Their periphery consists of spindle cells, epitheloid cells, lymphocytes, and sometimes giant cells. Some of these gummata undergo disintegration and caseation,

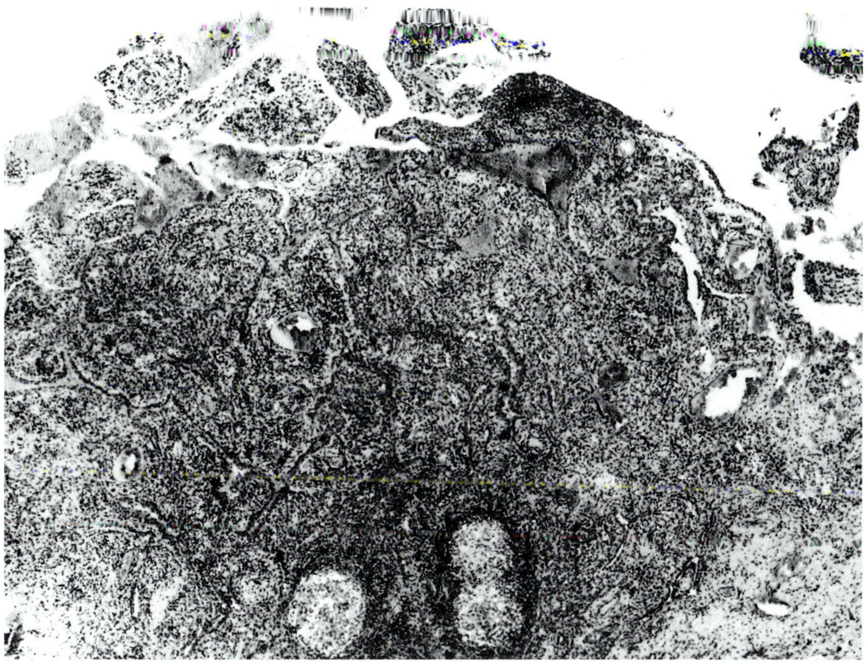

Fig. 140. The synovial membrane is raised in many villi which are close to each other. The subsynoviocytic tissue is extensively hypercellular with fibrocytes and chronic inflammatory cells. A few gummata lie in the depth of the synovial membrane

which expands much beyond the necrotic center and leaves a surrounding border of epitheloid cells and lymphocytes. Disintegration takes place concurrently in the articular cartilage by syphilitic granulations such as gummata. These proliferate from the epiphyseal marrow spaces and, penetrating through the subchondral bone, intrude into the cartilage at several sites (Fig. 141). Here the cartilage undergoes progressive destruction, resulting in defects in the cartilaginous surface (Fig. 141, 142). However, with subsequent proliferations of granulation tissue around the expanded gummata, some defects eventually become filled from the depth with dense connective tissue (Fig. 142). In the advanced chronic phase, synovial villi expand over the articular margin and as pannus erode the articular cartilage, causing defects in the epiphyseal surface. The resulting defects are progressively filled with maturing granulation tissue. Electron-microscopic examinations [1310] identified the presence of treponemalike bodies with typical coiling and characteristic longitudi-

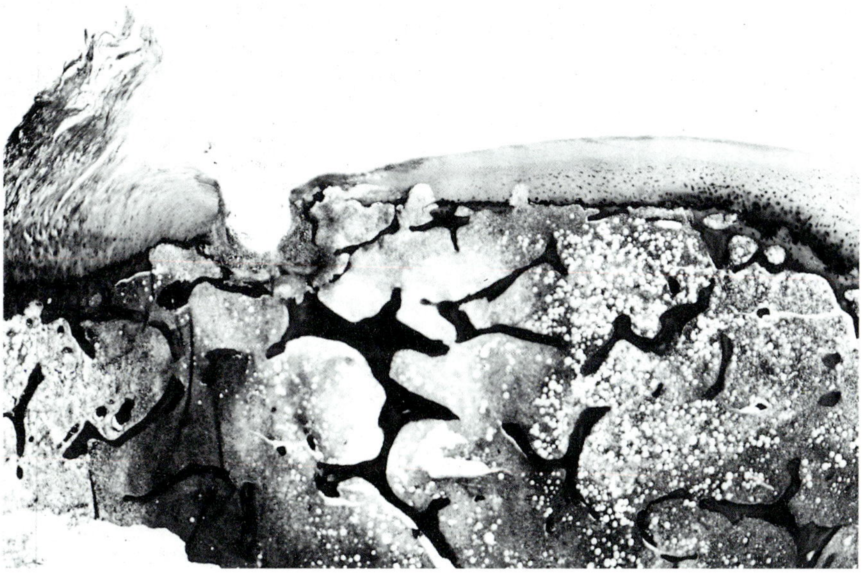

Fig. 141. A few gummata penetrate from the marrow spaces into the articular cartilage. A larger gumma, close to insertion of the joint capsule, has perforated into the joint space

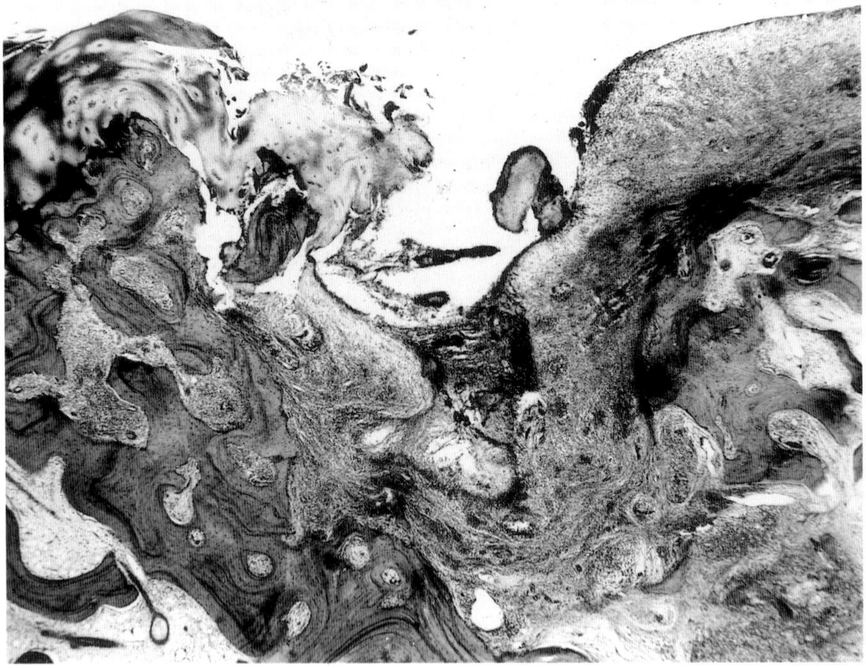

Fig. 142 Dense scarified connective tissue fills the defect in the articular surface penetrated by a gumma and also covers a part of the articular surface. The other part of the articular surface bears disrupted articular cartilage

nal filaments in areas of necrosis of the synovial membrane. This supports the concept of direct invasion of joints by spirochetes.

Syphilitic arthritis presents differential diagnostic difficulties since it simulates the clinical picture of other joint inflammations. The arthralgias in gonococcal infection are also fleeting and migratory in a few joints. Compared with rheumatoid arthritis, the negative response to salicyates is characteristic. The tuberculous fungus may be recognized by the early appearance of muscle atrophy, the roentgenographically observed osteoporosis, and the early tendency to stiffness. However, with an anamnestically reported genital infection, it is most important to ascertain a preceding or coincident skin rash and to exclude any other general disease etiologically associated with joint affections. The search for changes of internal organs helps to establish the proper diagnosis. The relevant serological tests provide conclusive confirmation.

Treatment with penicillin has proven very effective in all stages of syphilitic arthritis. Penicillin G in doses of 3,000,000 U–5,000,000 U are administered at 6-h intervals for 3 weeks; this is repeated after 6 weeks if the first series did not provide a distinct abolition of the symptoms. Due to massive disintegration of spirochetes by the penicillin, an allergic Herxheimer's reaction may occur. Penicillin treatment succeeds in reversing the VDRL test results in the blood to negativity usually 6–12 months later; similar changes may be obtained in the cerebrospinal fluid. In patients allergic to penicillin, effective substitutes include oxytetracycline, chloramphenicol, or erythromycin given daily in divided doses of 3.0–4.0 g and for a period of 3 months. However, these results are obtained only if medicamentous treatment is begun as soon as possible, after the symptoms become manifest, but not later than at the start of the second stage. The longer the initiation of treatment is delayed, the longer is the interval (12–20 months) until reversal of the serological test result to negativity and the less probable is such reversal. Nevertheless, the local organic symptoms partially regress. With advanced changes in a joint involving also the articular cartilage, the above treatments are not able to reverse these changes. Therefore, in addition to repeated physical therapy with shortwave diathermy and massage in two or three series of eight sessions, the ailing joints need support by semicircular braces or plastic splints with straps. In view of the poor healing tendency in syphilis, reconstructive surgical procedures on the ill-functioning joints are disadvised, even in the presence of serologically verified benefit by the medicamentous treatment.

Arthritis may also occur in congenital syphilis. This appears in children and adolescents and is usually manifested by symmetrical swelling of the knee and ankle joints. The dense swelling of the joint capsule is sometimes associated with a painless effusion, by which it may be distinguished from acute rheumatic or juvenile chronic rheumatoid arthritis. Also of diagnostic significance are the occurrence of keratitis, bossing of the frontal bones, notching of the incisor teeth, and roentgenographically observed changes [1448].

Among laboratory studies, the sedimentation rate is moderately elevated (25–35 mm/h). Once the suspicion of syphilitic affection has been raised, the Wassermann and VDRL tests on blood are performed; in the case of infection these yield strongly positive results. The synovial fluid contains an increased number (up to 15000) of lymphocytes but no microorganisms even on dark-field examination. Roentgenographs (Fig. 137) reveal thickening and densification of the joint capsule, broadening of the epiphyseal plates, and periosteal apposition at the metaphyses and diaphyses. The articular ends are irregularly delimited by erosion of the articular cartilage.

Histopathological examination [49] of the inner part of the joint capsule discloses thickening of the synovial membrane by proliferation of the superficial cells, diffuse edema, dilatation of all blood vessels, and extensive infiltration by lymphocytes. The inflamed synovial membrane encroaches upon the articular cartilage, which itself presents marked irregularity in the distribution of chondrocytes.

With the diagnosis established, treatment should begin without delay. Since parenteral treatment with penicillin G is not possible in young patients, semisynthetic penicillin 1.0 g should be given orally every 4 h in a protracted course of 2–3 months. If the penicillin is not tolerated due to allergy, oxytetracycline 2.0 g or erythromycin 2.0 g daily should be given in divided doses over a period of 3 months. In the rare situations in which oral antibiotic treatment does not provide an essential regression of the symptoms, the treatment must be intramuscular administration of penicillin G 5,000,000–8,000,000 U daily in divided doses over a period of 3–4 weeks, and is repeated if necessary after 2–3 months. Eventually the laboratory findings for syphilis may revert to negativity and the capsular changes subside. These joints can then function for the activities of daily life, but vigorous activities should be avoided. However, if the articular ends are very uneven, secondary arthritic changes and deformities are likely to ensue. These joints should be protected by splints and require physical therapy with diathermy, massage of the regional musculature, and a program of exercises. Surgical treatment is not advisable because of the poor healing tendency of all tissues in this condition.

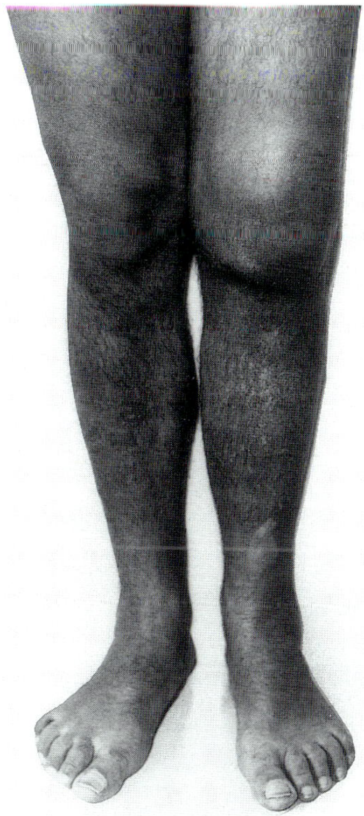

Fig. 143. The left knee is swollen with protrusion of the suprapatellar recessus by an increase in joint fluid. The quadriceps musculature is atrophic

14. Tuberculous Arthritis

With the dramatic decrease in overall incidence of pulmonary tuberculosis, the incidence of tuberculosis of the skeleton has also declined [474, 617, 1183]. The incidence of new active cases of pulmonary tuberculosis in United States was 14 per 100000 persons in 1975, while the incidence of skeletal tuberculosis was 2 per 100000 in 1976 [1661]. Since then the rates have declined further [1662]. The difference between these two figures indicates that not every case of pulmonary tuberculosis is followed by skeletal tuberculosis. On the other hand, not every case of skeletal tuberculosis can be traced to pulmonary tuberculosis; in more than 20% of the former condition, physical, sputum, and roentgenographic examinations do not reveal the presence of an active pulmonary infection. In such cases, the skeletal infection may have resulted by spread of mycobacterium tuberculosis from an asymptomatic pulmonary focus or from the gastrointestinal tract via the bloodstream or lymphatic system.

Although the concept of a primary tuberculous complex and its metastatic dissemination was corroborated by pathological-anatomical examinations, it is sometimes difficult to detect the organ of origin of the tuberculous infection by any modality of clinical examination. Identification of the spreading focus is often problematic because it may be scarified or healed when the infection of a joint becomes manifest. With hematogenous spread from a remote primary focus accepted as the mode of infection, tuberculosis of a joint may occur either as a primary synovial affection or as propagation from a primary epiphyseal focus [369].

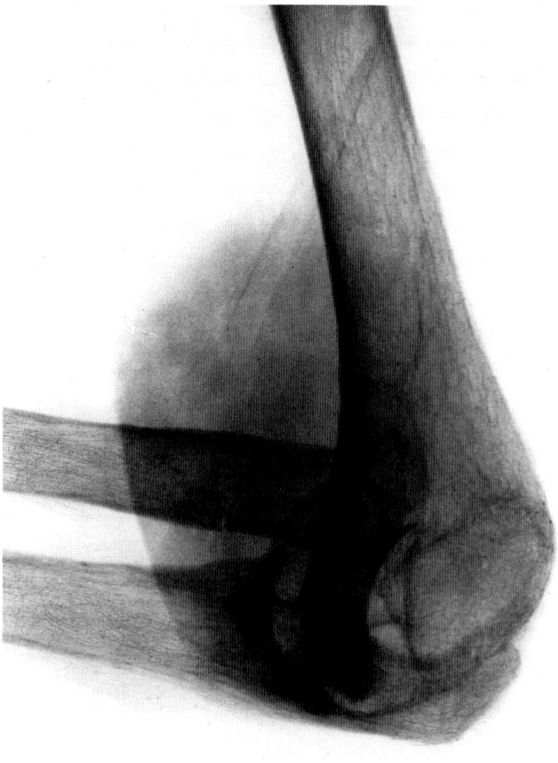

Fig. 144. Extensive erosion of the fossa trochleae of the ulna. The humeroulnar cavity is unevenly bordered and partly widened.

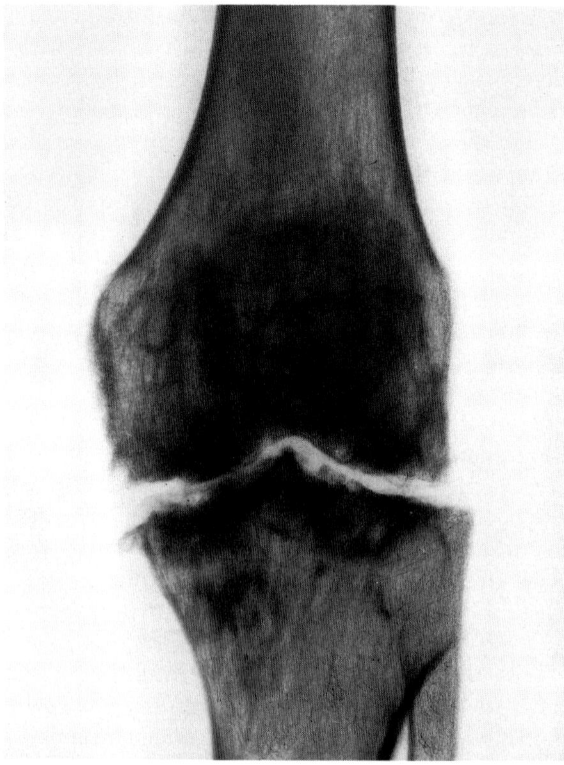

Fig. 145. The surfaces of the femoral and tibial condyles are eroded, and the joint space is unevenly bordered and partly narrowed. The tibial epiphysis and metaphysis are osteoporotic and of irregular structures

Tuberculosis of the joints [128, 371, 1094, 1779] most commonly affects adolescents and adults who have suffered of a preceding or concurrent tuberculosis of the lungs, or who have lived in economically disadvantaged conditions. Children develop it less commonly. Among the joints and bones those of the vertebral column are most often affected; these are followed in frequency, principally as monoarticular affection, by the knee, hip, ankle, wrist, shoulder, elbow, and interphalangeal joints. The joint disease begins insidiously and progresses slowly with impaired use of the limb and with pain. Examination discloses enlargement of the joint by a diffuse, doughy swelling, sometimes combined with increased joint fluid, chiefly in the knee (Fig. 143), ankle, elbow, and wrist, moderate increase in local temperature, diffuse tenderness, and concentric limitation of active movements. Conspicuous atrophy of the regional musculature sets in early. In advanced cases, the joint develops a contracture in faulty position and often one or a few draining sinuses from a cold abscess (Figs. 533, 534). On excessive swelling, expanding from the joint capsule into the periarticular structures, regional blood vessels become compressed, and the enlarged joint appears as tumor albus. On affection of the joints of the spine, the clinical signs are less obvious [62], being located in the depth of the musculature. Nevertheless, tenderness of the vertebral column both at the spinous processes and apophyseal joints and persistent defense of the regional paravertebral musculature point to a deep-seated involvement of the vertebrae and their joints. A gibbus deformity (Figs. 148, 149) often supervening in the middorsal or upper lumbar spine completes the clinical picture. This is complicated in 10%–15% of the cases by compression either of nerve roots, with more sensory than motor symptoms, or of the spinal cord, with resulting paraplegia. Another, more frequent complication is the descending cold abscess (Fig. 148) which is discharged through draining sinuses in the lower back and/or groin.

Among laboratory studies, the erythrocyte sedimentation rate (ESR) ranges between 16 and 35 mm/h at the beginning of inflammation and in the exudative forms. It increases when extensive granulomata are associated with destruction of cartilage and bone. Eventually the ESR may rise to 80 mm/h or higher when caseous disintegration, formation of cold abscesses, and marked drainage ensue. Similar high elevation of the ESR is noticed in primary osseous tuberculosis, when a tuberculous abscess expands into

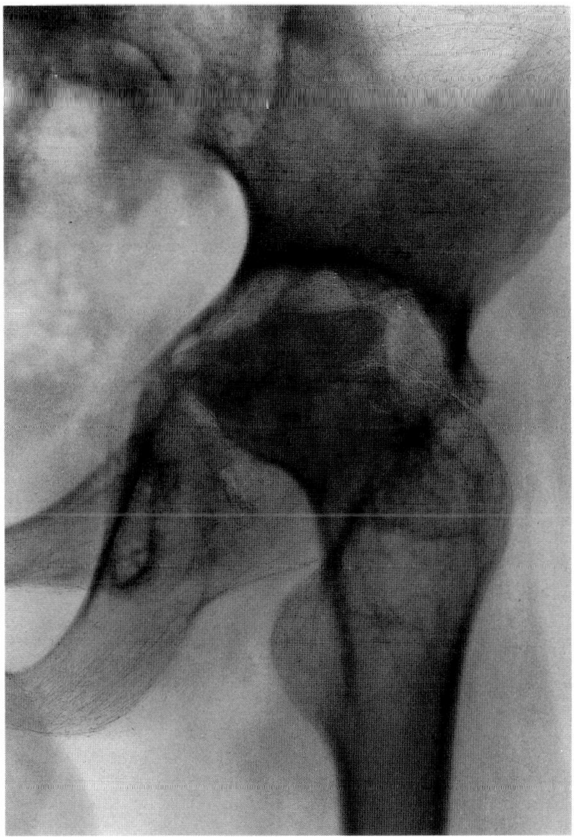

Fig. 146. The femoral head and acetabulum are extensively eroded, and the joint cavity is very widened and irregularly delimited. The dense structure of these epiphyses indicates healing of the process

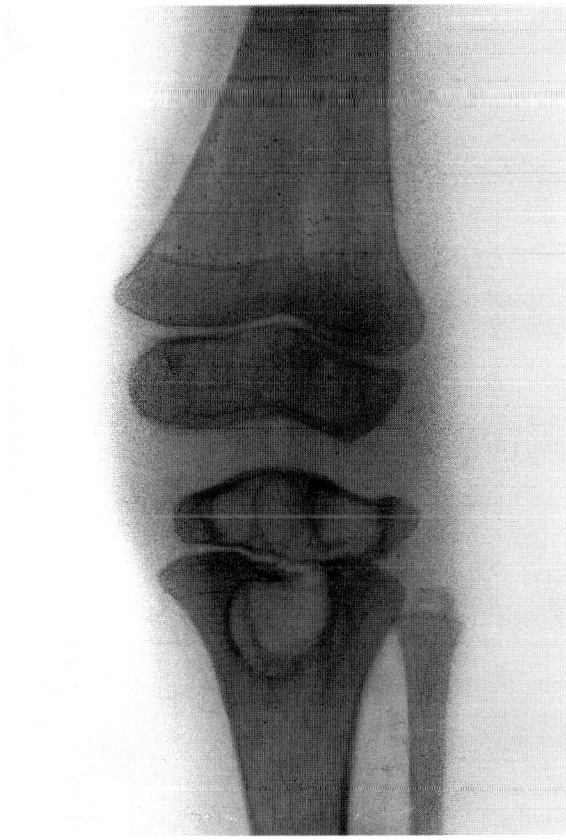

Fig. 147. An extensive but delimited destruction has penetrated the epiphysis and metaphysis of the tibia in a child

a joint. While the ESR does not have differential diagnostic value here, its importance lies in the realm of prognosis. Comparison of the ESR rates determined at intervals during the course of the disease permits an inference on the activity and phase of the tuberculous process. Similarly, the leukocyte count and differential count permit valuable inferences concerning the reactions of the body. On extensive destruction and formation of cold abscesses, polymorphonuclear neutrophilic leukocytes may be increased to 30000–50000/ml. On the other hand, increase of lymphocytes indicates overcoming of the infection. However, it is the predominance of monocytes which signals regression of the inflammation and the beginning of healing. A positive outcome on the tuberculin test in the skin onfirms that a tuberculous focus exists in the body, but it leaves open the possibility that the joint affection is not of tuberculous origin. On the other hand, a negative skin test result does not completely exclude a tuberculous nature of the joint affection.

Examination of the turbid joint fluid typically discloses an increase in white blood cells to 8000–25000/ml as well as increased total protein. Sugar is decreased to 50 mg%, which, while suggestive of the presence of a bacterial infection, is not sufficient to verify it conclusively. Therefore, the joint fluid should be stained in smear with carbolfuchsin to identify acid-fast microorganisms using the Ziehl-Neelsen method; it should also be cultured in Löwenstein-Jensen medium [163]. The acid-fast smear manifests the presence of tubercle bacilli in only 20%–30% of cases. Mycobacterium tuberculosis is a nonmotile rod which varies from coccoid to thin bacillary, curved or straight shapes. These are found in small clusters and at angles to one other. On the other hand, culture shows the presence of tubercle bacilli in 70%–80% of cases [769]. If the results of these tests remain negative, a biopsy from the affected joint by arthroscopy is indicated. Specimens of synovial tissue should be examined histopathologically for the presence of granulomata, stained for tubercle bacilli, and immersed in appropriate culture media. Löwenstein-Jensen culture of synovial tissue discloses the presence of tubercle bacilli in 50%–70% of cases [371, 769]. In involvement of the vertebral column, Caroit et al. [244] recommended needle aspiration of tissues from the affected

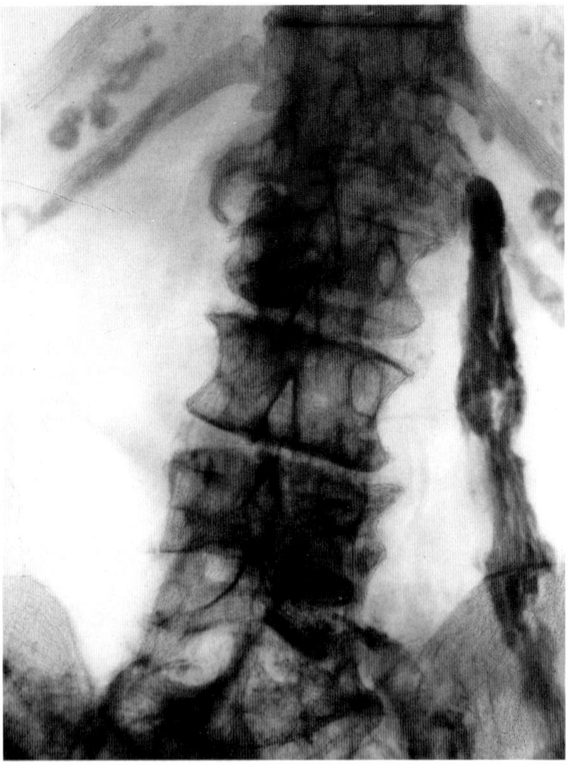

Fig. 148. The intervertebral space T12-L1 is completely obliterated secondary to fusion of these vertebrae. Marginal bridgings unite L1 and L2. A calcified paravertebral abscess descends from L1

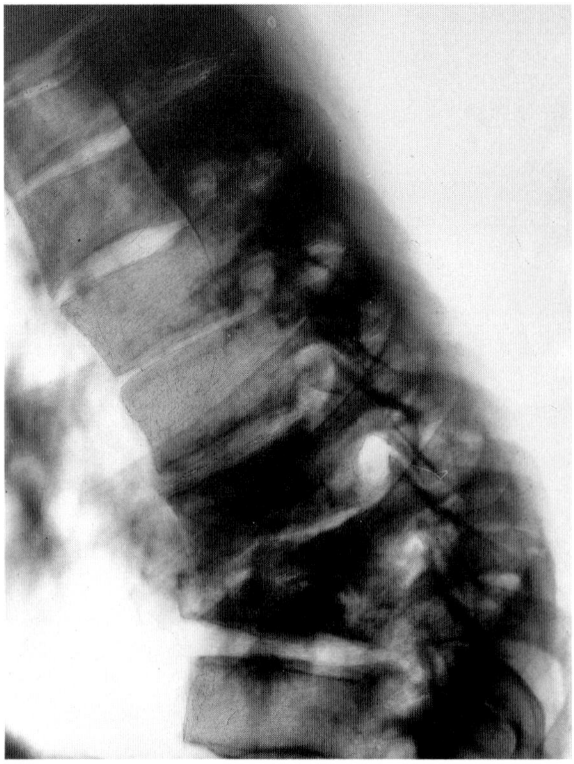

Fig. 149. Two thoracic vertebrae are united to a wedge-shaped block. The cranially situated vertebra slided ventrally above this wedge; the kyphosis of the dorsal spine is markedly increased

vertebrae and intervertebral disc. Examinations of these tissues by microscope and culture enable one in most cases to ascertain the etiology.

Roentgenographs of peripheral joints [875, 1346] reveal ballooning of the joint and widening of the cartilage space by increased joint fluid. Due to hyperemia and toxic influence, osteoporosis of the articular epiphyses soon results, with greater distinctiveness of their trabecular design (Figs. 144, 145). However, when the joint capsule becomes very infiltrated and dense, it obscures the articular ends; their structure becomes blurred, and the cartilage space is overshadowed. On invasion by synovial granulations the margins of the articular surfaces present the first sign of erosion. By progressive destruction of the cartilage, its space becomes substantially narrower. Proliferative granulations into the depth erode the subchondral bone, and cause its irregular jagged delineation (Figs. 144, 145, 146]. Destructive foci of primary osseous origin inside the epiphyses appear as roundish or ovoid areas of radiolucency, which may be bordered by normal or densified bone but lack regional periosteal apposition (Fig. 147). In other cases, necrotic, noncolliquating foci become impregnated with calcium salts and then present areas of density while the surrounding bone displays osteoporosis. If the tuberculous process has healed in its beginning stage, the cartilage space may be partly maintained; however, due to its incongruence sclerosed irregular articulating edges and marginal osteophytes develop (Figs. 145, 146). If abscesses occur in the areas of caseinification and are complicated by mixed infection, osteoporosis and sclerosis, extensive destruction and periosteal apposition alternate. A strange structure results here (Fig. 145) which conveys the impression of coccal osteomyelitis or sarcomatous destruction. Periosteal apposition at articular epiphyses or diaphyses, considered a sign of coccal osteomyelitis, is sometimes observed in osseous tuberculosis of the elbow or a digital phalanx (spina ventosa).

In roentgenographs of the vertebral column, two or sometimes three vertebrae are very irregularly delineated at their plates, and their intervertebral spaces are substantially narrowed (Fig. 148). A paravertebral abscess often descends from this level. The affected vertebral bodies are generally osteoporotic but reattain their structure and even sclerosis in the healing phase. Then, secondary to extensive destruction and loss of

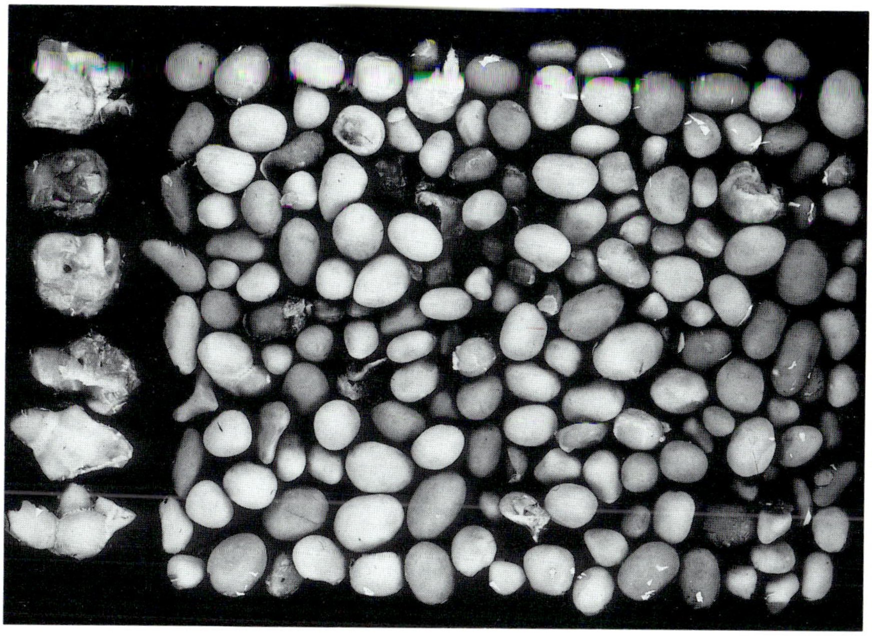

Fig. 150. Rice bodies from a knee joint. A few bodies have uneven shapes

substance, the vertebrae remain with wedge shape (Fig. 149) at obliteration of the intervertebral spaces and concurrent fusion of their bodies.

Gross-pathological examination of the affected joint discloses the following features.

1. Exudative inflammation with moderate edematous swelling of the inner part of the joint capsule, in addition to increased joint fluid. The latter is clear and greenish yellow and contains threads or clumps of fibrin. Sometimes numerous lentil- to ricegrain-sized white formations, rice bodies, are spread throughout the joint cavity (Fig. 150). By their elastic compressibility they may be identified as precipitates of fibrin, which by the movements of the joint have been molded into roundish or ovoid shapes [1127, 1327].

2. Proliferative inflammation associated with marked swelling of the inner part of the joint capsule, in addition to the formation of villi. The synovial membrane is a reddish spongy tissue which contains transparent gray nodules and fragile portions. Its expanding granulation tissue embraces the articular cartilage from the periphery, as pannus covers the cartilage, and penetrates it with tonguelike processes. Following the synovial erosion, the hyaline cartilage undergoes exten

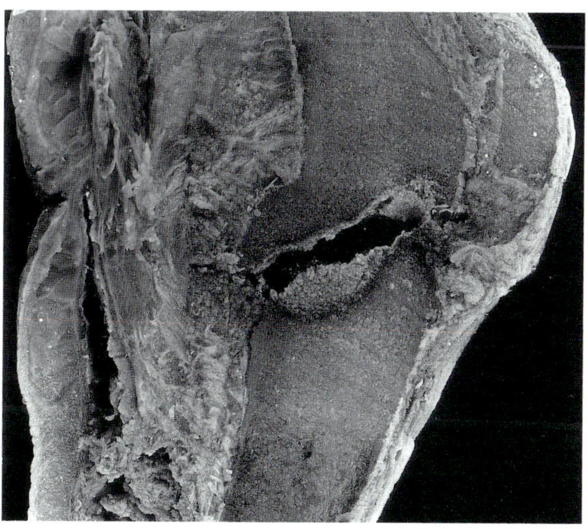

Fig. 151. The articular surfaces of the femur and tibia are extensively destroyed and replaced by granulation tissue. The joint cavity is very widenend. A descending cold abscess separates the calf musculature

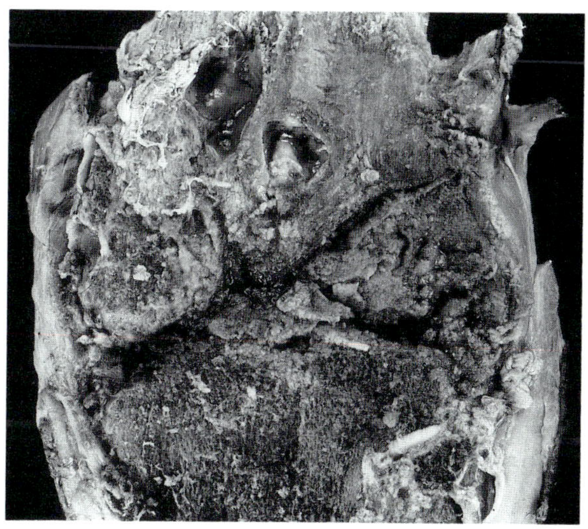

Fig. 152. Two large abscess cavities penetrate the femoral metaphysis, from which one condyle is separated. The articular surfaces are eroded and are separated by interposed fragments

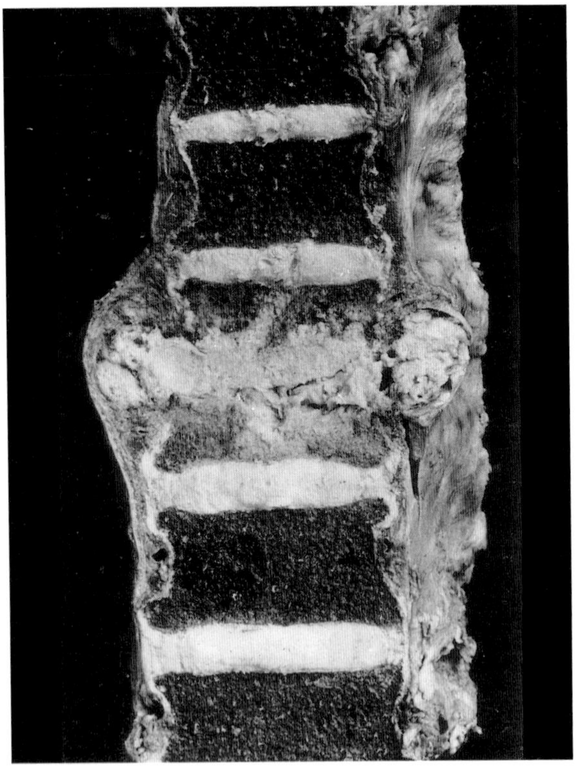

Fig. 153. An intervertebral disc is replaced by granulation tissue which erodes the contiguous vertebral bodies and expandes into the retrovertebral space

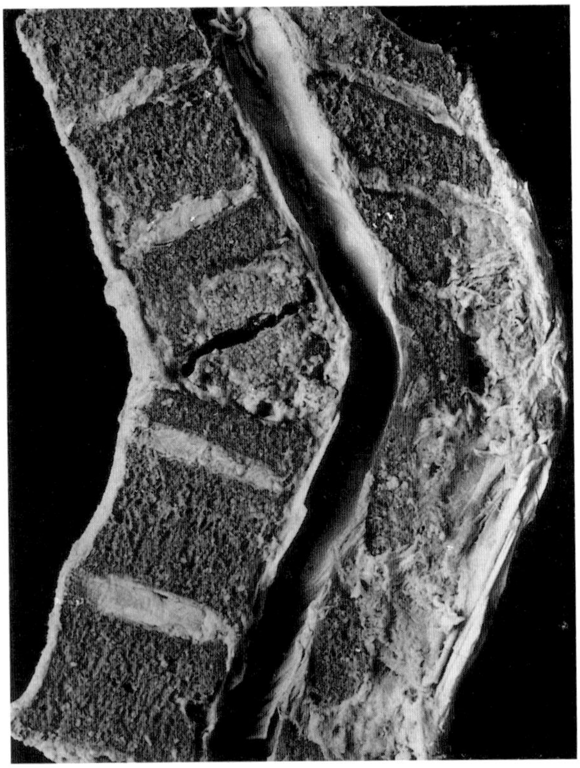

Fig. 154. Two vertebrae are eroded at their endplates, and one interposed vertebral body is eroded to wedge shape. Abscess cavities penetrate the latter vertebra. An abscess expands backward and descends caudally

sive destruction; it becomes detached in shreds. The yellowish red surface of the subchondral bone is exposed. The granulation tissue penetrates into the depth and there causes rarefaction and further destruction of the epiphysis (Fig. 151). In this phase the inflammatory foci may heal, and the proliferating tissue may shrink; a fibrous contracture then follows. However, with complete destruction of the cartilage cover and given immobilization of the joint, osseous ankylosis represents the final outcome. When larger areas of the articular cartilage have been maintained, and the joint cavity remains pervious, a secondary osteoarthritis with marginal osteopytes develops by continued mobility.

3. If the bacteria are very virulent, and/or the defensive powers of the patient's body are insufficient, a necrotizing joint inflammation arises from the proliferative form. It may also start primarily as a caseating-suppurative form. The joint is filled with thick greenish yellow pus which contains numerous cheesy crumbs. The inner part of the joint capsule is swollen and presents yellowish gray, softened portions. Some of these fungating granulations disintegrate in an ulcer-like way and may perforate outward through the peripheral joint capsule. This opens draining fistulae (Figs. 533, 534) which prepare the way for a mixed infection. The articular cartilage is extensively destroyed by advancing granulation tissue. Subsequently, expanding ossifications lead to osseous ankylosis.

4. A joint may become affected secondarily by an adjacent primary osseous lesion. The latter starts as extensive granuloma in the cancellous bone of the articular epiphysis and spreads into the articular cartilage and joint capsule. Similar changes in the joint cavity eventually result as in primary synovial tuberculosis. However, primary osseous tuberculosis is most often identifiable by the residual extensive destruction, necrosis, and abscesses in the epiphyses (Fig. 152).

5. The typical pattern of primary osseous tuberculosis is manifested also in the anterior part of a vertebral body (Figs. 153, 154), mostly of the lower thoracic spine or upper lumbar spine. It is initially of the granulomatous type and expands through the intervertebral disc into the directly adjacent vertebral body, where areas of caseous necrosis eventually follow [244]. These vertebrae then collapse and become contiguous with another by the disintegration of their intervertebral disc (Figs. 153, 154). This region of the spine assumes a ventrally concave curve. On occasional expansion of the necrotizing changes into the posterior parts of the vertebral bodies and the apophyseal joints,

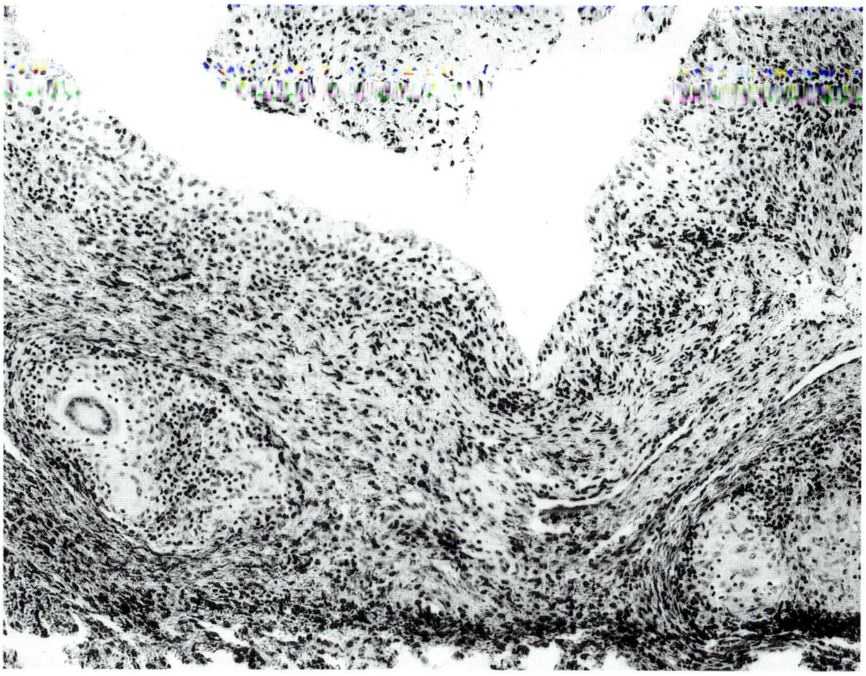

Fig. 155. The synoviocyte cover is slightly hypertrophic-hyperplastic, and the subsynoviocytic tissue is moderately hypercellular with fibrocytes, histiocytes, and lymphocytes. Two granulomata, one of them containing a Langhans' giant cell, are in the depth and are surrounded by marked hypercellularity

the vertebrae are approximated along their horizontal diameters. Caseated material accumulates in a paravertebral abscess along the lower thoracic and entire lumbar spine (Figs. 148, 153, 154).

Histopathological examination discloses three major features. (a) In the exudative serous type swelling of the synovial membrane with scant diffuse infiltration predominates (Fig. 155). Occasionally, nodules rich in lymphocytes occur here, covered by amorphous material which derives from degeneration of the superficial layer. In other places the synovial surface is overlain by broad precipitates of fibrin. The rice bodies are well-delimited formations of homogeneous acellular fibrin which stains specifically with celestine blue, acid fuchsin, or orange picric solution and is arranged in a characteristic network or honeycomb pattern (Fig. 156). (b) With duration of the inflammation, the lymphocyte nodules increase and permeate the synovial membrane. Specific tubercle nodules with a central necrosis surrounded by Langhans' giant cells,

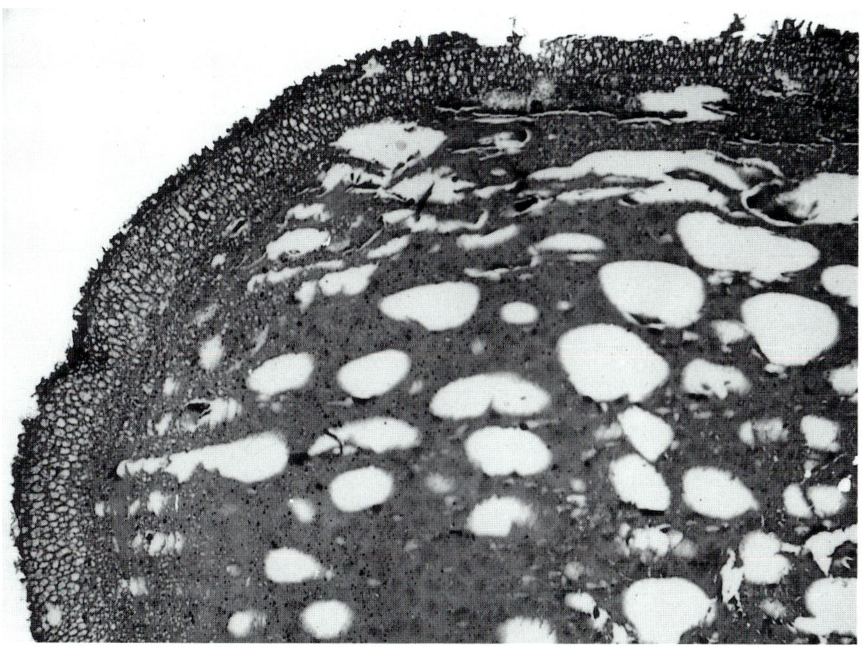

Fig. 156. The rice body has a finely serrated border with five to six rows of vacuoles which surround a homogeneous material perforated by many ovoid cavities

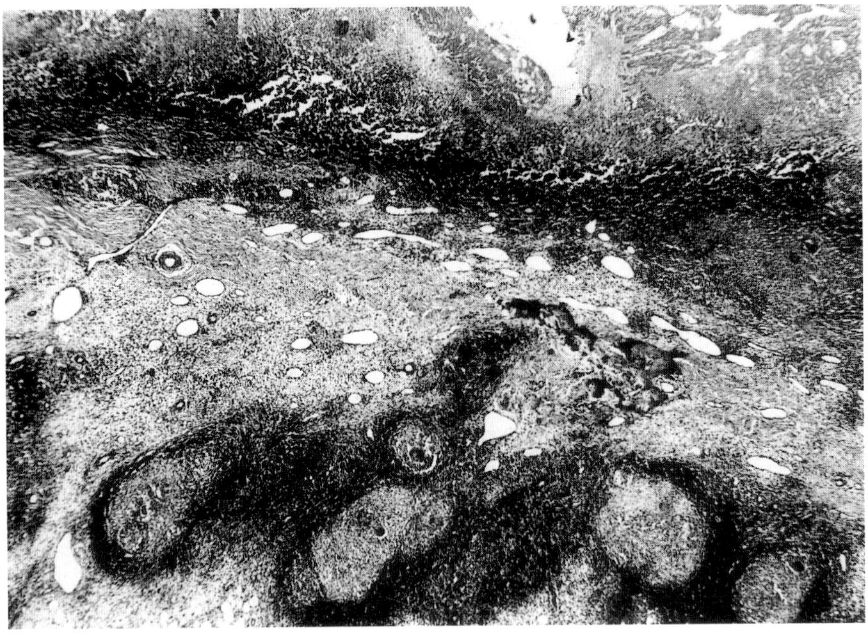

Fig. 157. The synovial membrane is covered by extensive deposits of fibrin which are organized to large parts. Several granulomata, containing Langhans' cells, lie in the deeper subsynoviocytic tissue and are surrounded by dense hypercellularity of fibrocytes, lymphocytes, and histiocytes

connective tissue fibrils, and epitheloid cells are scattered throughout (Fig. 157). In other cases, the synovial membrane presents fewer manifestations of specific inflammation but more nonspecific granulations rich in connective tissue cells and capillaries. The articular cartilage contains many widened lacunae left after necrosis of chondrocytes. Synovial granulations enter these lacunae, and advancing from them penetrate the zone of provisional calcification and further into the subchondral bone (Fig. 158). They then expand within the cancellous bone (Fig. 159). Similar changes are observed in the vertebral endplate, which is penetrated by granulation tissue emerging from the intervertebral space and expanding into the vertebral body. Less often, the granulation tissue originates in the vertebral body and invades the endplate secondarily, whereupon it spreads in the intervertebral disc. (c) Caseous necrotizing synovitis presents generally spreading granulomata and nodules with central foci of necrosis and surrounding Langhans' giant cells. Extensive areas of disintegration and necrosis lie in the synovial membrane, cartilage, and subchondral bone. It is difficult to

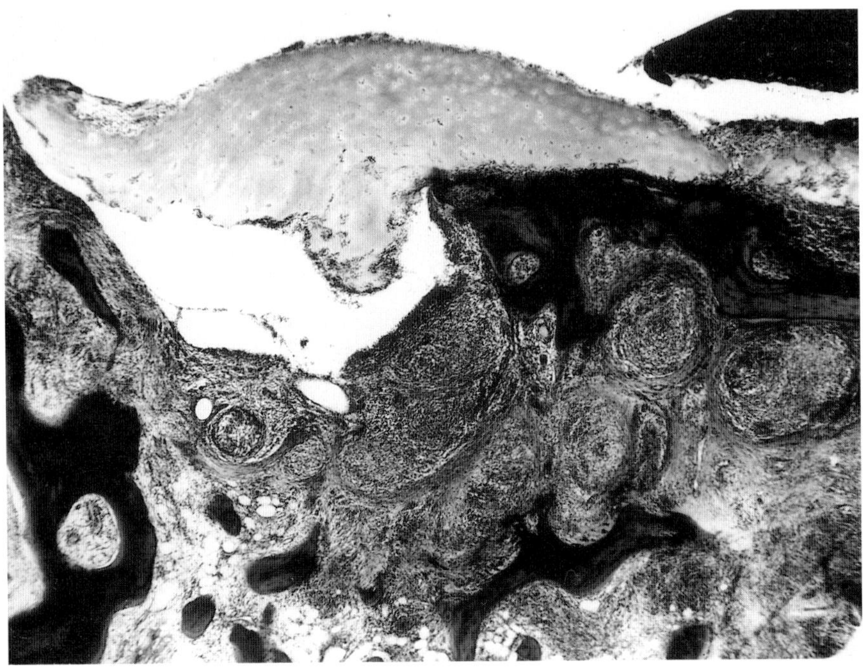

Fig. 158. Articular cartilage is partly separated from the subchondral bone by intervening granulation tissue which intrudes the subchondral subcortical marrow spaces and comprises several granulomata

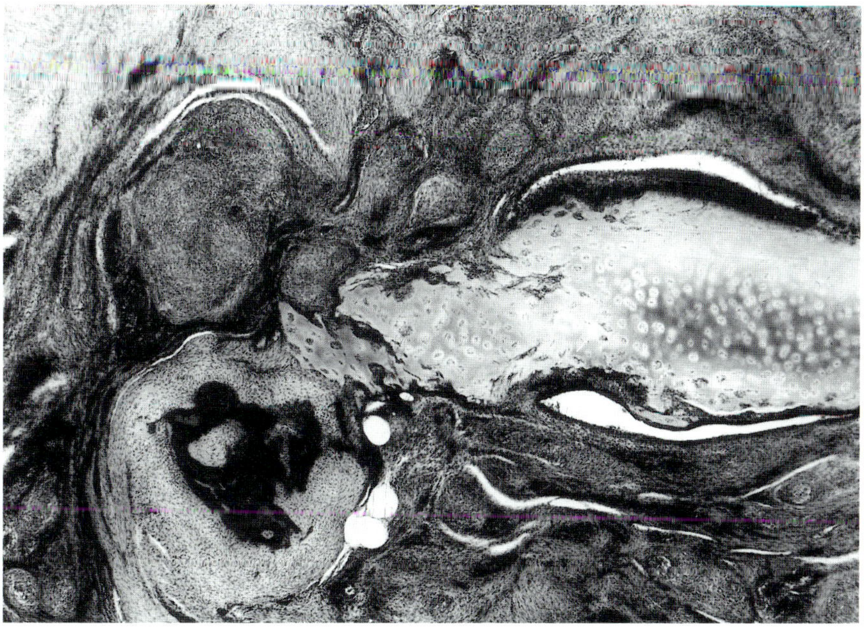

Fig. 159. Articular cartilage is in continuity with the subchondral epiphysis only in a small area, but it is otherwise entirely surrounded by dense granulation tissue which comprises several granulomata

decide here where the tuberculous granulomata originated.

Differential diagnosis [1686] in children includes synovitis secondary to any infectious disease of childhood and a beginning rheumatoid arthritis. In adults, beginning rheumatoid arthritis, syphilitic arthritis, and osteomyelitis in the articular epiphyses must be considered. Rheumatoid or syphilitic arthritis usually occurs symmetrically, but the former occurs multiarticularly and with pain and fever, while the latter occurs pauciarticularly and without pain or fever. The osteomyelitis causes characteristic roentgenographs, with ovoid or serrated foci of destruction surrounded by a sclerotic wall and neighbored by periosteal apposition.

Treatment of tuberculosis of the joints must be guided by the awareness that the joint disease is a local manifestation of a generalized disease. Therefore, all efforts should be directed at improving the general condition and thereby increasing the defensive forces of the body. Proper nutrition rich in proteins and vitamins, avoidance of strenuous activities, and frequent rest periods are essential. Similarly to cases of other bacterial inflammations, chemotherapy and antibiotic administration are applied in the treatment of tuberculosis of the joints. Of the medications thus far tested [551, 769, 1094, 1663] isoniazid has proven the most effective bacteriostaticum. It is administered daily at a starting dose of 5 mg/kg and is gradually increased to 10 mg/kg, but the dose should not exceed 300 mg daily. It is very beneficial in combination with rifampin 600 mg daily. Both medications are given for 9–12 months to obtain satisfactory subsidence of the osteoarticular lesions. Prior to rifampin, para-aminosalicylic acid 10 g daily was used in combination with isoniazid, but its benefits were uncertain. On the other hand, ethambutol 800–1000 mg daily has proven a very effective substitute to para-aminosalicylic acid and is given with isoniazid for 12–24 months in protracted skeletal affection. Similarly, streptomycin has proven to be a very effective antibiotic; it is administered in daily doses of 1.0 g, but for no more than 4 weeks. Whenever feasible, these medications are combined as triple therapy, and they effect healing of the tuberculous lesions in a significant percentage of the cases. In the rare situations of microbial resistance to isoniazid, rifampin is used as a substitute in the triple therapy. A substantial improvement in general condition is followed by radical changes in the condition and function of the affected joint. However, the shortcomings of these medications lie in the fact that each may be accompanied by very disturbing adverse effects. These include gastrointestinal and liver irritation by para-aminosalicylic acid, psychotic disorders and liver damage by isoniazid, severe liver damage and thrombocytopenia by rifampin, and toxicity to the acoustic nerve with resulting tinnitus, roaring sensation, and eventually permanent deafness by streptomycin. When any of these complications arises, the specifically noxious medication must be discontinued and only a part of the triple therapy continued. Whenever feasible, streptomycin should be omitted, especially in the treatment of children. Ethanbutol 700–1000 mg daily is also an effective chemotherapeutic medication and a supplement to isoniazid, but it may be given for only brief periods of time because of the potential decrease in visual acuity with higher dosage levels [769].

A very beneficial, and essential supplement to the medicamentous therapy is complete immobilization of the affected joint, as subsequently indicated. In the case of a draining sinus with mixed infection, antibiotics, as indicated by culture of the microorganisms participating in the infection, must be administered. By the combination of specific antituberculosis medications, antibiotics, and prolonged immobilization, arrest of the inflammation and the destructive lesions may be obtained in a significant percentage [45%–55%) of cases. This applies especially to children and adolescents, who generally attain a functioning, albeit sometimes moderately limited joint without surgical intervention.

However, some patients do not respond to medicamentous treatment or immobilization and remain with a continuously disabled or a draining joint [1759, 1760]. In addition, special topical modalities are necessary [1330]. The initial modality for the vertebral column consists of complete bedrest with immobilization of the body in a posterior plaster shell for 3 months. This is followed or may be started by a dorsolumbar plaster cast jacket for other 3 months or longer, depending on the extent and severity of the tuberculous process, with the patient ambulatory. The immobilization is continued by a dorsolumbar brace of leather and steel until the clinical and roentgenographic examinations demonstrate healing of the vertebral alterations. The healing period with these conservative modalities may last 1.5–2 years, but it can be shortened operatively by posterior spinal fusion using bone grafts removed from the iliac bone or tibia and apposed to both sides of the vertebral column. A paravertebral abscess must be treated by a broad posterior incision which permits evacuation of all decomposed tissues. If the thoracic spine is affected by such abscess, a costotransversectomy must be included in this operation [858, 1759]. However, the most severe complication is paraplegia caused by the pressure of a paravertebral abscess or intravertebral extradural abscess. The incident neurological symptoms may vary from paresthesias to complete loss of motor and sensory functions. Evacuation of the abscess and all necrotic tissue is the primary and indispensable step, but this does not always succed in restoring the neurological functions – nor does primarily or subsequently performed laminectomy or anterolateral decompression of the vertebral spine [241, 1453].

Of the peripheral joints, the shoulder generally presents moderate intraarticular changes. These can be treated successfully by immobilization with a chest-arm plaster cast which maintains the arm in 90° abduction and 30° flexion. After 3 months this treatment is followed by a leather-metal brace or one of plastic material until clinical and roentgenographic examinations reveal a satisfactory regression of the joint disease. The elbow joint is affected by deep erosion mostly of the proximal end of the ulna (Fig. 144) and less often at the proximal end of the radius. Immobilization with a plaster cast or plastic brace for 9–12 months succeeds in bringing regression of the articular alterations. A useable joint, although moderately limited in range of motion, is the result. On the other hand, in the rare situations of marked postinflammatory deformity of the olecranon or radial head associated with substantial limitation of motion, a limited resection of the affected articular end and extensive resection of the proliferated joint capsule substantially improves the function of the elbow joint. In the wrist joint with erosion of the radiocarpal surfaces, fibrous or osseous ankylosis often follows, provided that this joint is immobilized for 4–6 months. The proper functional position herefore is 15°–20° dorsal extension. With intense osteoporosis of the carpal bones and insufficient healing, a solid radiocarpal fusion can be obtained by limited resection of the articular surfaces combined with inlay of an arrow-shaped bone graft (Figs. 209, 210) removed from the radial shaft [1549].

The hip joint, if treated before extensive destruction of the femoral head has set in, responds well to ankle traction, with the leg in abduction to forestall an adduction contracture of the hip joint. It is often necessary to have the traction acting on the patient in supine position to prevent or correct a concomitant flexion contracture of the hip joint. Once the active inflammation regresses, the patient may be upright and ambulatory with the hip joint immobilized by a short hip spica plaster cast or a leather-metal brace until healing of the inflammatory alterations is observed. However, if destructive lesions expand into the femoral head and acetabulum, resection of the articular epiphyses may be indicated [1760]. These ends are then aligned in full extension and slight abduction and are fixed with steel staples [893]. Another procedure for a hip joint in which the triple treatment fails in preventing deep erosion into the femoral head and acetabulum is extraarticular arthrodesis as described by Trumble [1660]. Here a bone graft is inserted into a cleft in the ischial tuberosity and is passed into a cleft at the posterior aspect of the trochanteric area. Given the desire of young women to reattain mobility in an ankylosed hip joint, a total arthroplastic procedure may be performed, but this should be carried out only several years after the tuberculous process has completely healed, as corroborated by all relevant examinations [1033]. The knee joint greatly benefits from continuous traction for 2–3 months and subsequent immobilization with a plaster cast or a brace of leather and steel for this period of time, until all examinations indicate a distinct regression of the process. Subsequently, gentle mobilization of the knee joint by active exercises may be started, provided that the knee continues to be protected by a brace during walking periods. However, in cases with markedly fungating joint capsule and deep erosions of the articular ends or with destructive changes originating primarily from the subchondral bone, resection of the articular ends and wide excision of the inner part of the joint capsule is indicated [1660]. This is followed directly by immobilization with a plaster cast or by compression with clamps [279], metal plates, or an intramedullary nail [681, 1582]. The result is eradication of the disease process but at the price of mobility of the joint [666]. However, this price is not too high considering that the deep irregularities of the articular surfaces would never permit unlimited and painfree mobility of the knee joint. In an occasionally coincident flexion contracture of the knee joint, the hamstring tendons and dorsal portions of the joint capsule must be divided as an initial step in the operation; this is followed by commensurate resection and adaptation of the articular ends. Arthroplasty here is rarely applicable; it is discussed in "Rheumatoid Arthritis". As to the ankle joint, complete immobilization by a plaster cast is started without weight bearing. Gradual weight bearing is permitted depending on the degree of the regression of the disease process. A moveable, useful joint is restored in about 30% of cases. However, with deeply extending necrotic areas in the tibia or the body of the talus, resection of the distal articular surfaces of the tibia and fibula and of the proximal surface of the talus is combined with compression by staples [279]. Another effective modality for ensuring fusion of the resected articular surfaces consists of insertion of an arrow-shaped bone graft into the resected tibia and talus (Figs. 213, 214) and an early start of weight bearing on the ankle immobilized by a plaster cast [1549].

15. Mycotic Arthritis

The joints and bones of humans may become infected by pathogenic mycetes other than mycobacterium tuberculosis. These represent a small group from the large species of fungi of which more than 500 subspecies are known.

The radiating fungus actinomyces is a microorganism of bacterial size and shape but closely resembling fungi by its branching property and formation of spores. The species actinomyces Israelii is spread throughout the world, grows in the soil, and multiplies especially in moist, warm weather. It invades the human body by inhalation and remains initially in the oral cavity and/or upper resiratory tract. Once in the human body, it is very pathogenic [643]. The European species actinomyces cerevisiae grows on grasses and wheats; it may invade the human body through the oral cavity or through lesions of the skin. Actinomyces often affects persons who work in agriculture or gardening, and who expose themselves to contamination in the oral cavity by their habit of chewing grasses or wheat spicas. This fungus is facultatively anaerobic and develops especially in tissues with diminished blood supply and oxidative processes. Thus it multiplies in the crypts of tonsils, in inflamed gingiva, and in the maxilla or mandible, in which necrosis of local tissue follows deep caries of teeth.

From the peribuccal tissue the infection often spreads with hard infiltrates into the paravertebral tissue and adjacent vertebrae of the cervical spine and upper dorsal spine. There it causes slowly enlarging osteomyelitic abscesses with occasional formation of draining sinuses. On the other hand, the infection may expand from the throat into the chest, where it causes a pleurisy concurrent with pulmonary abscesses. From there it spreads into the ribs and dorsal spine, causing erosions, multiple osteomyelitic abscesses, and sometimes even meningeal irritations. The infection may also reach from the oral cavity the gastrointestinal tract and spread from there into the lumbar spine, causing osteomyelitic abscesses in two or three vertebrae, but without alteration of the interjacent discs [1321]. Under the toxic influence of regionally present and thriving saprophytes, an indurated swelling of the affected tissue develops, with expanding dense infiltration. The latter rarely results in scarified shrinking but most commonly in necrotic caseation and disintegration with ensuing abscesses and ulcerations. If an abscess perforates into the blood stream, the hematogenous spread of actinomyces leads principally to osteoarticular inflammation. Several years may elapse before the manifestation of a hematogenous focus. The prime site of articular inflammation is the synovial membrane, from which the inflammation expands into the hyaline cartilage and further into the fibrous capsule of the joint. The secondary site and manifestation of the infection is an epiphyseal osteomyelitis, which perforates through the osteocartilaginous surface into the joint.

Generalized actinomycosis starts insidiously with gradually increasing malaise and slight elevation in temperature. Symptoms such as persistent discomfort and sensation of stiffness are confined to the area of initial localization of the actinomycotic process. This is usually the cervical prevertebral area. Subsequently, the process shifts into the vertebrae. Affection of peripheral joints is a rather rare complication and occurs in about 5%–7% of these patients. It begins with vague and uncharacteristic symptoms. With aggravating inflammation of the joint, the pain becomes intense and may be very disabling because of its persistence. In

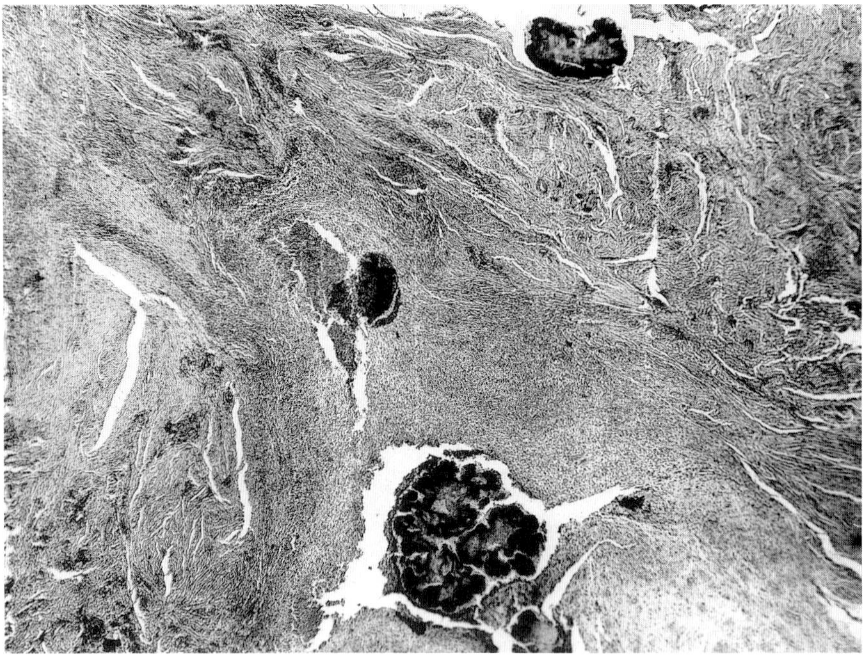

Fig. 160. A few roundish or ovoid agglomerations of branching filaments of actinomyces lie in the deeper and dense subsynoviocytic tissue

contrast to this are the rather pain-free infiltrates of soft tissue inside the body.

On physical examination, the enlargement of a joint of the extremities (shoulder, knee, hip, or elbow) is very conspicuous. The covering skin is tense but not discolored. The joint capsule is markedly thickened by dense infiltration and is tense because of increased joint fluid. If the inflammation spreads beyond the joint capsule, the entire extremity becomes swollen and its function very limited. Palpation discloses some very tender areas in the joint capsule and in the articular epiphyses of an extremity. By shrinking of the joint capsule and reflex-elicited contraction of the regional musculature, a contracture of a peripheral joint develops. Eventually a few sinuses perforate the skin and discharge thin fluid with small yellow sulphurlike granules. The more frequent affection is seen in the cervical spine, whose infiltrated and indurated paravertebral structures cause a thickening of the neck with moderate, localized tenderness. The range of active and passive motion of the cervical spine is significantly limited, and its paravertebral musculature is tense. The regional findings are similar when the dorsal or lumbar spine is affected.

Blood studies show lymphocytosis and simultaneous anemia; the sedimentation rate is invariably accelerated to 50–90 mm/h. Urine often contains an increased amount of protein. Microscopic examination of the aspirated joint fluid as well as of the yellow granules in the fistular secretion discloses numerous threads of molds which are sometimes radially arranged (Fig. 161) but more often form an irregular web in whose center lie fine granules. Actinomyces are Gram-positive, dichotomically ramified threads with clublike, enlarged ends. Their radiating filaments are Gram-positive, but the sporal clubs are Gram-negative. They grow on routine and anaerobic culture media in colonies which resemble creased skin.

Roentgenographs [1346] of the peripheral joints reveal no characteristic changes which would suggest a specific inflammation. Densification of the joint capsule causes overshadowing of the cartilage space and blurring of the structure of the articular epiphyses. On spread of the intraarticular granulation tissue and destruction of the hyaline cartilage, the cartilage space becomes narrowed or even obliterated. The adjoining epiphyses show irregular delimitation and deeply extending defects. Healing may result in fibrous ankylosis. Vertebral affections are manifested by multiple smaller and larger areas of radiolucency, representing osteomyelitic lesions, which are bordered by sclerosis. These are located within the vertebral bodies and often expand into the vertebral pedicles. However, even when two or three vertebrae are altered in this way, the intervertebral spaces retain their width, albeit irregularly delimited by eroded vertebral plates [1754]. A frequently accompanying anomaly is the regional paravertebral shadow, corresponding to a paravertebral abscess and/or indurated tissues.

Gross-anatomical examination discloses extensive thickening of the joint capsule with occasionally prominent, coarse nodules or broad adhesions. The synovial membrane is discolored yellowish gray and is swollen; its surface is elevated into villi, some of which encroach on the articular cartilage. In a few places the

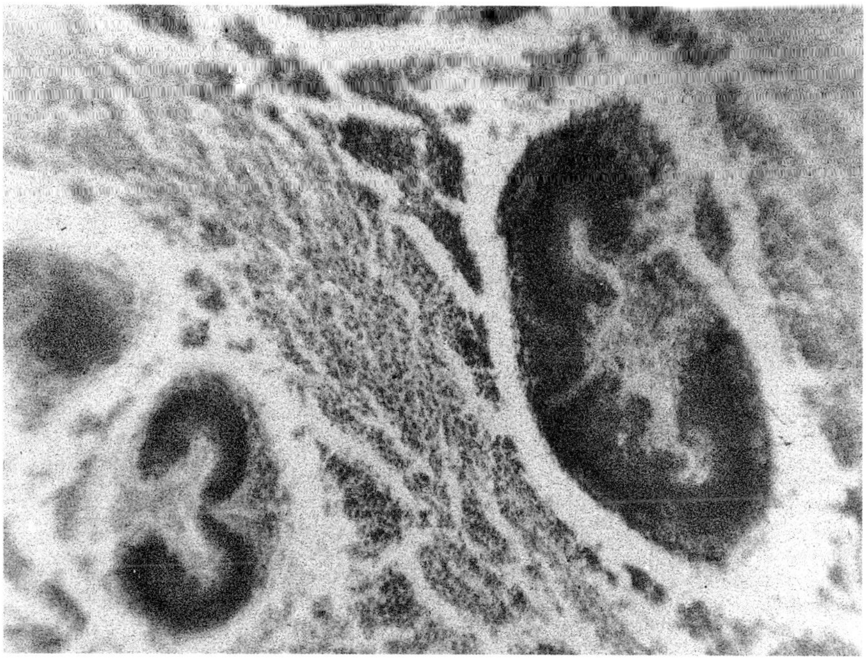

Fig. 161. The roundish or ovoid agglomerations consist of dense reticula of branching filaments which lie in characteristic radial arrangement and terminate in spores or clubs. The latter are larger than the filaments

synovial surface is perforated by small holes through which pus is discharged. By the confluence of such openings, extensive defects are formed which are covered with yellowish secretion. In other places the synovial tissue presents grayish white, dense scars. The articular cartilage is widely replaced by granulation tissue, which penetrates into the subchondral bone. The joint cavity contains increased serous fluid or often a thin, yellowish pus with small, yellow granules of 0.5–1.0 mm, the sulfur granules. The vertebral bodies of any region comprise cystlike areas within their hyperemic cancellous bone. Most of these cavities are filled with loose hyperemic granulation tissue, and a few of them contain yellowish tinted fluid. Some cavities merge with each other, and all of them are delimited by thickened osseous tissue. By expansion of some cysts to the borders of vertebral bodies, their marginal plates become very uneven.

Histopathological examination discloses edema of the synovial membrane and infiltration by polymor-

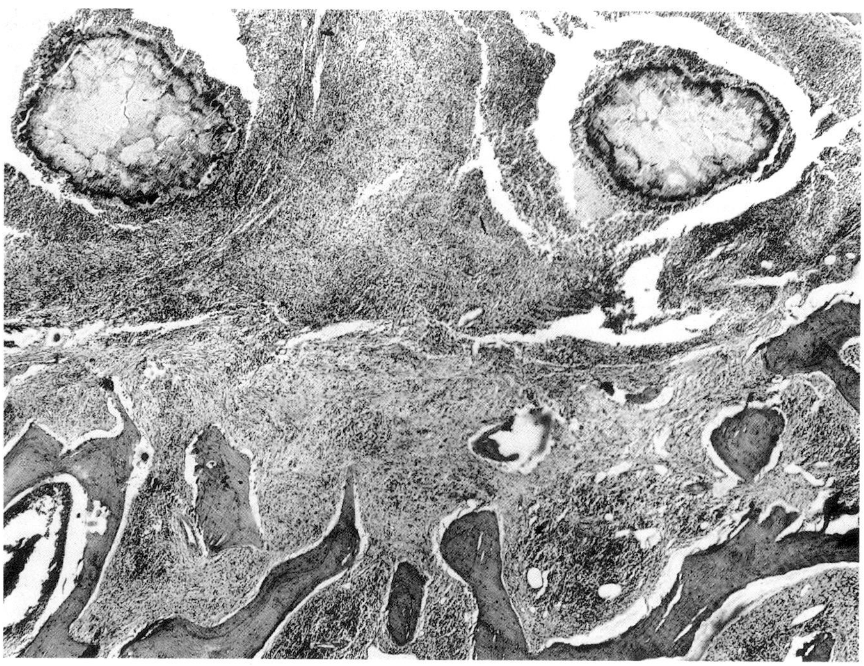

Fig. 162. Round agglomerations of reticula are located in the subchondral area of the epiphysis. These consist of branching filaments which terminate in less dense agglomerations of spores or clubs

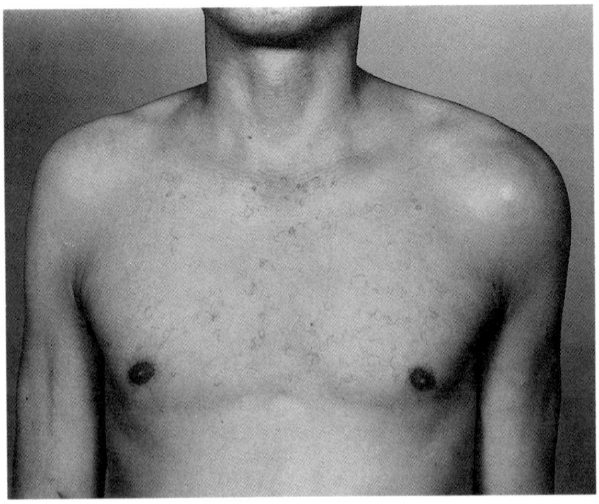

Fig. 163. Circumscribed swelling at the anterior aspect of the left shoulder by inflammation of the subacromial preglenoidal bursa

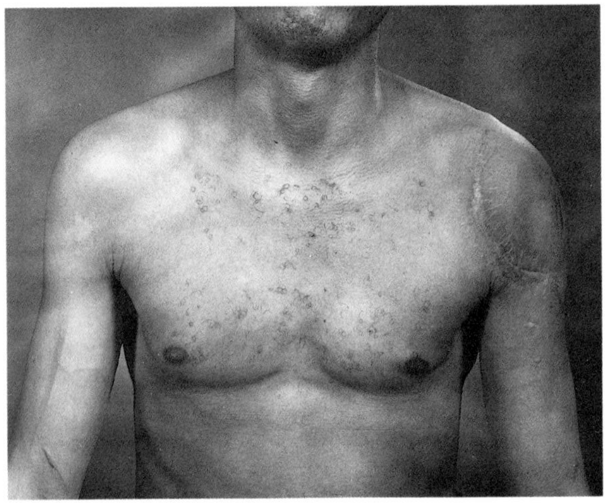

Fig. 164. Healing of the swelling secondary to wide excision and concurrent administration of amphotericin

phonuclear leukocytes and monocytes. In the superficial and deeper zones of the joint capsule, densified by substantially increased fibrocytes, histiocytes, and a few small giant cells, lie the characteristic, well-delimited, roundish agglomerations of delicate, branching filaments of actinomyces (Fig. 160). In other cases of probably more virulent strains, the filaments are surrounded by extensive and dense infiltrates composed predominantly of polymorphonuclear leukocytes and less so of lymphocytes. Small portions of acellular tissue are scattered between these, an indication of the necrosis taking here place. Among the infiltrates there also occur several areas of dense granulation tissue which comprises fibroblasts, epitheloid cells, and giant cells [1606]. In their centers lie round or ovoid formations, consisting of numerous multicellular filaments in characteristic radial arrangements terminating in clubs with spores (Fig. 161). The subchondral and marrow spaces in the articular epiphyses contain similar foci of dense granulation tissue composed of characteristically branching, delicate filaments (Fig. 162).

Differential diagnosis may cause considerable difficulty in the early phase of inflammation; actinomycotic arthritis resembles a tuberculous or syphilitic inflammation. However, by the sinuses discharging a secretion containing yellow granules and by identification of the mold threads in the fistular secretion and/or in the joint fluid, the diagnosis can eventually be established. The very commonly concurrent or even preceding alterations of any region of the vertebral spine and its ventrally located soft structures are diagnostically no less significant.

In the treatment of actinomycosis, penicillin G 5,000,000–15,000,000 U daily is given parenterally in divided doses either alone or in combination with sulfathiazine 2.0 g daily in divided doses, in a course over 3–4 months. Thereafter, oral penicillin 4.0 g daily is given for an additional 3 months. This therapy has proven very effective. In penicillin-resistant cases, tetracycline 3.0 g, erythromycin 3.0 g, or chloramphenicol 3.0 g provide similar therapeutic benefit, administered daily in divided doses over a period of 6 months. The adverse effects of tetracycline include gastrointestinal irritation and anemia; substantially more serious are those of chloromycetin – aplastic anemia, granulocytopenia, and thrombocytopenia. Regular blood studies are therefore necessary in these treatments. By its response to the customary antibiotic treatment, on the one hand, and by the lack of response to specific antifungal medications (amphotericin, griseofulvin) on the other, actinomyces manifests its biological nature of a bacterium rather than a fungus. For relief of the pain, mild warm compresses and traction for prevention or correction of a contracture are very beneficial. In persistent swelling of the joint capsule, a series of cobalt radiations with a total of 10–20 Gy provides regression of the swelling. Draining sinuses with much secretion respond well to irrigation with a solution of penicillin or of one of the other above antibiotics.

In extensive destruction of bone with severe pain and fever, the necrotic portions should be excised. This operation is often beneficial, merely by splitting the diseased tissue and providing an access of oxygen to the anaerobic molds. Beyond the local treatment, management of the patient's general condition by appropriate modalities should be included in the therapeutic program. If the antibiotic treatment is instituted in time, and the healing tendency is favorable, the patient's recovery and reattainment of articular function may be expected. If the mycotic necrosis affecting a joint is

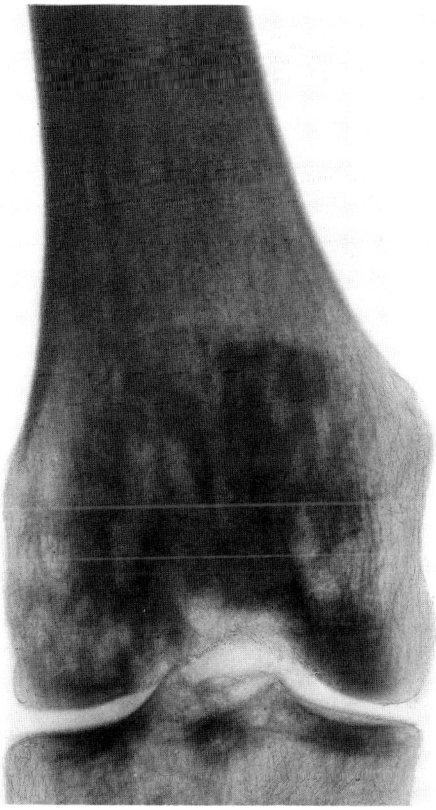

Fig. 165. The distal epiphysis of the femur and the proximal epiphysis of the tibia are penetrated by several areas of marked osteolysis surrounded by osteosclerosis. The joint cleft is partly widened

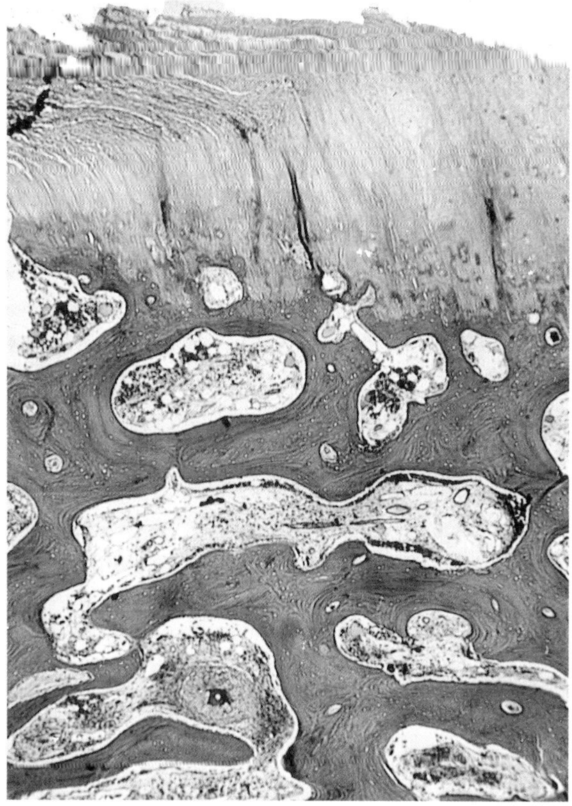

Fig. 166. The subchondral bone comprises, in a few marrow spaces, spherules of coccidioidomyces with doubly refractile walls surrounded by dense filaments

extensive, healing ensues with ankylosis of this joint. However, in the presence of mycotic foci in other organs and their disintegration followed by persistent suppuration, severe amyloidosis and intercurrent diseases may lead to death.

Among the numerous species of fungi, coccidioidomyces immitis has been identified as very pathogenic [1311]. It is a spherical, thickwalled microorganism which thrives as a mycelium composed of hyphae and spores on the soil. The spores are airborne; settling in the human body, they transform into spherules (Figs. 166, 167, 168) of 10–12 µm. These enlarge to 30 µm or more when multiplying and forming numerous endospores of 2–3 µm. The infection primarily causes, with concurrent erythema, an inflammation of the lungs. From there it is disseminated by the blood stream in 20%–30% of cases [671] to the bones and joints. In these, it causes multiple lesions after an interval of 4–5 years. Another frequent portal of entry of the fungus is the skin, from which it spreads by the lymphatic route into the body. Coccidioidomycosis rather often occurs in the southwestern United States, Central America, and South America [1311, 1652].

The most frequently affected joints are the knee, hip, shoulder (Figs. 163, 164), elbow, and ankle [94, 584, 671, 1557, 1634]. These are affected either primarily in their synovial membrane or secondarily by spread either from a paraarticular bursa or a focus in the subchondral epiphysis. Concomitantly with the different sources of the joint infection, the clinical picture varies. In primary hematogenous synovitis, the joint becomes gradually enlarged by swelling of the joint capsule and by increase in the joint fluid (Figs. 163, 164), but it is only moderately tender and not limited in its motion. However, on spread of an advanced inflammation from an osteomyelitic focus, the joint enlarges rather rapidly and becomes very painful, very warm, and limited in motion by the thickening of the joint capsule. On liquefaction necrosis of the joint capsule and perforation of abscesses through the skin, draining sinuses develop, through which a very malodorous and highly infectious secretion is discharged.

The joint fluid has a substantial increase in white blood cells (2400–9000), chiefly lymphocytes, among which a small number of coccidioides may be noted in the stained smear (Fig. 30). This fluid is also highly

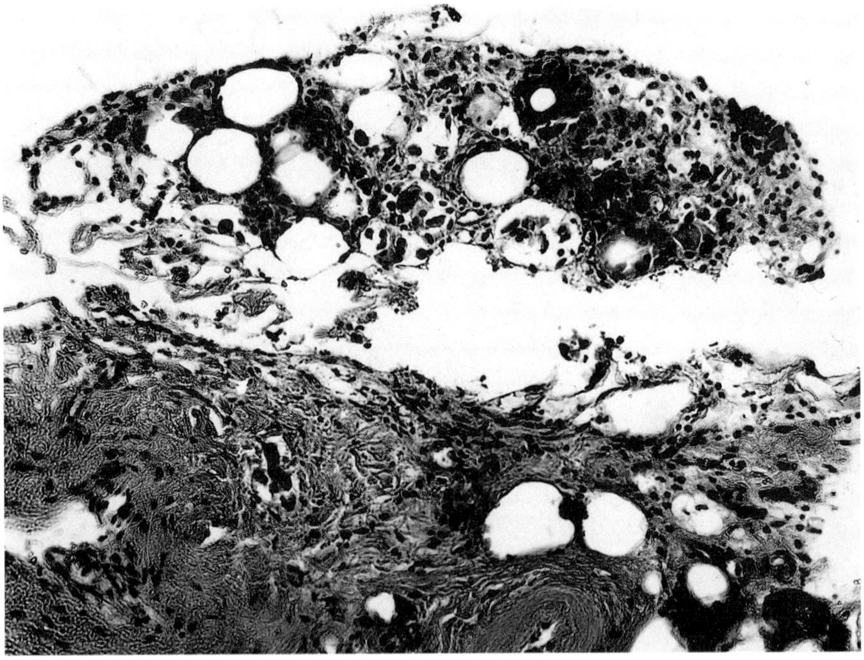

Fig. 167. The synovial membrane is moderately infiltrated by lymphocytes and large histiocytes and comprises three spherules of coccidioidomyces with doubly refractile wall

infectious [1311]. The diagnosis is established [436, 1331] by identifying the causative fungus: refractile thick-walled spherules of 8–10 μm in synovial fluid (Fig. 30) and/or in secretion from draining sinuses. Another diagnostic approach is to obtain a mycelium of widely mingling hyphae (Fig. 31) by culturing the suspicious fluids on Sabouraud's glucose-peptone medium. A serological test for complement fixation antibodies, positive at dilutions of 1:128–1:256 or higher, assists in this respect. Of similar significance is the coccidioidin skin test at the dilution 1:128. The culture from the joint fluid has a rather low yield, but that from the synovial tissue confirms the diagnosis in most cases [94, 1331].

Roentgenographs [149, 1065] reveal initially moderate thickening of the joint capsule and subsequent narrowing and irregular delimitation of the cartilage space by erosion of the articular epiphyses (Fig. 165). The structure in the depth of the latter is very irregular by many areas of radiolucency or osteoporosis alternating with sclerosis, indicative of osteomyelitic changes (Fig. 165).

Gross-anatomical examination [1634] discloses generalized thickening of the synovial membrane which is dark red, granular, and speckled in some places by small white bodies. In primary synovial inflammation, the articular cartilage becomes secondarily affected rather late and slowly. However, in all infections originating from epiphyseal osteomyelitis, cartilage damage sets in early and very extensively and is associated with deep bone erosions [1074].

Histopathological examination (Figs. 166, 167, 168) discloses that the subchondral marrow spaces and especially the synovial membrane are heavily infiltrated with lymphocytes, less so with polymorphonuclear neutrophilic leukocytes, and scantily with yeast spherules. The latter resemble the spherules of blastomyces dermatitidis and histoplasma capsulatum (Fig. 172); these decrease in number with the duration of the inflammatory process. In the chronically inflamed, deeper subsynoviocytic tissue, numerous granulomata are present which are composed of large epitheloid cells and foreign body giant cells. Several of the latter have within their cytoplasm doubly refractile round bodies, which are typical of the spherules of coccidioides immitis (Fig. 167). In conditions of longer duration many spherules of coccidioides are enlarged by intracellular budding of spores (Fig. 168) while other small spherules lie within giant cells of excessive size, measuring sometimes 100–160 μm (Fig. 168). Both these formations are surrounded by dense infiltrates composed of lymphocytes, polymorphonuclear neutrophilic leukocytes, histiocytes, and a few polymorphonuclear eosinophilic leukocytes. Scattered at distances, areas of amorphous or granular acellular material occur, indicative of local caseation necrosis, which is bordered by a wall of histiocytes and lymphocytes. Special stains for the presence of coccidioides or other fungi are periodic acid – Schiff and Gomori stain with methenamine – silver nitrate.

In view of the lack of response to routine antibiotic and chemotherapeutic agents, the antifungal antibiotic

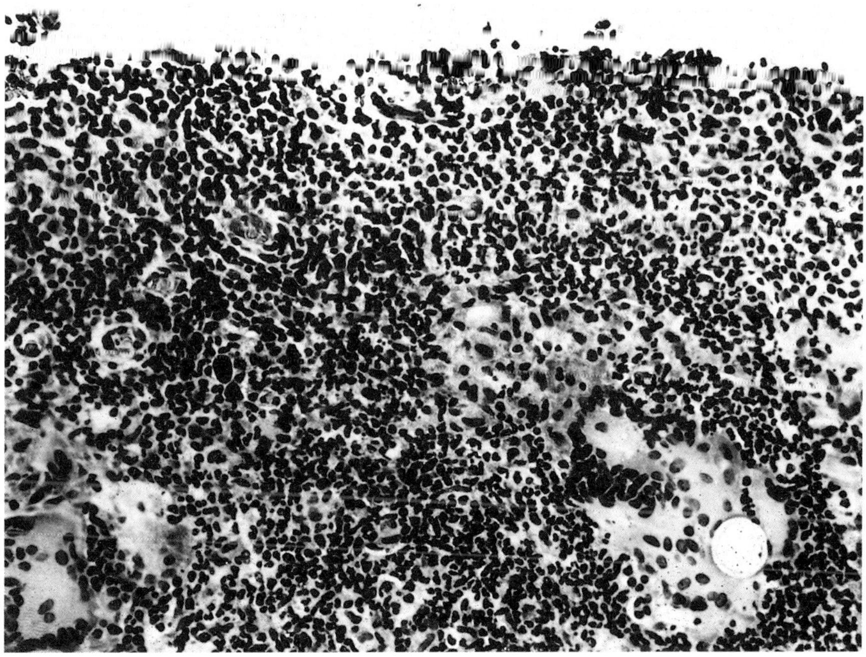

Fig. 168. The synovial membrane is extensively and densely infiltrated by lymphocytes, plasmacytes, histiocytes, and two giant cells. The larger of the latter comprises a spherule of coccidioidomyces with doubly refractile wall

amphotericin B has found increasing use [12, 748]. Amphotericin B is administered intravenously in daily doses of 100–150 mg for 3–4 months, until the total dose amounts to 4000–4500 mg. However, the potential adverse effects of amphotericin B are multiple: anorexia, hemorrhagic gastritis, liver damage, thrombophlebitis, anemia, leukopenia, granulocytopenia, impaired renal function with azotemia, oliguria or anuria, central neuropathies with blurred vision or loss of hearing, and peripheral neuropathies. Treatment with intravenous amphotericin B generally suffices in plain exudative synovitis, but it must be supplemented with intraarticular amphotericin B in cases of more advanced articular changes. Here, 50 mg amphotericin is administered daily in the joint for 3–4 weeks, then 3 times weekly for 1 month, then once weekly for 2 months, and finally once monthly for 6 months. Subsequently, synovectomy [1634] is indicated when the joint effusion recurs frequently or the joint capsule becomes progressively and irreversibly thickened. When extensive erosions have altered the articular surfaces, surgical treatment must be expanded to include wide excision. When osteomyelitic abscesses drain into the joint cavity, they must be eradicated by deep resection. If unrelenting suppurations affect the peripheral parts of extremities, amputation may be the only salvaging solution [1776]. The recently recommended treatment [257, 429] with the broad-spectrum fungostatic agent ketoconazole 400–800 mg daily for 6 months provides temporary suppression of the mycotic infection but is not able to eradicate it. The adverse effects of ketoconazole include nausea, liver damage, jaundice, and occasional fatality. Thus the prognosis is guarded, especially in cases with disseminated mycotic disease, manifested among other harm in infections of several bones and joints. When the vertebral column is affected, the outcome is usually fatal [1652]. The serious prognosis and limited efficacy of medications used so far is reflected in the statistics reported by Bayer et al. [94]. Their patients received antifungal therapy and surgical procedures; half of them either suffered recurrent synovitis or residual deformities or died.

The European blastomyces dermatitidis causes principally skin infections, whereas the American blastomyces dermatitidis [610] may cause wide dissemination, including to bones and joints. Gilchrist [610] described in skin sections a double-contoured fungal parasite which is observed in the yeast phase in tissues, and which in the mold or mycelial phase is composed of widely intertwining hyphae in culture. In the United States the disease occurs chiefly in the southeast and in the middle Atlantic states, where it is endemic. It may affect chiefly the skin and subcutaneous tissue by tuberculidlike lesions, as observed in Europe, or it may enter the body through the respiratory tract or gastrointestinal tract. Here it appears initially and most commonly as a pulmonary disease. After having produced necrotizing lesions in primary organs, it invades the bloodstream. Blastomycosis becomes localized in joints either primarily or secondarily by expansion from osteomyelitic foci in articular epiphyses. Most frequently affected are the knee, wrist, and elbow joints [1394]. They are warmer than the neighboring

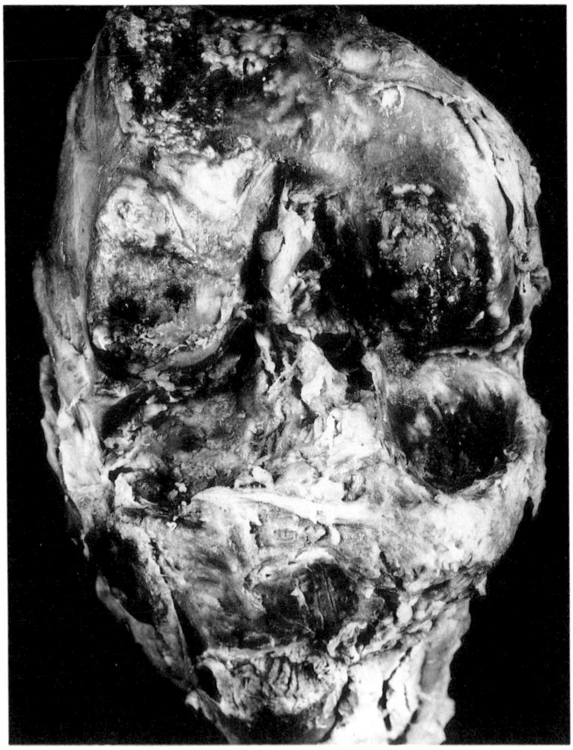

Fig. 169. The surfaces of the knee joint are deeply and extensively eroded in blastomycotic arthritis. One femoral condyle has partly retained its cartilage cover, but the other femoral condyle and one tibial condyle are penetrated by wide grooves

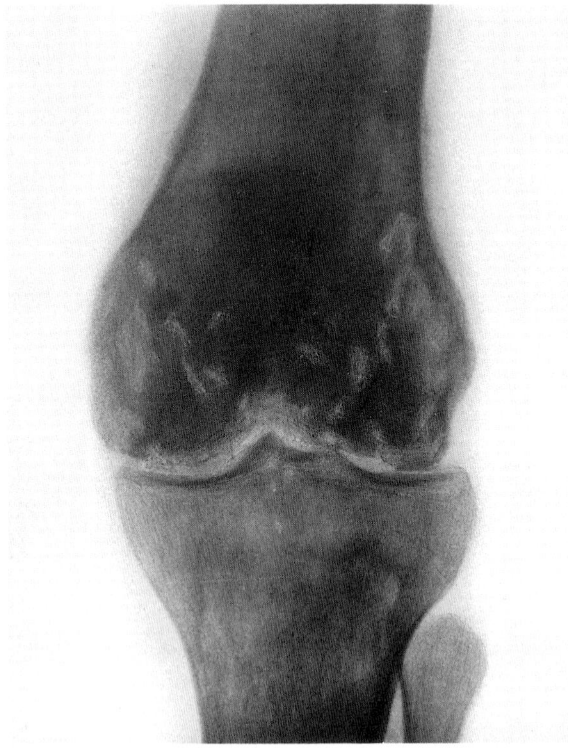

Fig. 170. The distal femoral epiphysis in cryptococcal arthritis presents extensive areas of marked osteolysis bordered by osteosclerosis. The articular surfaces of the femoral condyles are deeply eroded and very uneven

area and swollen and contain an increased amount of joint fluid [530, 594]. Pronounced malaise and high fever are associated with this arthritis [530, 557, 976, 1628]. On longer duration of the infection, the joints display marked thickening of the articular and periarticular soft tissues, intense pain, and contracture. In the case of suppuration, a much more frequent complication than in other fungal diseases [95], the joint effusion, unless drained in time, perforates outward and leads to formation of fistulae.

The aspirated joint fluid almost invariably contains blastomyces, identifiable as doubly refractile, thick-walled single yeasts of 8–15 μm (Fig. 171), on which smaller daughter buds are occasionally attached [95, 436, 594, 632, 1331]. Confirmation of the diagnosis is carried out by culturing the fluid on Sabouraud's agar and by obtaining a loose mycelial growth composed of intermingled branching hyphae which bear small spores at their ends. Confirmation of the diagnosis may also be obtained by skin tests with a blastomycin antigen or serologically by agglutination and/or complement fixation tests.

Roentgenographs of the joints reveal soft tissue swelling in the beginning stage, thereafter uneven delimitation of the directly subchondral bone due to erosion, and eventually deep epiphyseal areas of irregular structure with dissolution or osteoporosis and sclerosis due to osteomyelitis. Similarly, the long bones may present in their diaphyses multiple lytic areas delimited by sclerosis, indicative of osteomyelitic abscesses [356, 585].

Pathological-anatomical examination (Fig. 169) discloses that the inner part of the joint capsule is very thickened and generally scarified. The epiphyseal surfaces are extensively devoid of articular cartilage and are very uneven by deep erosions, which expand in a few places into the depth of the epiphyses. Large grooves are formed as the sequelae of abscesses.

Histopathological examination discloses granulations at the surface of the synovial membrane, resembling those of tuberculosis, and comprising double-walled blastomyces yeasts. In the subsynoviocytic tissue, granulomata are scattered (Fig. 171). Their centers consist of necrotic material and blastomyces as a single or a budding spherical cell of 10–15 μm with a thick refractile wall. While many yeasts of blastomyces are substantially enlarged by intracellular budding of spores, other yeasts are enlarged by extracellular budding of spores (Fig. 171). However, other yeasts are surrounded by numerous histiocytes, occasionally by a few small giant cells, and peripherally by a dense agglomeration of lymphocytes (Fig. 171). Rather large

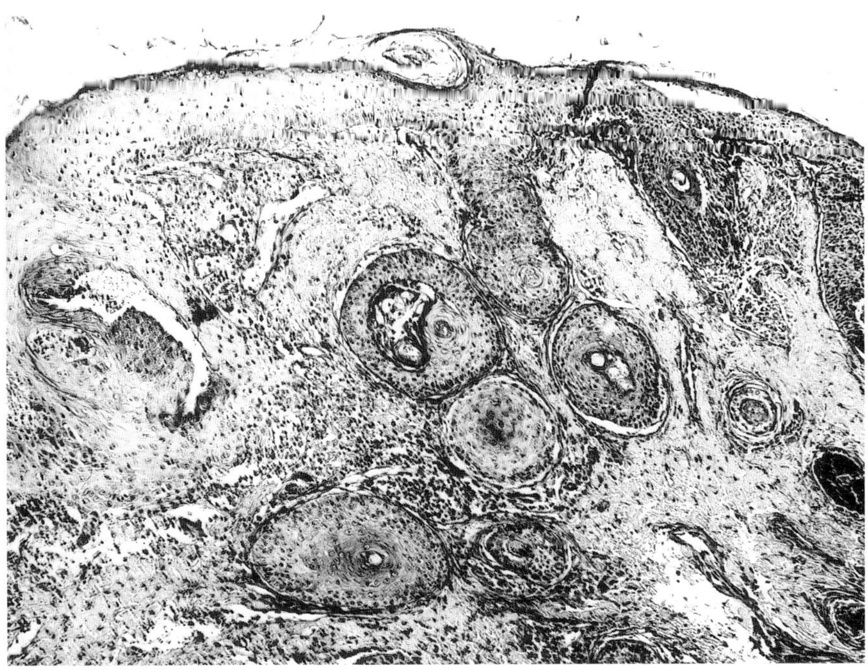

Fig. 171 The moderately infiltrated synovial membrane comprises several granulomata which have enclosed double-walled highly refractile yeasts of blastomyces

portions of amorphous, poorly stained material are occasionally scattered; these are devoid of cells but contain fragments of nuclei (Fig. 171), an indication of necrosis. At the periphery of these amorphous masses lies a wall of leukocytes, lymphocytes, and giant cells surrounded by histiocytes, collagen fibers, and newly proliferated blood vessels.

Medicamentous treatment is identical to that in coccidioidomycosis. Amphotericin B has proven in the recent past to be very effective in clearing the skin and systemic lesions [1394]. It is administered intravenously with 50 mg twice weekly to a total of 4000 mg over a period of 6–9 months. However, the adverse effects of amphotericin B include thrombophlebitis at the site of injection and several general effects of serious nature (see above). Ketoconazole, administered as in coccidioidomycosis, has also been used in blastomycosis [268] – 400–800 mg daily for 6 months and with similar results – but also with cases of intolerance to ketoconazole. Another medication used as a substitute for ketoconazole is hydroxystilbamidine, injected intravenously at 225 mg until a dose of 10–12 g has been attained [217]. In addition, the treatment often must include surgical evacuation of the suppurative processes in the joint and/or bones. Experience [95] indicates that blastomycosis is generally and locally more harmful than any other fungal infection, and despite all treatment modalities its mortality rate is about 10% [217].

Infection with the airborne and worldwide histoplasma capsulatum occurs primarily in the respiratory tract [1801]. It is manifested initially in moderate general symptoms such as weakness, fatiguability, elevated temperature, and breathing discomfort – simulating a common cold. If it remains confined to the lungs, it is a self-limited condition which eventually heals with spots of calcification in the lungs and enlarged regional lymphnodes. In less frequent cases it becomes aggravated into chronic pneumonia and/or pleurisy with chest pain and recurrent fever. Upon regression, an emphysema, mediastinal fibrosis, and/or pericarditis remains [650]. The liver and spleen are often enlarged.

However, upon invasion into the bloodstream, the fungus is disseminated in the body [373, 1515]. It then becomes localized, among other organs, very often in the diaphyseal marrow of long bones and less often in the articular epiphyses and their joints. Accompanying a concurrent skin affection such as erythema nodosum, the arthritic condition presents as synovitis [96, 295, 883, 1640] with moderate swelling and effusion of the serous type. The latter appears to result from a hypersensitivity reaction to the fungal antigen and responds satisfactorily to salicylates and/or antibiotics. In the rare cases of fungal infection expanding from lytic areas within the adjacent epiphyses, the joint is enlarged by very torpid, marked swelling of the joint capsule which substantially hampers the motion of the joint.

Microscopic examination [1331] of the discharged secretion from draining sinuses discloses, amid the pus cells, yeasts 2–5 μm in size and with refractile capsules. Scattered among them are large histiocytes and/or sporangia filled with such small capsules (Fig. 172). The culture on Sabouraud's agar yields

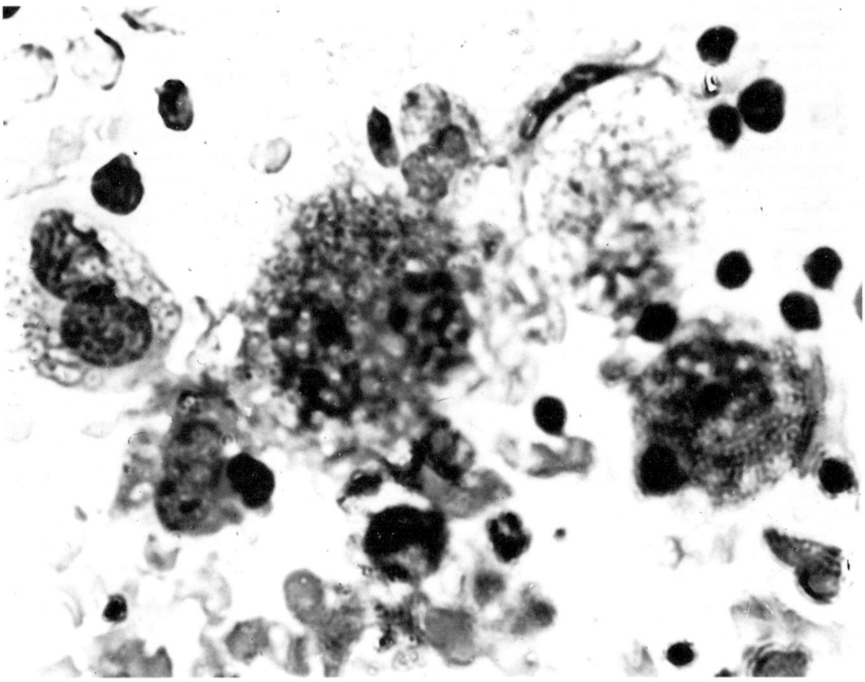

Fig. 172. A large histoplasma capsulatum is filled with many intracytoplasmic yeasts 1–3 µm in size. Two smaller histoplasmata lie in proximity

[436] a thin filament with ends enlarged by emerging spores. Serologically, the precipitation and complement fixation tests are of substantial diagnostic value if results are positive in a titer above 1:128. Skin tests with available antigen in decreasing concentrations yield positive results.

Roentgenographs reveal in the primary osseous affection multiple small, sharply delimited areas of distinct radiolucency lying within slight osteosclerosis in the epiphyses. The lungs display a variety of changes, manifested generally in irregular areas of density or calcification and a distended emphysematous pattern of the lobes.

Histopathological examination of the markedly thickened joint capsule discloses coarse plump villous proliferations on the inner surface and extensive infiltration of the subsynoviocytic tissue by lymphocytes. Among these, are scattered granulomata, composed of large histiocytes and giant cells. The latter have intracellular inclusions of microorganisms. In the depth also lie extensive agglomerations of histoplasma yeasts, readily identifiable by their thick capsules. Some of these are very large due to the great number of endospores comprised in them (Fig. 172). These agglomerations are surrounded by very cellular connective tissue which also contains a large number of histiocytes and lymphocytes and a few small giant cells.

Treatment of the serous joint effusions is managed effectively by the administration of salicylates 3.0 g, nonsteroidal antiinflammatory medications, or antibiotics (chloramphenicol 3.0 g, tetracycline 3.0 g, or erythromycin 3.0 g daily). On progressive thickening of the joint capsule, indicative of granulomatous formations, amphotericin B should be administered in the dosage described for coccidioidomycosis (see above). However, if amphotericin is not well tolerated, ketoconazole 400–800 mg given daily for 8–12 months is well tolerated although less effective. Medicamentous treatment [748] may have to be supplemented by synovectomy and resection of the articular surfaces when draining sinuses develop.

In addition to the fungi described above, cryptococcus neoformans, also spread worldwide, is a further possible causative agent of articular inflammation. It is an encapsulated budding microorganism which enters the human body through the respiratory tract [974, 1715] and is disseminated throughout the body after invading the bloodstream [632]. The liver, kidneys, lymph nodes, meninges, subcutaneous tissue and skin, bones, and joints then become affected [96, 507, 974].

Direct involvement of the inner part of the joint capsule is the least frequent manifestation of cryptococci. This is associated with moderate elevation in temperature and serous effusion in a joint, usually in the knee, elbow, or sternoclavicular joint. On the other hand, purulent effusion in a joint is the manifestation of a secondary infection resulting from perforation of the frequent juxtarticular osteomyelitic abscesses [970]. The onset of the articular disease is usually subacute [96] and is associated with mild or moderate symptoms. Little regional impairment is present.

Microscopic examination of the joint fluid and the discharge from a draining sinus discloses the presence of encapsulated, single or budding round microor-

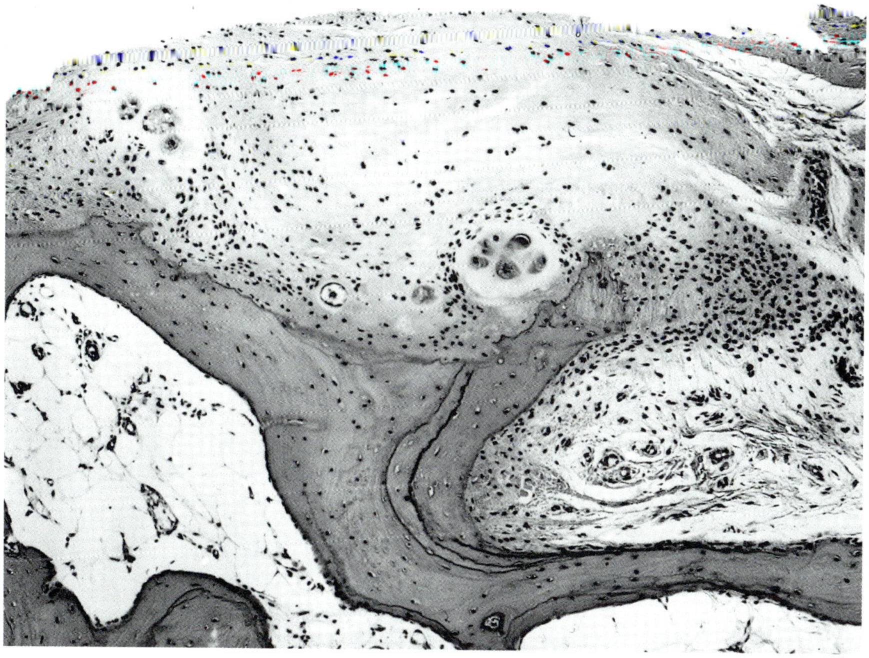

Fig. 173. The articular surface, covered by fibrocartilage, comprises a few sharply delimited agglomerations of encapsulated yeast cells of cryptococcus. The marrow spaces also comprise a few encapsulated cryptococci

ganisms 4–7 µm in size. Roentgenographs (Fig. 170) reveal, in cases of perforated multiple abscesses, narrowing of the cartilage space and erosion of the articular surface. Microscopic examination of synovial tissue discloses the presence of encapsulated round yeasts lying intercellularly and intracellularly. The articular surfaces (Fig. 173) merge with amorphous cartilage or fibrosed cartilage, which comprises a few isolated encapsulated round yeasts or a few agglomerations of encapsulated round yeasts. Similar encapsulated yeast cells lie in the directly subcortical marrow spaces, where they are close to granulomata or to very cellular granulation tissue.

Treatment by intravenous administration of amphotericin B, as described above for coccidioidomycosis, is supplemented with flucytosine 3.0–4.0 g daily in divided doses over a period of 6 months (but is contraindicated in preexisting renal impairment) [1671]. This produces a general and substantial improvement by regression of the inflammatory granulations.

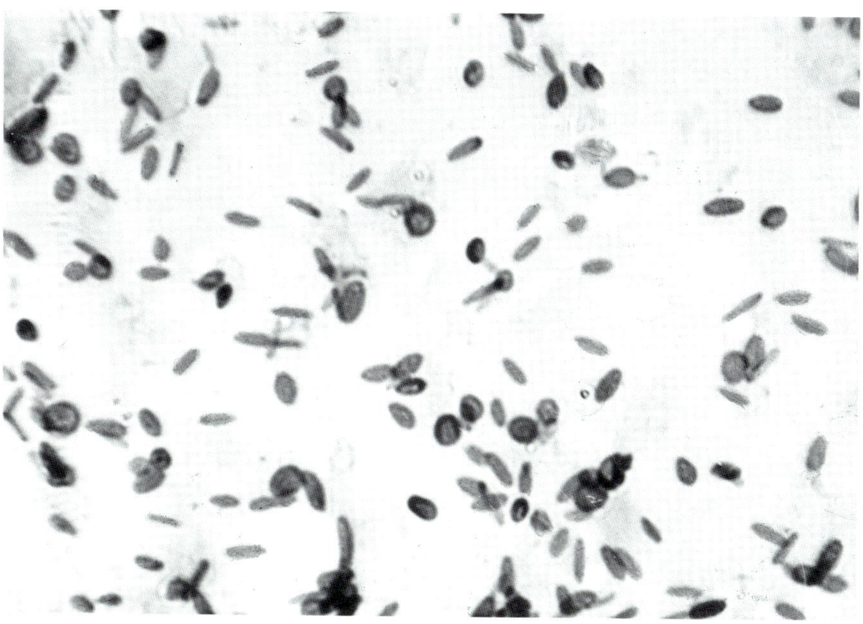

Fig. 174. Synovial fluid contains globular and ovoid shapes of sporothrix representing its mycelial phase and cigarlike shapes representing its yeast phase

Nevertheless, with suppurative joint inflammation or a draining sinus, arthrotomy is indicated for resection of the joint capsule and/or the articular epiphyses.

Another pathogenic fungus is sporothrix (or sporotrichon) Schencki, which grows on grass, moss, and other plants. It invades the human body through the respiratory tract and causes extensive infiltrates [1468], which heal with fibrosis. During the active phase of the pulmonary process, sporothrix spreads by the hematogenous route and may invade joints, although this is infrequent [389, 1468]. The most commonly invaded joints are those of the knee, elbow, wrist, or fingers. The affection is manifested in very active synovitis, with pronounced swelling of the joint and limitation of active motion due to pain. The joint fluid is sometimes increased. Eventually the articular cartilage becomes eroded, and mycotic destruction expands into the epiphysis.

Culture of the sputum or bronchial expectorate on Sabouraud's agar may yield budding cells in the shape of cigars or dots. The brownish yellow joint fluid contains microorganisms shaped like cigars or globules (Fig. 174), and conidiophores bearing spherical microconidia. In the absence of such examinations, the diagnosis can be established by intracutaneous injection of sporotrichial antigen. Roentgenographs reveal osteoporosis of the articular epiphyses; narrowing of the cartilage space supervenes on longer duration of the articular process.

Treatment should begin with the oral administration of amphotericin in similar doses as in coccidioidomycosis [12, 748] and may need to be supplemented with intraarticularly injected amphotericin [969]. However, if the articular condition deteriorates despite medication, and roentgenographs reveal expansion of the epiphyseal erosion, resection of the articular epiphyses is indicated.

IV. Allergic, Rheumatic, and Etiologically Unclarified Joint Inflammations

1. Seroanaphylactic Arthritis

Repeated parenteral administrations of serum, a protein foreign to the body, often lead to joint inflammation. This process may serve as a paradigm for the explanation of some inflammatory processes taking place in the joint capsule. Two to eight days after repetition of an intramuscular injection of serum against tetanus, some individuals experience swelling of joints associated with urticaria of the skin and exudation in body cavities. This syndrome ist termed serum sickness. Pirquet [1261] demonstrated that the concurrent changes represent an allergic phenomenon which is elicited as an anaphylactic reaction by some organs or structures to the injected foreign protein. The foreign serum or plasma is countered by antibodies, either already available or produced within a few days [131]. The resulting antigen-antibody complexes are deposited in the wall of blood vessels, the glomeruli of the kidneys, the reticuloendothelial cells of the liver and spleen, and the synovial cells of the joint capsules. The synovial cells thus manifest their similarity to reticuloendothelial cells and react with pronounced changes, namely seroanaphylactic arthritis.

The anaphylactic swelling of joints follows a few days after repeated serum injections against the disease. The circulating foreign proteins arrive as antigens in joints, where they are presumably encountered by antibodies produced by the synovial cells. The interaction of antibodies and antigens results in tissue responses which present the clinical picture of allergic seroanaphylactic arthritis. Pirquet et al. [1262] postulated an exudative phenomenon in the joints similar to that in urticaria of the skin. The joint inflammation developing upon the first or second administration of serum represents the prototype of allergic reactions of joints. It also explains the development of similar joint inflammations elicited by bacterial toxins or other toxinlike substances which act as antigens. Since serum arthritis does not occur in all persons treated with serum injections, one must presume an individual hypersensitivity manifested in an especially intensive reaction of tissues against substances of proteinic nature.

Serum arthritis usually appears after repetition of an injection of serum in the amount of 5–15 ml, but it may appear even after the first injection of a larger amount of 20–100 ml serum in predisposed individuals. The reaction usually develops 1–8 days after administration of horse serum and may also develop after injection of cattle serum. Similar allergic reactions with generalized symptoms may be observed after parenteral administration of some medications, especially antibiotics of protein or nucleoprotein composition in the treatment of infections. In the latter cases it is indispensable to determine whether the ensuing symptoms and arthritis are manifestations of serumlike sickness or complication of the underlying infection following inefficiency of the medications. Serum arthritis often appears concurrently with other allergic changes of the body such as urticaria, edema of the face, enlargement of lymph nodes, possibly splenomegaly, and albumin in the urine. The exanthem may be very discomforting by severe pruritus. The patient's general condition is often impaired by fever, malaise, and nausea.

Affection of the joints presents either as intensive arthralgia or as synovitis with acute swelling of the joint capsule, elevation in local temperature, and marked soreness. The latter condition is observed mostly in the knees, hands, elbows, and ankles. The moderately increased, yellowish, clear serous joint fluid contains up to 1500/ml polymorphonuclear leukocytes with a distinctly high proportion (5%–7%) of eosinophilic leukocytes and lymphocytes. Swift et al. [1616] demonstrated horse serum in the joint fluid by precipitin test. Roentgenographs of the joints do not reveal abnormal findings.

Histopathological examination of the specimens of synovial membrane obtained by punch biopsy discloses hydropic swelling of the superficial cell layers and extensive accumulation of interstitial fluid (Fig. 175). The collagen fibers of subsynoviocytic tissue are also hydropically swollen. Thin perivascular infiltrates are scattered scantly. A general serous inflammation characterizes the changes in the synovial membrane. Immunofluorescent studies reveal the presence of small granular accumulations of antigen in hypertrophic synoviocytes.

Differential diagnosis must consider any acute arthritis, especially that of rheumatic fever and gonorrhea. However, a recent injection of serum reported in the case history provides a direct clue to the etiology.

Prophylactically, apotoxins should be used, which are sera purified of protein substances eliciting anaphylaxis. Furthermore, in individuals with known vasolability or allergy, the serum should be injected in fractioned doses. When serum is to be injected for the second time, even after an interval of years, the fractional desensitization described by Besredka [131] is advisable.

When the serum disease with joint affection occurs fully, 10 ml calcium gluconate is injected intravenously and 1 ml 1% suprarenin solution subcutaneously, both twice a day. Diuresis by large amounts of tea and diaphoresis by salicylates, 0.5 g six to eight times daily, are very helpful. If the salicylates do not alleviate the articular pain, stronger analgesics should

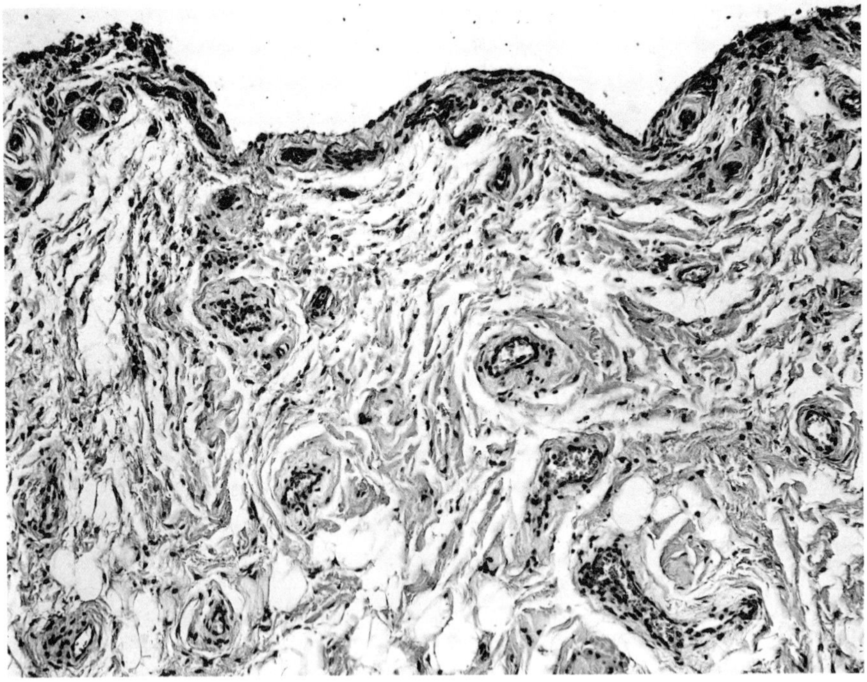

Fig. 175. The synovial membrane is extensively rarefied by interstitial edema, and all blood vessels are hyperemic

be administered. Nonsteroidal antiinflammatory medications are of similar benefit. Moist warm compresses applied continuously around the affected joints help to reduce the inflammation and pain. The symptoms usually subside within 8–10 days, and recovery of normal function in affected joints follows shortly thereafter with the help of shortwave diathermy in eight sessions. However, in the rare case in which no satisfactory regression of the condition is obtained, and the symptoms continue unabated, prednisolone 20 mg two or three times daily is advisable. The effect of corticosteroids appears to be determined by their suppressive influence on the receptor cells of the antigen-antibody complex. Regular application of an elastic bandage around the affected joint during the day is advisable in aftercare; this prevents recurrent swelling of the joint. The restoration of normal function in the joint may be explained by the reversible histopathological changes of the synovial membrane and by the lack of damage to the articular cartilage, as ascertained by roentgenographic follow-up examinations. Therefore the term synovitis is more appropriate for this form of joint disease than is arthritis.

2. Arthritis in Rheumatic Fever

Under the heading of rheumatism, derived from the Greek work rheo ("flow"), are included inflammatory affections characterized by a shifting from one region of the body to another or from one organ to another. Thus, ethymologically defined, rheumatic disease is a migrating process. Observations over the centuries have taught that the symptoms of this spreading or shifting condition are manifested primarily and distinctly in joints. Therefore, to refer to this joint affection as rheumatic arthritis emphasizes that its clinical picture represents the partial manifestation of a larger disease entity. On the basis of onset and course, manifestations, findings, and complications, the rheumatic disease may be differentiated into acute and chronic types. Acute rheumatic arthritis represents part of a wider clinical picture, that of rheumatic fever [1625, 1626, 1771].

The etiology of the latter, according to observations and experiences [135, 1594, 1615], lies in the concurrence of the following factors.

a. Predisposition due to congenital properties in the protoplasm or modifications in the connective tissue by circumstances during life appear to facilitate the occurence of rheumatic fever. One observes in some individuals, a susceptibility to rheumatic affections without identifiable outer causes. French experimental pathologists consider this predisposition to be a special diathesis of the connective tissue and designate it as arthritism. Allergy is implicated as a pathogenetically predisposing factor here [305, 1806]; this is plausible as acute rheumatic arthritis resembles in some features the arthritis which occurs in serum disease, and which is a response to allergy. Experimental confirmation was provided by Klinge [901], who produced morphological equivalents to the acute rheumatic nodules by repeated injections of serum alien to the body.

b. By mediation of the autonomous nervous system, a decreased blood flow is caused by some physical conditions as sudden exposure to cold, wetting of the body, or a period spent in moist surroundings. This is associated with decreased defense on the part of some tussues, which permits the localization of rheumatic disease. The greater incidence of rheumatic disease in northeastern Europe, in the United Kingdom, and in the northern United States may be related to the cold, moist climate in these areas [937, 1594, 1684]. However, with improved material conditions in the United States, Europe, and Japan the overall incidence of acute rheumatic fever has decreased dramatically [937, 1246, 1594, 1601].

c. Investigations [135, 936, 1752] and clinical observations [500, 852, 1246, 1594, 1625, 1806] indicate that streptococcal infections of the pharynx and/or throat precede acute rheumatic fever in about 80% of patients, and that prophylactic administration of antibiotics to larger, organized groups (school children, soldiers) has substantially reduced the occurrence of infections and rheumatic fever, Cecil et al. [265] cultivated streptococcus viridans from the blood of patients with acute rheumatic fever. However, Coburn et al. [305] demonstrated principally streptococcus hemolyticus A as the generally and most eliciting agent of acute rheumatic fever. Even in patients in whom a culture of throat smears failed to show positive results, Todd [1648] found antistreptolysin in their blood as an antibody against hemolytic streptococcus, but not in the blood of other patients. Another antibody, antihyaluronidase (against the hyaluronidase produced by the streptococci), was observed in 85% of patients with acute rheumatic fever [727]. The absence of microorganisms in the blood and joint fluid of these patients indicates that the streptococci do not penetrate from the portal into the bloodstream; however, they release substances and enzymes with antigenic properties [936] into the blood. These antigens are transported into joints and other organs such as the heart, lungs, and brain, where they elicit serous and/or proliferative inflammation [1752].

As a sequela of pharyngitis or any throat inflammation, fever sets in after an average latency of 5–10 days and then lasts between 8 and 20 days, depending probably on the virulence of the particular streptococci [500]. Concurrently, arthritis afflicts principally children and young persons [405], substantially less so adults, and has a different course in each age group. In children and adolescents, the acute rheumatic condition starts with fever, which may rise to 38.3–39.4°C. At the height of the fever, profuse malodorous outbreaks of sweat set in; the pulse rate often increases. A few days later, fleeting pain of varying duration appears in several joints of the extremities, until it finally becomes localized in a few joints – usually the knee, wrist, ankle, and/or elbow joints, less often in the hip or shoulder joints. The affected joints gradually swell and are often warmer than neighboring tissue. Because of pain these joints are held stiff, and their movement is avoided. If the swelling of soft tissues and the amount of joint fluid increase, the joint assumes an intermediate position which is usually that of moderate flexion. The latter symptoms are present chiefly in the multiarticular affections, which may last 6–10 weeks before they fully subside. In pauciarticular affection, the symptoms regress after 5–8 days in one joint and appear alternatingly in another joint until they too fully subside within 4–5 weeks.

Previously or concurrently, the skin of the trunk and proximal parts of the extremities often displays eruptions of the type of purpura rheumatica. However, the more frequent skin alteration is that of erythema marginatum [866, 1242, 1625], a rash of multiple, pink, nonitching papules with centers which fade away and normalize while the well-delimited outer margins expand. This persists for 3–6 weeks. Nontender nodules are occasionally palpated in the subcutaneous tissue of the head and on the extensor surface of the elbow and knee. They are rather firm, 1.5–2.0 cm in diameter, not adherent to the skin or underlying tissue and thus movable, and regress within 4–8 weeks. A complication of rheumatic fever may be chorea, a neurological disorder caused by affection of the basal cerebral ganglia. It is manifested by involuntary movements which subside during sleep or by muscular weakness.

However, the most serious complication is affection of the heart [167, 281], which appears in about 30–40% of patients in the 2nd–3rd weeks of rheumatic fever. This may be: (a) serous inflammation of the endocardium leading to shrinking or adhesion, most commonly of the mitral valve, and less often of the aortic or tricuspidal valve; (b) interstitial inflammation of the myocardium; or (c) serous inflammation of the pericardium with effusion. The resulting pathomechanics of the heart action is manifested in regurgitation or stenosis of the blood outflow, disorder in the rhythm of myocardial action, limited myocardial contraction or dilatation due to pericardial adhesions, and/or cardiac tamponade resulting in complete cardiac failure. The associated clinical symptoms are irregularity in heart beat and pulse, changes in heart sounds or heart murmurs, continuous pericardial rub or rales, enlarged heart shadow in roentgenographs, and significant changes in the electrocardiogram with prolonged P-R interval.

Acute rheumatic arthritis in adults is different [1059, 1243, 1594]. It begins with high fever, up to

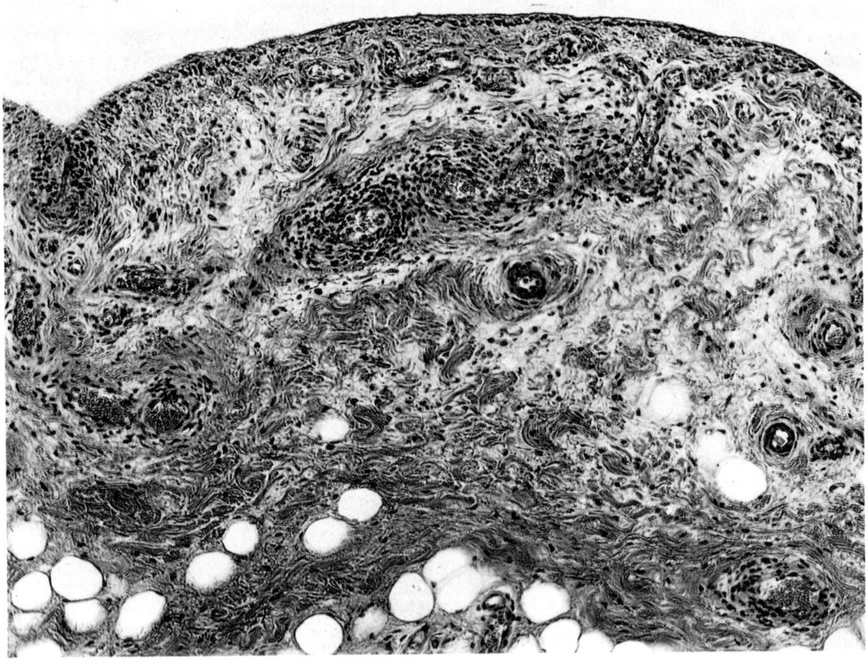

Fig. 176. The synovial membrane is moderately rarefied by interstitial edema. All blood vessels are hyperemic, and some of them are surrounded by infiltrates of lymphocytes and histiocytes

39.7–40° C, and full intensity of articular symptoms. The fever may show intermittent or remittent course; it may regress after a week and recur a few days later. In addition to the picture of marked involvement of the entire body, most joints present an acute and very active inflammation. The wrist, knee, and ankle joints are principally involved. Intense pain is associated with swelling of the joint capsules; increased joint fluid may further enlarge the joints. Movements of the joints are substantially limited. The clinical picture is that of severe inflammation of the joints. As complications, pleurisy, endocarditis, or abdominal pain due to mesenteric adenitis may occur.

Blood studies in children and adults disclose marked elevation (up to 75–85 mm/h) in sedimentation rate and increased leukocytes (to 12000–18000/ml) shortly after the onset of joint swelling. Examination of serum discloses the presence of antibodies [1751] directed against streptolysin, streptokinase, and streptohyaluronidase. These enzymes are produced by the strains of streptococcus A. Streptolysin-0 is a hemolysin, and its presence is manifested in an antibody titer of 150 Todd units or more. Such a titer is detected in 80% of children who recently had a streptococcal pharyngitis and in adults who suffered from a nonsuppurative infection [1366]. Antistreptokinase and antihyaluronidase are present in significant elevations in 20% of patients [135, 1243, 1366, 1751, 1752]. Similarly, cultures from the pharynx and throat secretions disclose the presence of streptococci in about 80% of patients. In the recent past, the agglutination test of sheep red cells coated with a mixture of streptococcal antigens has become available; this is very sensitive and yields positive results at a dilution of 1:200 in all patients [1625]. On the other hand, the outcome of the latex fixation test is negative. The test result for C-reactive protein is positive in 60%–70% of patients; its serial determinations indicate, besides the temperature curve, the response of inflammatory activity to the medications administered. The occasional exudate in the knee joint is a clear fluid containing 3%–5% protein and 500–10000 white cells/ml, with 60% polymorphonuclear leukocytes, 25% large mononuclear leukocytes, and 15% lymphocytes. The concentrations of complement components in the joint fluid are comparable to those in the serum [1608]. Neither staining of the sediment nor culture of the joint fluid discloses the presence of microorganisms.

Roentgenographs reveal moderate swelling of the soft articular tissues but no alteration in the articular epiphyses even on longer duration of the joint affection.

On gross-anatomical examination acute rheumatic arthritis is manifested chiefly by exudative alteration. The inner part of the joint capsule is reddened by hyperemia and swollen by edema. On its surface lie threads of mucin and flakes of fibrin which have been precipitated from the increased joint fluid. After repeated rheumatic attacks progressive formation of the intracapsular connective tissue ensues. However, no alteration in the articular cartilage is observed. On the other hand, the endocardium presents numerous excrescences occupying the surfaces and margins of the valves [901, 1786]. The following fibrosis and shrink-

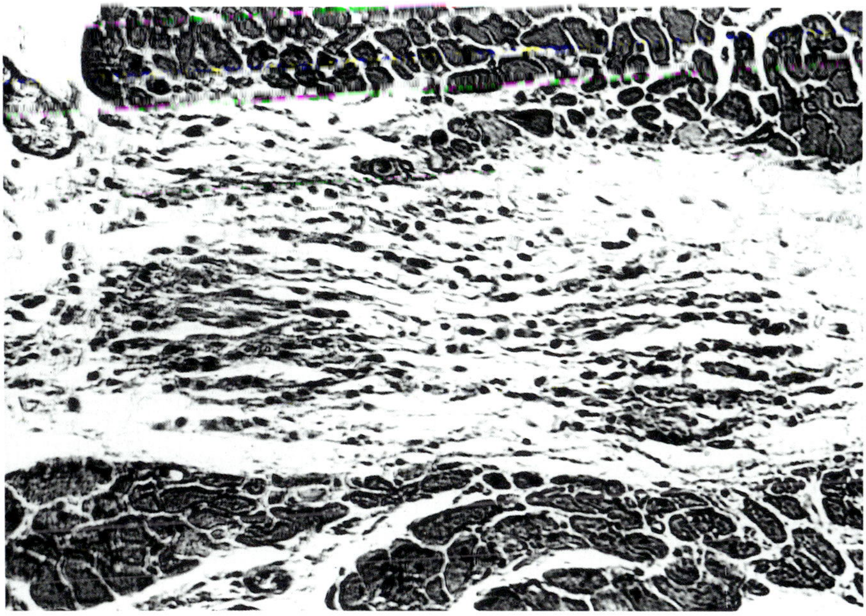

Fig. 177. Interstitial tissue between myocard bundles comprises rather extensive agglomerations of histiocytes and, less so, of fibroblasts. Between these, collagen fibers course, and a few lymphocytes are scattered

ing, also involving the chordae tendineae and rings, leads to retraction of the valves. On the other hand, stenosis of the valves may ensue by their contiguous adhesions and fibrotic rigidity. The myocardium is flabby and contains numerous local lesions, Aschoff's nodules [1397]. The pericardium is covered more extensively by verrucous excrescences than the endocardium; its visceral and parietal surfaces are fused in a few places [1786]. In less frequent cases, the pericardial cavity contains a serous effusion.

Histopathological examination (Fig. 176) discloses rarefaction of the synovial membrane by edema and desquamation of the synoviocyte cover in a few places covered by fibrin. In the subjacent zone the blood vessels are very hyperemic and are surrounded by thin infiltrates of inflammatory cells. In their vicinity lie focal agglomerations of polymorphonuclear neutrophilic leukocytes, lymphocytes, and plasmacytes. Histiocytes in small numbers participate in these infiltrates. A few fresh hemorrhages are scattered in the subsynoviocytic zone, where the fibrocytes are increased on longer lasting articular affection. However, the characteristic lesions of acute rheumatic fever, the Aschoff's [53] nodules, are detected chiefly in the myocardium [686, 941, 1161]. These (Fig. 177) are ovoid or longish lesions with numerous fibroblasts and lymphocytes which enclose a central core of degenerated collagen fibers and necrotic tissue. In their vicinity lie lymphocytes, polymorphonuclear neutrophilic leukocytes, eosinophilic leukocytes, histiocytes, and occasionally giant cells. Nodules of similar structure, although of much lower frequency, may be observed in the subcutaneous tissue, fascia, periosteum, and peripheral joint capsule.

In view of the marked involvement of the joints, an acute onset of chronic rheumatoid arthritis, a septic or metastatic bacterial articular infection in children, a gonococcal or other bacterial arthritis in adults must be taken in the differential diagnosis. Other systemic diseases occasionally associated with fever and swelling of joints, such as systemic lupus erythematosus or dermatomyositis, may present a similar picture, and should also be considered. However, the complete case history, especially with the report of an intense sore throat, the initial long phase of fever possibly accompanied by a skin rash, the relevant laboratory studies especially a high antistreptolysin titer, and possibly a supervening heart affection help to corroborate the diagnosis of arthritis in acute rheumatic fever.

As a very important measure in the treatment, the necessity of complete bedrest must be emphasized for the period at least until the temperature and pulse rate normalize, which may take 2–3 weeks. The observance of this requirement is indispensable for minimizing damage to the heart. In the event that such damage occurs, bedrest must be continued for 2–3 months. In view of the experience that a streptococcal inflammation of the pharynx causes the fever and arthritis, penicillin is the indicated antibiotic. It is given in a dosage to ensure a proper level in the blood. Thus 600,000–900,000 benzathine penicillin G are given intramuscularly to children and 1,200,000–2,400,000 to adults [499, 500, 1625]. If, nevertheless, the fever and general symptoms continue, and heart symptoms or arthritic symptoms set in, high daily doses are needed. Penicillin benzathine 1,200,000 U is injected intramuscularly every 4–6 h to adults for 10–14 days while children are given penicillin V 250 mg in tablet form every 4–6 h for 10–14 days. Those allergic or nonresponsive to penicillin receive erythromycin or cephalosporin 150 mg every 4 h for 10–14 days. On completion of the antibiotic treatment salicylates as acetylsalicylic acid or sodium salicylate are the next, and very efficacious, drug. The dose is 3.0–4.0 g in children or 6.0–8.0 g in adults, divided over 24 h for 2–3 weeks; this is increased or repeated if indicated by articular symptoms. Absorbed in the stomach, the salicylates are detected in measurable concentrations in the blood after 7–14 min and in the joint fluid after additional 18–30 min. The latter interval depends on the structural looseness of the inner part of the joint capsule [1542]. The beneficial effects of salicylate administration are noticeable in a few days by normalization in temperature and decreased pain and swelling of joints. Nevertheless, salicylates should be continued until the articular symptoms subside. In cases of poor tolerance to oral intake, the salicylates may be administered by enema, combined with sodium bicarbonate to prevent acidosis. If toxic effects such as persistent nausea, hemorrhages, hematuria, or hypoproteinemia occur, salicylates must be discontinued. Regular blood studies and administration of vitamin C and K are indicated. After the articular symptoms have subsided, and the sedimentation rate has normalized, the salicylates may be discontinued, but they must be resumed if these symptoms recur. This may occur after 6 weeks – 10 months, particularly in cases of primarily multiarticular joint affection [1821].

The affected heart, however, does not benefit from salicylates, but is strained by the concomitant changes in the general blood circulation. On the other hand, corticosteroids are able dramatically to reduce the acute rheumatic attacks [74, 997]; they also minimize the serous, infiltrative, degenerative, and productive alterations in the heart and other membranes [1771]. Even already discernible valvular noises diminish, and dilatation of the heart regresses. Therefore, the administration of corticosteroids should be instituted immediately at the slightest manifestation of cardiac affection, such as palpitations, dyspnea, irregularity of pulse, or cardiac arhythmia. Prednisone 40–60 mg daily is given in fractional doses for 3 weeks, and is then gradually diminished over the following 3 weeks under regular surveillance of heart function.

For regression of articular swellings, warm moist compresses should be applied regularly around the affected joints, which are additionally immobilized by splints or traction devices. The latter modality is indicated particularly in patients lacking sufficient discipline to observe prolonged bedrest. Subsequently, physical therapy with shortwave diathermy in eight to ten sessions to the affected joints, combined with massage for the regional musculature, is of benefit in restoring function of the extremities. Regular active mobilization exercises of the involved joints in a warm bath are of further benefit. If postinflammatory thickening of the joint capsule and limitation of motion persist in recurrent multiarticular cases, daily hot mud packs or a moist electric heating pad substantially help in decreasing the thickening of joints and restoring the normal range of motion.

Thus, the prognosis in acute rheumatic fever is favorable as long as only the joints are affected; however, the course of arthritis varies not only between children and adults but also among children. The duration of the joint inflammation and its primary complete subsidence or tendency to recurrence present distinct individual differences. The prognosis becomes very guarded in the approximately 40% of children who also develop an affection of the heart and require cardiac medications and prolonged limitation of physical activities. With an alteration in all heart constituents, pancarditis, acute cardiac failure leads in 8%–20% of these children to death [679, 1593, 1594].

3. Juvenile Rheumatoid Arthritis

Following the classic description by Still [1586], the view was held that essentially all arthritis in children – other than that in rheumatic fever, directly caused by microbial invasion, or concomitant with other system diseases – represents a single disease entity. However, increasing experience regarding the onset, general symptoms, clinical and laboratory findings, course and potential complications, has suggested the existence of three different types of rheumatoid arthritis affecting children aged 3–13 years [46, 225, 253, 1401, 1403, 1588]. These are: (a) the so-called pauciarticular type with involvement of only a few joints, (b) the type originally described by Still [1586] with acute arthritic onset and predominantly systemic features, and (c) the common type of multiarticular arthritis which clearly resembles the progressive rheumatoid arthritis in adults [511]. The age threshold of patients for distinguishing juvenile from adult rheumatoid arthritis lies at 14 years at the time when the joint disease begins. The changes in endocrine function at puberty appear to have an influence on the reaction of the body and on the course of the joint disease.

Differences in etiology exist between juvenile and adult rheumatoid arthritis. Although streptococcus viridans has been cultivated from the blood of children suffering from chronic rheumatoid arthritis, it is probable that an individually decreased defense ability in the infantile body plays a part in the occurrence and development of pronounced rheumatoid changes [89]. In view of the differences in tissue changes, course of

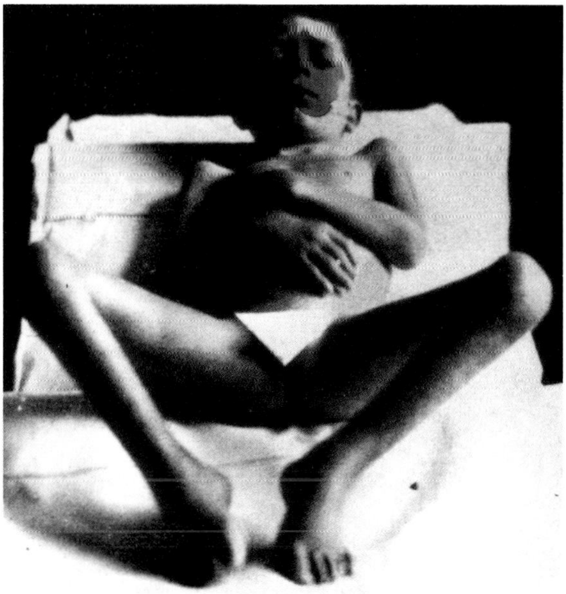

Fig. 178. An 11-year-old boy who had arthritis for the past 4 years without treatment. Flexion contractures developed in all major joints

the articular disease, and prognosis between rheumatoid arthritis in children and that in adults, separate descriptions of these are needed. As explained in "Rheumatoid Arthritis", the use of the term rheumatic is more appropriate than that of rheumatoid, and the former should therefore be used.

According to the initially indicated and generally accepted categorization of juvenile rheumatoid arthritis these types are described.

The pauciarticular type [253, 669] afflicting 30%–40% of children with juvenile rheumatoid arthritis, insidiously affects one to four joints and is accompanied by low-grade fever. The knee joint is chiefly affected, and at lower frequency the elbow, wrist and hand, ankle, and hip joints. The local pain is mild, and the swelling of the joint capsule is moderate; the knee joint occasionally presents an effusion. With longer duration of the joint affection and increasing thickening of the joint capsule, stiffness ensues; alterations in the articular epiphyses and residual deformities occur in 20%–30% of these cases. A very serious complication, chronic iridocyclitis, sets in in 20%–30% of these patients. The anterior chamber of the eye is affected by adhesions of the iris to the lens, with secondary glaucoma, degenerative alterations of the cornea, and cataract; all these in combination lead to severe impairment of vision or complete blindness [225, 254, 291].

In the systemic type, joint affection sets in mildly, but the general symptoms are very pronounced. The children are listless and in marked discomfort, weakness, and anorexia. The temperature is elevated to 39°–41°C and fluctuates daily over a wide range. A nonpruritic skin rash accompanies the fever episodes, with reddish evanescent small macules and larger papules on the face, trunk, and extremities, including the palms and soles. Multiple, moderately firm nodules appear in the subcutaneous tissue on the dorsal aspect of the elbow and forearm and in the flexor tendons of the wrist. The lymph nodes are also enlarged, as seen in the axilla and inguinal area; when the abdominal lymph nodes are enlarged, symptoms simulating an abdominal condition may set in. Concurrently, hepatomegaly and splenomegaly develop in about 70%–80% of these patients; liver function tests do not disclose any abnormality, but splenomegaly of conspicuous degree may simulate a serious abdominal condition. Another complication of lower frequency is pleurisy or pneumonia, which is also of much less severity than the equally frequent, serous pericarditis or interstitial myocarditis. The latter is associated with dyspnea, irregularity in pulse and heart action, enlargement of the heart shadow in radiographs, and changes in the electrocardiogram; these lead in 8%–10% of these patients to heart failure and death [1111].

The multiarticular type [46, 184, 223, 1401, 1403] involves 30%–40% of arthritic children. Also here, girls are affected more commonly than boys (Figs. 178, 179). It is manifested in gradually aggravating deformation in more than four joints of the extremities, most often the knee and wrist joints, and subsequently the hand, foot, ankle, elbow, hip, or shoulder joints, usually in a symmetrical way (Figs. 178, 179). In other children, the joint affection starts in the feet and hands and follows a centripetal course. The cervical spine is occasionally also affected, particularly in boys aged 10–14 years; its more profound alterations may lead to ankylosis [1404] and are appropriately discussed in "Ankylosing Spondylitis". Another rather rarely affected joint is the temporomandibular joint. The general symptoms are low-grade fever of up to 39°C and gradually increasing discomfort. The joints are moderately tender and present a diffuse swelling, which in the knee, ankle, and elbow joints may be compounded by an intraarticular effusion. Affection of the joint capsule expands in about one-half of these cases to the articular epiphyses, leading to profound alterations in the osteocartilaginous surfaces (Figs. 181, 182). Eventually marked deformation and limitation of motion of the joints ensue, possibly even ankylosis. Another sequel of long lasting inflammation of the joints is the disturbance of growth in the adjoining epiphyseal plates with resulting shortening and deformity by angular deviation (Fig. 182). However, the most disfiguring deformity is undoubtedly the occasional micrognathy

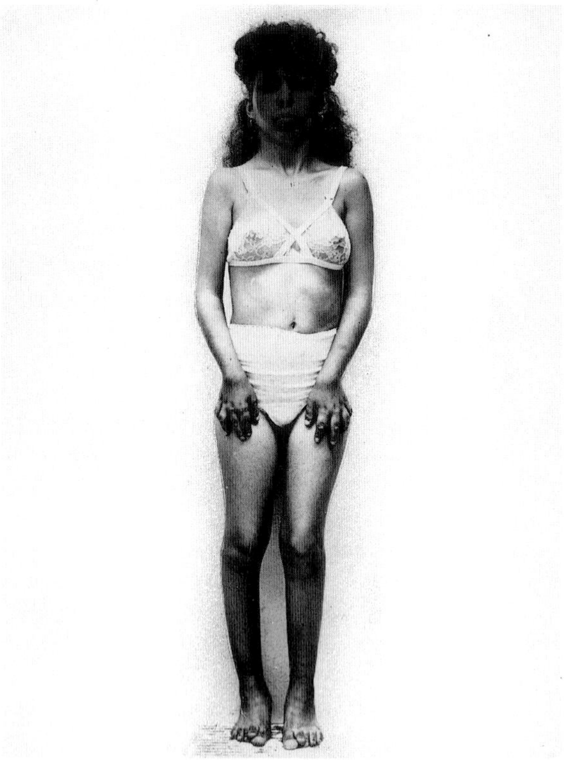

Fig. 179. A 17-year-old girl, conservatively treated for rheumatoid arthritis since the age of 6, attends a vocational school but needs crutches or canes on ambulation

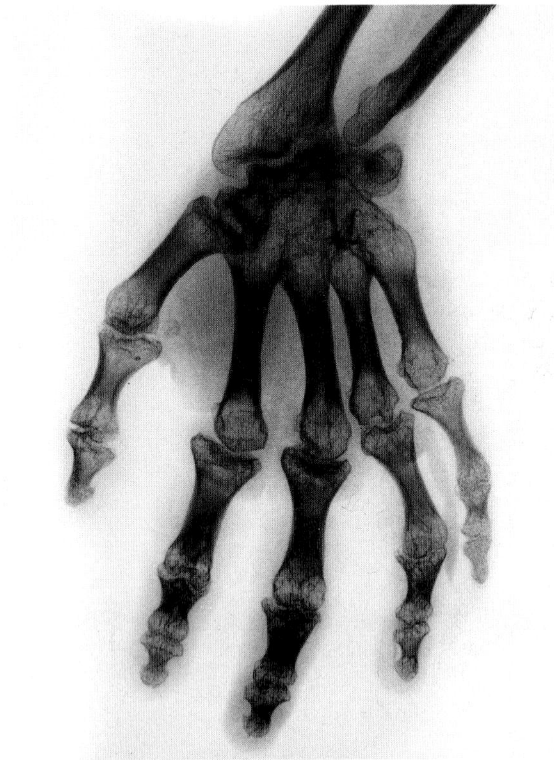

Fig. 180. The radiocarpal joint of the patient in Fig. 179 is moderately deformed and uneven, as are the metacarpophalangeal joints

of the mandible. Accompanying alterations include subcutaneous, rather firm nodules appearing mostly on the dorsal aspect of the elbow and forearm and sometimes on the hand. Splenomegaly and hepatomegaly may also occur in the multiarticular type, but at a distinctly lower incidence than in the systemic type. Similarly, affection of the heart is of much lower incidence and severity than in the systemic type.

Blood studies disclose moderate anemia, and in the systemic type principally a polymorphonuclear leukocytosis (20000/ml). The sedimentation rate is invariably elevated to 50–60 mm/h; comparison of several readings at intervals from one another provides a useful indication of the activity of the joint disease as well as the response to therapeutic agents. Of similar use is the test for C-reactive protein, which yields positive results in 50% of children with the systemic type. On the other hand, the test outcome for antinuclear antibodies is positive in 65%–80% [28, 109], principally in the pauciarticular type with chorioidoretinal complications. The test result for sheep cell agglutination and rheumatoid factor is positive in 12%–20% cases of the multiarticular type. In this type, the immunoglobulins are also increased [497, 1112, 1136], as demonstrated by serum protein electrophoresis. On the other hand, in the systemic type the soluble complexes are increased in proportion to the severity of the disease [497, 1136], as is the antistreptolysin titer [223, 1217, 1250]. The pale yellowish joint fluid contains a moderate or sometimes high number 2500–9000 of polymorphonuclear leukocytes and lymphocytes [1820].

Roentgenographs [1036] reveal thickening of the joint capsule and periarticular tissues, which due to overlapping blur the structure, and extensive osteoporosis of the articular epiphyses. Gradual narrowing of the articular cartilage space, irregular delimitation, and erosion of the epiphyseal articular surfaces with resulting deformities are evidenced (Figs. 180, 181, 182). On the other hand, accelerated growth and enlargement of the epiphyses may occur, as well as angular deviation in the metaphyses secondary to persistent hyperemia. Angulation may also be caused by retarded growth in the metaphyses (Fig. 182).

Gross-anatomical examination in the initial stage discloses edematous swelling of the joint capsule and periarticular structures. The synovial membrane is reddened and covered by a thick mucinous exudate. On continued inflammation the joint capsule becomes thickened and carries fibrin precipitates on its inner surface. From the latter numerous villous outgrowths

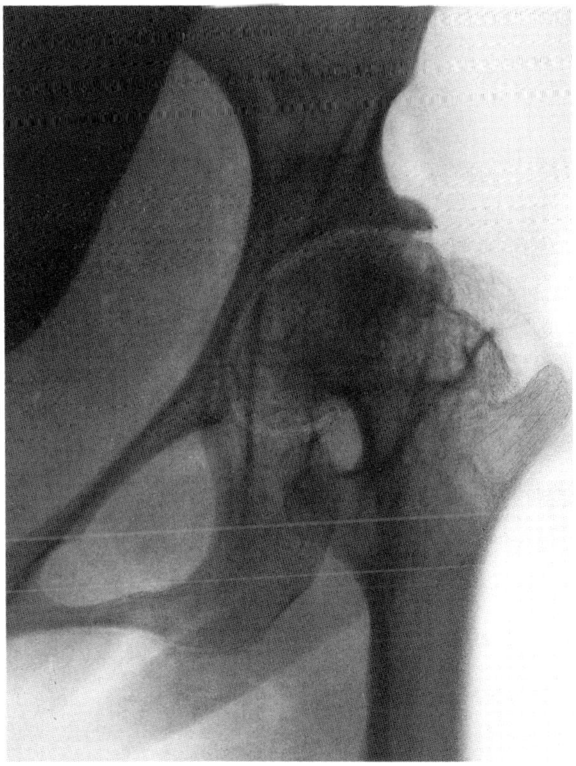

Fig. 181. The hip joint of the patient in Fig. 179 has a flattened femoral head and widened acetabulum at maintained joint space

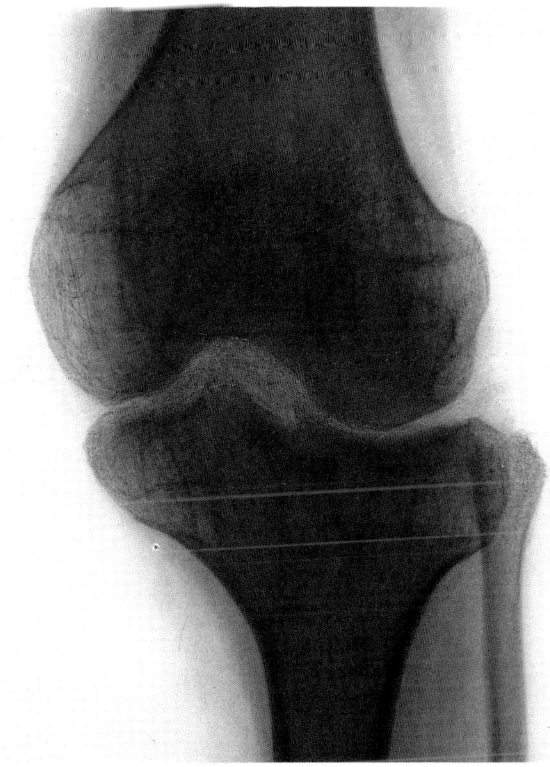

Fig. 182. The knee joint of the patient in Fig. 179 presents underdevelopment of the medial femoral condyle and of the lateral tibial condyle, but nevertheless congruence of the articular epiphyses. The lateral joint cleft is narrowed

protrude; some of these encroach upon the articular cartilage and erode it, eventually covering the defects with dense connective tissue. In the regional muscles the interstitial connective tissue is fibrosed. Sometimes a serous pericarditis or pleuritic thickening is also noted. The spleen may be enlarged and than contains hyaline degenerated tissue in the center of the follicles.

Histopathological examination [1543] of the synovial membrane in the early stage discloses that all smaller blood vessels are hyperemic; some are surrounded by narrow infiltrates, while the interstitial tissue is rarefied by edema. Subsequently, focal agglomerations of lymphocytes, plasmacytes, and histiocytes are scattered throughout and lie amid proliferating fibroblasts and a growing number of fibrocytes. By this hypercellularity extending to the surface, numerous villous excrescences of moderate size are formed (Fig. 183). When the infiltrates of inflammatory cells substantially regress, an increase in the amount of collagen fibers takes place. General fibrosis characterizes the end of inflammation. The articular cartilage also undergoes changes. Chondrocytes are hypertrophic or hyperplastic in some areas, while chondrocytes and the intercellular matrix disintegrate in others (Fig. 184). Pannus expands into the latter from synovial granulation tissue and penetrates to the subchondral bone. Here the articular cartilage is extensively replaced (Fig. 185). The subchondral bone becomes denuded in a few places. However, the articular cavity is only rarely obliterated by synovial proliferations.

In the pauciarticular type the arthritis evolves gradually with moderate symptoms and resembles arthritis of other etiology, such as tuberculosis, viral or mycotic infection, Lyme disease, or leukemia. Arthritis in the systemic type is diagnostically no less challenging; the local findings associated with high fever are very suggestive of acute arthritis in rheumatic fever or of septic arthritis. On the other hand, multiarticular affection with symmetric distribution makes the diagnosis rather easy, especially when the test result for rheumatoid factor is positive, which occurs maximally in 20% of these cases.

Treatment consists of complete bedrest and a diet rich in proteins, vegetables, and fruit [46, 47, 223]. Spending time in a region with dry and warm climate is beneficial. All infections and inflammatory foci in the body should be treated and eradicated. As long as the diagnosis is uncertain, and septic arthritis is a reasonable explanation, antibiotics (ampicillin 1.0–1.5 g or cephalosporin 1.5–2.0 g daily in divided doses) are

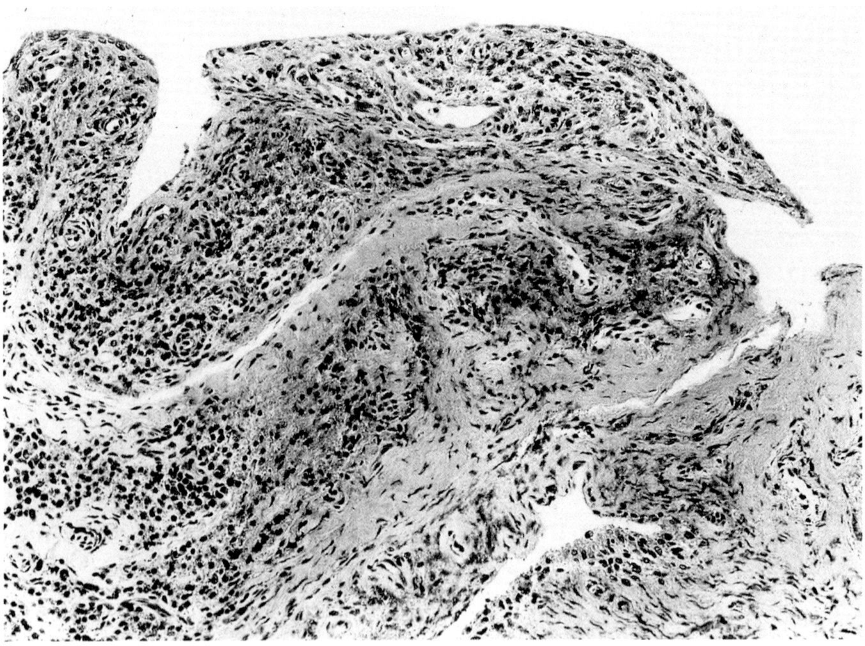

Fig. 183. The synovial membrane is raised in plump villi and is hypercellular with fibrocytes, fibroblasts, and histiocytes. Moderate diffuse infiltrates composed chiefly of lymphocytes and less so of plasmacytes are scattered in the subsynoviocytic tissue

advisable for the beginning phase of articular affection. However, once the diagnosis of rheumatoid nature has been established, salicylates [400, 985], preferably buffered, should be given without delay. In children with body weight up to 25 kg salicylates 100 mg/kg are given four times daily in divided doses, while in children with more than 25 kg body weight the therapeutic dose is 2.5–3.5 g daily in divided doses. Experimental studies [1542] indicate that salicylates enter the bloodstream 7–12 min after ingestion and admix with the joint fluid after an additional 8–15 min depending on the density and alterations of the inner part of the joint capsule. This brings analgesic, antiinflammatory, and antipyretic effects and is therefore of therapeutic benefit. This treatment should be continued in intervals for 2–3 years, in the awareness that prolonged intake of salicylates may be associated with adverse effects. These include gastrointestinal irritation, sometimes even gastrointestinal bleeding, which can be minimized by taking the salicylates together with milk, soft food, or antacids. Since the prothrombin level can drop on salicylate intake, regular determinations of the pro-

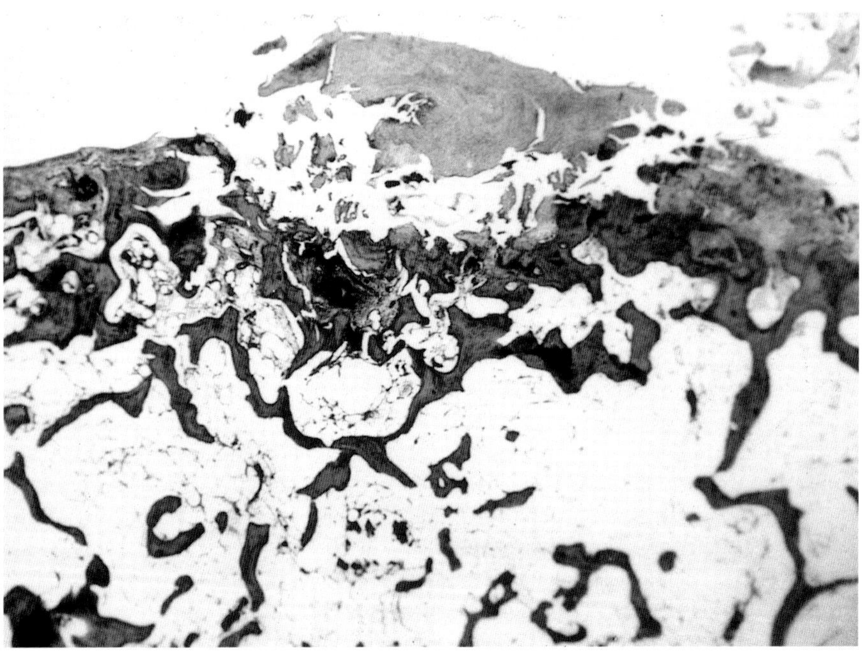

Fig. 184. The articular cartilage is disrupted in a few areas, and fragments are separated from it. The subchondral bone is thickened

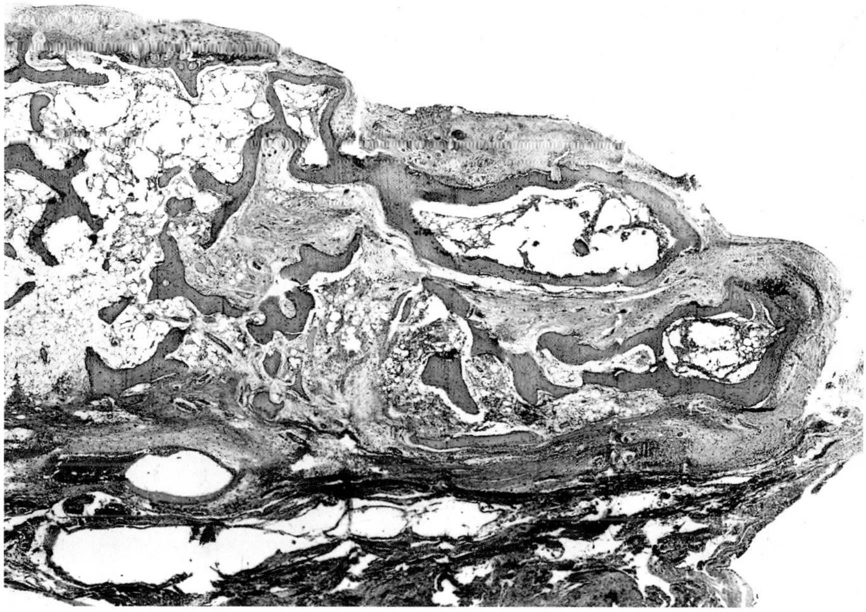

Fig. 185. The articular surface is uneven and is covered partly with articular cartilage and partly with fibrosed tissue. The subchondral bone is thinned. A broad osteophyte rises at the margin

thrombin level are indicated. Salicylate overdose may result in acidosis, hyperventilation, tinnitus, and nervousness; these adverse effects can be corrected promptly by temporary discontinuation of the salicylates.

If salicylate treatment does not provide substantial benefit in reducing the articular symptoms within 6 months, and the swelling of joints continues at concomitant decrease in mobility, gold salts should be administered intramuscularly. Their initial dose of 5 mg is followed once weekly, and if well tolerated twice weekly, by a gradually increasing dose to 0.75 mg/kg administered for 6 months. If the results of this regimen are satisfactory, as has been reported [185, 607, 971], the gold salts are continued at the last dose for 3 months at intervals of two weeks and for 3 more months at intervals of three weeks. However, if the gold salts do not result in improvement within 6 months, they should be discontinued. They should also be promptly discontinued if toxic symptoms such as dermatitis, depression of bone marrow, or nephritis develop. Regular blood studies with leukocyte count and urinalysis for protein level are required in this treatment. Antimalarial drugs have been used [1587] with improvement, albeit less than obtained by gold salts in the multiarticular type of juvenile rheumatoid arthritis. The potential complications of retinopathy and keratopathy drastically curtail the use of antimalarial drugs.

In cases of uncontrollable aggravation and progressive joint alterations, corticosteroids represent the ultimate resource. However, this medication does not provide permanent subsidence, only temporary remission of inflammation in the joints. Thus, corticosteroids should be used for only a limited period of time. Prednisone is given in the initial dose of 10–20 mg and subsequently in divided daily doses of 20–40 mg until no further improvement in swelling and mobility is obtained. Prednisone is then gradually tapered off and eventually discontinued, when salicylates should be resumed. Discontinuation of prednisone is indicated especially once symptoms of hypercorticism occur. On the other hand, prednisone is indispensable in cases of iridocyclitis, which develop principally in children suffering the pauciarticular type. The participation of an ophthalmologist is also indispensable in the management of eye complications. This treatment must be started without delay and requires prolonged topical and systemic administration of prednisone in higher doses. Eventually, surgical correction of the eye complications may be indicated.

In addition to medicamentous treatment of the arthritis, local management is required [47, 1402] initially in the form of moist warm packs applied two or three times a day around the joints. Support for these joints by splints of plaster or polymeric material and straps is highly advisable, even indispensable, for preventing deformity. If a deformity has already developed, traction, especially to the joints of the lower extremity, often succeeds in correcting it. This treatment should be followed by the use of rigid plastic or leather-metal splints to maintain the proper position. When the inflammation regresses to the chronic phase, as indicated by clinical signs (absence of locally elevated temperature, decrease in pain and swelling) and laboratory findings (decreased sedimentation rate, leukocyte count, and C-reactive protein), physical therapy with shortwave diathermy and massage in series of ten sessions repeated over a period of a few years is highly beneficial [944, 1613]. Mobilization of the joints by active and passive exercises is equally beneficial.

Nevertheless, despite the use of all prophylactic and conservative modalities, contractures may persist in the joints of the upper and lower extremities. Such contractures are observed mostly as adduction contracture of the shoulder joint and/or as flexion contracture of the elbow, wrist, hip, knee and/or ankle joint. Their treatment, indicated in any phase of childhood or adolescence, is discussed in "Contracture of Joints." Additionally, synovectomy may be indicated in cases of marked thickening of the joint capsule, which without alterations in the articular epiphyses limits movements of the joints [487, 661, 815, 1610]. Angular deviations develop mostly in the weight-bearing joints due to overgrowth or retarded growth in the femur and/or tibia (Figs. 181, 182). The treatment of these growth deformities at the hip, such as coxa vara or coxa valga, or at the knee, such as genu varum or genu valgum, should be postponed until growth is completed. The indicated osteotomies, discussed in "Osteoarthritis" may then be performed. For this period of time, the eventually necessary arthroplasties [1511] or arthrodeses [279, 1549], as discussed in "Rheumatoid Arthritis" and "Osteoarthritis" should be deferred.

In the meantime, some 8%–10% of the young patients do not recover from their generalized weakness and internal complications, and eventually succumb to these or to intercurrent infectious diseases. The other patients go through puberty and enjoy a more vigorous appearance, improvement in general condition, increase in body weight, and normalization in blood picture. Puberty also often brings local changes in the affections of joints, and attainment of satisfactory functions of the joints is probable in the majority of these patients (Fig. 179). Thus, the prognosis in regularly supervised and treated juvenile rheumatoid arthritis is fair [253, 722, 1402, 1590]. However, in about 20% of cases, the alterations in the joints have proceeded too far and continue with further aggravations into adulthood; here a clinical situation results identical to that in rheumatoid arthritis of adults. The conservative and operative treatments are then those described in "Rheumatoid Arthritis."

4. Rheumatoid Arthritis (Rheumatic Arthritis)

The designation rheumatoid arthritis, given by Garrod, is a misnomer, but continues to be used in the English-language literature. (The Greek suffix "oid" to rheuma means "rheuma-like.") If this is applied to the progressive and severely disabling joint disease, the question arises what other, more severe joint disease is the truly rheumatic arthritis. In fact, the so-called rheumatoid form of arthritis is the most disabling disease known among the chronic joint inflammations. In view of this, the term rheumatoid should actually be replaced by that of rheumatic, as used in continental European medical literature.

Primary chronic rheumatic arthritis [901] in its typical course is easily discernible by clinical signs, physical findings, laboratory studies, and progressive aggravation from the acute arthritis in rheumatic fever, which afflicts children more frequently than adults. This differentiation can be made primarily by the fact that the etiology of rheumatic fever is related in most cases to a previous streptococcal infection. However, between chronic juvenile rheumatic arthritis and chronic adult rheumatic arthritis exist borderline cases which, as in the entire rheumatic spectrum, represent transitions from one disease entity to the other. The etiology of neither juvenile nor adult rheumatic arthritis has yet been fully clarified [1245]. Nevertheless, the differentiation between these two entities is possible in the great majority of cases on clinical grounds.

Chronic rheumatic arthritis in adults was formerly regarded as a sequela of infection. This was suggested by Coburn et al. [305], who demonstrated hemolytic streptococci in the blood of patients with chronic rheumatic arthritis, and by Braun [180], Dawson et al. [378], and Kalbak [843], who noted in their patients an increased agglutination titer for hemolytic streptococci. However, in other patients [115, 726] neither anamnestically nor clinically and serologically did an indication exist of streptococcal infection, which militates against such infection as the prime cause of rheumatic arthritis. Also supporting this are the facts (a) that the treatment of streptococcal foci in the throats of patients with chronic rheumatic arthritis does not provide an improvement in the joint affection, and (b) that other individuals suffer of a hemolytic streptococcal infection in an organ for years, without ever incurring an inflammation of joints.

On the other hand, the findings of significantly increased immunoglobulins and immune complexes [45, 468, 522, 535, 1682] in the serum of such patients strongly suggest that an immunological reaction elicits the inflammatory response in the joints. Thus, antigens originating from other microorganisms have been implicated in the etiology of rheumatic arthritis [26]. Olhagen et al. [1204] identified clostridium abundantly in the feces of patients and regarded this as the etiological agent, whereas Stewart et al. [1583] found diphtheroid organisms in the synovial membrane and joint fluid, and Person [1245] isolated mycoplasma from the synovial membrane and joint fluid. In addition, research has discovered intrasynovial viruslike particles [1436] from which the formation of immune complexes in the blood presumably results. Other observations [29, 1493] indicate that viruses such as the Epstein-Barr virus are lymphotropic and are able to initiate the production of antibodies. The combination of these and resulting immune complexes is thought to elicit a reaction in the synovial tissue. Whereas infection with viruses is able to cause arthritis [25, 844, 1436, 1629], this type of arthritis, as noted by its regression, is completely different from the unrelenting course of rheumatic arthritis.

In view of the variety of microbiological agents implicated in the causation of rheumatic arthritis in some individuals while remaining harmless in other individuals, it appears that an individually inherent factor is responsible for the production of primary or secondary antibodies. These are identifiable by the presence of formed immune complexes. Thus Steffen [1573] regards rheumatic arthritis as a collagen autoimmune disease elicited by synovial collagenase and followed by formation of collagen-anticollagen immune complexes associated with inflammatory effects. The individual factor probably determines the excessive response and hyperergy in the host's synovial tissue [115, 1822] as well as the concurrent damage to other organs of the body. This view has been confirmed by the findings of HLA-DR4 factor in the serum of the majority of patients with rheumatic arthritis [855, 1076, 1182, 1407]. A strong indication is thereby given that genetic components account significantly for the occurrence of chronic rheumatic arthritis.

External factors also participate in the etiology of rheumatic arthritis. Common colds act either by enhancing susceptibility to inflammation, activating inflammatory foci, or harming vasomotor structures with impairment of the peripheral circulation and decrease in the defense mechanisms. Thus, chronic rheumatic arthritis occurs more frequently in individuals living in cold, humid quarters or regions, such as northern Europe the northern United States. Similarly, physical stresses, frequent fatigue, or emotional upheavals impair the defense mechanisms of the body and facilitate the development of chronic rheumatic arthritis. By these occasional circumstances, silent inflammatory foci or circulating antigens may become active and harm mesodermal organs, especially the joints. Another conclusive fact for the etiology lies in the observation that chronic rheumatic arthritis occurs at a distinctly greater frequency in women, especially those of preclimacteric age. This points to the participation of hormonal factors in the etiology. It is probable that ovary dysfunction influences the adrenal cortex and by dyscorticism causes a decreased defensive ability of the connective tissue system. This results in a susceptibility to antigenic substances. Furthermore, the articular symptoms in chronic rheumatic arthritis show regression in young women during or shortly after pregnancy.

The evidence of occasionally decreased defensive ability upon initiation of chronic rheumatic joint disease, raises the question regarding the explanation of the adaptation syndrome. This has been answered by Selye [1462, 1463]. Following exhaustion or dysfunction of the hypophysis and adrenal cortex, which control defense reactions, inadequacy of the defense mechanisms may occur with weakening of the alarm and resistance phases. Harm to these two endocrine glands by external factors or by dysfunction of other endocrine glands results in a dyscorticism, which with the coincidence of hyperergy permits the establishment of chronic rheumatic arthritis as an adaptation syndrome to harmful factors.

The occurrence of rheumatic articular inflammation can be explained on the basis of all the above factors, which include a preexisting constitutional allergy or a dispositional hypersensitivity of the connective tissue system to toxins or antigenic substances, and probably also a decreased defense ability. However, the characteristic course of this disease and its tendency to expansion and aggravation of the tissue inflammation have not yet been explained. Therefore, in contrast to the acute arthritis in rheumatic fever, which remits completely in the joints, one must also assume that the elicited hyperergic action of the connective tissue continues inexorably [703, 704]. Lansbury et al. [942] suggested that a disturbance in immunity also to substances of noninfectious nature exists in chronic rheumatic arthritis. Probably following some toxic affection, the connective tissue is influenced antigenically by adsorbed radicals of various nature and is maintained constantly in a state of hyperergy. Accordingly, Lansbury et al. [942] demonstrated in the blood of patients with chronic rheumatic arthritis precipitins which yield a positive antigen-antibody reaction with extracts of connective tissue from both healthy individuals and patients with rheumatic arthritis. It appears plausible that, following antigenic affection, the connective tissue is so altered that it is maintained in a state of hyperergy and reacts allergically with a perpetual or a repetitious process [726]. The events, evolving as immune responses to penetrating or internal antigenic substances, represent in the articular tissues the general manifestation of inflammation [726]. These reactions are readily discernible by clinical, morphological, and immunobiological examinations.

Chronic rheumatic arthritis affects women more than men, primarily those aged between 30 and 45 years and those in poor general condition. The joint disease starts

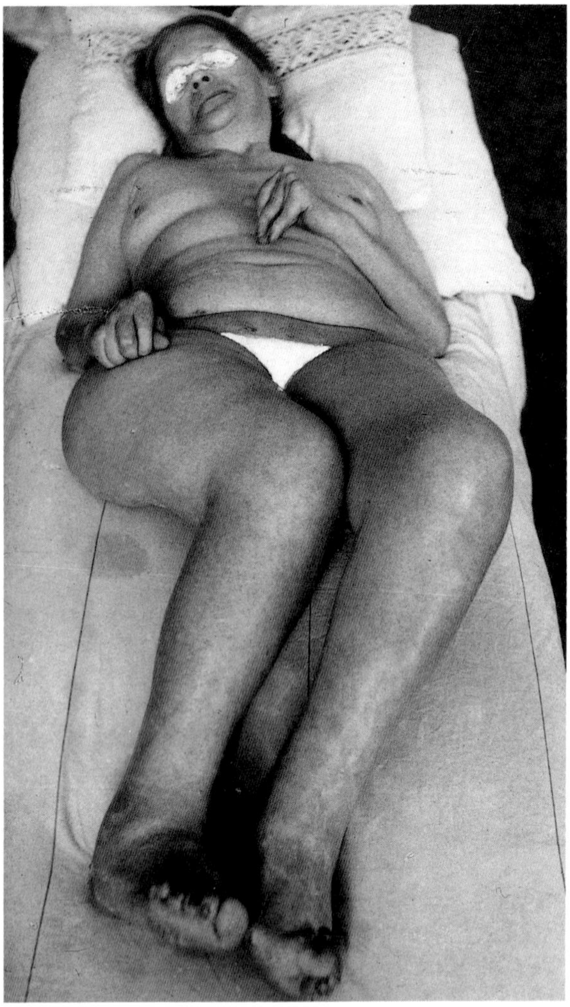

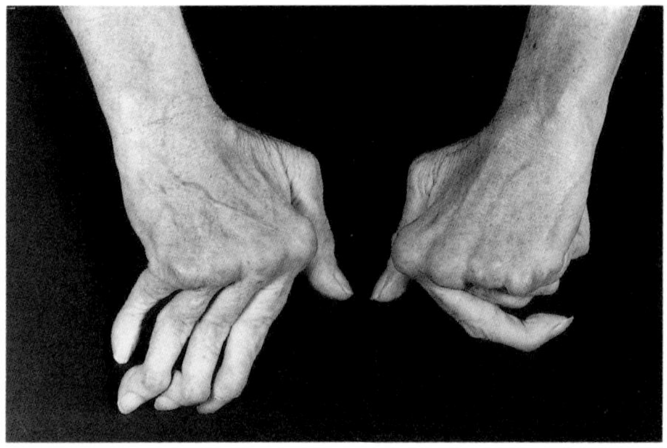

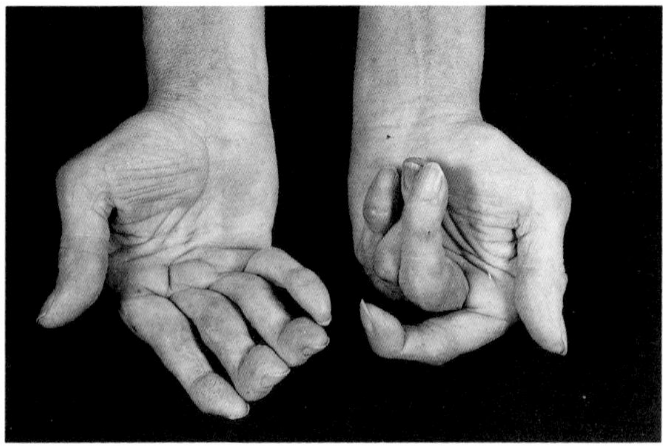

Fig. 187. Dorsal view **Fig. 188** volar view. Flexion deformities and ulnar deviation of the fingers and adduction contractures of the thumbs in rheumatoid arthritis

Fig. 186. A 60-year-old woman with rheumatoid arthritis since age of 28 has contractures in all minor and major joints of the extremities and also subluxations in some of these joints

insidiously. The temperature is elevated to 37.5°–38.2° C in the acute phase of joint swelling, and decreases after 2–3 weeks, assuming an irregular course; it may become elevated again on increase in swelling and development of effusion. Pallor of the skin, caused partly by anemia and partly by toxic influence, is often noticed, as well as yellow-brown patches on the face and extremities. The skin is always moist because of increased sweating. The peripheral circulation is impaired, and hands and feet are cold. The joint disease [984] usually begins symmetrically in the fingers and toes, thereafter affects the wrists and ankles, extends centripetally to the elbows and knees, and finally affects the shoulders and hips (Fig. 186). Variations from this course are often observed, with some joints affected more prominently, and others only slightly or moderately. Joints of the mandible and vertebral column are affected much less often. Slowly and gradually aggravated, sometimes intensified by a few episodes of exacerbation, this affection eventually leads to deformities and destruction, particularly of peripheral joints and sometimes the uppermost part of the cervical spine.

The following three stages may be discerned in the course of chronic rheumatic arthritis [1766].

a. The prodromal stage in the joints is associated with radiating, not clearly localized pain which may be interpreted as myalgia, neuralgia or bursitis.

b. The stage of manifest joint disease is associated with diffuse swelling of the joint capsule, occasional increase in joint fluid, tenderness of the entire joint, and distinct elevation in local temperature. The increased joint fluid is usually resorbed spontaneously, while the joint capsule becomes thicker and denser. The motion of affected joints is limited in the extreme degrees. Because of intensified pain on ambulation, the patient needs bedrest most of the time and avoids using the joints. Due to the general inactivity, the musculature of the extremities becomes atrophic unless the muscles and tendon sheaths themselves are also affected by rheumatic inflammation, in which case they swell. The beginning deformation of the joints is already noticeable. Nevertheless, the rheumatic process in the joints may heal in this stage, being followed by secondary osteoarthritis (Figs. 191, 219, 220).

c. The final stage is that of irreversible deformities. Due to shrinking of the joint capsule, contracture of the regional musculature, and deviation of the eroded articular epiphyses, the joints are ultimately deformed in a way which is chracteristic for each individual joint. The fingers are hyperextended at the distal interphalangeal joint due to overaction of the intrinsic muscles and are flexed at the proximal interphalangeal joint (buttoniere deformity) due to detachment of the long extensor tendon and palmar retraction of the lateral bands of the extensor hood by the eroding joint capsule. In another type of deformity due to imbalance of the intrinsic muscles, the fingers are flexed at the distal interphalangeal joints and hyperextended at the proximal interphalangeal joints (swan-neck deformity; Figs. 186, 187, 188). The metacarpophalangeal joints are very swollen, deviated ulnarward, and always flexed by shortening of the flexor muscles and tendons; they are sometimes flexed to such an extent that the fingers are clutched in the palm (Figs. 186, 188). On persistent flexion and ulnar deviation of the first phalanx of the four fingers, distension of the collateral ligaments and instability of the metacarpophalangeal joints ensue. The thumb is contracted in adduction at the metacarpophalangeal joint and is hyperextended at the interphalangeal joint. The wrist joint is pulled by the volar forearm muscles into volar flexion and radial deviation, which aggravated the ulnar deviation of the fingers by the concomitant ulnar shift of their extensor tendons (Figs. 186, 187). The deformation of the wrist joint is invariably associated with diffuse thickening of the joint capsule and often also with concurrent marked swelling of the inflamed flexor or extensor tendon sheaths (Fig. 536). On erosion of the intraarticular fibrocartilage, the cohesion between radius and ulna is substantially weakened, whereupon the radius subluxates volarward and the ulna subluxates dorsally. The elbow joint is stiffened in flexion contracture (Fig. 186) and deviated into valgus position due to pull of the flexor muscles of the elbow and fingers, and by erosion of the radial head. The shoulder joint is often contracted in adduction, and its external rotation is concurrently limited.

The toes are dorsally subluxated at the metatarsophalangeal joints (Fig. 186) and stiffened in flexion contracture at the first interphalangeal joint (hammertoes). Previously or concurrently, the metatarsal heads are deviated plantarward, from which results a plantar convexity of the metatarsal arch (Fig. 186). This deformity is very painful since the soft tissue padding has been diminished due to atrophy of the plantar musculature. The feet are deviated at the midtarsal and subtalar joints, into varoadductus position (Fig. 186) more often than into valgus. The ankle joint is usually stiffened in plantar flexion by shortening of the Achilles tendon, and the ankle is often deformed at its anterior aspect by proliferative swelling of the extensor tendon sheaths. The knee joint is contracted in pronounced flexion position (Fig. 186), which is often associated with valgus deviation and posterior subluxation of the tibia at tightness of the hamstring tendons (Fig. 190). The hip joint is contracted in flexion-adduction position (Fig. 186), often associated with internal rotation, due to tightness of its flexor and adductor muscles.

In rheumatic affection of the vertebral column, which occurs less often than that of the joints of the extremities, the upper cervical spine requires special attention because of the potential of very serious complications. Instability of the head and marked discomfort are experienced as well as radiating pain into the back of the head or along the neck. The neck is held stiff usually in upright attitude, and any movement is anxiously avoided. The cervical paravertebral musculature is very tense, and the affected area is very tender. Major problems arise here on expanding synovial erosion into the articular facets; the atlantooccipital junction becomes unstable and may subluxate. This may compress the emerging nerve roots and the basilar artery. However, as Villiaumey et al. [1693] emphasize, the more serious prognosis of the atlantooccipital erosion lies in the danger of complete dislocation of this joint, followed by compression of the medulla oblongata and death. Of similarly serious consequence may be the erosion between the odontoid process and the transverse ligament, which is often concomitant with erosion between the lateral apophyseal articulations (Fig. 194). Subluxation at the atlantoaxial joint and of the odontoid process may then follow, leading to compression of the spinothalamic tract, manifested in radiating pain or numbness. On compression of the pyramidal tract, muscular weakness or spasticity occurs. However, the most serious consequence of marked dislocation of the ondontoid process is, as Fielding [509] and Ranawat et al. [1304] have emphasized, compression of the medulla oblongata and death. Thus the extensive erosions in the uppermost two cervical vertebrae carry the ominous potential of intervertebral dislocation compounded by compression of the medulla oblongata and death. The affection of the middle or lower part of the cervical spine (Figs. 193, 194) is associated with steady discomfort, substantially impaired mobility, and occasionally pronounced neurological symptoms (Figs. 298, 299).

Rheumatic arthritis of the lower part of the vertebral column affects the lumbar area and the lumbosacral junction. This area is tender and limited in its movements in all directions. The attempt passively to increase the range of movements is countered by increased tenseness of the regional paravertebral musculature. However, the more impairing features are, according to Caroit [246], the frequently associated neurological symptoms caused by pressure on the lumbosacral plexus. The persistent radiating pain is very bothersome; it sometimes expands (Figs. 300, 301) into the anterior aspect of the thigh but more commonly into the gluteal area and along the posterior aspect of the thigh, corresponding to the course of the sciatic nerve. Changes also occur here in the reflexes of the lower extremity.

In all above listed deformities of the extremities, the malposition of the articular ends, determined by their incongruence and muscular contracture, partially accounts for the limitation of motion. Narrowing of the joint cavity by synovial pannus further accounts for the decreased range of motion. Therefore, in most of these deformities, especially those of the lower extremities, the patient is not able to move around and to carry out activities of daily life. The patient is often confined to bed, and the general condition gradually, although slowly deteriorates. This limitation in the mobility of the extremities is sometimes (in about 5%–8% of the seropositive patients) aggravated by concurrent affection of the cervical and/or lumbar spine. There, in adition to the concomitant limitation of motion, the rather frequent pressure on nerve roots represents a substantial impairment in the general condition. Especially in the upper cervical spine, the potential compression of the medulla oblongata casts a very serious aspect to this local affection.

Rheumatic arthritis is invariably associated with extraarticular manifestations [385, 793, 1485, 1666] by affection of other structures and organs. Subcutaneous nodules [377] are the most frequent alterations and are noticed as 0.5- to 2.0-cm-large, rather firm, indolent thickenings; they develop principally on the dorsal aspect of the elbow and forearm. Less frequent, though more extensive sites, chiefly in seropositive patients, are the occipital, cervical, and scapular areas and sometimes the anterior aspect of the lower leg or the ankle. The nodules may regress or rarely necrotize and then break through the skin, causing draining wounds. Other thickenings in the depth of the subcutaneous tissue are regional lymph nodes, which swell in areas proximal to inflamed joints; the enlarged lymph nodes are usually in the cubital and popliteal fossa and inguinal area. Of the internal organs, the lungs may be affected by interstitial fibrosis or a pleurisy with moderate effusions and subsequent adhesions. Similarly, the heart may develop [167, 829, 895, 1243] pericardial effusion with subsequent friction rales or interstitial myocarditis. Affection of the heart occurs much less often in rheumatic arthritis of adults than in juvenile rheumatic arthritis. Of more serious concern are the affections of the eye, such as iridocyclitis, leading to intraocular adhesions and progressive impairment in vision up to blindness, and episcleritis with formation of painful, longer lasting nodules. Other affected structures are the middle-sized and small blood vessels, which by thickening of their media and/or adventitia account for the diminished trophics and function of internal organs, especially of the nerves.

In accordance with the pale appearance of the patient, laboratory studies regularly show hypochromic normocytic anemia, with hemoglobin decreased to 8–10 mg%. On the other hand, the leukocytes count may be increased to 14000, but also may be decreased in very toxic conditions. The sedimentation rate is invariably elevated to 45–55 mm/h, even to 80–90 mm/h, and declines in quiet phases to 25–35 mm, but rises again promptly when the inflammatory changes in the joints become exacerbated or reactivated. Determination of the sedimentation rate does not help diagnostically to differentiate chronic rheumatic arthritis from other joint diseases; however, comparison of several rates obtained at longer intervals provides instructive clues as to the course, therapeutic response, and prognosis of the disease. Similarly, the test for C-reactive protein does not offer a differential diagnostic clue, but its quantitative determination at longer intervals permits an inference as to aggravation or regression of the joint disease. The test result for antinuclear antibodies is distinctly less frequently positive than in systemic lupus erythematosus and is thus of differential diagnostic value [1060]. Serological studies [271] also disclose that IgG and IgM are present at considerable concentrations [293, 770] and IgA and IgE at lower concentrations. Antibodies (rheumatoid factors) to certain determinants of IgG, IgM, and IgA [251, 264, 265, 496, 498, 909, 910, 911, 1060] appear in the serum; these can be ascertained at the considerable titer of 1:160 or beyond by the red cell agglutination and/or latex fixation test [1505]. Results of these tests are positive in 80%–85% of patients who present articular and extraarticular affections in a more aggravating course than in seronegative patients [15, 18, 454, 1371, 1372]. The outcome of the sheep cell agglutination test is positive in about 80% of the former patients [1699, 1812, 1813]. On the other hand, the positive outcome of the test for rheumatoid factor does not represent unequivocal confirmation of rheumatic arthritis; this is also positive, although at the significantly lesser incidence of 5%–8%, in other arthritides [80], especially in tuberculous arthritis, syphilitic arthritis, and other granulomatous arthritides. Equally, antibodies to degenerated collagen can be detected in the serum [45]. The sera of 73% of seropositive

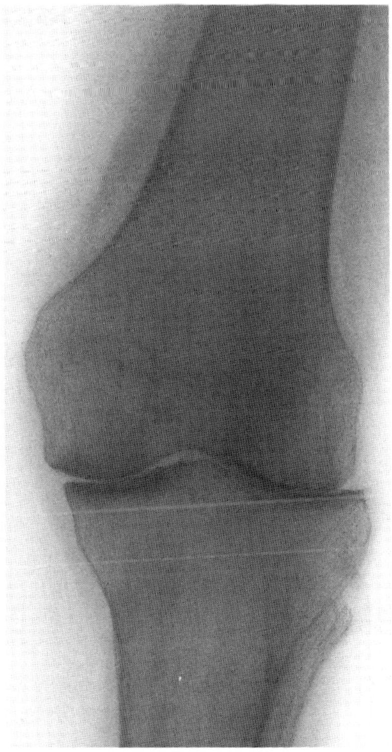

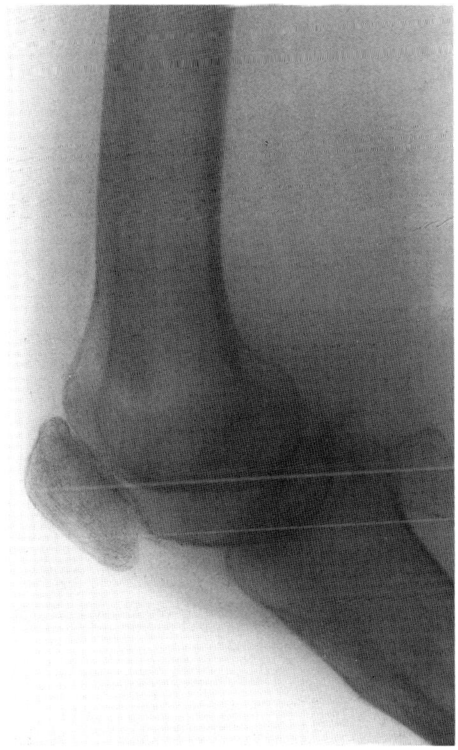

Fig. 189. The joint cleft is very narrowed especially at the lateral aspect, and the tibia is laterally deviated. The adjoining epiphyses and metaphyses of the femur and tibia are osteoporotic

Fig. 190. The knee joint is held in flexion contracture, and the tibia is dorsally subluxated. The articular surfaces of the patellofemoral joint are eroded, and the adjoining areas are osteoporotic

patients also manifest a positive precipitin reaction with streptococcal substances [91].

The increased joint fluid is yellowish and slightly turbid and contains numerous fibrin flakes as well as enzymes (protease, collagenase, elastase). The cell count yields 1000–4000/ml polymorphonuclear leukocytes [1819], in contrast to their paucity in the synovial membrane. The cell count may be as high as 10000/ml in very active inflammation but then shows a major percentage of lymphocytes. The stained smear (Fig. 27) and culture of the joint fluid disclose no microorganisms. Immunological studies reveal the pres-

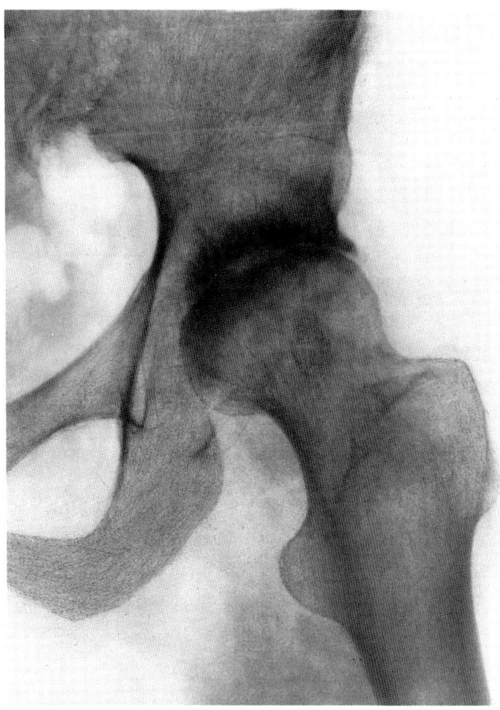

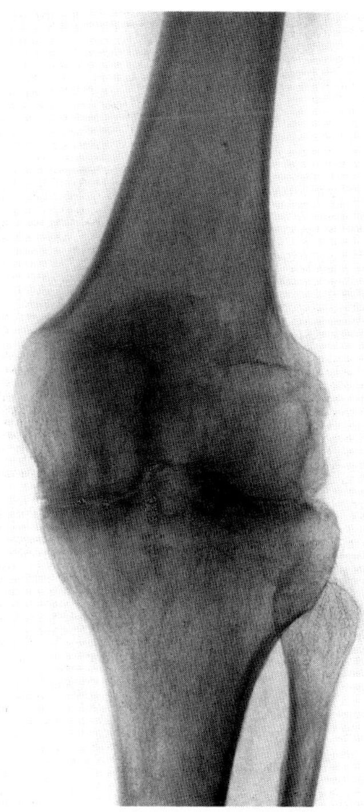

Fig. 191. The articular surfaces of the hip joint are extensively eroded and sclerosed; the joint cleft is uneven and narrowed. The adjoining bones are extensively osteoporotic

Fig. 192. The joint cleft of the knee is completely obliterated, and the articular epiphyses are fused. The trabeculae pass from one to the other epiphysis

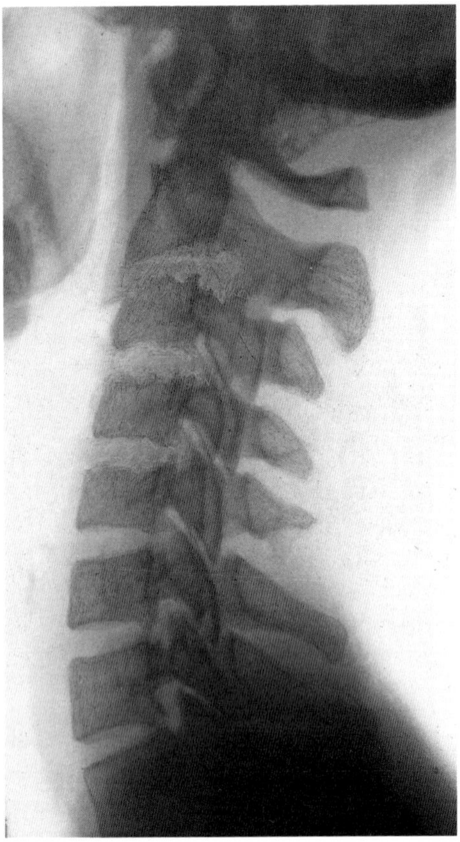

Fig. 193. The odontoid process is well maintained, and adequate alignment exists between C1 and C2. The endplates between C2 and C5 are eroded, and subluxation occurred between C2 and C3

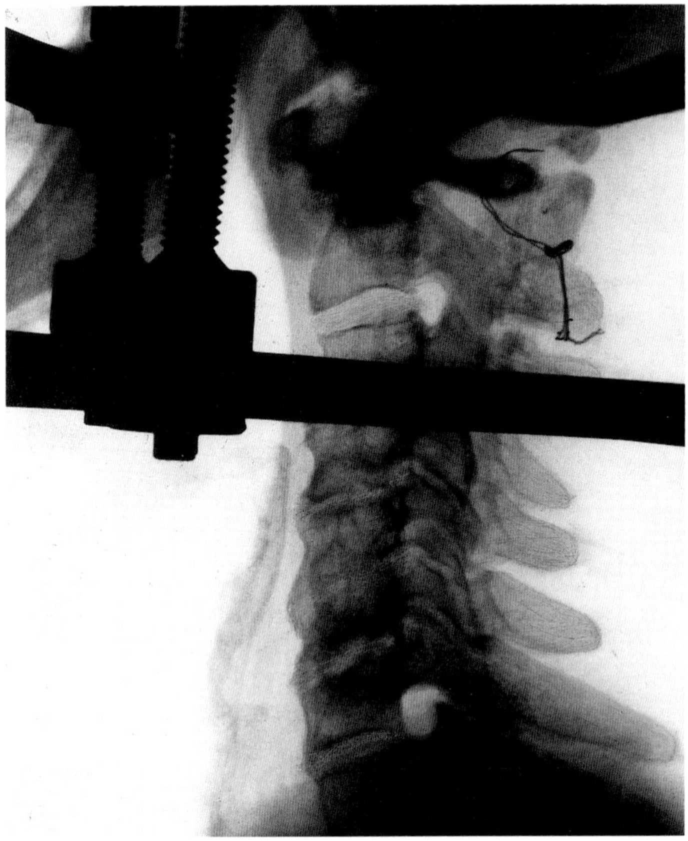

Fig. 194. The odontoid process is very eroded, and dislocation followed between C1 and C2, whose posterior arches have been wired. A loop of the wire is disrupted, and a stabilizing halo has been applied. The endplates between C5 and C7 are very uneven

ence of antibodies to IgG, IgM, and IgA, produced by synoviocytes and becoming associated with consumption of complement in the joint cavity [710, 911, 1371, 1650].

Roentgenographs reveal the stages of progression of the joint disease. Osteoporosis of the articular epiphyses characterizes the onset of the disease, being caused partly by inactivity and partly by inflammatory influence with consequently more distinct osseous catabolism. However, with increasing thickening of the joint capsule, the fine structure of the articular ends becomes blurred. Nevertheless, the irregularity in the intraarticular outlines of these ends is discernible; the articular margins of the epiphyses appear eroded (Figs. 207, 211, 219) and may display small indentations. The cartilage space becomes gradually narrower (Figs. 189, 190, 191, 220) until the opposite articular margins become possibly contiguous with each other. In other cases the articular epiphyses change their configurations by the deepening of defects at the articular border and by the outgrowths of osteophytes at the margins (Figs. 191, 223). Here the articular epiphyses partly lose contact and may deviate into angulation or subluxation (Figs. 189, 207). Unless ankylosis supervenes (Fig. 192), the uneven articular margins become sclerosed (Figs. 191, 219, 220) under the continued motion of the joint, and the marginal osteophytes become larger. The alterations of secondary osteoarthritis are present here. Roentgenographs of the cervical spine (Figs. 193, 194) reveal extensive erosions of the lateral masses of the atlas and of the atlantooccipital and/or atlantoaxial articulation, anterior subluxation of the atlas on the axis, and upward displacement of the ondontoid process into the foramen magnum [1304]. Fielding [509] and Ranawat et al. [1304] demonstrated that in the cases with additional erosion of the odontoid process the intervertebral spaces are also eroded and narrowed, and that the subluxation of the atlas is then substantially more pronounced. In contrast to these marked changes, the rheumatic arthritis of the middle and lower cervical spine is limited to irregular outlining of the vertebral endplates, osteoporosis of the vertebral bodies, and moderate to marked narrowing of the vertebral interspaces (Fig. 194).

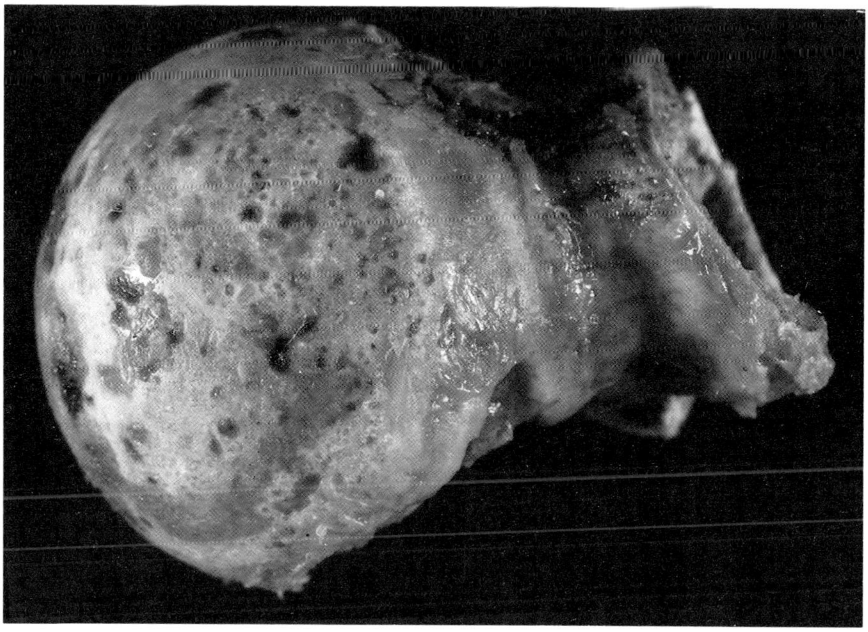

Fig. 195. The articular surface of the femoral head is uneven by numerous small and deeper erosions. A part of the articular surface is worn off; articular cartilage is maintained in a small area

On gross-anatomical examination [568, 570] in the early phase, the inner part of the joint capsule is reddened, swollen, and edematous. Its thickening becomes gradually more pronounced by concomitant outgrowth of villi. The joint fluid is moderately increased in amount, and here numerous small, roundish, white formations (rice bodies; Fig. 150) are occasionally scattered in the joint cavity. Their elastic compressibility and smooth surface indicate that they probably originated from precipitated fibrin and have been shaped in this way by joint movements [282]. The villi gradually increase in length, whereupon they protrude into the articular cavity and substantially narrow its extent. Concurrently, the articular cartilage loses its shiny and smooth surface in places; whitish gray streaks appear in it. Expansions of the swollen inner joint capsule encroach upon the articular cartilage and erode it on increasingly larger areas (Figs. 195, 196). From these defects the synovial granulations penetrate into the depth of the subchondral bone (Figs. 196, 197). When opposite areas of articular cartilage are similarly invaded by granulation tissue, the contiguous articular surfaces may become fused with each other by intervening connective tissue; fibrous ankylosis results ((Fig. 197). By concurrent metaplastic ossification, osseous ankylosis may result (Fig. 192). However, in most situations no ankylosis develops, but the joint capsule shrinks. By additional shrinking of the periarticular tissue and contraction of the regional musculature, the articular ends are pulled into faulty alignment; a contracture of the joint with subluxation of the articular ends results (Fig. 479).

Histopathological [322, 494, 495, 570, 587, 588, 589, 630, 891, 1531, 1543] and histochemical examinations [577, 586, 590, 770, 1822] disclose the events evolving in the articular tissues. In the initial phase of inflammation the small and medium size blood vessels of the synovial membrane are dilated and hyperemic. A few polymorphonuclear leukocytes and numerous lymphocytes are interspersed. The leukocytes migrate into the joint cavity. The lymphocytes, initially accumulated around the blood vessels, multiply and spread throughout the subsynoviocytic tissue [1674]. By the action of histiocytes (megakariocytes [494, 495, 1527] in the subsynoviocytic tissue antigens are presented to the lymphocytes, which produce immunoglobulins and swell to plasmacytes [570, 784, 910, 1527, 1811, 1812]. Thus in the progressive phase of inflammation (Fig. 198) the subsynoviocytic tissue comprises large accumulations of plasmacytes which also contain antibodies to the produced immunoglobulins. Concomitantly, the synoviocytes enlarge (Fig. 198) and produce more hyaluronate and lactate and also produce enzymes such as protease and collagenase [589, 590, 1093, 1371]; they subsequently increase in number [890]. Fibrocytes and fibroblasts also increase in the subsynoviocytic tissue. The fibroblasts contain thin cytoplasm and a very pale nucleus with one or two nuclei and a few chromatin particles (Fig. 199). Due to the paucity of cytoplasm and chromatin and to their unusually large size, these fibroblasts appear as "phantom cells" [1543], a feature not observed in any synovitis of other etiology. Giant cells with 2–20 nuclei occasionally occur beneath the synoviocytes and among the

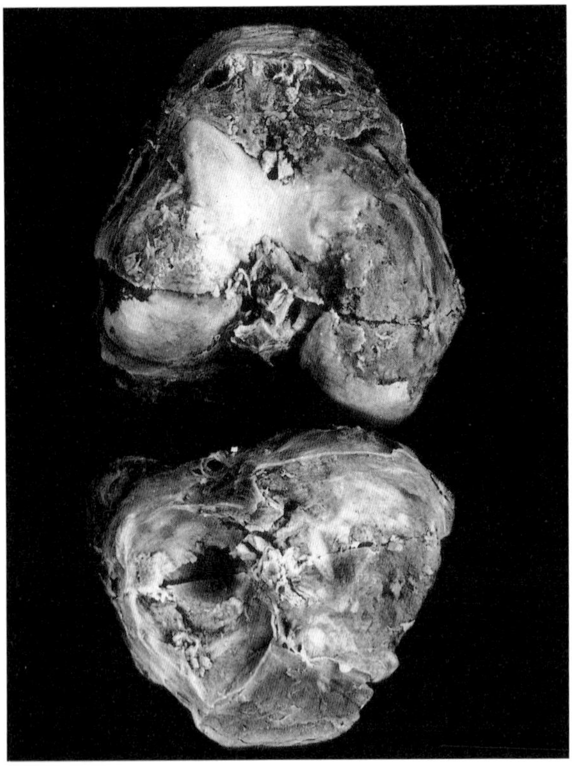

Fig. 196. The articular surfaces of the femoral condyles and tibial condyles are extensively eroded; deep grooves penetrate into the tibial condyles. A part only of the femoral condyles has remained with articular cartilage

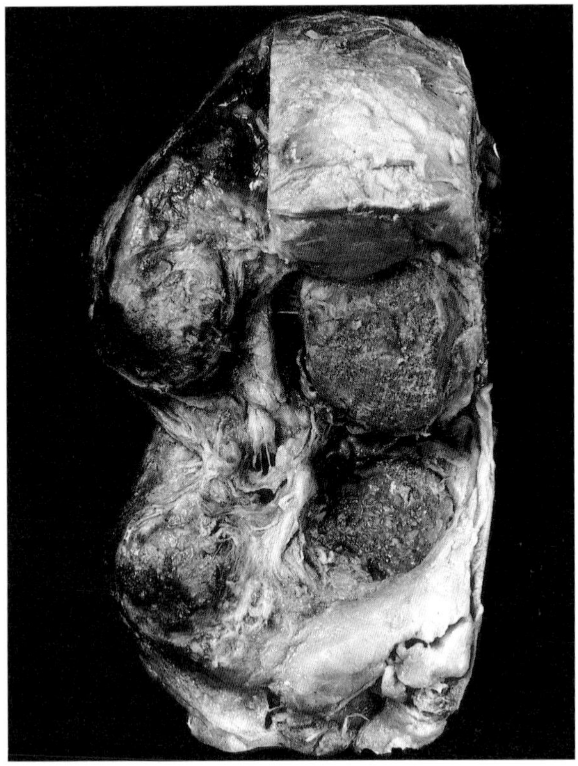

Fig. 197. The articular surfaces of the femoral condyles and tibial condyles are completely eroded. Scarified connective tissue extensively fills the intercondylar space, and the patella is fused with the femur. A fibrous ankylosis has partly occurred

fibrocytes and fibroblasts. By the reaction of the synoviocytes, fibrocytes, and fibroblasts as well as in the transformation of lymphocytes to plasmacytes, the pathogenetic role of the immunoglobulins is manifested. Excessive proliferation and perpetuation of inflammatory changes characterize the chronic process in the joints [726].

By the multiplication of the synoviocytes and by the increase in subjacent infiltrates, numerous elevations, villi, are formed (Fig. 200). Larger masses of fibrin are often deposited on the synovial membrane, and their organization forms additional villi. The villi protrude into the articular cavity, come close to the articular cartilage, and intrude into it with tonguelike processes [822, 1093, 1478, 1479] (Figs. 201, 202). In the articular cartilage (Fig. 202) some chondrocytes are ballooned and pale, and other chondrocytes are shrunken, leaving around them large lacunae. Other chondrocytes are disintegrated at concomitant fragmentation of their nuclei; empty lacunae are the result [1478, 1740, 1744, 1814]. Concurrently, synovial granulation tissue encroaches from the margin of the articular cartilage, and other synovial granulation tissue undermines the articular cartilage. By these tonguelike processes and by the intruding villi, all of them containing protease, the synovial tissue splits the proteoglycans of the articular cartilage and dissolves them further by carbohydrase and sulfatase [730, 1736, 1740, 1814]. Concurrently, the fibers of the cartilaginous matrix are dissolved by the collagenase and elastase of the synoviocytes [76, 913, 1783]. In this harmful effect [426] the polymorphonuclear leukocytes also participate by their enzymes [1128, 1207, 1813, 1814]. Eventually the articular cartilage is replaced from a few sides by the intruding synovial granulation tissue, which subsequently becomes fibrosed and sometimes resembles fibrocartilage. The expanding substitution of the cartilage cover is compounded from the depth by granulation tissue, which originates from inflammatory reaction in the marrow spaces and advances from the subchondral marrow toward the surface by eroding the subchondral bone [1796]. This granulation issue merges in a few places with the pannus on the surface. Nevertheless, the dense fibrous cover becomes progressively worn off on continued functional use of the joint (Fig. 203). Thereupon the subchondral bone is

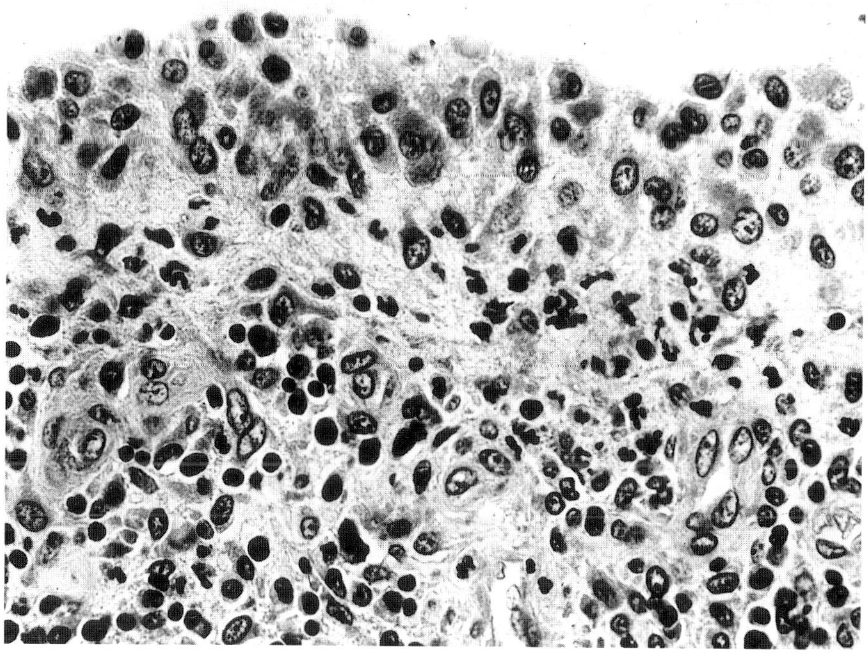

Fig. 198. The synoviocytes are markedly hypertrophic hyperplastic, and the subsynoviocytic tissue is very cellular with plasmacytes, lymphocytes, histiocytes and with a smaller number of large fibroblasts

denuded to a large extent, and it is also worn off. Streaks of cancellous bone are exposed on the articulating ephiphyseal surface (Fig. 204).

In the depth of the synovial membrane granulomata are sometimes noticed. They contain a core of necrotic tissue surrounded by a serrated border of histiocytes and fibrocytes arranged in a palisadelike manner. While such granulomata are rather characteristic for rheumatic arthritis, their rare incidence (2%–4% of cases) in the synovial membrane lends them a limited diagnostic significance [494, 630, 984, 1544]. In contrast, the subcutaneous nodules invariably contain granulomata (Fig. 205) composed of a core of necrotic tissue, bordered in a serrated line by histiocytes and fibrocytes arranged in a palisadelike way (Fig. 205) and surrounded by loosely agglomerated lymphocytes. Rice bodies are occasionally present in the joint cavity, and these consist of homogeneous material arranged in a plump network or in a honeycomb (Fig. 156). Their staining with celestine blue or orange picric solution

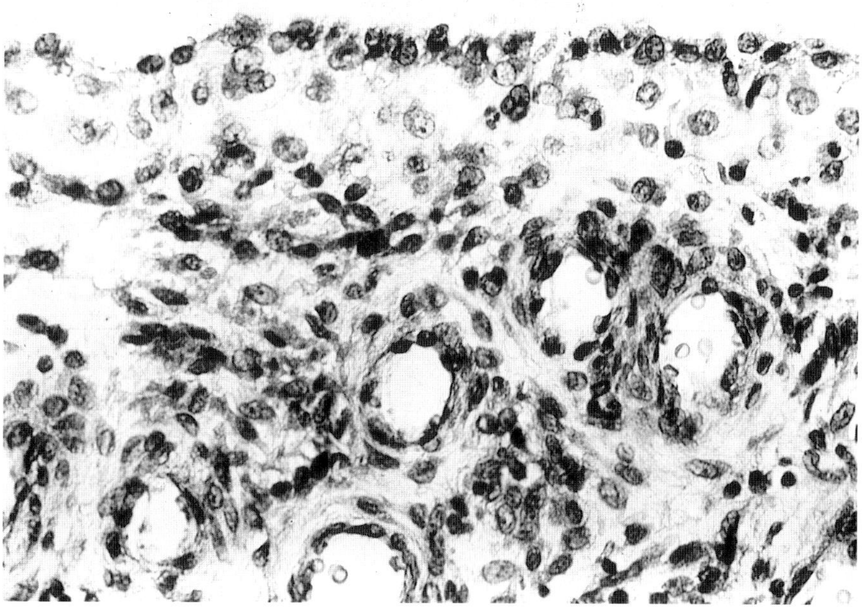

Fig. 199. The subsynoviocytic tissue in extensively permeated by large fibroblasts, of which many contain large pale nuclei

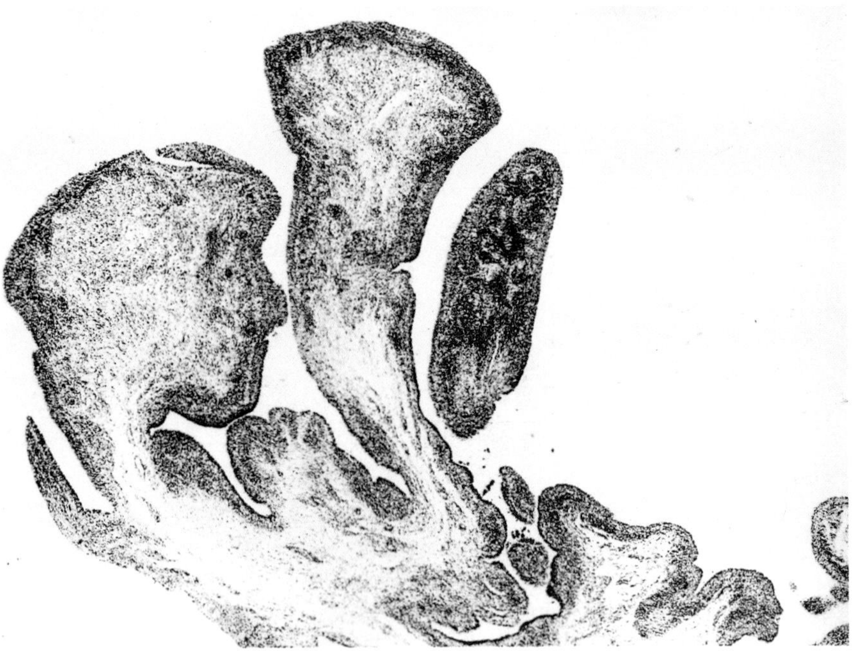

Fig. 200. The synovial membrane is raised in many villi of various length and thickness. Their synoviocytes are moderately hypertrophic-hyperplastic, and their subsynoviocytic tissue is moderately hypercellular with lymphocytes, fibrocytes, and fibroblasts. Few villi only are hypercellular by extensive infiltrates

[122] indicates that they are composed of fibrin and fibronectin. They sometimes contain a nucleus of collagenous material or necrotic tissue, with fragmented nuclei originating from disintegrated synovial tissue.

Immunofluorescence studies [586] disclose the presence of IgG, IgM and IgA in the synoviocytes and subsynoviocytic plasmacytes, which also contain antibody-immunoglobulin complexes.

Electron-microscopic examinations [603, 605, 796, 1195] disclose that the synoviocytes (Fig. 206) extend several broad filopodia, enclosing formed particles, to all sides. The intracellular rough endoplasmic reticulum is very enlarged and comprises dilated cisternae which contain electrondense proteinaceous material. Similarly, the lysosomes are increased in number and size 1736, 1740] and are filled with either dense homogeneous material or fine granules representing acid enzymes. On the other hand, the Golgi complex is rather atrophic in some cells which comprise a few membranous stacks and vacuoles. Numerous micro-

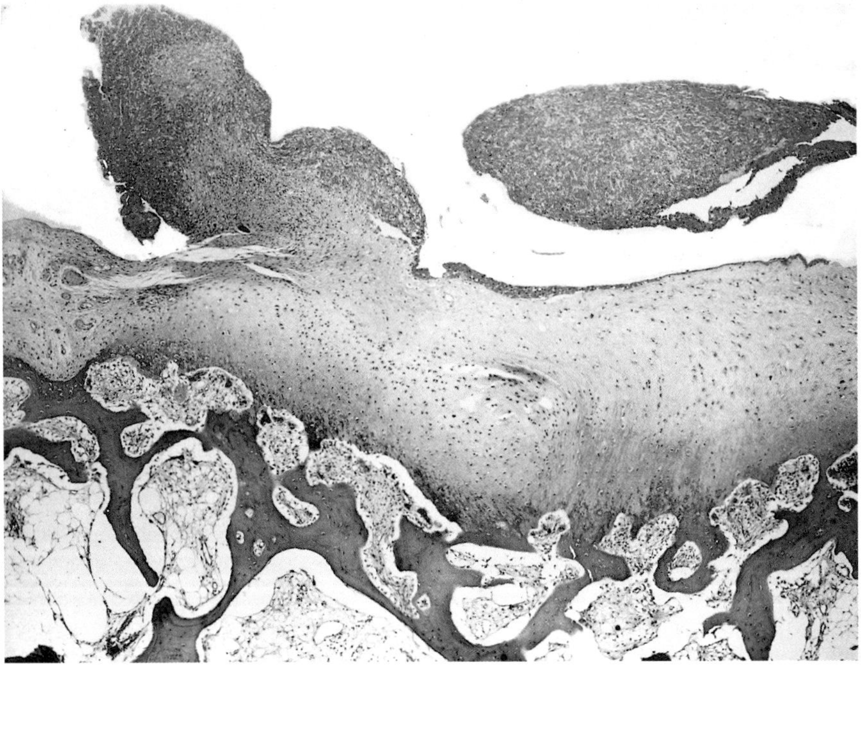

Fig. 201. Some villi are close to the articular cartilage, expand along its surface, and intrude it

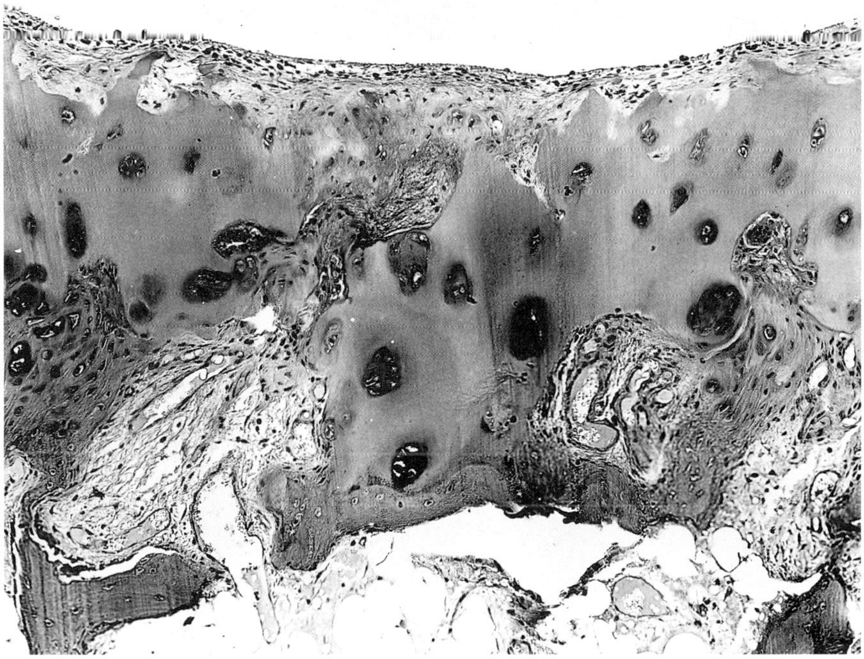

Fig. 202. Granulation tissue expands along the surface of the articular cartilage and intrudes it with tonguelike processes. Very vascular granulations penetrate the subchondral bone from the marrow spaces and expand into the articular cartilages. In the latter, some chondrocytes are necrotic, and others are hypertrophic or hyperplastic and are surrounded by broad halos of increased ground substance

pinocytotic vesicles are scattered, as are swollen mitochondria. Ferritin particles, probably the residues of hemorrhages, have also been observed [1157]. Further electronmicroscopic examinations [72, 495, 905, 1195] disclose marked hypertrophy and hyperplasia of the synoviocytes. Among them those of the A type participate more distinctly, containing a great number of lysosomes and vacuoles. Those of the B type contain an enlarged and dense ergastoplasm; those of the intermediate C type contain only a few lysosomes with numerous filopodial protrusions. Histochemical analyses [1736, 1740] show that a substantial amount of enzymes (cathepsin, acid phosphatase) is produced by the lysosomes.

The clinical picture of the fully developed chronic rheumatic arthritis [725] is so characteristic (Fig. 186) in most situations that the diagnosis cannot be missed. However, in the initial phase the possibility of infec-

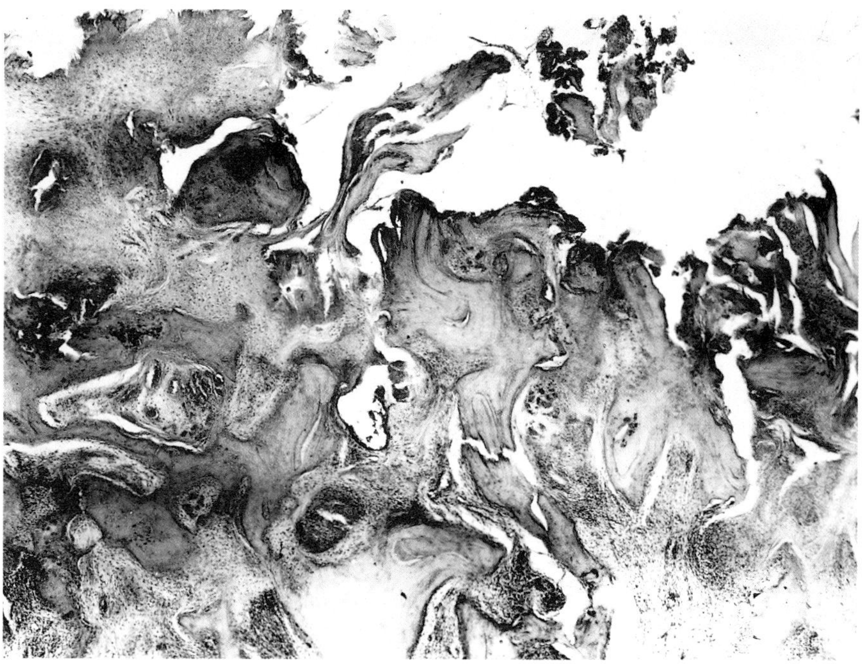

Fig. 203. The articular surface has remained with worn-off cartilage in a small area. In the other part of the surface denuded trabeculae are fragmented and disrupted. Connective tissue extensively expands from the marrow spaces into the subchondral bone

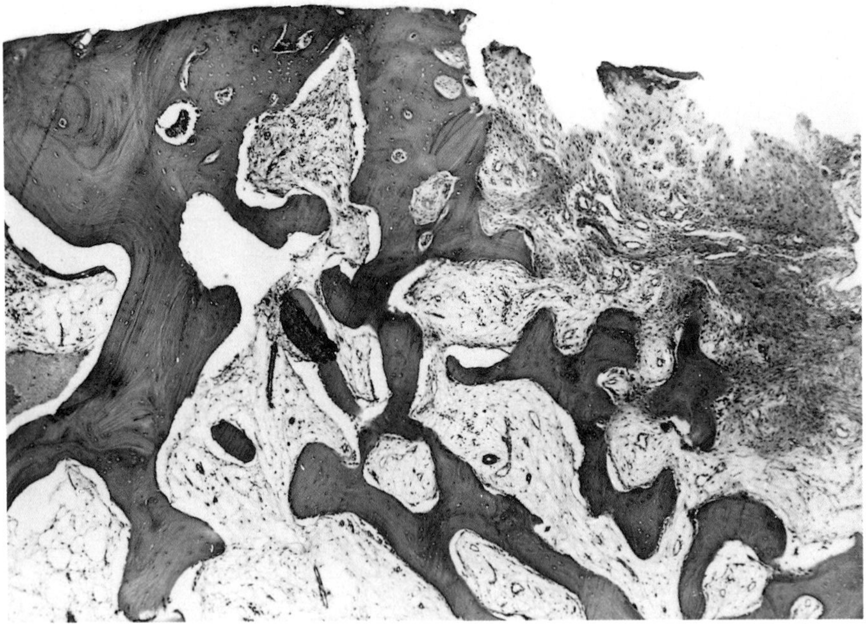

Fig. 204. A part of the articular surface is invaded by vascular granulation tissue (pannus). The other part of the articular surface is denuded and sclerosed

tious arthritis, tuberculous arthritis, syphilitic arthritis, mycotic arthritis, or arthritis in rheumatic fever or in gout must be taken into the diferential diagnosis. Laboratory studies as well as the slow but relentless progression to deformities clarify the diagnosis. The features adopted by the American Rheumatism Association [1116] have been accepted as criteria to aid in establishing the diagnosis of chronic rheumatic arthritis.

Treatment of rheumatic arthritis [979, 1370] requires much patience and endurance from the patients as well as from those responsible for their care. A thorough explanation of the nature and course of the joint disease to all involved persons is indispensable. The therapeutic benefit depends substantially on the understanding cooperation of the patient – here more than in most other types of arthritis. At the beginning, continuous bedrest is necessary until regression of the acute inflammatory signs, when out-of-bed activities may gradually be resumed according to tolerance. Concurrently, nutrition should be rich in proteins, vegetables,

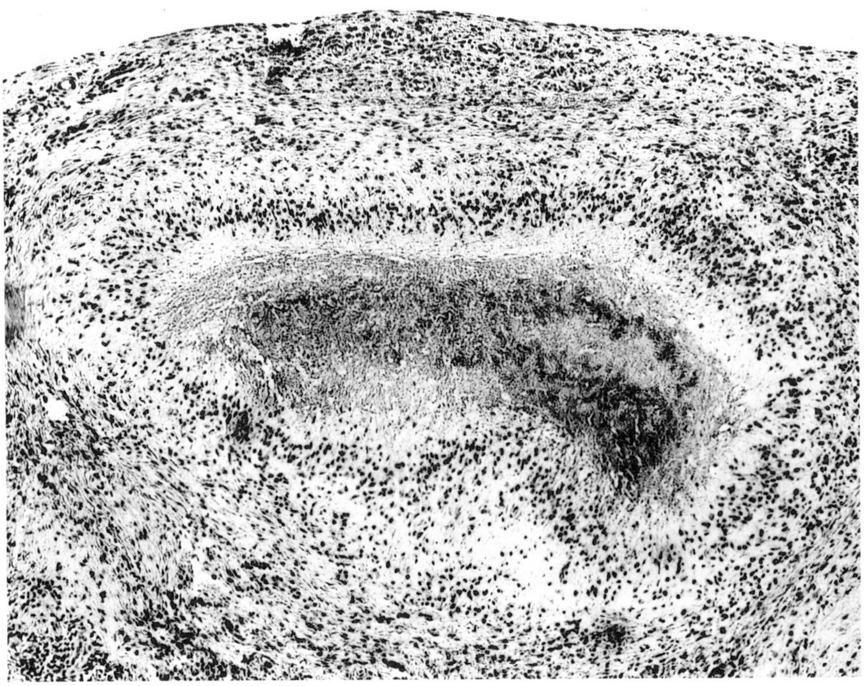

Fig. 205. The center, consisting of necrotic cellular material and disintegrating nuclei, is surrounded by palisadelike, densely positioned fibrocytes. The adjacent tissue is hypercellular with fibrocytes and, less so, with lymphocytes and histiocytes

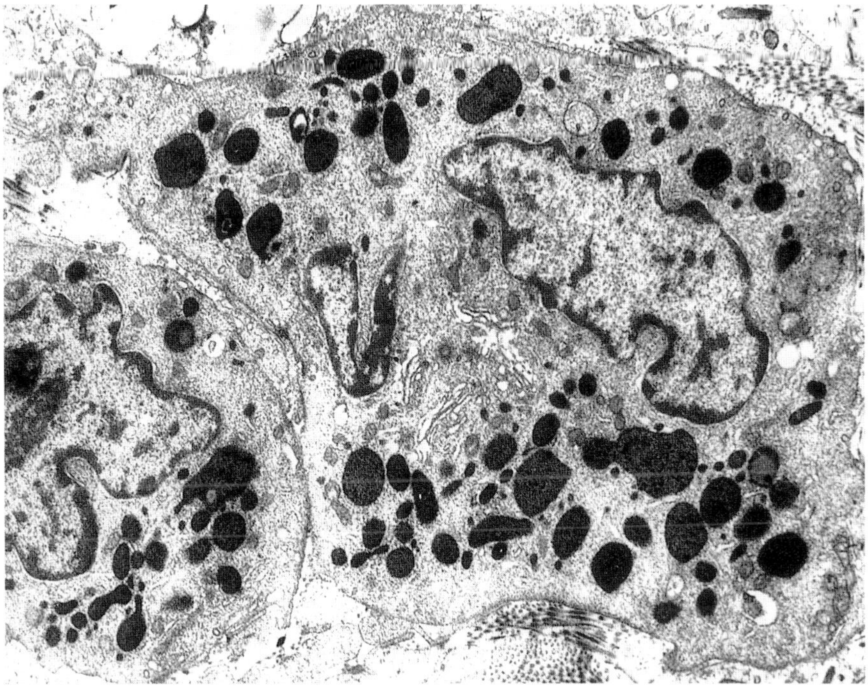

Fig. 206. Electron microscopy of the synoviocyte type a (Fig. 9) discloses that it contains numerous primary and secondary lysosomes. Some of these are homogeneous, and others are loosened by small vesicles. The Golgi complex is prominent

fruit, and vitamins, but no diet special in composition essentially influences the course of rheumatic arthritis. An indispensable adjunct is the local application of moist warm compresses in the early phase of rheumatic arthritis. Their technical use is discussed in "Osteoarthritis." These applications improve the local circulation [1212], aid in the absorption of the swelling, and relieve the pain in the joint as well as the spasm of the regional musculature. Otherwise, the reflexive teneness of the regional musculature pulls the articular ends into deviation and initiates a deformity. Highly useful devices are splints made of plaster cast or plastic material, which are individually molded in middle or functional position and prevent an individual joint from angular deviation. They hold the elbow in midposition, the wrist in 10°–15° extension, the fingers in midposition, the knee in full extension, and the ankle in midposition. While securing the proper alignment, the splints should be temporarily taken off twice daily to permit mobilization exercises of the joint and massage of the regional musculature. Hereby the performance of active and passive movements is facilitated, and it helps to separate adhesions and to correct or prevent contractures.

The concept of attaining mobility after a not excessively long immobilization does not apply in rheumatic affection of the cervical spine. The prevailing sensation of instability of the head here, associated with marked discomfort and with or without neurological symptoms requires initially prolonged immobilization. This is obtained by complete bedrest and cervical traction. Upon regression of the symptoms ambulation may be resumed, with the provision of continued reliable immobilization of the neck by a plaster cast resting on both shoulders, snugly molded around the neck and supporting the chin and occiput. Another modality for reliable immobilization, while ambulatory, is a halo of metal and plastic material which rests on the shoulders and firmly carries the chin and the occiput (Fig. 194) als long as no pronounced subluxation in the upper cervical spine exists. This suffices in the majority of patients [509, 1519], but it must be used for a longer period of time, as determined by roentgenographic followup examinations. These modalities are well indicated in view of the conclusions by Fielding [509] that the cervical spine in rheumatic arthritis rarely needs fusion, and that its fusing tendency is insufficient. Ranawat et al. [1304] reported insufficient results, however, in half of their patients who underwent posterior fusion for subluxation of the upper cervical spine. The arthritic lumbar spine almost never needs operative treatment and responds satisfactorily to prolonged bedrest and pelvic traction, followed by immobilization with a firm lumbosacral belt reinforced with metal stays (Fig. 51). In the situations of lasting nerve root symptoms, shortwave diathermy, ultrasound, and/or longitudinal galvanization provide the desired benefit.

In view of the frequent deformities of the feet, manifested principally in valgus deviation of the heels, marked flattening of the longitudinal arches and metatarsal arches, and hammer toes, the patient should be fitted with proper shoes. These shoes should have [1631] firm counters, high waists and uppers, and soft high toe boxes; the heels should have Thomas extensions. Soft, broad metatarsal pads of foam rubber should be inserted in the shoes, or metatarsal bars of leather should be attached to the soles. Of the routine modalities of physical therapy [608, 944, 1613] shortwave diathermy applied at longer intervals in two to four series of eight to ten sessions provides local benefits for the ailing individual joints by temporary hyperemia, regression of the soreness, and increase of mobility, especially when combined with massage of the regional musculature. Atrophy of the musculature is minimized, and its motor power is increased. A similar purpose is served in very chronic cases by spas, where medicamentous and physical treatment are carried out in a systematic and regular way. A curative factor not to be underestimated in these situations is the change of environment and the improved psychological outlook which contribute to the healing tendencies of the body. Additional modalities used in some spas and curative institutions are hot mud packs, which are highly effective in chronic cases by providing – albeit after intervals of 2–4 months – long-lasting or even enduring regression of the pain and substantial increase in mobility [170, 1301]. The overall effect of the locally applied hot mud packs on inflammatory articular changes is also evidenced by the subsequent decrease in sedimentation rate and in C-reactive protein [338]. The penetration of the joints with galvanic current or the transcutaneous electric treatment is of temporary benefit in relieving local pain. The application of ultrasound [687] at an intensity of 2.5–3.0 W/cm^2 relieves pain by a direct effect on the sensory nerve endings [1541] and also improves the local blood and lymph circulation, which leads to regression of swelling in the joint capsule.

Concurrently with the external local modalities, treatment [426] should begin with salicylates which are the basic medication and are given in doses of 0.5–1.0 g every 4–6 h. In more severe cases, especially those of protracted course, the daily dose may have to be increased to 8.0–10.0 g, until gastrointestinal irritation, dizziness, or ringing in the ears appears. In view of the frequent irritation of the gastrointestinal tract arising on intake even of smaller doses, salicylates should be swallowed with milk or soft food; of greater benefit are buffered or enteric-coated salicylates. Salicylates are detectable 6–8 min after ingestion in the blood and 8–15 min later in the joint fluid [1542]; they reach maximum concentration in the joint fluid 115–150 min later. Variations in the time interval for diffusion of salicylates into the joint fluid depend on the coincident structural changes in the synovial membrane. Repeated intake of salicylates during the day ensures the persistence of maximum concentration levels in the blood. The therapeutic effect of salicylates on inflamed joints is not as dramatic as in rheumatic fever, but also here they have antipyretic and analgesic effects which expedite resumption in the use of the joints [3]. In cases of more severe pain, 0.5–1.0 g acetaminophen [847] or codeine 0.3 g is indicated. Salicylates have an antiinflammatory effect [148] on the joints by controlling swelling, presumably due to the suppression of prostaglandins, the mediators of inflammation [473, 1131, 1334, 1737, 1738]. In this way salicylates render their effects within 3–4 weeks of regular intake, and they should be continued for months or years if necessary.

However, if salicylates or their modifications are not tolerated from the start of their administration or have no effect or no more effect on progression of the articular process, nonsteroidal antiinflammatory medications with presumably stronger antiinflammatory effect should be administered [3, 183, 205, 256, 379, 531, 658, 795, 846, 848, 849, 900, 1737]. Depending on their chemical composition, these belong to the following groups (each available in commercial brands and in specific doses): pyrazole with its derivates oxyphenbutazone and phenylbutazone 200 mg daily, oxicam with its derivate pyroxicam 20 mg daily, phenylalkanoic acid – propionic acid with their derivates fenoprofen 400–600 mg daily, ibuprofen 800 mg daily, naproxen 500–1000 mg daily, fenamic acid with its derivates meclofenamate 100–200 mg daily and mefenamic acid 100–200 mg, and diclofenac sodium 100–200 mg. Further details regarding these medications are discussed in "Osteoarthritis." Comparison of their effects with those of salicylates indicate that the former sometimes provide faster regression of the capsular swelling, and thus earlier attainment of the mobility of the joints. Nevertheless, their adverse effects resemble those of salicylates but are often more severe. These consist primarily of gastrointestinal irritation with nausea, frequent diarrhea, occasional constipation, or gastrointestinal bleeding. Other untoward effects characteristic for only some of the nonsteroidal antiinflammatory medications are: nephritis with proteinuria and hematuria, hepatic damage, anemia, granulocytopenia, thrombocytopenia, and visual and acoustic disorders. Therefore, clinical examinations and blood and urine analyses are indicated at frequent intervals during their use [183, 459, 531, 649, 846, 848].

If the signs of inflammation in the joints and paraarticular structures, such as tendon sheaths and bursae, are not influenced by any of the nonsteroidal antiinflammatory medications, the administration of gold salts is advisable. Following an initial intramuscular dose of 3–5 mg, gold salts in a dose range of 20–50 mg depending on body weight are administered intramuscularly once weekly until a total dose of 1.0–1.2 g has been attained. Thereafter they are continued in 50 mg doses once a week for 4–6 months and subsequently in 50 mg doses once every 3 weeks for 4–6 months. The benefits of this medication, administered in the active phase of joint inflammation, may be seen in a gradual decrease in the soreness and swelling of affected joints as well as the paraarticular structures. Concomitant improvement in function is obtained in about 60%–70% of patients [324, 325, 549, 1325]. These effects can be explained by blocking the reaction of the connective tissue, especially the macrophages in which deposits of gold salts can be identified. However, about 30% of patients experience adverse reactions to the gold salts, such as exfoliative dermatitis with severe itch, granulocytopenia, pancytopenia, anemia, nephritis, and/or hepatitis with icterus, leading to death in 1% of those treated. Therefore, patients with preexisting skin conditions or nephritis present distinct contraindications to the administration of gold salts. Regular blood and urine examinations are indispensable in all patients receiving injections of gold salts [1007]. Immediate discontinuation of their administration is indicated at the slightest signs of complications. In these, corticosteroids (prednisone 40–60 mg) may be given daily in divided doses until subsidence of the complications. In cases of grave complications, blood transfusions and administration of British antilewisite (BAL), which combines with the gold to a complex salt and is eliminated, are urgently indicated. In view of the potentially pronounced adverse effects following intramuscular administration of gold compounds, such compounds for oral administration (auranofin 3, 6, or 9 mg daily) have recently come in use. While their potential complications are thus lessened, so are their therapeutic effects. This shortcoming appears due to the probability that orally administered gold salts do not enter the bloodstream in concentrations as high as those administered parenterally. Consequently, the macrophages are less extensively and less intensively influenced.

Next in the line of antirheumatic medications are antimalarial agents (chloroquine and hydrochloroquine 200–300 mg daily in divided doses), used for their inhibition on the release of the enzymes which are so harmful in joint inflammation. However, a percentage, although small, of these patients [1822] develop blurred vision by opacities in the cornea and abnormal pigmentation in the retina, vertigo, acoustic disorders with tinnitus and deafness, and neuromuscular disorders with ataxia, and absence of deep reflexes. This experience essentially limits the use of these medications [130, 742]. On the other hand, immunoregulatory drugs (azathioprine 50–100 mg daily for 1 week, mercaptopurine 100–200 mg daily for 2 weeks, cyclophosphamide 40–150 mg daily for 1 week, methotrexate 2–3 mg daily for 1 week) have been used for their suppressive effect on the immunodefensive mechanisms. These mechanisms appear overactive in rheumatic arthritis and are regarded as responsible for the manifestation of excessive proliferative changes [59, 324, 353, 713, 1053, 1669, 1757]. Besides the gastrointestinal symptoms with nausea, vomiting, diarrhea, and enterocolitis, other frequent adverse effects of immunoregulatory drugs include blood disorders with anemia, leukopenia and thrombocytopenia, hypersensitivity reactions with urticaria, pleural effusion, and pericarditis, also toxic harm to the liver and kidneys, and infertility in both sexes sometimes [384, 1369]. The question arises here of whether the general suppression of immunodefense mechanisms and antibody formation may not occasionally prove a great shortcoming, when intercurrent inflammation of other etiology supervenes. Another disease-modifying agent, penicillamine, given at 200–500 mg daily, is effective in cases of both seronegative and seropositive rheumatic arthritis not responding to conventional therapy [819]. However, it also has numerous and serious adverse effects, such as skin rash, oral ulcers, gastrointestinal irritation with nausea and diarrhea, pneumonitis and hemoptysis, renal damage with proteinuria and hematuria, and severe suppression of the bone marrow with anemia, leukopenia, and thrombocytopenia [208, 563, 1575, 1734].

Since corticosteroids have been recommended in cases of pronounced untoward effects arising from the intramuscular administration of gold salts, they may also be used in cases of severe general impairment and systemic symptoms following the administation of the above medications. In these, they succeed by relieving the frequent critical symptoms. Moreover, when the treatments with antiinflammatory medications and gold salts are no longer able to provide further benefit, or serious adverse effects have developed, prednisone 20–40 mg daily is given in divided doses until a distinct change toward improvement is attained.

Corticosteroid medications obtain a dramatic effect by decreasing or eliminating the pain in all affected joints, reducing their swelling and stiffness, and substantially increasing their mobility. This brings the feeling of well-being. The beneficial effect of corticosteroids observed [667, 997, 1027, 1578] in larger series of patients may be explained, according to Hench et al. [741] and Selye [1463], by restoring a balance between the secreted mineralocorticoids and glucocorticoids. In the joint capsule, systemically administered corticosteroid medications diminish the proliferation of fibroblasts and fibrocytes as well as the formation of villi and granulation tissue [1553]. This effect of corticosteroids in chronic rheumatic arthritis can be explained by the suppression of mesodermal proliferation. It also corroborates the concept that most articular changes in rheumatic arthritis are due to a hyperergic reaction of the connective tissue. Other beneficial effects of corticosteroids include decrease in elevated temperature and normalization of the sedimentation rate by restoration of the globulin-albumin ratio in the plasma. However, hypopotassemia, retention of sodium with tendency for edema, and hyperglycemia are noted in the plasma as adverse effects. General adverse effects include pigmentations, acne, hirsutism of the skin, moonlike face, hypertension, and diabetes. Therefore, the administration of corticosteroids should gradually be tapered off once an optimum therapeutic effect on the joints is obtained. While corticosteroid treatment must not be regarded as the only or permanent modality of treatment, it definitely represents a possibility for influencing, although temporarily, the pathological process of the connective tissue by hormones. These change the course of the rheumatic process [773]. On the other hand, the intraarticular administration of hydrocortisone, as described by Hollander [773] and others, is not advisable. Although the symptoms are relieved for a period of time, but the alterations of the joint rapidly become aggravated to substantial deterioration [16, 121, 1018, 1149, 1577]. Mohr [1125] demonstrated that intraarticular injections with corticosteroids are followed by local necrosis and formation of granulations.

Detrimental effects were not observed after synoviorthese in which osmium tetroxyde, alkylating agents, or radioactive isotopes [394, 685, 1007, 1216, 1644] were injected intraarticularly. These temporarily and partially suppress the proliferative synovial changes, but do not completely or permanently eliminate the changes.

If, despite all medications and protective splintings, the joints tend to deviate into faulty alignment, additional application of Buck's traction is of benefit for the elbow, hip, and knee joint to obtain lengthening of the contracted muscles and shrunken joint capsule. Once the contracture has been corrected by these conservative methods, the proper alignment is secured by immobilizing the joint with a plaster cast or a rigid brace for a period of 4–6 weeks. Temporary immobilization of the joint is then continued, mainly over night, in corrected position either with a bivalved plaster cast or a molded splint of polymeric material. Active and passive mobilization exercises of the joint are practised during the day.

However, if the joint capsule and periarticular structures are thickened and shrunken to the degree that conservative treatment is of no further benefit, the surgical treatment [1644] with one or another of its procedures is indicated. These are:

a. Synovectomy [689, 691, 1030, 1285, 1302, 1303] consists of the widest possible excision of the thickened inner part of the joint capsule. Tissue portions interfering with movements are removed, and expansion of the villous granulations over the articular cartilage is prevented. Synovectomy is thus indicated and of benefit chiefly in the stage in which roentgenographic examination discloses maintenance of the articular cartilage space and integrity in the outline of the articular epiphyses. Excision of bulky tissue portions and uneven marginal portions of the osteocartilaginous surfaces [1003] permits reattainment of or at least increase in the range of motion. Arthroscopic synovectomy suffices only in cases of limited synovial thickenings. If more extensive thickening of the inner part of the joint capsule develops, arthrotomy for extensive synovectomy is indicated. The inner part of the joint capsule is capable of restructuring, and displays about 6 months later a reorganized synovial membrane (Fig. 218). Unless the rheumatic process is no longer active and has come to a definite standstill, the synovial membrane may again develop changes of chronic rheumatic arthritis [808, 1125, 1302], although at distinctly lesser intensity.

b. If in longer lasting arthritis the regional muscles become reflexly contracted and eventually shortened on one side of any joint, this joint assumes a deviation deformity principally in flexion position, typical for each joint. Therefore, the tendons of the contracted muscles must be Z-wise lengthened, whereby release from the malposition, is obtained. No additional transposition or transference of other tendons is necessary, but combination of the initial tenotomy with synovectomy may be indicated to remove the intraarticular impediment. Details of this deformity and its treatment are discussed in "Contracture of Joints."

c. Formerly, arthroplastic resection of the articular ends was practiced, when these epiphyses became so deformed following invasion by pannus or possibly secondary osteoarthritic changes that no congruence with each other remained. In the resection the articular ends are shaped smoothly, and apposed to each other with concurrent interposition of a flap of fascia lata and adipose tissue. Except for the elbow joint, this procedure has been replaced by more extensive and more effective operations such as arthroplastic insertions.

d. In conspicuous angular deviation at metaphyses, osteotomy [159, 335, 412, 805] close to the joint, is indicated to obtain proper alignment of the articular ends (Figs. 279, 280, 283, 284). While this restores right axial statics, a possibly coexistent incongruity is not corrected.

e. In partial destruction of an articular end, insertion of a metallic substitute is used for partial arthroplasty in the knee joint [299, 1070, 1071] (Fig. 266). However, a complete resurfacing substitute is used in the hip joint [40, 239, 1656, 1657, 1702] (Fig. 267).

f. Total arthroplasty [227, 278, 320, 683, 1275, 1651] is carried out when the articulating surfaces are so eroded that no smooth contact remains between them (Figs. 208, 212, 221, 223). Their mechanical deployment is hampered and is associated with constant pain. Hence, the contiguous articular ends are resected, and replaced by endoprosthetic inserts of metal or metal combined with polymer which are glued tightly by a cement of methylmethacrylate within the marrow cavity. In the last few years arthroplastic inserts with sintered porous surfaces have been used to permit ingrowth of osseous trabecula; this eliminates the need for methacrylate cement. Longer follow-up examinations are necessary in the latter modality to evaluate the final results [198]. A postoperative complication not rare (1%–4%) [920] in arthroplasty is infection, which, if not eradicated, requires removal of all arthroplastic inserts. Loosening of the arthroplastic inserts may ensue as late complication, especially if the cancellous bone is porotic and does not always provide firm support for the arthroplastic inserts; exchange for broader stem endoprostheses may be indicated. Details of total arthroplasty are discussed under the major peripheral joints as well as in "Osteoarthritis" and "Ankylosis of Joints."

g. In advanced deformation of the articular ends associated with malalignment of the joint and persistent pain on motion, when none of the above surgical procedures is applicable or after having been applied, was followed by a failure in function or in healing fusion of the joint, (Fig. 217) represents the ultimate solution [279, 402, 555, 1069, 1421, 1549]. Thus, arthrodesis is indicated when total arthroplasty was followed by infection, and all arthroplastic inserts had to be removed and could not be reinserted at a later date. Arthrodesis is also advisable when the skin and soft tissues surrounding a severely impaired joint are so atrophic and scarified that infection following a plastic operation appears an unavoidable complication. At the arthrodesis, the articular ends are exposed by arthrotomy and are resected to the extent that their defective cartilage surface is fully removed (Fig. 213), and that an angular deviation is corrected. The denuded articular ends are then apposed to each other in functional position and immobilized with a well-molded plaster cast until roentgenographs show fusion to have been attained; this requires a period of 3–4 months. With such immobilization, internal or external compression by metallic devices is unnecessary. These devices often do not provide adequate fixation due to postoperative osteoporosis and/or catabolism. Sufficient compression is obtained in the joints of the lower extremities immobilized by a plaster cast on weight bearing during normal upright standing. On the other hand, when the plaster cast is not accepted, immobilization by internal or transcutaneous metallic fixation devices is carried out. Local infection may follow here. On achieving fusion, stabilization of the joint is attained, and pain is eliminated. However, the resulting lack of motion cannot be compensated at advanced involvement of the neighboring joints; arthrodesis is therefore not advisable in such cases. In view of these shortcomings, arthrodesis has been applied as a practical modality only for some peripheral joints such as the interphalangeal, wrist, or ankle joints (Figs. 209, 210, 217).

In full evaluation of an established deformity of any joint, the following components should be considered: degree of malalignment of the articular ends, limitation of motion of the joint, pain arising on its use, gross-pathological alterations, and extent of tissue changes. Accordingly a surgical procedure is used individually in each involved joint, keeping in mind its participation in the movements of the body as well as the sex and occupational requirement of the patient.

In the fingers with flexion contracture (buttonhole deformity) of the proximal interphalangeal joint and hyperextension deformity of the distal interphalangeal joint, the disrupted long extensor tendon is surgically reattached to the first phalanx together with the lateral bands of the extensor hood. This directs the extensor forces to the first phalanx and relieves the hyperextension in the distal interphalangeal joint. At a swan-neck deformity with hyperextension in the proximal interphalangeal joint and flexion contracture at the distal interphalangeal joint (Figs. 187, 188), the connecting transversal bands of the extensor hood are divided so that its lateral slips are separated from its central slip. The latter then exerts an extension effect only on the first phalanx, and hyperextension in the metacarpophalangeal joint is corrected; the freed lateral slips now act only on the distal interphalangeal joint in the direction of extension. In longstanding rheumatic arthritis, synovial granulations erode into the tendinous insertions of the hand and finger muscles. The resulting imbalance in the regional muscles causes ulnar deviation of the fingers (Figs. 187, 188) and contracture of the metacarpophalangeal joint into flexion or hyperextension. For correction of pronounced ulnar deviation, the third and fourth dorsal interossei muscles should be detached at their insertions and transferred onto the dorsoradial aspect of the metacarpals. The tendon of the abductor digiti quinti should be similarly treated, whereupon a rebalancing of muscular forces is obtained.

Independently of malalignment or contracture, the proximal interphalangeal joint may be very enlarged

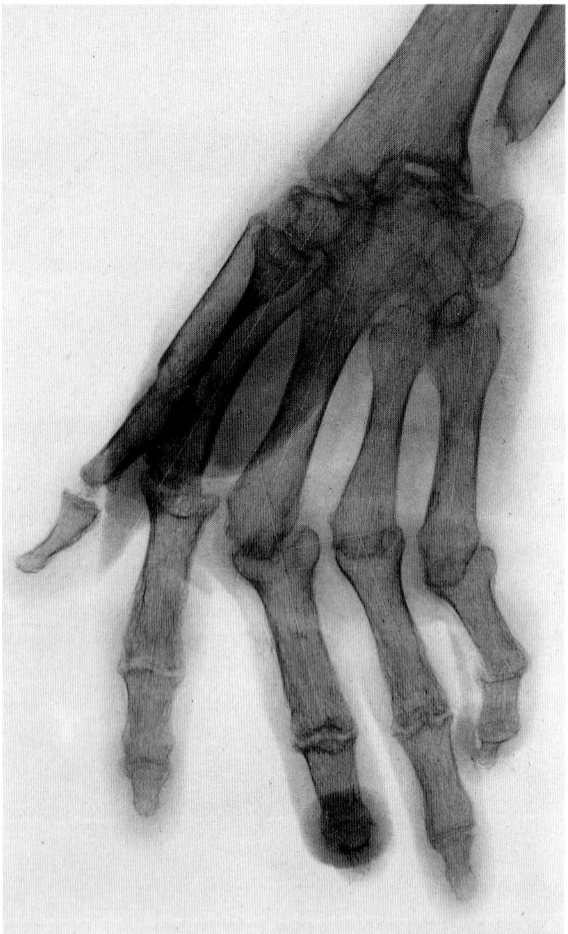

Fig. 207. The epiphyses of the metacarpophalangeal joints are very uneven and are subluxated ulnarward. The articular ends of the radiocarpal joint are deeply eroded and very uneven

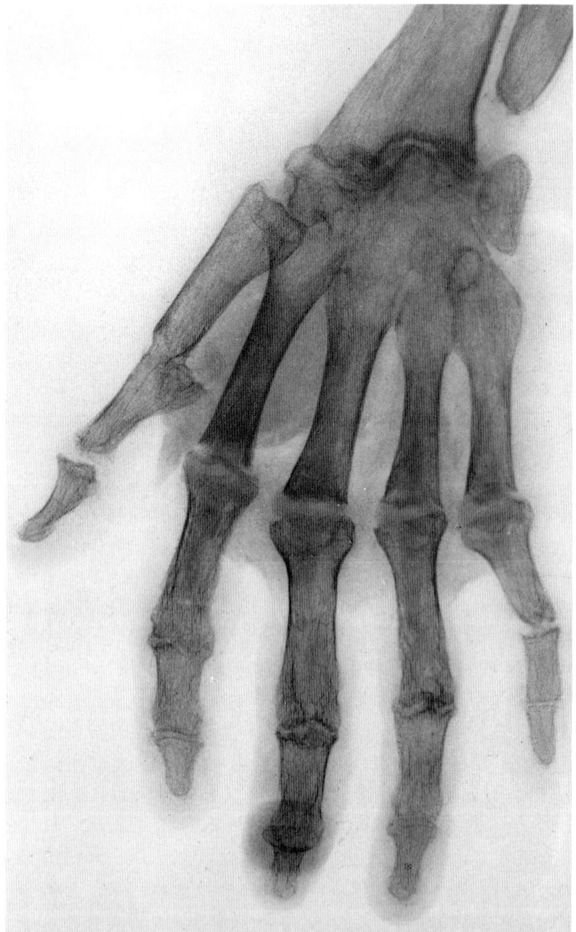

Fig. 208. The metacarpophalangeal joints have been resected and have been replaced by arthroplastic implants. Normal alignment of these joints has been attained

due to capsular thickening; synovectomy here normalizes the configuration and corrects disruption of the inflammatory process at least for a period of time. On the other hand, when this joint is limited in its motion due to alterations in the articular ends, these ends may be excised and substituted by endoprosthetic inserts of silicone rubber, silastic [1109, 1611]. Silastic implants may also be inserted in the metacarpophalangeal joints [519, 1109, 1611] after flat resection of the articular ends (Figs. 207, 208,). Reconstruction of the ligaments and joint capsule is also necessary here to provide stability of the joint [1109]. However, loosening or breaking of the silastic implants presents a serious shortcoming of this treatment. Another procedure for restoring the mobility of interphalangeal joints is the wedgelike resection and smoothening of the articular epiphyses, followed by reinforcement of the joint capsule. Improvement in articular function is entrusted here to the modeling forces. The arthroplastic procedures can also be used with the distal interphalangeal joints; however, stability is here of greater necessity. Resection of the articular surfaces followed by transfixation with wires ist therefore the preferred procedure here for attaining osseous fusion in moderate flexion position. Arthroplastic resection also appears indicated for the metacarpophalangeal joints which are contracted in marked flexion or ulnar deviation. Wedge-shaped resection of the metacarpal heads permits full extension and flexion, and should be followed by regular mobilization exercises. The almost invariably concurring ulnar deviation in the metacarpophalangeal joints requires reefing of the extensor hood of the fingers on the radial side. Other procedures, such as transference of intrinsic muscles at this deformity, are less sucessful because of the supervening adhesions which limit the ability of the transplants to function properly.

The tumb [1030], differently from the other fingers, is contracted in marked adduction at the carpometacarpal joint, in flexion at the metacarpophalangeal joint, and hyperextended at the interphalangeal joint. Therefore, the

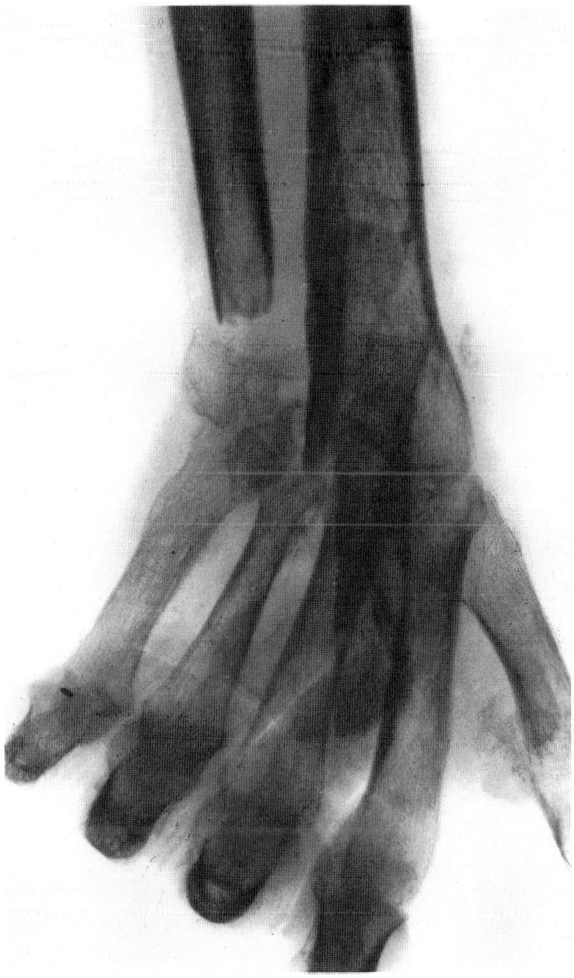

Fig. 209. The distal end of the ulna has been elsewhere resected. An arrow-shaped (Figs. 215, 216) bone graft has been inserted into the resected distal end of the radius and into the proximal parts of the second and third metacarpals

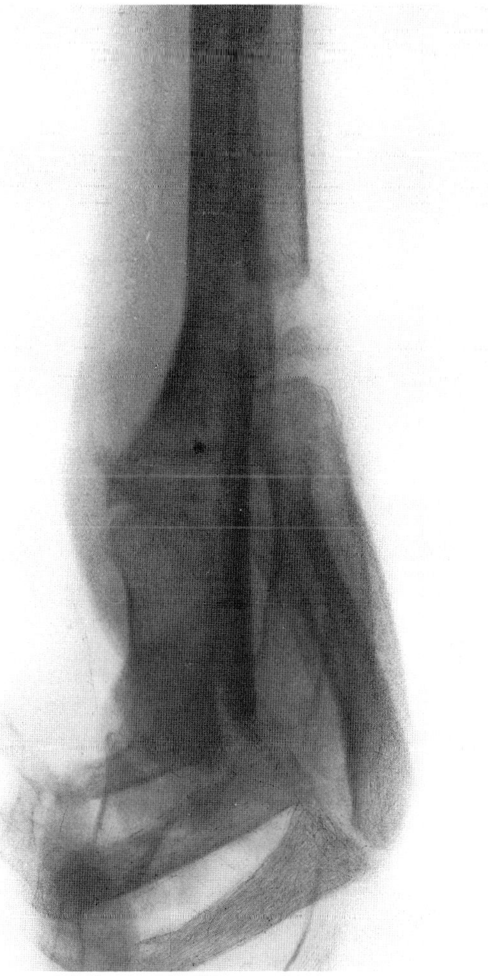

Fig. 210. An arrow-shaped bone graft has been inserted into the resected distal and of the radius and into the second and third metacarpals

adductor tendons should be detached from the first metacarpal, and all other shortened structures, including the intrinsic muscles, between the first and second metacarpal bones should be individually lengthened. Interposition of a short bone graft as a block between the first and second metacarpal bones or excision of the trapezoid is necessary to maintain the thumb in abduction-opposition. Additionally, the metacarpophalangeal joint or the interphalangeal joint of the thumb should be fused in flexion to ensure an effective pinch between the tip of the thumb and the other fingers.

The wrist joint is a gratifying object of synovectomy, which permits correction of the ulnar deviation by reefing of the fibrous capsule at the radial side. Synovectomy of the wrist joint is also indicated in a later stage, when it may be combined with excision of the often concurrently inflamed and swollen tendon sheaths (Fig. 536) on the dorsum and/or volar aspect of the wrist. Their alterations and treatments are discussed in "Tenosynovitis". Resection of the distal ulnar end has generally been recommended for advanced articular alterations to increase the otherwise restricted motion of the wrist joint. However, this procedure is of controversial value; by removal of the supportive buttress on the ulnar side, the wrist eventually deviates substantially to the ulna. The ultimate loss in motion by such deformity is greater than the initial gain. However, in cases with advanced erosion of the articular surfaces, pronounced deformity, and pain on motion, arthrodesis of the wrist joint should be performed after resection of the articular surfases in 20%–25% dorsal extension and midposition between radial and ulnar duction. The outcome of arthrodesis is ensured by insertion of an arrow-shaped inlay bone graft extending from the radius through the carpus into the third metacarpal bone [1549] (Figs. 209, 210).

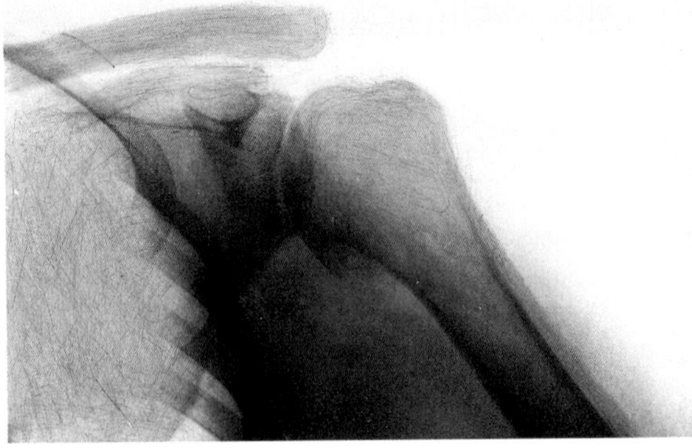

Fig. 211. The articular surfaces of the scapula and humeral head are eroded, uneven, and sclerosed. The joint space is substantially narrowed

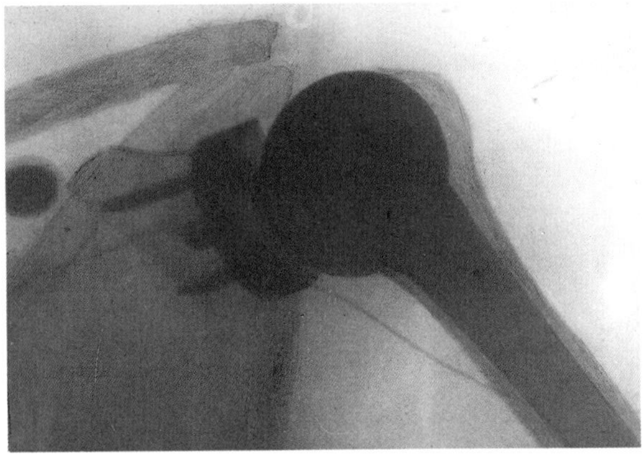

Fig. 212. Arthroplastic components of the unconstrained type have been inserted into the resected glenoidal area and proximal humeral metaphysis

With the expanding application of arthroscopy, arthroscopic synovectomy has also been used in the elbow joint for circumscribed swelling of the joint capsule. While the postoperative disability is mild, the benefit obtained is of short term. On the other hand, the elbow joint benefits well from a wide excision of the markedly thickened synovial membrane in stage II of rheumatic arthritis [463]. The elbow joint is also affected rather often by erosive changes in the articular ends followed by deformation of the joint. Such changes are more pronounced and more frequent in strongly seropositive patients [1210]. In addition to the synovectomy, arthroplastic resection of the radial head may be indicated if the latter is very deformed [803]. Yet such resection must be very economical, lest instability or pronounced valgus deviation of the elbow follows, even if the articular surfaces of the medial humeral condyle and trochlea ulnae are not altered.

Therefore, in more extensive erosion confined to the radial head or one of the humeral condyles, substitution of the individual articular end by a prosthetic insert of polymeric material may be indicated. In far-reaching involvement of all articular ends of the elbow joint, these ends are excised and replaced by the components of a total arthroplasty. The following replacement devices in this arthroplasty are available: (a) the nonconstrained implants [484, 917, 988], whose stability is achieved by the configuration of their surfaces and by the reefing of surrounding tendons; (b) the semiconstrained implants [320, 804, 1412], which have full flexion and extension and are secured in their medial and lateral movements by a snap-fit device which diminishes the torque forces across the cement bond; and (c) the totally constrained implants [387, 690], which are hinged metal-to-metal and are used mainly in extensive bone defects. The semiconstrained implants (Fig. 499) are used more frequently. The results, however, are similar in these three procedures in terms of providing satisfactory relief from pain and increasing the range of motion. The final results of these arthroplasties [1141] depend in terms of stability on preserving the articular ligaments and the joint capsule, as well as on the firm seating of the prosthetic implants, not diminished by bone resorption around these implants. The extent of active movements depends on the intactness and reeducation of the regional musculature. As in other joints, the end results of total arthroplasty of the elbow may be marred by loosening of the implants, subluxation or dislocation, or infection. A less complicated procedure, but possibly providing almost as effective a restoration of mobility, is arthroplastic economic resection of the articular ends supplemented by interposition of a flap of fascia-adipose tissue. This operation is now seldom performed, and it necessitates prolonged physical therapy with mobilization exercises. It relieves the pain but may be followed by instability and heterotopic bone formation [903, 1672].

The shoulder joint [1645] may present, in addition to swelling of the joint capsule, a conspicuous swelling of the sheath of the long biceps tendon and the neighboring bursae. Therefore, excision of these swellings concurrently with that of the accessible inner part of the joint capsule is indicated only initially, as long as no deep erosions or cystic radiolucencies are noted in the humeral head. A possibly slight erosion of the humeral head does not essentially impair the function of the shoulder joint. However, at pronounced incongruence between the articular ends (Fig. 211) and persistent soreness in the shoulder joint, excision of the humeral head and its substitution by a metallic long-shaft endoprosthetic insert (Fig. 212) is indicated with reattachment of the rotator cuff. The latter is well maintained in the majority of cases. Hereby, a pain-free motion over a greater range is restored. Due to non-weight-bearing

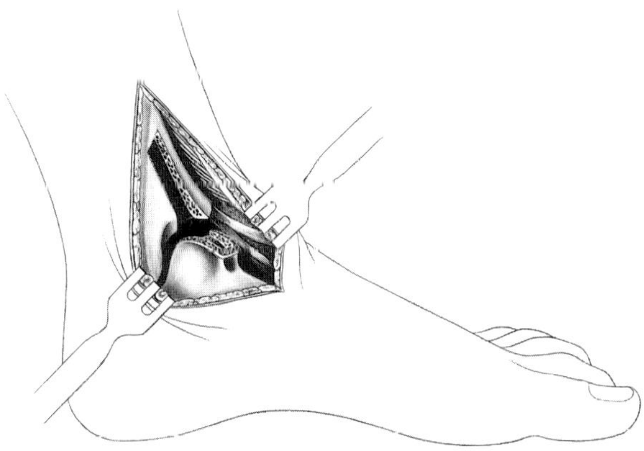

Fig. 213. The articular surfaces of the tibia and talus have been resected, and an arrow-shaped bone graft has been removed from the tibia

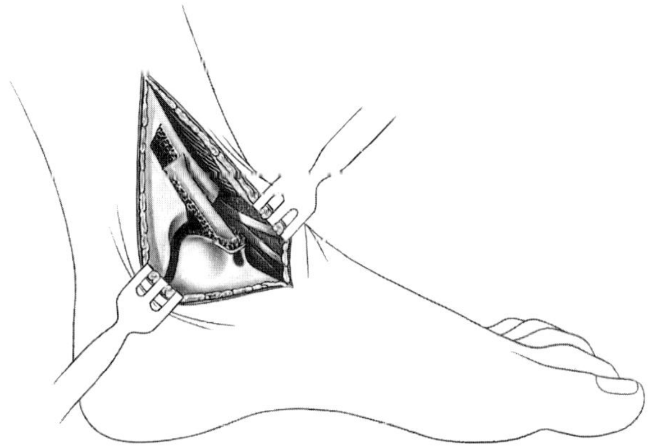

Fig. 214. An arrow-shaped bone graft has been inversely inserted into the grooves made in the tibia and talus

function of this joint replacement of the glenoid cavity by a polyethylene insert [1179] is not absolutely necessary, but it is almost always carried out when pronounced unevenness of the glenoid cavity coexists. For these situations, total arthroplasty sets are available in three modifications: (a) the unconstrained set [1179] (Fig. 212), with components cemented separately into the bones and held together by the repaired joint capsule and rotator cuff, (b) the semiconstrained type [683], with the pear-shaped glenoid cavity preventing superior subluxation of the humeral head, and (c) the constrained arthroplastic set [1275], with components secured by a self-locking ring and not dependent on repair of the soft structures (especially the rotator cuff) but imposing greater stress on the cement bond [803]. In view of the possibility of endoprostheses, especially the acetabular component, becoming loosened, the nonconstrained set is used most often. In all these systems, the patients receive a postoperative program of gradual mobilization and reattain a satisfactory range of motion within 2–3 months.

Affection of the acromioclavicular joint is a separate entity. On impingement with pain and limitation both of abduction and rotation, excision of the clavicular end, or possibly a part of the acromion, is the advisable procedure [1178].

The toes of the rheumatic foot [1030] are usually deformed into hammertoes, with flexion contracture at the interphalangeal joints, and subluxated to the dorsum of the metatarsal heads (Fig. 186). The transversal arch of the front of foot then sags into plantar convexity (Fig. 186). The herefore recommended resection of metatarsal heads [299] does not carry the promise of lasting benefit because the distal ends of the metatarsal shafts protrude plantarward, and the toes eventually resubluxate dorsally. Concurrently, the skin on the sole of the forefoot continues to be covered with extensive calluses, and the toes develop corns on their dorsal aspects. Therefore, the first palanx of the toes should be resected, whereupon the toes can be brought into proper alignment with the metatarsal heads. The latter should be raised by arch supports with high metatarsal pads; a metatarsal bar on the sole of the shoes is also indicated, and diligent passive plantar flexion exercises of the toes are indispensable. A rather frequently associated deformity is hallux valgus, developing as the sequela of the splayfoot and its compression by improper footwear. If corrective shoes do not help to relieve this condition, an operation [1552] designed to correct the components of the hallux valgus (Fig. 270) is indicated.

The midtarsal and subtalar joints, apart from being thickened by capsule swelling, are pulled by muscle tenseness into faulty alignment and remain deviated either in valgus or less often in varoadductus position. A wedge resection of the deformed subtalar joints for subtalar arthrodesis or, preferentially, triple arthrodesis is indicated [299, 556]. This restores the proper alignment between the tarsal bones. Combination with immobilization by a plaster cast for 3 months with concurrent weight bearing ensures the fusion of these joints and satisfactory function of the foot, as long as the ankle joint is well maintained.

In the ankle joint [1724] synovectomy is often indicated [299], especially when marked swelling of the tendon sheaths on the dorsum of the ankle occurs simultaneously and requires treatment by excision. On the other hand, extensive articular synovitis may be associated with shortening of the Achilles tendon; then ventral and dorsal synovectomy is combined with lengthening of the tendon. This procedure renders satisfactory results as long as the articular surfaces are intact. However, on deeper erosion of the articular cartilage, function in the ankle joint essentially becomes

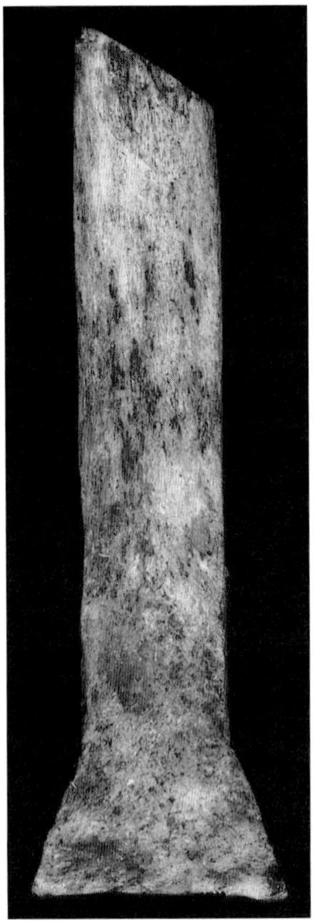

Fig. 215. Frontal view of the bone graft, pointed at its proximal end and broadened at its distal end

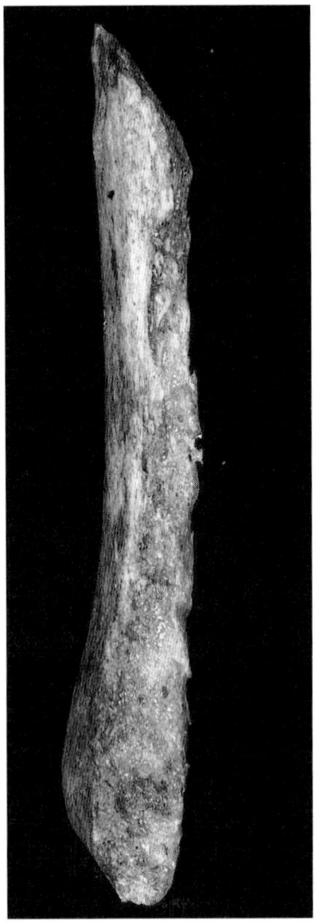

Fig. 216. Lateral view of the bone graft, thinned and sharpened at its proximal end

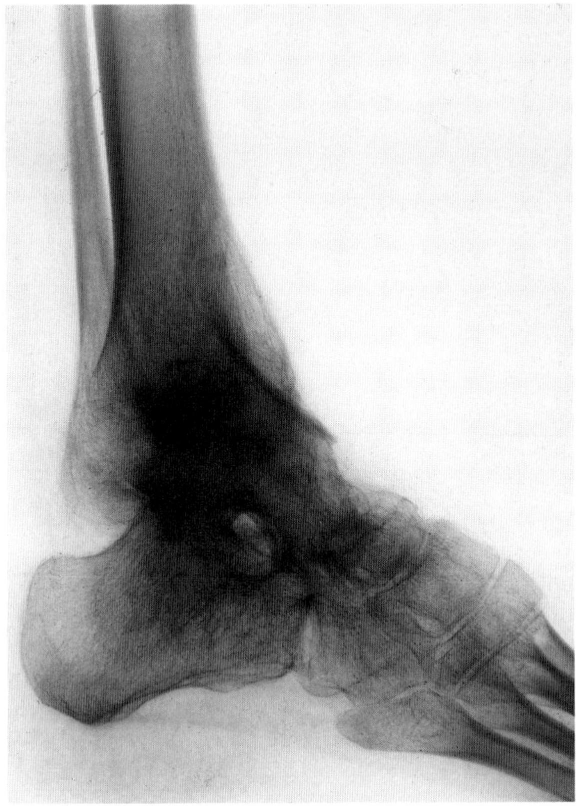

Fig. 217. Fusion of the talotibial joint has been attained by resection of the articular surfaces and by insertion of a bone graft. The cartilage spaces of the talocalcaneal joint and talonavicular joint are uneven and narrow

impaired, being limited and continuously painful [299]. Therefore, considering the sex and type of professional activity, the ankle joint can be restored in men with a sedentary type of work and in women by total arthroplasty with endoprosthetic inserts of high-density polyethylene connected with high-strength metal alloys (Figs. 273, 274). The geometric design of their articulating surfaces accounts for the degree of stability of these implants. They can be made to be constrained against rotation, anteroposterior and/or mediolateral movements. Thus unconstrained implants [1184], semiconstrained implants (Figs. 273, 274) [1723], and constrained implants [1392] are in use. In addition, the intactness of the articular ligaments and the firmness of the joint capsule account largely for the stability of the ankle joint. However, total arthroplasty of the ankle joint is fraught with a significant failure rate due to loosening of the arthroplastic implants and instability, subluxation, or infection. In these situations the implants should be removed. Another arthroplasty may be attempted after a longer period of time [1651], or an arthrodesis may solve the instability and pain, yet at the loss of motion. Therefore, apart from cases of occupational limitation, total arthroplasty should be carried out mainly in situations of concurrent arthritic limitations of motion in the subtalar and midtarsal joints. Because of the frequent loosening of the cemented arthroplastic implants, the recent designs of these implants employ coated porous stems which permit ingrowth of bone and thus offer a good chance for reliable fixation. On the other hand, in heavy laborers, arthrodesis [1549] of the ankle joint by denudation of the articular surfaces and inlay of a sliding bone graft (Figs. 213, 214, 215, 216) is the more advisable procedure. This is combined with immobilization by a plaster cast for 3 months with concurrent weight bearing; the fusion provides (Fig. 217) permanent freedom from pain. Another procedure for arthrodesis of the ankle joint is resection of the articular surfaces and their compression by a clamp [279] until fusion is completed or resection combined with intraarticular immobilization by screws (Figs. 275, 276). The occasional drainage at the site of the pins of the clamp is a serious shortcoming of this procedure. Earlier removal of the pins and immobilization with a plaster cast at concomitant weight bearing until completed fusion

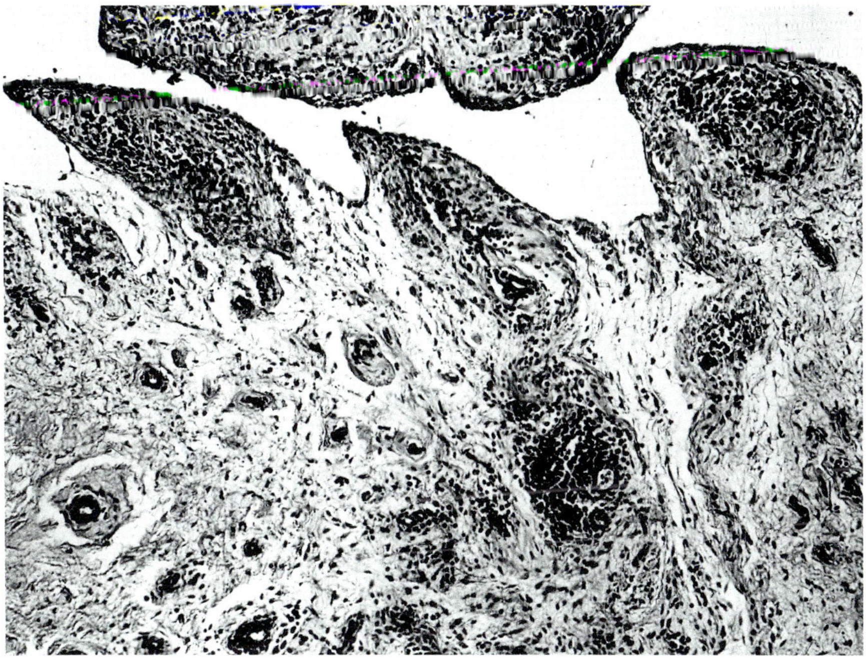

Fig. 218. The surface of the synovial membrane, 2 years after synovectomy, is raised in moderate-sized villi filled by agglomerations of lymphocytes. Similar agglomerations, but in smaller numbers, lie in the subsynoviocytic tissue, which is moderately hypercellular with fibrocytes

minimize this problem. However, before deciding for arthrodesis of the ankle joint, the function of the subtalar and midtarsal joints must be ascertained. Only with maintained mobility of these joints can arthrodesis of the ankle joint succeed in improving the use of the foot.

The knee joint, is a frequent object of treatment. In the initial or gradually progressing stage and with marked swelling of the joint capsule, synovectomy by an anterior approach may prove beneficial. Further swelling of the joint capsule, recurrence of effusions, and overstretching of the ligaments are thus prevented or at least minimized in about 70%–75% of patients [949, 1303]. However, this result decreases somewhat within 2–3 years by moderate proliferation of the regenerated synovial membrane [689, 691, 1302] (Fig. 218). In the other operated patients and in nonoperated patients swelling of the joint capsule increases, with concomitant erosion of the ligaments and the articular cartilage. It is questionable whether arthroscopy, even when performed through a few portals, permits extensive and even excision of the inner part of the joint capsule. Similarly, it has not yet been established that the chemical influence of intraarticularly injected substances (alkylating agents, osmium tetroxyde, or radioactive isotopes) provides lasting regression of proliferative synovial changes [394, 685, 1007, 1216]. Loss of the articular cartilage, as evidenced by pronounced radiographic changes and marked instability of the knee joint, present contraindications to the synovectomy. Synovectomy is beneficial in more advanced rheumatic arthritis when thickening of the joint capsule is associated with marginal osteophyte formations. Here, synovectomy should be combined with debridement of the articular surfaces [1030]. A substantial shortcoming particularly of early synovectomy is the experience that thickening of the inner part of the joint capsule (Fig. 218) recurs in about 25%–30% of cases due to reactivation of the rheumatic process. Since a flexion contracture often develops in the late cases of rheumatic arthritis, lengthening of the hamstring tendons and posterior capsulotomy are necessary to restore the extension ability. In view of the concurrent shortening of the popliteal blood vessels, it appears here as a mandatory, immediately postoperative precaution to check the circulation of the lower leg and foot hourly and to diminish the corrective alignment at the slightest sign of impaired circulation. On restoration of normal peripheral circulation, the straightened knee joint is kept immobilized with a brace in fully corrected position until active extension can be fully carried out. Active flexion is concurrently practised.

Since in the course of the rheumatic disease the trophics of the articular epiphyses or juxtarticular metaphyses of the knee is often impaired, these areas eventually become misshapen. The deep erosions by the expanding synovial granulations contribute substantially to deformation of the articular condyles (Figs. 219, 220). Axial malalignment at the knee results from this more often in the direction of genu valgum than in that of genu varum. Correction of these deformities aiming at restoration of proper axial weight bearing in the knee joint can be obtained by osteotomy

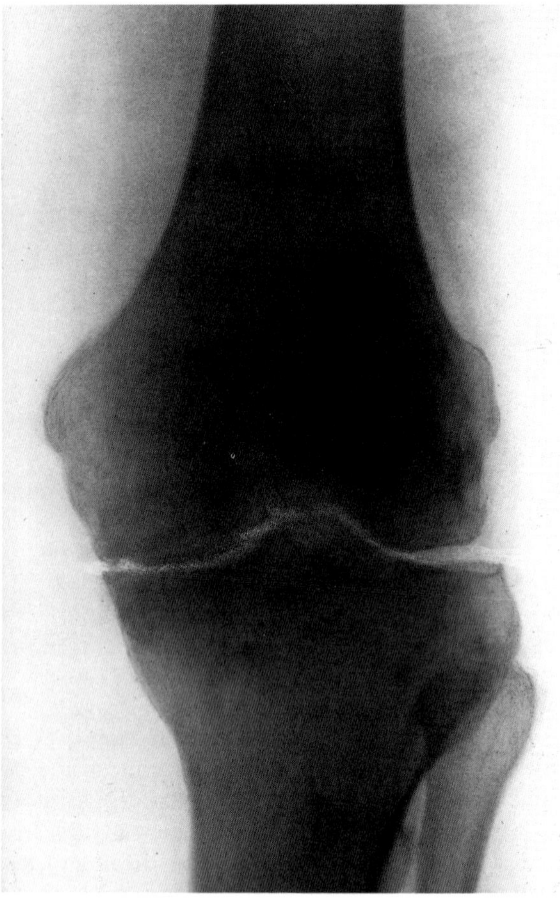

Fig. 219. The cartilage space of the knee joint is unevenly delimited and is narrowed at its medial part. The medial articular epiphyses are sclerosed, and the tibia is deviated medially

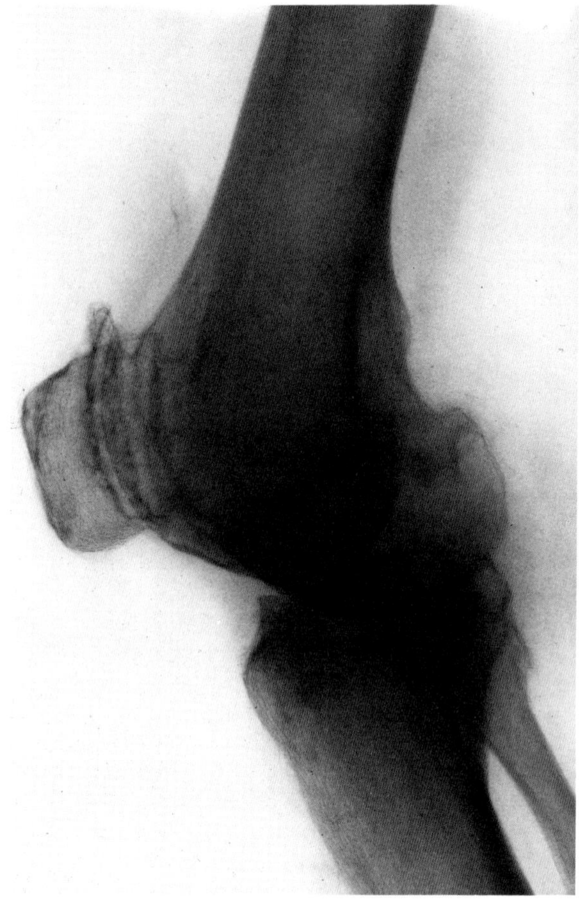

Fig. 220. The contiguous articular epiphyses of the femur and tibia are uneven, and the cartilage space between them is narrowed. The articular surfaces between femur and patella are also uneven

at the site of angular deviation [335, 805]. However, the rheumatic process remains unaffected by the osteotomy; the alterations and symptoms in the knee joint continue unabatedly. Thus the use of osteotomy for correction of malalignment in rheumatic arthritis is limited principally to the situation of distinctly extinguished inflammation. The technique and the types of osteotomy (Figs. 279, 280, 283, 284) in which osteotomy has a substantially wider use are described in "Osteoarthritis". On the other hand, when an articular end has been eroded at one of its condyles only, and the knee deviates axially within the joint cavity, the thickness of this articular condyle can be substituted by a polymeric or metallic plate of proper thickness (Fig. 266) [999, 1071].

Finally, in far advanced erosion and deformation of all articular ends (Figs. 219, 220), extensive thickening of the joint capsule and persistently painful impairment in the use of the knee joint, total arthroplasty (Figs. 221, 222) is indicated. Its purpose is to provide an adequate range of motion with stability and freedom from pain. A promising prerequisite for the success of this operation is a functioning extensor and flexor musculature unencumbered in its contracture and relaxation by adhesions or extensive scars. Considering the various factors in the resulting deformity of the knee joint, different types of total arthroplastic implants, varying in constituent materials and mechanical performance, have been designed to suit individual needs corresponding to the organic situation [316, 483, 779, 807, 806, 1507, 1721, 1722]. The articular implants used are made of stainless steel or of steel-titanium, or cobalt alloys, coated on their surfaces with high-density polyethylene, and cemented by methylmethacrylate with their shafts into the marrow cavities of the long bones. However, the shortcomings – subsequent or late loosening of the endoprostheses due to fragmentation of the cement or resorption of bone – led to the use of noncemented endoprostheses fitted tightly into the marrow cavities. As further improve-

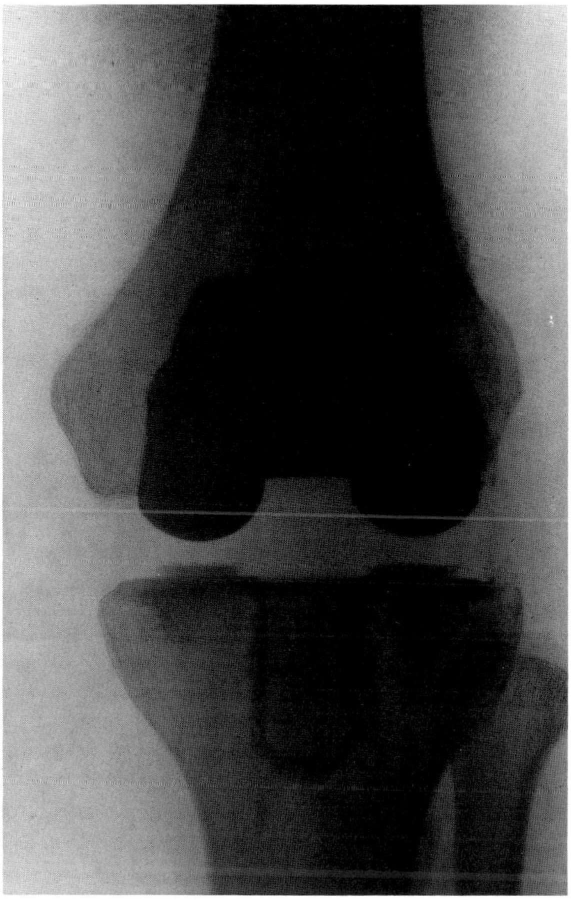

Fig. 221. Status after total arthroplasty with insertion of the components of the condylar total replacement type into the distal part of the femur and into the proximal part of the tibia

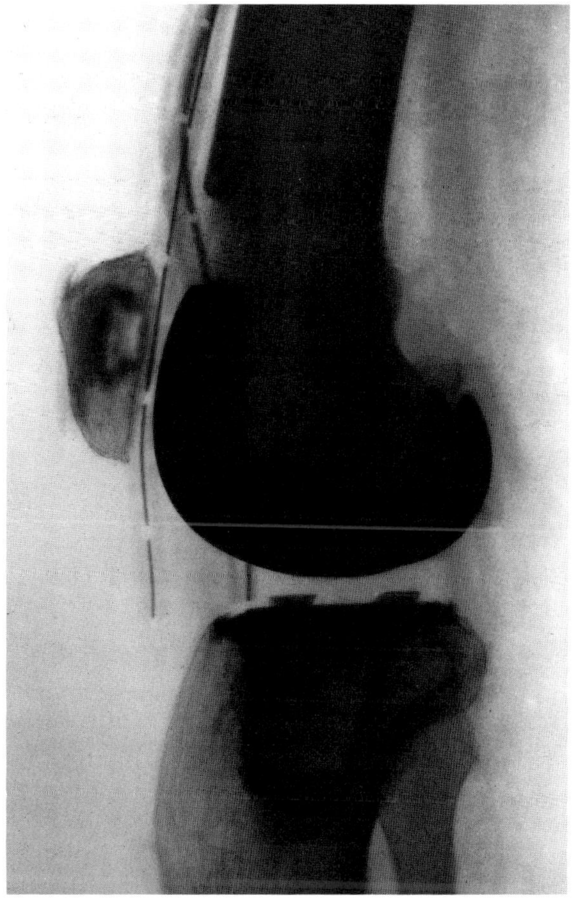

Fig. 222. Status after concentric insertion of arthroplastic components of the total condylar replacement type into the femur, patella, and tibia

ment with the aim of obtaining lasting fixation, the stems of the implants have been coated with porous sintered metal components which permit the ingrowth of osseous trabecula from the surrounding bone. Concurrently, the articulating surfaces have been designed geometrically to provide congruence and an increased range of motion; the greater their congruence, the greater is their inherent stability and the less their attrition [1651]. The tricompartmental implants, which encompass articulation of all compartments of the knee joint, can be classified as: (a) the unconstrained implants [1657], which provide full motion but have little stability and depend on the firmness of the surrounding soft tissue; (b) the semiconstrained implants [807] (Figs. 221, 222), whose design provides increased stability and relies partly on the ligaments; and (c) the fully constrained implants [926], which have rotating hinges permitting rotation in addition to extension-flexion but are exposed to increased attrition. On uncomplicated postoperative course, mobilization of the knee joint is carried out systematically by assisted active and passive exercises. Ambulation is then started with partial weight bearing and using the support of crutches.

While arthroplasty succeeds in substantially increasing the range of motion and relieving or diminishing the pain in a significant percentage of cases, its potential complications must not be disregarded. The postoperative course as well as the late afterperiod may be fraught with: delayed healing and/or superficial infection of the wound, phlebitis and thromboembolism, loosening or breakage of the implants, fracture of the bone, or incomplete attainment of the normal range of motion. Yet the most worrisome complication, occurring in 3%–5% of patients with rheumatic arthritis [682, 1651], is deep infection, which subsides after intense and prolonged antibiotic treatment only in a small percentage. In the other cases, removal of the implants is unavoidable. The subsequent modalities of salvage are support of the knee by a brace with hinges or the attempt at another implantation of arthroplastic inserts possibly years later after the suppuration has

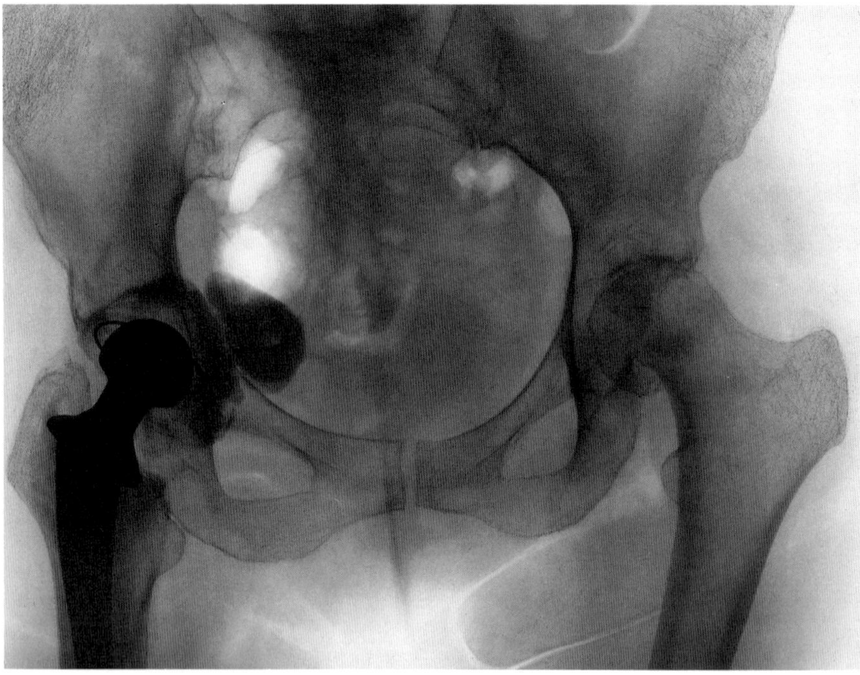

Fig. 223. The joint cleft of the left hip joint is substantially narrowed and unevenly delimited especially at the acetabular roof area. The right hip joint underwent a cemented total arthroplasty with a plastic acetabulum

completely healed, or the rarely practised solution of arthrodesis of the knee joint. Consequently, in view of the great potential of complications following arthroplasty, all other modalities of treatment should be attempted before embarking on arthroplasty.

For those patients needing absolute stability and painfree use of the leg in their occupational activity, arthrodesis for fusion of the knee joint may be the preferable and ultimate solution. This sometimes applies as a salvage procedure in cases of infected total arthroplasty in which all implants were removed, marked instability of the knee joint resulted, and the chances for successfully repeating a total arthroplasty are nonexistent. After resection, the articular epiphyses are apposed to each other and held tightly by the Charnley [279] compression clamp for 2 months. Immobilization with a plaster cast follows, with concurrent weight bearing. Prerequisites for establishing the indication for arthrodesis of the knee joint are satisfactorily functioning hip joint and ankle joint.

The hip joint usually and gradually assumes a flexion-adduction contracture (Fig. 186) which is often compounded by external rotation. If prolonged traction does not succeed in correcting the deformity, the shortened adductor and flexor tendons are exposed and divided. Without additional intervention on the joint capsule, but possibly by additional manipulation, the hip joint is then brought into proper alignment and secured by applying a plaster cast or brace. After discontinuation of the immobilization device diligent mobilization of the hip joint by active and passive exercises is indispensable. However, if the rheumatic alterations extensively involve the articular ends, and substantial impairment in the function of the joint ensues with persistent soreness, improvement in the articular function can be attained by the following procedures [298, 1563, 1564]. Angulation osteotomy at the intertrochanteric level realigns the femoral head and neck in their relation to the femoral shaft in the sense of valgization or varization (Figs. 289, 290). The proper angulation is determined by the roentgenographically ascertained areas of overloading in the femoral head, and attains a redistribution of the gravitational and weight-bearing stresses. While preferentially used in younger individuals with well-maintained acetabulum and only partly altered femoral head [127], angulation osteotomy [702, 1229] has also found acceptance in elderly patients with not overly advanced alterations in the hip joint and quiescent inflammatory process. Nevertheless, its application is rather limited in rheumatic arthritis; it is of substantially wider use in osteoarthritis and is therefore discussed in "Osteoarthritis".

On the other hand, arthroplasty as an intraarticular operation has received increasing applications in view of its treating the alterations in the articular ephiphyses as well as those in the joint capsule. Arthroplasty of the hip joint can be performed as surface replacement arthroplasty (Fig. 267), as hemiarthroplasty, or as total arthroplasty (Figs. 223, 292). The indications for these modalities depend on the predominant location of arthritic alterations, whether affecting only the femoral head or also the acetabulum, and on the degree and extent of the alterations. Surface replacement arthroplasty [38, 40, 239, 1656, 1702] removes only the altered part of the femoral head and, if necessary, the acetabulum. Thus it largely maintains the anatomy of the hip joint. The defect of the femoral head is replaced by a shell of titanium alloy or ceramic secured by a stem impacted into the neck, and the defect of the acetabulum is replaced by a cemented shell also of titanium alloy (Fig. 267). The procedure proves very beneficial in abolishing the pain and restoring motion. However, late follow-up examinations [732, 995] have disclosed loosening of the femoral and/or acetabular component and aseptic necrosis of the femoral area under the cap. The shortcoming of loosening or displacement of the femoral cap can be avoided by using a femoral cap coated on the inside with porous polyethylene, which allows the ingrowth of osseous trabeculae. The indication for resurfacing arthroplasty has been narrowed basically to cases of moderate and bilateral affection of the hip joints. Hemiarthroplasty [100] is applied in extensive alterations confined to the femoral head, which is excised. A femoral component of vitallium is used; its head fits the dimensions of the acetabulum, its collar provides a snug fitting onto the calcar femoris, and its long stem has been preoperatively determined in its cross-section to fit the dimensions of the femoral medullary cavity. The implant is secured within the femoral shaft by methylmethacrylate cement. However, this procedure has limited application since its organic prerequisite of an unaltered acetabulum is rather rare.

In view of the shortcomings of the above procedures, and after exhaustion of all modalities of conservative treatment, total arthroplasty of the hip joint (Fig. 292) as described by Charnley [278, 280] has received wide acceptance [270, 1563, 1564]. Its basic components are the femoral implant of head and stem, made of stainless steel or titanium or cobalt alloy, and the acetabular cup, made of ceramic or polyethylene reinforced by a metal shell. These implants are cemented into their bases by methylmethacrylate. However, because of the rather frequent loosening of the implants due to fragmentation of the cement and resorption of the bone, the noncemented implants are finding increasingly use. The femoral stem and acetabular cup are tightly press-fitted into the marrow cavity. As further improvement for enduring fixation, the femoral stem and acetabular cup are coated with porous sintered polyethylene alloy which allows the ingrowth of osseous trabecula [198]. This substantially enhances the chances for reliable fixation, but the implants must be protected from excessive strain and load for a reasonable period of time. Charnley's total arthroplasty [278, 280] has been designed as a low-friction torque arthroplasty which also decreases the total load on the hip joint; it uses an anterolateral approach to the hip joint. On the other hand, Moore [1135] used a posterolateral approach to the hip joint, Mueller [1152] a posterior, and Amstutz [38] a lateral. A special modification is the bipolar endoprosthesis of Bateman [86] and Gilberty [611], which employs a polyethylene liner on top of the metallic acetabular cup. This carries the motion out also between the liner and the acetabulum and increases the range of motion. Following all these arthroplasties and upon uneventful postoperative course, during which the hip joint is kept in abducted traction, the hip joint is gradually mobilized by active exercises and subsequently by assisted passive exercises. After a satisfactory range of motion has been attained, partial weight bearing is started with the support of crutches. Strengthening of the musculature by active exercises, massage, and faradic stimulation is carried out until satisfactory function of the hip joint is attained. Whenever feasible, regular swimming is of great benefit for strengthening of the musculature and mobilizing the hip joint.

However, this extensive operation may be followed by serious complications [227], some of which are of general surgical nature and others particular for this type of operation. The general complications are phlebitis or thrombosis, injuries to the sciatic or femoral nerve, superficial infection and/or delayed healing of the wound, and protracted deep infection. The latter is very feared and is caused mostly by staphylococcus, streptococcus, Escherichia coli, or pseudomonas [1792]. According to Calandruccio [227] it occurs more often (5%) in patients with rheumatic arthritis and especially in those treated with steroids. Buchholz et al. [203] also cultivated various other microbes in deep suppurations. Treatment of these consists of widening the wound for unimpeded drainage and prolonged administration of antibiotics. This leads to subsidence of the infection and closure of the wound in 20%–30% of cases [227]. In the other cases, the infection continues and requires removal of all implants, including the cement, if used. Since marked instability of the hip joint follows, stability may be improved or restored after an adequate period of time following the healing of the suppurative area. One of the possibilities in this Girdlestone-like [613] situation is subtrochanteric abduction osteotomy [1546], in which the weight of the pelvic bone is carried on the aligned proximal fragment of the femur. The stability is improved, but the substantial shortening of the leg continues. The procedure, which restores the length of the leg and permits proper weight bearing and motion of the hip joint, consists of a revision of the operated area and insertion of another complete set of arthroplastic implants. The necessity of removing the arthroplastic implants upon persistent suppuration is regarded by Calandruccio [227] as a very strong indication for revision of the arthroplasty.

The other reasons for this revision, according to Calandruccio [227], include loosening or fracture, irreducible dislocation or recurrent subluxation of a component, all of which are specific complications of total arthrosplasty. A specific complication is also the shortly postoperative dislocation of the hip joint [1781], which requires immediate, usually closed reduction and immobilization with a spica plaster cast in abduction. Turner et al. [1667] also regard loosening or dislocation of an arthroplastic compound and fracture of the femoral stem or femoral shaft as the major specific complications which require revision. Scheller et al. [1406] advised in the failure of the femoral stem a longer femoral compound of high-strength superalloy. Bierbaum [133] recommended on loosening of the acetabular compound another properly oriented and thicker socket. On the basis of pathological-anatomical examinations, Thurner [1642] demonstrated the occurrence of erosions on the surface of the implants as the cause of many of their failures. These erosions are manifested by areas of unevenness which lead to weakening, subluxation, dislocation, or fracture of the metallic implants. With many years' experience now in the use of total hip arthroplasty, it has become evident that at the latest 10 years following the operation loosening of the femoral component occurs in 30%–50% of patients and loosening of the acetabular component in 10%–20% [1563]. Details as to arthroplastic treatment of the hip joint are also discussed in "Osteoarthritis". Operative arthrodesis of the hip joint [73] is rarely advisable in rheumatic arthritis in view of the usually impaired mobility of the neighboring joints.

While the joints of the extremities, deteriorated by advanced rheumatic changes are often treated by operative procedures, surgical treatment is not routinely used in the vertebral column. This applies especially to the cervical spine, in which the fusing tendency is insufficient due to extensive osteoporosis, and operation carries a great mortality risk [342, 1304]. On the other hand, in gradually aggravating subluxation of the uppermost cervical vertebrae, fusion of these vertebrae may be necessary [1304]. By posterior approach, the upper three cervical vertebrae are united by wiring with the skull (Fig. 194), and bone grafts are tightly packed in [428, 1091, 1098]. In very grave subluxation of the upper cervical vertebrae and threatening compression of the medulla oblongata [1098, 1646], laminectomy combined with arthrodesis may be indicated as an emergency procedure. The rheumatic changes of the lumbar spine, often causing impaired function, are adequately treated by the conservative modalities indicated above, as are the occasional symptoms arising by compression of the nerve roots of the lumbosacral plexus.

5. Arthritis in Sjögren's Syndrome

Sjögren's [1506] syndrome, originally described by Mikulicz [1104] is a set of symptoms characterized mainly by diminished secretions of the lacrimal and salivary glands. Other exocrine glands may also be affected in this syndrome [857, 1599]. The sicca complex [1595] occurs in combination with rheumatic arthritis but may also occur as a separate entity.

While the cause of this complex has not yet been clarified, it appears that the glandular insufficiency is the outcome of infiltration by lymphocytes and plasmacytes in the parenchyma of these glands and around their ducts. The associated harm to the epithelium of these ducts probably manifests an autoimmune process. This process appears [1618, 1619] to originate from the activity of specific antigens and the resulting response of immunologically regulatory lymphocytes. The frequent concurrent findings of certain histocompatibility antigens of the HLA group indicate that individual susceptibility and/or reactivity has a bearing on the occurrence and development of these changes. The events in the evolution of the glandular lesions may be interpreted as the recognition of antigen and its damage to glandular tissue by lymphocytes and plasmacytes migrating into these areas [1043, 1599, 1746, 1748].

The sicca complex [144, 1746, 1748] occurs predominantly in women aged between 50 and 60 years. Their complaints are a frequent itching sensation by a foreign body or a burning sensation in the eyes, diminished tearing, impaired visual acuteness, dryness in the mouth with abnormality or loss of the taste sense, difficulty in chewing, and persistence of food crumbs in the mouth. Dryness is also experienced in the nose, with concurrent abnormality of smell. Dryness may occur in the pharynx, with difficulty in swallowing, and/or in the larynx, with difficulty in phonation. Frequent need of coughing, sometimes even tightness of the throat, and difficulty in breathing are experienced.

Examination of these elderly women discloses marked redness of the eyes due to conjunctivitis, and occasionally small ulcerations and opacities in the cornea (keratoconjunctivitis sicca). Similarly, the lips, tongue, and mucosa of the cheeks are dry (xerostomia), crusty, and often disfigured by cracks, chronic ulcerations, and angular stomatitis. The floor of the mouth is bare of saliva [1746, 1748]. The parotid glands are enlarged and sensitive in the majority of these patients, as are the mandibular glands. In addition to the salivary glands, the sweat glands and sebaceous glands are affected over large areas. Herewith are associated dryness, rigidity, and tenderness of the skin, with tendency to frequent cracking. In these cases the intestinal glands and the pancreas may also be affected, but rarely the

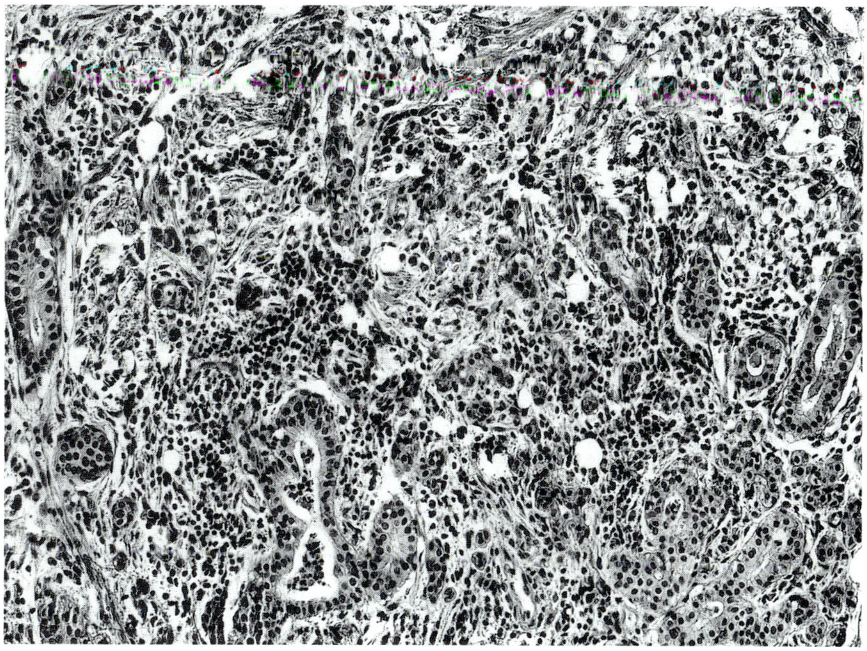

Fig. 224. The structure of the parotid gland is partly maintained upon rather diffuse infiltration by lymphocytes and plasmacytes. Concomitant atrophy of the acini results

kidneys. The regional lymph nodes and spleen are enlarged in about 30% of patients.

The often associated affection of the joints [14] corresponds to the clinical picture of moderate rheumatoid arthritis with symmetrical involvement of the hands, wrists, elbows, ankles, and knees. The frequent episodes of soreness and aching in these joints are associated with thickening of the joint capsule and moderate limitation in the ranges of their motion but not pronounced contracture. About one-half of the patients with the sicca syndrome present such articular changes. The other half lack articular changes but present the sicca syndrome to a much more pronounced and extensive degree.

The functional test of the lacrimal glands [1410] is carried out with standard filter paper strips, measuring the amount of drained lacrimal fluid within a unit of time. Slit lamp examination of the eyes, detecting corneal ulcerations and/or filamentous keratitis, corroborates the diagnosis of keratoconjunctivitis sicca [1599]. Sialograms of the parotid glands show gross distortion of the duct arrangements.

Laboratory studies disclose moderate anemia and moderate leukopenia in about 30% of patients, and equally so eosinophilia. Immunoglobulins especially IgA, IgG and IgM are increased in the serum of most patients, as are antinuclear antibodies and rheumatoid factor, even in patients without arthritis. These findings indicate the overall increase in antibodies [27, 213, 447, 515, 694, 1023, 1474, 1748].

Histopathological examination [242, 285, 1009, 1139, 1619] discloses the spread of focal infiltrates of lymphocytes and plasmacytes in the parenchyma (Fig. 224) of the salivary (parotid, submandibular and palatinal) glands. Other exocrine glands such as those of the respiratory and gastrointestinal tracts [1746, 1748] display similar changes. Gardner [570] demonstrated that the architecture of the salivary glands is maintained, while acinar atrophy is present as the result of the extensive lymphocyte infiltration.

Diagnosis is based [352] on the sicca complex in the eyes and mouth with correlated local symptoms, occasional enlargement of the parotid gland, almost regular increase of immunoglobulins in the serum, frequent increase in autoantibodies, and biopsy of the minor salivary glands of the lips. Enlargement of the oral salivary glands is not necessarily confirmation of Sjögren's syndrome, because this may be elicited by bacterial or mycotic infections or may also occur in other affections of the connective tissue [14, 15].

Treatment is directed at replacing the lacking ocular fluid by ophthalmic solution [1742, 1768]. Consultation with an ophthalmologist should be obtained in any situation of corneal lesion. Replacement of the deficient oral fluid by frequent intake of fluids devoid of sugar is advised, as well as minimizing the intake of sweet food. Regular mouth hygiene and thorough dental care must be emphasized [899]. Immunosuppressive medications may be used to decrease glandular infiltrates and to improve exocrine glandular function in patients with severe renal and/or pulmonary manifestation [1599]. Treatment of the concurring arthritis is discussed in "Rheumatoid Arthritis".

6. Ankylosing Spondylitis

Ankylosing spondylitis, also known as spondylitis ankylopoetica or Bechterew's [99] disease, has sometimes been regarded a rheumatoid variant. However, reconsideration of its predominant features indicates clearly that ankylosing spondylitis is a distinct clinical entity quite separate from rheumatoid arthritis [146, 232, 1044, 1064, 1130]. Its features are the notable 10:1 involvement of men versus women [1470], the primary affection of the axial skeleton with less frequent and not necessarily symmetrical affection of the peripheral joints, the pronounced tendency for fibrous or osseous ankylosis of the affected joints, and the usually negative outcome of laboratory tests characteristic for rheumatoid arthritis. Beyond these, other laboratory tests without significance for rheumatoid arthritis have a high specificity for ankylosing spondylitis [1676].

Nevertheless, the etiology of this condition has not yet been clarified, although trauma, intensive stresses, and/or inflammation, especially nonspecific urogenital infections, have been linked to the occurrence of ankylosing spondylitis [1044]. More recent studies [186, 187] point out the familial incidence of ankylosing spondylitis or of its specific features and indicate the possibility that hereditary factors may have a bearing on individual reactivity to noxious agents. Hereby the development of ankylosing spondylitis is facilitated. This is suggested by the recessively transmitted and strikingly frequent histocompatibility antigen HLA-B27 [186, 187, 230, 233].

The characteristic affections are manifested primarily in the sacroiliac joints, lumbosacral joint, lumbar spine [146, 1605], somewhat less often in the dorsal spine, and distinctly less often in the cervical spine. Much less frequent (12%–18%) affections are manifested in the hip, shoulder, and knee joints. Alterations generally begin in the sacroiliac joints, with intraarticular granulation tissue which invades the hyaline cartilage and subchondral bone. Hereby erosions of varying depth are caused. With further erosion of the sacroiliac borders, on one hand and expanding reactive new bone formation, on the other, partial or complete fusion of the sacroiliac joint ensues. Very extensive alterations also occur in the intervertebral fibrocartilages. From these areas, metaplastic ossification spreads beyond the confines of the annulus fibrosus into the vertebral endplates, contiguous anterior longitudinal ligament and lateral and posterior intervertebral ligaments. Identical substitution of the articular cartilage and obliteration of the joint space by dense fibrous tissue is followed by ossification in the vertebral apophyseal joints, costovertebral joints, and sternoclavicular joints. Similar histopathological changes may lead to osseous ankylosis in the major joints of the extremities. The synovial changes in the major peripheral joints [1543] resemble in their initial phase those of rheumatoid arthritis. However, dense fibrosis follows in ankylosing spondylitis, accompanied by extensive ossification. The contact of the denuded articular surfaces results in fusion of the joint to an osseous block. This general tendency to ossification may be related pathogenetically to a constitutional predisposition, associated with the presence of the histocompatibility antigen HLA-B27.

Ankylosing spondylitis [232, 725] involves mostly young men aged between 20 and 25 years. It also may be seen in boys between 9 and 14 years of age who were initially regarded as having juvenile rheumatoid arthritis. Eventually they were properly classified in view of the pain and tenderness becoming confined to the lumbosacral spine and sacroiliac joints [929, 1349, 1404]. The disease usually starts insidiously, with pain most commonly being localized in the lower back and buttocks, sometimes also involving the thoracic and cervical spine and rarely starting at the anterior aspect of the chest. Easy fatiguability and diminished mobility of the vertebral spine gradually set in, sometimes combined with impaired breathing ability. Subsequently, soreness of the pelvis and pain arise, radiating from the lumbar spine to the thighs. The pain increases through the day commensurately with the duration of activity. Radiating pain from the upper cervical spine to the occipital and temporal region may also occur. Eventually, complete stiffness ensues; this is associated with very debilitating limitation of respiratory excursions. Symptoms then also develop indicating cardiopulmonary complications. Finally, the joints of extremities may become affected by unrelenting gradual aggravation leading in severe conditions to ankylosis.

Examination [146, 728] in the initial stage discloses localized tenderness of the lumbar spine, lumbosacral junction, and both sacroiliac joints, associated with moderate tenseness in the regional paravertebral musculature. Movements of the vertebral column are very limited in ventral and lateral flexion and in dorsal hyperextension out of proportion to the moderate degree of muscle defense. Lateral or oblique compression of the pelvis elicits pain in the affected sacroiliac joints. In cases with involvement of the dorsal spine, the anterior chest cage is tender especially at the costosternal junctions. Respiratory excursions are distinctly limited on measuring the midchest circumference at maximal inspirium and maximal exspirium. On aggravation of the alterations in the lumbar spine and by compression of nerve roots or the cauda equina, neurological signs appear along the lateral femoral cutaneous and sciatic nerves. Paresthesia und hyperesthesia in the lower extremities and depressed ankle reflex may be pronounced. On the other hand, incontinence of the urinary bladder and rectum and paresthesia in the perineum rarely occur. In affection of the cervical spine, persistent neuralgias sometimes develop along the occipital nerves or along the branches of the cervical and/or brachial plexus. In instability of the upper cervical spine secondary to ankylosis of the lower cervical spine, compression not only of the posterior roots but also of the spinal cord may occur [1381]. On eventual complete stiffness, active and passive movements are absent in any direction, either of the entire vertebral column or particularly, of the lower half of the thoracic spine, entire lumbar spine, and lumbosacral junction. The trunk becomes stiff, generally in excessive kyphosis of the entire vertebral column (Fig. 225). The head is then inclined downward, and looking upward is not possible. Similarly, turning the neck to the side is not possible, requiring the entire body to be turned. In cases with unrelenting progression to generalized ankylosis, the hip, knee, and shoulder joints also become stiff in 30%–40% of patients.

Other organs too may become affected, as Villiaumey [1690] emphasized. Iridocyclitis occurs in about 15%–20% of patients and may be aggravated by depigmentation and severe visual impairment. Due to the limited expansion of the chest cage the lungs develop interstitial pneumonitis and fibrosis, with eventual dense shrinking of their parenchyma and thickening of the pleura. Cardiovascular symptoms may appear, with heart block, cardiomegaly, and aortic insufficiency due to shrinking of the aortic valves [141, 243].

Of the laboratory studies [877, 1687], the sedimentation rate is elevated, in the very active phases not beyond 60 mm/h. IgA and IgG are increased distinctly throughout the activity of the disease and decrease with regression of the disease paralleling the sedimentation rate. Langness et al. [940] demonstrated that a hydroxyproline-containing protein, derived from the degradation of collagen and related to the progression of ossification, is increased in the blood. Brewerton et al. [187, 189] reported a significant increase (96%) in the incidence of the antigen HLA-B27 in the blood of patients with ankylosing spondylitis; similar findings were reported by others [230, 232, 884, 1416, 1681]. This antigen is an inherited autosomal dominant tissue antigen [104] which occurs in 4%–8% of the normal white population [187, 189]. With its essentially increased incidence, suggesting a genetically transmitted special reactivity in patients with ankylosing spondylitis, a serological test of diagnostic sensibility thus seemed to have been detected. Nevertheless, the advisability of routinely performing the test for HLA and the clinical as well as practical usefulness of this test have been disputed by Calin [230] and Vasey [1681]. Upon

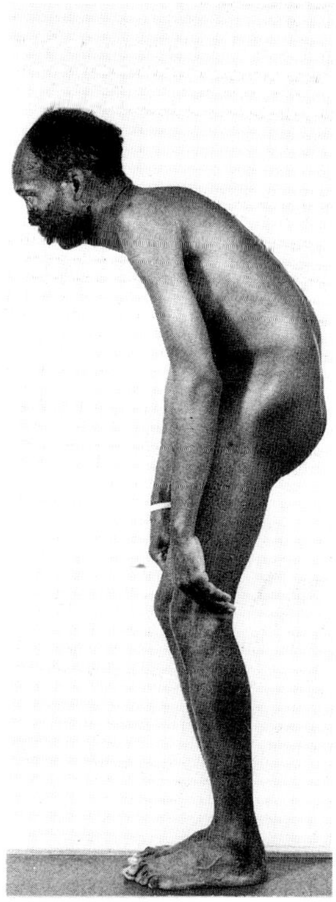

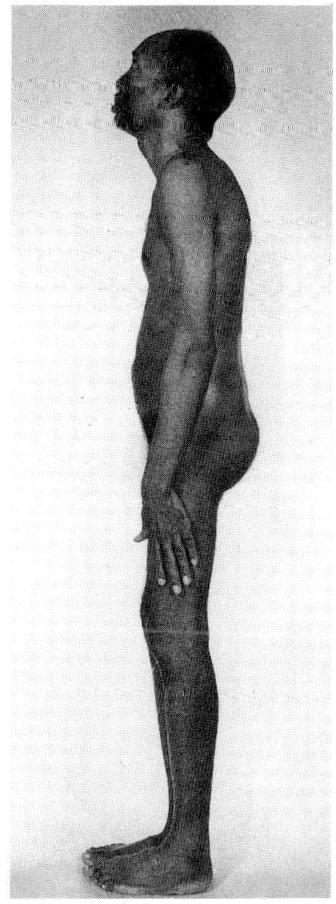

Fig. 225. The spine is stiff in marked kyphosis, and the patient is not able to look upward

Fig. 226. Following vertebral osteotomy (Fig. 233) the spine is straight, and the patient is able to look upward

evaluation of data obtained in patients with ankylosing spondylitis, Gerber et al. [597] concluded that in diagnostically questionable cases a positive test for HLA-B27 has little diagnostic validity. Testresults for rheumatoid factor are positive in only 6%–9% of patients with ankylosing spondylitis.

Roentgenographic examination [181, 1318] of the vertebral column and pelvis often reveals changes in the sacroiliac joints before the spine becomes affected [1130]. The beginning inflammation of the sacroiliac joints is characterized by irregular erosion of the joint cleft and hazy structure of the adjoining areas of the sacrum and iliac bone. In these bones osteoporosis and small spots of sclerosis subsequently appear; eventually the sacroiliac joint space becomes obliterated and partially or completely ankylosed (Fig. 227). The adjacent metaphyses contain larger areas of sclerosis and condensation. Bone proliferation “whiskering” may also be seen in the iliac crests at the attachment of tendons and ligaments (Fig. 227). More pronounced bone formation is noticed in the thoracic and lumbar spine, whose ossified anterior ligaments account for the straightening of the normally concave anterior contour of the vertebral bodies (“squaring of the vertebrae”; Fig. 232). The ossified peripheral ligamentous connec-

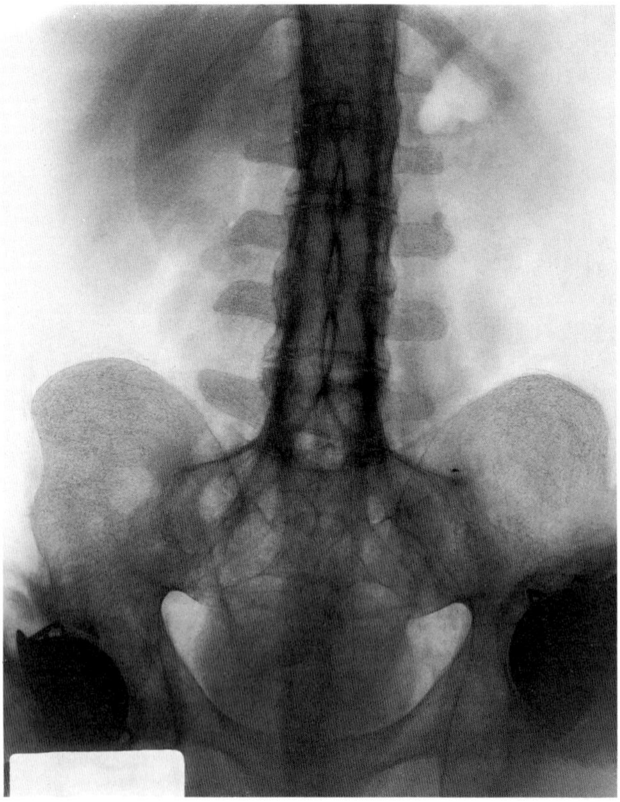

Fig. 227. The lower thoracic spine, entire lumbar spine, and upper part of the sacrum are fused by dense ossifications extending along the apophyseal joints and interspinous ligaments. Most of the intervertebral spaces and both sacroiliac joints are fused. Both hip joints underwent cup arthroplasties

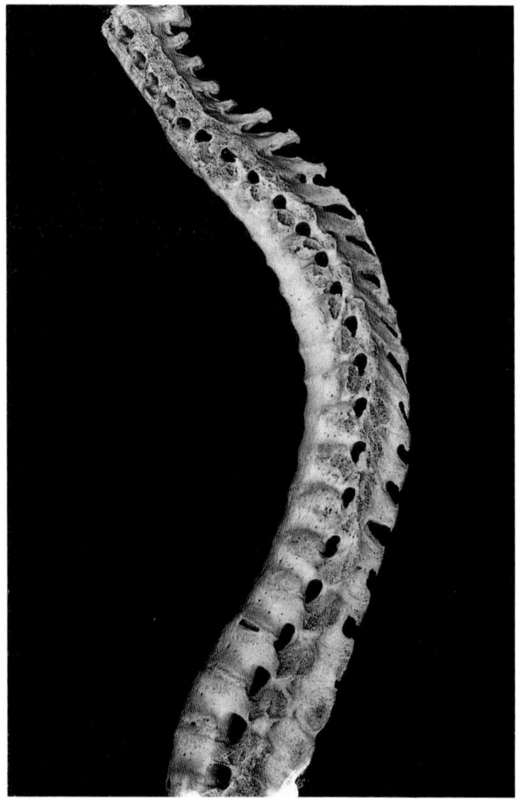

Fig. 228. The entire spine is fused at the intervertebral spaces and apophyseal joints in pronounced kyphosis

tions with the annulus fibrosus present curved syndesmophytes which expand upward and downward to the neighboring vertebrae and eventually bridge the intervertebral spaces ("bamboo" appearance, Fig. 227). In contrast to the fusion of the lumbar spine established here (Figs. 227, 232) and that of the lower or entire thoracic spine (Fig. 227), the cervical spine may display atlantoaxial subluxation. Similar subluxation may occur at lower levels of the spine at the transition between its ankylosed and nonankylosed parts. Regarding the joints of the extremities, irregular delimitation of the articular ends occurs with progressive narrowing of the cartilage space; eventually the latter disappears, and the contiguous articular ends are fused. Such changes occur chiefly in the hip joint (Fig. 227).

Gross-anatomical examination [350] carried out in the advanced stage of ankylosing spondylitis discloses extensive ossification of the paravertebral ligamentous connections, as well as fibrous or osseous ankylosis of the apophyseal joints (Fig. 228). Even more extensive ossifications are noticed in the peripheral areas of the intervertebral discs, whose ossified tissue merges with the ossified paravertebral ligaments. Thus osseous bridges are formed around and between the vertebral bodies. The sacroiliac joints are partly filled with dense granulation tissue which has eroded in several areas the adjacent articular surfaces of the sacrum and iliac bone. In the very advanced phase, these surfaces are fused to each other partly by dense connective tissue and mostly by osseous bridges (Fig. 228). The gradual changes into ankylosis are sometimes also observed in the larger joints of the extremities, such as the hip joint. Its joint capsule is substantially swollen and extensively erodes the hyaline cartilage of the articular epiphyses by villous proliferations. This causes gradual obliteration of the cartilage space and joint cavity and leads to fusion of the denuded articular surfaces by the interposed pannus. Eventually fibrous ankylosis transforms into an osseous ankylosis.

Histopathological examination of the joint capsule [1320, 1543] from the hip joint discloses in the early stage marked hyperemia of most blood vessels, whose walls show partly both segmental loss in structure and infiltration by inflammatory cells. Concurrently, the

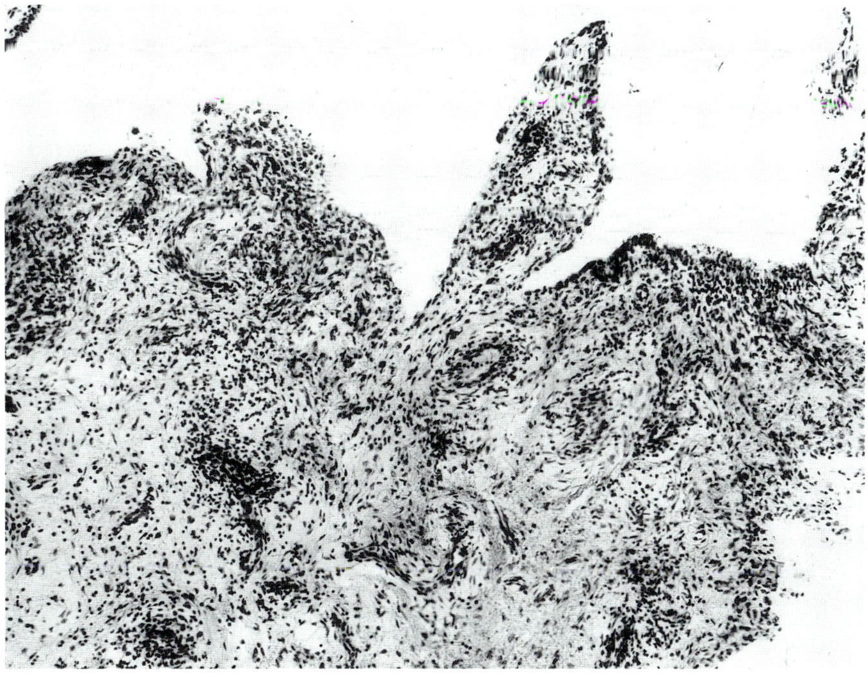

Fig. 229. Villi similar in structure to the synovial membrane rise from the latter. The hypercellular subsynoviocytic tissue contains an increased amount of collagen fibers

synoviocytes are hypertrophic and hyperplastic, while in the subjacent tissue fibroblasts proliferate, and fibrocytes are substantially increased. Extensive and dense fibrosis follows here. Secondary to superficial hypercellularity, villi are formed (Figs. 229, 231) which protrude into the joint cavity and expand over the articular cartilage by concurrently penetrating it. Eventually the contiguous articular epiphyses are united to a fibrous ankylosis which becomes ossified. The apophyseal joints of the vertebral column are similarly fused to fibrous (Fig. 230) and subsequently to osseous ankylosis. The perivertebral and paravertebral ligaments display fibrosis. The dense connective tissue of the ligaments undergoes cartilaginous metaplasia, which is followed by extensive ossification. Other areas of the ligaments directly undergo ossification. Concurrently, clones of chondrocytes appear in the fibrocartilage of the intervertebral disc and progressively enlarge to interstitial areas of hyaline cartilage (Fig. 231). The latter undergo metaplastic ossification, concurrently with the

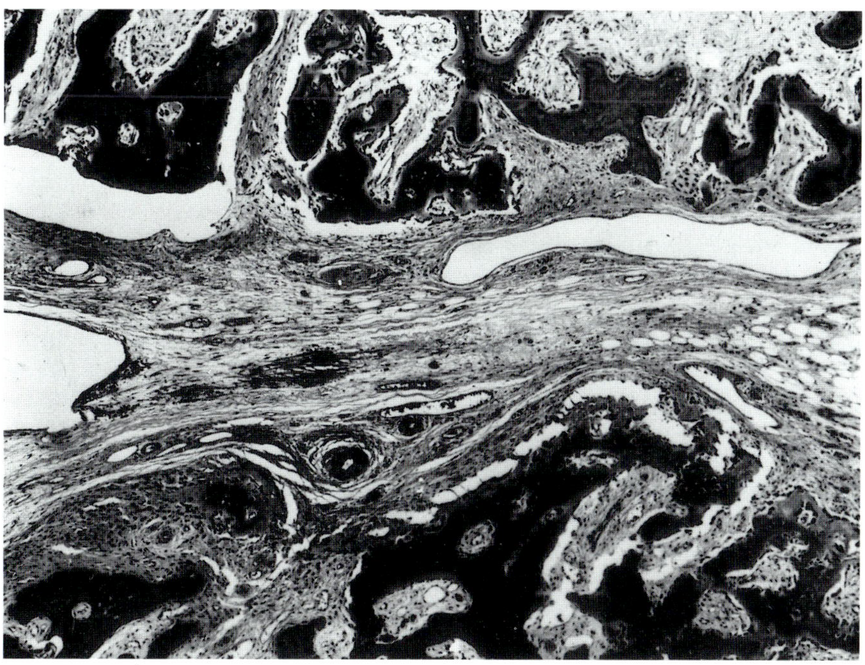

Fig. 230. The articular surfaces of the vertebral apophyseal joints are bare of their cartilage cover which has been invaded by dense connective tissue. The latter fused these articular surfaces

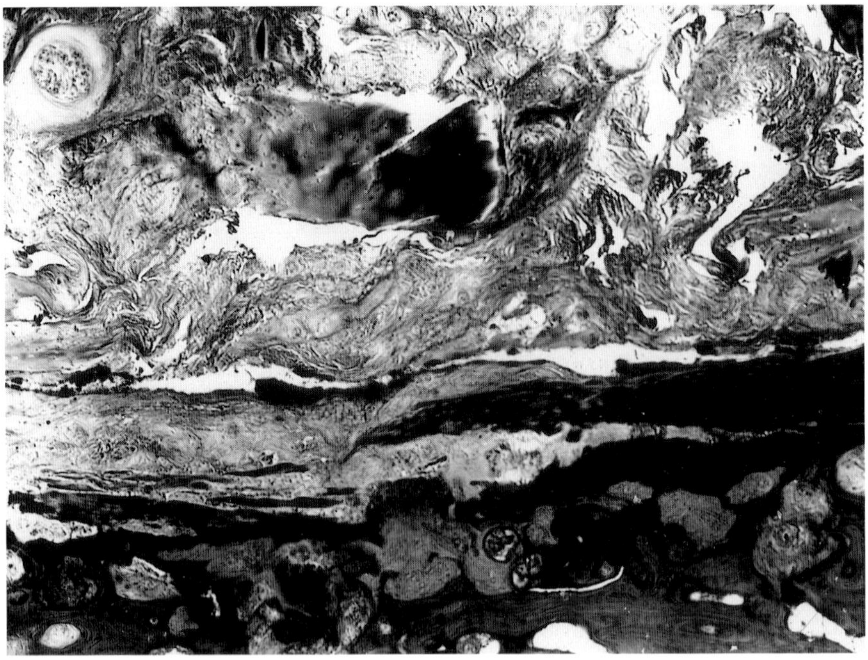

Fig. 231. The fibrocartilage of the intervertebral disc has undergone extensive metaplasia into hyaline cartilage and osteoid

ossification of the perivertebral ligaments. By expansion of these ossifications the entire intervertebral disc and its surrounding ligaments are transformed into osseous tissue.

While considered a separate entity, ankylosing spondylitis also appears in association with inflammatory diseases which primarily affect other organs of the body but may subsequently be complicated by affections of peripheral, sacroiliac, and vertebral joints. These diseases are Reiter's syndrome (Fig. 111), psoriasis (Figs. 234, 235), ulcerative colitis (Fig. 340), and regional ileitis. Results of tests for HLA-B27 are less often positive in the latter entities as long as the affection is confined to the primary extraskeletal organs but are significantly more positive (50%–60%) when the vertebral column becomes affected [187, 189]. Nevertheless, it is not reasonable for practical purposes to request the rather expensive test for HLA-B27 as a routine study [230, 1681]. Diagnosis should be based on the history, clinical examination, significant symptoms, and roentgenographic findings [232]. Rheumatoid arthritis also affects the vertebral column, but far less often than the peripheral joints, and when it does, then mostly the cervical spine (Figs. 193, 194). However, no ankylosis develops here [1470].

Treatment should be started as soon as the suspicion of ankylosing tendency has been raised. This consists primarily in education of the patient in those exercises and activities which prevent and/or correct deformation of the trunk and major peripheral joints. Regular active stretching of the vertebral column is essential, especially in cases in which a ventral flexion curve, the most frequent deformity of the vertebral column, is beginning. Active and passive stretching exercises also must be applied to the hip, shoulder, and knee joints. Proper posture must be maintained throughout the day and should be continued at night by sleeping flat on a firm mattress without a pillow, preferably in prone position. Regular swimming, especially with the breast stroke, is of great benefit because of its systematic utilization of the entire musculature of the body and concomitant deep respiration. Such breathing should be practiced daily to minimize the stiffening tendency of the costovertebral and sternocostal joints. Adherence to this program is elementary for maintaining adequate posture and continued working ability.

Of benefit are also physical therapy with supervised mobilization exercises and ultrasound of 2.5–3 W/cm^2 in one or two series of eight to ten sessions. Frequent application of moist hot packs reduce the local soreness and sensation of stiffness. Among medications, salicylates at higher doses are helpful in beginning or moderate cases. At longer intervals they should be replaced by phenylbutazone 100 mg twice daily for 1–2 weeks. Thereafter blood studies should be carried out for possible depression of bone marrow manifested by leukopenia and/or anemia [1145]. On such adverse effects, other nonsteroidal antiinflammatory medications may be used. Corticosteroids do not essentially decrease the stiffening tendency and, in view of their potential systemic complications, should be used only topically for inflammations of the eyes. Roentgenotherapy is also not advisable, considering the risk of following aplastic anemia and myelogenous leukemia [332, 1517], as

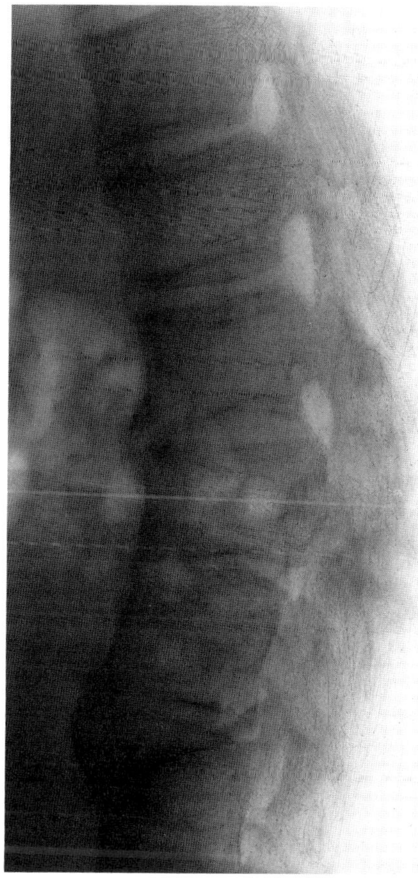

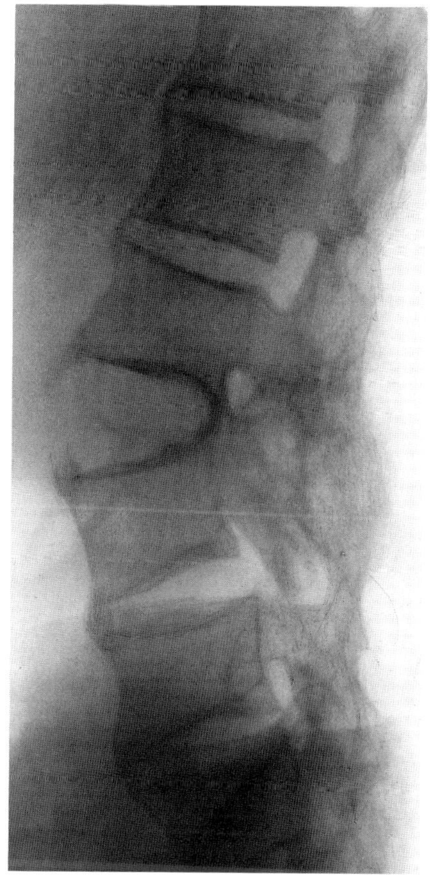

Fig. 232. The lumbar spine is fused in kyphosis by ossification of the anterior intervertebral ligament and by osseous ankylosis of the apophyseal joints

Fig. 233. The intervertebral space L2-L3 is extremely widened secondary to osteotomy and resection of the interjacent apophyseal joints. Lordosis of the lumbar spine in Fig. 232 is obtained

well as lung complications such as extensive interstitial pneumonitis. However, by adherence to the above outlined modalities a substantial deformation of the vertebral column can often be prevented, and sufficient function can be maintained. This provides most patients a satisfactory private life and adequate occupational mobility [243].

Despite all therapeutic measures, stiffening of the vertebral column occurs in 15%–20% of patients. If ankylosis developed in proper alignment secondary to postural exercises and affects only a part of the spine, these patients are able to function adequately. However, when ankylosis of the lumbar spine combined with that of the thoracic spine occurs in one arc of kyphosis (Fig. 230), and the entire body is deeply bent forward (Fig. 225), correction is necessary for functional needs. Correction is even more indicated in those situations in which the cervical spine is also ankylosed and joins the thoracic spine in marked kyphosis. The head is held in downward flexion, and the patient is not able to look forward (Fig. 225).

Operative correction appears the only modality able to restore adequate posture of the body. In this operation [1073, 1452] the patient is placed prone on the operating table, which is flexed at its junctions in such a way that it is entirely adapted in the sagittal plane to the kyphosis of the vertebral column. The latter is approached on the dorsal aspect of its midlumbar area, and a wedge – whose location and size have been predetermined on paper tracings of the roentgenograph – is excised by broad thin osteotomes. The excision starts from the spinous processes and advances through the laminae into the articular processes, which are removed as well. After inspecting the nerve roots and freeing them from surrounding scarified tissue, the operation table is gradually and very slowly straightened out under visual and palpatory inspection at the site of operation. Hereby the apex at the area of the wedge excision becomes the fulcrum of the straightening motion, and the two operated vertebrae become separated at the ventral portion of their intervertebral plates (Fig. 233), obviously by yielding of the ossified anterior longitudinal ligament. Lordosis of the lumbar spine is obtained which compensates the thoracically remaining kyphosis and provides the straightening of the body (Figs. 226, 233). To ensure such consolidation the excised wedge should be divided sagitally and applied as bone grafts onto both sides of the osteotomy. In the immediately postoperative course the patient must be watched for vital signs and neurological complications. On resumption of ambulation, a body plaster jacket or at least a thoracolumbar brace should be worn until full consolidation at the site of the wedge excision.

Fusion may also be indicated as atlantooccipital fusion in cases of atlantoaxial subluxation in which traction and rigid shoulder-head support do not provide sufficient relief. Stabilization here can be obtained by fusion with a bone graft which extends from the occiput to the fourth and fifth cervical vertebrae after inaugurating the operation with wiring.

In about 30%–40% of patients the ankylosing process also affects peripheral joints such as the hip (Fig. 227), shoulder, and knee joints, which in the phase of marked inflammation and swelling of the joint capsule develop a flexion contracture. In this phase, continuous traction and diligent mobilization exercises may succeed in averting complete stiffness of the joint. However, when ankylosis has become the outcome, only total arthroplasty – as described in "Rheumatoid Arthritis" (Figs. 222, 223) and "Ankylosis of Joints" (Figs. 500, 501) – succeeds in restoring the mobility of the joint. Even here the possibility of repeated ankylosis exists, unless the joint capsule has been totally excised.

7. Arthritis in Mediterranean Fever

Persons native from countries around the Mediterranean Sea (North Africa, Arabian countries, Israel, and Turkey) are known [457, 738, 749, 1215, 1528] to manifest a disease characterized by recurrent episodes of fever associated with attacks of pleural and/or abdominal pain and affections of joints.

The etiology of this disease has not yet been clarified. It is known [738, 749, 1486] only that it often occurs in the members of particular families. Thus being transmitted by autosomal recessive genes [1528], it afflicts siblings usually in childhood or early adolescence. The primary and predominant symptom is fever, which may be elevated to 39.5°–40° C and lasts a few hours for several days to 2 weeks, yet without marked prostration.

Episodes of pulmonary atelectasis sometimes concur with the bouts of fever [179]. However, the frequent thoracic pain is almost invariably associated with abdominal pain. Both these symptoms are caused by polyserositis [1484], and are sometimes so severe that the latter symptom simulates a serious abdominal condition; laparotomy has therefore sometimes been mistakenly performed. Another frequent symptom is joint affection, which involves asymmetrically the knee, hip,

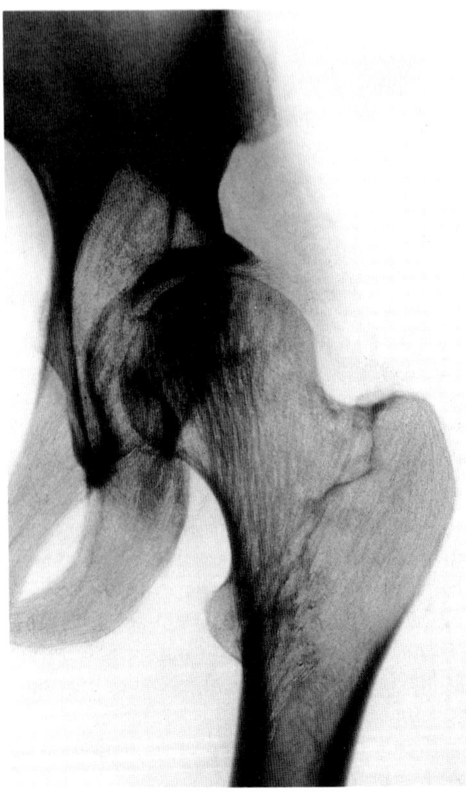

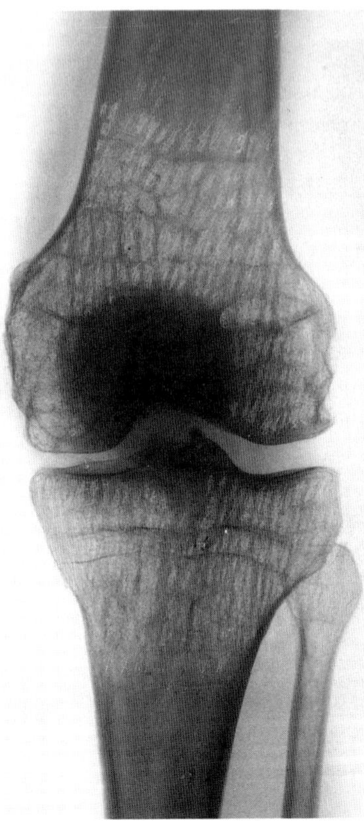

Fig. 234. The supraacetabular area presents an extensive, delimited area of marked osteoporosis. Such osteoporosis also involves the femoral head, neck, and intertrochanteric area. The joint space is narrowed but widened in one area due to uneven erosion of the femoral head. A large marginal osteophyte expands from the acetabulum

Fig. 235. The distal femoral epiphysis and metaphysis and the proximal tibial epiphysis and metaphysis are very osteoporotic. The vertical trabeculae are concomitantly very pronounced, and transverse trabeculae are abnormally present. The medial joint space is narrowed, and a marginal osteophyte expands laterally

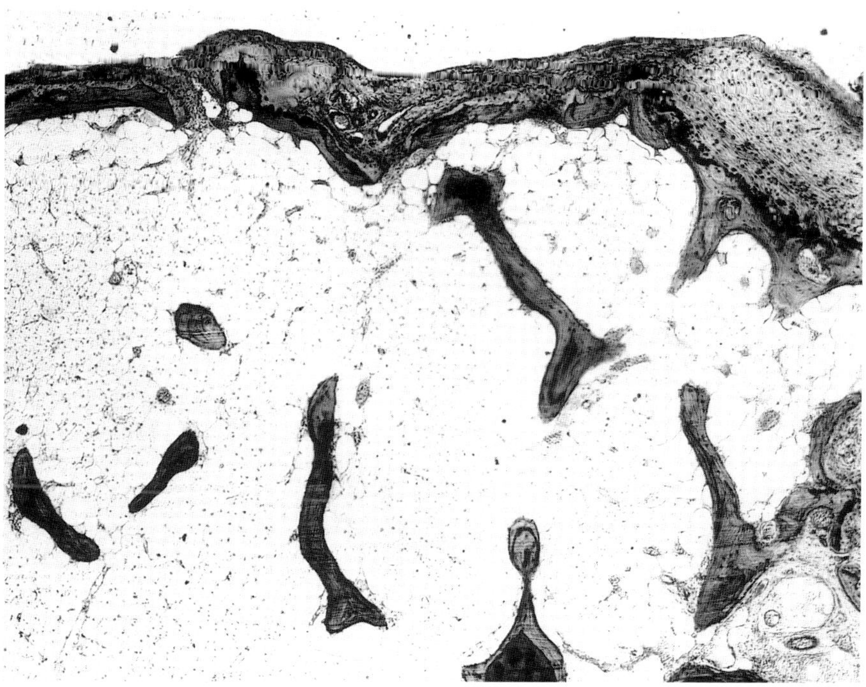

Fig. 236. The articular surface has a cartilage cover only to a small extent, and is covered otherwise by fibrosed tissue. The subcortical osseous tissue comprises very few and very thin trabecula

ankle, shoulder, and/or sacroiliac joint. According to Ehrlich [457], Heller et al. [738], Makin et al. [1008], and Siguier [1486], it may appear in the following clinical pictures.

a. Fleeting arthralgia, occurring after strain and migrating from one to another joint, is associated with mild fever and subsides after a few days of bedrest.

b. Acute, brief attacks with moderate or high fever, usually involving one joint are always associated with distinct swelling of the joint. The latter is often held in midposition by muscle tenseness. The concomitant pronounced pain is aggravated by movements of the joint. This condition resolves within 1–4 weeks.

c. Protracted attacks lasting several weeks to several months with repeated bouts of fever up to 40° C involve joints and are associated with persistent, intense pain and swelling. Joint fluid is often increased. Especially in the hip joint erosive changes of the articular epiphyses may lead to limitation of motion and function. Secondary to lasting tightness of the regional musculature and shrinking of the joint capsule a contracture of the joint may develop in a faulty position. Due to lack of function the articular epiphyses, of the hip and knee, undergo osteoporosis, which may sometimes be aggravated by a partial or complete fracture. During the protracted course of advancing articular changes, symptoms of progressive amyloidosis become manifest in enlargement of the spleen and aggravated impairment of kidney function.

Laboratory studies disclose a moderate elevation in the sedimentation rate and an increase in globulins, while the albumin and the erythrocyte counts are decreased. Gamma globulin is increased in the bouts of fever, as are the levels of circulating immune complexes [972]. On the other hand, Matzner et al. [1048] reported the deficiency of a complement-related protein in the synovial fluid and peritoneal fluid on inflammation of these cavities. Results of tests for rheumatoid arthritis are negative.

Roentgenographs [1528] reveal juxtarticular osteoporosis, less pronounced in the shoulder and elbow but very distinct and extensive in the articular epiphyses of the hip (Fig. 234) and knee (Fig. 235). In the latter two, the osteoporosis expands to the subcortical zone and is associated with almost cystic widening of the spongiosa in the femoral condyles and femoral head. Here the subchondral cortical bone is thinned to resembling an eggshell. The longitudinal trabeculae, very distinct in osteoporosis, are crossed by transversal trabeculae, an indication of disturbance in enchondral ossification during the age of growth. The cartilage space is moderately narrowed and bordered by small osteophytes.

Histopathological examination [457, 1528] discloses edematous swelling of the synovial membrane, with moderate hyperemia of the small and middlesized blood vessels and diffuse infiltration by lymphocytes, plasmacytes, and histiocytes. Infiltrates regress in the late phase, when fibrocytes proliferate at concomitant thickening of the joint capsule. The articular epiphyses merge on their surfaces with very thinned, fibrosed articular cartilage. The very wide spaces in the spongiosa of the articular epiphyses (Fig. 236) are sparingly filled with fibrosed marrow.

On the basis of the clinical picture and roentgenographic findings, this condition may be confused with arthritis in rheumatic fever, rheumatoid arthritis, or tuberculous arthritis.

Treatment so far has been only symptomatic by administering analgesics during episodes of pain. In situations of longer lasting symptoms and joint swelling, nonsteroidal antiinflammatory medications and physical therapy with shortwave diathermy in eight to ten sessions are applied. It appears on the basis of recent experiences [635, 644] that colchicine 0.6 mg given four to six times a day is able to decrease the frequency and the severity of febrile attacks.

Heller et al. [738] and Siguier [1486] indicated that even protracted attacks may resolve, if slowly, but completely and without special treatment. However, Hernes et al. [749] and Sohar et al. [1528] pointed out that in a small percentage of patients, especially those in whom roentgenographs reveal narrowing of the cartilage space, a secondary osteoarthritis develops. When followed by substantial limitation of motion and deformity, chiefly in the hip and/or knee joint, reconstructive operations are recommended [749, 1528] for improving or restoring adequate function to the joint. However, general life expectancy is substantially shortened by the expanding amyloidosis and worsening kidney function. It is hoped [1305] that regular administration of colchicine will prevent or at least diminish the incidence and extent of amyloidosis. Brauman [179] observed subsidence of pulmonary atelectasis following the intake of colchicine. On the other hand, Simmons [1503] reported a fatal complication secondary to the intake of colchicine.

V. Degenerative Changes of Joints

1. Chondropathia Patellae

Degenerative changes of peripheral joints appear most frequently in the lower extremities, and are sometimes observed primarily and distinctly in the articular surface of the patella [806]. The cause of these changes may lie in injuries or mechanical disuse, particularly in young adults who do not manifest changes in any other joint. Not only are unequivocal traumata adduced as causes of this condition but, as Buedinger [210] noted, more commonly mechanical stresses associated with vertical pressure and tangential friction. Such stresses are produced by appositional tenseness of the contracting quadriceps muscle. In this context, Karlson [854] described cases in which alterations in the patellar articular cartilage were observed secondary to repeated minor traumata. These directly posttraumatic alterations are classified as idiopathic chondropathia patellae due to the nature of the observed pathological changes. Injuries involving other parts of the knee joint, such as the menisci or cruciate ligaments, may also lead to disuse of the patellofemoral articulation, which is followed by early attrition of the patellar cartilage. The prevailing affliction of the patella in comparison with other articular epiphyses may possibly also be related to the phylogenetically and ontogenetically later appearance of the patella [1537]. Finally, malalignment such as patella alta, or lateral deviation of the patella in knock-knee or in laxity of the medial retinaculum, are invariably followed by attritional changes in the articular cartilage of the patella [414, 508, 648, 806, 833, 907, 1024, 1294, 1755]. Similar changes occur on the contiguous surfaces of the femoral condyles.

Symptoms usually begin without a directly preceding injury, but with discomfort localized around the patella. The most often reported symptoms are vague radiating pain at the final degrees of extension or flexion, insecurity within the knee, and quick fatigue. In the more advanced stage discomfort is also experienced behind the patella [328, 1630]. This sensation is aggravated to pain upon vigorous extension of the knee joint by forceful contraction of the quadriceps muscle. In very advanced alterations even episodes of buckling or brief locking in the knee joint may be experienced at normal walking.

Physical examination occasionally discloses moderate swelling of the joint capsule around the patella or slight enlargement of the entire joint due to an effusion. Thickening of the joint capsule is more pronounced in advanced cases, when the quadriceps muscle becomes atrophic secondary to prolonged limitation in the use of the knee joint. On palpation, the circumference of the patella is tender, and this tenderness extends into the medial or more rarely into the lateral joint space. Contraction of the quadriceps muscle upon concurrently pressing the patella onto its femoral bed elicits pronounced pain. Similarly, passively moving the patella on the femoral condyles cranially and caudally or medially and laterally elicits even more pronounced pain, often associated with audible crepitation or rattling noise. The range of active flexion is usually diminished, and the attempt of forced passive full flexion elicits pain in the areas of cartilage alteration [648]. Yet the most distinctive sign is direct tenderness at the areas of cartilaginous alteration within the articular surface of the patella. This can be tested by palpating the posterior patellar surface. With the patient in the supine position, the knee joint is brought into hyperextension by placing a pillow beneath the heel; hereby the quadriceps muscle is fully relaxed. The patella is pushed from its lateral border medially beyond its contact with the femur, making the medial articular facet palpable through the soft tissues. For palpation of the lateral articular facet, the patella is pushed from the medial border laterally beyond its contact with the femur. The circumscribed tenderness thus tested is a significant pathognomonic sign for chondropathia patellae.

Roentgenographs reveal a few, small, irregular areas of radiolucency sometimes bordered by sclerosis in the articular surface of the patella (Fig. 237) in a progressing phase. Conspicuous irregularity and sclerosis of this surface, bearing osteophytes at the margins and deformation of the patella (Fig. 238), are noticed in a very advanced phase. Similar changes are conspicuous in the contiguous articular surfaces of the femoral condyle.

Pathologic-anatomically the following stages may be discerned in the patellar articular cartilage. (a) In the initial stage one observes swelling and an elevated area of yellow discoloration and soft consistency leading to the designation of this as chondromalacia patellae [907]. Within the elevation, a shallow gap (Fig. 239) is filled with fragments of cartilage. (b) In the second stage, several small areas of the articular cartilage are uneven, being disrupted by fissures or clefts (Figs. 239, 243). (c) Upon expansion of the latter on the surface and at depth, fragments of cartilage are separated from the articular surface, and deep defects result in it (Fig. 243). (d) The subchondral bone is denuded over wide areas, and also partly eburnated. The articular surface is very uneven (Figs. 240, 243) small osteophytes arise at its margin. The patella has become plump (Figs. 238, 243). The medial articular facet of the patella is affected by these changes almost as often as the intermediate ridge. The lateral facet of the patella

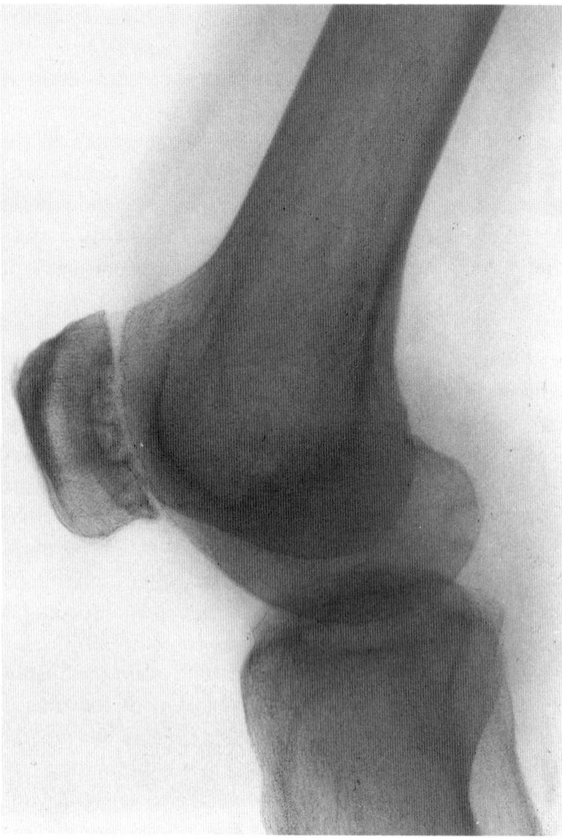

Fig. 237. The articular surface of the patella contains several small areas of radiolucency in the directly subcortical zone

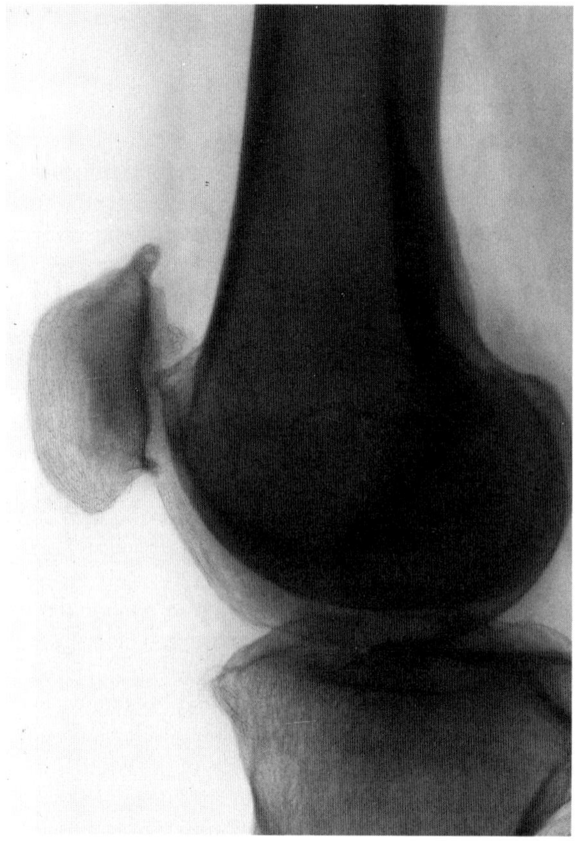

Fig. 238. The articular surface of the patella is very sclerosed and uneven. Marginal osteophytes rise on its cranial and caudal borders. The contiguous areas of the femoral condyles are also very uneven

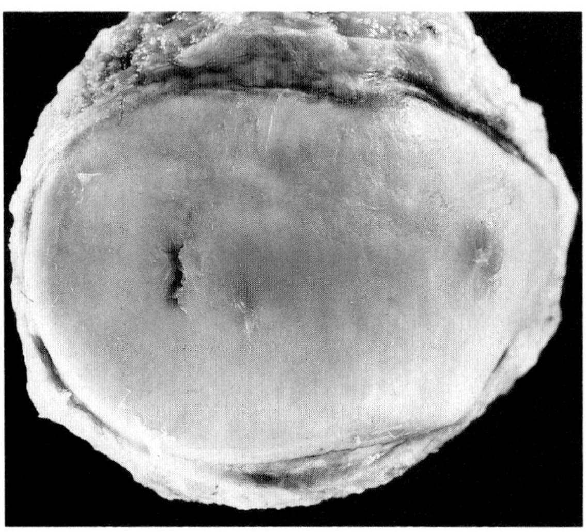

Fig. 239. The articular surface of the patella presents a few small areas of unevenness and discoloration and a deep cleft

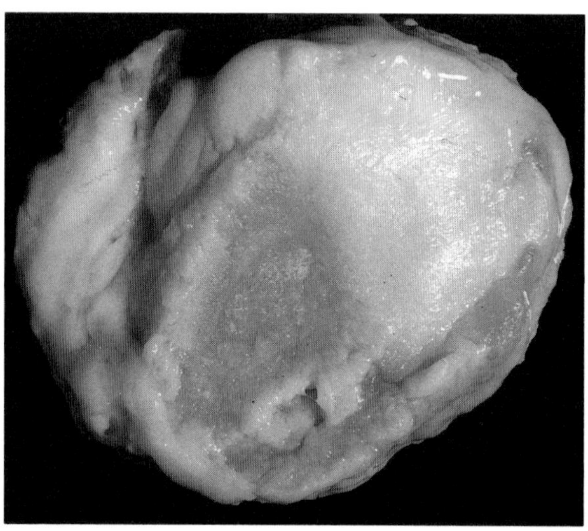

Fig. 240. The articular surface of the patella has retained its hyaline cartilage only partially. The larger part of the surface is bare of cartilage and is uneven. A marginal part is separated by a deep and long cleft.

is affected less frequently – usually in the advanced stage, when pathological changes have expanded over the entire articular surface of the patella. Similar changes are usually noticed in the contiguous articular surfaces of the femoral condyles.

Histopathological examination [120, 1080, 1082] discloses in the initial phase a changed, patchy staining pattern and disintegration of the intercellular ground substance of the articular cartilage of the patella (Fig. 241). Concurrently, chondrocytes in a few areas contain fragmented or pyknotic nuclei, while in other areas chondrocytes are enlarged or are hyperplastic to agglomerations of four to eight cells. Following unmasking of the collagen fibers, portions of the cartilage are separated along these vertical and horizontal fibers (Figs. 241, 242); defects in the articular cartilage result. The provisional calcification line (tide line) is disrupted here, and the subchondral bone is exposed. In neighboring areas the tide line is duplicated or even multiplied. Histochemical studies [760] reveal decreased and altered content of proteoglycans in the articular cartilage in the areas with beginning degeneration. Changed metachromasia by staining with toluidine blue or safranin is noted. Biochemical analyses [287, 1482] disclosed the presence of significant concentrations of beta-glucuronidase and cathepsin-D, probably responsible for the enzymatic degradation of the proteoglycans in chondropathia.

Differential diagnosis must consider injuries to the menisci and/or cruciate ligaments, loose joint bodies, or beginning osteoarthritis of all articular surfaces of the knee joint [2, 1080]. An arthrogram helps to ascertain an internal derangement which, nevertheless, does not exclude the coexistence of alterations in the patellar cartilage. Therefore, arthroscopy permitting the direct visualization of all present pathological articular components, including those of the patellar articular surfaces (Fig. 35), succeeds in clarifying the diagnosis.

With the diagnosis established [328], treatment attempts to alleviate the soreness by regular application of moist hot packs, avoidance of vigorous activities, wearing of an elastic knee cap throughout the day, physical therapy with diathermy in a series of eight to ten sessions, and systematic quadriceps exercises. Salicylates and other nonsteroidal antiinflammatory medications are of brief benefit. In habitual malalignment of the patella, transposition of the tibial tuberosity may improve the position of the patella and may min-

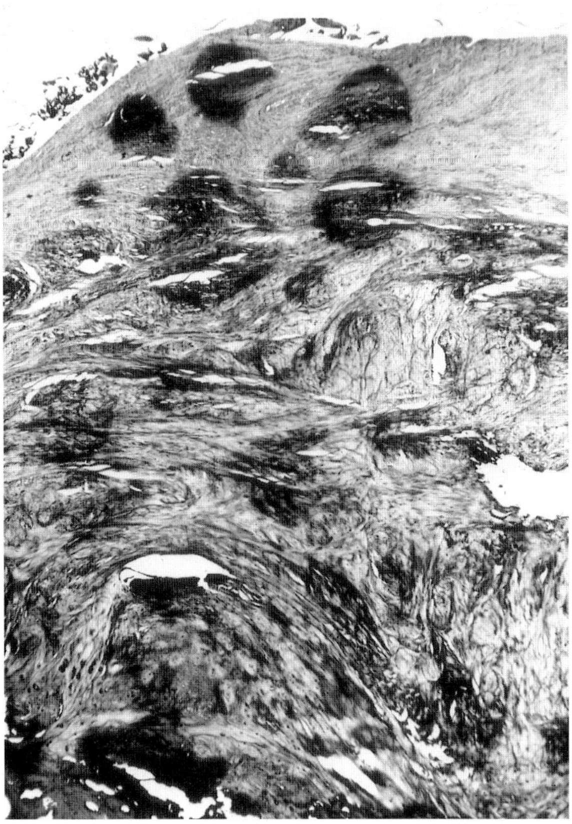

Fig. 241. The articular cartilage of the patella presents several spots of abnormal staining, indicative of changes in the ground substance, and clefts and dehiscences

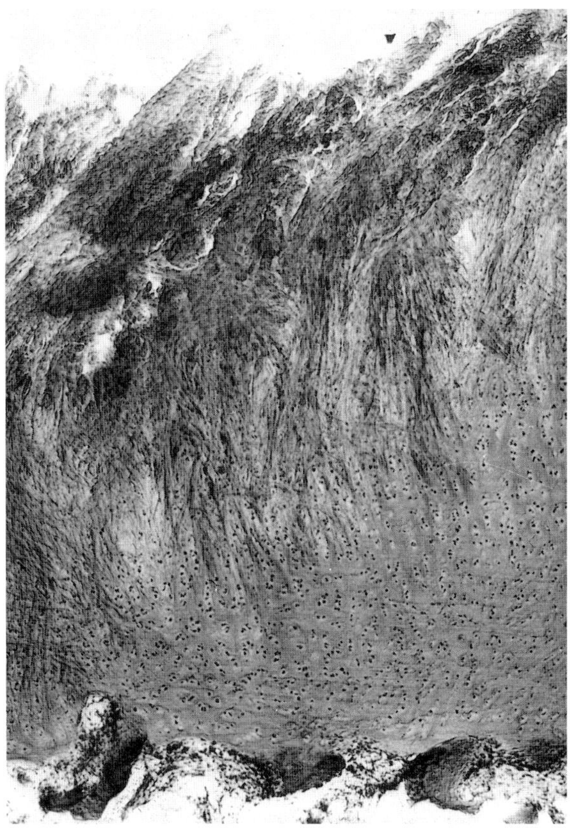

Fig. 242. The articular cartilage of the patella presents extensive unmasking of the fibers and cleft formation on the surface

imize its further attrition, but it is not able to restore the integrity of the articular surface. Therefore, with persistent or aggravated symptoms indicating expansion of the lesion of the cartilage, flat excision of the superficial defect and surgical smoothening of its edges are performed [932]. In this way healing may be obtained in the early lesions by fibrous metaplasia of the superficial cartilage, with evidence of scattered chondrocyte division and reproduction [400, 403]. In a defect of the articular cartilage extending to the bone, a deep excision through the subchondral bone is made at concurrent gradual bevelling of the margins of the defect [1755]. The rationale for this procedure is the expectation that granulation tissue will grow from the subchondral space and will fill the defect in the cartilaginous surface. The smoothening of the cartilage defect is considered a treatment which succeeds in alleviating or suppressing the symptoms at least for some time. It is also thought to prevent premature development of osteoarthritis of the entire knee joint [1755]. However, the eventual outcome of the latter does not refute the value of partial chondrectomy. Chondropathia patellae in these cases may be the primary manifestation of generalized osteoarthritis, which understandably cannot be prevented by a patellar chondrectomy. With increasing use, arthroscopy has also been applied for shaving off the cartilage in defects of chondropathia. The therapeutic outcome is similar to that obtained by the smoothening in arthrotomy, but the morbidity and the potential for complications have been significantly decreased by arthroscopic shaving [1294].

In those cases in which the above procedures fail, or the alterations of the cartilage are too extensive and/or too deep to permit a probable cure, by partial chondrectomy, total patellectomy is carried out [119, 758, 973, 1755]. The result is satisfactory regarding the symptoms related to the cartilaginous defect. However, the shortcomings of this procedure have become obvious: habitual lateral gliding of the quadriceps tendon and insufficiency of the extensor mechanism [859, 1607] due to lack of the patella. The latter transfers the force of the quadriceps muscle onto the patellar ligament. The motor effect of the quadriceps muscle is substantially diminished due to its impaired lever action. Along with it the stability and reliability of the knee joint is decreased. Therefore, the substitution of the patella by a prosthetic metallic device [400, 806, 1784] has been recommended. However, the gliding of this substitute is not always even and smooth, and this impairs the undisturbed movement between femur and tibia. Similarly, the resurfacing procedure by Insall et al. [806], although maintaining the organic connection between the patella and its tendon and ligament, does not provide adjustable articulating due to the metallic surface of the patella, and may be associated with painful crepitation against the femoral condyles.

It therefore appears more physiological to retain the patella and to make it more serviceable by an operative procedure which provides an organic articulating surface. After having exposed and shaven the defective areas of the articular surface (Fig. 243), the entire articular surface of the patella is covered with one or two pedunculated flaps of synovial and adipose tissue derived from the infrapatellar and suprapatellar inner parts of the joint capsule (Fig. 244). In aftercare, active and passive mobilization exercises of the patella and the knee joint as well as isometric strengthening exercises of the quadriceps muscle are necessary. Follow-up examinations after this operation diselose subsidence of the soreness behind and around the patella, its smooth and noiseless gliding on the corresponding surface of the femur, moderate limitation of its medial and

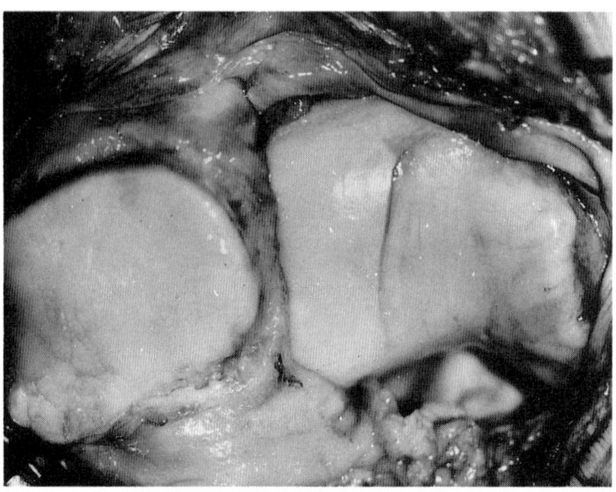

Fig. 243. On arthrotomy, the patella has been laterally subluxated. The patella presents a large area of unevenness. The lateral femoral condyle presents a long and deep cleft, and the medial femoral condyle is uneven

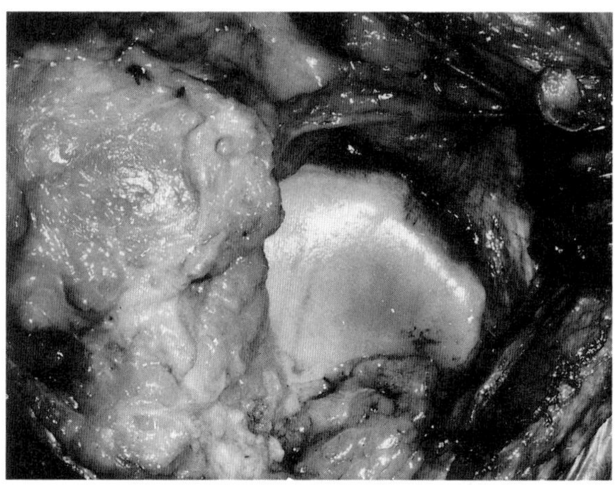

Fig. 244. The surface of the lateral femoral condyle is partly visible. The patella is completely covered with a flap of connective-adipose tissue

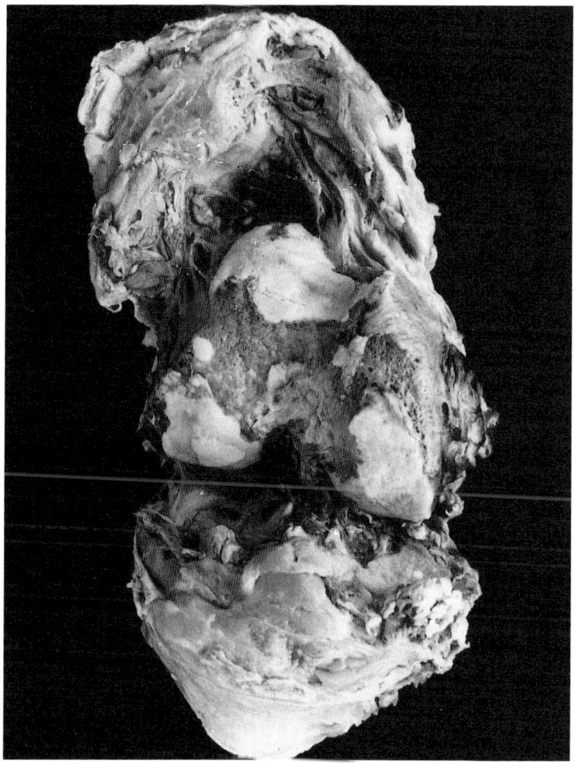

Fig. 245. The articular cartilage of the knee joint is worn off upon sharp delimitation and on a larger extent. The articular surfaces are penetrated by indentations; small osteophytes protrude at their margins

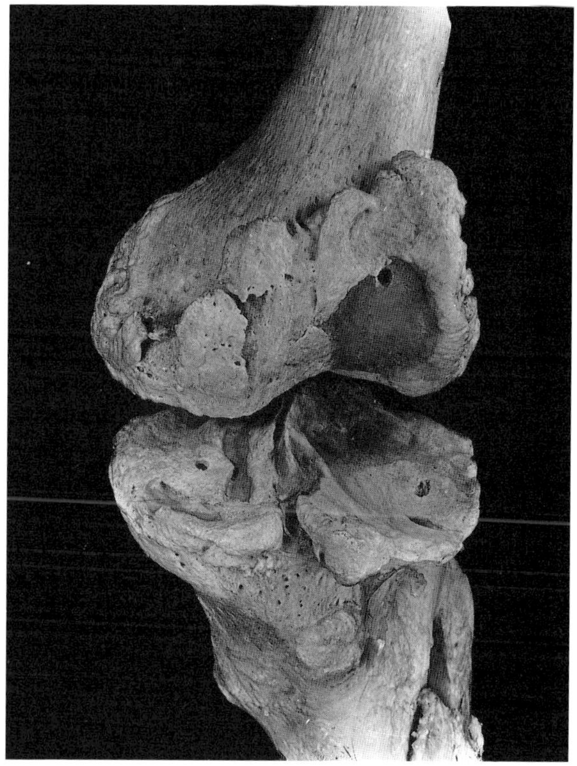

Fig. 246. The articular surfaces of the knee are completely denuded and worn off; grooves and small cavities expand into their depth. Broad, marginal osteophytes rise around these surfaces

lateral excursion, and almost full reattainment of the contractile force of the quadriceps muscle.

2. Osteoarthritis

Among the joint diseases, osteoarthritis has drawn increasing attention owing to the recognition that it is the most frequent joint disease. This condition develops either as a primary disease in most elderly persons or as a secondary disease as a sequela to injuries, discongruities, inflammations, or most other ailments of joints. The National Arthritis Data Workgroup reported that 12% of the adult population of the United States had osteoarthritis in 1989. Accompanying the substantially increased life expectancy among the elderly, the percentage of adults suffering from osteoarthritis can be expected to increase. Wagenhaeuser [1700] reported a frequency of degenerative joint changes in central Europe comparable to that in the United States. Since it has also been realized from numerous publications that the articular cartilage manifests the initial osteoarthritic changes, its pathology [174, 736, 1293] should be discussed as an introduction to osteoarthritis, thus clarifying the etiology and pathogenesis of this disease.

In beginning osteoarthritis of the peripheral joints [1125, 1532] the hyaline cartilage of the articular surfaces macroscopically has partially lost its shiny smooth bluish white surface. It presents irregularly delimited, uneven areas which lie below the level (Figs. 245, 247) and are discolored yellowish. These areas become more extensive by confluence and subsequently display a striping which assumes an asbestoslike coarse fibrillation, gradually expanding into the depth. By further disruption of the cartilage, the underlying bone becomes exposed (Fig. 245). The denudation is followed by indentations in the central areas of the articular surface (Figs. 245, 247), while small spurs grow out at the margin of the articular surface (Fig. 246) and gradually enlarge to plump elevations. These osteophytes have a smooth surface with a cartilaginous cover which may also display areas of fibrillation and/or facets of attrition. Similar facets, resembling the traces of cartwheels, sometimes traverse the articular surfaces (Fig. 246). In the latter, the subchondral bone is denuded in places; it has become sclerosed (Figs. 246, 248), smooth, and shiny like polished ivory (eburnation). Such changes follow in other areas of the surface (Fig. 246). However, in a few places the denuded bone is thin and osteoporotic and is often disrupted by discontinuities through which

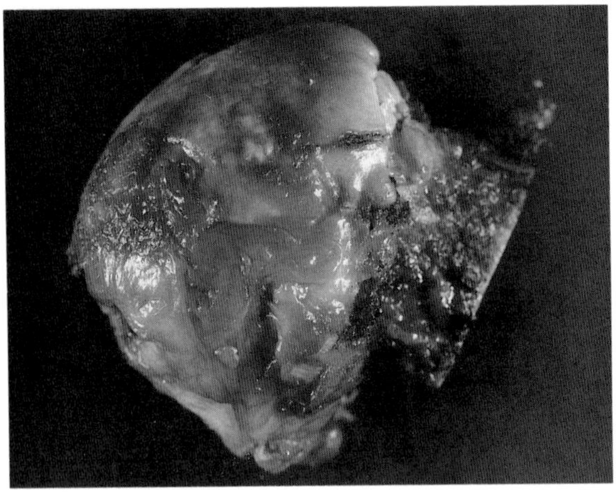

Fig. 247. The articular cartilage of the femoral head is worn off chiefly in the central area. The articular cartilage in the peripheral area is very uneven, and is disrupted by deep indentations and clefts.

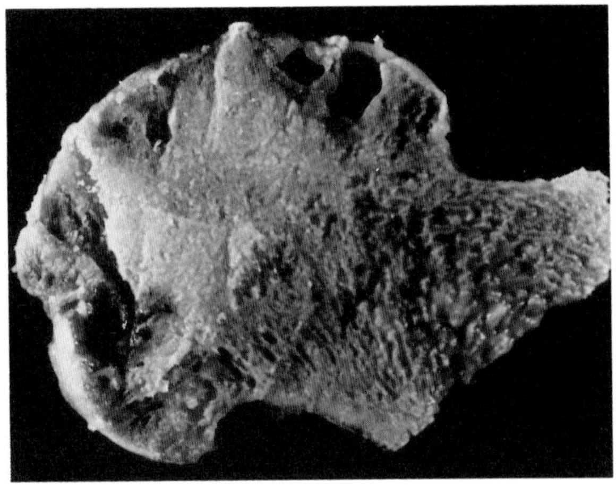

Fig. 248. The femoral head is very uneven particularly at its central area, and the articular cartilage is worn off over the entire surface. Several large cysts lie in the subcortical area. The osseous tissue beneath one extensive cyst is very sclerosed

hyaline cartilage sometimes expands from the surface into the subcortical marrow spaces (Fig. 248). In other instances, these spaces are rather wide and are filled either with myxomatous or loose connective tissue which is bordered by a rim of thickened bone (Fig. 248). The increasing growth of the marginal osteophytes, the mirrorlike grinding down of the opposing articular ends, and the expanding attrition of the more central parts of the cartilaginous surfaces (Fig. 247) effect a far-reaching transformation of the articular ends (Fig. 246). The latter have lost either in protruding convexity or in indented concavity, followed by attritional flattening of their surfaces, but they have increased in latitude by marginal apposition (Fig. 246). Eventually they assume mushroomlike shapes in extreme cases. In view of this deformation, also involving the subjacent bone, the term osteoarthritis is used in the English-language literature for the hypertrophic arthritis, while that of arthrosis deformans is preferred in most European publications to indicate the degenerative nature of this joint condition.

The concurrent changes in the joint capsule initially involve the synovial membrane, which is moderately reddened and swollen but gradually becomes dis-

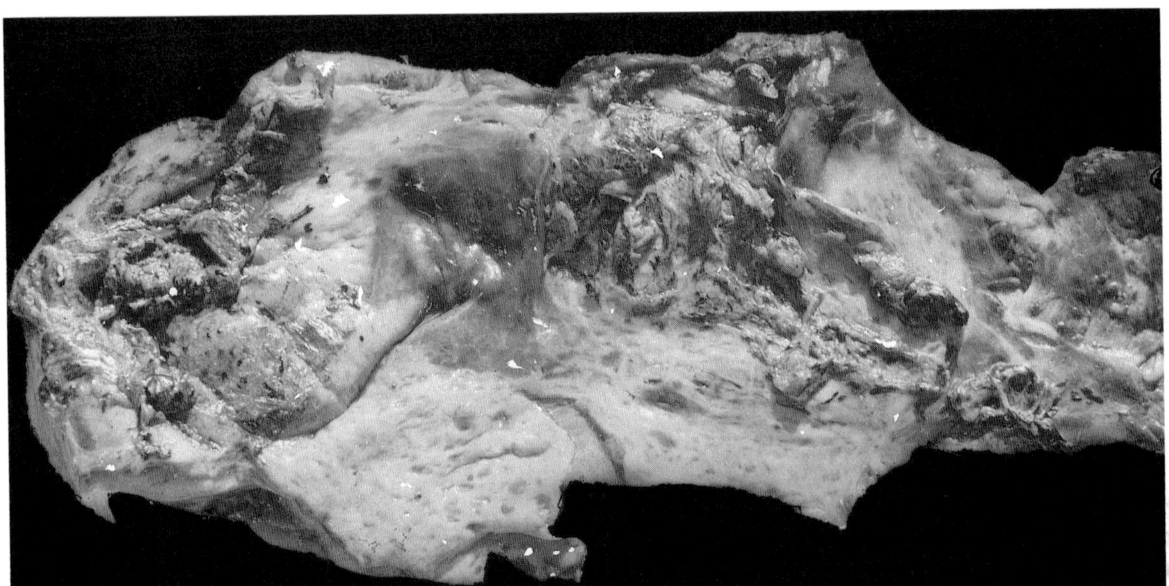

Fig. 249. The inner part of the joint capsule is uneven in the central area by plump villi, nodular elevations, and thick folds. The remainder of the tissue is rather even and very dense

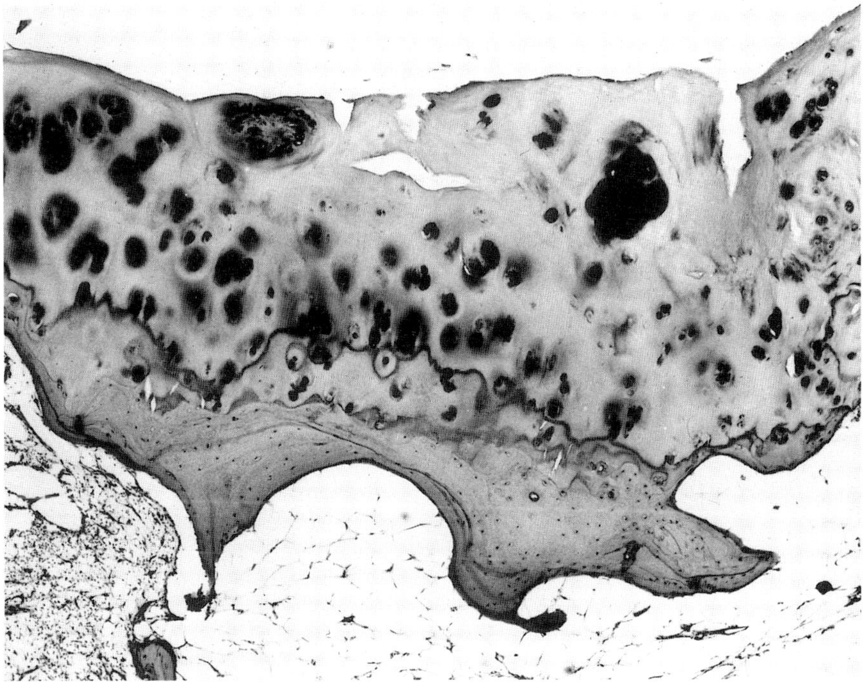

Fig. 250. The surface of the articular cartilage is disrupted by short vertical and horizontal clefts. A few chondrocytes are necrotic or have small, fragmented nuclei, but the majority are hypertrophic or hyperplastic and are surrounded by large halos of intensely stained ground substance. The tide line is duplicated

colored grayish and more dense (Fig. 249). In this phase the inner surface of the joint capsule is uneven by the outgrowth of short plump elevations (Fig. 249) which narrow the joint cavity. These villi and folds often border small outpouchings, which sometimes contain free bodies stemming from fractured marginal osteophytes, detached portions from the articular ends, or torn-off calcified villi. In advanced cases, the densification expands into the outer layer of the joint capsule and produces substantial thickening and hardening of the latter.

Histopathologically [261, 1079, 1080, 1082, 1314, 1351, 1352, 1530, 1532] the changes in the articular cartilage are initially observed in a changed staining pattern. The ground substance comprises spots of irregular staining (Fig. 241) or irregularly delimited areas of decreased basophilia on hematoxylin-eosin-phloxin-safran-staining. Similar irregularities may be observed on safranin or metachromatic staining. Mallinger et al. [1012, 1013] pointed out that the proteoglycans of the articular cartilage undergo structural changes with advancing age; the keratansulfates are increased in the interterritorial matrix. With this the staining as well as the mechanical properties of the articular cartilage are changed. The chondrocytes present shrinking of their cell bodies and retraction from the surrounding ground substance, with a widening of their pericellular lacunae. Their nuclei are smaller and very dense or fragmented or completely absent (Fig. 250). Areas with tombs of chondrocytes, Weichselbaum's lacunae [1727], then appear. In their neighborhood, viable chondrocytes have become hypertrophic and hyperplastic in clusters by clonal growth and are surrounded by broad halos of markedly intensified basophilic-staining ground substance, indicative of increased production of proteoglycans (Fig. 250). In other areas the basophilia decreases, the ground substance becomes disintegrated [1351, 1352], and the collagen fibers are separated and distinct – they are "unmasked". Then, starting with the superficial horizontal fibers [1253] and subsequently involving the vertical fibers, the hyaline cartilage assumes a striped structure which follows the arcade arrangement of the interstitial fibers (Figs. 5, 7, 251). By further decomposition of the binding ground substance, the interfibrillar dehiscences widen to clefts which by confluence separate flakes of cartilage (Fig. 250). Defects result, with poorly stained cartilage cells at their base or with complete denudation of the underlying cortical bone.

In such attritional furrows, the denuded bone becomes smoothened and sclerosed secondary to substantial thickening of its trabeculae (Fig. 254). In the neighboring area, the zone of calcified cartilage expands toward the surface into the residual hyaline cartilage, whereupon the tideline multiplies (Figs. 250, 252). However, in other areas osteoclastic activity prevails, and the trabecula become thinned. This bone surface suffers discontinuities; subjacent marrow spaces are opened, and cavities are formed by lacunary resorption. Through the discontinuities, portions of hyaline cartilage may be displaced from the surface into the depth,

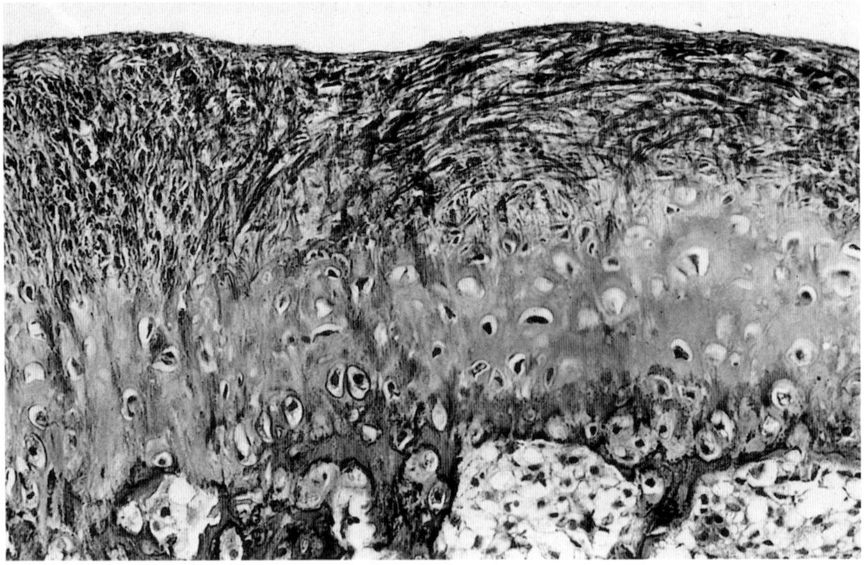

Fig. 251. The ground substance in the superficial zone is completely missing. The interstitial collagen fibers are unmasked, and their arcade course is manifest. Some chondrocytes have fragmented nuclei, and several lacunae from chondrocytes are scattered

where they proliferate due to maintained vitality (Figs. 252, 253). In other instances [1108, 1375] synoviocytes and fibrocytes are dislodged from the articular cavity through discontinuities in the subchondral bone into the subcortical marrow spaces (Fig. 255). There they either multiply and form masses of loose or dense connective tissue (Fig. 255), or they undergo mucoid degeneration and assume stellate shape (Fig. 256). Due to growth and expansion of these formations, the surrounding cancellous bone initially undergoes osteoclastic resorption, until eventually by reactive new bone formation a delimitation of these cystic cavities by sclerosed bone follows (Figs. 255, 256).

The subchondral bone marrow, stimulated in a few areas beneath thinned cartilage cover, sometimes proliferates into the layer of basal cartilage cells at concurrent multiplication of the tideline (Fig. 252). The vascularization from the subchondral bone marrow and the multiplication of the tideline cause progressive thinning of the cartilage cover from its basis (Fig. 254). On the other hand, the in the marginal areas of the articular surface under the stimulus of intermittent

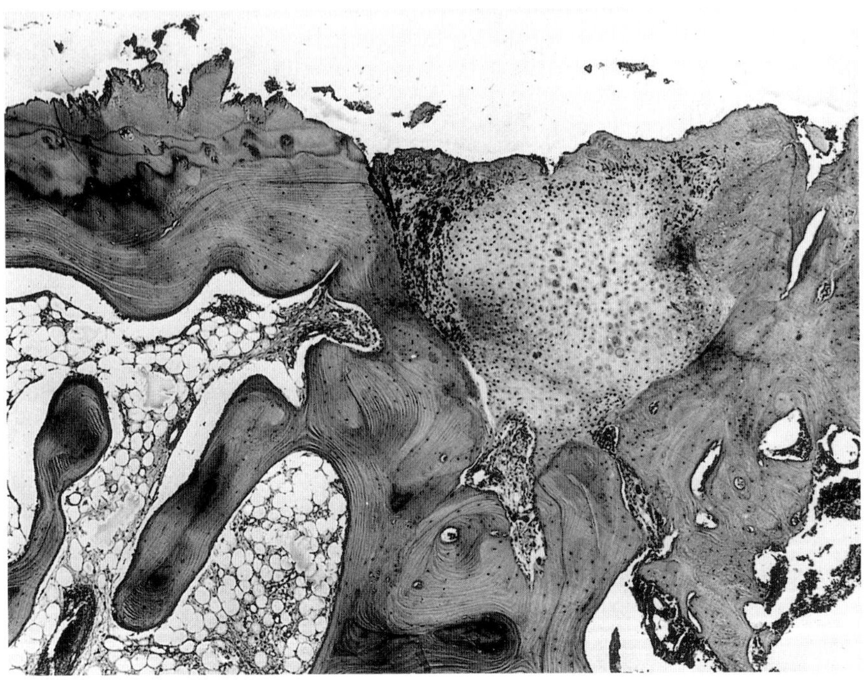

Fig. 252. The articular cartilage is very thinned in one area and is absent in another area. In the latter, a large clump of hyaline cartilage is deeply displaced through a gap in the subchondral bone. The latter is markedly thickened

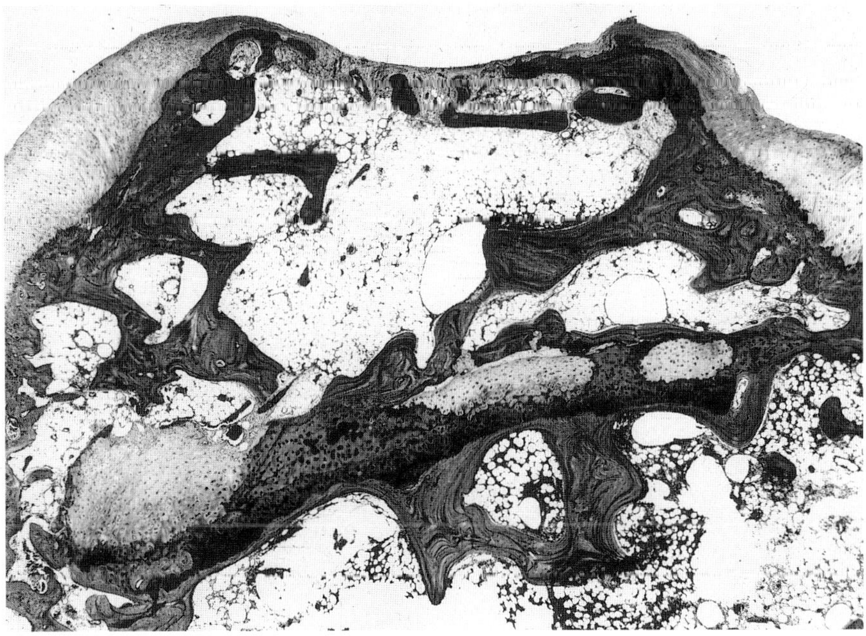

Fig. 253. The central area of the articular surface is bare of articular cartilage and has a thin cover of fibrosed tissue. Portions of articular cartilage are displaced into the depth, where they fuse with the metaphyseal plate

pressure. Secondary to local enchondral ossification, these cartilage elevations develop to marginal osteophytes (Fig. 257) which have lamellar structure and a cap of hyaline cartilage. Thus atrophic and sclerosed portions of the articular surface alternate with each other; on disintegration of the articular cartilage, reparative processes set in from the subchondral bone (Fig. 254). The combination of the changes is characteristic for the histopathology of osteoarthritis.

Electron-microscopic examinations [1079, 1080, 1589, 1735] disclose that the chondrocytes extend a few cytoplasmic processes. On the inner side of their cell membrane lie micropinocytotic vesicles (Fig. 258). The rough endoplasmic reticulum consists of regularly aligned membranes enclosing moderately dilated cisternae. The Golgi complex (Fig. 258) is composed of lamellae which enclose vacuoles and large vesicles. In addition, separate vacuoles and vesicles are scattered

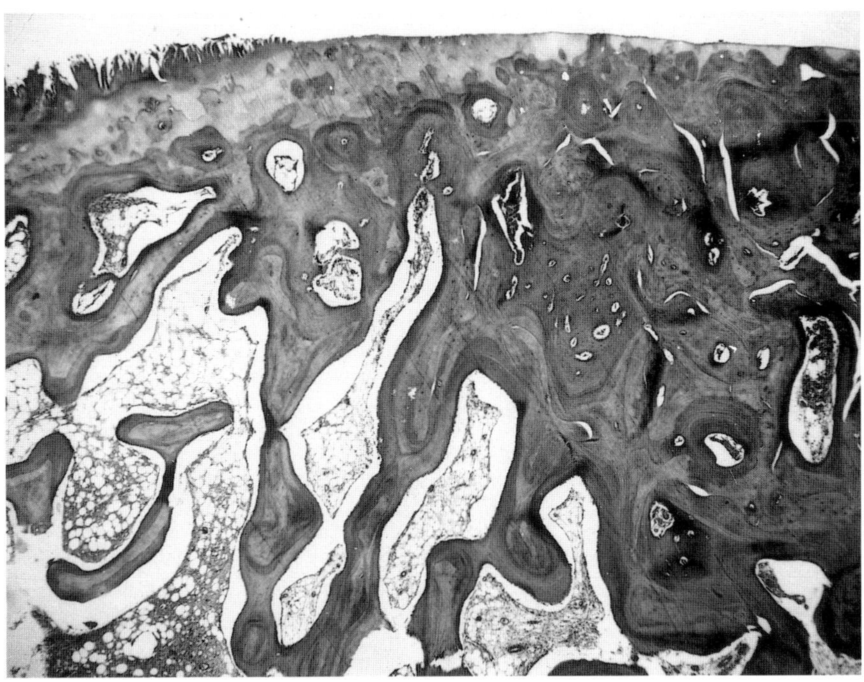

Fig. 254. The articular surface has remained over a short extent with articular cartilage, which is very thinned and disrupted by many vertical clefts. In the area bare of articular cartilage, the subchondral bone is extensively thickened and sclerosed

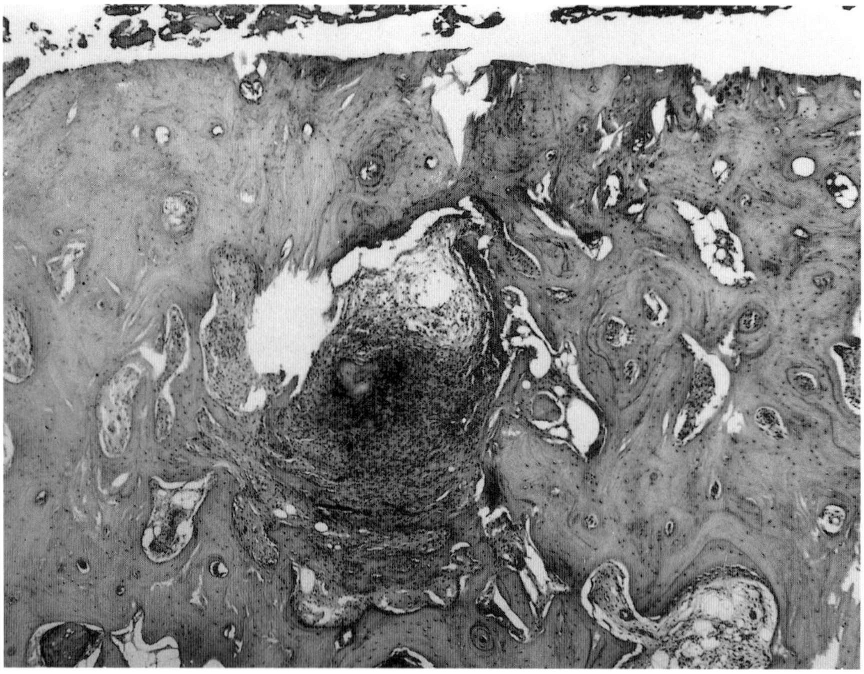

Fig. 255. Dense connective tissue is displaced into the depth through a gap in the denuded and sclerosed subchondral bone. The surrounding bone is partly resorbed and partly more sclerosed; a cystic cavity has formed

throughout; some of the latter contain a dense material. Many chondrocytes also contain fine filaments and ovoid bodies of an electron-dense material. The nucleus of indented outline is delimited by a double membrane and contains a nucleolus and chromatin-dense granules. In advanced age, many chondrocytes become disorganized with formation of membranous remnants, granular particles, and lipidic debris. Similar disintegration occurs in the nucleus by fragmentation and densification of the nuclear membrane, nucleolus, and chromatin.

The inner part of the joint capsule histopathologically [603, 630, 633, 797, 1368] manifests in the beginning phase [1543] moderate hypertrophy of the synoviocytes and slight to moderate hyperemia as well as moderate edema of the subsynoviocytic tissue (Fig. 259). The latter contains a small number of focal infiltrates composed chiefly of lymphocytes and less so of plasmacytes and

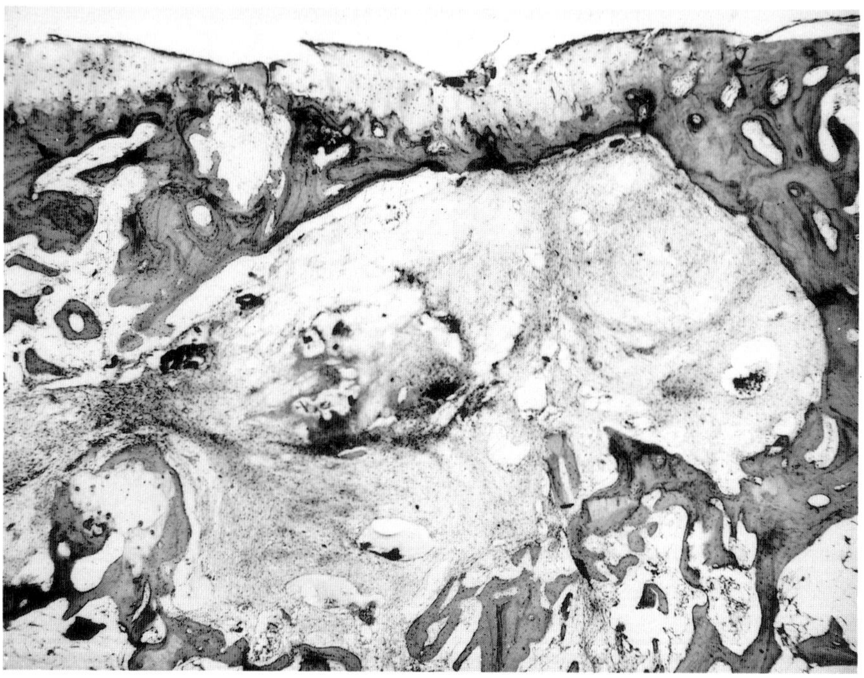

Fig. 256. Connective tissue beneath a partly disrupted and partly sclerosed articular surface is extensively transformed into mucinous tissue. A cystic cavity bordered by sclerosed bone has formed

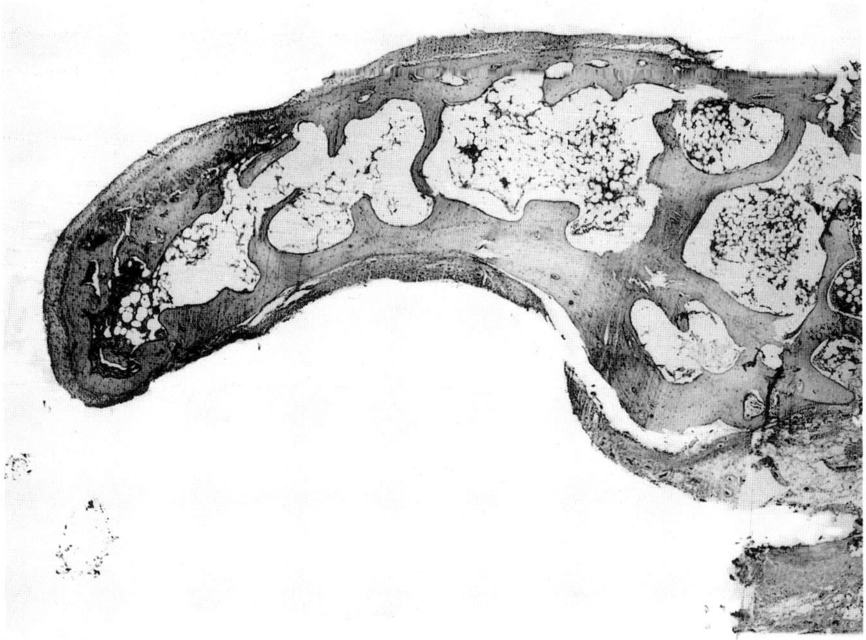

Fig. 257. A marginal osteophyte expands from the articular surface. It merges on its surface in some places with articular cartilage and in others with dense connective tissue

histiocytes. In a few instances the hyperemia, edema, and inflammatory infiltrates are more extensive and diffuse. Subsequently the subsynoviocytic tissue becomes more cellular in fibrocytes and a few fibroblasts (Fig. 260). Eventually, the synoviocytes multiply in the progressing phase and form a cover two to four rows thick (Fig. 261). Beneath them the fibrocytes also increase. Due to its hypercellularity the subsynoviocytic tissue rises together with the synoviocytes in villi of considerable thickness (Fig. 261). The amount of broad collagen bundles increases concurrently and assumes an overwhelming proportion (Fig. 261) which appears to compress the regional cells and blood vessels. In cases of long duration and following conspicuous increase in fibrocytes, the fibrosis extends from the subsynoviocytic tissue to the outer layers and causes marked thickening of the entire joint capsule. Occasionally, portions of articular cartilage and subchondral bone, obviously separated from the articular surface, are lodged in the subsynoviocytic tissue.

Electron-microscopic examination of the synovial membrane [630, 797, 1364] discloses that the synoviocytes are roundish or plump cuboidal and extend a few filopodia. Their cytoplasm contains a small amount of

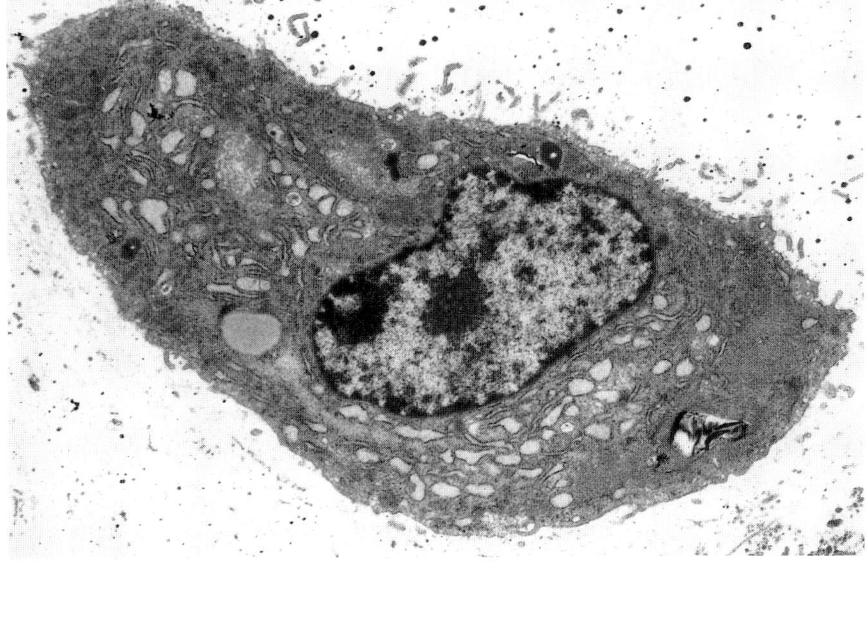

Fig. 258. Electron microscopy of a chondrocyte from a femoral head in osteoarthritis discloses that, compared with a chondrocyte from a normal joint (Fig. 6), it contains more abundant ergastoplasm and very pronounced organelles of the Golgi complex in larger quantities

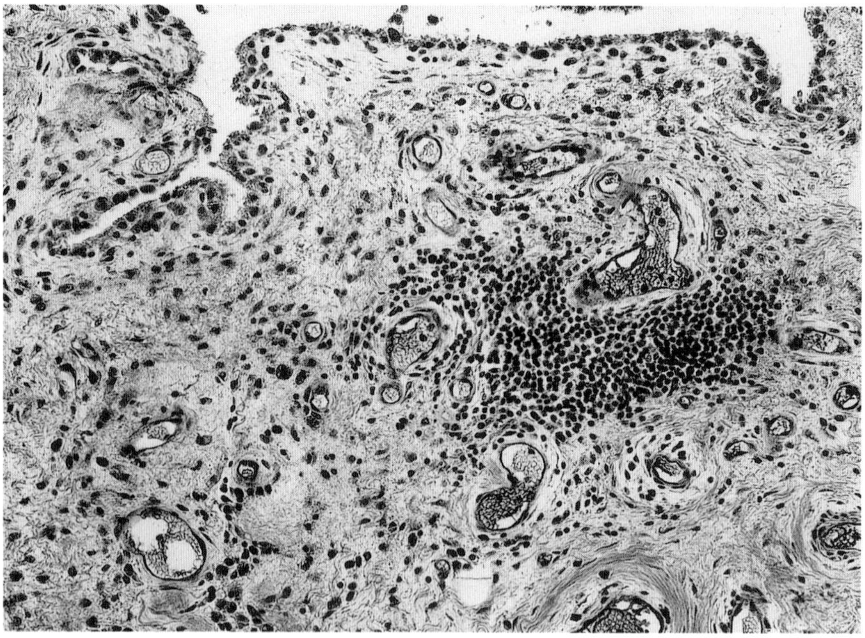

Fig. 259. The synovial membrane has moderately hypertrophic synoviocytes and is elevated in small and flat villi. The subsynoviocytic tissue is moderately hypercellular with fibrocytes. All blood vessels are moderately hyperemic. A large accumulation of lymphocytes surrounds a larger blood vessel

special organelles. The rough endoplasmic reticulum has thin trabecular stacks; its cisternae are very dilated and contain a scant electron-dense material of granular or fibrillar precipitates. The lysosomes are in small number and contain electron-dense granules and lipid droplets. The mitochondria are very short and have flattened cristae.

The changes of the synovial membrane comprise several, although slight to moderate features which characterize inflammation [587, 589, 590, 630, 633, 980 B, 1543]; these justify the designation of arthritis [30, 32, 458, 596], in contrast to the term arthrosis, as suggested by Mueller [1151]. The latter term is used mostly in the European medical literature to indicate the degenerative character of this entity. However, since this joint disease is initiated by degeneration of the articular cartilage, the use of the term chondrosis appears very descriptive. Thus it is appropriate to refer to this entity as chondrosarthritis [1556]. This designation also appears etiologically justified because experimental studies of George et al. [596] indicate that substances from hyaline cartilage injected into the joint cavity elicit an inflammatory reaction of the synovial membrane. However, no justification can be adduced

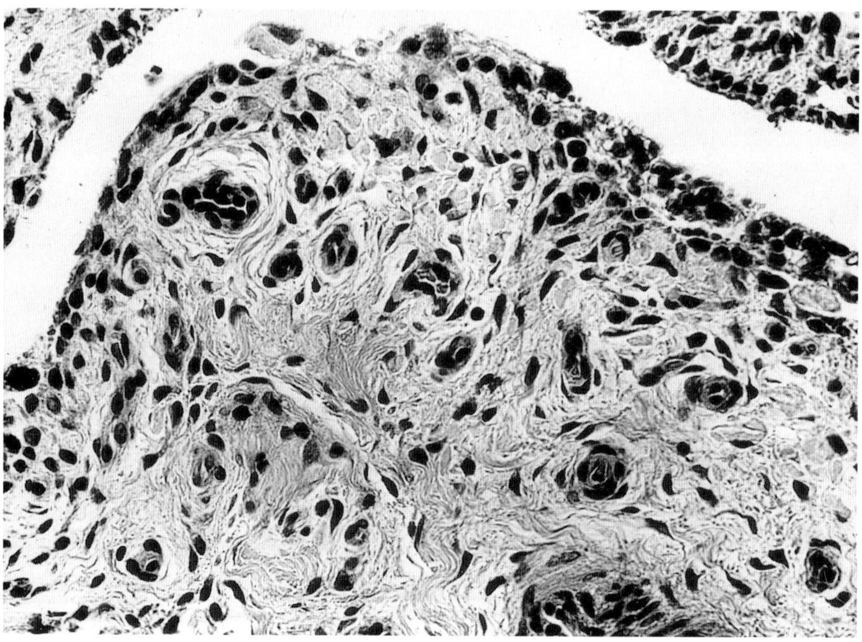

Fig. 260. The synovial membrane has moderately hypertrophic hyperplastic synoviocytes and is moderately hypercellular with fibrocytes and fibroblasts in the subsynoviocytic tissue. The collagen fibers are moderately increased

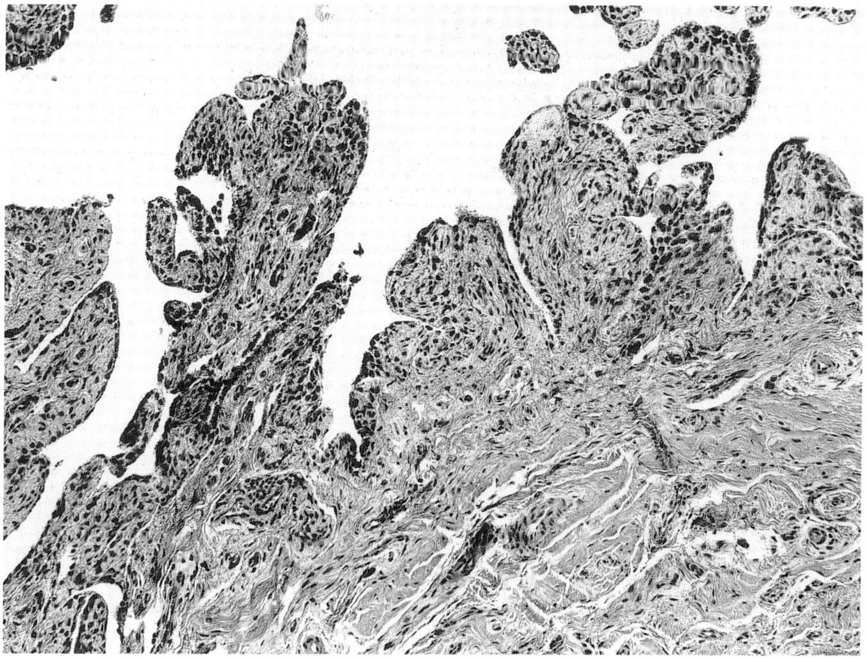

Fig. 261. The synovial membrane is raised in many, rather large villi, some of which are ramified. The subsynoviocytic tissue contains moderately increased fibrocytes and is very dense by substantial increase of the collagen fibers

for the prefix "osteo-" (osteoarthritis) since no research so far has established this type of joint disease to originate from osseous tissue or even to involve it particularly. Nevertheless, the term osteoarthritis is maintained in this treatise due to its conventional use in the English-language medical literature. It is hoped that consideration of the underlying tissue changes will eventually lead to the use of the proper designation chondrosarthritis.

The histopathological changes in the articular cartilage, proliferations in the subchondral marrow, and conspicuous marginal osteophytes provided the basis for Pommer's functional theory of osteoarthritis. Pommer [1270] emphasized the mechanical importance of the hyaline cartilage, which by virtue of its structure is able equally to distribute oncoming pressure and to protect the subjacent bone from undue stress. However, the altered articular cartilage, impaired in its elasticity, is no longer able to fulfill its buffering function. Subsequently, all normal stresses are transmitted as insults to the depth and cause irritation of the subchondral bone marrow. The latter protrudes into the basal layer of the articular cartilage and contributes from the depth to its further thinning. The subsequent changes eventually lead to deformity of the articular surfaces. The pathogenesis of osteoarthritis [154, 155, 458, 460, 596, 802, 1016, 1020, 1034, 1155, 1395, 1532] is herewith explained, but not its etiology. The attempt of Heine [736] to incriminate the mere function of joints as the etiology of osteoarthritis is inadequate. This cannot explain why osteoarthritis appears in some individuals at early age and in others at late age despite vigorous use of their joints. Thus additional factors inherent in the body or joints must be taken into consideration; these are presumably general constitution and local disposition of the articular tissues.

Therefore, osteoarthritis originating from not yet fully identified factors is designated as primary and that following diseases or conditions known to inflict damage to the articular cartilage as secondary. Statistical surveys of the incidence of primary osteoarthritis show unequivocally that this ailment does not occur in young or middle-aged adults, but that it starts in the fifth decade of life and is noticed thereafter with sharply increasing frequency in the sixth, seventh, and finally eighth decade of life. Thus, the aging process appears to essentially affect the biology of the chondrocytes by altering their function and thereby the chemical structure of their produced proteoglycans [850]. If one acknowledges that the cells of other organs (brain, eye) undergo senescent changes, one must concede that the cartilage cells of the joints are also liable to undergo senescent degeneration, especially since they are subjected to intense mechanical impact even under physiological use. In this sense Melanotte [1085] points out that primary osteoarthritis is a biological senescence phenomenon which does not necessarily appear at old age but individually and commensurate with aging.

Histochemical and biochemical studies are able to shed a light on the initial alterations taking place in the osteoarthritic articular cartilage. Sylven et al. [1617] demonstrated that with advancing age the content of proteoglycan decreases within the articular cartilage. Meyer et al. [1097] noted that the proportion of the various types of chondroitinsulfate changes with age; chondroitinsulfate H decreases, while the chondroitinsulfate C and keratansulfate increase. In accordance, further studies [23, 31, 76, 113, 154, 157, 178, 287, 596, 781, 802, 954, 962, 1016, 1019, 1020, 1079, 1080, 1236, 1352, 1353, 1395, 1689, 1778] point out that the early changes in osteoarthritic articular cartilage are associated with a decrease in the concentration of glycosaminoglycans, a basic component of the ground substance, as well as with their degradation. Some of the chondroitinsulfate subunits are distinctly diminished, while keratansulfate is often increased. These changes are accompanied by a shortening of the chain length of the glycans attached to the protein core. Hereby the great binding capacity of the interstitial ground substance for water is essentially diminished, as well as the elasticity and shock-absorbing ability of the articular cartilage [154]. This provides an explanation of the etiology of the individually varying setting in the disorganization of the articular cartilage.

Howell [781], Leppelmann [962], and Mankin et al. [1019] related the decrease in proteoglycans, which may amount to 50% of their normal concentration, to the histological severity of cartilage lesions. Staining with metachromatic dyes shows a varying depletion of mucopolysaccharides starting from the superficial zone and extending into the depth. Similarly as with hematoxylin-eosin-phloxin-safran, the intercellular material of the cartilage stains less basophilic or pale grayred, an indication that the composition of the intercellular material has changed. Some authors [287, 802, 1253, 1689, 1740] regard the action of enzymes (protease, chondrosulfatase, cathepsin) produced by lysosomes in the chondrocytes and synoviocytes as the cause of the breakdown of the protein-polysaccharide unit. The findings [1398] that the chondrocytes produce proteoglycanase and cathepsin [1696], which contribute to the disintegration of proteoglycans, must not necessarily be interpreted as the primary etiological factors in osteoarthritis. These are, rather, pathogenetic factors manifesting the perverted function of senescent chondrocytes after their ability to produce normal proteoglycans has been altered. No change in the content of collagen has been noticed [582, 583, 1016, 1019].

Explanation is provided for the pathogenesis of chondrosarthritis in the fact that the degenerating hyaline cartilage has lost its elasticity and is no longer able to act as a buffer, which protects the articular ends from pressure and shock imposed by the normal function. However, no elucidation has yet been provided of the factors which elicit the primary changes in the metabolic function of the chondrocytes.

Since individually varying senescent changes in the function and structure of the articular cartilage probably account for the observed primary alterations in the degenerative arthritis [546], it is appropriate to term the disease chondrosarthritis. This means a primary affection of the articular cartilage without known causes, at concomitant inflammatory changes of the synovial membrane [32, 458, 1556]. In distinction from it, secondary chondrosarthritis may be related to [56] or initiated by the following: (a) unequal use of articular ends due to congenital deformity [701], to deformity following disturbance of growth, to acquired and faulty statics in a weight-bearing joint, or to a malunited extraarticular fracture; (b) excessive stress to a joint or joints at work or in extraneous physical activities; (c) injuries to joints such as contusion, sprain, dislocation, or intraarticular fracture [1190, 1191, 1432]; or (d) frequent intraarticular disuse by a loose meniscus or a loose joint body. Thurner [1641] expanded these factors to include the following potential conditions: (e) paraarticular injury affecting the epiphyseal subchondral bone; (f) rheumatic joint disease with inflammation of the synovial membrane which affects the articular cartilage [590, 1740] and the subchondral bone; (g) specific bacterial or bacteriotoxic articular inflammations which inflict extensive destruction to the hyaline cartilage or cause gradual decomposition of its intercellular substance and subsequent disintegration of the cartilage cover; (h) metabolic disorders (gout, ochronosis) and blood disorders (hemophilia); and (i) hormonal disorders (of the pituitary, thyroid, adrenal, or sex gland).

In this sense, Hackenbroch [701] pointed out that these joint alterations resulting from primary disorders and elementary lesions of the structure of the articular cartilage should be acknowledged as primary osteoarthritis. On the other hand, all types of osteoarthritis developing as sequelae of identified factors, which lead to impaired trophic or disturbed mechanics, must be considered as secondary osteoarthritis. Cotta et al. [329, 330] emphasized that a large variety of factors, including those of traumatic, enzymatic, inflammatory, metabolic, or hormonal nature, which cause alterations of the articular cartilage, eventually lead to secondary osteoarthritic changes.

The symptoms of primary osteoarthritis [1146] appear insidiously in individuals of advanced age, most of them older than 40 years. It cannot be disregarded that women, chiefly those of overweight, are particularly affected by osteoarthritis. Associated with the latter, these patients may have a hormonal imbalance which is also manifested in osteoporosis of the vertebral column and by the Heberden's [734] and/or Bouchard's nodes in the fingers [1565, 1566]. Apart from this, the generally observed transformation of the articular ends by the decrease in protective cartilage cover no longer provides frictionless movements in the joints. Pain arises in the joints on the initiation of movements or after their longer continuation; static discomfort often also appears in the vertebral column and lower extremities. Thus the pain in osteoarthritis is experienced characteristically at the start of movement, in sudden change of posture of the body, or on shifting of the position of an extremity. The cogwheel-like articular ends are then put into motion and engage each other until a certain fitting has been established, which suffices as long as the mechanism is being used in the middle ranges of motion. Pain also arises due to frictional irritation after prolonged use of a joint. Similarly, pain arises when a joint is moved to the final degrees of excursion; the marginal osteophytes of the opposing articular ends come into contact and rub against each other as well as against the joint capsule. Another sign of advanced osteoarthritis is manifested in the unilateral or concentric limitation of motion which is rather typical for each individual joint. This limitation resides primarily in the incongruence of the articular ends and secondarily in the thickening of the joint capsule and periarticular structures, less often in tenseness of the regional musculature. The rather characteristic limitations of motion in each joint are described below together with other characteristic symptoms at each individual joint.

On longer duration of this condition, the increasing plumpness of the articular ends causes their obvious deformity to be readily perceived, where they lie close beneath the skin (Fig. 262) and are sometimes compounded by malalignment. Correspondingly, the joint capsule on palpatation presents a rather dense thickening, which differs from the soft swelling in acute inflammatory condition, and a moderate tenderness which relates principally to the joint cleft and uneven articular ends. On expanding changes of the articular constituents, the motion in the joint no longer evolves without friction and is often associated with a fine, silklike rustle by rubbing of the hardened joint capsule against the articular ends. In other patients, the noises vary from slight grating to coarse crepitation by friction of the uneven articular surfaces against each other. These sensations can be perceived either by the palm placed on the joint in motion or by auscultation with a stethoscope.

In extreme deformation of the articular ends with substantial narrowing of the cartilage space, the movements have very limited ranges. In rarer cases the joint is enlarged by an increase in joint fluid; then the motion is almost free or only moderately limited because the joint cleft is widened, and the friction is minimized. The local temperature is usually not elevated. In the majority of patients one has the erroneous impression due to cracking noises that the joint fluid is decreased, and that the joint is dried up. Thus osteoarthritis appears as a progressive degenerative joint disease which usually and clinically lacks general and local inflammatory manifestations. However, Ehrlich [458] described a polyarticular osteoarthritis which involves chiefly the small joints of the hands and is manifested in swelling and increased local warmth. Similar observations can sometimes be made in the shoulder, knee, and ankle joints, with frequent effusions in the knee joints. The clinical impression of distinct signs of inflammation of the joints in about 24% of patients with osteoarthritis are supported by histopathological findings [1543]. In view of these observations and on the basis of the histopathological synovial findings, which meet the criteria formulated by Geiler et al. [589], the basic designation of arthritis appears justified.

Laboratory studies in primary osteoarthritis do not disclose any essential or specific abnormal findings. The sedimentation rate lies in the normal range in most cases; however, it is elevated beyond 30 mm/h and even to 70 mm/h in about 24% of patients. These are principally those with extensive swelling of the joint capsule of the hip, knee, or shoulder joint. Results of the test for rheumatoid factor are false positive in about 6%–7% of patients, but they may suggest in a few cases an antecedent episode of rheumatoid arthritis affecting mostly the hip joint. Such positive outcomes should initiate investigation as to the possibility of previous rheumatoid arthritis. Examinations of the synovial fluid [374] sometimes disclose a substantially increased content of desquamated synoviocytes, presenting the majority of the 200–800 cells/ml. Independently of it, the concentration of proteoglycans is increased in advanced cases, these being released from the disintegrating hyaline cartilage in proportion to the extent of its alterations. Concomitantly, the viscosity of the synovial fluid may be increased to 160–280 units as determined by the viscometer. In some rare cases crystals of calcium pyrophosphate or hydroxyapatite are observed [420, 421, 441, 1117, 1439, 1442].

Roentgenographs are much more informative since they reveal the osteoarthritic changes starting from a rather early phase. Once the thickness of the cover of hyaline cartilage decreases, the width of the cartilage space diminishes (Figs. 263, 264), until it eventually becomes an irregular hairline cleft (Fig. 265). However, with increased joint fluid and despite worn-off cartilage the cartilage space may appear widened and actually corresponds to the joint cleft; it is then clearly discernible, being sharply delimited by the sclerosed subchondral bone. Sometimes the sclerosis extends rather deeply into the cancellous bone (Figs. 263, 264, 265). In the majority of the cases, the sclerosis of the subchondral bone is disrupted by smaller and larger, ovoid or roundish areas of radiolucency corresponding to subchondral cysts (Fig. 264). In this phase the articular surfaces show loss of evenness due to attrition (Figs. 263, 264) or very

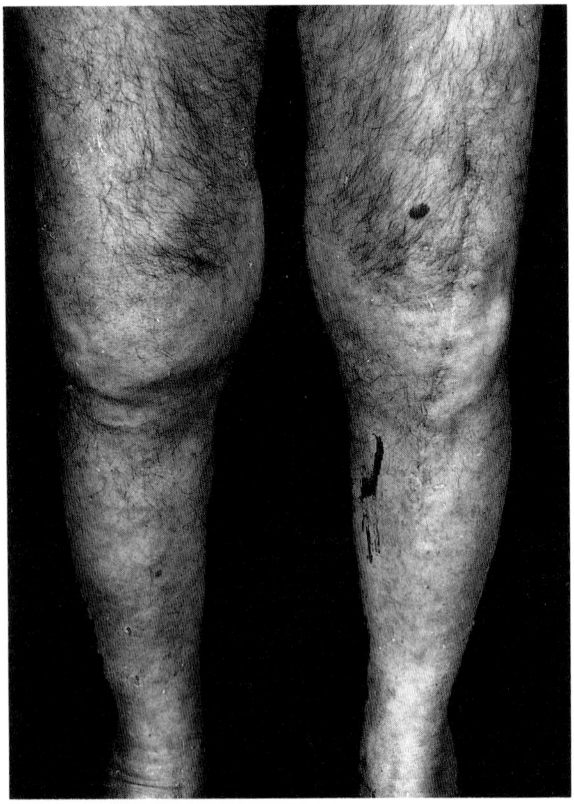

Fig. 262. Both knees, the right more than the left, are very enlarged by thickening of the joint capsule. An oblique scar extends on the anterior aspect of the left knee secondary to an arthrotomy

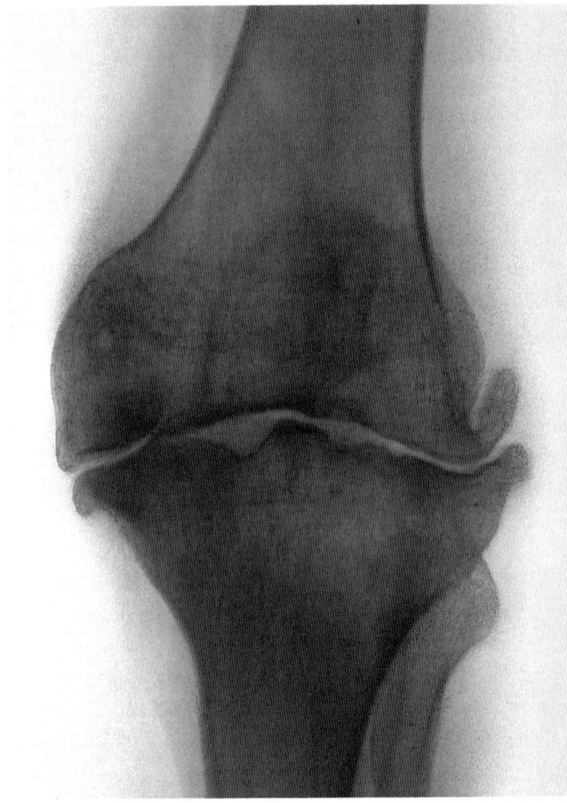

Fig. 263. The femoral condyles are worn off and have lost their convexities. The joint cleft is narrower and irregularly delimited by sclerosed articular surfaces. Large osteophytes rise from the margins of the articular condyles

often to formation of protruding marginal osteophytes of beak or spur shape (Figs. 263, 264, 265). Eventually the articular epiphyses, no longer have their original outliness (Figs. 246, 291). The surrounding joint capsule sometimes becomes discernible, being sclerosed and densified tissue.

Differential diagnosis should consider primarily the case history, paying special attention to any antecedent episode of injury, generalized inflammation, or infection, to any metabolic disorder, concurrent generalized or localized bone disease, or to any other preceding direct involvement of the affected joint. Upon elimination of all potentially etiological conditions in joint affections and with regard to the age of the patient the laboratory and roentgenographic findings, the diagnosis of primary versus secondary osteoarthritis or of any distinctly traumatic or inflammatory condition may be correctly inferred.

Independently of general and local signs free of inflammatory changes, each joint presents its individual changes on physical and roentgenoraphic examination and thus requires adjustment of the local treatment corresponding to the specific needs. Nevertheless, the general treatment [175, 1144] takes precedence.

One of the prime concerns is the frequent overweight which must be corrected to minimize further disuse of the worn-out joints. The diet should be low in fat and carbohydrates but rich in protein to help correct an often coincident osteoporosis of the vertebral spine and pelvis. For similar reasons, multivitamin tablets are prescribed containing particularly vitamin C, which assists in assimilating protein into the matrix of the connective tissue and bones, vitamin D, which helps in incorporating calcium into the newly formed osteoid tissue, and vitamin E, which generally improves the trophics of all tissue. As to medications, acetylsalicylic acid should be given 0.6 g three to five times daily for its analgesic effect and antiinflammatory influence [460, 795, 848] on the connective tissue by inhibiting the prostaglandin inflammatory mediator. The latter also contributes to disintegration of the articular cartilage by degradation of the proteoglycans [288, 1502]. Experimental studies [1542] disclose that acetylsalicylates appear in the blood at an average of 7.7 min after ingestion and reach their maximum concentration at an average of 40 min after ingestion. They are then transported, commensurately with the hyperemia and thickening of the synovial membrane, at an average of

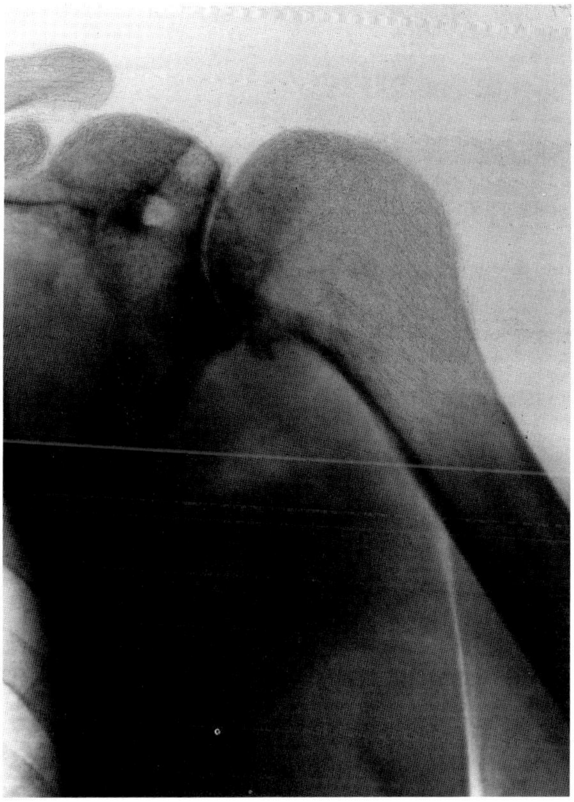

Fig. 264. The glenoidal joint cleft is narrowed, and the adjoining articular surfaces are sclerosed and uneven. An exostosis rises from the caudal border of the humeral head, and two cystic areas lie in the depth of the glenoid

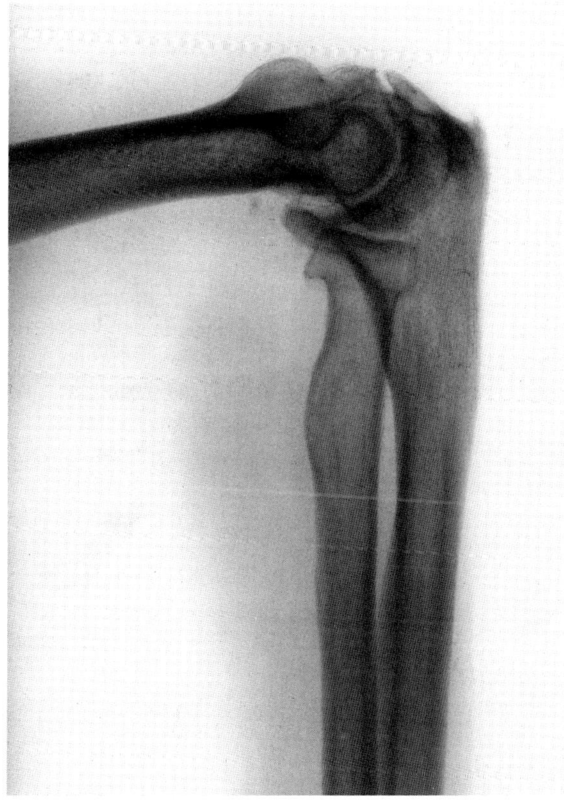

Fig. 265. The articular surfaces of the humeral condyle and the fossa olecrani of the ulna are uneven and sclerosed. Broad osteophytes rise from the margins of these epiphyses

11.7 min into the joint fluid, where they attain their maximum concentration at an average of 39.5 min. When regularly given and in adequate dosage, salicylates often suffice therapeutically, especially in cases with swelling of the joint capsule and substantially increased sedimentation rate. While it is generally assumed that acetylsalicylate by virtue of its acetyl component is more potent in suppressing the inflammatory enzymes [1502], its antiinflammatory influence continues after deacetylation, which occurs in the joint fluid 120–145 min after ingestion [1542]. Therefore, plain salicylates are of equal value although presumably with less initial antiinflammatory effect. If salicylates do not reduce or suppress the pain, stronger analgesics – propoxyphene 65–130 mg, acetaminophen 500 mg, up to codeine 30–60 mg – may be necessary. In such acute situations muscle relaxing medications – methocarbamol 750 mg or cyclobenzaprin 10 mg – can also ease the painful reflectory tenseness of the regional musculature.

However, in cases of persistent symptoms nonsteroidal antiinflammatory medications are necessary [88, 245, 442, 794, 846, 849]. While varying in degree from patient to patient, these often prove effective in suppressing pain, reducing inflammatory changes, and improving function. Depending on their chemical composition, these medications may be classified [846, 849] in the following groups: pyrazole, with its derivates oxyphenbutazone and phenylbutazone; oxicam, with its derivate pyroxicam; indolacetic acid, with its derivates indomethacin, sulindac, tolmeten; phenylalkanoic acid–propionic acid and their derivates: fenoprofen, ibuprofen, naproxen, naproxen sodium; and fenamic acid, with its derivates meclofenamate, mefenamic acid, and diclofenac sodium. The dosage differs for these medications. In addition to their action, like the salicylates, inhibiting the synthesis and release of prostaglandins, they also inhibit neutrophilic leukocytes in releasing lytic enzymes [3]. Thus nonsteroidal antiinflammatory medications probably have an effect on proteoglycan metabolism [1221]. The above list does not claim to be complete. The omission of other available medications must not be interpreted to suggest that they are not effective; it indicates only the insufficient experience with them. As with salicylates, any antiinflammatory medication may be accompanied by adverse effects. These arise principally either from the gastrointestinal tract, ranging from nausea, diarrhea, constipation to severe bleeding due to harm to the gastrointestinal mucosa, or from the blood (substantial decrease in leukocytes and/or erythrocytes) due to suppression of the bone marrow. Other occasional complications are headache, nephrotic syndrome with salt and water retention due to harm to the kidney parenchyma [794, 795, 846, 849], and icterus due to harm to the liver. The patient must be alerted to such possibilities and the need instantly to discontinue the use of the medication should adverse effects arise. In view of the frequent gastrointestinal irritation, it is advisable to take these medications together with food. A noncustomary medication for lasting symptoms particularly of the vertebral column and nonresponsive to the above medications is colchicine. While specifically used in gout, it sometimes proves helpful in osteoarthritis, although neither the clinical examination nor the laboratory tests offer any suggestion of gouty etiology in these conditions. In the light of recent findings [420, 441, 1117, 1439, 1442] of calcium crystals in the joint fluid in primary symptomatic and asymptomatic osteoarthritis of elderly persons, this medication appears well indicated. Colchicine is prescribed here with doses similar to those in gout, 0.3–0.6 mg three to five times daily until regression of the symptoms.

A very beneficial treatment is the topical use of moist heat, performed in its simplest form by applying a towel soaked in hot water to the ailing region once daily for 30–60 min and surrounding it with a nylon sheet; despite this insulation, the towel cools off fast. Therefore an effective heating device is the electric moist heating pad which is supplemented with an inserted wet sponge and stays warm as long as desired and at a regulated temperature. Another modality for applying moist heat is the natural mud, composed partly of anorganic material from the local soil and 25%–40% organic material originating from the decomposition of microfauna. Particularly the latter accounts for the therapeutic affects: increased range of motion in the affected joints and regression of the spinal nerve root symptoms. Accompanying these is a decrease in the sedimentation rate and C-reactive protein [170, 338]. These mud packings are usually applied in two series of five to six sessions at an interval of a few days, depending on the individual tolerance. It takes 2–3 months thereafter to develop the full therapeutic benefit. Mud applications are practiced in several European spas, and among these applications the fango packings are highly effective [170, 338]. The benefit experienced following local application of moist heat, especially hot mud packs, can be explained in the following points. (a) Warmth has a soothing effect on the sensory nerve fibers and thus decreases the local soreness; however, in excessive degrees it irritates the nerve fibers and may intensify the pain. (b) Probably secondary to the soothing of sensory nerves and possibly by direct softening effect on muscle fibers, the spasm of the regional musculature regresses, and better mobility ensues. (c) By dilatation of the small and medium-size blood vessels and by regionally increased blood flow, yet without emigration of leukocytes, restructuration of the regional tissue is initiated and especially a softening of the fibrosed tissue by ingrowth of blood vessels. (d) By dilatation of the lymph vessels inflammatory infiltrates are resorbed, and the swelling regresses. (e) Ott et al. [1212] additionally postulate the liberation of inflammatory modulators which contribute to the regression of the inflammation.

On application of hot mud packs, hyperthermia develops in the tissue to a depth of 5–7 cm and can be measured there by needle-copper thermocouple as a temporary elevation in the temperature to 40°–42°C. This activates the local metabolism. The effects of the proper moist heat application cannot be simulated by other modalities. The commonly practiced submersion of the entire body into a warm bath dilates the blood vessels of the entire body and thus dissipates the effect in areas which do not need treatment.

Another effective local modality is physical therapy with shortwave diathermy [944, 1613] and/or ultrasound [687, 1541], applied in one to three series of eight sessions. These may be combined with massage of the regional musculature, and all are helpful by eliciting local hyperemia and diminishing the local tenseness. Ultrasound, when used at higher intensity (3.5–5.0 W/cm^2) also has a direct effect on the sensory and motor nerve fibers [1541]. A valuable adjunct [1188] to the modalities of physical therapy are active exercises which the patient is instructed to carry out by himself. These exercises have the purpose of strengthening the regional musculature, to prevent osteoporosis and maintain the range of motion. However, they are not able to influence inflamed articular tissues or to smoothen uneven articular ends; when carried out to excess, they accelerate the attrition of the joints. At pronounced weakness of the musculature secondary to long inactivity, strengthening of the musculature can be attained effectively by galvanic and/or faradic stimulation over a period of 3–6 months.

In the rare cases in which none modalities succeed in suppressing or relieving the persistent soreness of a joint, periarticular or intraarticular injections with hydrocortisone have been recommended [773, 1466, 1572, 1600], since they provide marked relief lasting for weeks or months. However, the potential for local infections [1316] and especially for subsequently rapid deterioration in the condition of the cartilage of a joint [105, 121, 269, 552, 655, 663, 1149, 1389, 1577] requires very judicious use of intraarticular steroid injec-

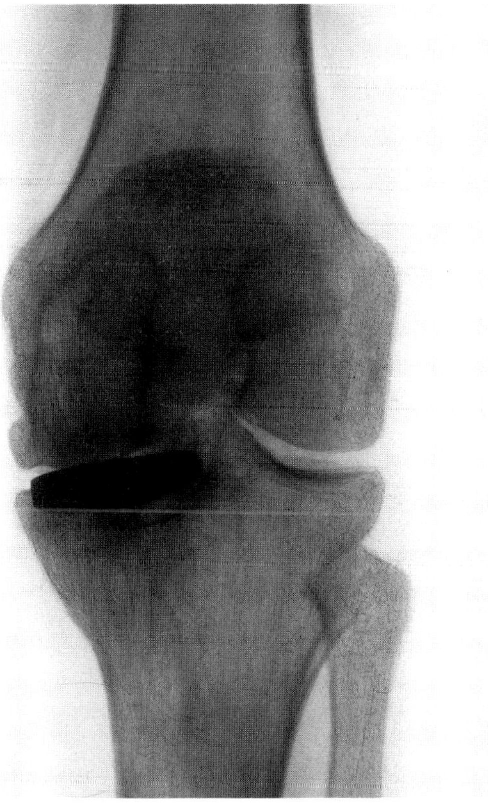

Fig. 266. Hemiarthroplasty of the knee joint by insertion of a metal plate into the medial tibial condyle. The articular surface of the medial femoral condyle is uneven and sclerosed and bears a marginal osteophyte

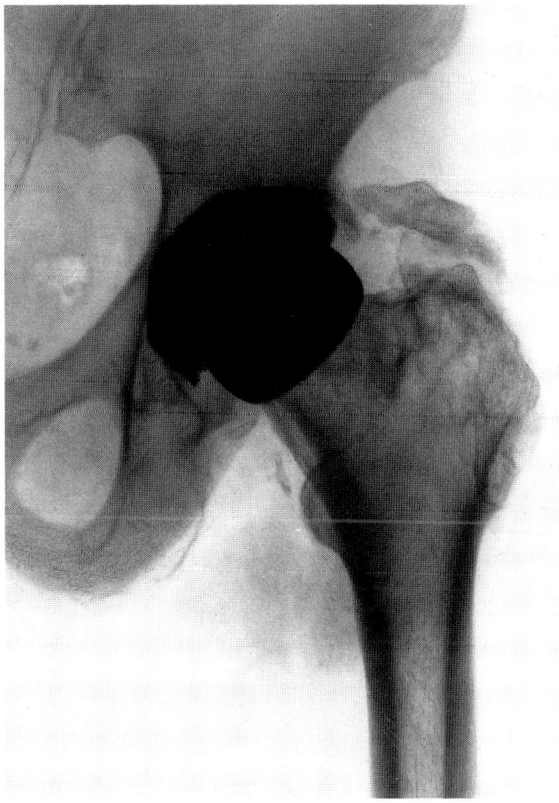

Fig. 267. Resurfacing arthroplasty of the hip joint. The subjacent bone in the femoral neck is not osteoporotic. An osseous shadow, indicating myositis ossificans, expands cranially to the femoral neck and trochanter

tions and only in cases of symptoms remaining unaffected by any other modality. Mankin et al. [1018] concluded, on the basis of the changes following intraarticular injections of cortisone into rabbits, that cortisone causes a decrease in the synthesis of proteoglycans. Mohr [1125] demonstrated that the intraarticular injections of corticosteroids are followed by local necrosis and formation of granulation tissue. In addition to the limitations in their intraarticular use, corticosteroids should also not be used systemically in osteoarthritis because of the potential for generalized osteoporosis and for adverse effects on the metabolism and other endocrine glands.

In addition to the generally and locally applied conservative treatment modalities, various surgical procedures and techniques are used. These depend on the degree of deformity and malfunction observed in any joint of the extremities or in the joints of certain segments of the vertebral column. These procedures are used [1646] taking into consideration the sex, age, occupational activity, and involvement of neighboring joints. The procedures are also discussed in "Rheumatoid Arthritis".

Synovectomy [689, 691, 1030, 1285, 1302, 1303, 1644] endeavors to excise as widely as feasible the thickened inner part of the joint capsule. Since this thickening is not always as pronounced in osteoarthritis [1429] as in rheumatoid arthritis, the indication for a concurrent synovectomy arises when hindering marginal osteophytes and/or irregularities of the articular surfaces must be removed by a débridement [1003].

Synovectomy may also have to be combined with tenotomy when the periarticular tendons become tense and shortened, and a contracture develops. Such situations may occur in the knee joint as a flexion contracture with tightness of the hamstring tendons or in the ankle joint in an equinus contracture with tightness of the Achilles tendon. Lengthening of the tendons is indispensable in operations on these contractures.

In the frequent alterations of the articular surfaces, sometimes a part of one articular epiphysis (a condyle) becomes profoundly worn off while the contiguous epiphysis remains more or less intact. The correction can be obtained by hemiarthroplasty in which the one-sided defect is compensated by insertion of a metal plate of corresponding thickness [998, 999, 1070, 1071]. This procedure is applied exclusively in the knee joint (Fig. 266).

When, on the other hand, the entire articular surface of an epiphysis becomes altered, without extending into the depth, resurfacing arthroplasty may be indicated. It is performed principally in the hip joint [40, 239, 1656, 1657, 1702] using a shell of metal or ceramic to replace the surface of the femoral head (Fig. 267) and possibly also the acetabulum.

When, beyond the alterations of the articular epiphysis, the juxtarticular metaphysis is also affected, axial angulation ensues at the site of the metaphysis, most commonly at the hip and/or knee joint. This deviation can be corrected by osteotomy [159, 335, 412, 702, 805, 1077, 1229, 1312], which can minimize the one-sided attrition of the articular surfaces (Figs. 279, 280, 283, 284, 289, 290).

In cases of extensive and profound attrition of contiguous articular surfaces, with concurrent impairment in the function of the joint, total arthroplasty is indicated [227, 278, 280, 320, 683, 804, 1275, 1651]. Here these articular epiphyses (Figs. 271, 272, 285, 286, 291) are excised and replaced (Figs. 273, 274, 287, 288, 292) by implants of stainless steel or cobalt or titanium alloy. The concave implants are made of polyethylene or ceramic. All types were initially secured within the bone by methylmethacrylate cement. However, these implants became loose in about 40%–50% of cases due to resorption of the surrounding bone and fragmentation of the cement, and became subluxated or dislocated. Therefore, types of implants have been designed which are tightly press-fitted into the marrow cavity. To ensure lasting fixation, newer endoprostheses have been designed with stems coated with sintered porous metal, polymer, or ceramic which permits ingrowth of bone. As further modifications, the articulating surfaces of the implants have been shaped with various degrees of congruence, and they are also held together by various technicalities. This allows various degrees of constraint in terms of ranges and axes of motions.

An operation applicable in extensive and profound alterations of the articular epiphyses of the wrist (Figs. 209, 210), hip, knee, or ankle (Figs. 275, 276) joint is arthrodesis [555, 1549]. Here the remainders of the articular surfaces are evenly excised, and the denuded epiphyses are approximated under compression by metallic devices [279, 402, 1421]. Although the alterations are brought to a standstill, the resulting complete elimination of mobility is such a shortcoming that arthrodesis is accepted chiefly by men and only after all other surgical possibilities have been tried and have failed.

The above surgical procedures are performed with regional variations and specific indications for each joint of the extremities. They are discussed below specifically in the context of individual joints.

While primary osteoarthritis involves preferentially the weight-bearing joints, one exception is the involvement of the fingers at their distal and proximal interphalangeal joints with nodular protrusion at the bases of the phalanges (Figs. 468, 469). These Heberden's [734] and Bouchard's nodes correspond to proliferations of synovial connective tissue into the bases of the distal and second phalanges. They are manifested roentgenographically (Fig. 470) in cystic enlargements and/or deep erosions of the articular surfaces with narrowing or widening of the cartilage space. The invariably associated swelling of the joint capsule is often accompanied by increased local temperature, which relates osteoarthritis to the group of inflammatory joint diseases [458]. Another particular feature here is the predominant occurrence of these changes in women of menopausal age, about 20–22 times as often as in men, which makes this type of osteoarthritis appear a hormone-related autosomal disease. Conservative treatment with moist hot packs usually suffices; resection of excessively protruding, very large nodes may sometimes be necessary. In cases of marked limitation of motion in an interphalangeal or metacarpophalangeal joint due to advanced alterations of the articular ends, these ends may be excised and replaced by endoprosthetic inserts of silicone rubber silastic [519, 1109, 1611] (Fig. 208). However, loosening or breaking of the implants presents a serious shortcoming of this treatment. Another procedure for restoring the mobility of these joints is the wedgelike resection and smoothing of the articular epiphyses, followed by reinforcement of the joint capsule.

The carpometacarpal joint of the thumb is affected secondarily to constant overuse in occupational activities. Regular splinting is necessary whenever compatible with the work. Otherwise, arthrodesis [1030] secured by cross-wires and a small inlay bone graft in functional abduction position provides painfree use of the thumb. Another effective procedure is excision of the navicular bone, which restores full mobility of the thumb.

The wrist joint is rarely the site of pronounced primary osteoarthritis but often that of osteoarthritic changes which develop secondarily to extensive intraarticular fractures or severe inflammations involving the distal end of the radius and the carpal bones. Concomitantly the joint capsule is very thickened, but motion is not as limited as roentgenographs would indicate by the degree of deformity of the articular ends and by the narrowing of the joint space. Therefore, in addition to local moist heat applications and physical therapy with shortwave diathermy in eight sessions, the wrist joint should be restricted either by a firm wristlet or a plastic splint. However, on persistent intense pain or in persons whose occupational demands expose them to heavy strains on the wrist joint, arthrodesis at 15°–20° dorsalextension with denudation of the articular surfaces and insertion of a sliding bone graft [1549] (Figs. 209, 210) provides reliability and freedom from pain, although excluding motion in this joint.

The elbow joint is affected by osteoarthritis and, lying close beneath the skin, readily displays its deformity, due to which rotation and flexion become limited more than does extension. In accordance, roentgenographs (Fig. 265) reveal deepening of the olecranon fossa, with protrusion of the elongated olecranon and coronoid process and plumpness of the radial head. All articular surfaces are very uneven. This condition often responds to conservative local measures; application of moist hot packs and physical therapy with manipulations and massage provide a substantial benefit. Otherwise, arthroplastic resection of the deformed articular ends, chiefly of the humeral condyles or radial head, with interposition of a fascial flap and adipose tissue, helps substantially to increase the range of motion. In cases of extreme deformity and persistent pain, total arthroplasty with insertion of metallic and polymeric components may represent the last solution. For this purpose three types of arthroplastic implants consisting of metal and/or polyethylene are available. These types are: the unconstrained prosthesis [484, 917, 988], the semiconstrained prosthesis [320, 804, 1412] (Fig. 499), and the totally constrained prosthesis [387, 690]. These are also discussed in "Rheumatoid Arthritis" and "Ankylosis of Joints". Aftercare requires about 3 months; long-term follow-up examinations are necessary to evaluate the final results.

The shoulder joint is often affected by soreness on motion. It is enlarged due to deformation of its articular ends and thickening of the joint capsule, and is tender along its circumference especially at the anterior aspect. Its movements are often limited in the direction of external rotation and especially in the direction of abduction and elevation. This is often followed by an adduction contracture with substantial limitation of even of passive abduction. Any movement is associated with palpable crepitation. Roentgenographs correspondingly reveal flattening of the glenoid cavity and humeral head with thickening and sclerosis of their subchondral bone. The cartilage space is invariably narrowed and uneven (Fig. 264). The loss of roundness of the articular surfaces accounts for the diminished mobility. Therefore, the arm should be positioned as often as feasible in abduction to prevent shrinking of the joint capsule and periarticular structures. Two or three peri- and intraarticular injections of 1% anesthetic, administered in intervals of 1–2 months, may succeed in suppressing substantially the soreness of the joint. Mobilization exercises as described in "Contracture of Joints" should be performed diligently to increase the range of movements. However, if an adduction contracture develops, forced manipulation of the shoulder joint under general anesthesia, as described in "Contracture of Joints", may restore the range of motion.

In the cases of marked incongruity of the glenoid cavity and humeral head and persistent pain even at the limited motion, arthroplasty is indicated. In view of the advanced erosion of the articular margins, confined principally to the humeral head, excision of the latter and its substitution by a metallic long-shaft endoprosthetic insert (Fig. 212) is carried out. The rotator cuff is hereto attached. A pain-free, substantially increased range of motion is thereby restored. Due to the non-weight-bearing function, replacement of the glenoid cavity by a polyethylene [1179] or metallic insert is not absolutely necessary, but is always done when pronounced deformity of the glenoid cavity coexists. For this situation total arthroplasty sets are available in three modifications: the unconstrained [1179] (Fig. 212), the semiconstrained [683], and the constrained type [1275]. Their specifications are described in "Rheumatoid Arthritis" and "Ankylosis of Joints". Following satisfactory healing, the patient is placed on a program of mobilization exercises and reattains a satisfactory range of motion in 2–3 months. The indications, contraindications, and complications of total arthroplasty are generally discussed in this chapter in the context of total arthroplasty of the knee joint. Since the shoulder joint is a non-weight-bearing joint, primary osteoarthritis rarely produces conspicuous deformation, but secondary osteoarthritis following intraarticular fracture or a severe inflammation may do so. Excessive deformation occur more frequently still in neuropathic arthropathies, especially syringomyelia (Fig. 455). The decision regarding surgical treatment must consider the primary etiology.

The big toe sometimes, especially upon fallen metatarsal arch, displays advanced osteoarthritic changes with marked narrowing of the metatarsophalangeal joint. This substantially limits its motion, and the condition is therefore referred to as hallux rigidus; use of the big toe in the deployment of the foot is very hampered. Another disturbing feature is the associated dorsomedial enlargement of the metatarsal head (bunion) which often becomes irritated by the pressure of the shoe and develops an overlying chronic bursitis. As conservative treatment, passive plantar mobilization exercises at the metatarsophalangeal joint are advised, as is widening of the top leather of the shoe into which an arch support with a broad metatarsal pad is inserted. If these modalities do not provide improvement, excision of the exostosis of the metatarsal head

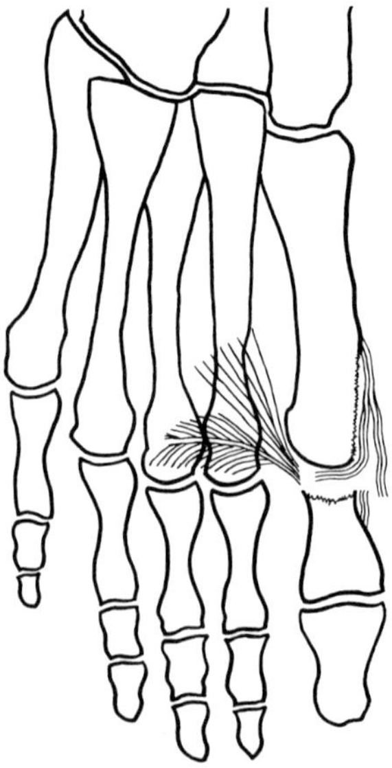

Fig. 268. Deformation and misalignment at the metatarsophalangeal joint of the big toe can be corrected by resection of the basis of the first phalanx, excision of the exostosis of the metatarsal head, and interposition of a part of the abductor hallucis tendon

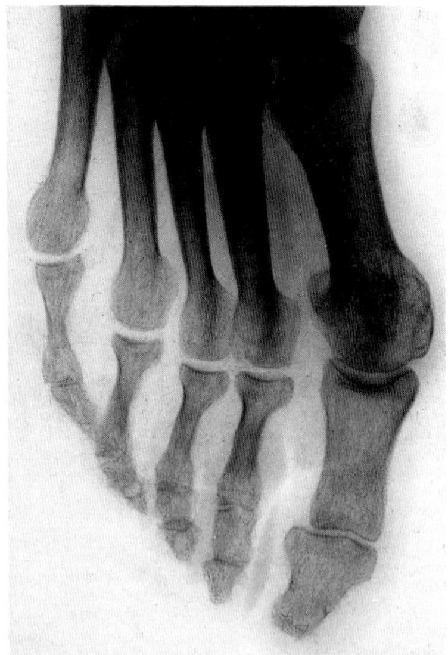

Fig. 269. The first metatarsal is deviated into valgus, and its head is enlarged. The adjoining phalanx is deviated into varus position. This metatarsophalangeal joint is uneven, and its articular surfaces are sclerosed

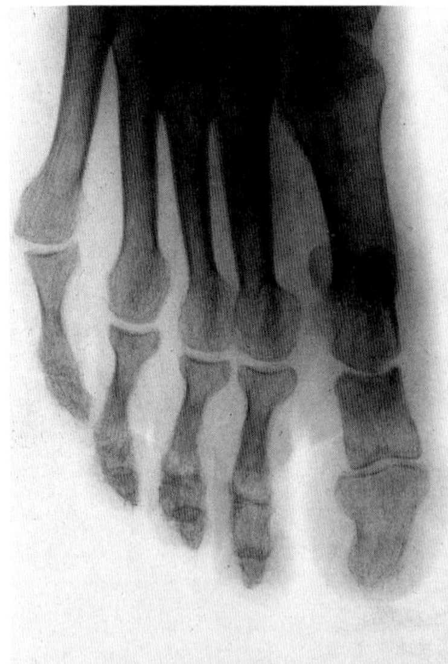

Fig. 270. The exostosis of the first metatarsal has been resected, and its valgus deviation has been corrected. The basis of the first phalanx has been resected, and proper alignment of the metatarsophalangeal joint is attained

and resection of the basis of the first phalanx with optional insertion of a capsular flap are designed [1552] to reshape the metatarsal head and restore the motion of this joint (Figs. 268, 269, 270). Regular, active and passive plantar flexion of all toes is of elementary necessity in the aftercare.

Osteoarthritis of moderate degree in the subtalar and midtarsal joints responds well to arch supports, physical therapy with diathermy and massage, and firm shoes; that of severe degree is treated effectively by subtalar or triple arthrodesis. However, such arthrodesis must be considered carefully in the case of coex-

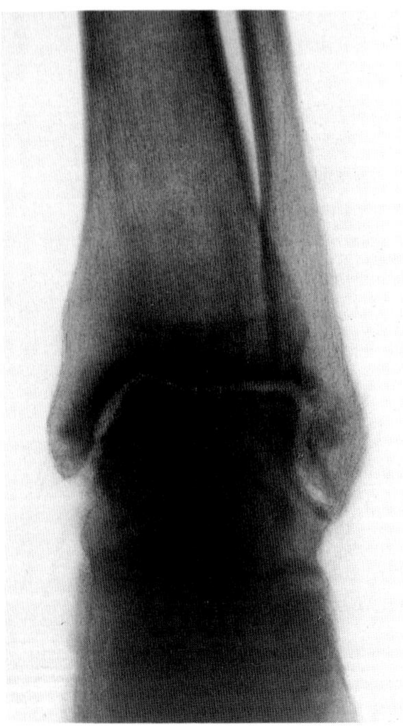

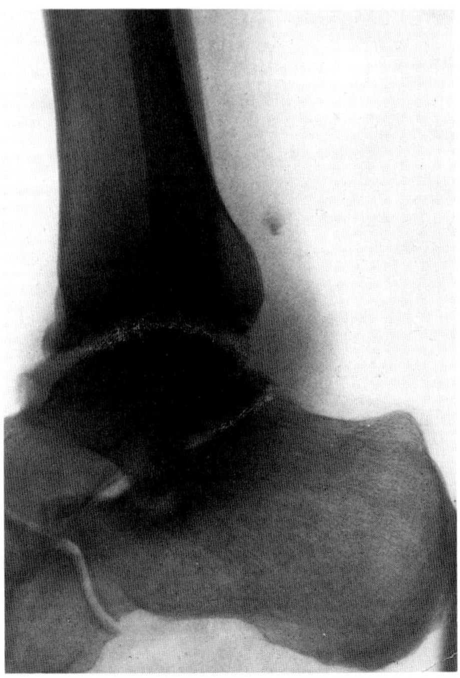

Fig. 271. The tibiotalar joint space is uneven and oblique at concomitant varus deviation of the talus

Fig. 272. The tibiotalar joint space is wider at its anterior area, and narrower at its central area. Marginal osteophytes expand from the anterior edge of the tibia and from the neck of the talus

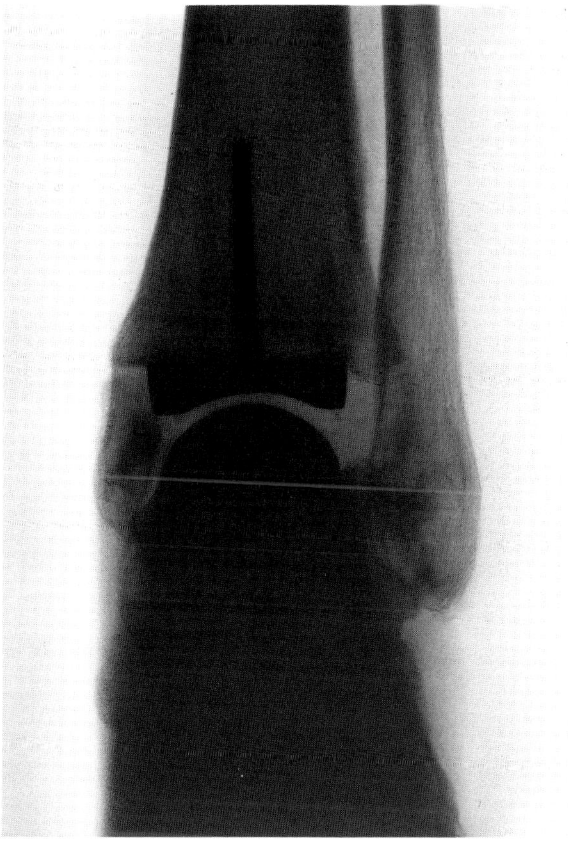

Fig. 273. Arthroplastic components of the semiconstrained type have been centrally inserted into the distal part of the tibia and the body of the talus

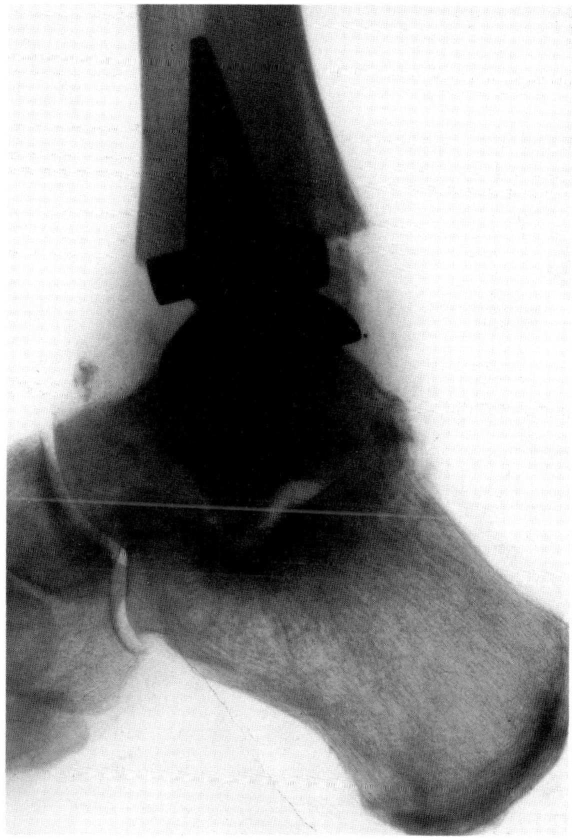

Fig. 274. Arthroplastic components of the semiconstrained type have been centrally and perpendicularly inserted into the distal part of the tibia and the body of the talus

istent osteoarthritis of the ankle joint in view of the limited motion in the latter joint. Elimination of motion of the subtalar joints may impose excessive strain on the inadequate ankle joint.

Proper treatment for osteoarthritis of the ankle joint varies with the degree of involvement of this joint and with the sex and occupation of the patient. In primary osteoarthritis, which generally remains within moderate degree, topical application of moist hot packs and diathermy are of value; elastic compression with an ACE bandage or anklet minimizes the strain to this joint. Firm high shoes or boots often complete the treatment. However, in secondary osteoarthritis, which is commonly of posttraumatic etiology and invariably of more pronounced degree in symptoms and roentgenographic appearance, an operation is often needed after exhausting the conservative modalities. The first choice of operative procedure, especially in women, is replacement arthroplasty [1723, 1724] by excision of the articular surfaces of the tibia and talus and cementing of a metal-polymer component into the distal end of the tibial shaft and a metal component into the talus (Figs. 271, 272, 273, 274). This restores mobility of the ankle joint for several to many years, but not always to the full range. A greater inconvenience than that of decreased motion lies in the rather frequent loosening, especially of the tibial component. This inconvenience has been averted in the recent past by using components with porous-coated stems whereby ingrowth of bone can be secured following immobilization for about 6–8 weeks. Follow-up examinations indicate that arthroplasty of the ankle joint is generally satisfactory and remains so for a long period of time in individuals aged over 55–60 years and who place only moderate stress on the ankle joint. However, if this procedure does not render a satisfactory result or becomes progressively unsatisfactory in the range of motion and freedom from pain, the possibility of converting such artificially mobilized and insufficient joint into a stiff joint by arthrodesis remains open (Figs. 275, 276).

In men, especially those of overweight or heavy laborers, arthrodesis of the ankle joint is the primary alternative. Arthrodesis may also be performed as a

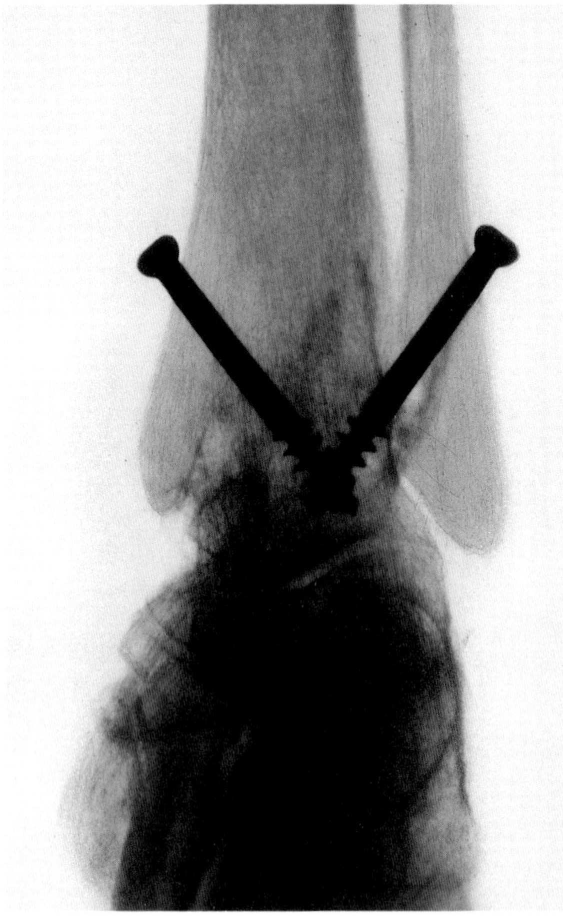

Fig. 275. Arthrodesis of the ankle joint by denudation of the articular surfaces and compression-immobilization with two screws. The distal part of the tibia presents areas to osteoporosis and sclerosis, suggestive of osteoarthritis

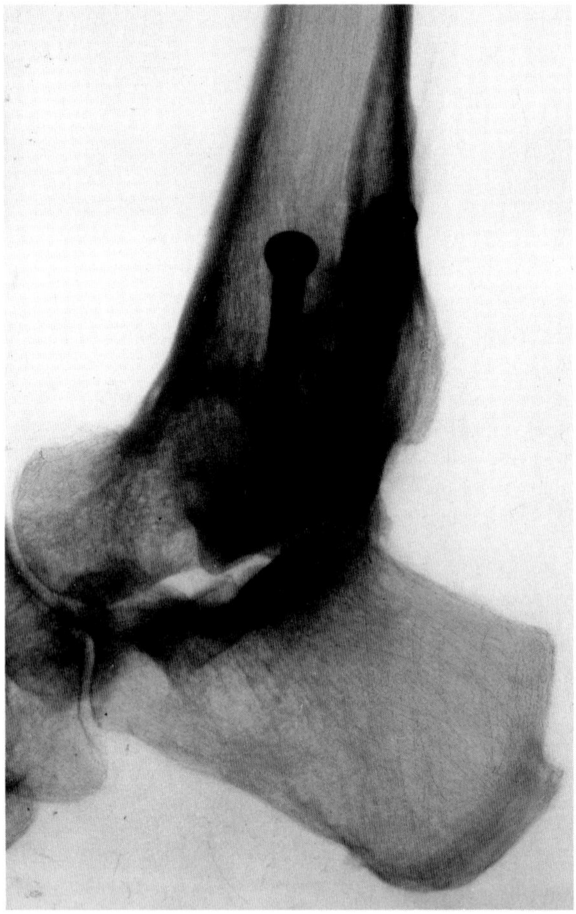

Fig. 276. The surfaces of the distal end of the tibia and the body of the talus are fused together by arthrodesis and immobilization with two screws. Osseous trabecula pass from one to the other articular epiphysis

primary procedure in young patients and in adults who place considerable stress on the osteoarthritic ankle joint at professional work. Arthrodesis is performed by denudation of the articular surfaces followed by fixation with a sliding bone graft [1549] (Figs. 213, 214, 215, 216) with screws (Figs. 275, 276), or with a compression clamp [279]. Arthrodesis in slight (5°) plantar flexion facilitates walking, and while it eliminates the motion of the ankle joint, this shortcoming is compensated partly by the motion in the subtalar joints. If desired, the fused ankle joint can be converted into a moveable joint by arthroplasty after reaching 55–60 years of age.

The knee joint is the most commonly involved joint by primary or secondary osteoarthritis, and it manifests its affection conspicuously by thickening of the fibrosed joint capsule, circumscribed tenderness along the joint cleft and peripatellar area, and coarse crepitation on motion. This is moderately limited in the final degrees of flexion. On the other hand, the knee joint may sometimes present instability to any side, being often associated with axial deviation. Women are more often affected, especially those of overweight and sometimes manifesting signs of hormonal disorder. In men, on the other hand, the history reveals significant injuries to the articular epiphyses and/or soft structures or strenuous activities in work or sport. In all these situations, a densely woven ACE bandage, elastic knee cap with metal hinges, rigidly enforced felt splint, or short brace supplemented with locks provides improved stability and economic utilization of the knee. Administration of antiinflammatory drugs combined with physical therapy may provide improved use of the knee joint for longer periods of time. Due to its position close beneath the skin, the knee joint responds satisfactorily to all modalities of physical therapy [687, 944, 1541, 1613]; thus heat by an electric moist heating pad should be applied regularly and may be alternated with shortwave diathermy or ultrasound in series of eight to ten sessions.

When the inner part of the joint capsule is excessively thickened, and roentgenographs reveal only moderate involvement of the articular surfaces of the knee (Fig. 245), synovectomy [689, 1302, 1303] may provide benefit of longer duration. When loose joint bodies, osteophytes, or circumscribed unevennesses of the articular surfaces impair the function of the knee joint, these are removed by débridement [1003] in combination with synovectomy. Where thickening of the synovial membrane is not extensive, and osseous irregularities are small, synovectomy and débridement can be achieved by arthroscopy through one or two portals. The effect of synovectomy may be explained by the fact that a large part of the inflamed inner part of the joint capsule and thereby the substrate of the soreness has been excised. However, the synovial membrane regenerates (Fig. 55) and may redevelop inflammatory changes and symptoms unless disuse of the joint can be avoided.

On the other hand, in some patients irregularities in the articular surfaces are associated with narrowing of the cartilage space and malalignment of the articular epiphyses, such as in genu valgum (Fig. 277) or genu varum (Fig. 281). This deviation may be the result of faulty development during childhood and was thus noticeable in adolescence. In other patients the axial deviation (apart from the cases with deviation secondary to a fracture) developed gradually during mature age without specific identifiable causes, unless intense use of the knees in certain private or work activities could be considered so. Corresponding to the site of skeletal deviation, either a supracondylar femoral osteotomy (Figs. 279, 283) or an infracondylar tibial osteotomy (Figs. 280, 284) succeeds in restoring normal alignment in the metaphyseal area [335, 805, 1703] (Figs. 277, 278, 282). This osteotomy should preferably be carried out in the shape of a dome, a V, or an inverted V (Figs. 279, 280, 283, 284). This permits any corrective angulation at the indicated level and at the same time provides broad stable contact between the fragments. Unless the deviation is located distinctly in the proximal third of the tibia, the osteotomy should preferentially be carried out through the directly supracondylar area of the femur (Figs. 279, 283). Otherwise, the osteotomy through the directly infracondylar area of the tibia must invariably be combined with an oblique osteotomy through the middle third of the fibula (Figs. 280, 284). Without the latter osteotomy, forcing the osteotomized tibia into corrected alignment may compromise the posterior tibial blood vessels or elongate the peroneal nerve. It is also advisable to immobilize the osteotomized bones by a plaster cast, which by its wedging permits any desired correction should postoperative roentgenographs reveal unsatisfactory alignment. The operative fixation with metallic devices does not allow any postoperative correction and, if applied

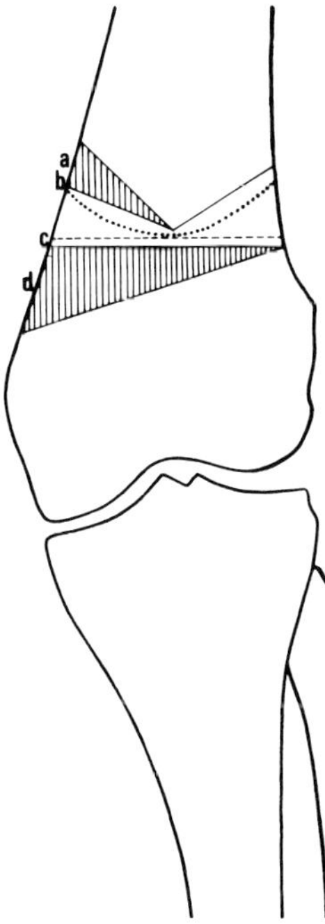

Fig. 279. Modalities of supracondylar correction of genu valgum: *a*, V osteotomy with excision of a medial wedge; *b*, dome-shaped osteotomy, *c*, transversal osteotomy; *d*, wedge osteotomy with medial basis

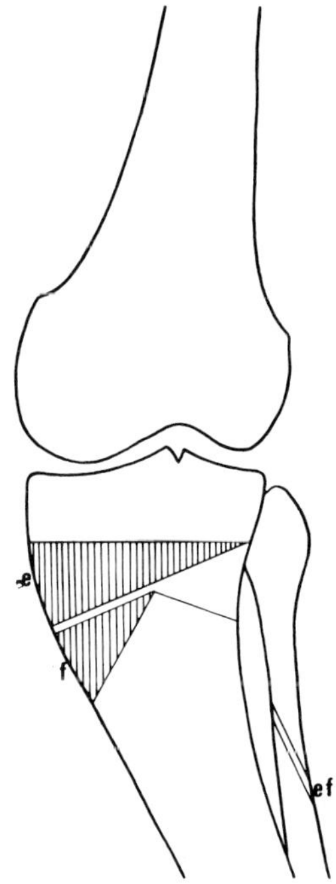

Fig. 280. Modalities of below tibial tuberosity correction of genu valgum: *e*, wedge osteotomy with medial basis; *f*, V osteotomy with excision of a medial wedge. These types of osteotomies are combined with an oblique osteotomy through the middle third of the fibula

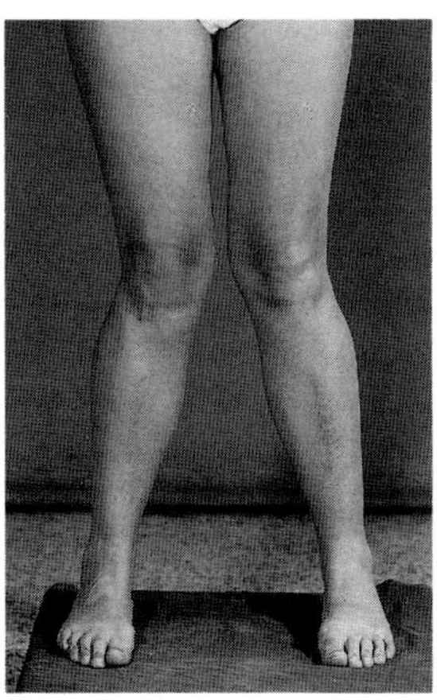

Fig. 277. Knock knees with 18° valgus deviation, especially in the right leg, and distance of 30 cm between the medial malleoli

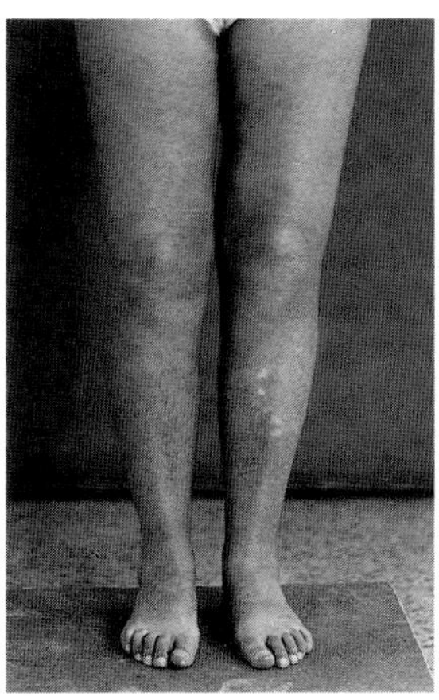

Fig. 278. Full correction of the deviation in both legs (Fig. 277) by supracondylar osteotomy

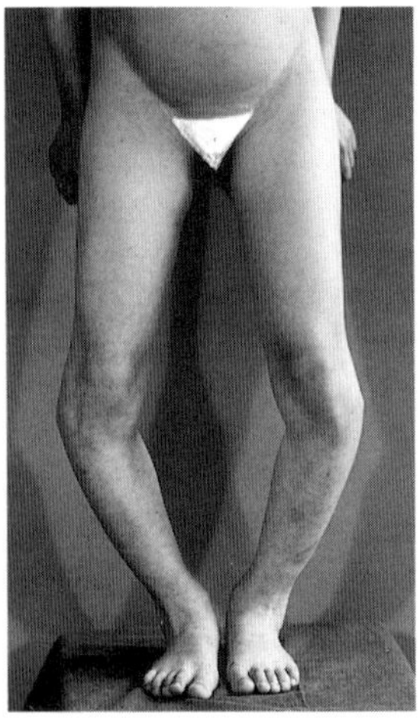

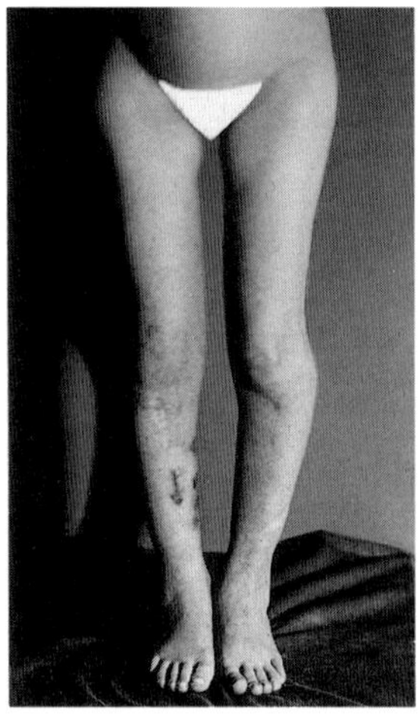

Fig. 281. Bowlegs with the knee joints completely out of the vertical axis between the hip joint and ankle joint. The distance between the anterior edges of the tibiae is 35 cm

Fig. 282. Adequate correction of the bowlegs by infratuberositary V osteotomy of the tibiae and oblique osteotomy of the fibulae

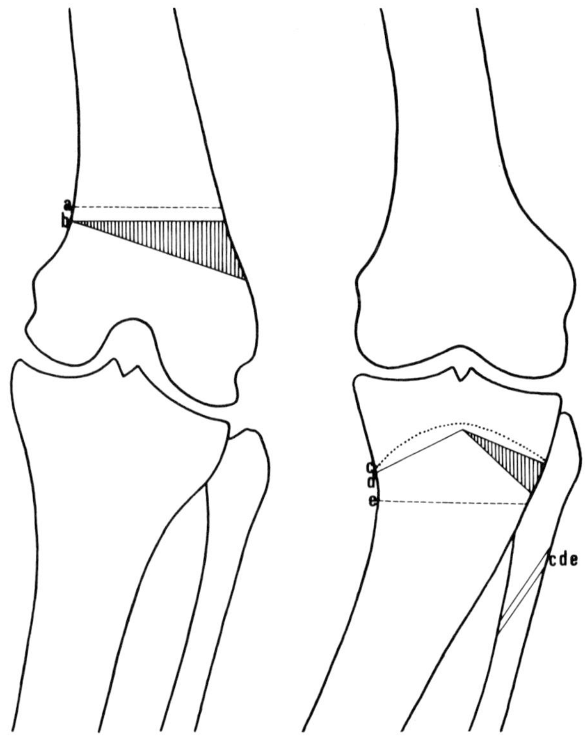

Fig. 283. Supracondylar modalities of correction of genu varum: *a*, supracondylar transverse osteotomy; *b*, supracondylar wedge osteotomy with resection of lateral basis

Fig. 284. Infratuberositary modalities of correction of genu varum: *c*, dome-shaped osteotomy; *d*, V osteotomy with excision of a lateral wedge; *e*, transverse osteotomy. These osteotomies are combined with an oblique osteotomy through the middle third of the fibula

with adequate alignment, does not allow approximation of the fragments after bone resorption at the osteotomy site. Thus, delayed union or nonunion may follow here. On the other hand, with the operated leg without internal fixation but merely immobilized by a plaster cast the patient is instructed to put weight on this leg soon after the operation; consolidation at the osteotomy site is obtained in 3 months. This provides satisfactory function of the knee joint for a long period of time.

In the cases in which the articular surface of one tibial condyle has been markedly worn off, while the articular surface of the other condyle is well maintained, a one-sided defect can be compensated by a metal plate of adequate thickness (Fig. 266) [472, 999, 1071]. The plate is secured by screws into the depth of the condyle and reestablishes equal load bearing on both tibial condyles. However, this method is effective only with maintained collateral and cruciate ligaments; it then delays further attrition of the articular surfaces for 5–7 years. In more extensive, but not deep alterations, the resurfacing arthroplasty of Townley [1657] can be used.

When these procedures do not provide lasting benefits (Figs. 246, 285, 286), total arthroplasty of the knee joint (Figs. 287, 288) may eventually be indicated. This arthroplasty is indicated beforehand in cases with marked unevenness of the articular surfaces and substantial narrowing of the cartilage space [274] (Figs. 285, 286) at persisting symptoms and disturbing inpairment in the use of the knee joint [545, 1445]. Arthroplasty follows the same principles as in total arthroplasty of the hip joint, designed by Charnley [278], by inserting articulating components into the femoral shaft and tibial shaft from which the defective articular ends were excised. However, in view of the complex mechanics and more precarious stability of the knee joint, the design of adequate prosthetic substitutes in the knee is more complicated. The models of the polycentric endoprosthesis [696] and geometric endoprosthesis [334] have been further modified for reciprocal coordination and function of their components. Three types of tricompartmental arthroplastic implants are in use: (a) the unconstrained endoprosthesis [1657], which has a satisfactory range of motion in all axes but depends on the integrity of the ligaments for stability of the knee joint; (b) the semiconstrained endoprosthesis [483, 807, 1031] (Figs. 287, 288), which has some restraint by the design of the articulating surfaces but relies partly on the ligaments; and (c) the fully constrained endoprosthesis [383], which is interconnected by hinges and is constrained in two

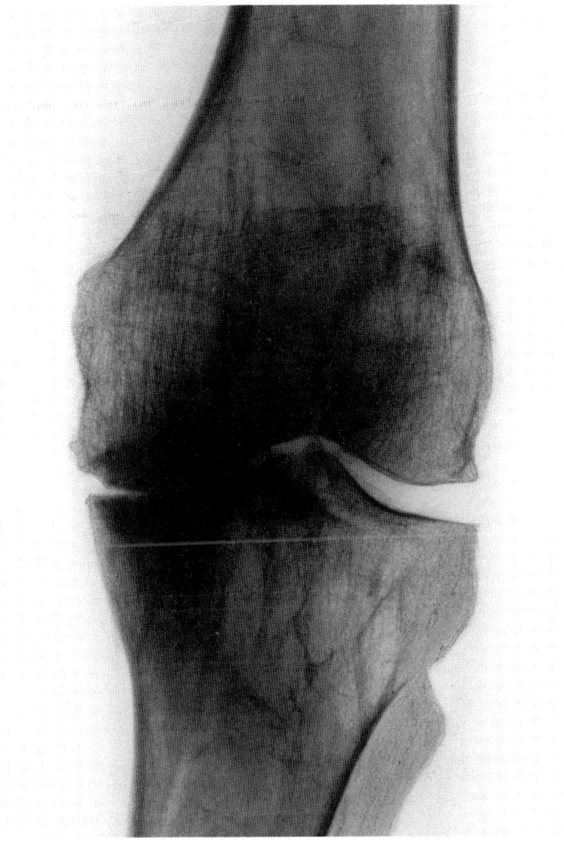

Fig. 285. The articular epiphyses are sclerosed and their borders are uneven. The medial joint space is very narrowed, and marginal osteophytes expand from both medial epiphyses. The tibia is deviated into varus

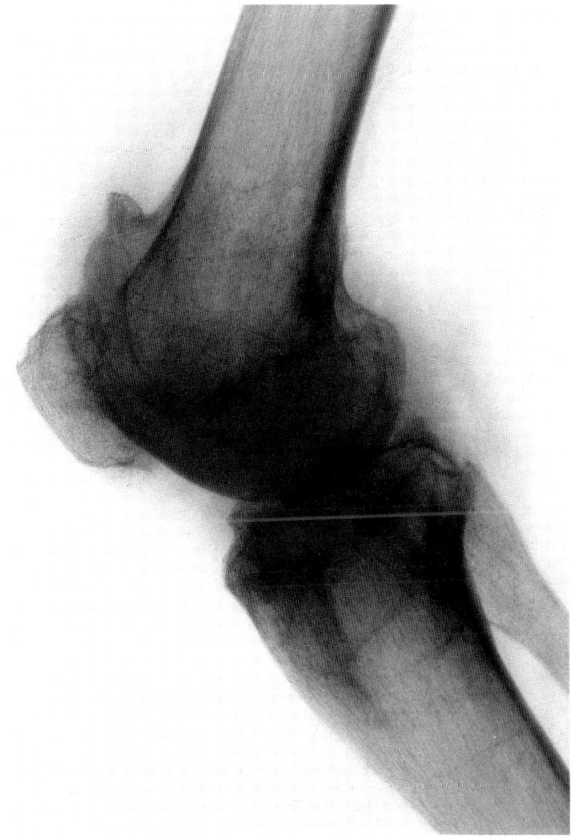

Fig. 286. The articular epiphyses are unevenly delimited, as is the joint space between the femoral condyles and the patella. Large osteophytes rise at the cranial aspect of the patellofemoral joint

planes. The latter is indicated primarily in conditions with substantial loss of bone and marked instability. The advantages and shortcomings of each of three types are rather distinct and have been demonstrated by comprehensive follow-up examinations [807, 1031, 1770, 1809]. Nevertheless, independently of its design and degree of constraint, one basic requirement must be fulfilled by any implant into the knee joint: the realignment of its articulating cleft with the weight-bearing axis. For this purpose, it is sometimes necessary to release the medial or lateral soft structures so that the implants may articulate horizontally.

The construction principles of most endoprostheses types for the knee joint are the same in that the femoral condyles are substituted by convex components of high-strength metal alloys with cobalt or titanium, while the tibial articular surfaces are substituted by hemispherical sockets of high-density polyethylene, as is the patella, if necessary. These basic materials provide weight-bearing surfaces with optimal low-friction [1651]. All components are fixed to the bone by a cement of methylmethacrylate. However, in view of the rather frequent (about 40%) loosening of the implant stems cemented into the bone, press-fitted endoprostheses were designed which immediately attain reliable fixation and dispense the cementing. Another improvement to ensure lasting fixation is the coating of implants with sintered porous metal which permits the ingrowth of surrounding bone. An important prerequisite for total arthroplasty is adequate function of the quadriceps muscle and absence of flexion contracture. Otherwise, the full extension cannot be attained, especially since the range of extension and flexion usually remains slightly decreased after total arthroplasty. At preexisting flexion contracture of the knee joint, the tedious surgical release of the popliteal soft tissue can be spared by excision of an adequately thick portion of bone from the proximal tibial metaphysis. On uneventful postoperative course, which is substantially secured by preoperative administration of anticoagulants and broad-spectrum antibiotics, the knee joint is gradually mobilized by active exercises supplemented with assisted passive exercises. On attainment of a satisfactory range of motion, ambulation with partial weight bear-

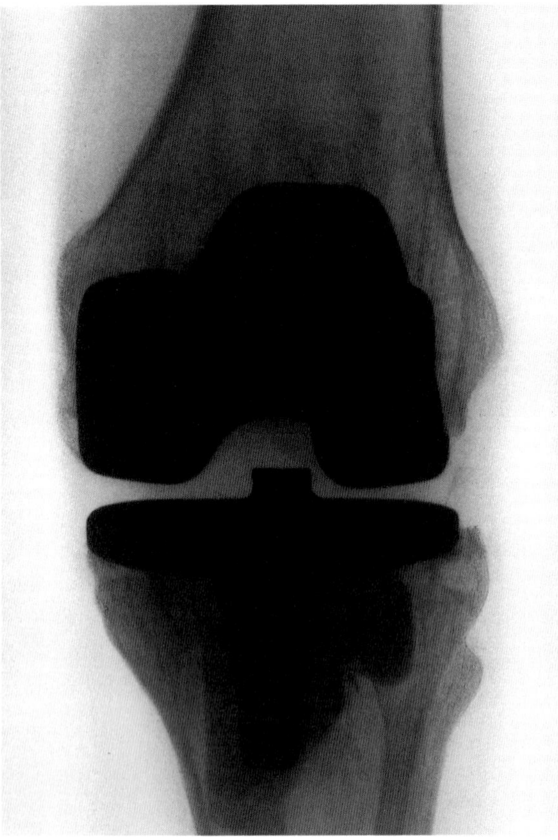

Fig. 287. Total unconstrained arthroplasty by insertion of substitutes into the femoral condyles, tibial condyles, and patella

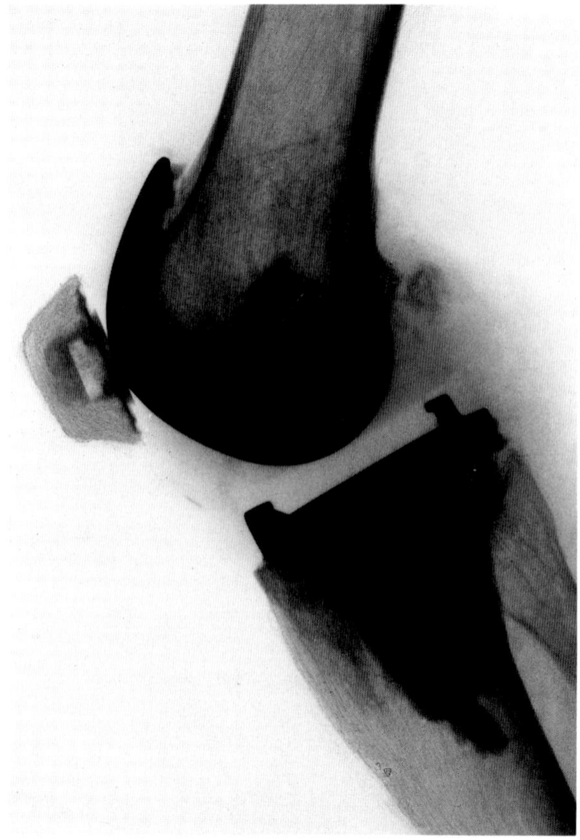

Fig. 288. Total unconstrained arthroplasty by insertion of substitutes into the femoral condyles, tibial condyles, and patella

ing is started, and muscle strengthening exercises are instituted commensurately.

However, the postoperative and late courses are rather often (7%–12% of cases [1809]) marred by complications, some of which jeopardize the outcome. These complications are phlebitis and/or thromboembolism, injury to the peroneal nerve, loosening, subluxation or dislocation of the implants, and fracture of the bone. Removal of the prosthetic implants and insertion of other implants may be necessary in most of these complications. The most worrisome complication is deep infection, which occurs in about 1%–1.5% of cases and requires wide débridement and administration of broad-spectrum antibiotics for about 2 months. Healing may be obtained in about 40%–50% of these cases [1809]. In other cases of unabated infection the implants must be removed and the antibiotic treatment be continued until closure of the wound. Subsequent possibilities for treatment are protection of the leg by a brace with/or without hinges, or arthrodesis [194], which is a salvage procedure by restoring a pain-free and stable knee joint, albeit at the price of mobility. Another insertion of prosthetic implants may be attempted after an 18- to 24-month period free of local inflammatory alterations.

Thus, arthrodesis of the knee joint is occasionally performed as a secondary procedure after failed arthroplasty or upon extensive destruction and insufficiency of the articular epiphyses. On corrective resection of these epiphyses, their compression may be obtained by a clamp in the situations of diminished inflammation or by a plaster cast and weight bearing in cases of persistent suppuration. Arthrodesis of the knee joint as a primary procedure is rarely accepted, and then only by men, especially heavy laborers.

The hip joint is very often affected by osteoarthritis which causes pain and marked impairment in walking due to the progressive limitation of internal rotation and abduction. These limitations are associated with the loss of roundness of the femoral head and with narrowing of the cartilage space. On longer duration and greater extent of the epiphyseal attrition, the joint capsule and pericapsular tendons are irritated. The regional musculature consequently assumes a reflex contracture. An adduction or adduction-flexion contracture of the hip joint often develops due to which the posture of the entire body becomes distorted, with concomitant obliquity of the pelvis and relative shortening of the leg. This results in a severe handicap in the activities of daily life. Since these changes in primary osteoarthritis are very pronounced with advanced age, they have been termed malum coxae senile. Regular active and passive mobilization exercises – extension, abduction, and internal rotation – are of elementary necessity for restoring the normal range of movements. Locally applied moist warm packs and physical therapy with diathermy and massage in repeated series are equally necessary. A cane in the opposite hand is used at ambulation to diminish the weight load on the ailing extremity. Bedrest on a firm mattress, preferentially in prone position, is also advisable. If the flexion contracture of the hip joint nevertheless persists, this can be corrected by pelvic and ankle traction, or, if unsuccessful, by tenotomy of the iliopsoas and adductor tendons. This should be combined preferably with immobilization in a plaster spica cast or in a lumbofemoral brace for 6–8 weeks in corrected position, which is full extension, slight abduction, and slight internal rotation (inversion).

When despite the absence of contracture the walking ability is impaired and pain arises on any activity, roentgenographic examination may reveal abnormal alignment of the femoral head and neck, with the femoral shaft at an angle greater or smaller than the physiological angle of 120°–130°. McMurray [1077] advised here a transposition of the weight-bearing line by subtrochanteric osteotomy. This shifts the femoral shaft medially beneath the femoral neck, which becomes adducted, and other areas of the femoral articular surface are brought into contact with the acetabulum. As a variant of this procedure, especially in young patients without excessive involvement, Bernbeck [127] recommended intertrochanteric transposition osteotomy for correction of rotational and valgus deviation. Pauwels [1229] emphasized the deviation of the femoral neck in the direction of varus or valgus, with associated caudal or cranial protrusion of the femoral head beyond the acetabulum, as a frequent etiological factor in osteoarthritis. The unequal contact is associated with unequal weight bearing between the acetabulum and the femoral head and thus also with one-sided excessive attrition. Therefore, Pauwels [1229] recommended abduction osteotomy in cases of coxa vara (Fig. 289), whereby the femoral head is raised toward the upper edge of the acetabulum. On the other hand in coxa valga, adduction osteotomy (Fig. 290) was recommended, whereby the cranially protruding femoral head is brought caudally and concentrically into the acetabulum. These osteotomies restore equal weight bearing on the femoral head, as is seen by the equal width of the cartilage space. The benefit provided is evidenced by a decrease in subchondral cystic and/or sclerosed areas [159, 310, 412, 762, 1312]. Hackenbroch [702] emphasized the corrective value of transposition osteotomy at the proximal end of the femur in those cases in which clinical signs

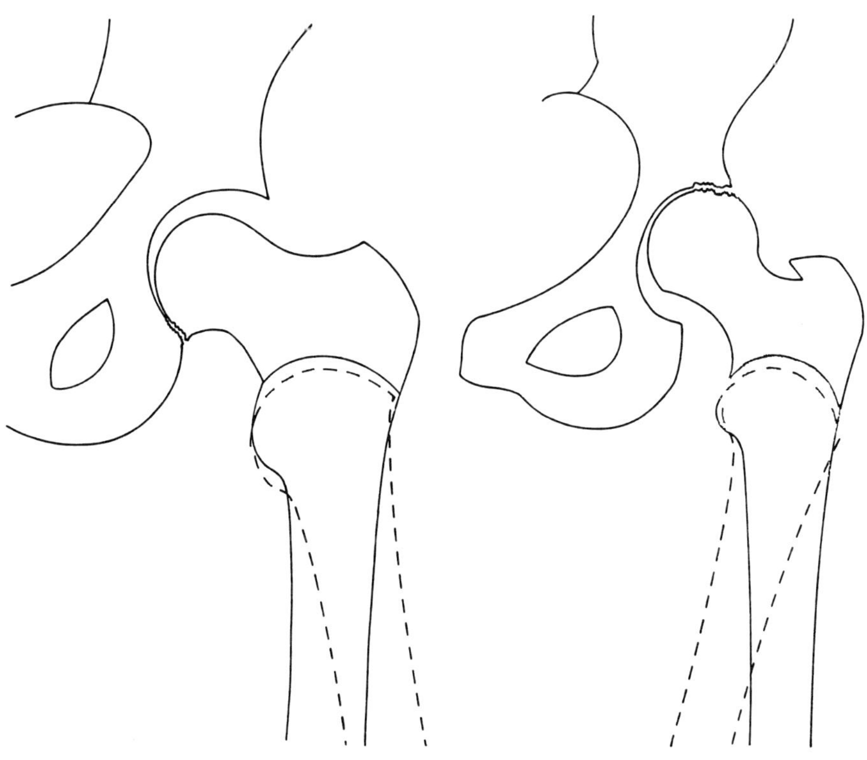

Fig. 289. In coxa vara, a subtrochanteric dome-shaped or V osteotomy with alignment of the peripheral fragment at the proper angle of abduction restores the proper angle between femoral neck and shaft and the concentric position of the femoral head

Fig. 290. In coxa valga, a subtrochanteric dome-shaped or V osteotomy with alignment of the peripheral fragment at the proper angle of adduction restores the proper angle between femoral neck and shaft and the concentric position of the femoral head

and roentgenographically confirmed alterations indicate the necessity of operation [145]. In difference from Pauwels' recommendation [1299] to excise a wedge at the site of the osteotomy, the necessary angulation can be carried out by an intertrochanteric osteotomy of reversed V type or dome shape, by which no osseous substance is removed, and reliable contact is maintained (Figs. 289, 290). Additionally, internal fixation by a metallic plate and screws is necessary, whereupon the mobilization of the hip joint can be started at an early date. Nevertheless, satisfactory results are not obtained in all cases by this intertrochanteric osteotomy. The shortcoming is seen in cases in which corrective osteotomy was performed too late, and deep alterations were already present in one sector of the femoral head at the time of the osteotomy.

In the osteoarthritic alterations involving only the surface of the femoral head and possibly the acetabulum, resurfacing arthroplasty (Fig. 267) [40, 239, 1656, 1702] is indicated. Here a shell of metal or ceramic is secured by a stem into the debrided femoral head, and a plastic shell is cemented onto the acetabulum. While the postoperative results are very satisfactory, apart from occasional myositis ossificans (Fig. 267) or phlebitis, loosening of the implants or aseptic necrosis of the femoral head beneath the shell may occur later. It is probable that the use of implants with porous coated surfaces will minimize or eliminate some complications. Nevertheless, resurfacing arthroplasty has maintained its indications in cases of bilateral moderate osteoarthritis of the hip joint and coincident osteoarthritis of the knee joints and lumbar spine.

In advanced alterations of the femoral head and acetabulum, especially when one-sided and confined chiefly to the hip joint, total arthroplasty (Figs. 291, 292) is indicated [38, 86, 101, 1135]. It is also discussed in "Rheumatoid Arthritis", but the pathological-anatomical alterations in osteoarthritis differ; the articular ends are larger and sclerosed in the latter condition, and the joint capsule has no invasive tendency. The arthroplastic implant for the femur is made of stainless steel, titanium alloy, or cobalt alloy and is inserted by its stem into the femoral shaft (Fig. 292). The acetabulum is supplemented with a cup (Fig. 292) of polyethylene or ceramic cemented into its site by methylmethacrylate, as is the femoral stem. Follow-up examinations disclosed that in about 40%–50% of cases the cementing provides lasting fixation for 10 years or more, but in the other cases loosening or subluxation of the endoprosthetic implants occurs after 1–4 years due to resorption of the surrounding bone and fragmentation of the cement. Therefore, new types of implants for the femoral shaft and acetabulum have been designed which are tightly press-fitted into the marrow cavity. Another recent modification provides the stems of the inserts and the cups with a porous coating of sintered metal, ceramic, or polyethylene, making the ingrowth of bone into the implants possible and hereby increasing the probability of a lasting fixation [198]. The total arthroplasty as originated by Charnley [278] is a low-frictional torque arthroplasty which decreases the total load on the hip joint. Whereas Charnley used an anterolateral approach to the hip joint, Moore [1135] used a posterolateral, Amstutz [38] a lateral, and Mueller [1152] a posterior. On uncomplicated postoperative course, the operated hip joint is held by traction in abduction and is gradually mobilized by assisted active and passive exercises. The musculature is subsequently strengthened by diligent contractions and massage, and the patient regains a satisfactory range of motion in the hip joint within 3–5 months.

Nevertheless, immediate postoperative and late complications may occur, some of them specific for the type of treatment and others of a general surgical nature. Sometimes 1–2 days after the operation the femur completely dislocates, requiring immediate reduction under general anesthesia and thereafter immobilization of the hip joint by plaster cast in abduction and internal rotation for 4 weeks. After 1–4 years the implants may become loose, subluxated, or dislocated, wherefore their removal and replacement is necessary. On the other hand, heterotopic ossifications may develop and become rather extensive, limiting motion substantially; radical excision of all ossified tissue is necessary here. General surgical complications include superficial infection, which can be treated satisfactorily by dressings and antibiotics, phlebitis and thromboembolism, which are often fatal, injury to nerves, or deep extensive suppuration, which occurs in about 1.3% of cases [227, 1181, 1792]. Preoperative initiation of treatment with broad-spectrum antibiotics and anticoagulants is a wise precaution. Deep suppuration is caused mostly by staphylococcus, streptococcus, Escherichia coli, and pseudomonas [227], but it may also result from any other microbe [203]. Treatment [791] consists of debridement of the wound and administration of antibiotics, as indicated by the culture and sensitivity tests, for a duration of about 2 months. Closure of the wound and salvage of the implant arthroplasty are attained in 20%–30% of these cases [227]. In the other cases with persisting infection, removal of all arthroplastic implants, including the cement, and thorough revision of the wound are mandatory [136, 502, 1251]. The antibiotic treatment is continued until complete closure of the wound. Subsequent possibilities of management include: (a) stabilization of the completely unstable hip joint by orthosis, which provides support for the pelvis and permits motion in the hip joint; (b) subtrochanteric support osteotomy [1546], whereby the proximal frag-

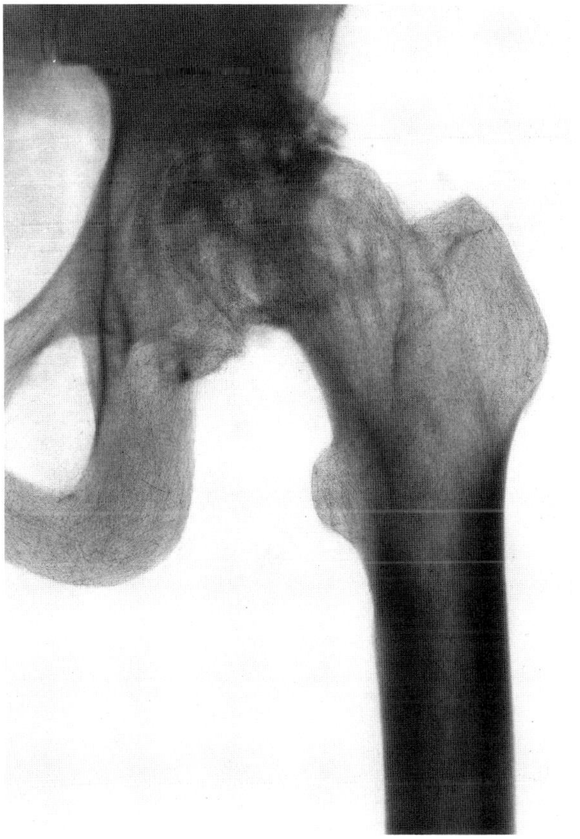

Fig. 291. The femoral head is no longer round, but ovoid. The joint space is narrowed and uneven, especially at the cranial area, where the femoral head and acetabulum are very sclerosed. A marginal osteophyte protrudes there. Several large cystic radiolucencies penetrate the femoral head, neck, and acetabulum

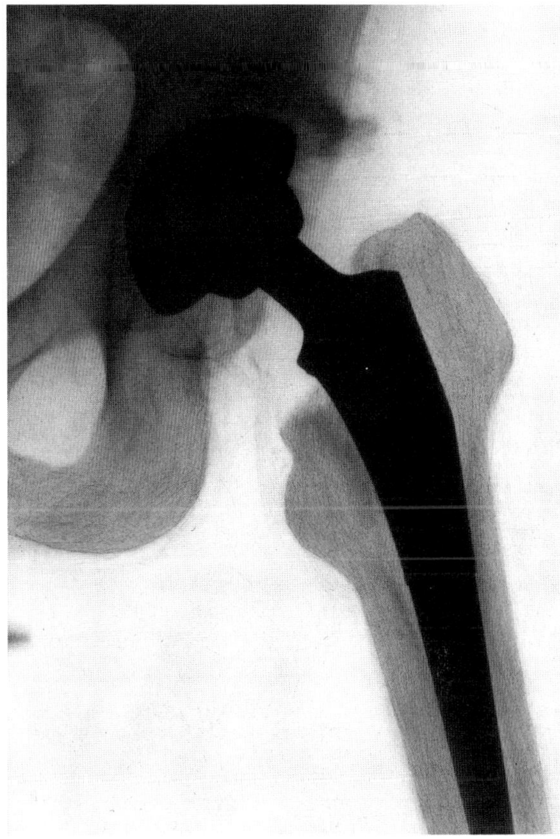

Fig. 292. A total noncemented arthroplasty was performed in the hip joint in Fig. 291 with central insertion of a metallic cup and of a metallic long stem femoral head

ment is aligned along the iliac bone, the sagging of the pelvis is minimized and stability is substantially increased at maintained mobility; and (c) revision of the healed wound after 18–24 months and insertion of a complete set of arthroplastic implants with concurrent administration of broad-spectrum antibiotics.

While Calandruccio [227] regards deep infection as the most cogent reason for revising the operative area, other reasons include: loosening, subluxation, or dislocation of the implants, fracture of the stem or shaft, and extensive heterotopic ossification. Turner et al. [1667] also emphasized loosening or dislocation of the femoral compound, fracture of the femoral shaft, or failure of the femoral stem as important late complications. Revision in these untoward situations is fraught with complications, but it also renders rewarding results by enduring fixation of the endoprosthetic components [1667]. Scheller et al. [1406] advised wide exposure in fracture of the femoral compound, extraction of this compound, and reconstruction with a longer femoral compound of high-strength superalloy. After removal of the loosened acetabular compound, Bierbaum [133] advised bone grafting of the deficient socket and insertion of an adequately thick socket. In explaing some of the complications which occur with arthroplastic implants, Thurner [1642] pointed out that these implants often present areas of unevenness on the surface. These changes are the results of decomposition of the constituent metals due to localized electrochemical processes. These changes therefore also present the potential for subluxation and displacement. Another result of corrosion is decreased mechanical resistance of the metallic implants, whereupon their fractures may occur [1642]. In addition, mechanical factors such as disproportionate stresses may also play a role in the occurrence of fractures of the metallic implants [1642].

Arthrodesis of the hip joint is rarely accepted by patients due the resulting complete loss of mobility. However, it may sometimes be the unavoidable ultimate solution, especially in those cases in which after failed total arthroplasty a brace with pelvic support and hinges at the level of the hip joint does not provide satisfactory function. Thus arthrodesis of the hip joint is generally applied as a secondary procedure or, rarely,

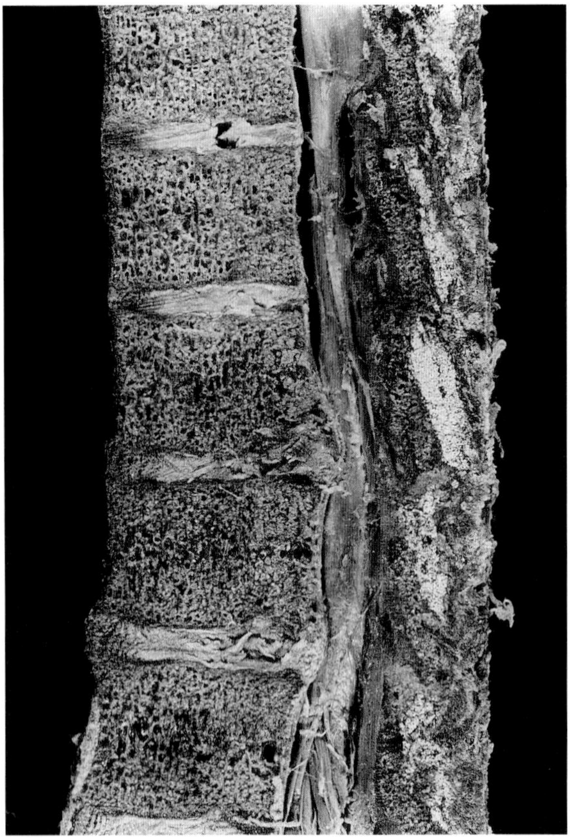

Fig. 293. The upper two intervertebral discs are locally disrupted by clefts. The caudal two intervertebral discs are extensively disintegrated, and their fragments are displaced dorsally, compressing the spinal cord. The retrospinal soft tissue is extensively calcified

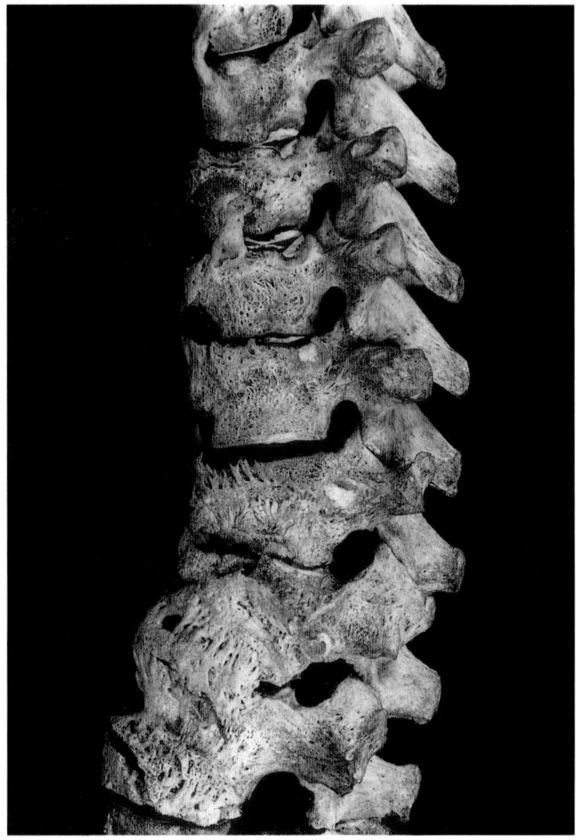

Fig. 294. Several vertebrae are worn off and are very uneven at their endplates, from which extensive osteophytes rise. Some apophyseal joints are also very uneven. The lowermost two vertebrae are fused to a single block

as a primary procedure in secondary osteoarthritis; it is then carried out for fusion in extension or 10° flexion, 10°–15° abduction, and neutral rotation. Since fusion of the hip joint puts increased stress on the ipsilateral knee joint, contralateral hip joint, and lumbar spine, it is advisable only with satisfactory function of the latter joints. For women, fusion of the hip joint is not acceptable, even with one-sided confined deficiency. Persistent indications for arthrodesis of the hip joint include osteoarthritic conditions which develop in spastic conditions, especially in cerebral palsy [1340].

In contrast to most joint diseases, either of inflammatory etiology or related to a systemic disease and primarily involving the peripheral joints, osteoarthritis often and primarily involves the vertebral column. The reason for this prevalence lies in the special anatomy determining frequent and early changes. In addition to its diarthrodial apophyseal joints, the vertebral column is characterized by the intercalation of amphiarthrodial joints, comprising elastic fibrocartilages, the intervertebral discs (Figs. 1, 2).

Anatomical studies (Schmorl and Junghanns [1420]) disclose that the intervertebral disc, composed of annulus fibrosus and nucleus pulposus, undergoes degenerative changes at an age much earlier than the joints of the extremities. The height of the intervertebral disc diminishes, as does the density of the annulus fibrosus and nucleus pulposus. This loosening is more pronounced in the central zone than in the peripheral zone bordering the vertebral plate (Figs. 3, 293). Portions of discolored amorphous tissue occur in the disc and sometimes portions of crumbled calcified material. These changes are more pronounced in the nucleus, which has lost its resilience. The distinction between the annulus fibrosus and nucleus pulposus disappears. Eventually this disrupted mass is no longer held reliably in the intervertebral location due to concurrent disruption of the surrounding connective tissue and is liable to prolapse out of the intervertebral confinement. When protruding dorsally into the intradural space (Fig. 292), the disc may exert pressure on the spinal cord or nerve roots. However, before or without prolapse, the weakening of the intervertebral disc causes substantial impairment in the mechanics of the contiguous vertebrae, which secondary to the disuse develop attrition of the hyaline cartilage in the apophyseal joints and osteophyte formations at the vertebral bodies (Fig. 294). Eventually the attritional changes come to a standstill, but general unevenness and fibrosis result (Fig. 294). Beyond this, the hypertrophic changes of the vertebral bodies and apophyseal joints may sometimes exert pressure on the emerging nerve fibers, similarly as a prolapsed intervertebral disc.

The annulus fibrosus consists physiologically of 80 % water and 20 % organic substances. The latter comprise 15 %–20 % collagen and 80 %–85 % proteoglycans [5, 1155, 1156], among which chondroitin sulfate predominates, and hyaluronic acid is the smaller proportion. However, physical and chemical changes are noticed by the age of 25–30 years [761, 1360], and these include: decrease in water content, hyaluronic acid, and chondroitin sulfates, and increase in keratan sulfate [1639], with concurrent increase in collagen fibers [486, 1427]. Similar, but more pronounced changes characterize the nucleus pulposus. Upon dehydration, structural alterations set in [1617]. Histopathological examination [726, 761, 823] (Figs. 295, 296) discloses that the ground substance of the intervertebral disc has lost its physiological staining properties, staining irregularly with increased or decreased basophilia over larger areas. Concurrently, a substantial number of the chondrocytes in the fibrocartilage are blown up, and fibrocytes in the nucleus pulposus are disintegrated with pyknosis or fragmentation of their nuclei (Figs. 295, 296). The collagen fibers are disrupted and distributed irregularly in areas of mucinous degeneration. With a substantial decrease in the number of the cells, the intercellular substance also decreases. Rarefied areas with cavitation [645] result, in which only the interstitial collagen fibers, delimiting empty spaces, are left (Fig. 297). In other areas, fibrosis prevails.

Symptoms develop insidiously and often without any identifiable external cause, on change in the posture of the body, at the start of motion, or after prolonged daily activities. They may also appear suddenly, elicited by a sprain or strain at work or at presumably innocuous movements of the vertebral column [968]. When the cervical spine is very affected, the patient is perturbed by a sensation of abnormal friction which may be associated with cracking noises propagated to the ears. The symptoms are commonly localized in the lumbar spine (lumbago), which is more subjected to stress and pressure by weight bearing, and appear distinctly earlier in the vertebral column than in joints of the extremities [1167]. While in some patients an external incident is incriminated in provoking a painful episode, in others, mostly women, an instability of the vertebral column caused by constitutional ligamentous insufficiency or developmental variations in the configuration of the vertebrae [1189] contribute to the incidence and manifestation of chronic symptoms of the vertebral column. The general symptoms are sensations of stiffness or lameness on rising. These sensations regress after limbering up and permit activity for

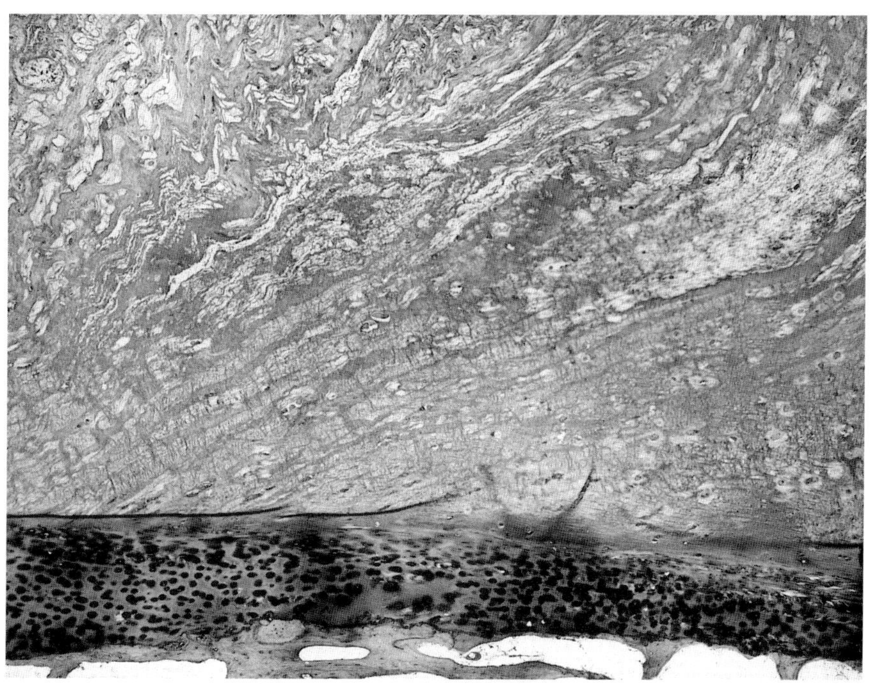

Fig. 295. The intervertebral fibrocartilage is extensively loosened by interstitial edema, which widely separates the collagen bundles

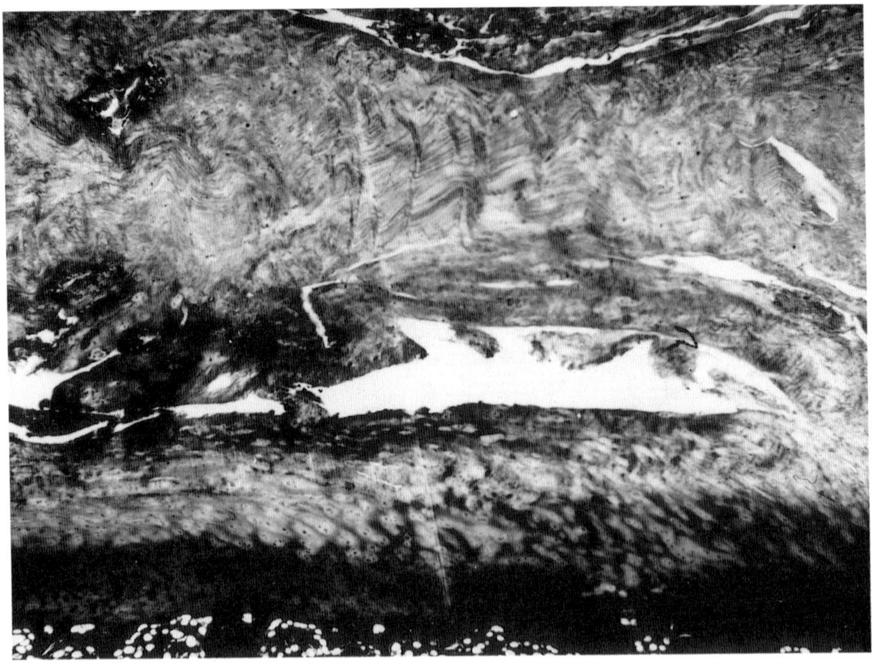

Fig. 296. The intervertebral fibrocartilage is placevise sclerosed due to densification of the collagen bundles but is generally rarefied by the disintegration of the ground substance. Consequently, large dehiscences and gaps have formed in the intervertebral disc

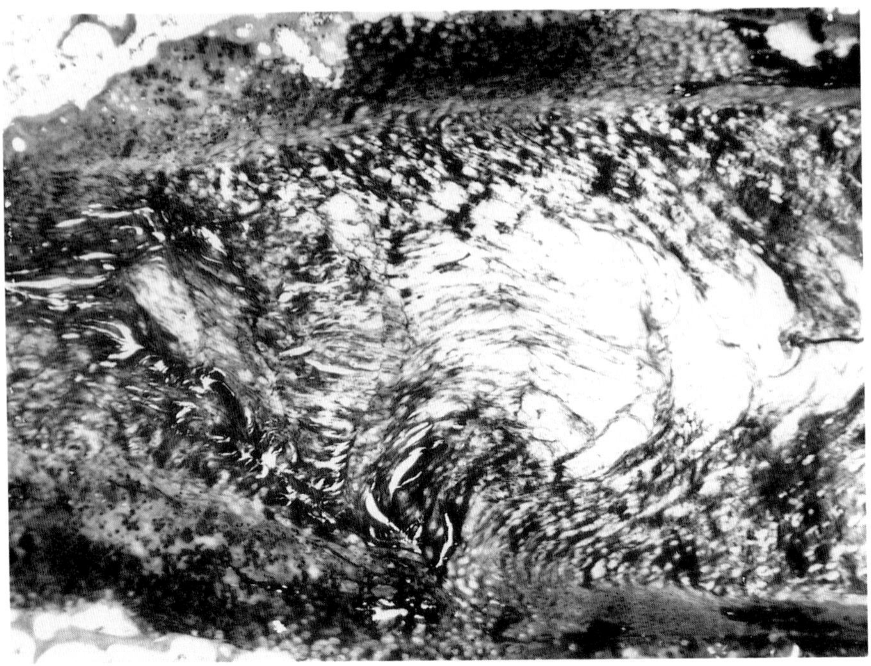

Fig. 297. On extensive disintegration of the ground substance, large cavities result in the intervertebral disc. Only a few interstitial collagen fibers persist in these cavities

an individually varying period of time, but they then return with increased intensity, pain, and impairment of function.

Corresponding to the affected area, the vertebral column [331, 550, 1167, 1420] is tender at the midline along the spinous processes and on both sides along the apophyseal joints. Reflectory tenseness of the regional paravertebral musculature, which is sensitive or tender, accompanies the acute irritation and pain. Active and passive movements of the vertebral column are limited commensurately in the directions of ventral flexion and lateral flexion, sometimes also in that of extension [656]. On regression of muscle irritation, the passive motion of the vertebral column normalizes, while the active motion remains limited for a longer period until full subsidence of the painful irritation of the vertebral joints. More disturbing are the neurological signs [341, 830], caused by the pressure of a prolapsed disc or less often by the deformed apophyseal joints. Sensory, motor, and reflex changes become manifest, related to the site of the pressure. Electromyographic examination is of essential help in determining the severity of neurological impairment [778, 939].

The most common distribution of neurological symptoms is as follows. Pressure by the cervical spine [809, 810] at C1–C3 causes pain radiating to the back of the head, anterior and posterior aspects of the neck, and posterior aspect of the shoulder (Figs. 298, 299). Pressure at C4–C5 causes pain radiating to the anterior and posterior aspects of the shoulder, anterolateral aspect of the chest, and lateral aspect of the forearm (Figs. 298, 299). Pressure at C5–C6 causes root symptoms with pain and/or sensory disturbance along the anterolateral aspect of the upper arm and forearm, as well as at the volar aspect of the wrist and first three fingers (Figs. 298, 299). The biceps tendon reflex may be depressed at concomitant atrophy of the biceps muscle. Pressure at C6–C7 causes pain radiating into the suprascapular area and axilla, tenderness and/or sensory disturbance at the posterior and anterolateral aspects of the shoulder, and tenderness and/or sensory disturbance at the posterior aspect of the upper arm extending along the dorsoradial aspect of the forearm to the dorsoradial aspect of the hand and first three fingers (Figs. 298, 299). Depression of the triceps reflex may occur, as well as weakness and/or atrophy of the triceps muscle. Pressure at C7–T1 causes pain and paresthesia at the medial aspect of the upper arm, extending from there distally into the anteromedial and posteromedial aspects of the forearm and farther into the fourth and fifth fingers (Figs. 298, 299). Weakness in active motion of the fingers also occurs. Pressure on nerve roots in the thoracic spine causes intercostal neuralgias chiefly in the lower chest cage.

In the more frequently involved lumbar spine, pressure on nerve roots at L3–L4 is manifested in pain at the anterior aspect of the thigh, and anteromedial aspect of the lower leg (Figs. 300, 301). The quadriceps reflex is depressed, and atrophy of the quadriceps muscle occurs. With pressure at L4–L5 tenderness is noticed along the posterolateral aspect of the thigh and lateral aspect of the lower leg (Figs. 300, 301). Weakness of the extensor hallucis concurs. On pressure at L5–S1 tenderness is noticed along the posterolateral aspects of the thigh and of the lower leg (Figs. 300, 301). Upon weakness or absence of the ankle reflex, atrophy of the hamstring and/or calf musculature occurs. The combination of arthritic symptoms in the lumbar spine with the complicating regional neurological symptoms has been termed "low back syndrome".

The local neurological picture, changing from tenderness and hyperesthesia to paresthesia and depression of the reflex, depends on the degree and duration of nerve compression. On incipient and mild pressure, irritation of the nerves causes pain and distributional

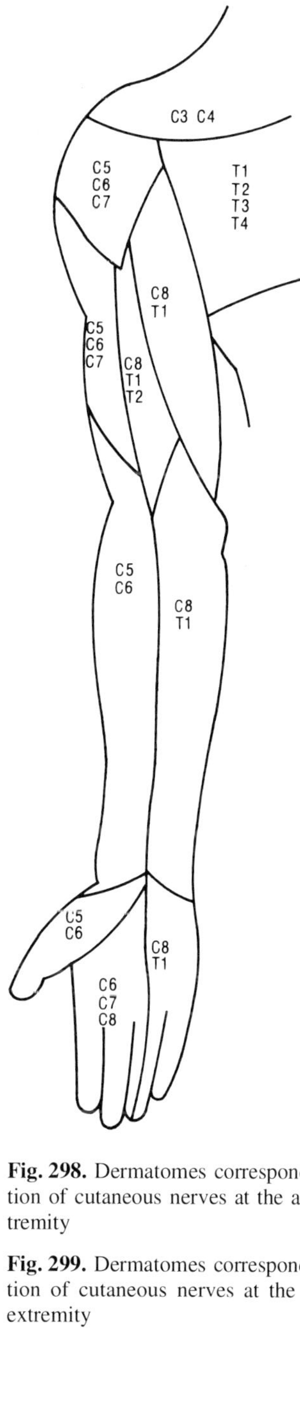

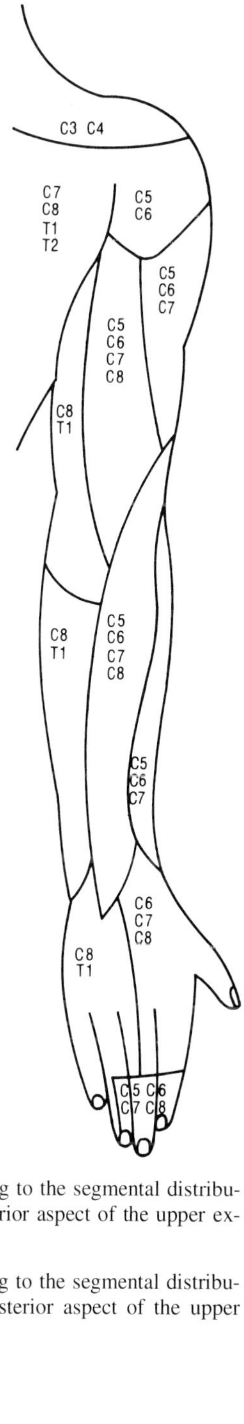

Fig. 298. Dermatomes corresponding to the segmental distribution of cutaneous nerves at the anterior aspect of the upper extremity

Fig. 299. Dermatomes corresponding to the segmental distribution of cutaneous nerves at the posterior aspect of the upper extremity

tenderness, while prolonged and more intense pressure causes degeneration of the nerves, with resulting paresthesias or loss of sensation, weakness or absence of reflexes, and muscle atrophy. Thus the clinical picture and the findings are sequential and depend on the localization, duration, and degree of disc pressure.

Roentgenographs indicate the changes in intervertebral discs by narrowing of the intervertebral spaces, especially if they are associated with irregular delinea-

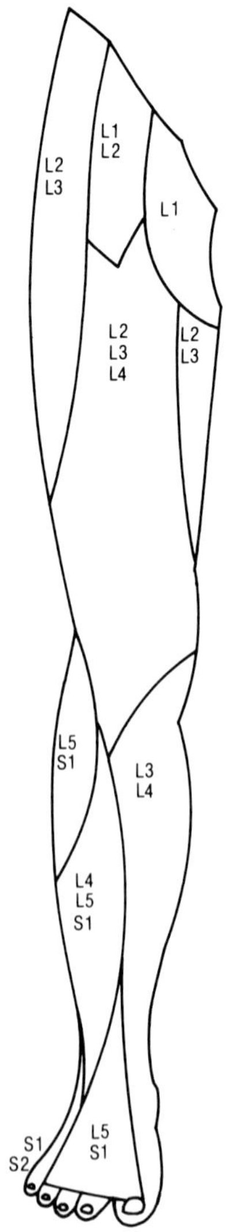

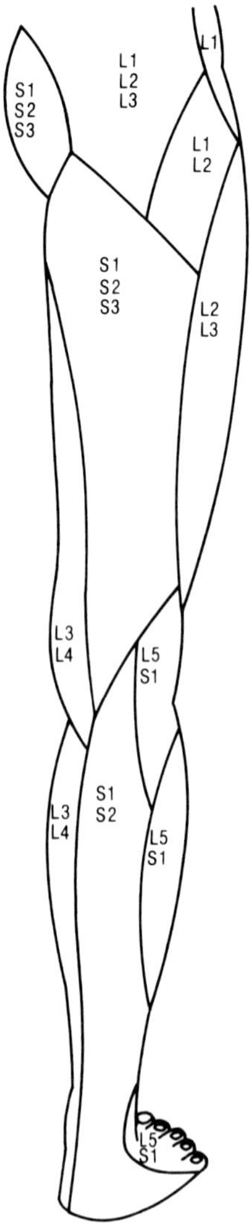

Fig. 300. Dermatomes corresponding to the segmental distribution of cutaneous nerves at the anterior aspect of the lower extremity

Fig. 301. Dermatomes corresponding to the segmental distribution of cutaneous nerves at the posterior aspect of the lower extremity

tion of the adjacent vertebral plates and/or with their eventual thickening and sclerosis (Figs. 302, 303, 304). Concurrently, the ventral edges of these plates may be worn off, while in other cases marginal osteophytes of various sizes extend from there and face similar osteophytes from the neighboring vertebrae (Figs. 302, 303, 304). Less pronounced changes are noticed dorsally in the apophyseal joints, whose spaces are substantially narrowed, and whose facets are sclerosed. Similarly, the intervertebral foramina delineating the exit of nerves are often narrowed (Figs. 303, 304). A rather rare change, upon sclerosis of the vertebral endplates, is abnormally increased radiolucency of the intervertebral space (Fig. 305), the cavitation phenomenon [645], due to accumulation of air in the meshes of the disintegrated intervertebral disc (Fig. 297). Additional special studies for verifying the site and degree of compression of the spinal cord and nerve roots include computed tomography (CT) and electromyography. The former is used routinely in cases of spinal neurological complications and has widely replaced myelography. The latter was formerly used in neurological symptoms presumably resulting from compression by a herniated intervertebral disc, but this was occasionally followed by the complication of symptoms of meningeal irritation. Computed tomography permits visualization of the intervertebral disc in its relationship to the neighboring spinal cord and spinal nerves (Figs. 21, 22) and makes it possible to ascertain a compression of these structures. This test has recently been partly replaced or supplemented by the magnetic resonance imaging (MRI) as discussed in "Radiological Examination" (Figs. 23, 24). MRI has been shown to be very informative in lesions of the spinal cord, assumed to be caused by compression by an intervertebral disc; it is able to reveal a bulging or a prolapse of the intervertebral disc [267, 512, 513, 1122].

Due to its proximity to other important organs, osteoarthritis of the cervical spine may have special clinical implications [809, 810]. A number of mimicking conditions must be considered in the differential diagnosis of cervical radiculopathy. Suddenly radiating severe pain into the anterior aspect of the chest and left arm by pressure in the lower cervical and upper thoracic spine simulates cardiac angina by coronary insufficiency [372, 1168]. This can be clarified by examination of the cervical nerve roots and by electrocardiogram, enzyme studies, and a trial with nitroglycerine. A syndrome elicited by pressure of the cervical spine on nerve fibers supplying the vertebral arteries is insufficiency of the cerebral basilar artery. This may also be caused by direct compression of these arteries and is manifested in frequent, longer lasting episodes of dizziness, nausea, vertigo, and occipital headache. Another, and very impairing symptom may be caused by direct pressure of conspicuously protruding ventral osteophytes on the esophagus, with resulting dysphagia [1281, 1307].

In view of the painfulness of the vertebral column, confined to its upper or lower part or along its entire extent, and the often associated episodes of general fatigue, a complete bedrest lying flat on a firm mattress or on a bedboard with both thighs elevated on pillows is necessary. Administration of analgesics and muscle relaxants is also required. The types of medications – salicylates and nonsteroidal antiinflammatory drugs – and their dosages are described in context of osteoar-

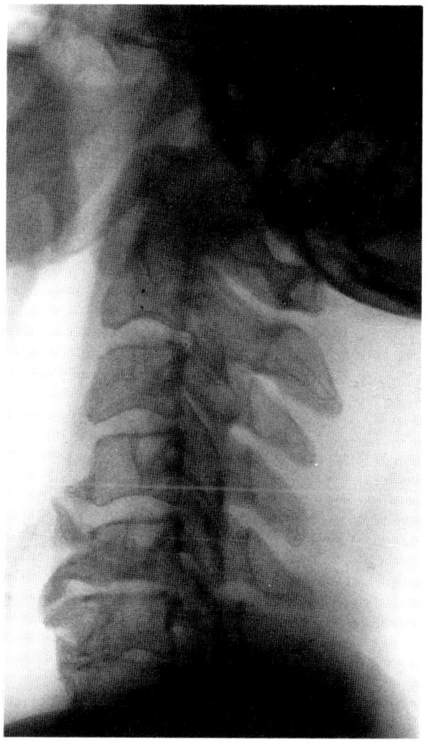

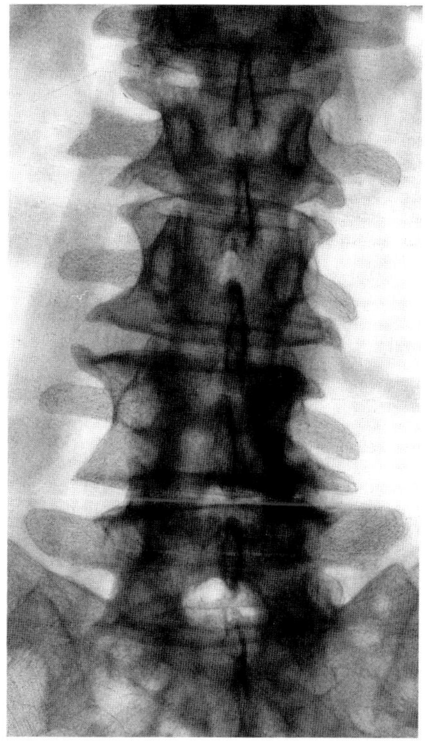

Fig. 302. The caudal vertebral plates between C2 and C4 are very concave. Large osteophytes expand from the ventral aspect from C4 to C7. The intervertebral spaces of C5–6 and C6–7 are narrowed and unevenly bordered

Fig. 303. Large marginal osteophytes expand from all lumbar vertebrae. The vertebral plates of L4 and L5 are sclerosed, and their interspaces are onesidedly narrowed

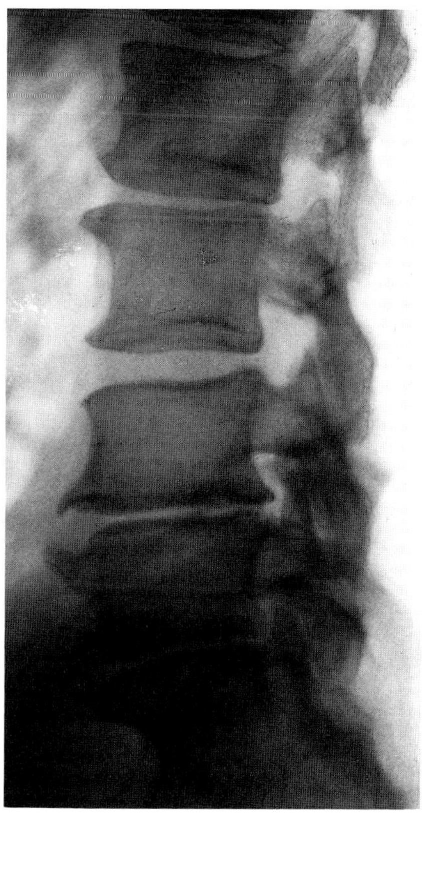

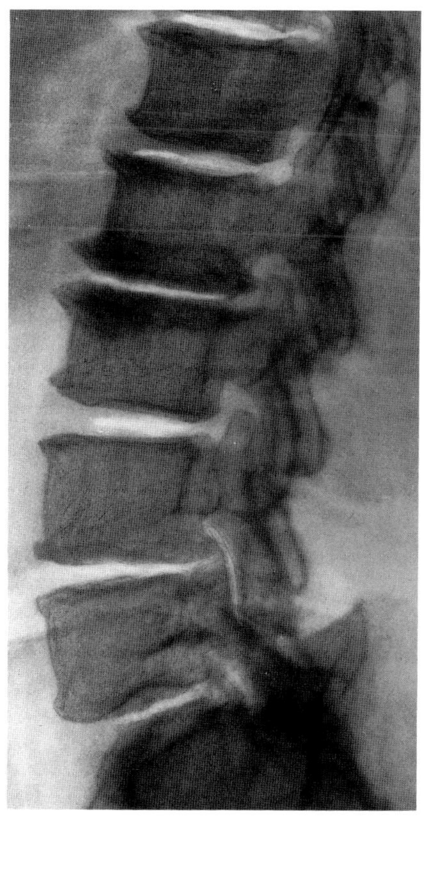

Fig. 304. Marginal osteophytes expand from all lumbar vertebrae. The cranial plate of L4 is worn off and sclerosed, as are the contiguous plates of L4–L5 and L5–S1 at marked narrowing of their interspaces

Fig. 305. Small marginal osteophytes expand ventrally from all lumbar vertebrae, whose endplates are uneven and sclerosed. All lumbar intervertebral spaces comprise delimited areas of marked radiolucency due to cavitation of the intervertebral discs

thritis of the extremities. However, osteoarthritis of the vertebral column requires more and prolonged administration of muscle relaxants two or three times daily; benefit is also often obtained from a 2- to 3-week course of colchicine administration. Regular topical use of moist heat is of basic benefit, supplied by an electric moist heating pad or, more effectively, by hot mud packs [1377]. If these modalities do not suffice, as manifested in persistent regional muscle defense and unabated neurological signs, hospitalization for traction of the cervical and/or lumbar spine is indicated, especially when reflectory symptomatic scoliosis (Fig. 49) with tilt of the trunk develops in affection of the lumbar spine. In the latter condition, the hip joints must be held flexed so that the traction can act on the straight lumbosacral spine; otherwise, the lumbar spine is held by muscle tenseness in hyperlordosis. Subsequent application of a plaster body jacket or leather jacket is useful for maintaining the lower part of the vertebral column in straight alignment; thereafter a belt or corset (Fig. 51) is indicated. Regular posture exercises are an essential factor in the aftercare for attaining adequate muscle strength and self-support. On the other hand, if no complete bedrest or traction are needed, ambulation may be resumed with a plastic cervical collar (Fig. 50) or a lumbosacral belt of firm canvas with metal stays (Fig. 51) to be worn in all activities. In advanced lumbar osteoarthritis, a leather-metal brace provides adequate support in all activities in private and occupational life which impose a strain on the vertebral column. Nevertheless, these activities may be pursued as long as the patient's general health permits. Physical therapy with ambulatory cervical or pelvic traction, shortwave diathermy, and massage in two or three series of eight to ten sessions expedite the process of recovery. In long-lasting conditions, ultrasound treatment in eight sessions of 2–3 W/cm^2 is very beneficial [687, 1541]. When faulty posture of the vertebral spine develops, causing frequent fatigue and probably aggravating the osteoarthritic changes in the vertebral column, an exercise program for improvement of posture is indicated. If feasible, combination with regular swimming is able to restore sufficient muscle strength to carry the vertebral column in a balanced posture.

While the tenderness of osteoarticular tissues gradually subsides, as manifested in regression of the defense of the regional paravertebral musculature, the possibly concomitant nerve root symptoms last much longer and require additional modalities of treatment. Transcutaneous longitudinal galvanization provides satisfactory results. However, in cases of unabated nerve root symptoms, persisting as painful neuralgias but without sensory or motor deficit, one to three intraparavertebral nerve blocks with 1% anesthetic solution provide a substantial subsidence of the radiating pain. No systemic corticosteroids may be prescribed. Nonsteroidal antiinflammatory medications are often also indicated. Eventually, at the completion of treatment, patients are instructed in strengthening exercises of the abdominal and back musculature for improvement of posture. On the other hand, no mobilization exercises for the vertebral column should be practised because they aggravate the attritional alterations in the joints and may cause the recurrence of neurological symptoms. Similarly, athletic activities should be avoided as they impose strain on the vertebral column.

Subsidence of the symptoms and significant improvement is obtained in 90%–95% of patients by the above modalities. However, in the other patients, neurological signs continue despite all conservative modalities, an indication of pressure by excessive degenerative changes at the apophyseal joints or by a nonregressing prolapsed disc. This can be ascertained by electromyography, computed tomography, or magnetic resonance imaging. In such situations, operation is indicated, with a partial laminectomy which permits adequate visualization and removal of the compressing structures, especially of a herniated disc. On this occasion, a thorough search should also be carried out in the neighboring intervertebral spaces for separated and possibly dislodged fragments of degenerated intervertebral discs. Therefore, an exploration at two or three levels is usually indicated. The question arises here whether the ailing part of the vertebral column should be stiffened by either an intertransverse fusion or an anterior interbody fusion. Since the operative exposure for the removal of one or two discs is not very extensive, topical arthrodesis is not strictly necessary, especially because fusion of one part of the vertebral column imposes increased strain on the directly neighboring parts. This may aggravate an already existing osteoarthritis of the neighboring areas. However, such fusion is indicated in cases of extensive and advanced osteoarthritis of the vertebral column complicated by persistent neurological symptoms which cause disabilities in the activities of daily life and occupational requirements.

VI. Trophic Alterations of Joints

1. Osteochondritis Dissecans

Osteochondritis dissecans is the term given by Koenig [907] to a joint ailment in which a fragment of cartilage and subchondral bone becomes separated from an articular surface. Its cause was viewed [907] as trauma to an area of the joint which was either mechanically very stressed or perhaps previously weakened by inflammation of the bone and cartilage, thus the designation of osteochondritis. Axhausen [57] emphasized that the weakening of the articular cartilage and its subchondral bone was predetermined by local necrosis of these tissues. The cause of these changes was considered [57] to be occlusion of the regional blood vessels in the subchondral bone either by bland mycotic emboli or secondary to injuries of the vascular wall. On disruption of the local blood supply, infarction and necrosis follow. This view has been supported by Platzgummer [1265] and others. On the other hand, Burckhardt [214] postulated that momentary disturbances in the function of a joint by sudden, uncoordinated muscle action expose its articular surfaces to violent impact, separating a fragment from the articular surfaces. As support for this view, Burckhardt [214] described young athletic patients whose vigorous musculature probably caused either injury to the regional blood vessels or direct separation of a portion of the articular surface. However, to these patients can be opposed legions of athletes who, despite vigorous musculature and abundant occasions for injuries, continue their activities without any disruption in the osteocartilaginous surfaces. Therefore, in addition to trauma as an eliciting cause, preexisting weakness of the osteochondral surface must be assumed, either by toxic harm or occlusion of the nutrient blood vessels with following aseptic necrosis. Thurner [1641] pointed out that osteochondritis dissecans, whose initial alteration is aseptic necrosis of directly subchondral bone, is related to the large entity of aseptic necrosis of metaphyseal bone – in which, however, no dissection evolves.

A necrotic focus in osteochondritis dissecans may become organized by the surrounding tissue and may heal. In other cases, the already weakened tissue, being crushed by an additional injury, becomes further devitalized; it loses the capacity to resume continuity with the adjacent osseous tissue. Because of disintegration of the marginal bony trabecula, the residual portion becomes separated as a foreign body from the surrounding tissue. A minor injury or an uncoordinated movement then suffices completely to sever the already loosened aseptic fragment. Therefore, one discerns in osteochondritis dissecans a stage of necrosis, another of sequestration or dissection, and finally one of traumatic separation. The lack of complete immobilization and the continuation of articular movements are responsible for the further course because the possibilities of reparatory organization and healing are prevented. The extruded sequestrum as well as its bed eventually become smoothed by grinding activities of the articular surfaces.

Osteochondritis dissecans [11, 981, 983, 1022, 1123, 1223] appears predominantly in adolescents and young adults. Distinct injuries or significant faulty movements are seldom recorded in the history. The presence of bone dissection is introduced by a long phase of undefined symptoms in the joint. With continued activity, diffuse soreness develops which limits the range of movements. On longer use and after prolonged duration, the joint capsule becomes diffusely swollen. The joints principally affected by osteochondritis dissecans [286] are, in order of frequency, those of the knee [1123], elbow, hip, and ankle. Certain areas of their articular epiphyses are preferentially involved: in the knee it is the medial femoral condyle, in the elbow the capitellum humeri, in the hip the cranial surface of the femoral head, and in the ankle the trochlea tali. When a joint of the lower extremity is involved, early fatigue sets in. With separation of the sequestrum, usually caused by a strenuous activity, the symptoms of a loose joint body eventually become manifest. Intense pain is then experienced at well circumscribed locations. These may change to other locations on migration of the loose body, expecially when it resides temporarily in a recessus or outpouching of the joint capsule (Fig. 322). Therefore, episodes of marked pain may be followed by longer phases (even a few months) of freedom from pain or discomfort. Eventually, an episode of entrapment of the loose body within the joint cleft and with locking of the joint may occur, repeating itself at varying intervals. Most patients learn to shake out the entrapped fragment by certain active or passive movements of the joint. However, on frequent repetition of the locking episodes, severe impairment in the use of the joint arises.

Physical examination discloses a moderate, circumscribed tenderness without limitation of motion, as long as the sequestrum remains in its original location. On its detachment and migration, the pain shifts and becomes propagated to various areas at the surface corresponding to the present site along the transient course of the loose body. The joint capsule becomes more swollen and sometimes distended by increased joint fluid. Concurrently, the regional musculature becomes atrophic, with the joint appearing more thickened and deformed. However, the range of its movements remains rather undiminished, except for

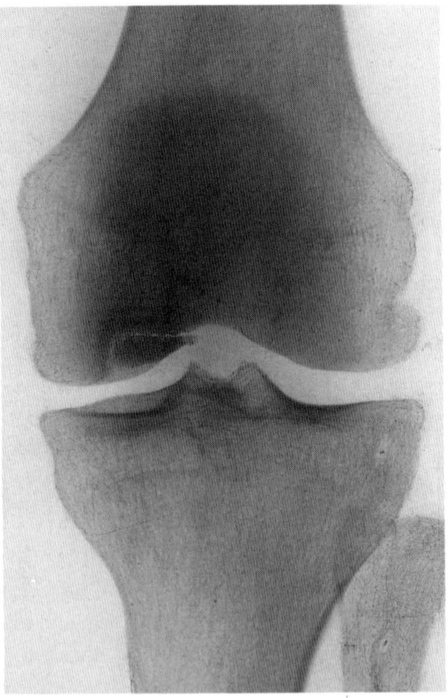

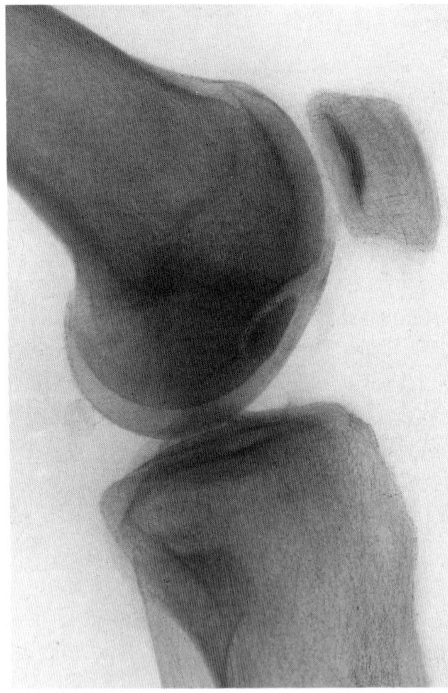

Fig. 306. An area of densification within the articular surface is separated from the surrounding medial femoral condyle by a narrow zone of radiolucency

Fig. 307. An ovoid densified area within the articular surface is partly separated from the surrounding femoral condyle by a zone of radiolucency

a phase of entrapment or when a contracture (rarely) sets in.

Roentgenographs [1107] initially reveal only a small ovoid area of radiolucency which may sometimes escape detection. When necrosis of the subchondral bone becomes more extensive, the sequestrum appears as an area of circumscribed densification surrounded directly by a narrow zone of osteoporosis, thus of lesser density and peripherally to this by normal bone; it lies like "an egg in a nest" (Figs. 306, 307, 315). After the sequestrum has been completely separated and detached, it can be followed roentgenographically in its migration tract. Its empty bed can be discerned for a long period of time, until it eventually becomes shallow partly by being filled up from the depth and partly by being ground off on the surface through articular action.

Osteochondritis dissecans in the initial stage, with the sequestrum in situ, is gross-anatomically [10, 1107] noticeable by a small, circumscribed area of whitish hyaline cartilage, contrasted against the bluish white glistening hyaline cartilage of the surroundings. The former cartilage cover is also conspicuous by its difference in level because it is a little deeper than the surrounding cartilage and can be pushed deeper by digital or instrumental pressure. This indicates the presence of interposed compressible tissue. The latter granulation tissue becomes obvious after elimination of the sequestrum because it covers the residual defect, which is sharply delimited by a steep margin, and extends rather deeply into the subchondral cancellous bone. Prior to its elimination the separated sequestrum lies in its bed and is connected to it by a stalk of cartilage and connective tissue, but it can easily be lifted out from the bed. The sequestrum (Fig. 308) has the shape of a lens, a length of 0.8–2.4 cm, and a width of 0.5–1.2 cm. One of its surfaces bears whitish cartilage; the other (Fig. 309) is yellow due to denuded, sometimes uneven, but more often friction-smoothened bony trabeculae. These are covered scantily with connective

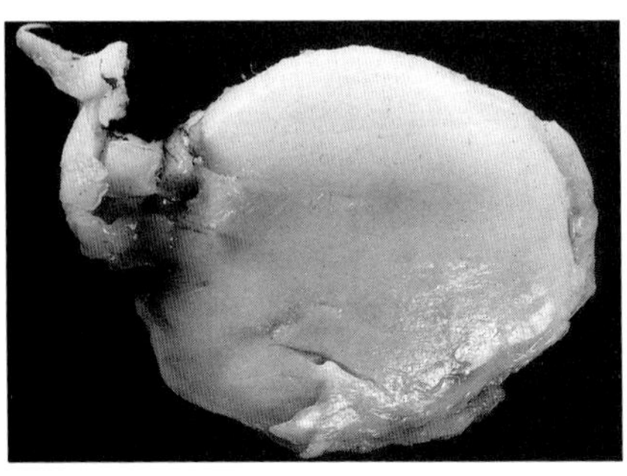

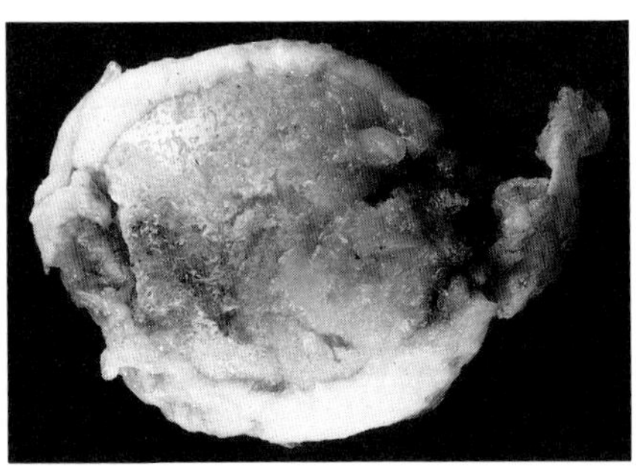

Fig. 308. A lens-shaped tissue portion is entirely covered by articular cartilage on one surface

Fig. 309. The other surface of the tissue portion in Fig. 307 is smoothened cancellous bone

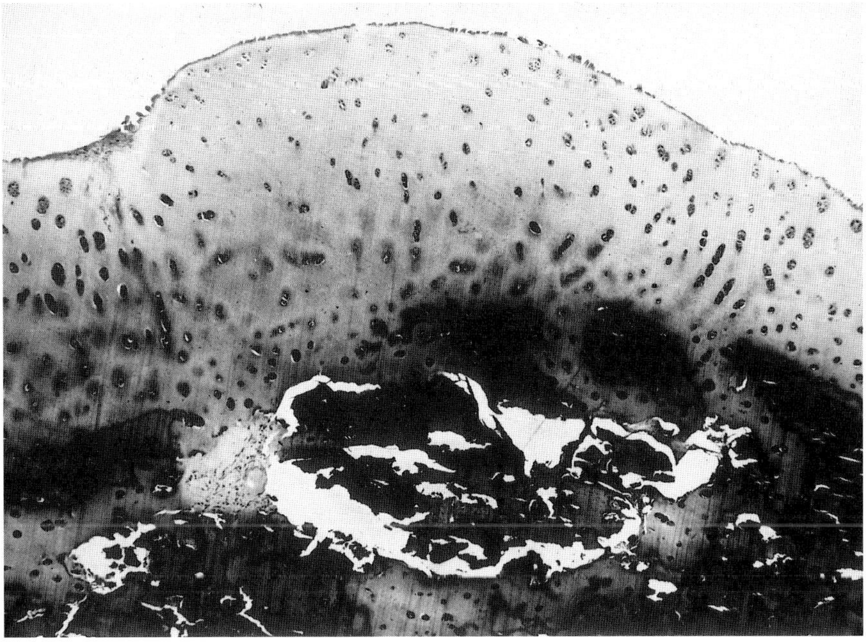

Fig. 310. A portion of articular cartilage and its subjacent bone is necrotic and is separated by empty spaces from the adjacent viable cartilage and bone

tissue and are usually bordered along their margin by a rim of hyaline cartilage. After longer duration, the margin of the defect becomes even by attrition, and its ground is filled with dense connective tissue. The free sequestrum then no longer fits into its bed.

Histopathological examination [1107] in the initial stage discloses an area of the directly subcartilaginous bone being completely necrotic (Fig. 310) and presenting numerous lacunae bare of osteocytes, with maintained trabecular structure. The regional blood vessels are obliterated. In a subsequent stage, a thin, rather even line of separation courses at the base of this portion (Fig. 311) and eventually widens to a broad zone which causes a complete separation of the necrotic bone from the underlying, normally structured bone. Granulation tissue expands from the marrow spaces of this cancellous bone into the zone of separation, and partly fills it (Fig. 313). The freed sequestrum (Fig. 312) is covered [284] at the surface by sometimes normally structured hyaline cartilage but which more often is disrupted by horizontal and/or vertical clefts. This hyaline cartilage, nourished by diffusion, remains

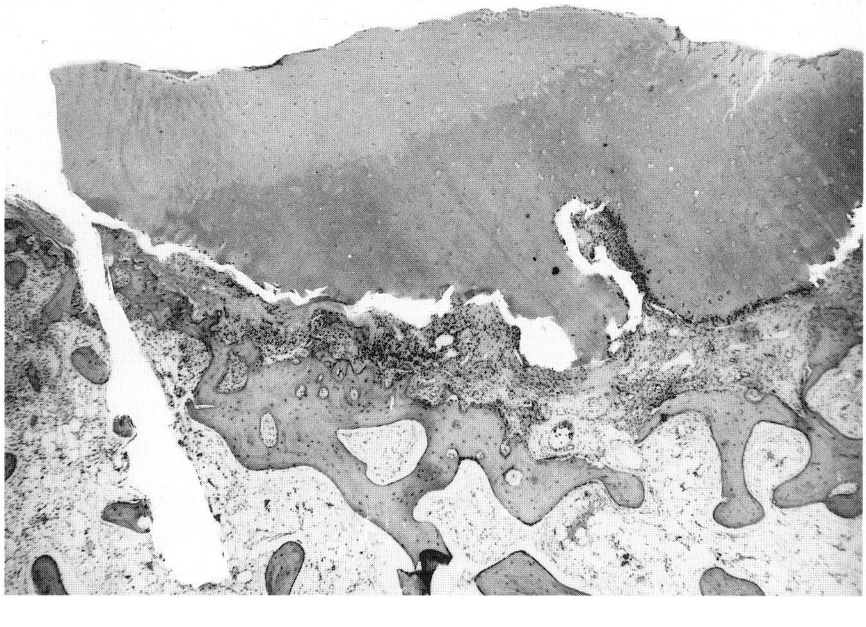

Fig. 311. A portion of articular cartilage is partly separated by granulation tissue from the underlying cortical bone. The latter is partly separated from the surrounding bone

viable and presents only in small areas a changed staining pattern and a few lacunae with pyknotic or fragmented nuclei. The cartilage cover sometimes expands over the lower margins of the sequestrum and forms here a rim (Fig. 309) in the stage of separation. Beneath the articular cartilage of the sequestrum lies a thin layer of subchondral cortical bone merging with a broader layer of trabeculae of cancellous bone. The latter is necrotic to its greatest extent and comprises many empty tombs of osteocytes. The surface of the sequestrum toward the metaphysis in partly covered by a thin layer of connective tissue (Fig. 312) which expands from the underlying healthy cancellous bone. This granulation tissue on the lower surface causes lacunary resorption of bony substance and thereby separation in a plane. Nevertheless, before its complete separation, the sequestrum remains connected with the epiphysis by a few thin bridges of connective tissue, until these too are disrupted.

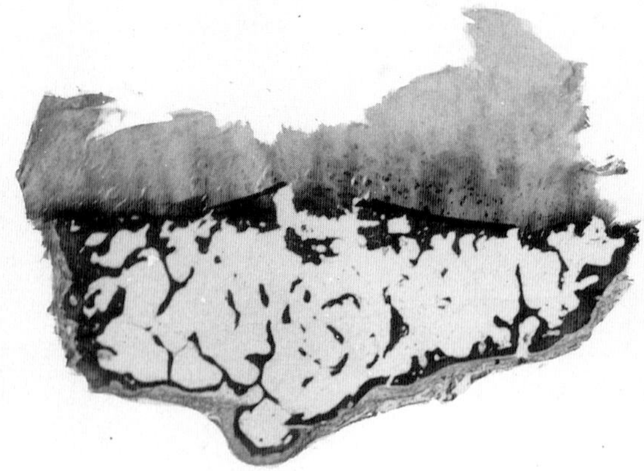

Fig. 312. A portion of partly worn off articular cartilage together with the subjacent cortical and a small zone of cancellous bone is comletely separated and is loose

On longer duration of the condition, the synovial membrane presents a thickening of its most superficial layer by three- to fourfold hyperplasia of the synoviocytes and irregularity in its surface by formation of numerous small villi. The subjacent zone displays a distinct paucity of inflammatory cells, but numerous small blood vessels with conspicuous thickening of their walls by hyaline apposition and fibrosis of the surrounding tissue are present (Fig. 314). The subsynoviocytis tissue also often comprises a few smaller or larger, sharply delimited portions of viable hyaline cartilage (Fig. 314), obviously fragments separated from the articular surface.

Differential diagnosis must consider loose joint bodies of other etiologies, especially broken-off marginal osteophytes, severed calcified portions of the inner part of the joint capsule, and chondromata. However, these formations are mostly roundish, longish, or of irregular shape (Fig. 517), but not of lens shape, and are usually multiple, in contrast to the single sequestrum in osteochondritis dissecans. They also do not leave an empty bed or nest in the articular surface. In the knee joint with absence of a roentgenographically detectable, isolated bone shadow, an injury to a meniscus must be considered as a possible cause if episodes of locking of the joint occur.

Once the diagnosis of osteochondritis dissecans is established, and the cartilage-bone sequestrum is still lying in its original indentation, reorganization and complete healing of the sequestrum is possible, even probable. Therefore, treatment should start without delay. The joint should be completely immobilized, whenever feasible, by a plaster cast for 3–4 months to preclude any traumatization and disruption of the healing process. Subsequent protection of the joint by a firm strapping or brace is indicated. Hereby the complete organic incorporation of the sequestrum can be obtained, especially in adolescents (Figs. 315, 316). Conservative treatment is usually fully sufficient in this age group. However, if this management does not

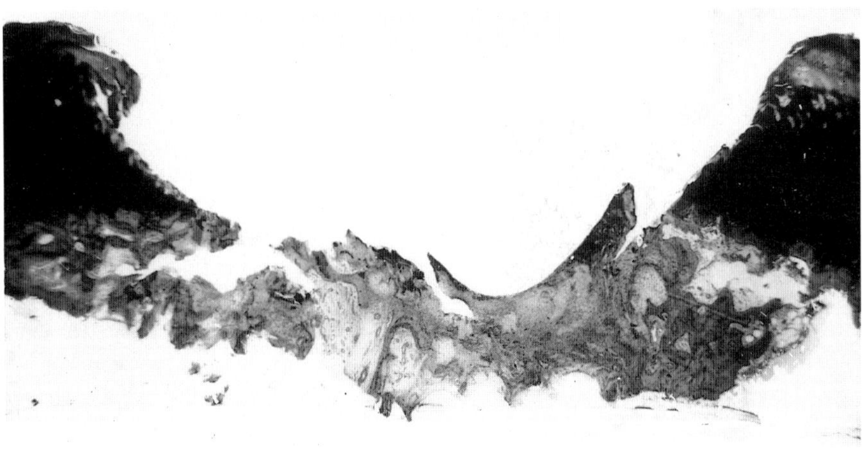

Fig. 313. The articular cartilage and its subjacent cortical and cancellous bone present an extensive smooth defect caused by separation of a large portion from this surface

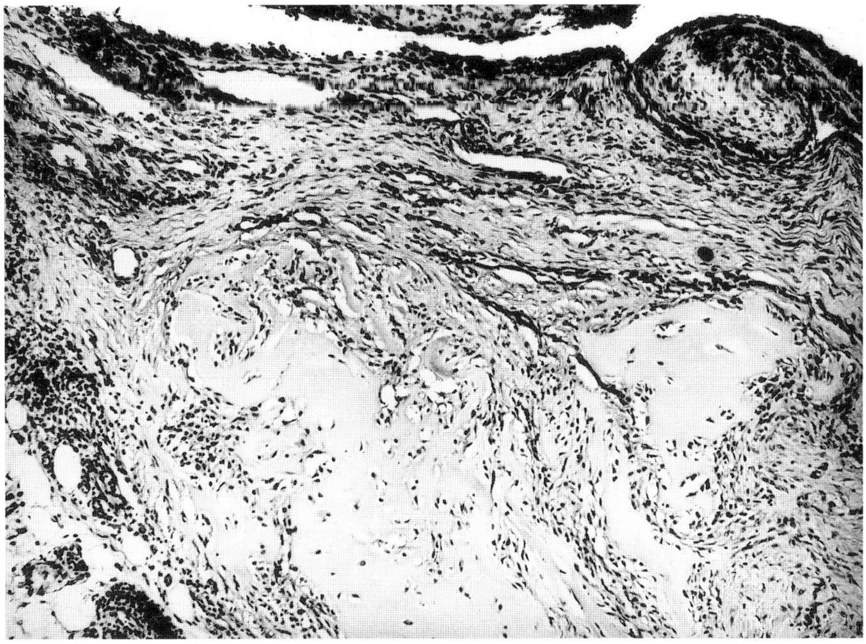

Fig. 314. The synovial membrane is rather densely hypercellular in its subsynoviocytic area secondary to an increase in fibrocytes. Within the latter lie two large fragments of hyaline cartilage intruded by granulation tissue

succeed in adults, then the revioal of the sequestrum, if still lying in its niche, and of its bed can be implemented. With a thin drill bit, a few canals are drilled extending through the sequestrum into the subchondral bone. Reorganization of the sequestrum from the depth may thus be obtained [292, 1022, 1701]. With the recently demonstrated versatility of arthroscopy, such drilling can be accomplished in an arthroscopic exploration [693]; arthrotomy is no longer necessary. It is not advisable then to stabilize the sequestrum in situ by a screw, which disrupts the articular evenness, as long as it remains in the joint; moreover, the screw leaves a hole after its removal. Nevertheless, it is indicated after the arthroscopic drilling to immobilize the joint by a plaster cast or brace until progressive reorganization of the sequestrum is noticeable in roentgenographs.

On the other hand, in cases in which the sequestrum has been eliminated from its niche and migrates in the joint cavity, it should be removed [292, 1022]. Depending on its size and ultimate location, its removal in entirety can be achieved either by arthroscopy or by arthrotomy. The latter uses a direct and thus the short-

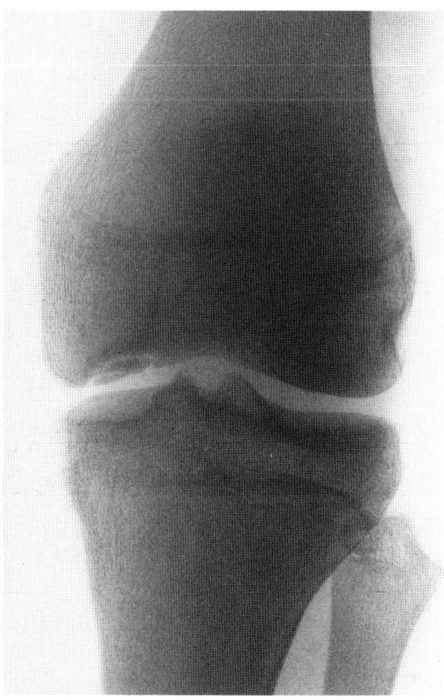

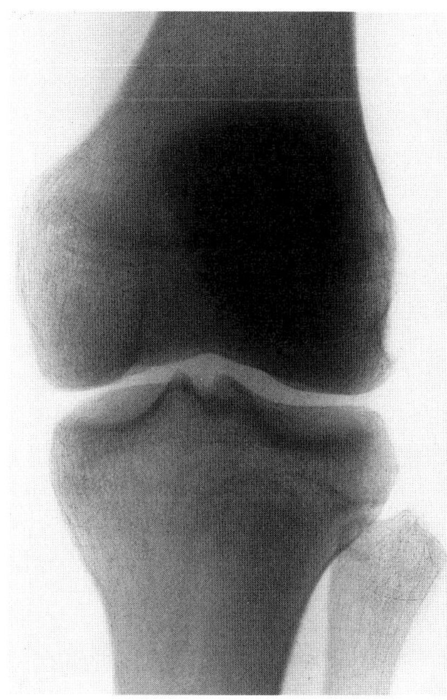

Fig. 315. The articular surface of the medial femoral condyle presents a delimited area of radiolucency within which a dense ovoid shadow lies like an egg in a nest

Fig. 316. The previous area of radiolucency in the articular surface of the medial femoral condyle (Fig. 315) is almost fully restructured

est approach to the location of the displaced sequestrum. It is also indicated here to curette the connective tissue lining the ground of the defect in the articular surface. Hereby filling of the defect is initiated from the depth with granulation tissue which, under the influence of resumed function of the joint, undergoes transformation into dense connective tissue and fibrocartilage. Nevertheless, even with responsive filling of the curetted defect, the smooth surface of the articular epiphysis cannot be fully restored. The later development of osteoarthritic changes in this joint is therefore a frequent outcome. Such sequelae may also be observed in the joints of adults with less advanced and conservatively treatable osteochondritis dissecans [1123].

2. Loose Joint Bodies

The undisturbed function of a joint depends to a great degree on its smooth articular surfaces and its unobstructed joint cavity. However, if firm bodies of a certain minimal size are interposed within the joint cavity and especially between the articular surfaces, they elicit a functional disorder which may entail substantial impairment.

Koenig [906] explained the etiology of the loose joint bodies by direct trauma or as a late sequela of trauma to healthy articular cartilage and subjacent bone. Nevertheless, previous bland infarcts or inflammatory processes may also lead to such occurrences by ischemic necrosis of circumscribed areas of cartilage and bone. These become separated by subsequent strain or minor trauma. Similarly, developmental inferiority or local predisposition secondary to degenerative processes may diminish the resistance of the osteocartilaginous surface to damage by normal function. Consequently, small portions of this surface become separated. Whereas Koenig [906] ascribed an important role to trauma in the etiology of loose articular bodies, Barth [82] and Kappis [853] regard trauma as the sole cause of loose joint bodies. According to Barth [82], any blunt or open injury of a joint may elicit the direct separation of fragments of cartilage and bone or the compression of soft tissue and its blood vessels. If necrosis of circumscribed areas of tissues follows, portions of these become demarcated and detached as sequestra. Histopathological findings, similar to those in fractures, and the absence of inflammatory changes, may be regarded as support for the primary traumatic etiology [214]. Accordingly, Thurner [1641] concluded that trauma plays a great part in the etiology of the loose bodies stemming from the articular surfaces, either by direct separation of fragments or by creating the conditions for subsequent detachment. On the other hand, Axhausen [57] emphasized the primary dystrophic pathogenesis of loose joint bodies by bland thrombosis leading to ischemia of circumscribed tissue areas. The resulting necrotic tissue portions are separated from their grounds by the mechanical stresses of normal joint function.

In addition, loose bodies of other well-explainable pathogenesis may be found. Intense inflammations of the synovial membrane lead to exudation and precipitation of fibrin. Flakes of fibrin become clumped together (Fig. 150) by the joint function and come to lie between folds or in outpouchings of the joint capsule. Into these organic nuclei calcium salts may be deposited; the hardened material is eventually eliminated into the free joint space, where it is shifted around depending on the range of movements. Similar events accompany traumatically separated portions of the joint capsule. On gaping of the joint cleft upon wide-range movements, villous portions of the capsule become entrapped and sheared off between the articular epiphyses; these become necrotic and subsequently encrusted with calcium salts (Fig. 394). More common are protruding marginal spurs and other unevennesses of the articular epiphyses being broken off (Fig. 265) in primary or secondary osteoarthritis (Figs. 444, 447, 452, 453, 455). Similarly, after healing of destructive processes in the epiphyses such as osteomyelitis or metastatic suppuration, the remaining mobility causes evenness of the articular surfaces by cracking off all prominences and elevations.

Independent of traumatic origin are benign new formations in the joint capsule which may be found as loose bodies in the articular cavity. Predominantly, solitary (Fig. 515) and multiple chondromata or chondroosteomata (Figs. 321, 516) enter the joint cavity after their separation from their areas of origin in the synovial membrane. More rarely, a small fibroma (Fig. 508) or lipoma (Fig. 510) loses its pedunculated connection to the inner joint capsule and is shifted back and forth in the joint cavity.

The types of loose joint bodies may be classified in terms of their respective etiology, als follows:

Primarily traumatically caused loose joint bodies

Fragments of cartilage and/or bone from articular epiphyses

Sheared-off villi from the inner joint capsule

Torn-off menisci

Chipped-off marginal osteophytes or surface unevennesses

Traumatic separations in trophic disorders of the articular epiphysis

Necrosis of articular cartilage secondary to occlusion of blood vessels

Osteochondritis dissecans

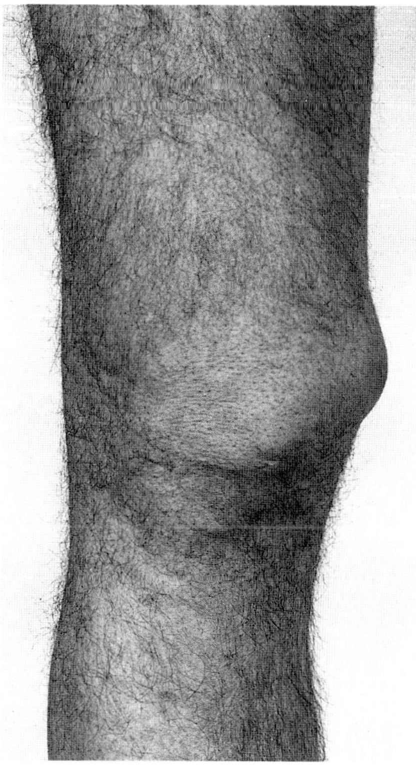
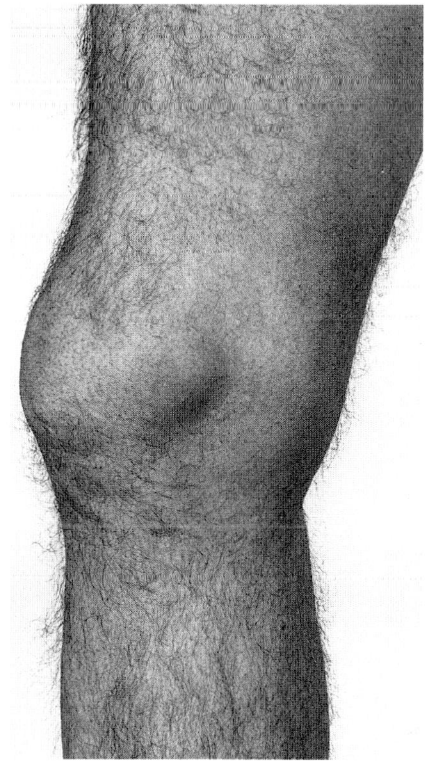

Fig. 317. A circumscribed elevation protrudes on the medial aspect of the right knee

Fig. 318. The elevation on the medial aspect of the right knee is well circumscribed and of globular shape

Neuropathic arthropathies in diabetes, tabes, syringomyelia

Loose joint bodies formed secondarily to inflammation

Coagulation of fibrin deposits: rice bodies
Calcification of fibrin precipitates from exudates
Calcification of separated necrotic villi
Sequestration after inflammatory destruction of the cartilage-bone surface (empyema, osteomyelitis, tuberculosis etc.)

Loose joint bodies from detached benign new formations

Fibroma
Lipoma
Chondroma, solitary or multiple
Chondroosteoma, solitary or multiple

The joint most frequently affected by loose bodies is that of the knee (Figs. 317, 318). It is affected in about 70% of cases, more often than the elbow, shoulder, hip, or ankle joint.

When questioned about possible causes, some patients indicate a distinct and marked trauma which occurred months or years ago while others recall only an insignificant sprain. In many other cases, even very discerning patients are not able to indicate a factor in the origin of their loose bodies. The symptoms caused by these bodies are vague, at least initially, and depend chiefly on the position of these bodies within the joint cavity. In addition to a slightly radiating pain, whose emananting site cannot always be accurately indicated, patients often experience a disturbing sensation within the joint. This sensation is rather vague as long as the loose body remains attached to the joint capsule or to the osteocartilaginous surface or is located in an outpouching. However, once it becomes completely separated, it causes pronounced symptoms such as localized soreness or marked discomfort. On its shifting, the loose body is liable to enter between contiguous articular epiphyses when they are disengaged from each other at a certain angle of motion. Thereupon invariably follows a locking of shorter or longer duration of the joint. Since at another angle of active or intentional passive motion the entrapped joint body may become liberated, it may resume its migration in the joint cavity, with the result that it appears at the next occasion in another place. Thus, the term "joint mouse". If several loose bodies exist concurrently in various locations, they may elicit alternating episodes of locking. However, characteristic for the joint mouse are its solitary existence, its polished pathway, and, for the patient, its well-known locations. Chronic irritation of the joint with frequent discomfort arises from the friction of the joint capsule. The patient is also aware of the joint becoming locked by the interposition of the migrating joint body. He learns with time to release the locking of

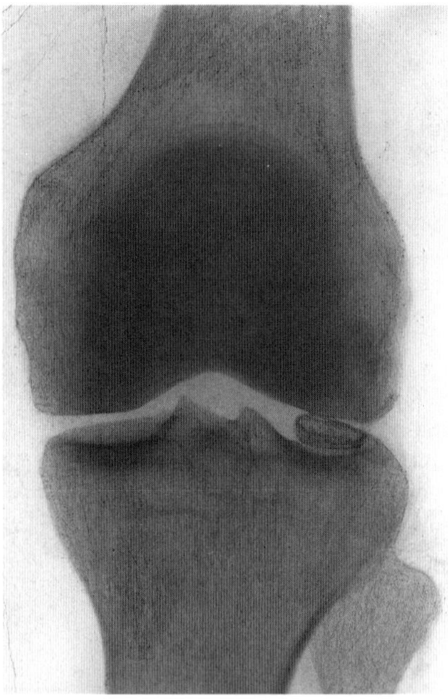

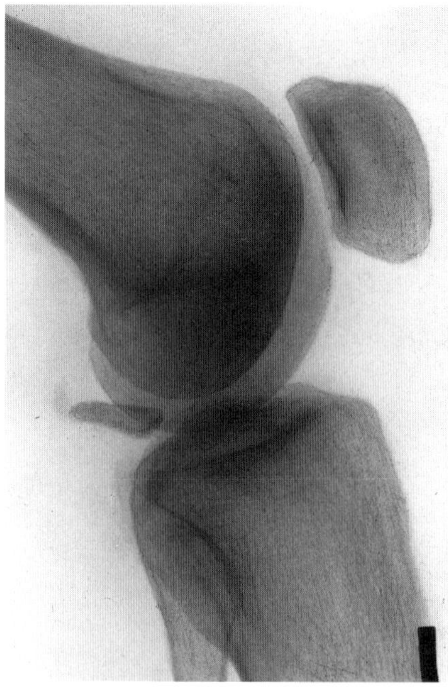

Fig. 319. A flat rather thick shadow of bone density lies in the lateral joint space

Fig. 320. The shadow of bone in Fig. 319 lies in the posterior joint space, almost entirely retrocondylarly

the joint by certain active or passive manipulations which shake the loose body out. Nevertheless, its persistent presence, aggravates the functional disturbance in the joint. Eventually a significant impairment in the use of this joint ensues in daily activities, work, and sport.

Clinical examination discloses atrophy of the regional musculature, which becomes more conspicuous by contrast with the thickening of the joint capsule (Figs. 317, 318). Within the joint, free bodies of hard consistency are often palpated; these are sharply delimited and movable. When superficially located and close to the skin, they are observable by presenting a protrusion foreign to this region (Figs. 317, 318). The mobility of the joint is generally not diminished unless an entrapment occurs, but any movement is associated with crepitation. Auscultation of the joint discloses abrupt cracking.

Roentgenographs reveal, close to or between articular epiphyses (Figs. 319, 320), one or several loose bodies of osseous density; the configuration may provide a clue as to its or their provenance. Ovoid discs (Figs. 306, 307, 315) are fragments separated by osteochondritis from the articular epiphyses which most often present a defect at the site of separation. Edgy multiangular pieces are fragments of bone broken off by a trauma (Figs. 319, 320, 447). Jagged or mulberry-shaped shadows are osteomata or detached necrotic capsular portions impregnated with calcium salts. Similarly, several jagged or roundish homogeneous densifications scattered throughout the joint correspond to multiple chondroosteomata (Fig. 514). On longer persistence of the loose bodies, the articular epiphyses display changes of attrition.

Gross-anatomical examination of the inner part of the joint capsule discloses chronic inflammatory changes; it is reddened and thickened. Its villi are elongated, and most are very vascular. The synovial fluid is increased, serous clear, and brownish yellow. Within the joint cavity (Fig. 321), sometimes connected with the synovial membrane or lodged in an outpouching of the joint capsule (Fig. 322), lie loose bodies. Their most frequent location is the folding at the attachment of the inner part of the joint capsule onto the articular epiphyses. They are very often single (Figs. 508, 510, 515), but in a substantial number of cases they are multiple (Figs. 150, 321, 322, 516, 517). They are of various shapes and sizes: roundish and lentil- or pea-shaped (Fig. 515), longish and flat like pebblestones (Fig. 517), polyhedral with many facets (Fig. 515), or curved like a coral growth. Some have a shiny white

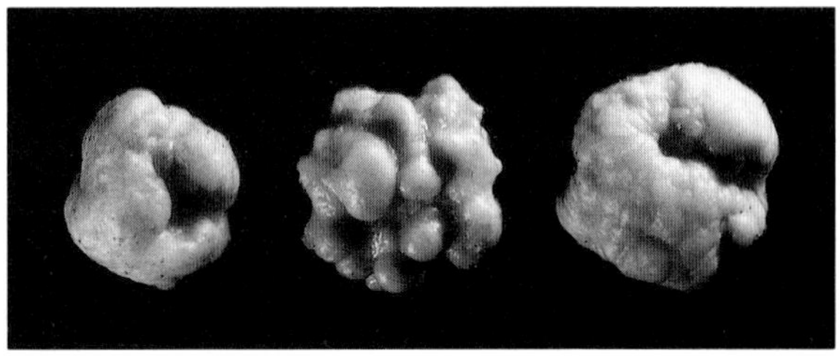

Fig. 321. A few joint bodies are loose. Their rather nodular surface and hard consistency indicate that they are chondroosteomata

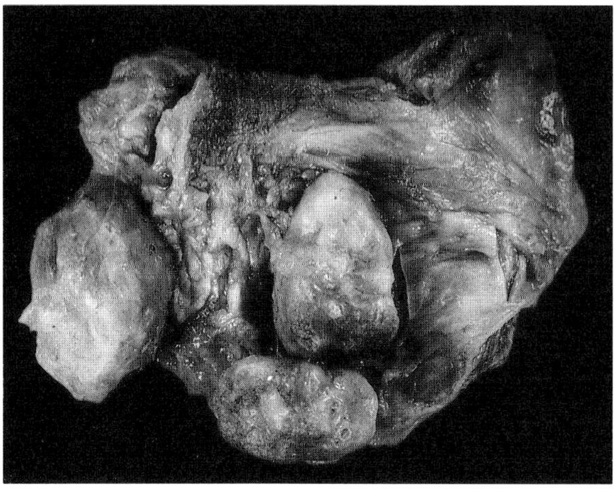

Fig. 322. Two loose joint bodies lie free on the inner surface of the joint capsule, and another loose body lies in an outpouching of the joint capsule

cover of hyaline cartilage on one surface and bony trabecula with yellow gray cover of connective tissue on the other (Figs. 308, 309). Others have a glistening bluish white cartilage cover on all sides and a hard core of bone (Fig. 321), and still others are irregularly shaped composites of connective tissue with a hard core (Fig. 510) of amorphous calcified or osseous material.

On microscopic examination, free bodies (Fig. 323) stemming from the articular epiphyses display on top a rind of hyaline or fibrocartilage in which lie pale stained cells surrounded by halos. Beneath follows bony tissue (Fig. 323), whose trabeculae are thin and sometimes necrotic by presenting empty lacunae; the marrow spaces contain partly fibrosed tissue. Other loose bodies originating from the joint capsule comprise dense connective tissue or fibrocartilage which forms a broad cover around a core either of large islands of chondrocytes and a few thick osseous trabeculae (Fig. 519) or of necrotic and calcified connective tissue. The area at which the free body was connected to the joint capsule is indicated by an expansion of cellular connective tissue (Fig. 323). Other free bodies are composed of lobules of variedly structured cartilage differing in the composition of its ground substance and the shape of its cells (Figs. 519). Most of these lobules consist of hyaline cartilage, with chondrocytes surrounded by basophilic halos. Others display regressive changes by vacuoles and fragmentation of nuclei of chondrocytes and mucinous disintegration of the ground substance with the appearance of lacunae and larger cavities. In other lobules, precipitations of calcium salts as well as formation of osteoid and osseous tissue took place.

Differential diagnosis is difficult in the initial stage, especially when the loose body is not yet completely detached or is not ossified or calcified. In these cases a contrast arthrogram or magnetic resonance image may detect a loose joint body that does not yet cast a shadow. Especially in the knee joint, these radiological modalities are able to distinguish between a lesion of a meniscus and a loose joint body. Differential diagnostic benefit may also be expected from arthroscopy,

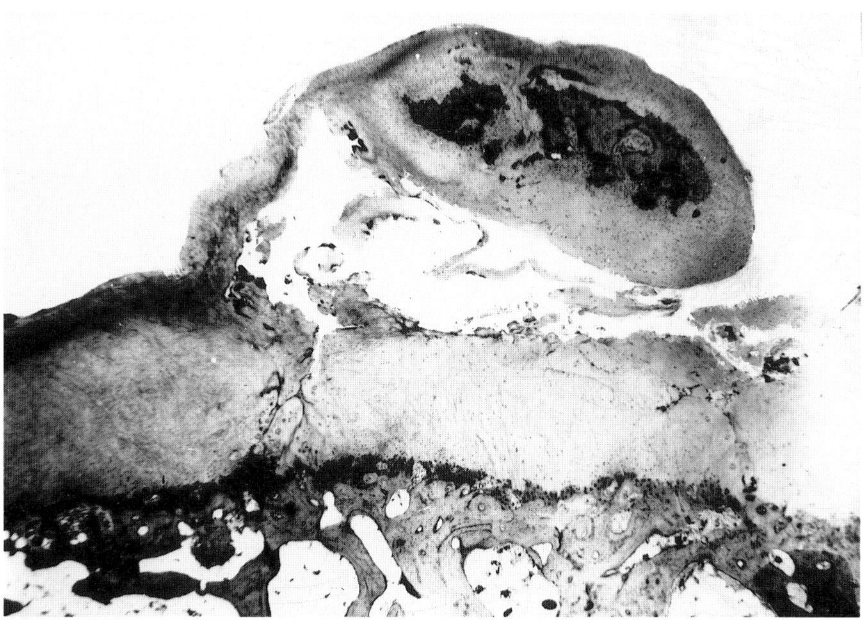

Fig. 323. Loose joint body of osteocartilaginous structure is connected by a cartilaginous stalk with the partly disrupted articular cartilage

which by varying the direction of the scope can provide a survey over a larger extent of the joint cavity.

Treatment endeavors in the stage of acute locking to release the entrapment by separating the articular ends by longitudinal traction or, if this maneuver does not succeed, by added adductional, abductional, or rotational manipulations. One should not rush at the first locking episode to surgical removal because other loose bodies may follow and thus necessitate repetition of the operative intervention. However, if follow-up symptoms and roentgenographs confirm constance in the clinical findings, the loose joint body or bodies should be removed. This procedure can be performed simply and accurately when the loose body is entrapped, and its location can be precisely determined by palpation. In such cases a thick injection needle inserted through the skin and joint capsule may succeed in harpooning and stabilizing the loose body. This obviates its displacement during the preparatory steps for operation and a search during the operation. The approach to the loose body should, if possible, follow the direct route. This may be carried out by arthroscopy if the loose body or bodies are very small. Otherwise, arthrotomy is necessary for extensive inspection of the joint cavity and for removal of the loose bodies, as well as for detection of loose bodies hidden behind capsular folds. Determining the proper moment for arthrotomy depends on experience and is important for the prognosis. With premature intervention, the necessity of additional arthrotomies may follow. On the other hand, long postponement of the intervention may lead to usuration of the articular surfaces, followed by secondary osteoarthritis.

VII. Joint Affections in Systemic Diseases

1. Joint Affections in Skin Diseases

a. Arthropathy in Psoriasis

Bourdillon [168] described in 1888 the coincidence of psoriasis and arthritis and postulated an etiological relationship between them. This connection was subsequently discounted by Gribble [678] and Margolis [1026] who interpreted the arthritis in their cases as rheumatoid arthritis occurring incidentally in psoriasis. Coste [326] also considered the joint affection in psoriasis as rheumatoid arthritis but with its features modified by a psoriatic background. However, distinct differences in certain clinical traits and laboratory findings led Bennett [117], Dawson et al. [378], DeSeze et al. [408], Moll et al. [1129], and Wright [1789] to consider the joint changes occurring in psoriasis as a disease of its own, and basically related to psoriasis.

Indeed, statistical surveys point out that peripheral rheumatoid arthritis occurs in about 1.5%–2.5% of the general population [304], whereas peripheral arthritis occurs in 7%–15% of patients with psoriasis [668, 953, 1203]. While the causal relationship between psoriasis and concomitant arthritis appears established, the temporal relationship in the onset of these two diseases varies. Roberts et al. [1333] reported that psoriasis preceded the arthritis in 84% of patients; however, they as well as Wright [1789] also found arthritis to precede the skin lesions in 16%. The psoriatic lesions [1099] represent an excessive proliferation of the epidermis resulting from an imbalance in the cyclical nucleotides. The prime cause of these changes may be mediated by genetic factors [1099]. Indeed, psoriasis appears as an inherited disease in about 10%–12% of patients, being transmitted as a dominant non-sex-linked trait, as is the case in concurrent arthritis. The fact that the extent and degree of the arthritis vary greatly with the severity of the skin disease, and that episodes of exacerbation of the skin lesions are usually followed by aggravation of the arthritic symptoms indicates that the primary psoriasis and incident arthritis are related to the same pathomechanism.

The skin of the hands and feet in psoriatic patients is covered with pustules which extend into the nailbeds (Figs. 324, 325); the nails are deformed by pitting or are crumbled by lytic necrosis. The underlying skin in the nailbeds is hyperkeratotic. In these cases, the tips of the fingers are shortened while the soft tissues of the middle and proximal parts of the fingers are thickened ("saucerization," Fig. 324). The skin alterations in other areas vary [1129] from small scaling lesions on the dorsal aspect of the elbow and ventral aspect of the knees (Fig. 326) to extensive exudative and exfoliating erythrodermias on the back and abdomen.

With the fingers and toes, including their nails, being deformed (Figs. 324, 325), the diagnosis of arthritis concurrent in psoriasis is readily established in severe cases [845]. However, also in cases of less severe psoriasis, arthritis can be ascertained as a condition related to the skin alterations and not as rheumatoid arthritis occurring incidentally in psoriasis. Psoriatic arthritis starts as a more painful condition than rheumatoid arthritis, in young persons usually early in their third decade, and it involves men and women almost equally. The affected joints are principally and primarily the distal interphalangeal joints of the hands and feet. From there other joints are centripetally affected, especially the wrist, ankle, and knee joints, less often the shoulder and hip joints, but usually not in symmetrical distribution. No subcutaneous nodules are palpable. These joints are distinctly enlarged by thickening of the joint capsule (Fig. 326) as well as by plumping of the articular epiphyses. Their movements are associated with coarse crepitation; these are moderately limited in the wrist and ankle joints but more so in the hip joints. Yet no contracture develops in any of the peripheral joints except for the distal interphalangeal joints, which often become even ankylosed. The larger joints are painful on motion and prolonged use but are rarely as continuously painful as in rheumatoid arthritis [1129]. Even after long duration of the affection, the major peripheral joints (shoulder, elbow, hip, and knee joints) do not become as contracted as in rheumatoid arthritis. However, with limitation of motion, they present rather the clinical picture of secondary osteoarthritis. Also in contrast to rheumatoid arthritis, in 25%–40% [820, 935, 1789] of cases of advanced psoriasis, the sacroiliac joints and those of the lumbosacral spine are affected. They are painful at the start of motion as well as after prolonged activity and are very tender. The lumbosacral joints are limited in their movements in all directions. Sometimes the active and passive movements of the lumbar spine are completely abolished, without concurrent tenseness of the regional paravertebral musculature, an indication of ankylosis in this part of the spine. No neurological signs are noticed. The cervical spine may be similarly affected, although less frequently.

In surveying the general distribution of affected joints, a certain grouping pattern according to the prevalently affected joints may be noticed: (a) severe affection of the interphalangeal joints with conspicuous deformation of the hands and feet, decreasing intensity of the affliction toward the centripetally located joints, and extensive skin alterations; (b) rheumatoidlike af-

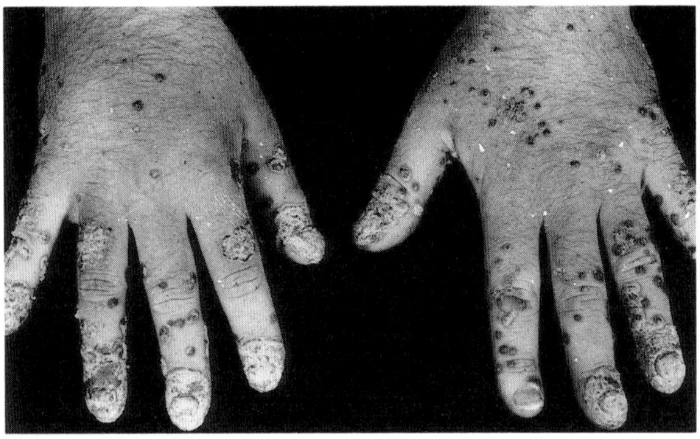

Fig. 324. The skin of the hands and fingers is extensively covered with crusts and pustules. Some of the latter are exulcerated and expand into the nailbeds

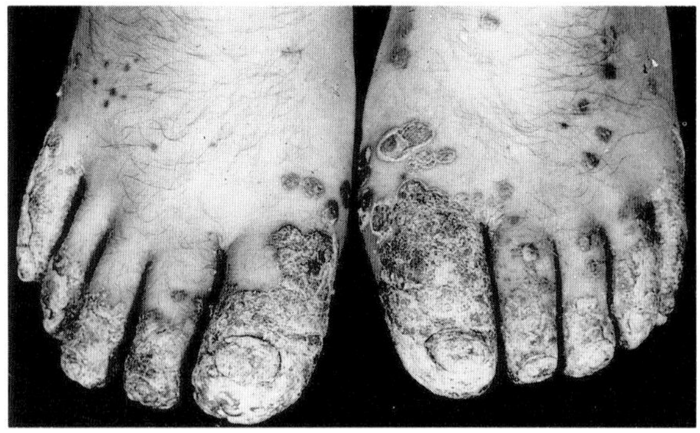

Fig. 325. A few pustules lie in the skin on the dorsum of the feet. Extensive ulcerations on the dorsum of the toes expand onto the nailbeds. The nails are crumbled or completely fallen out, leaving crusty or ulcerated nailbeds

fection of the smaller and larger peripheral joints with similar distribution and moderate intensity, yet without the tendency of aggravation to very advanced deformities; and (c) oligoarticular involvement with moderate changes in the fingers and toes and a few larger peripheral joints, but with pronounced affection of the sacroiliac joints and especially the vertebral column.

Laboratory studies disclose an increased sedimentation rate of 45–60 mm/h in cases with involvement of the spine or major joints of the extremities and as long as the joint capsule of the latter is swollen. Electrophoretic studies reveal an abnormal A/G ratio, with decreased albumin and increased gammaglobulin. A characteristic finding is the increased presence of the antigens HLA of various B groups, especially B27, as ascertained by typing with selected sera [668]. This finding is noticed in (73%–78%) of the patients with marked alterations in the sacroiliac joints and/or ankylosing changes of the vertebral column [480, 935, 1095, 1382, 1750]. No less characteristic is the negative outcome of tests for sheep cell agglutination and latex fixation (90%–93%) of patients with psoriatic

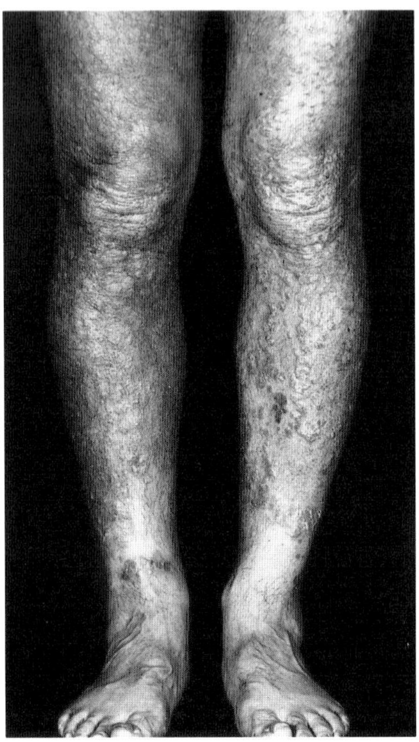

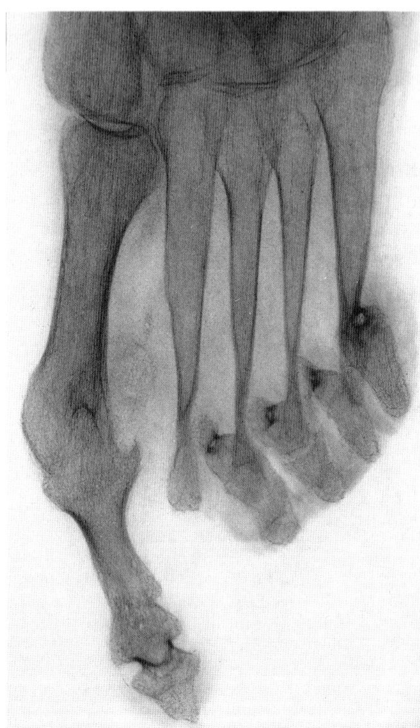

Fig. 326. The left knee is enlarged beyond the suprapatellar area and presents two healing ulcers at the prepatellar area. The skin of both lower legs is covered by many pustules and also presents large scaling lesions

Fig. 327. The first metatarsophalangeal joint is very deformed, and the second to fifth metatarsals are pencil-like sharpened. The metatarsophalangeal joints of the second to fifth toes are dislocated

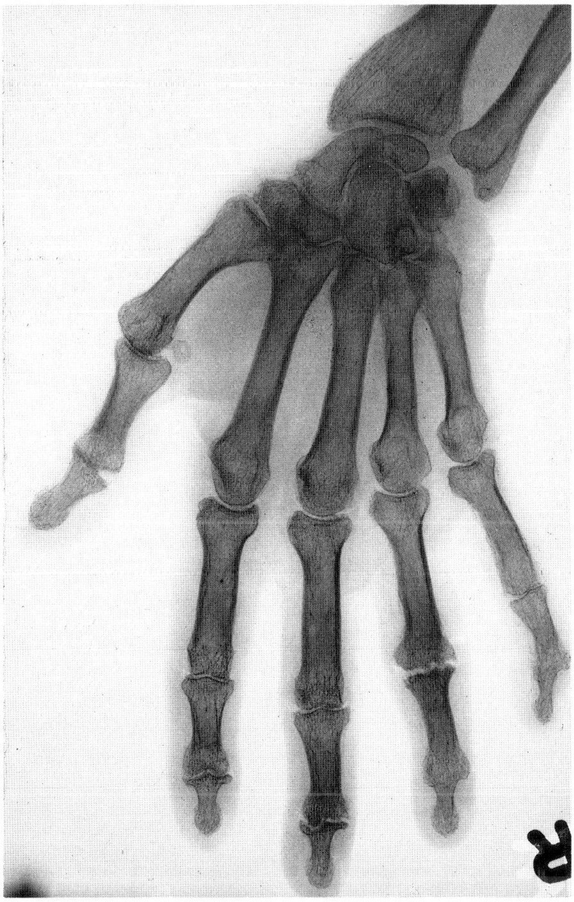

Fig. 328. The distal interphalangeal joints of the first, fourth, and fifth fingers are ankylosed. The other distal interphalangeal joints are very uneven, as is one proximal interphalangeal joint

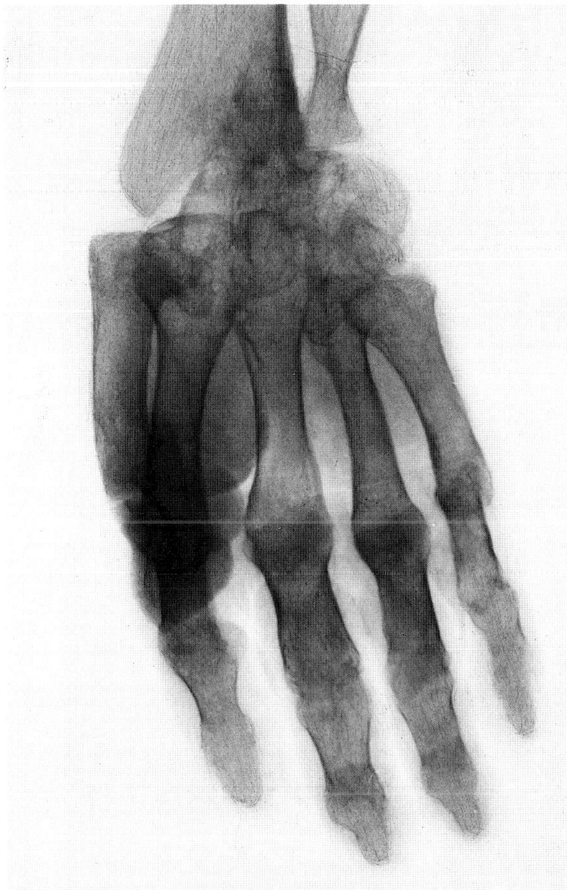

Fig. 329. The distal interphalangeal joints and proximal interphalangeal joints of the second to fifth fingers are ankylosed, and their metacarpophalangeal joints are subluxated. The carpometacarpal joint of the thumb is ankylosed in adduction

arthropathy [156, 1063, 1789]. The occasionally positive outcome of tests for rheumatoid factor may be ascribed to the increased levels of IgG antiglobulins [783].

Roentgenographs reveal the constant involvement of the distal interphalangeal joints, with irregular limitation of the narrowed cartilage space by uneven and often subluxated articular epiphyses (Fig. 328). More commonly, hovewer, the distal interphalangeal joint space is substantially narrowed or completely obliterated by fusion of the adjoining articular epiphyses (Figs. 328, 329). The endphalanx is substantially decreased in size by erosion (whittling). The proximal interphalangeal joint may display similar changes (Figs. 328, 329). The base of the proximal phalanx is broadened ("cupping"). The distal part of the metacarpal or metatarsal shaft is sometimes very thinned ("pencil sharpening;" Fig. 327). The larger joints of the extremities (Figs. 330, 331) present persistent, although altered joint spaces. These are unevenly narrowed in some areas and slightly widened in others and are bordered by sclerosed articular epiphyses bearing marginal osteophytes (Figs. 330, 331). Similarly, the vertebrae, especially those of the lumbar spine (Figs. 332, 333), are broadened by marginal osteophytes; their endplates are sclerosed and irregularly outlined by wavy indentations. The intervertebral spaces are very uneven. Ankylosis of the lumbar spine is manifested, in rarer instances (5%–8%), in marked narrowing of the lumbar intervertebral spaces and bridging by ossification of the anterior longitudinal ligament or connection of the lumbar vertebral bodies by lateral paravertebral ossification. Similarly, in 3%–5% of patients ankylosis occurs of the small apophyseal joints and/or larger intervertebral joints of the cervical spine (Fig. 332). The sacroiliac joints present pronounced changes in about 30%–40% of cases, especially in those with extensive erythrodermias, ranging from spots of osteoporosis, broader areas of sclerosis, hazy structure of the adjoining epiphyses, and irregular

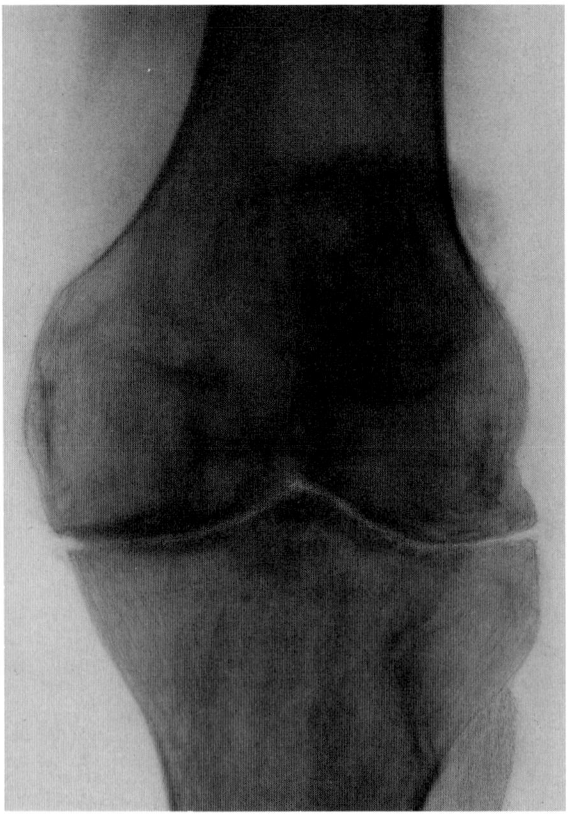

Fig. 330. The joint space of the knee is narrowed and unevenly delimited. Marginal osteophytes expand from the epiphyses

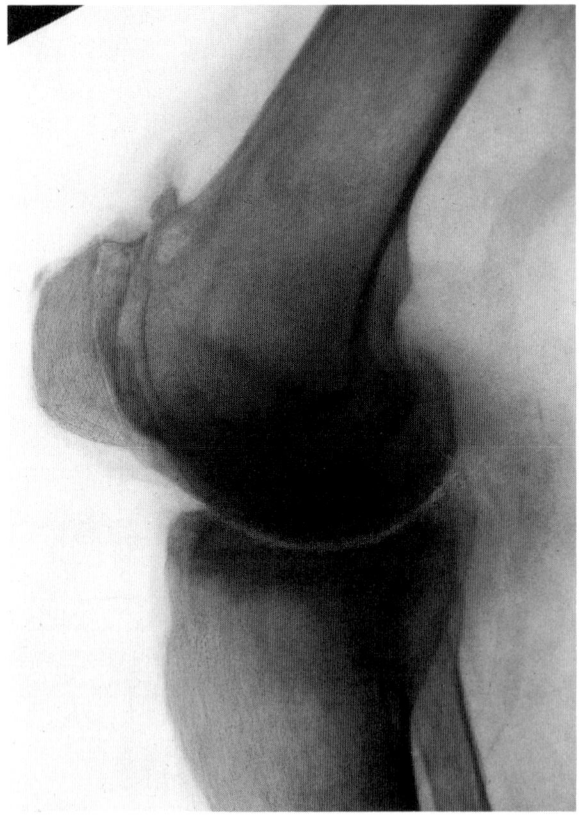

Fig. 331. The joint space between the femoral condyles and tibial condyles is narrowed and slightly uneven. Similar changes are noticed in the patellofemoral joint

narrowing of the joint space sometimes up to its complete obliteration.

Gross-anatomical examination discloses pronounced inflammatory as well as degenerative changes, with the former prevailing in the joints of the fingers, toes and, vertebral column and the latter in the larger joints of the extremities (Figs. 334, 335). The joint capsule in all cases is swollen and is thickened by villous excrescences. The latter expand as pannus into the interphalangeal joints of the fingers and toes and erode the articular cartilage, replacing it with inflammatory and eventually scarified connective tissue. Obliteration of the articular cavity is the outcome in the joints of the fingers and toes, often also in the joints of the spine and sacroiliac area. This is caused by fibrous ankylosis which often progresses to osseous ankylosis. In the larger joints, such as the elbow, wrist, hip, knee, and ankle, the inner part of the joint capsule is also swollen and thickened. The synovial granulation tissue only superficially involves the peripheral margins of the articular cartilage. On wide extents the central areas of these articular surfaces (Fig. 334) display loss of glistening, yellowish discoloration, unevenness and attrition of the hyaline cartilage, or complete denudation with sclerosis of the exposed osseous surfaces (Fig. 335). Concurrently, marginal spurs form in the weight-bearing joints. The vertebral column displays, especially in its lumbar segment, advanced changes of varied nature. In the majority of these cases, the vertebral bodies carry conspicuous and bizarre marginal exostoses, which sometimes extend from the anterior and lateral aspects to the neighboring vertebrae but without fusing with them (Figs. 332, 333). In other cases extensive ossifications of the intervertebral ligaments are associated with ankylosis of the lumbar apophyseal joints and with erosion and partial fusion of the sacroiliac joints.

Histopathological examination [495, 1543, 1551] of the synovial membrane of larger peripheral joints discloses in the initial stage of inflammation (Fig. 336) hypertrophy of synoviocytes, moderate hyperemia, and infiltrates composed of lymphocytes, histiocytes, and especially plasmacytes. Some of the latter are conspicuously larger and contain either two nuclei or homogeneous globules, Russel's bodies. In the progressive stage, fibroblasts proliferate in the subsynovio-

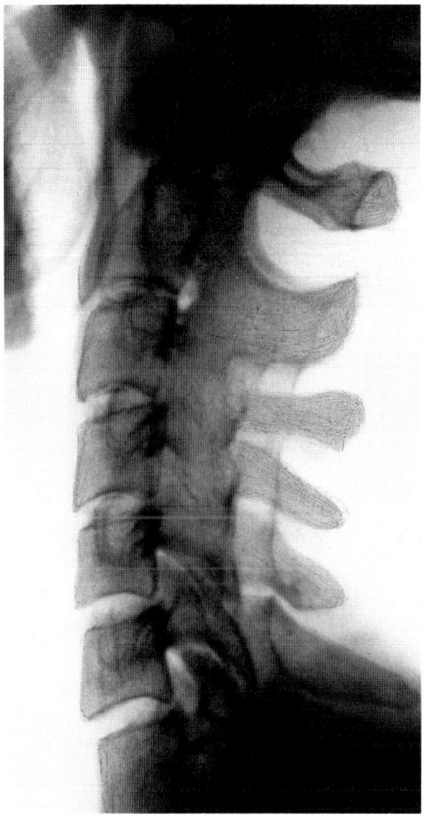

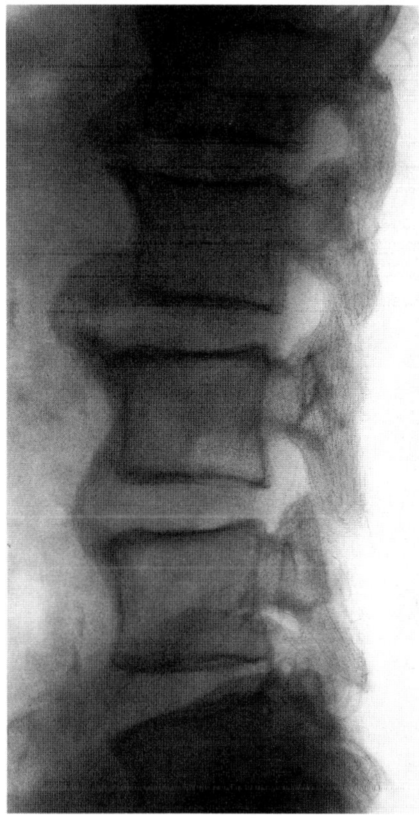

Fig. 332. The apophyseal joints from C2 to C5 are ankylosed, and the intervertebral spaces C2–3 and C3–4 are unevenly delimited

Fig. 333. Large osteophytes expand cranially and caudally from the anterior aspect of lumbar vertebrae and fuse these vertebrae

cytic tissue. Some blood vessels in the superficial and deeper zones display regressive changes. The capillaries and venules have hyaline apposition; the arterioles, small arteries, and small veins have narrowed lumina by thickening of their walls secondary to an increase in fibrocytes and fibrosis in onion-skin-like apposition (Fig. 337). On spreading of the inflammatory infiltrates and increase in fibroblasts and fibrocytes, the synovial membrane is raised in villi. This expands as granulation tissue over the margins of the articular surface and intrudes into the cartilage, eventually penetrating to the subchondral bone (Fig. 338). Larger areas of the articular cartilage are completely replaced here by granulation tissue which subsequently transforms into dense fibrosed tissue. Such changes are observed principally in the interphalangeal joints. In the larger and major weight-bearing joints the articular cartilage manifests a decrease in basophilia, extensive necrosis of chondrocytes, and horizontal and vertical clefts with fragmentation and separation of flakes. The articular cartilage, although largely thinned in most cases, is sometimes sufficiently maintained. The subchondral bone becomes thickened where it is denuded. Conspicuous enlargements are noted at the margins of the articular surfaces, where subsequent enchondral ossification (Fig. 339) results in formation of broad osteophytes. Examination of the synovial tissue [948] by immunofluorescence and immunoperoxidase tests discloses deposits of immunoglobulins and complement components. Probably as sequelae of the wide spread of plasmacytes in synovial tissues and their considerable production of immunoglobulins, deposits of amyloid were observed by Ferguson et al. [504] and Friedman et al. [553] in gastrointestinal and vascular walls. Similar deposits, ascertained by metachromasia on crystal violet stain, occasionally also occur in the synovial membrane [553].

Differential diagnosis poses problems in these cases in which the joint alterations precede the skin alterations, and in which the primary affection of the distal interphalangeal joints with maintenance of a narrowed and irregularly delimited cartilage space suggests primary osteoarthritis. In the presence of inflammatory skin and vertebral alterations, Reiter's syndrome must be considered, but this can be disregarded in the absence of urethral inflammation.

Treatment of psoriatic arthritis should be associated primarily with that which is specific for the skin condition. While regression of the latter is not necessarily followed by regression of the former, experience in follow-up examinations indicates that aggravation of the skin condition is commonly followed by exacerba-

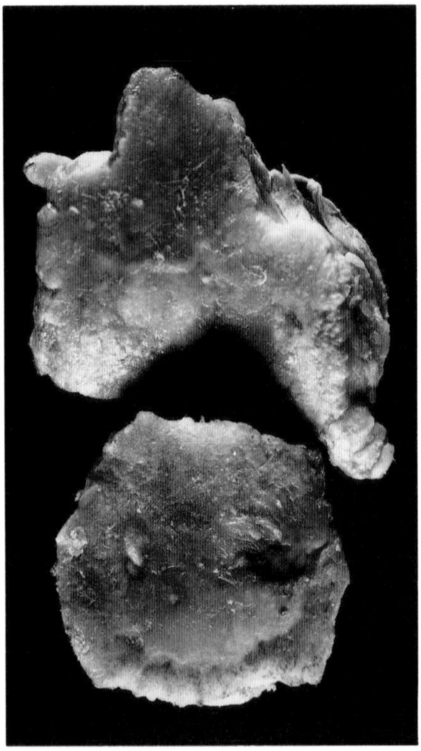

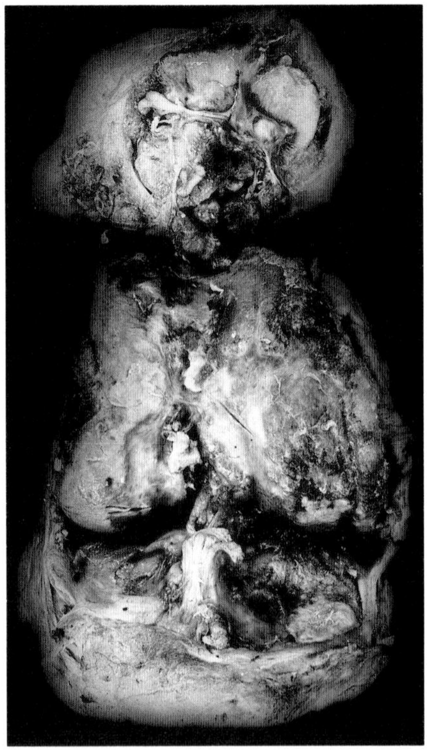

Fig. 334. The articular cartilage, resected from the femoral condyles and tibial condyles, is thinned and very uneven secondary to extensive attrition. The cartilage from the tibial condyles has two central deep defects

Fig. 335. The articular surfaces of the knee joint are covered by articular cartilage to only a small extent and are worn off in the other areas. Deep defects expand into the patella, one femoral condyle, and one tibial condyle

tion of arthritic symptoms. Regularly taken salicylates 3.0–4.0 g daily often suffice to provide relief of the arthritic symptoms even on long range, especially in cases with an elevated sedimentation rate. In cases with pronounced swelling of the joint capsule, nonsteroidal antiinflammatory medications (as indicated in "Rheumatoid Arthritis") are able to reduce the local inflammatory changes as well as soreness in the joints. However, in nonresponsive cases corticosteroids (prednisone 25–40 mg daily) should be used with slowly tapering doses, a treatment also often benefiting the skin condition. However, the potential complications on longer use of steroids should be kept in mind. Similarly, cytotoxic [90, 452] drugs improve the skin lesions as well as the articular alterations [1733]; of these, methotrexate due to its depressive effect on the

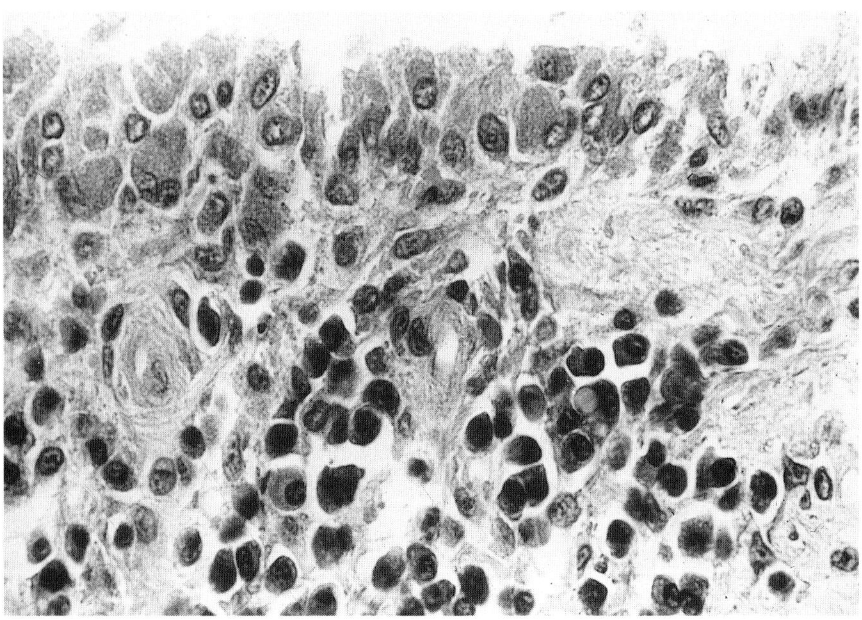

Fig. 336. The synoviocytes are very hypertrophic and moderately hyperplastic. The subsynoviocytic tissue is extensively infiltrated chiefly by plasmacytes

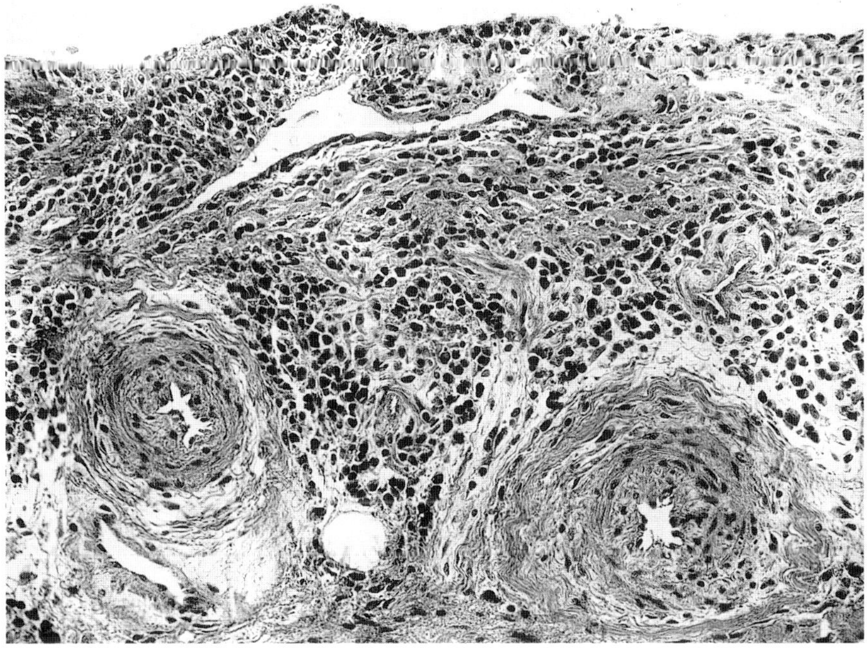

Fig. 337. The subsynoviocytic tissue is very cellular, partly by an increase in fibrocytes and partly by accumulation of plasmacytes and lymphocytes. Some middle-sized arteries have very thickened walls by an increase in the cells in the media and adventitia

increased metabolism of nucleic acid in the epidermal cells is used at 5 mg daily for 1 week, repeated after 1–2 weeks interval. The potential complications (alopecia, gastrointestinal ulcerations, hepatotoxic effects, and pancytopenia) advise caution in the use [274] of cytotoxic medications and suggest limiting them to short periods of time. Furthermore, methotrexate has been administered intraarticularly (synovioorthesis [709]) in the expectation that is immunosuppressive effect will influence the inflammatory changes in the inner part of the joint capsule. Follow-up controls by punch biopsies and histopathological examinations [1551] revealed that the expectations placed in this treatment are not completely fulfilled. By analogy to rheumatoid arthritis, intramuscular injections with gold salts have also been used in psoriatic arthritis [439] with similar toxic effect, especially as to skin lesions, but with distinctly less satisfy-

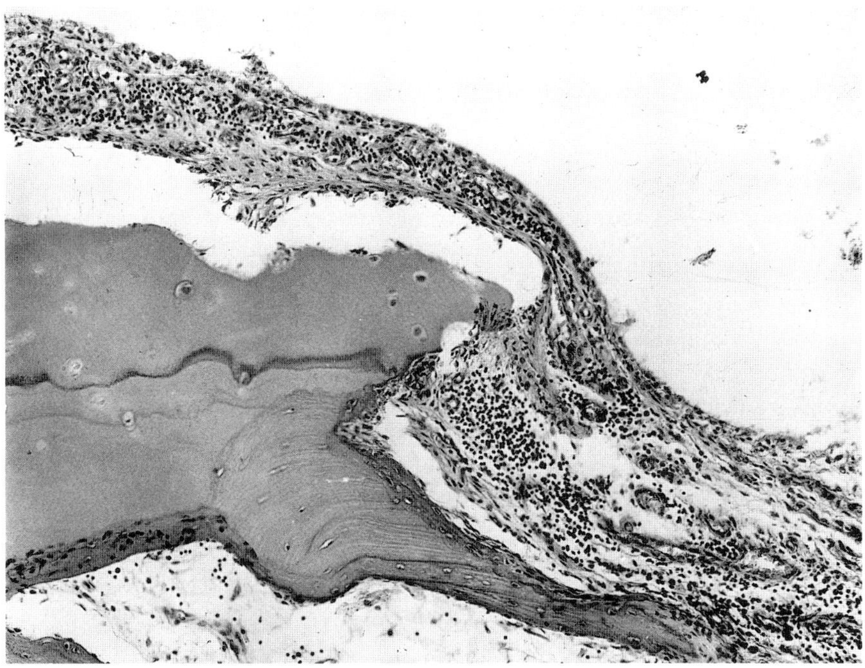

Fig. 338. Articular cartilage of an interphalangeal joint is extensively invaded and eroded by synovial pannus, which also contains extensive infiltrates of inflammatory cells

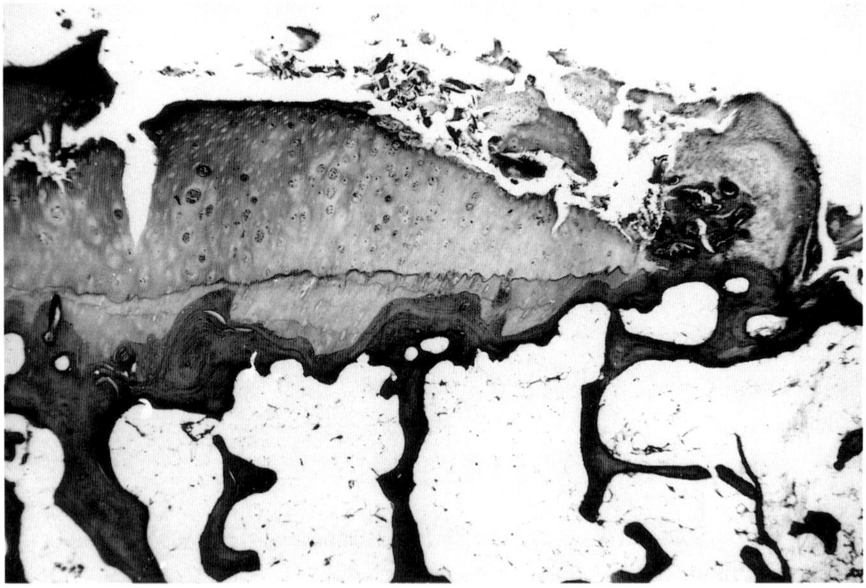

Fig. 339. Articular cartilage of a knee joint is disrupted by a few clefts and is very thinned toward the edge of the articular surface, where a marginal osteophyte is developing. Fragments of disintegrated cartilage are separated

ing therapeutic effects than in rheumatoid arthritis. This observation also indicates that the etiopathogenetic mechanism in psoriatic arthritis is different from that in rheumatoid arthritis.

Thus, synovectomies are indicated in the rare cases of excessive thickening of the joint capsule of the wrist or knee joint, and arthroplastic procedures may be indicated for the joints of the fingers, and other small joints with advanced attrition of the articular surfaces. However, such extensive operations are seldom needed for the larger joints because their alterations and symptoms are usually within the range of moderate osteoarthritis [920]. In the rare situations of very deformed hip and/or knee joint, total arthroplasty as discussed in "Osteoarthritis" may provide the desired benefits. A precautionary attitude to avoid or to minimize surgical procedures is imposed by the often coexistent inflammatory alterations in the regional skin and the consequently high probability of postoperative infections. The experience prevails that psoriatic arthritis of the joints of the extremities carries a much better prognosis than does rheumatoid arthritis. Similarly, the alterations in the vertebral column, although sometimes very pronounced, need no surgical treatment, but frequent physical therapy repeated at intervals of 2–3 months. Shortwave diathermy in two or three series of eight sessions each proves effective for the vertebral column and for the joints of the extremities. Ultrasound of 2.5–3.0 W/cm^2 in two or three series of eight sessions and massage are of greater benefit for the vertebral column [687, 944, 1613]. Additionally, a firm lumbosacral belt with metal stays (Fig. 51) may be needed as a support for the lumbar spine or a firm collar for the cervical spine (Fig. 50). Another very effective modality for all joints is the application of moist hot packs, which, however, must not be used in the phase of active inflammation. This helps greatly in the longer range to diminish soreness, to reduce thickening, and to restore mobility of joints.

2. Arthropathies in Intestinal Inflammations

Joint inflammations have been reported [70, 346, 503, 524, 1062, 1064, 1545, 1677, 1790] as extraintestinal complications in ulcerative colitis and regional ileitis. The fact that such involvement occurs far more frequently (about 15%–40%) in patients with intestinal diseases than rheumatoid arthritis occurs (2%–4%) in the general population [304] suggests that it is not rheumatoid arthritis merely coinciding with, but a joint involvement related to the intestinal diseases. Indications of the differences from rheumatoid arthritis are also presented by the localization, clinical signs, laboratory findings, and course of the joint affections in both ulcerative colitis and regional ileitis. While the latter two affections have many characteristics in common, their separate descriptions are indicated for the sake of completeness and identification.

a. Arthropathy in Ulcerative Colitis

Joint symptoms in ulcerative colitis [68, 196, 505, 1062, 1361, 1790] are considered to be related to this intestinal disease because of their manifestation in close temporal relationship to the latter, and because of the absence of any other disease which could be followed by arthritis. The diagnosis of ulcerative colitis is corroborated by roentgenographs of the gastrointestinal tract, sigmoidoscopy, and occasionally by operative findings and pathological examination. Barium enema studies of the colon and sigmoid show irregularities with fine serrations or moth-eaten appearance and small filling defects of the mucosal outline. Additional findings may include shortening and tubelike narrowing and a leadpipe appearance of the colon, with failure to contract. Sigmoidoscopy discloses reddening and friability of the mucosa, which easily bleeds with pinpoint hemorrhages, diffuse granulomatous inflammation, and small ulcers covered with yellow exudate. Gross examination of surgical specimens discloses swelling of the colonic mucosa, which is studded with numerous abscesses and irregular ulcers scattered over the inner surface; the wall of the colon is thickened and indurated.

The average incidence of peripheral arthritis in ulcerative colitis is 12%–17% [68, 196, 503, 505, 1361, 1790]; an even higher incidence of almost 50% was reported by McEwen et al. [1062]. About two-thirds of patients are men aged 16–56 years; among women the group aged of 20–26 years predominates. Articular involvement starts in about 10% of patients shortly after onset of the intestinal disease, in most patients between 3 and 12 months after onset and in another 10% between 12 and 24 months after onset. The affections recur in the same joints or freshly involve other joints in a close temporal relationship to the onset of to exacerbations of ulcerative colitis in 65%–72% of patients. The joint affections of the extremities often regress after regression of the colonic disease or completely subside after excision of the diseased colon. However, the joint affections remain uninfluenced by colonostomy.

Articular complications appear as subacute attacks of aches mostly of polyarticular type. They begin in a larger joint of an extremity and migrate to other joints or, more frequently, involve a few joints simultaneously but not necessarily in symmetrical distribution. The affected joints present diffuse arthralgias which regress after 2–4 weeks and possibly recur in the same manner or with swelling. However, more commonly the joint disease appears primarily as swelling with tenderness and increased local warmth, sometimes associated with intraarticular effusion. The latter complication is generally observed in the knee and ankle joints, rarely in the elbow joint. Nevertheless, any other peripheral joint may be affected, such as the metacarpophalangeal or interphalangeal, wrist, shoulder, metatarsophalangeal, hip, sternoclavicular, and temporomandibular joints.

Inflammations of the joints of the extremities in ulcerative colitis usually cause less pain than those in rheumatoid arthritis, but in a few cases the elbow, wrist, finger, or knee joint is so painful that movement is temporarily limited by regional muscle spasm. Morning stiffness is experienced in long-standing joint affections. The peripheral type of joint involvement subsides after 1–8 months but lasts longer in the shoulder, hip, and knee joints and may recur one to six times. However, a different course characterizes affection of the vertebral column, which occurs at a lower frequency (7%–25% [503, 672, 1062, 1823]) than in the extremities and 1–6 years after onset of the intestinal disease. Starting usually in the sacroiliac joints, this condition subsequently and principally involves the lumbar and lower thoracic spine and is associated with less tenderness than in the peripheral joints but with early stiffness of the vertebral column [1001]. It is rarely mitigated by episodes of remission but follows its independent, although slow course of aggravation despite regression or eradication of the disease of the colon. In these situations, coincident inflammatory changes of the shoulder and especially hip joints are more extensive and profound.

Laboratory studies show a sedimentation rate elevated to between 38 and 90 mm/h and positive outcome for C-reactive protein in 25%–40% of patients. Test results for antinuclear antibodies are negative, but those for rheumatoid factor are positive in 6% of patients with peripheral arthritis, consistent with the average population, but are negative in patients with affection of the vertebral column [1062]. On the other hand, the outcome of the test for HLA-B27 is quite characteristically positive in 53%–75% of patients with ulcerative colitis and ankylosing spondylitis [390, 799, 1170]. Circulating anticolon antibodies were found in a significant titer in the serum but were not always present [398]. The increased and slightly turbid joint fluid contains 2000–12000 leukocytes, among which polymorphonuclear neutrophilic leukocytes predominate.

Roentgenographs of the larger joints of the extremities reveal in long-standing affections thickening of the joint capsule, narrowing of the cartilage space with irregular outline of the articular surfaces, and osteoporosis alternating with cysts and sclerosis of the subchondral bone. The apophyseal joints of the lower dorsal and entire lumbar spine are indistinct or obliterated, and the anterior longitudinal and lateral paravertebral ligaments are partly ossified [1062]. In other cases, the thoracic and lumbar vertebral bodies are completely united by bony bridges (Fig. 340). The sacroiliac joints are poorly delineated or fused, and the adjoining bones are sclerosed (Fig. 340).

Gross-pathological examination of the enlarged joints discloses thickening of the joint capsule with hyperemia and formation of numerous villi in cases of

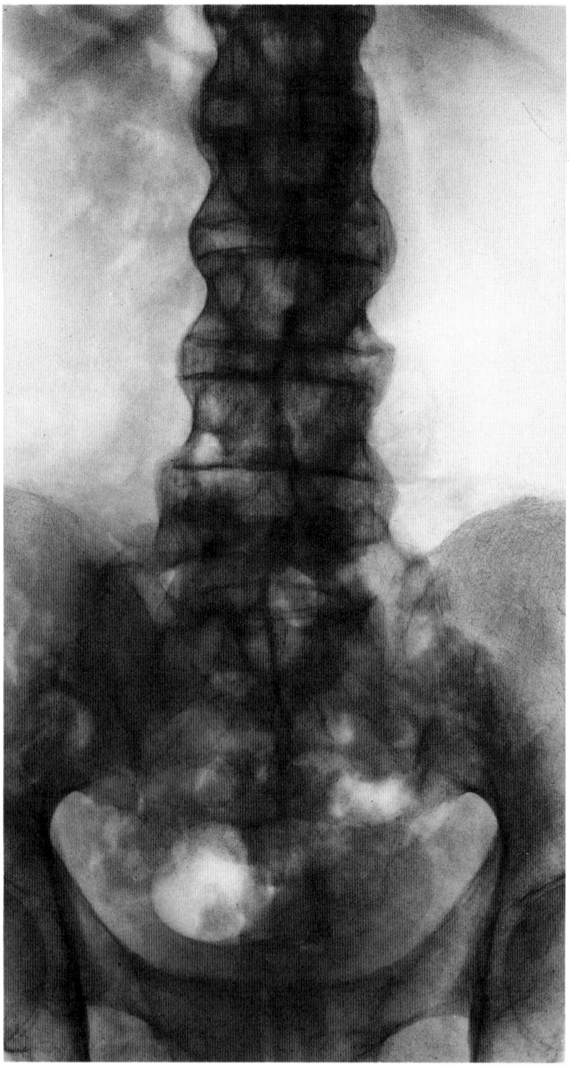

Fig. 340. The 12th thoracic vertebra, all lumbar vertebrae, and the first sacral vertebra are fused together by ossification of the lateral intervertebral ligament. The interjacent intervertebral spaces are obliterated by ossifications. The sacroiliac joints are ankylosed

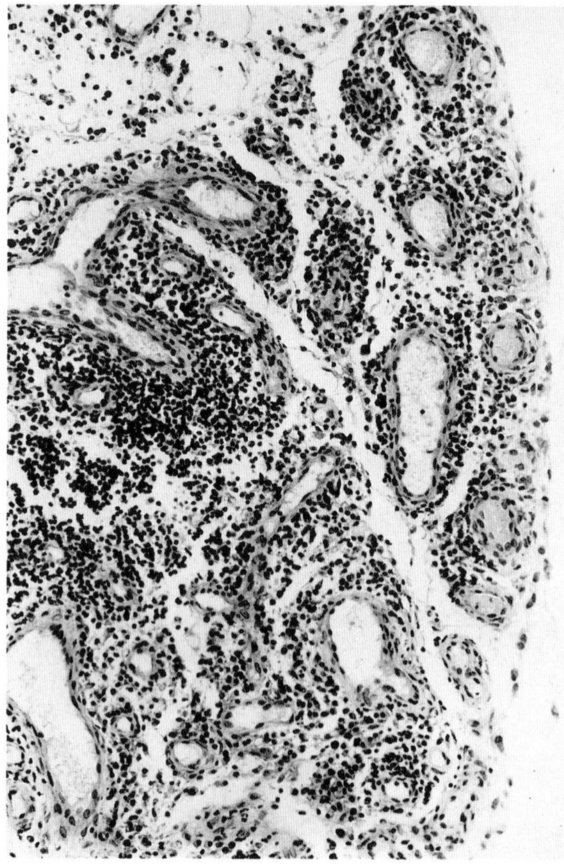

Fig. 341. The synovial membrane is extensively rarefied by interstitial edema. All blood vessels are widened and are surrounded by broad accumulations of lymphocytes and histiocytes and a few plasmacytes

longer duration and advanced changes. The articular cartilage is thinned, uneven, discolored yellowish, and devoid of luster in some areas. The joint cavity is narrowed concentrically by the swelling of the joint capsule. Histopathological examination discloses moderate focal hypertrophy of the synoviocytes. The subsynoviocytic tissue is diffusely infiltrated by lymphocytes, plasmacytes, and histiocytes (Fig. 341). By increase of the infiltrates, the bulk of the synovial membrane enlarges, and numerous villi are formed (Fig. 342). After regression of the inflammatory infiltrates, hypercellularity with fibrocytes and moderate fibrosis take place in the subsynoviocytic tissue.

Treatment in cases with thickening of the joint capsule of the extremities consists, in addition to frequent rest, of regular application of moist warm packs and possibly aspiration of the increased joint fluid combined with elastic compression of the joint. Antibiotics and especially sulfadrugs (sulfathiazole, sulfamethoxazole, sulfisoxazole, or sulfaguanidin) often prove of benefit for the intestinal condition as well as for the joint affection. They should be given in higher doses for a period of 2–3 months. If these measures do not provide a substantial regression, mainly of the inflammation of the colon, excision of the colon is indicated. This may bring substantial regression of the articular symptoms. In the very rare case of metastatic bacterial spread and purulent inflammation of a joint, the complete treatment must be instituted as in any suppuration of a joint. On the other hand, in the uncomplicated course symptoms subside; in the majority of affected joints of the extremities additional physical therapy with shortwave diathermy administered in two or three series of eight sessions each is indicated. In some joints (sternoclavicular, elbow, finger, knee, ankle) persistent thickening of the joint capsule results, but

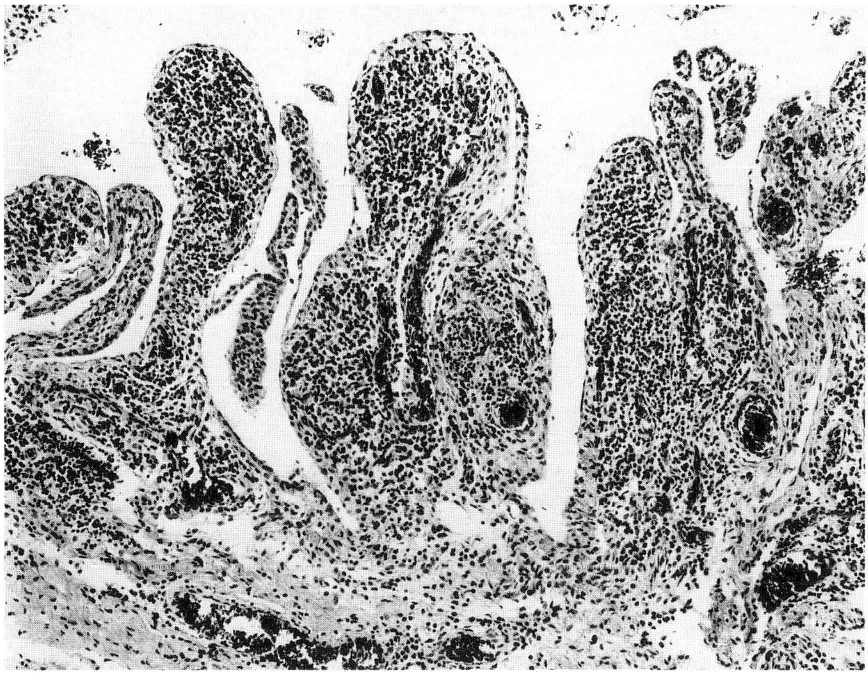

Fig. 342. The synovial membrane is elevated in many large villi which are extensively infiltrated by lymphocytes and histiocytes

with maintenance of normal motion. Narrowing of the cartilage space with irregular outlining of the articular surfaces and substantial impairment in the function of the joint is the outcome in 30%–35% of affected joints (shoulder, hip, knee, ankle). On progression of these joint alterations, synovectomies possibly combined with tenotomies are indicated. However, total arthroplasty as described in "Rheumatoid Arthritis" may represent, under continuous protection by antibiotics, the final solution in rare and far-advanced alterations with extensive deformation of the articular surfaces and painful impairment in the movements of a joint.

That the joint involvement results from intestinal substances is indicated by the relatively short interval between onset or reactivation of ulcerative colitis and manifestations of articular symptoms in the majority of the patients, as well as by the frequently observed parallel between exacerbations of colitis and recurrences or new occurrences of joint affections. The harmful substances are released from the diseased intestinal wall and transported by the blood stream, affect the synovial membrane, and provoke an inflammation there. Ferguson et al. [504] reported the parallel pattern in the course of the intestinal disease and joint involvement in 60%–70% of patients. The presence of numerous small abscesses in the intestinal wall and the high titer (up to 2000 U) of antistreptolysin-0 in the blood of 8 of 14 patients tested herefore suggest that bacterial toxins probably affect the joints. Two other explanations for the etiology of the described joint affections may be offered. (a) The joint affections in temporal and clinical relationship to the intestinal disease are aspects of a single clinical entity and are caused by a common etiological factor. However, the lower incidence of joint affections suggests the participation of additional factors in it. (b) The joint affections are of rheumatoid nature and have been activated by antigens emitted from the ulcerative colitis. However, militating against this are the localization and clinical features of the peripheral joint affections, their overall lack of tendency to progressive deformation, the ankylosing changes of the spine, the absence of rheumatoid nodules, and the general absence of rheumatoid factor.

b. Arthropathy in Regional Ileitis

The peripheral articular involvement in regional ileitis [70, 410] exceeds the frequency of 2.5% reported by Crohn et al. [346]; Greenstein et al. [672] reported one of 14%. It is probable that the actual frequency is even higher, approximately 20% [728]. Ankylosing spondylitis and sacroiliac arthritis occur in 4%–6% of patients with regional ileitis, a lower frequency than in ulcerative colitis.

The intestinal disease is corroborated by studies with barium contrast, which evidence that the lumen of the ileum is irregularly delimited and narrowed over longer extents. In a few areas small, marginal streaks of barium are also deposited. In cases of long duration the intestinal lumen is substantially narrowed and delimited by straight outlines of tubelike appearance.

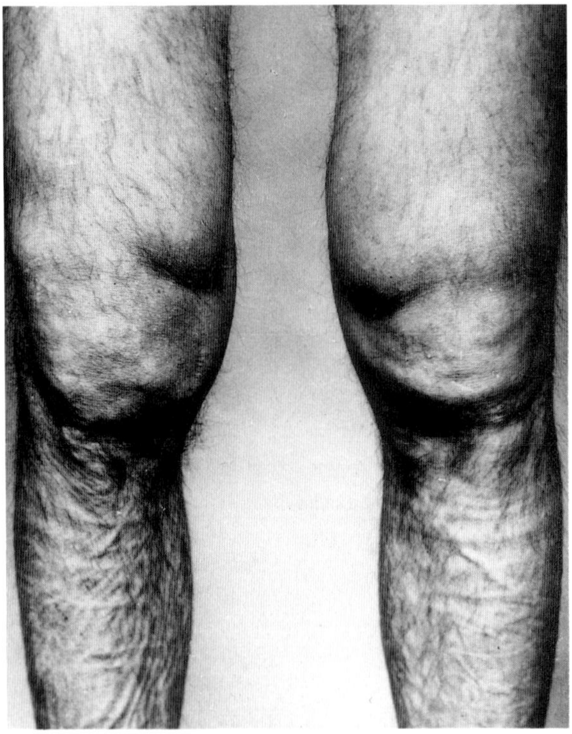

Fig. 343. Both knees are very enlarged to above the suprapatellar recessus by a marked increase in the joint fluid and by thickening of the joint capsule

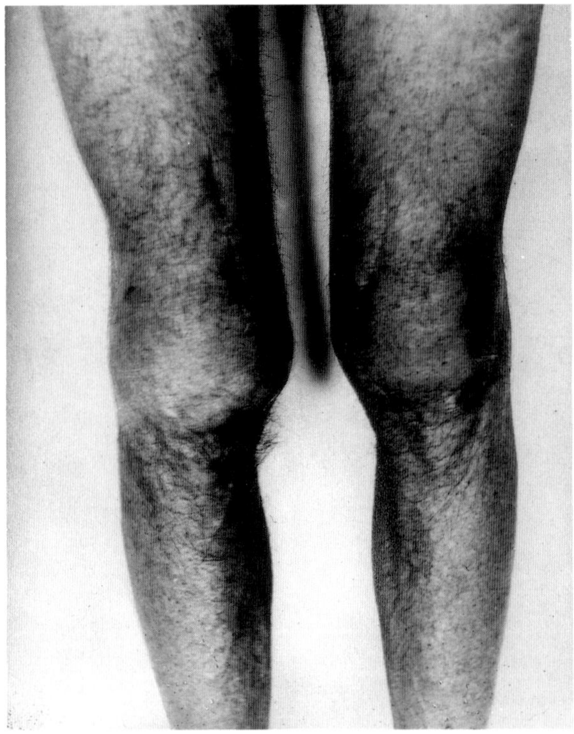

Fig. 344. The enlargement of the knees (Fig. 343) has substantially diminished secondary to extensive synovectomies (Fig. 345), as suggested by the incisional scars on the anteromedial aspects

Transection of the ileum and ileotransverse colonostomy are the generally applied treatment [346]. Grossanatomical examination [346] of the resected intestine discloses that its wall is thickened, coarse, and no longer pliable in some circumscribed areas. The mucosa of these areas is discolored dark-red and is uneven due to polypous elevations. These present in their center an ulceration expanding into the submucosa and, rarely, expanding to the thickened and fibrosed serosa. Histopathological examination discloses that the mucosa neighboring the ulcer is substantially thickened and very uneven from plump elevations. The submucosa is focally and intensely infiltrated by large histiocytes and lymphocytes.

The joint affection [1545] starts in some patients several months and in others 1–3 years after onset of the intestinal disease, but not necessarily correlated in degree with the severity of the latter. Initially one major joint (knee, elbow) and gradually a few other joints of the extremities (shoulder, wrist, ankle) are involved. The affected peripheral joints present either arthralgias with diffuse tenderness or arthritis with conspicuous swelling of the joint capsule (Fig. 343) and circumscribed tenderness, but without substantial limitation of motion. Intraarticular effusions are observed in the knee joint (Fig. 343), and pronounced periarticular edema is also observed in the wrist and ankle joints. The inflammations of the joints of the extremities appear as subacute or chronic processes and slowly subside either spontaneously or as the result of medicamentous and physical therapy. However, they recur and subside again depending on the course of the intestinal disease. In most (75%–82%) patients a close relationship is noted between the activity of the intestinal disease and the peripheral articular symptoms. The exacerbations of the intestinal disease are accompanied by recurrences of previous or by manifestations of recent joint involvements. New appearances of joint symptoms indicate reactivation or further spread of the intestinal disease. Inflammation of the peripheral joints does not subside completely unless the intestinal disease subsides, or the entire diseased ileum is excised. However, the affection of the vertebral column advances independently of the course of the intestinal disease [410] at slow speed but at lower intensity and lesser extent than in ulcerative colitis; this involves chiefly the lower part of the lumbar spine and the sacroiliac joints. Nevertheless, stiffness of the lumbar spine also results here, but without concomitant severe involvement of the hip and shoulder joints.

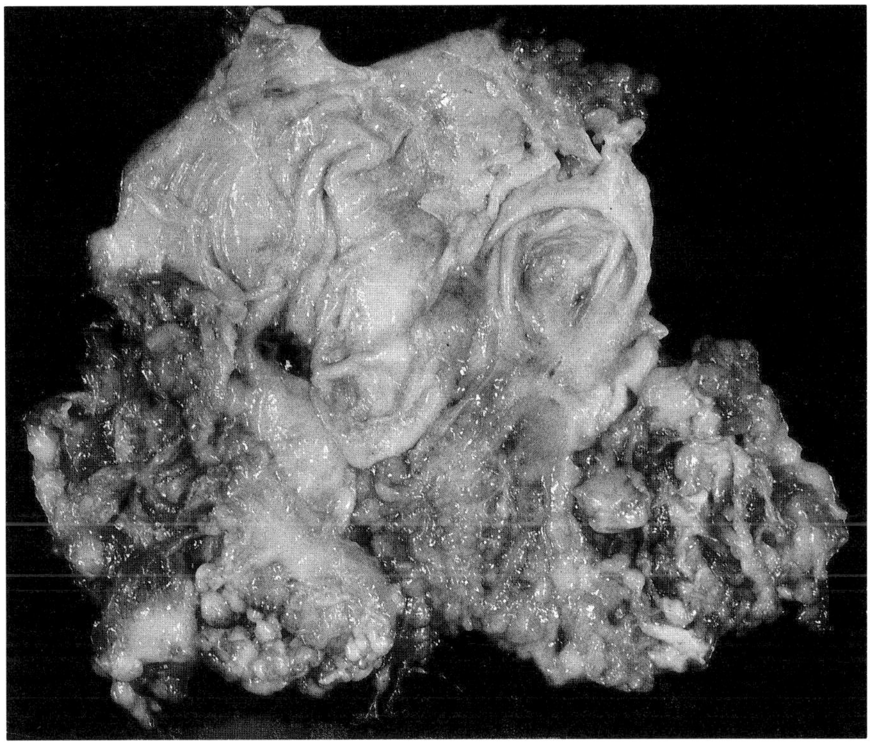

Fig. 345. The excised inner part of the joint capsule is rather smooth but rich in folds in the upper area. The lower area is very uneven by many large villi and thick plump nodes

Of the laboratory tests, the sedimentation rate is elevated to 35–55 mm/h; the test result for C-reactive protein is positive in the majority of patients, and that for rheumatoid factor is positive in 6%–8%. Tests for HLA-B27 antigen yield a positive outcome principally in patients with regional ileitis and concomitant involvement of the sacroiliac joints and vertebral column [390, 744, 816].

Roentgenographs of the initial joint involvement reveal marked swelling and density of the joint capsule but no changes in the cartilage space. In advanced cases moderate narrowing of the cartilage space and irregular delimitation of the adjoining epiphyseal surfaces ensue in the knee, ankle, elbow, and hip joints. After several years of joint involvement, the articular surfaces become eroded in 15%–20% of patients. Similarly, the apophyseal joints of the lumbar spine have a blurred structure and are sometimes obliterated; the intervertebral ligaments are ossified and connect the adjacent vertebrae. The sacroiliac joints then present more distinct alterations by partial or complete obliteration of the joint space, with irregular structure alternating between osteoporosis and sclerosis of the contiguous epiphyses.

Surgical exploration of the knee or ankle joint reveals marked thickening of the inner part of the joint capsule, with conspicuous unevenness of its inner surface by rather broad-based villous protrusions (Fig. 345). The articular cartilage is generally intact except in advanced joint affections but presents yellowish discoloration and loss of glistening appearance in a few extensive areas. Microscopic examination [1543, 1545] discloses that the synovial membrane, delimited by moderately hypertrophic synoviocytes (Fig. 346) is elevated in numerous villi (Fig. 347) by extensive accumulations of lymphocytes, plasmacytes, and histiocytes. These inflammatory cells also infiltrate the deeper subsynoviocytic tissue, either diffusely or in nodules. A moderate increase in fibrocytes and collagen fibers in the deeper zone (Fig. 346) indicates gradual fibrosis of the joint capsule.

At follow-up examination affected joints of the extremities are found to be slightly to moderately tender but not deformed, with the exception of the knee joints, which may remain with thickened joint capsules. The return of most joints of the extremities to adequate function even after several years of involvement indicates that only the joint capsule was affected while the articular cartilage was spared. However, in patients with additional involvement of the lower part of the vertebral column, substantial limitation of motion in the lumbar spine may ensue due to ankylosis of the apophyseal joints and/or ossification of the intervertebral ligaments.

Treatment is based primarily on suppression or eradication of the intestinal disease by resection of the ileum and secondarily on administration of salicylates and antiinflammatory medications for the affected

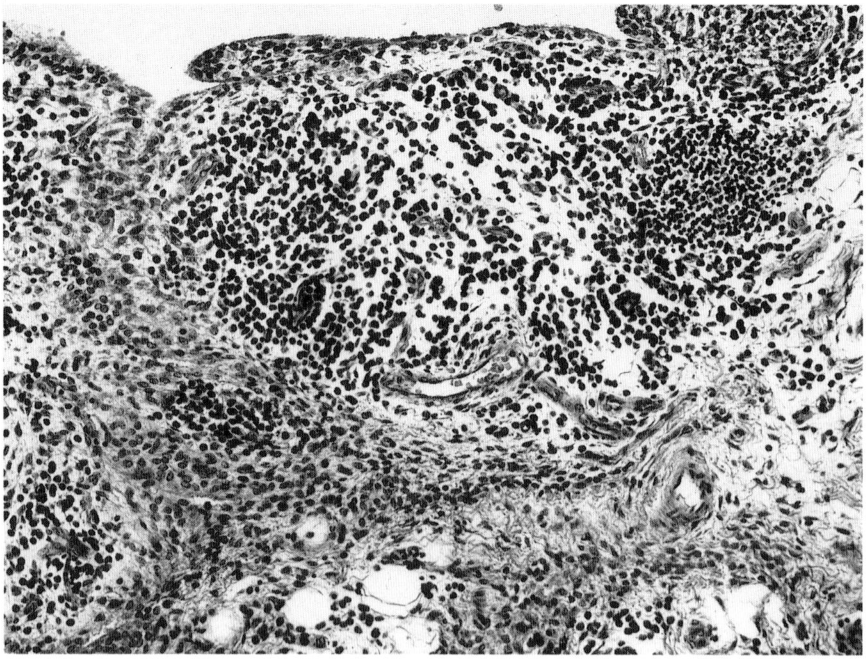

Fig. 346. The synovial membrane is extensively infiltrated by lymphocytes, histiocytes, and plasmacytes and is dense by an increase in fibrocytes and collagen fibers

joints. Physical therapy with shortwave diathermy in one or two series of eight sessions is of substantial benefit for these joints. Corticosteroids provide episodes of remission as long as they are administered, but these are followed by recurrences after their discontinuation. Wherever marked thickening of the joint capsule persists, total synovectomy (Fig. 345) restores the normal configuration (Fig. 344) and facilitates joint movements. On stiffening of the column, diligent posture exercises and regular protracted physical therapy with moist hot applications, ultrasound at 2.5–3 W/cm^2 [687], and massage provide substantial benefit.

While the etiology of regional ileitis has not yet been clarified, the following possibilities of the etiology of the accompanying joint affections may be considered. (a) The disease of the intestine is caused by an as yet

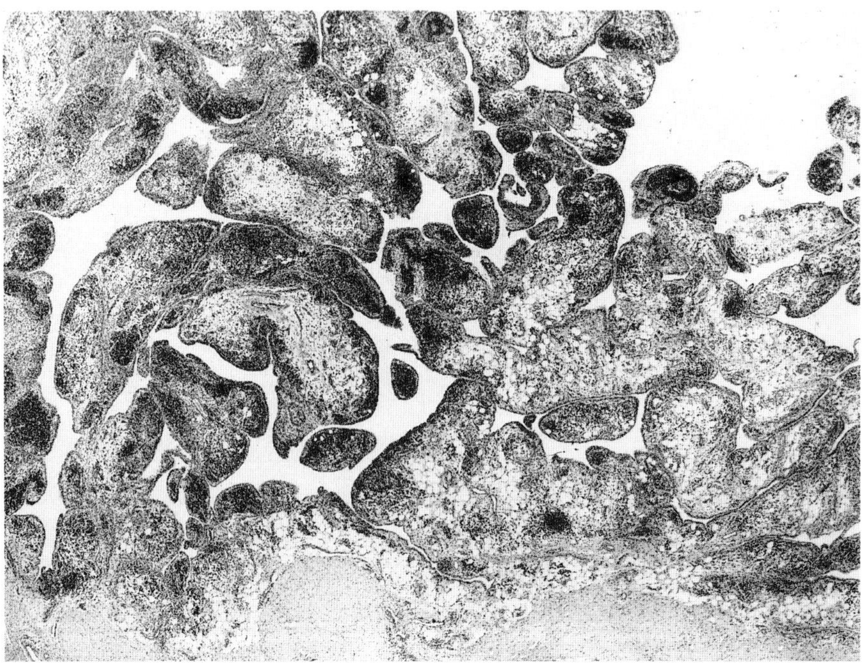

Fig. 347. The synovial membrane is raised in numerous villi of substantial height. Some villi are branched, and most villi are extensively infiltrated by lymphocytes and histiocytes

Table 2. Comparison of joint affection in ulcerative colitis and regional ileitis

	Ulcerative colitis	Regional ileitis
Diagnosis of intestinal alteration corroborated by	Contrast roentgenographs, colonoscopy, examination of excised colon	Contrast roentgenographs, examination of excised ileum
Age of patients	16–55 years	20–50 years
Sex of patients	Men prevailing	No difference
Interval between inception of intestinal disease and joint involvement	1 month–8 years	10 months–10 years
Incidence of peripheral joints involved	17%–50%	20%–24%
Frequency of peripheral joint involvement	Four to six times	Three to five times
Peripheral joints involved	Knee, ankle, elbow, shoulder, wrist, hip, fingers, sternoclavicular	Knee, elbow, ankle, shoulder, wrist
Incidence of spinal involvement	7%–35%	4%–7%
Laboratory tests	ESR 38–90 mm/h, C-reactive protein +ve in 25%–40%, antistreptolysin-0 titer elevated in a few patients, rheumatoid factor +ve in 6%, HLA-B27 +ve in 66%–72% of patients with spondylitis	ESR 35–55 mm/h, C-reactive protein +ve in 33%, rheumatoid factor +ve in 4%–7%, HLA-B27 +ve in 52% patients with spondylitis
X-ray findings in peripheral joints	Thickening of joint capsule, narrowing of cartilage space, irregular delimitation of articular surfaces, chiefly in shoulder and hip joints	Marked swelling of joint capsule, narrowing of cartilage space, osteoporosis of articular epiphyses
X-ray findings in spine	Osteophytes bridging adjacent vertebrae, ossification of paravertebral ligaments with bambooing of spine, ankylosis of sacroiliac joints and hips	Extensive osteophytes bridging lumbar vertebrae, irregular delimitation and partial obliteration of sacroiliac joints
Response of peripheral joints to conservative treatment	In 65% of affected joints	In 80% of affected joints
Response of spine to treatment	In 15%–20% with limitation of motion in those without roentgenographic evidence of ankylosis	In 45%–50% with substantial limitation of motion in those without roentgenographic evidence of ankylosis
Permanent regressive changes in peripheral joints	In 30%–35%	In 15%–20%
Permanent regressive changes in spine	In 50%–85% of those with involved spine ankylosis results	In 30%–45% of those with involved spine ankylosis results

unclarified infection which may also affect the joints. (b) The disease of the intestine and the affections of the joints are aspects of a single entity. (c) The diseased intestinal wall releases antigenic substances which are transported by the bloodstream to the joints. The parallelism between exacerbations of regional ileitis and occurrences or recurrences of joint involvement supports the latter view.

Table 2 summarizes the features of joint affections observed in ulcerative colitis and those in regional ileitis, their essential signs and the common and distinctive features.

3. Joint Affections in Metabolic Disorders

a. Arthropathy in Gout

Arthropathy in gout [576] is an unequivocal and the prime example of metabolically induced joint alterations. The causative factor is uric acid, a normal product of purine degradation which, when excessively increased, becomes deposited in articular and other tissues. Thus, characteristic for gout is the increased concentration of urates (sodium urate and uric acid) in the blood and their subsequent deposition in various organs. The causes of increased urate levels in the blood (hyperuricemia) are increased urate production, or decreased renal elimination of urates, or a combination of the two.

Considering these anomalies, the condition with increased production of urates as the initial cause is defined primary gout, occurring in some patients by genetic factors. The overproduction of urates can be ascertained on a regular purine diet by determining the excreted amount of urates in a 24-h period; an excess of 1000 mg urates is considered abnormal [1711]. The cause of overproduction of urates in primary gout is seen [868, 869, 870, 1797] in an accelerated rate of purine biosynthesis which is not secondary to another condition. Three specific defects appear as the responsible factors for this overproduction: deficiency in hypoxanthine-guanine-phosphoribosyl transferase, overactivity of phosphoribosyl-pyrophosphate synthetase, and deficiency in glucose phosphatase [868, 869, 870]. Of these, the increased activity of phosphoribosyl-pyrophosphate synthetase appears the main cause of the increased rate of phosphoribosyl-pyrophosphate and thus as the prime factor in the overproduction of urates [1559]. Deficiency in transferase and increased synthetase activity are transmitted by autosomal factors in inherited primary gout [1142].

On the other hand, hyperuricemia,which results from decreased excretion of uric acid due to reduced glomerular or tubular function in nephropathies, is defined secondary gout. A frequent external cause of secondary hyperuricemia is the chronic administration of diuretics, followed by their effect in decreasing urate clearance, and in enhancing the tubular reabsorption of secreted urates [417]. Other causes of secondary hyperuricemia are neoplastic disease of the kidneys and chemotherapy.

Wyngaarden [1797] regards aberration of metabolism with increase in the enzyme amidoribosyl transferase, which catalyzes purine biosynthesis, as the prevailing cause of hyperuricemia. On the other hand, Diamond et al. [417] maintains that diminished renal clearance of urates due to a lower glomerular filtration rate accounts for hyperuricemia in the majority of patients. Gutman [698, 699] views the lack of the enzyme uricase in the presence of overproduction of urates as a prime factor in the causation of hyperuricemia; decreased renal clearance of uric acid due to tubular dysfunction contributes to the persistence of hyperuricemia. Thus the cause of gout is an abnormal metabolism [1621] resulting in increased production of purines appearing in the blood and not compensated by degradation in the intestine and/or adequate elimination through the kidneys. The result is an increased pool of purines and urates in the blood and tissues.

The urates in the serum are monosodium urate and uric acid, with the latter being almost insoluble above a serum concentration of 7.0 mg%. The increased urates arriving in the tissues interact with the local proteoglycans and undergo an exchange of anions and cations. Sodium ions diffuse into the ground substance of the connective tissue, and urates precipitate in the interstitial spaces between the collagen bundles [676]. Thus the bursae, tendon sheaths, joint capsules, and subcutaneous tissue become prime depots of urates. The latter are imparted from the joint capsule to the joint fluid and are eventually also deposited in the articular cartilage. Chemical, osmotic, and hydrodynamic factors are responsible for this. The deposition of urates occurs initially in the superficial layer of the articular cartilage and progresses gradually into its depth with concurrent involvement of the entire thickness of the joint capsule and periarticular structures.

Gouty arthritis affects men more than women, predominantly those of mature age, who are well nourished and indulge in alcohol; vegetarians are considerably less affected. Other clinical findings often associated with gout are obesity, diabetes, hypertension, and arteriosclerosis. Arthritis may appear either as acute oligoarthritic swelling or as chronic polyarthritic thickening.

The classical acute gouty attack is characterized by certain prodromal symptoms. After an opulent meal, excessive alcohol intake, or intensive physical strain follow dizziness, nausea, vomiting, dyspepsia, and frequent micturition. The next morning the patient is awakened by severe pain which may last many hours unless calmed by strong analgesics. Gout usually starts in the small peripheral joints; those of the big toe (Fig. 351), fifth toe, and thumb (Figs. 349, 350) are principally and characteristically involved. The ankle, knee, wrist, and elbow joints are commonly and secondarily involved. The area of the affected joint is swollen, discolored dusky red, and much warmer than its surroundings. The acute attack is often associated with temperature elevated to 39.5°C which is commensurate with the regional inflammatory changes. The local tenderness is very intense, sometimes to such degree that the patient cannot tolerate the weight of the

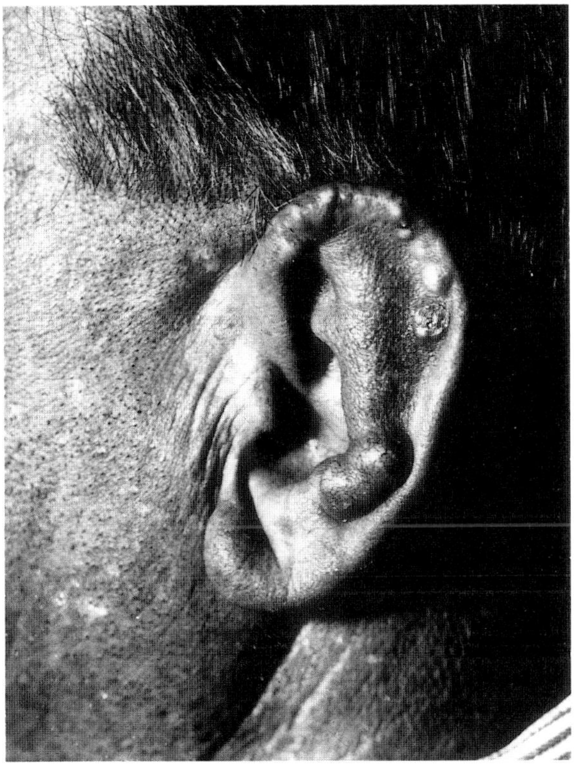

Fig. 348. Nodular thickenings (one of them exulcerated) protrude in the skin covering the cartilage of the external ear

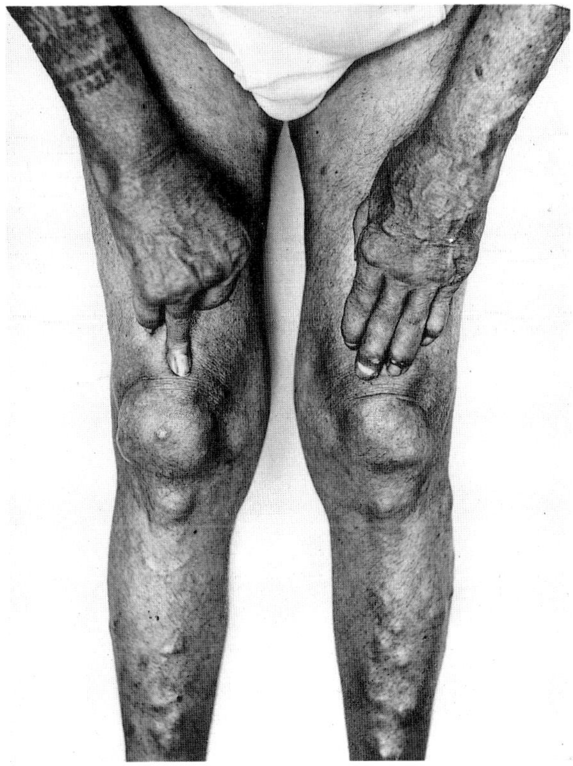

Fig. 349. The fingers are contracted and deformed by nodular thickenings. Larger thickenings protrude at the anterior aspects of the knees and lower legs

blanket. The examination for motion of the affected joints causes pain, and thus the patient avoids any motion. The pain decreases in 1–3 days, the local inflammation regresses, and the mobility of the joint normalizes, unless the acute attack repeats itself after a few weeks or several months. In other cases gout takes a chronic course from the first episode, with intermittent and more painful episodes of exacerbation of the swelling. Eventually the affected small, middle-sized, or even large joints become unevenly thickened (Fig. 349). Where nodular urate masses, termed tophi, attain large sizes in the fibrous capsule of the joint, they may perforate the skin. However, such outcome is more characteristic of the subcutaneous tophi, which upon exulceration (Fig. 348) cause draining sinuses with discharge of a white cheesy material. When larger and multiple [1172], the tophi located in bursae and/or tendon sheaths form protrusions around joints. Together with subcutaneous tophi, they cause deformities, especially of the fingers (Fig. 349), as well as substantial impairment of motion in their joints. Since the urates can be deposited in any cartilage in addition to the articular cartilage the helix and antihelix of the external ear may be similarly affected (Fig. 348).

Of the laboratory studies, the colorimetric or spectrophotometric determination of uric acid in the serum is of prime importance. In the appropriate clinical setting, an elevation of uric acid beyond 10 mg% in men and 8 mg% in women is highly suggestive, and that beyond 11 mg% is definitely indicative of gout [698, 699]. The excreted amount of uric acid in urine decreases during an acute attack on average from 0.7 to 0.3–0.4 g% and resumes normal levels 3–4 days after termination of the acute attack. Examining joint fluid by polarized light, McCarty [1051] and Hollander [774] identified negatively birefringent, needle-shaped urate crystals – either located intracellularly in leukocytes or freely floating – as a pathognomonic sign for the presence of urates in joints. Indeed, urate crystals located in leukocytes or freely floating can be seen in the joint fluid of gouty patients, even in periods without acute attacks. The milky joint fluid contains 3000–4000 leukocytes, among which polymorphonuclear leukocytes predominate. Therefore, the joint fluid should be examined by smear with Gram stain to exclude the presence of microorganisms, although an infection is here very rare. The urates discharged through sinus openings can be identified by the murexid test and by negative, strong birefringence under polarized light. By crystallography the sodium urate can be identified as needles of the monocline system and the uric acid as right-angular tablets or amorphous deposits.

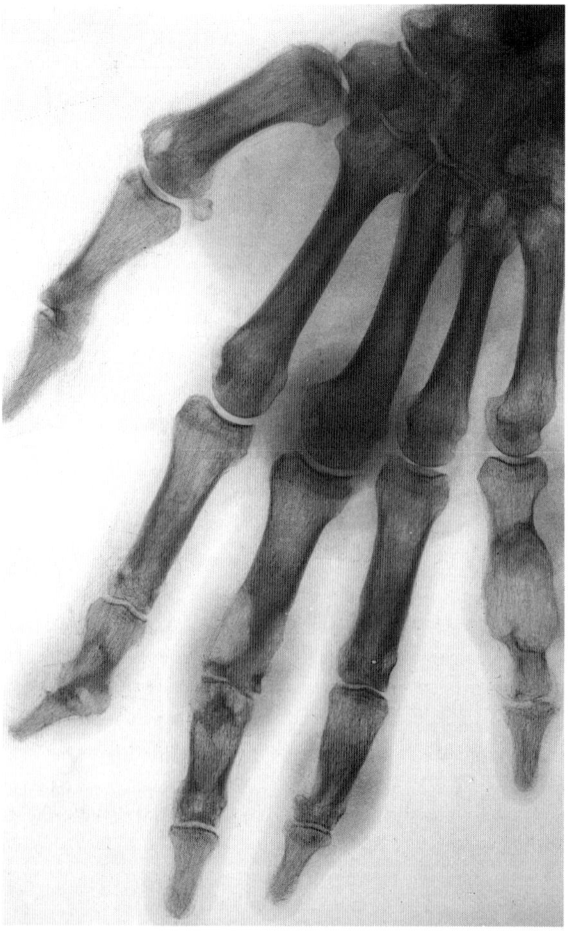

Fig. 350. The phalanges of the fingers comprise delimited areas of pronounced radiolucency. The proximal phalanx of the fifth finger is blown up by such radiolucency. The soft tissue around the third metacarpophalangeal joint is densified

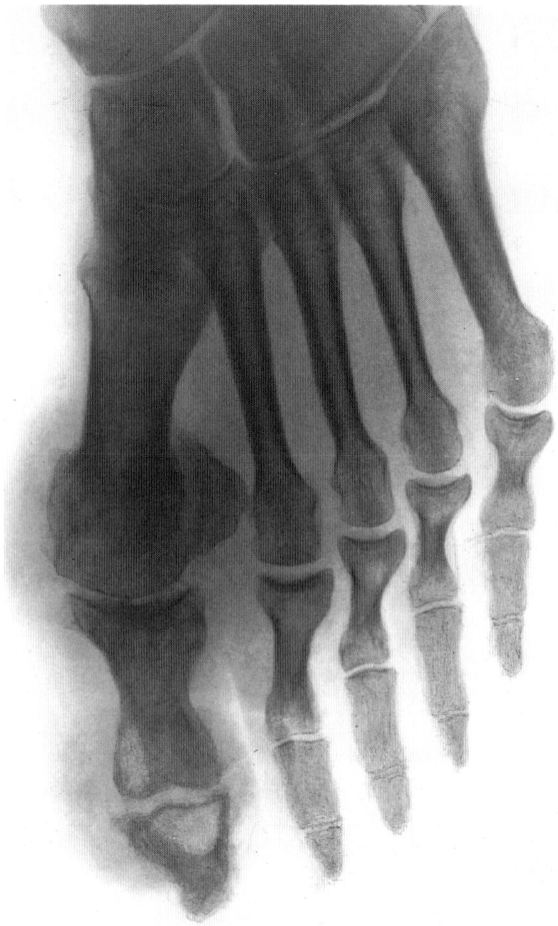

Fig. 351. The phalanges of the big toe comprise large, well-delimited areas of radiolucency. The periarticular metatarso-phalangeal tissue of the big toe is very densified

Furthermore, patients should undergo a metabolic test to ascertain a probable tendency for retention of urates. In healthy individuals given a meal with 400 g roast beef after a few days of purine-free diet the total uric acid excreted rises in the first 24 h to 1.0–1.2 g% and returns in the following day to the normal level of 0.5–0.7 g%. By contrast, in the gouty patient the excretion of uric acid is delayed by 2–3 or more days.

Roentgenographic examination reveals conclusive changes after the urate deposits have caused lytic lesions. These appear as punched-out areas in the phalangeal epiphyses or metaphyses and are sharply delimited by a border of sclerosed bone (Figs. 350, 351). Similar lesions may be noted in the subchondral bone of middle-sized joints (wrist, elbow, ankle). The cartilage space becomes narrowed and irregularly defined where the articular cartilage is eroded by pannus and especially where the subchondral bone has also been invaded by inflamed connective tissue or by deposits of urates (Figs. 350, 351). Tophi of long existence in the joint capsule or periosteal or subcutaneous tissue may appear as shadows of increased density (Figs. 350, 351) due to formation of reactive, dense fibrous encapsulations.

Gross-pathological examination of the metacarpo phalangeal or metatarso-phalangeal joints discloses swelling of the joint capsule with grayish white discoloration of the surface and increase in joint fluid. The articular cartilage has in places lost its smooth, glistening surface due to fine white stipplings or larger and deeper defects which are filled with white dense material. The subchondral bone comprises a few cystic areas also filled with white material. On progressive swelling the synovial membrane sometimes invades the articular cartilage from the margin. On expansion of the urate deposits the inner surface of the joint cavity eventually appears as if smeared with chalk. Similar changes are noticed in the larger joints, especially those

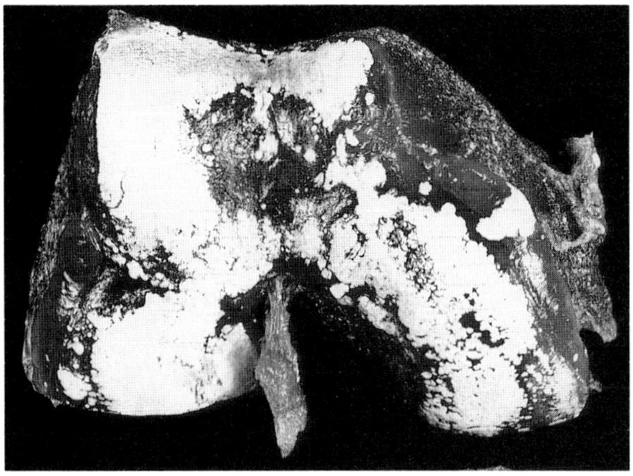

Fig. 352. The articular surfaces of the femoral condyles are extensively permeated by white amorphous material

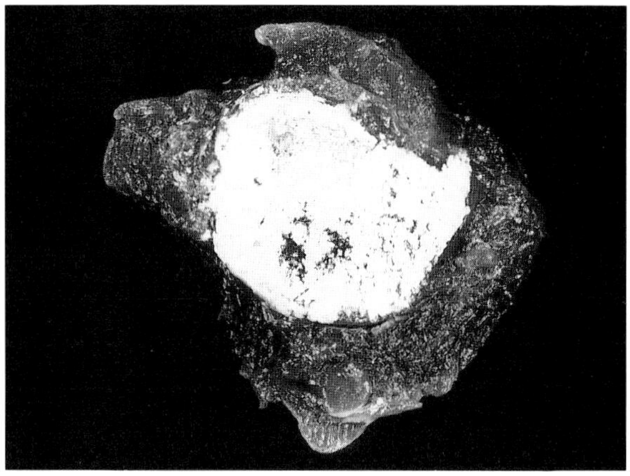

Fig. 353. The articular surface of the patella is almost completely permeated by white amorphous material

of the wrist, elbow, knee (Figs. 352, 353), and ankle. Eventually their joint capsules become substantially thickened, and they may obliterate the joint cavity. This initiates contractures of these joints. Urates are also deposited in periarticular structures. In bursae [238] (especially subdeltoid, olecranon, prepatellar) the urate masses fill the cavities; the thickened bursal capsules become adherent to the underlying bones. In tendon sheaths the urate deposits produce irregular thickenings which by expansion along the sheaths produce conspicuous deformities, especially of the hands and feet. In the subcutis the tophi form nodules situated principally on the extensor surfaces of the extremities. These tophi consist of a capsule originating from the local connective tissue and contain a cheesy material. They are often subdivided into lobules by septa of connective tissue which account for their occasional firmness. By expanding pressure the tophi may cause necrosis and ulceration of the covering skin, leading to unrelenting draining sinuses.

Histopathological examination of the synovial membrane at an early phase of gout shows the synoviocytes to be markedly hypertrophic (Fig. 354). The deeper subsynoviocytic tissue contains areas of disintegration which are filled partly with amorphous masses (Fig. 354) or with needles of urates (Fig. 355). These

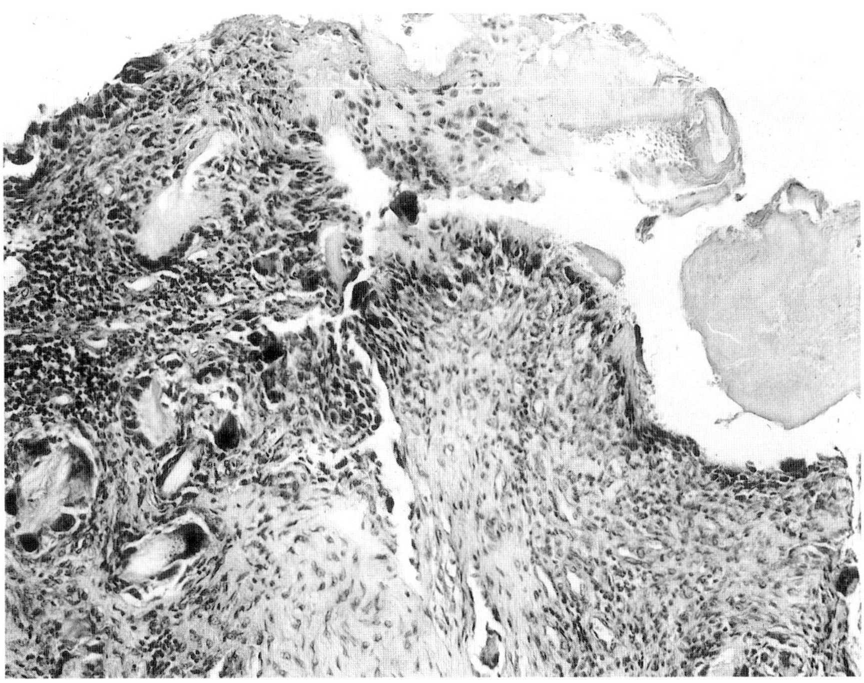

Fig. 354. The synovial membrane is partly covered by a thin layer of amorphous material and is overlain by clumps of such material. The subsynoviocytic tissue is hypercellular mostly with fibrocytes and in a few areas with lymphocytes. Several granulomata lie in the deeper subsynoviocytic tissue

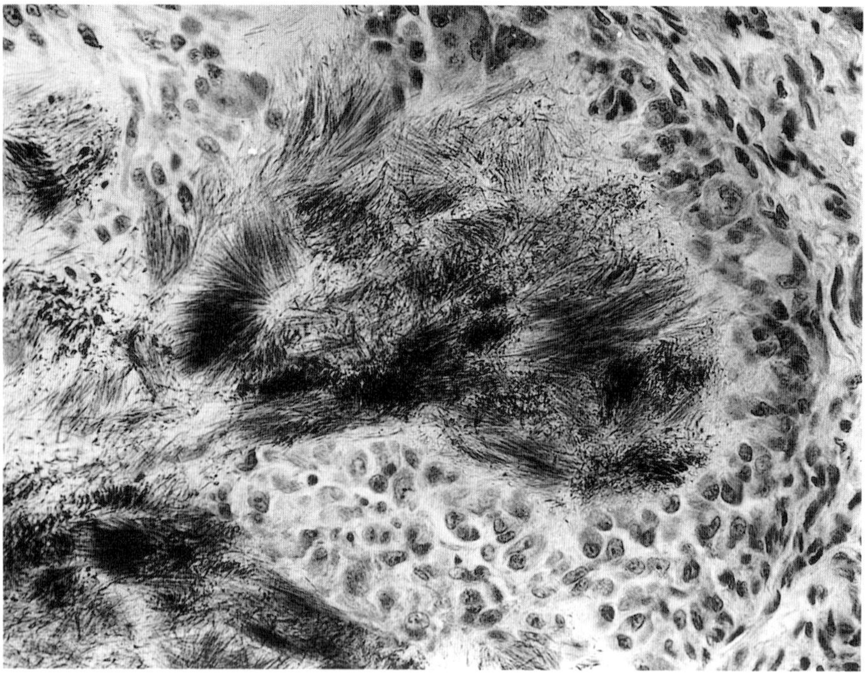

Fig. 355. Some granulomata comprise accumulations of needlelike sharp thin crystals

contents are bordered by histiocytes, a few giant cells, and collagen bundles (Fig. 354). In the articular cartilage, amorphous material and/or negatively birefringent needle crystals, verified by polarized light, are deposited (Fig. 356) in halos and lacunae close to necrotic chondrocytes. The intercellular ground material is decreased, and the provisional calcification line is multiplied. Into these areas hyperemic synovial pannus invades the articular cartilage and replaces the latter, providing the ground for additional deposition of urates. Other pannus approaching from the articular margin undermines the articular cartilage at the junction with the subchondral bone. By expansion this pannus eventually merges with the superficial pannus and thus completely replaces the articular cartilage. In these areas large encapsulations take place comprising either amorphous urate deposits or needlelike crystals arranged in a radial pattern. Similar deposits occur in the

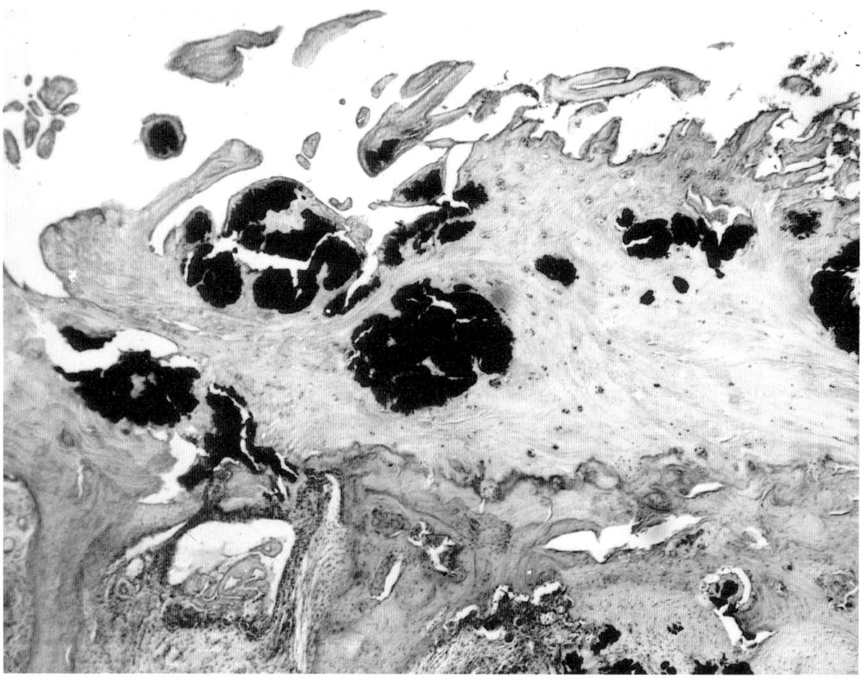

Fig. 356. The articular cartilage is extensively disrupted and fragmented on its surface. Several large accumulations of intensely stained amorphous material lie in its deeper zone, where the chondrocytes are distinctly diminished, and many lacunae are scattered. Accumulations of amorphous material also lie in the marrow spaces of the subchondral bone

articular epiphyses (Fig. 356) of small and middle-sized bones, in which they are surrounded by a border of sclerosed bone. The tophi [1437] are very extensive deposits, more frequently of amorphous urate masses than of urate crystals, in active or necrotic connective tissue. These deposits are delimited by a wall of histiocytes, fibrocytes, lymphocytes, a few giant cells, and bundles of collagen fibers.

The pronounced local symptoms associated with intense painfulness in a joint during an acute gouty attack resemble those in septic arthritis, acute episode of rheumatoid arthritis, or arthritis in gonorrhea. Differential diagnostic problems arise especially if the wrist, ankle, or knee joint is affected, and the swelling diffusely expands beyond the joint capsule. Nevertheless, a history of habitual consumption of purine-rich food, determination of uric acid concentration in the serum, possible presence of tophi, and chemical and polarized microscopic identification of urates in the mesodermal tissue help to ascertain the gouty nature of the condition. The aspiration of fluid from the swollen joint and the detection of urate crystals or microorganisms in the joint fluid further assist in differentiating between gouty and septic arthritis. On the other hand, an increased level of uric acid in the blood without acute arthritic changes or tophi need not necessarily be related to primary gout. This may be caused by underexcretion of uric acid in renal disease or by overproduction of uric acid in leukemia, erythrocytosis, or other blood disorders. An inherited blood disorder with the absence of the enzyme hypoxanthine-guanine-phosphoribosyl transferase is associated with increased production of uric acid and results in gouty arthritis [1456]. Drug-induced hyperuricemia, such as following prolonged intake of antihypertensive medications or intake of potent diuretics, should also be considered in the differential diagnosis. Furthermore, a tophus-resembling acute bursitis may be caused by deposition of calcium crystals; their identification in the bursal fluid by crystalographic scheme and positive birefringence confirms the etiology.

Treatment of gouty arthritis is systematical and according to its clinical phase. In the acute gouty attack complete bedrest, immobilization of the involved joint by a splint, and continuous application of cold or lukewarm compresses greatly help to relieve the pain. The medication of choice, especially in the tophaceous attack, is colchicine [273, 1455, 1803], which is given in hourly doses of 0.6 mg up to a total dose of 6.0 mg in the 1st day, and is continued at half of this dose for the next few days until the painful attack regresses [1803]. If moderate articular symptoms continue, nonsteroidal antiinflammatory medications are indicated. In such cases salicylates in daily doses of 4–6 g are very beneficial because of their analgesic, antiinflammatory, and uricosuric effects. On subsidence of the acute attack the patient should be placed on a weight-reducing and low-purine diet and be given detailed instructions as to which types of food should be avoided. These are: meat soups, sweetbreads, liver, brain, kidney, sardines, anchovies, lobsters, oysters, and roasted meat. Equally, mushrooms, asparagus, lentils, cauliflower, and spinach should also be avoided or at least limited. During the attack-free period a baseline management should be established upon repeated determinations of the serum uric acid levels as well as upon the uric acid excretion in 24-h urine collections. On a regular diet with the normal amount of purine intake, the normal concentration of uric acid in 24-h is 7–9 g%. If the output of urates is less than 700 mg in 24 h, the patient is a hypoexcretor; a uricosuric drug [492] (probenecid 250 mg two or three times a day or salicylates 0.6 g four times a day), which partly inhibits the proximal tubular resorption, should be given. However, these two drugs may not be given concurrently because salicylates block the effect of probenecid. If the patient is an overproducer or hyperexcretor of urates, allopurinol (100 mg three or four times daily) should be used. This inhibits xanthine oxydase and thus the conversion of hypoxanthine to xanthine; consequently, the levels of uric acid in both serum and urine are lowered [1376]. Adverse effects of allopurinol may be dermatitis and gastrointestinal irritations. Nevertheless, this is preferable in most situations to the uricosuric drugs, which enhance the concentration of the eliminated uric acid and thereby increase the potential danger of kidney stones forming (10%–25% of patients [699]). Further complications from uricosuric intake are progressive nephropathy and eventual kidney failure, a frequent cause of death in gout. While on the allopurinol or uricosuric drugs, daily intake of large amounts (2500–3000 ml) of fluid is very necessary.

With all modalities of treatment observed, uric acid levels in the blood should be monitored at intervals to ascertain whether a change in medication is indicated. Upon persistent high concentrations of uric acid in the serum, concurrent administration of colchicine [1803] is indicated for prevention of acute attacks of gouty arthritis. In cases of recurrent and pronounced swellings of the joint capsules, phenylbutazone 100 mg twice daily for 2 weeks may be very beneficial; concomitant blood studies are necessary because of potential depression in bone marrow and granulocytopenia. Nevertheless, despite diet and medications tophi develop in about 7%–10% of patients, however of smaller sizes than observed without medications. These tophi are large enough to be unsightly, especially when involving the hands or superficial bursae, and to cause functional impairment when involving the tendon sheaths or joint capsules. Wide excision of such tophi from the joint capsule is indicated when the motion of the joint is limited. Thereafter, satisfactory results are observed in an increased range of motion and restoration of the normal configuration of the affected limb. Excision becomes even urgent when the tophi lead to necrosis and exulceration of the overlying skin, followed by a persistently draining sinus; aseptic and enduring closure of such wounds may be obtained [946, 1602]. In addition, resection of the deformed articular epiphyses may be indicated to restore or improve the motion of the joints.

While the familial type of gout generally derives from an inborn faulty metabolism, a similarly increased concentration of uric acid in the serum may result from excessive breakdown of normal blood cells or from normal breakdown of excessively formed blood cells. The resulting excessive quantity of nucleic acids is metabolized to urates, which in their high concentration encounter limited excretion and cause a secondary gout [573, 698]. As such blood disorders, Talbott [1620] lists, among others: polycythemia vera, polycythemia and leukemia, leukemia, multiple myeloma, hemolytic anemia, and sickle cell anemia.

With its concentration in the serum of secondary gout increased, the precipitation of uric acid in articular tissues is a frequent sequela. It is often also the very first symptom which requires laboratory studies into the underlying cause. These studies include total blood count, leukocyte differential count, stained smear of the blood and bone marrow, protein electrophoresis, and that of Bence-Jones substance in urine. The concomitant elevation in uric acid concentration may be even higher than in primary metabolic gout, but the affection of the joints, bursae, tendon sheaths, and subcutaneous tissue is very similar. However, the urate deposits are not as extensive as in primary gout due to timely treatment of the primary blood disorder. Equally to primary gout, colchicine is used in the acute arthritic attacks, and allopurinol is used with equal dosage and effects in the chronic phase.

b. Arthropathy in Ochronosis

Ochronosis is the term given by Virchow [1695] to extensive alteration of hyaline cartilage, fibrocartilage, and dense connective tissue to a yellow-ocher appearance. Subsequently, Wolken et al. [1780] identified homogentisic acid as the substance deposited in the mesodermal tissues and also eliminated in the urine causing its black discoloration on the addition of alkaline substances; therefore, the other term alkaptonuria. Further studies [930, 931] revealed that phenylalanin and tyrosin, contained in the protein of food, is catabolized in ochronosis only to homogentisic acid and not further to acetoacetic acid, which becomes incorporated into the citric cycle. Eventually, LaDu et al. [930, 931] ascertained that the absence of homogentisic acid oxydase, an enzyme physiologically present in the liver and kidneys, accounts for the lack of further breakdown and for the circulatory presence of homogentisic acid. The latter becomes deposited [559] in the pericardium, blood vessels, kidneys, prostate, skin, sweat glands, sclerae, cartilage of the ears, nose and larynx, and articular tissues of peripheral joints and vertebral column.

Ochronosis may occur spontaneously without precedence in the family. Recent studies [904] on family trees indicate that ochronosis is inherited as a simple autosomal trait. A consanguine marriage is able to convert this inborne recessive trait into a dominant one and to bring ochronosis to manifestation [904]. The clinical picture [1198] often comes into evidence in triangular bluish gray (slate) discoloration of the sclera between limbus corneae and epicanthus. In elderly persons, the pigmentation of the skin may be so far advanced that it causes dark staining of the forehead, cheeks, and around the eyes; the lower part of the face has a normal coloring. The pigmented skin, especially in the axilla and groin, releases brown sweat which causes brownish discoloration of the shirt. The urine also becomes discolored brownish on longer duration. Increasing pain in the lumbar spine, starting at the rather early age of 35–40 years, presents the overture to the expanding involvement of the entire spine, knee, hip, shoulder, and elbow joints [411, 1465]. The lumbar spine is very tender and substantially or completely limited in its movements in all directions. Eventually the lumbar lordosis is lost and may merge into kyphosis with the dorsal spine. On further deterioration of the intervertebral discs root neuralgias appear, but without profound motor or sensory deficit. The larger joints of the extremities are sore and present crepitation in their movements. Weakness and stiffness are experienced in these joints at a distinctly earlier age than usually experienced in primary osteoarthritis. Pronounced thickening of the capsule of the knee joints ensues, with limitation of motion. Similar changes are noted in the shoulder and hip joints. Eventually stones, resulting from insufficiency of tubular excretion and/or reabsorption may develop in the kidneys and prostate.

In laboratory studies, enzymatic assay studies [931, 1198] of the blood and urine disclose the presence of homogentisic acid (5.2 mg per 100 ml); blood urea nitrogen ranges between 15 and 20 mg%. The urine turns black after standing 2 h in open air or on addition of an alkaline substance and strongly reduces Fehling's solution. The total homogentisic output, amounting normally to 120–140 mg in 24 h, is increased to 400–500 mg, as determined by paper chromatography, io-

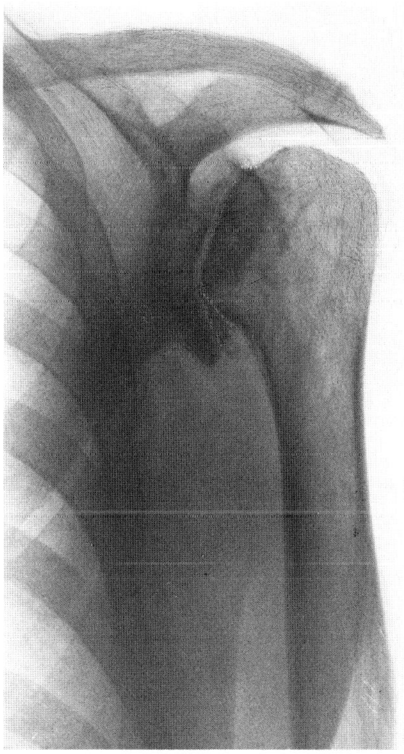

Fig. 357. The joint cleft is narrowed and uneven. The glenoid cavity and the humeral head are worn off and sclerosed. A large osteophyte expands from the lower border of the glenoid cavity

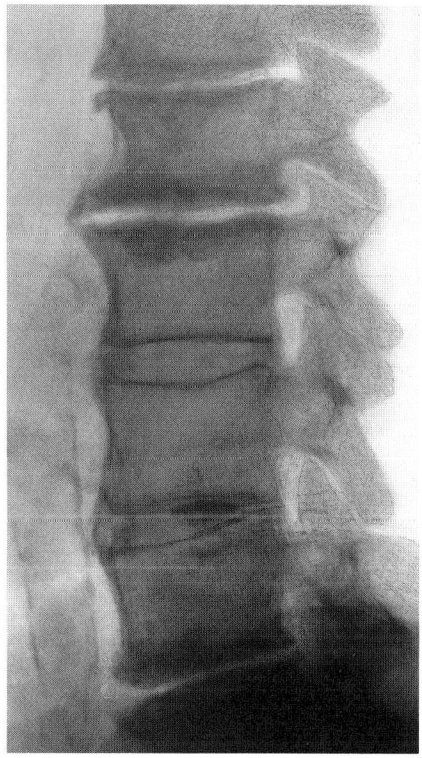

Fig. 358. The upper lumbar vertebrae have marginal osteophytes, whereas the lower lumbar vertebrae are united by ossification of the anterior ligament. The latter intervertebral spaces are obscured by deposition of homogentisic acid, while the intervertebral space L2–3 has abnormal transparency due to cavitation

dometry, and colorimetry [1153, 1465]. Examination of the occasionally increased and dark yellow discolored joint fluid discloses floating particles and small fragments of dark brown cartilage appearing like ground pepper [792]. Similar minute particles have been phagocytosed by polymorphonuclear leukocytes and monocytes in the joint fluid, while other leukocytes contain crystals of calcium pyrophosphate [1441].

Roentgenographs reveal in the joints of the extremities similar changes to those in pronounced primary osteoarthritis. These changes are manifested (Fig. 357) in substantial narrowing of the cartilage space and in deeply extending subchondral sclerosis in the articular epiphyses [1211]. In other cases these epiphyses show a partial duplication of their outline due to calcinosis of the fragmented articular cartilage. The subchondral bone often contains delimited lesions of radiolucency corresponding to cysts. The intervertebral spaces of the thoracic spine and especially of the lumbar spine are narrowed. Extensive calcification of the intervertebral

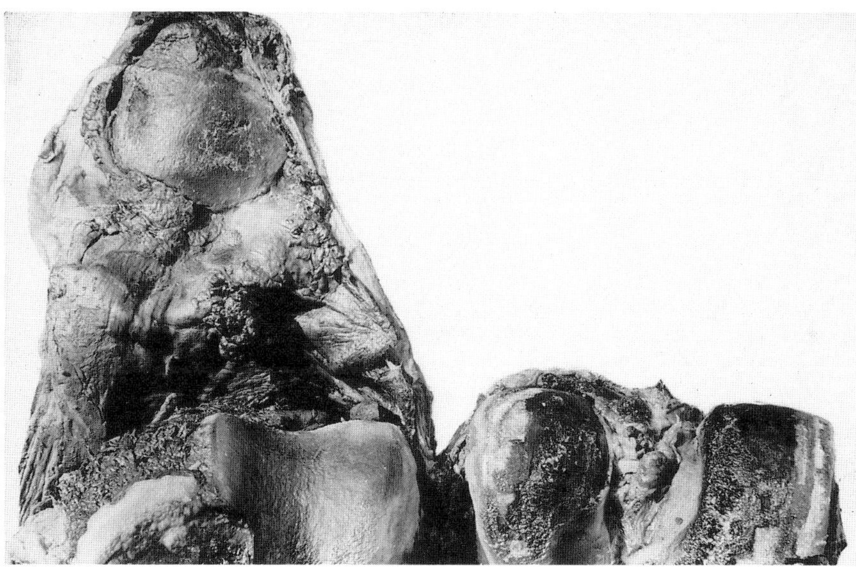

Fig. 359. The articular surfaces of the femoral condyles are partly worn off. The residual articular cartilage on the femoral condyle and on the patella is discolored black

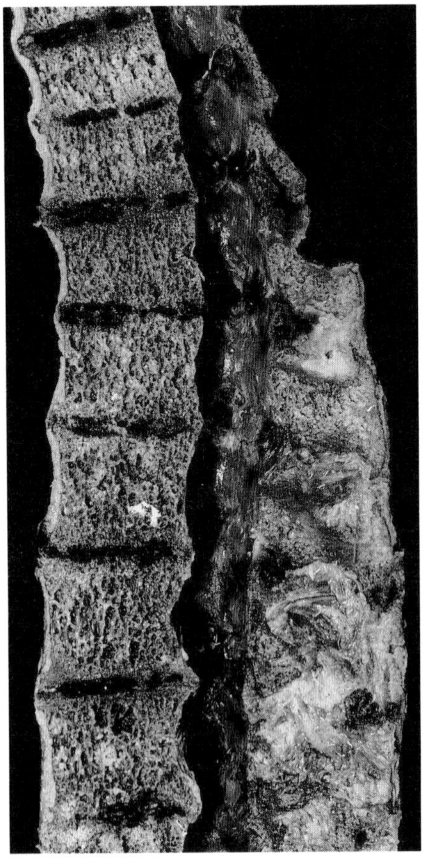

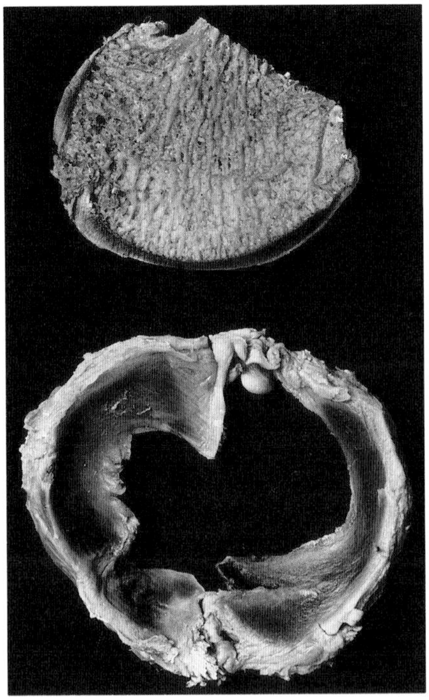

Fig. 360. The articular cartilages of the femoral condyle and both menisci are extensively discolored black

Fig. 361. The intervertebral fibrocartilages and the tissues adjacent to the apophyseal joints are discolored black. The intervertrebral spaces are unevenly delimited, some of them are narrowed, and others are partly widened

discs occurs at several levels (Fig. 358), as well as sclerosis of the adjacent vertebral plates and formation of marginal osteophytes. Mueller et al. [1153] emphasized the vacuum phenomenon, the presence of air-containing large clefts in the intervertebral discs (Fig. 358), as a pathognomonic radiological feature of this disease. In other cases no calcification or vacuum formation in the intervertebral discs is observed. The cervical spine has less narrowing and less calcification of its intervertebral discs but more irregular delimitation of its vertebral plates, more pronounced marginal osteophytes, and frequent calcification of the paravertebral soft structures [448]. The sacroiliac joints are occasionally affected by irregular borders and sclerosis.

Gross-anatomical examination discloses that the articular epiphyses of the joints of the extremities lack the bluish white glistening of their surfaces; their hyaline cartilage is brownish and comprises a few areas of grayish black discoloration (Figs. 359, 360). The smoothness of the cartilage cover has been partly lost due to striplike fibrillation and roughness. In addition, the cartilage in the center of the articular surfaces is worn down, with subsequent denudation of the subjacent bone (Fig. 359). Consequently, marginal osteophytes have formed. The subchondral bone presents grayish cystic spaces containing minced fragments of hyaline articular cartilage (Fig. 360). Other fragments of articular cartilage lie loosely in folds of the synovial membrane, which is discolored blackish brown and substantially thickened in its entire extent. It is placewise elevated in hard villosities. The intervertebral discs are discolored blackish brown at their fibrocartilage and nucleus pulposus [559, 977, 1220] (Fig. 361). This tissue is extensively cleaved and fragmented, with substantial decrease in the height of the discs. These are also calcified in places, as noticed by their dirty whitish discoloration. The adjacent vertebral plates are very sclerosed, and osteophytes rise from their margins.

Histopathological examination [923] discloses extensive dark brown discoloration of the articular cartilage (Fig. 362) by deposition of fine pigment granules in the ground substance, which has become decomposed. The interstitial fibers are then unmasked and separated. The cartilage cells show degeneration or necrosis, with fragmentation or loss of the nuclei. Inside the cells and at their peripheries are large lacunae in which fine dark pigmented granules are deposited [1126, 1309]. In some cases the cartilage is necrotic over larger areas and is heavily impregnated with calcium salts [1055]. These altered cartilage areas have

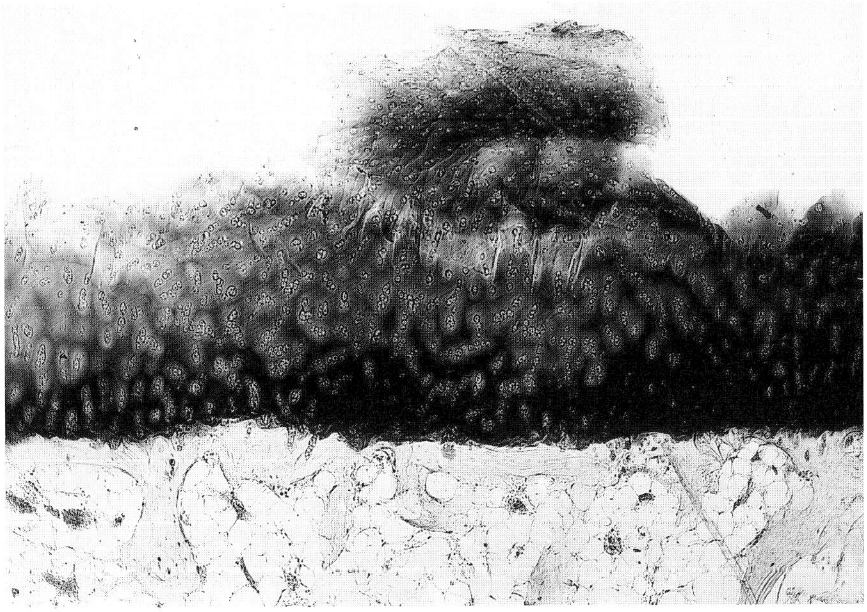

Fig. 362. In this unstained tissue section, the articular cartilage obtained its staining by deposition of homogentisic acid

become disintegrated and fragmented; portions of them are separated (Fig. 362). Into the resulting defects blood vessels proliferate from the subchondral marrow. In other places the line of provisional calcification is disrupted, and portions of pigmented cartilage are displaced into the depth of the subchondral bone, where they lie in cavities. The synovial membrane is elevated in broad villi. Its subsynoviocytic stroma is hypercellular with fibrocytes and histiocytes, and contains numerous granules of pigmented material as well as small and larger fragments of pigmented cartilage (Fig. 363). Some of these cartilage fragments are undergoing lacunar resorption, and others are surrounded by foreign body reaction. Granules of brown pigment are accumulated in neighboring histiocytes [923, 1127]. Most cartilaginous endplates of the vertebrae are intensely dark stained and slightly disrupted at the zones, where they merge with the intervertebral discs. The latter contain a few dark-stained tissue portions over a small extent, but otherwise are disrupted in thinner and thicker fibers, which are neighbored by an extensive area completely bare of tissue (Fig. 364) – cavitation.

In addition to these osteoarticular lesions, gross-anatomical and histopathological examinations [977,

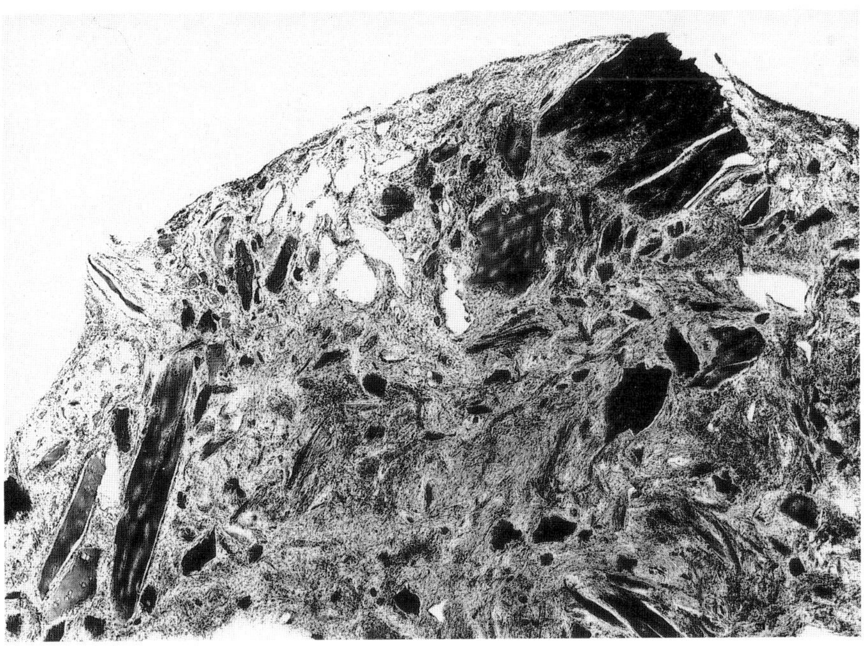

Fig. 363. The synovial membrane is very densified by a marked increase in the fibrocytes throughout. Many fragments of black cartilage, some necrotic and others viable, are deposited in the superficial and deeper tissue

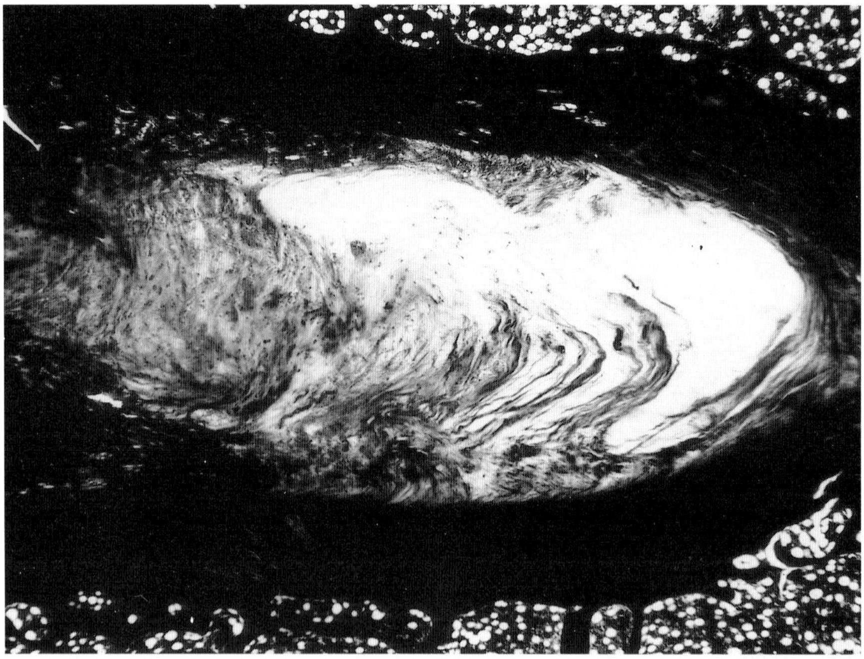

Fig. 364. The hyaline cartilage of the vertebral plates is stained intensely black. The intervertebral disc is bare on a great part of its tissue, and a cavity has been formed. The remaining tissue consists mainly of widely separated fibers

1220] disclose extensive deposits of homogentisic acid particularly in the media of arteries, all layers of the heart, and tubules of the kidneys.

In view of the fact that the urine gives a strong reducing reaction with Fehling's solution, diabetes may be suspected as the causative factor of the articular symptoms. However, the probable presence of darkly pigmented areas in the eyes or in the skin of the face and ears and the spontaneous blackening of urine provide clues to the underlying condition. The early manifestations of osteoarthritic changes in major peripheral joints assist in the diagnosis, as does the calcinosis of the vertebral column.

Treatment of ochronotic arthritis cannot be etiological as long as the missing enzyme for homogentisic acid cannot be replaced. Also, no possibility exists for decreasing the concentration of circulating homogentisic acid by reducing the intake of the necessary minimum of protein in the diet. Therefore, the management of ochronotic arthritis is for the time being confined to avoidance of vigorous activities of the entire body so as to minimize attrition of the joints. Regular application of moist hot packs and shortwave diathermy in a number of distanced series of eight to ten sessions provide substantial relief to the painful joints. Similarly, the intake of salicylates and/or nonsteroidal antiinflammatory medications is indicated in the episodes of soreness. In view of the frequent concomitant deposition of calcium crystals [1441], administration of colchicine 0.6 mg every 2–3 h is very beneficial for the first 5–7 days of painful attacks. Lustberg et al. [991] recommended intake of high doses of ascorbic acid, which experimentally reduces the binding of homogentisic acid to connective tissue. A brace or firm high lumbosacral belt (Fig. 51) provides substantial support for the ailing spine. Otherwise, arthroplastic operations may represent the ultimate solution for the shoulder and hip joints; their techniques are discussed in "Osteoarthritis". A brace in the early stage and total synovectomy combined with removal of free bodies in the late stage, as discussed in "Rheumatoid Arthritis", prove beneficial for the knee joint. However, the general prognosis is very guarded because the life expectancy is substantially curtailed in the presence of extensive deposits of homogentisic acid in the heart and arteries.

c. Arthropathy in Gaucher's Disease

Disorders of the lipid metabolism [1257] may be associated with joint ailments secondary to extensive local accumulation of abnormal metabolic products. One of these intermediary metabolites is kerasin, a glucocerebroside resulting from faulty breakdown of glucolipids due to absence of the normally participating enzymes glucocerebrosidase and glucosidase [542]. These catalyze the hydrolytic cleavage of the glucolipids [172, 206, 1338, 1633]. The other intermediary metabolites occurring here are galactocerebroside and a polycerebroside. The deficiency in this disorder is congenital and transmitted by autosomal dominant or by recessive genes, as suggested by its occurrence in parents and their offspring [1338, 1633].

On extensive spread of histiocytes laden with these intermediary metabolites, the spleen, liver, and lymph nodes become markedly enlarged, primarily by the ac-

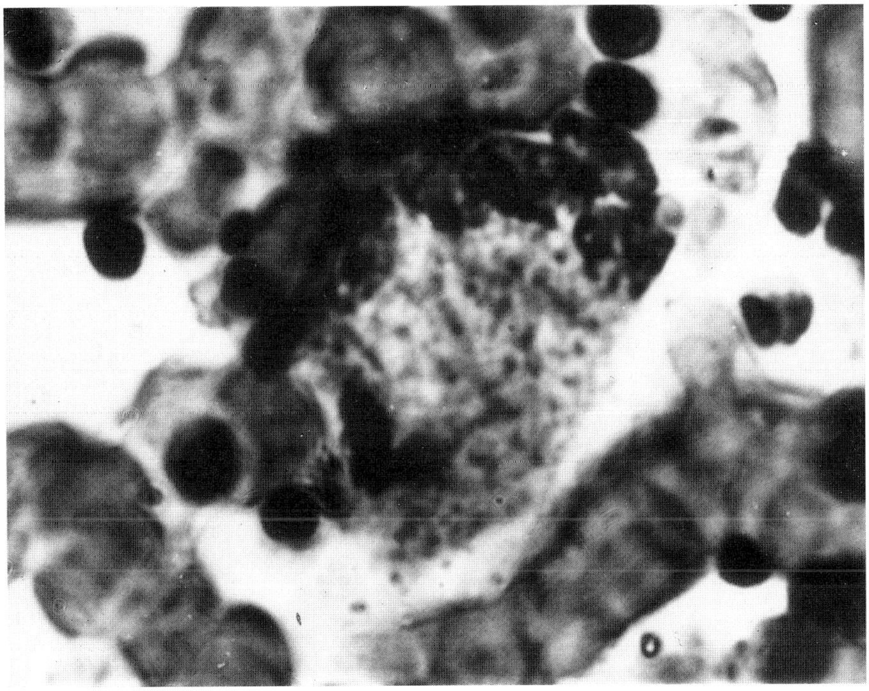

Fig. 365. Large multinuclear cells of 30–65 μm lie in the aspirate from bone marrow. They comprise a network filled with homogeneous lipidic material

cumulation of these histiocytes and secondarily due to thickening of the interstitial connective tissue. As originally described by Gaucher [580], this storage disease expands by large accumulations of the characteristically blown-up histiocytes within the bone marrow of the epiphyses and metaphyses [1496]. Such areas with rarefaction of bone and compression of blood vessels, followed by local necrosis, are sites of decreased structural support. Repeated minor fractures occur here. Indentations remain in articular surfaces as the sequences of spontaneous intraarticular fractures and despite their refilling with callus. Displaced articular cartilage sometimes proliferates here. These indentations result in articular incongruence which eventually leads to osteoarthritis. The deposition of Gaucher's cells occurs predominantly in the proximal and distal ends of the femur and is then followed by involvement of the hip and knee joints. The proximal part of the humerus is affected distinctly less often than the femur and is followed by secondary involvement of the shoulder joint. Similarly, the vertebral bodies are less often affected, and then become compressed.

Gaucher's disease [1247] can appear in infants and children, in whom the prognosis is very grave, especially when it starts in the 1st year of life; this leads to early death. Otherwise, when it appears in young adults, it usually expands over several decades, with a good part of these years spent in fair working conditions. Nevertheless, the frequent anemia causes weakness and sometimes submucosal and subcutaneous bleedings. Gradually the skin assumes a patchy grayish brown or yellow-brown coloring, especially on the abdomen and lower extremities. Besides the frequent episodes of malaise or weakness, the local symptoms depend on the prevailing sites of accumulation of lipid-laden histiocytes. These initially may affect either the visceral organs or the bones, more rarely and simultaneously both systems. The spleen is enlarged, protrudes beneath the lower ribs, and may extend to the iliac bone. The liver may also be enlarged, causing distension of the abdomen. The superficial lymph nodes are usually enlarged and palpable. However, the persistent discomfort and aches in the extremities and vertebral column may sometimes be the predominant symptoms [1494, 1496]. The affected areas in the proximal and distal epiphyses of the femur are associated with limitation of rotation and abduction in the hip joint and with enlargement and coarse crepitation on motion in the knee joint. The shoulder joint, affected by infiltrates in the humeral head, is enlarged, tender, and limited in its rotation and abduction. The accumulation of glycolipids in vertebral bodies may be followed by collapse of these vertebrae and compression of the spinal cord or, more often, of the nerve roots. The neurological signs elicited are hyperreflexia, hypertonicity, and rigidity. Similar symptoms may be elicited by a glycolipidic epidural mass, which can be identified by magnetic resonance imaging [747].

On massive infiltration of the bone marrow, the temperature is elevated, and the number of erythrocytes and leukocytes is decreased. The sedimentation rate is invariably elevated to 45–60 mm/h. Serum globulin is

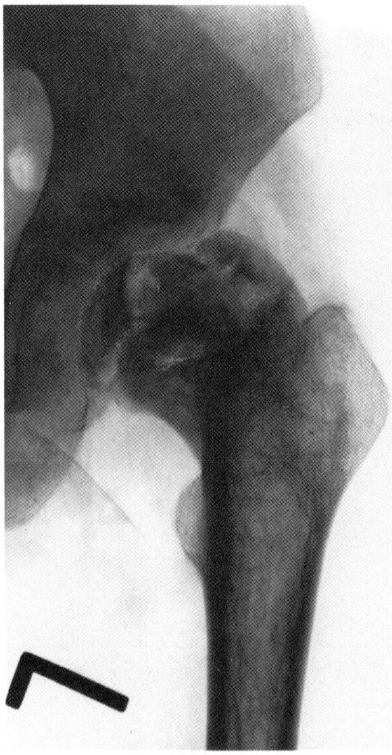

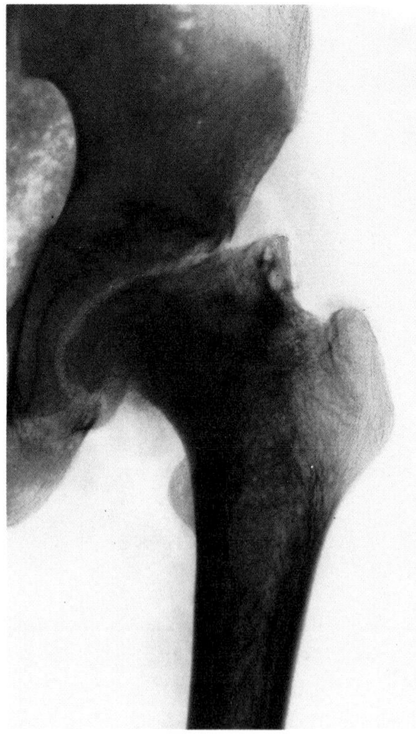

Fig. 366. The proximal femoral ephiphysis is uneven and is subdivided by a few areas of radiolucency, as is the area of the femoral neck. The line of the metaphyseal plate is not yet ossified

Fig. 367. Ten years later, the femoral epiphysis is compressed to a thin uneven plate which is fused with the femoral neck. The cleft of the hip joint is very irregular

increased [1278], as is the level of angiotensin-converting enzyme [1494]. B-lymphocytes were found increased in the majority of patients, as was the serum IgG level [1040]. The diagnosis is established by identification of Gaucher's cells (Fig. 365) – 30 to 60 μm-sized, mononuclear or multinuclear cells with a vacuolated cytoplasm – in the aspirate from the sternal marrow or the spleen. Testing leukocytes in the blood for glucocerebrosidase and glucosidase activities [918, 1268] is also of diagnostic value.

Roentgenographic examination of children reveals rather extensive, delimited lytic areas, mostly in the proximal ends of the humerus and femur (Fig. 366). With weight bearing on the latter, collapse and disorganization of the femoral head and neck (Fig. 367) may follow. In adults, the kerasin-laden histiocytes expanding in the long bones, especially in those of the lower extremities (Figs. 368, 369), may occupy vast areas of the osteoporotic marrow cavity. From here they encroach upon the cortex, which becomes scalloped [39, 965, 1525]. Thus, Moseley [1143] pointed out that extensive osteoporosis of the distal end of the femur is probably the earliest and most consistent change. On further expansion of the histiocytic infiltration, the thinned cortex bulges outward and assumes a convex contour. In this way the distal half of the femur becomes broader, and the femoral shaft presents a club or bottle shape (Fig. 368), "Erlenmeyer's flask," appearance [516]. The rather homogeneous osteoporosis of the marrow cavity often changes by reactive bone formation to a variegated pattern. Numerous lytic areas are surrounded by borders of dense bone with a "worm eaten" appearance (Fig. 369). Such changes are observed principally in the proximal and distal half of the femur and in the proximal half of the tibia (Fig. 369). Due to these changes small fractures and indentations of the articular surfaces occur; the epiphyses are irregularly outlined. In the course of the subsequent attrition the cartilage space becomes narrowed and is partly delimited by sclerosed bony margins. In other long and short bones the cortex may become thickened by endosteal and/or periosteal apposition which causes narrowing of the medullary cavity.

Gross-anatomical examination discloses enlargement of the articular epiphyses of the lower extremities. On dissection [357] of the softened bone, the marrow is permeated by whitish semitransparent nodules which are distinct by their color and consistency. Many trabeculae are replaced by a yellowish gray soft material surrounded by thickened trabeculae. Thus, softened and hardened tissues alternate with each other. In some cases this material is spread diffusely to the cortex, which therefore becomes scalloped from the inside and substantially thinned. In other cases the cortex becomes substantially thickened by endosteal and periosteal reaction which eventually narrows the marrow cavity. In the epiphyses lie cysts containing soft tissue. The articular cartilage, bare of luster, is roughened, uneven, and worn off in several places, exposing the directly subjacent bone. The inner part of the joint capsule is trans-

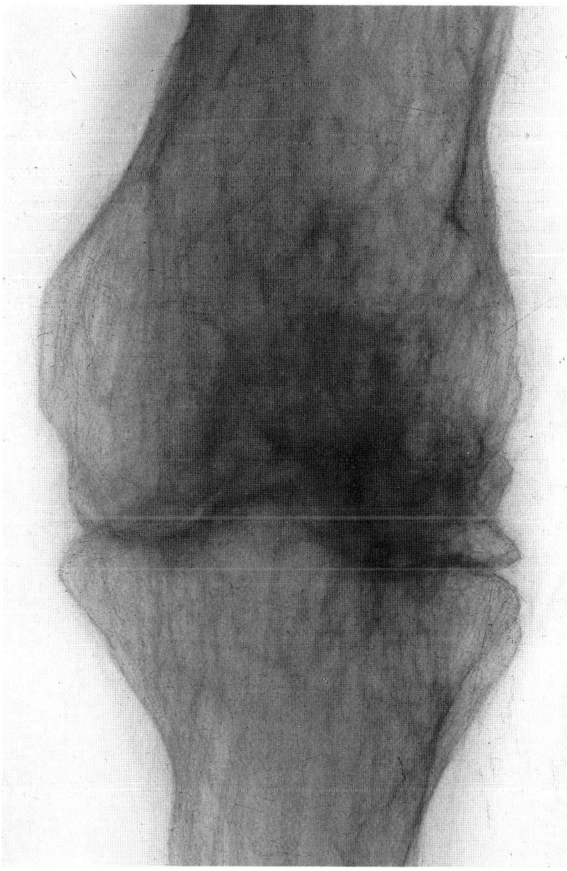

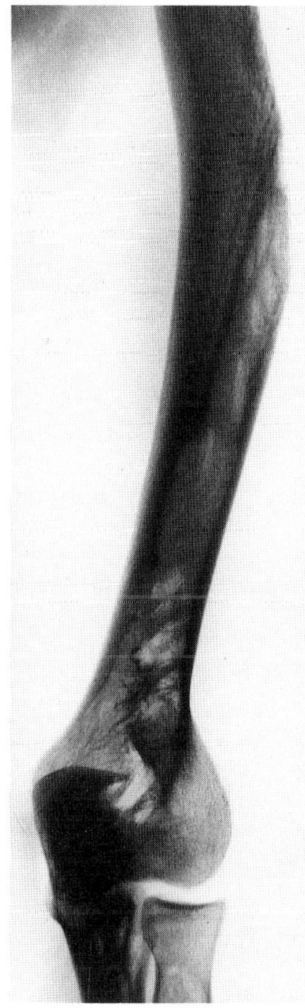

Fig. 368. The femur and tibia are extensively permeated by large areas of radiolucency, between which thin trabeculae course. The distal part of the femur is distinctly broader, and the joint space is very narrow and uneven

Fig. 369. Areas of radiolucency, some of them bordered by sclerosis, are scattered in the humerus

formed into a scarified tissue containing fragments from the cartilaginous surface.

Histopathological examination [50] discloses deep-reaching fibrosis of the synovial membrane, as well as extensive fibrillation, and in places thinning of the articular cartilage (Fig. 370] down to the subchondral bone. The latter displays some appositional thickening as a sign of repair, but mostly areas of osteoid tissue expanding from the depth with widened marrow spaces [357]. Here the Gaucher's cells lie densely accumulated, compressing each other and assuming longitudinal or rectangular shapes. However, at the margins of the accumulations, these cells are roundish or ovoid and have a diameter of 35–55 μm and one or a few nuclei (Fig. 371). Their cytoplasm comprises a thin fibrillar network whose spaces are filled with a homogeneous, clear, lipidic material which stains red with Sudan dye, but is otherwise extracted during routine staining. Glycolipids were identified and structurally determined by chromatography and spectrometry [921] in most organs of the patients with Gaucher's disease.

The presence of the enlarged spleen and the enlarged lymph nodes raise the possibility of an infectious disease or hematological disorder and require relevant laboratory investigations. The clinical findings of marked circumscribed tenderness of a long bone of an extremity with regional swelling and increased local warmth and roentgenographs showing numerous lytic areas may convey the impression of other blood disorders or of osteomyelitis with far-reaching involvement of the neighboring joint. The final diagnosis rests on the examination of aspirates from bone marrow and the identification of Gaucher's cells (Figs. 365, 371) in it, as well as on the verification of glucocerebroside in leukocytes of the peripheral blood.

Due to the lack of the enzyme responsible for the occurrence and persistence of an intermediary product in the lipid metabolism, the treatment is confined to restricting the intake of fat-containing food and to supporting the patient by a diet rich in vitamins. Beyond this, the search for substitution of the missing enzyme is the key point in all therapeutic endeavors. Datta et al. [366] experimentally obtained the formation of increased levels of glucosidase in animals in which Gaucher's disease was provoked experimentally. They thus expressed the hope that by injecting phosphatidylserine the low-level glucosidase could be stimulated to catabolize the stored glycolipids. The traditional attitude to remove an enlarged spleen, which comprises an excessive deposit of the noncata-

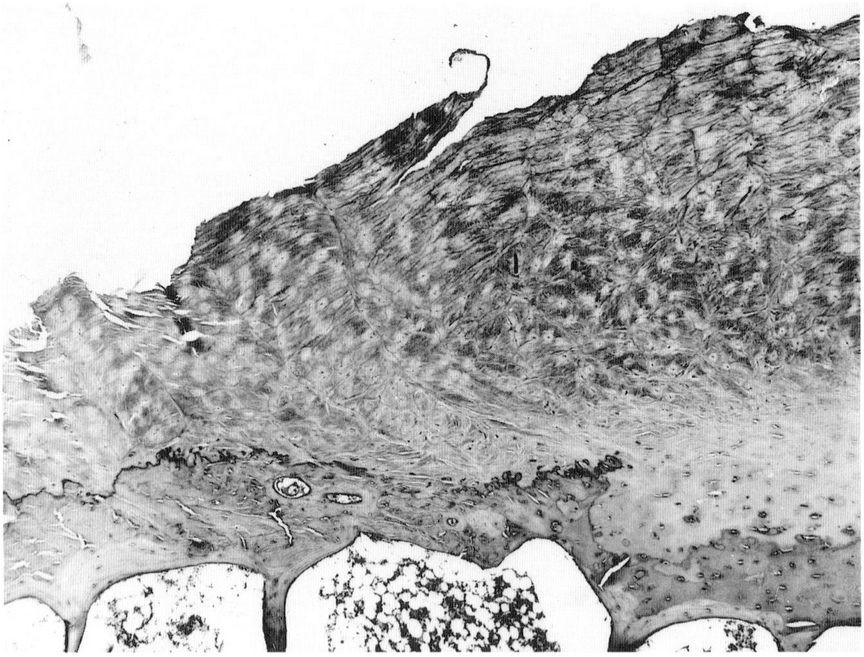

Fig. 370. The articular cartilage is in places uneven and disrupted by horizontal clefts. The ground substance contains many small areas of abnormal staining. The marrow spaces contain accumulations of large cells

bolized glucokerasin, may be counter productive [1476] because it diverts the formation of Gaucher's cells into the marrow of long bones. This enhances the potential for osteoarticular complications including pathological fractures. In cases with advanced bone changes, radiation with 8–10 Gy in six to eight sessions may prove of benefit by causing involution of the histiocyte laden-bone marrow and reformation of the osseous tissue. When the joint alterations are far advanced, especially in the hip joint secondary to necrosis of the juvenile femoral head and neck, total arthroplasty may be indicated [928]. This technique is discussed in "Osteoarthritis".

d. Arthropathy in Hyperlipoproteinemia

Hyperlipoproteinemia is a disorder characterized by an excessive concentration of cholesterol or triglycerides in the serum. Therefore, Thannhauser [1633] divided hyperlipoproteinemia into (a) cholesterolemia and (b)

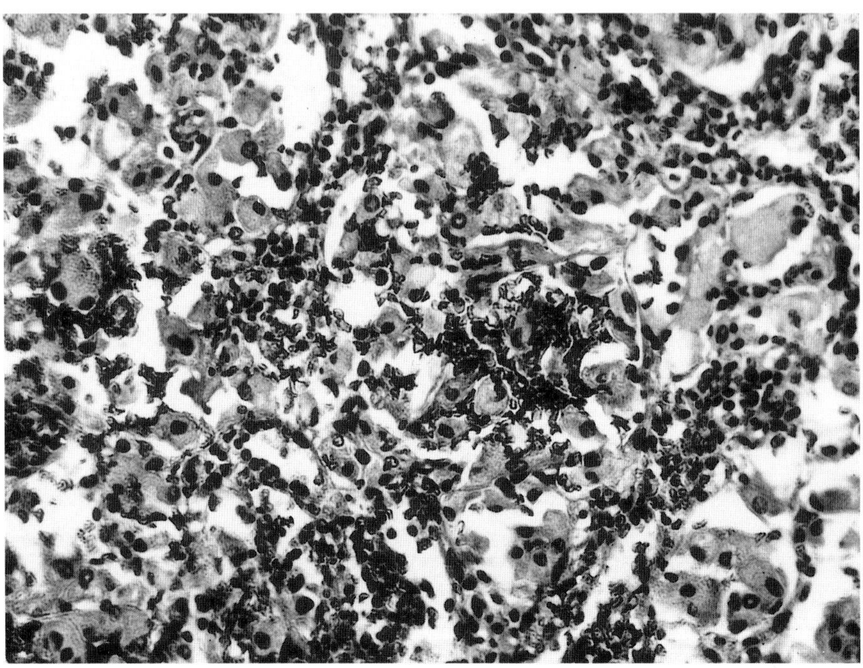

Fig. 371. The bone marrow in the widened subcortical spaces contains, amid numerous histiocytes, large cells which comprise a cytoplasm of lipidic material and a few nuclei lying mostly at the margin

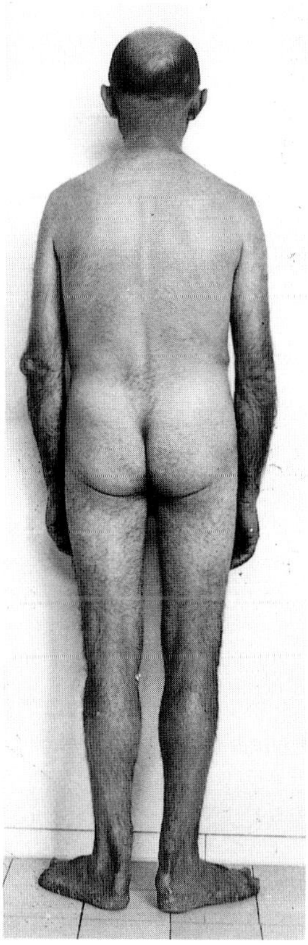

Fig. 372. A large node protrudes at the dorsal aspect of the left elbow. Two similar nodes protrude at the dorsal aspect of both heels. The transitional areas of the Achilles tendons to the calf muscles are very thickend and deformed

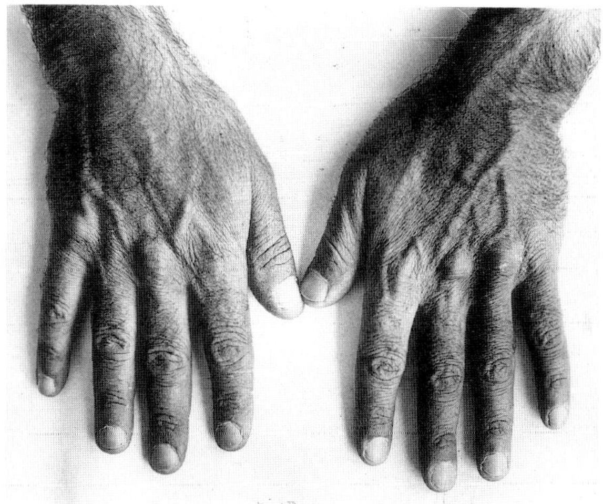

Fig. 373. Moderate-sized nodes protrude on the dorsal aspects of the metacarpophalangeal joints of both hands

total lipemia with substantial increase of cholesterol, neutral lipids, and phospholipids.

The disorder [1338, 1339] appears in men and women of two to three generations of a family, evidently being transmitted by autosomal dominant non-sex-linked genes [7, 763]. The histories of these patients disclose that multiple nodules and protrusions (Fig. 372) have developed over various parts of the body at an age over 20 years. Upon their gradual enlargement these nodes mechanically interfere with the motion of the adjacent joints, which themselves are usually not yet affected. Nevertheless, the joints are exposed to friction and aching irritation by the overlying nodes. Subsequently, episodes ranging from moderate soreness to pronounced pain are experienced in the joints. These joints are distinctly tender and slightly red and warmer, but the symptoms regress within 3–4 weeks [206, 1338, 1339]. The knee and ankle joints are occasionally enlarged by a moderate increase in joint fluid. However, the motion of these joints is not substantially impaired unless the joint capsule becomes thickened, and/or the adjacent bursa and tendons comprise nodules. A moderate contracture of the joints then ensues. Occasionally associated diseases with this lipid disorder are: hyperthyroidism, obstructive hepatic disease, and nephrotoxicity [543, 544].

The characteristic alterations of this disorder are manifested in nodules in the submucosa, subcutis, tendons, and articular tissues. The submucous nodules are papules in the lips, tongue, nasal and bucal cavity, and pharynx. The rather soft nodules beneath the skin appear in the face, scalp, neck, and extremities; they may enlarge or regress and are thus different from rheumatoid nodules. The more prominent subcutaneous nodules are designated according to their structural composition and configuration as xanthoma planum, nodosum, or tuberosum [1260]. The latter type, composed of a few larger nodes, occurs chiefly in the trunk, back, buttocks, and in the proximity to extremities. The spread and multiplicity of the nodular and tuberous xanthomata vary with the degree of the individual lipid disorder. Eventually nodules appear in the tendons of the shoulder, triceps tendon (Fig. 372), extensor tendons of the wrist and fingers (Fig. 373), quadriceps tendon, Achilles tendon (Fig. 372), extensor tendons of the foot and toes, and tendons in the sole of the foot. Upon expansion of these nodes the triceps, quadriceps, and calf muscles are partly substituted by platelike, flat xanthomata which occupy the transitional areas between muscles and tendons. These structural changes cause rigidity of the muscles and lack of mobility of the adjacent joints. The ligaments of the knee and ankle are similarly affected. By concurrent infiltration of the articular tissues the joints of the extremities (fingers, hand, elbow, shoulder, knee, and ankle) are enlarged. The deformities of the joints become more pronounced on additional involvement of paraarticular structures such as the olecranon or prepatellar bursa [641].

By the symmetrical involvement, progressive limitation of the motion of joints, and the presence of subcu-

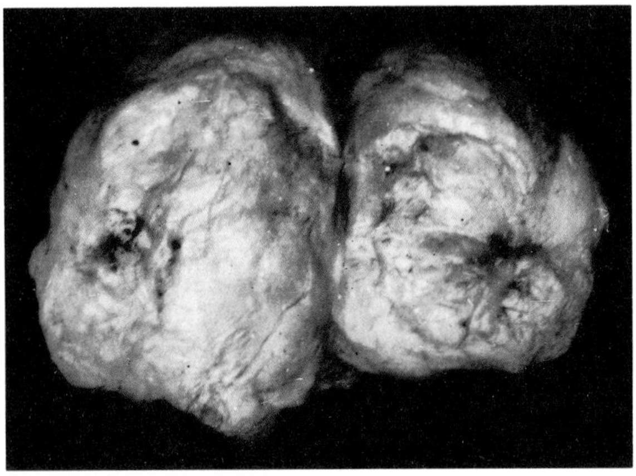

Fig. 374. Hemisection of the node excised from the left elbow evidences that the node is composed of yellowish grey compressible tissue

taneous nodules, the deformities of the joints resemble those in rheumatoid arthritis. Upon expansion of the xanthomatous infiltrates into the outer capsules of the joints, the ranges of motions are increasingly limited, although with slight tenderness of the joints. The contiguous or neighboring bursae, becoming the depots of rather hard tuberous xanthomata, are often adherent to the adjacent tendons, fasciae, or ligaments and then cause substantial impairment of motion. However, the lipid deposits are of more serious consequences when occurring in the endothelium of larger blood vessels and in the endocardium.

Laboratory studies yield false-positive results for rheumatoid factor in about 15% of these patients. The sedimentation rate is invariably elevated to 40 mm/h or above. More significantly [712], total lipids are increased to 850–1200 mg% with participation of all low-density fractions such as cholesterol 220–420 mg%, phospholipids 100–150 mg%, and triglycerides 300–550 mg%; blood urea nitrogen is 20.5–26 mg%, albumin 3.7–4.5 g%, and globulin 2.8–3.5 g%. Liver function tests (serum glutamic-oxalacetic transaminase and serum glutamic-pyruvic transaminase) usually do not reveal abnormal findings. The electrocardiograph most frequently shows deviation in the TS segment and depression of the T wave in leads I, III, and V. Roentgenographs reveal densification and thickening of the joint capsule, no alterations of the bone at the subchondral level, but occasional marginal erosions at the cortex of the epiphyses and diaphyses.

On the basis of the laboratory findings of anomalies in the concentration in each of the lipid components, Frederickson et al. [543, 544] divided the biochemically ascertained disorder of lipid metabolism into a number of types. They classified as type II hyperlipoproteinemia this one, in which the beta-lipoproteins, representing the triglycerides, are substantially increased, as is the cholesterol. This is the most common type of disorder of fat metabolism manifested by the above clinical features. The laboratory findings relate to it.

Gross-anatomical examination of the xanthomatous tissue excised from a bursa or tendon discloses a dense node in the size of a walnut or up to that of small apple, with uneven surface, and of a very dense consistency. On transverse section (Fig. 374), the ocher- to clay-stained, rather homogeneous tissue is traversed by whitish bundles of connective tissue. The dry substance of these nodes consists of 22%–30% lipids, of which 7.8%–10.0% are cholesterol, 8%–12% triglycerides, 1.5%–2.2% unsaturated fatty acids, and 2.2%–3.0% phospholipids.

Histopathological examination [1540] discloses two different components of the xanthomatous tissue which, although neighboring, rarely transgress into each other. Some extensive areas consist of large histiocytes (Fig. 375) with polygonal contours where they lie close to each other, but otherwise they have irregular contours; they have a foamy or fine-vacuolated cytoplasm (foam cells) and an indented or ovoid nucleus with particles of chromatin (Fig. 375). A substantial number of capillaries and a few giant cells with four or five central nuclei are scattered throughout. These areas are divided by bundles of collagen fibers which also surround areas of a different structure in the vicinity. Agglomerations composed chiefly of nests of fibrocytes and a few interspersed foam cells alternate here with ovoid or longish, empty, sharply pointed spaces which are aligned in thin tracts or rosettes (Fig. 376). These are cholesterol clefts. Differential staining can be accomplished for cholesterol using acetic acid and sulfuric acid, for neutral fat and fatty acids by Nile blue sulfate, and for lipoids by potassium-ferrocyanide-borax. On examination with polarized light the areas of foam cells remain predominantly dark, an indication that they contain lipids; the areas of cholesterol clefts display positively birefringent needles and long crystals.

Histochemical examination of the connective tissue from unaffected areas discloses no alterations or abnormal composition as a potential predisposition for the accumulation of lipids. Thus an inability of the normal connective tissue to metabolize an excess of circulating lipids must be assumed. The increased lipids, including cholesterol, in the serum represent a physicochemical imbalance which accounts for the precipitation of solved and dispersed substances within certain areas of the connective tissue. Correspondingly, multiple formation of xanthomata results in patients with hyperlipoproteinemia. The histological and histochemical examinations of the xanthomata indicate that the

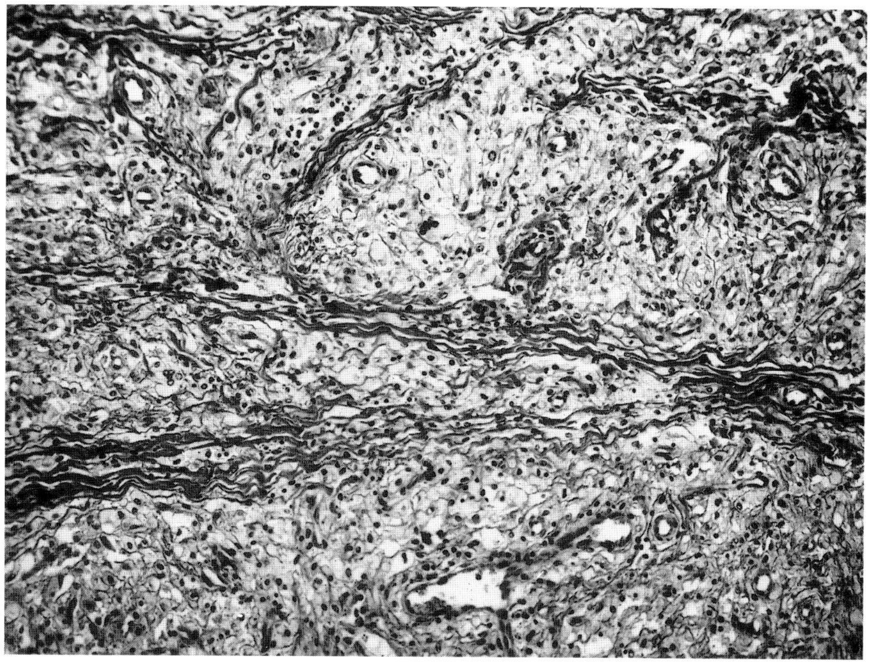

Fig. 375. One part of the excised node (Fig. 374) is com posed of many accumulations of large cells completely filled with adipose material

excesses of products derived from the lipid metabolism are being absorbed principally by histiocytes which accumulate in large agglomerations. The stimulated fibrocytes also proliferate and eventually produce abundant collagen fibers with gradual local densification. This explains the coexistence of two different tissue structures. The metabolites of neutral and acid lipids are readily absorbed by the connective tissue cells. However, the barely or entirely nonsoluble cholesterol remains precipitated mostly in crystals and undigested within nests of fibrocytes and dense connective tissue. The resulting dense and scarified tissue indicates that a partial or complete resorption of the xanthomata cannot be achieved.

The underlying disorder of metabolism in hyperlipoproteinemia cannot be corrected since no enzymatic deficiency has yet been identified as a possible cause. In view of this, the treatment endeavors to restrict the intake of fat in the diet, especially of foods containing cholesterol. Hereby the concentration of circulating

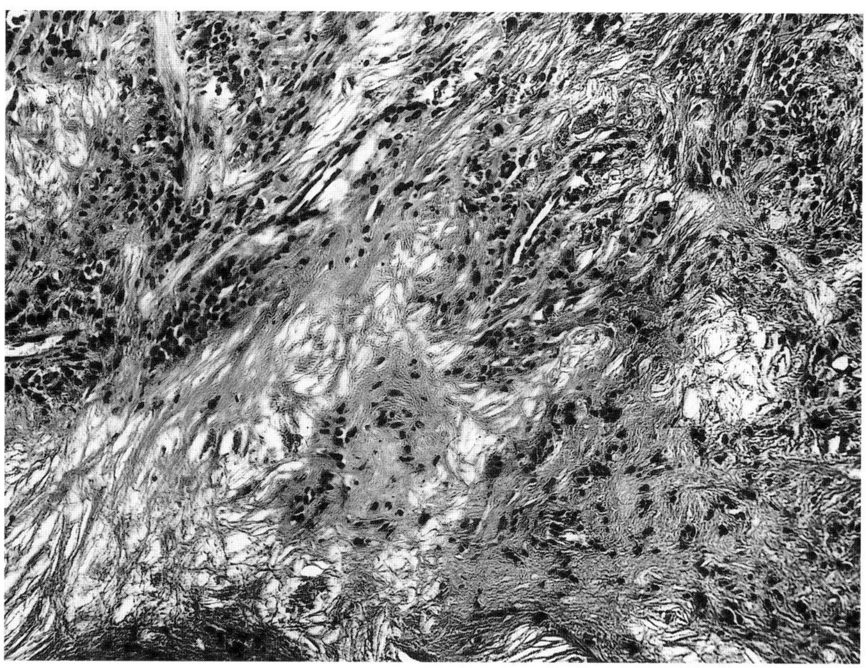

Fig. 376. The other part of the node (Fig. 374) consists of dense, very cellular, and very fibrosed connective tissue which comprises many empty spaces, mostly in rosette arrangement

lipids in the blood is decreased. The intake of carbohydrates should also be limited for a similar consideration which applies to the intake of alcohol. As to medicamentous treatment [543, 544], thyroxin lowers the cholesterol level by increasing its metabolism but inhibits the release of free fatty acids from adipose tissue. Chlorophenoxyisobutyric acid lowers hyperglyceridemia, but no sufficient experience has as yet been gathered regarding this matter. On the other hand, Rifkind et al. [1328] recommended the intake of nicotinic acid, and Golding [638] recommended the intake of clofibrate, which reduces the levels of low and very low density lipids in the blood. Indeed, the regular intake of 500–1000 mg nicotinic acid per day has a very beneficial effect on the concentration of lipids and especially on cholesterol, as ascertained by laboratory studies. The impaired function of the limbs can be improved by gentle massage as well as by active and passive mobilization exercises of the joints. In cases of conspicuously protruding or mechanically interfering nodes, excision provides a satisfactory correction of the musculoskeletal symptoms. Thereafter a series of physical therapy with diathermy and massage is indicated. However, in the foreground of all considerations is the concern for potential affections of the cardiovascular system (coronary sclerosis and arteriosclerosis), which in severe disorder of lipid metabolism cast a very serious shadow on the prognosis and on all therapeutic endeavors.

e. Arthropathy in Reticulohistiocytosis (Lipoid Dermatoarthritis)

Lipoid dermatoarthritis [77, 108, 462, 623, 1206], a systemic disease of as yet unclarified etiology, belongs to the lipid storage diseases which also affect articular tissues. It occurs predominantly in women at a proportion of 1 : 2 or 1 : 3 versus men [206] and principally in those of middle age. No heredity or affliction by other family members has been recorded; it appears that this condition is not gene transmitted.

The disease usually starts with moderate fever up to 38.5°, pronounced general weakness, and diffuse aching in the muscles of the extremities and/or back. Eventually these symptoms also become manifest and more intensified in the joints of the extremities. The affection of the joints is the initial manifestation of this condition in a substantial number of patients. However, simultaneous affection of joints and the appearance of nodules in the soft tissues occurs in the majority of patients. This explains the term multicentric reticulohistiocytosis [77, 108, 462, 548, 612, 623]. In addition to these patients, others are characterized by the appearance of nodules preceding by several months to 2 years the affection of the joints [646, 915, 1010, 1089, 1206].

These changes in the skin and subcutis [77, 78, 108, 646, 1206] are invariably multiple, often accumulated in a greater number, and varying in size from 2 to 20 mm. They are either nodules (Fig. 377) elevated above the level of the skin and/or papules within the skin (Fig. 377); their color is yellowish brown to reddish brown, and they are of rather soft consistency. These changes appear on the dorsum of the hands, around the beds of the fingernails (which become deformed, discolored yellowish grey, thickened, and very uneven), on the scalp, behind or in the ears, and on the wings of the nose. They are sometimes associated with pruritus. When appearing in excessive amount, they cause conspicuous deformation of the face (facies leonina [77, 78]). Extensive brownish discoloration and thickening of the skin such as xanthelasma may affect the eyelids and/or the face. Nodules in the skin and subcutis also appear on the neck, trunk (Fig. 377), over the shoulder blades and pelvic bones, and on the extensor surfaces of the upper and lower extremities. The changes in the mucosa and submucosa are less elevated but broader, and appear as flesh-colored papules inside the nose at the nares, in the lips, and in the pharynx and larynx. Less frequently nodules also involve the tendon sheaths on the dorsum of the wrist and ankle. These papules and nodules may occasionally enlarge or regress in the course of the disease, and may eventually completely disappear.

In contrast, the articular changes invariably progress, leading to deformation and impairment in the function of the joints, usually in symmetrical distribution. The most frequently and characteristically affected joints are the distal interphalangeal joints; thereafter follow in frequency the other finger joints, the wrist, elbow, knee, shoulder, ankle, and hip joints. The joints of the cervical spine, rarely of the thoracic or lumbar spine, costosternal joints, and temporomandibular joints may also be affected, but at a substantially lower frequency. The ailing joints are sore, sometimes very painful, and invariably deformed by thickening of the joint capsule occasionally associated with an increase in the joint fluid. On expansion of the alteration into the articular cartilage and subchondral bone, the ranges of motions increase into unphysiological excursions; impairing laxity and further deformation of joints result. These situations apply mainly to the finger and toe joints, less to the wrist, elbow, and ankle joints. Such is the outcome (arthritis mutilans) in about 30%–35% of patients after a slow, but unrelenting course of 8–10 years' duration, when the arthritic alterations and symptoms eventually come to a standstill. By that time the fingers have usually become conspicuously deformed, being thickened in a way resembling

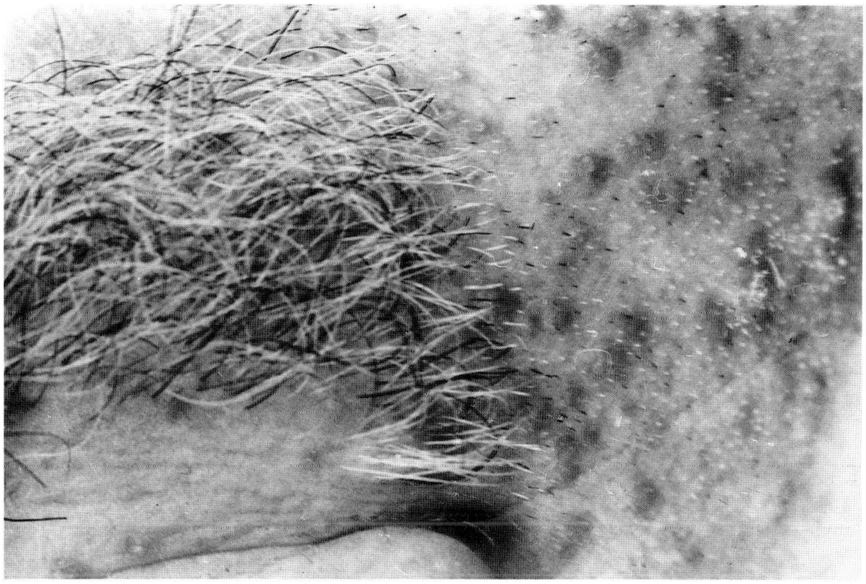

Fig. 377. Inflamed nodules rise in the skin at the anterior aspect of the shoulder close to the axilla. Flat papules are interspersed

sausages and flabby; they are also shortened, but may become elongated by traction and then return to their shortness upon cessation of the traction (telescoping). Sometimes, to the contrary, flexion contractures involve the finger, wrist, and elbow joints. The thickening of the wrist and ankle joints is usually compounded by swelling of the tendon sheaths on their dorsal aspect. Eventually contractures in the knee, shoulder and hip joints may ensue.

Laboratory studies disclose elevation in the sedimentation rate to 45 mm/h, but elevations as high as 60–120 mm/h and reversal of the albumin-globulin ratio have been reported [462, 1010]. The latex fixation test usually shows negative results, as does the test for antinuclear antibodies. On the other hand, the results of lipid quantifications in the serum vary. Albert et al. [20] reported a substantial increase in total lipids and a moderate increase in phospholipids and total cholesterol, whereas Ehrlich et al. [462] reported normal ranges of lipids, triglycerides, and cholesterol. In 48% of the patients of Barrow et al. [77, 78] the sedimentation rate was significantly elevated and so were the total lipids, triglycerides, and free and esterified cholesterol in the serum of 33%; similarly, total lipids, triglycerides, and total cholesterol were increased in the tissue extracts of these patients. The joint fluid [548] shows a poor mucin clot and contains a moderate to substantial (2000–8000 cells/ml) number of lymphocytes and monocytes. Also a few, 35- to 60 μm-large, bizarre cells with a large nucleus and numerous granules containing cytoplasm occur here.

Roentgenographic examination [462, 623, 1010] discloses densification of the joint capsule surrounding articular epiphyses, being deformed following deep erosion of the articular surfaces and loss of subchondral bone (Fig. 378). The joint space becomes irregularly delimited and widened, an alteration noticeable particularly in the interphalangeal joints (Fig. 378) and less so in the metacarpophalangeal and wrist joints. In the other joints, the joint space is partly narrowed due to thinning of the articular cartilage or is widened and irregularly delimited by epiphyses which present several subchondral defects (Fig. 379). Similar rather sharply delimited defects are noticed in the metaphyses and diaphyses of smaller and larger bones, such as the metacarpals, metatarsals, radius, and ulna, and in the distal humeral epiphysis without periosteal apposition or neighboring osteoporosis (Figs. 378, 379). In very advanced cases, the head of the humerus, the head of the femur, and the proximal end of the tibia present extensive lytic changes, and narrowing throughout of the adjoining cartilage space secondary to erosion of the articular epiphyses. A rare and rather characteristic involvement is the affection of the atlantoaxial part of the cervical spine [623], with erosion of the vertebral plates.

Gross-anatomical examination of the subcutaneous nodules discloses easily compressible, small lumps of 3–18 mm diameter, with a peripheral layer of whitish gray connective tissue and traversing thin strips of similar connective tissue. A yellowish to light-brown material of soft consistency is interspersed between the latter. Similarly to the nodules, the capsules of the interphalangeal, elbow, and knee joints contain areas of yellowish coloring and soft consistency. The inner surface of the joint capsule of the larger joints is uneven due to broad-based villous elevations.

Histopathological examination of the nodules discloses in a stroma of normal and larger fibrocytes, accumulations of polygonal histiocytes containing a

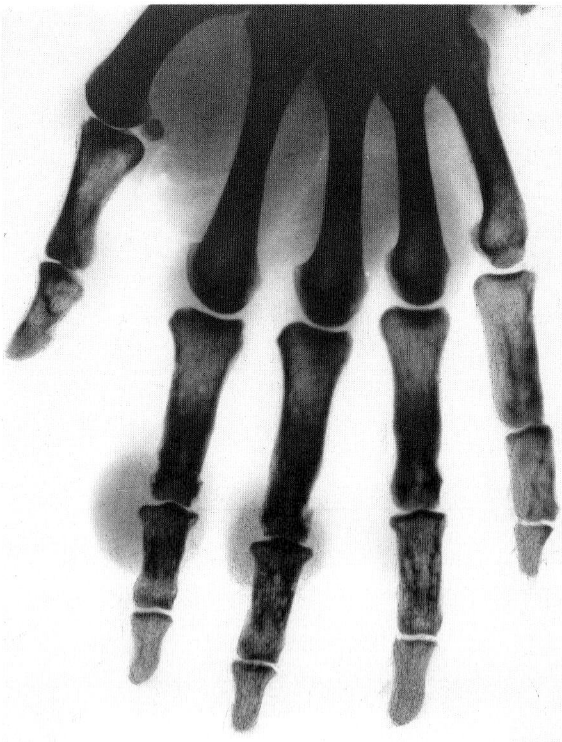

Fig. 378. The phalanges of the thumb and other fingers are rarefied by smaller and larger, rather well-delimited areas of radiolucency. The periarticular tissue is densified at some interphalangeal joints

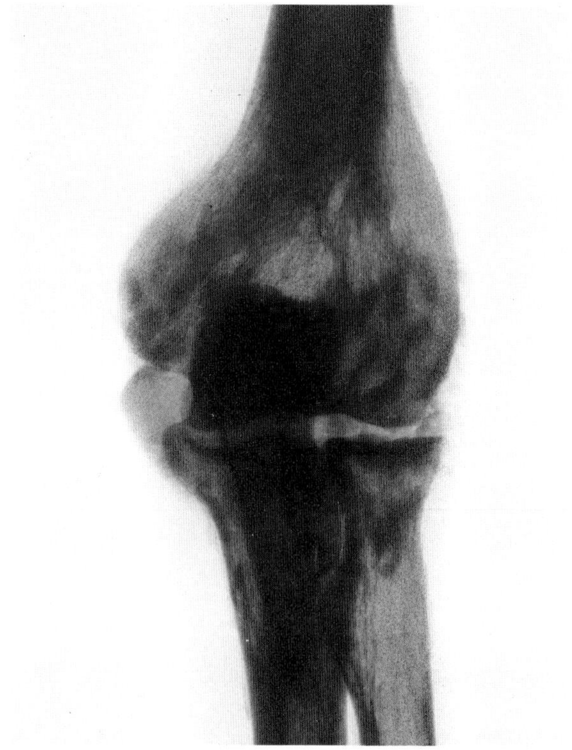

Fig. 379. The humeral condyles are broadened by large areas of radiolucency. The proximal part of the radius is also extensively rarefied

large ovoid or round nucleus and a great amount of eosinophilic cytoplasm which appears finely granular, foamy, or like ground glass (Fig. 380). These accumulations are surrounded and traversed by thinner and thicker bundles of collagen fibers. Among the histiocytes are scattered roundish giant cells with a diameter of 35–70 μm, 2–20 darkly stained and irregularly or peripherally dispersed nuclei, and a cytoplasm of

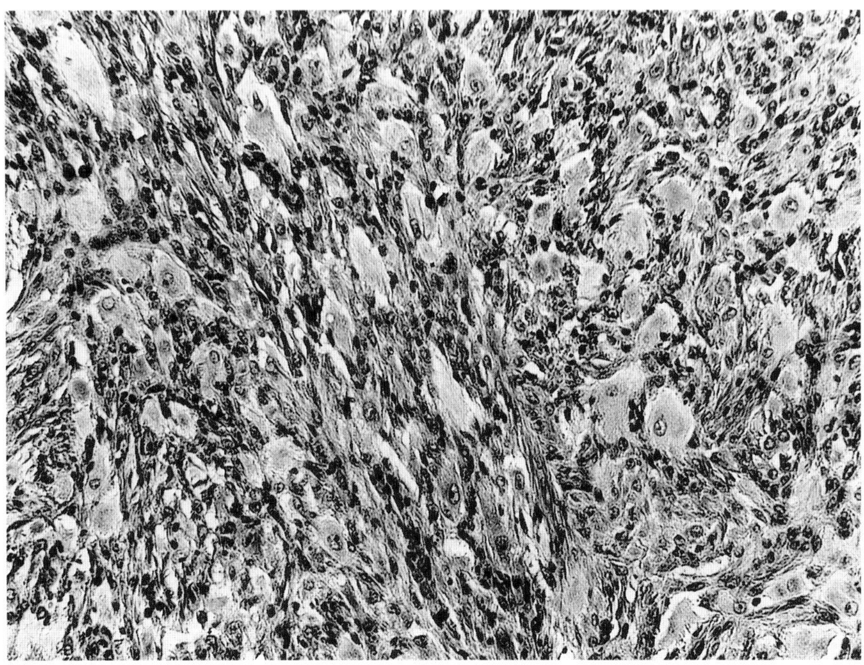

Fig. 380. Tracts of large histiocytes with finely vacuolated cytoplasm are scattered in the subcutaneous connective tissue

similar appearance as in the histiocytes (Fig. 381). Eventually, in conditions of longer duration (Fig. 382), the giant cells are substantially decreased in number and size. Similar although less conspicuous changes affect the histiocytes. On the other hand, dense broad bundles of collagen fibers (Fig. 382) course between these cells, which appear as if being compressed by the bundles. Thus, fibrosis characterizes the late stage of many of these nodules. The inner part of the joint capsule [548, 915, 1089] contains beneath hypertrophic synoviocytes areas with accumulations of histiocytes, similar to those observed in the nodules. Loose infiltrates of lymphocytes and plasmacytes are scattered among the histiocytes; a few hyperemic capillaries, arterioles, and venules course along with the traversing thin bundles of collagen fibers. More conspicuous, however, are the giant cells which contain an abundant eosinophilic cytoplasm with fine granules positive on periodic acid Schiff test or pale vacuoles and 2–15 darkly stained nuclei [20, 915, 1010]. The proportion of giant cells among the histiocytes appears to increase with the duration of the joint affection (Fig. 383) but

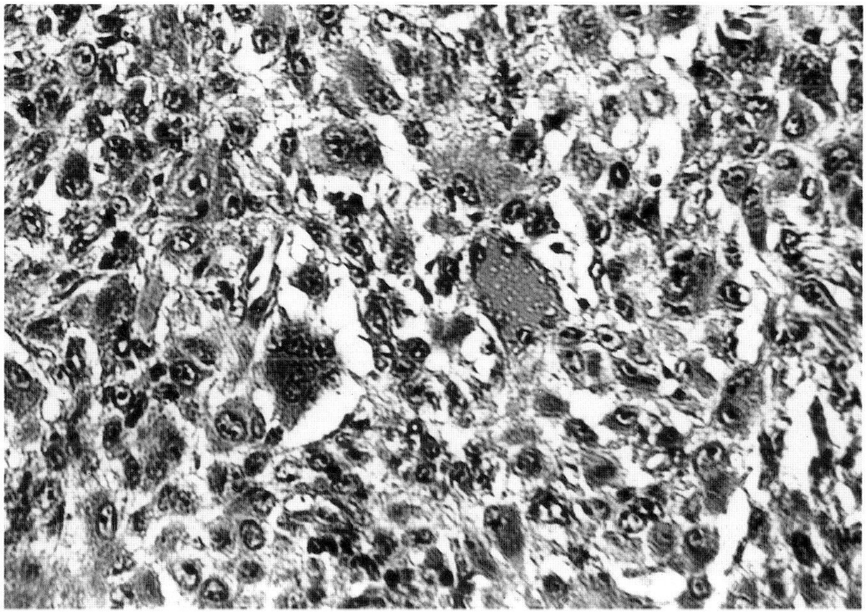

Fig. 381. Giant cells with two to eight nuclei and a cytoplasm resembling that of the neighboring histiocytes are scattered in the connective tissue

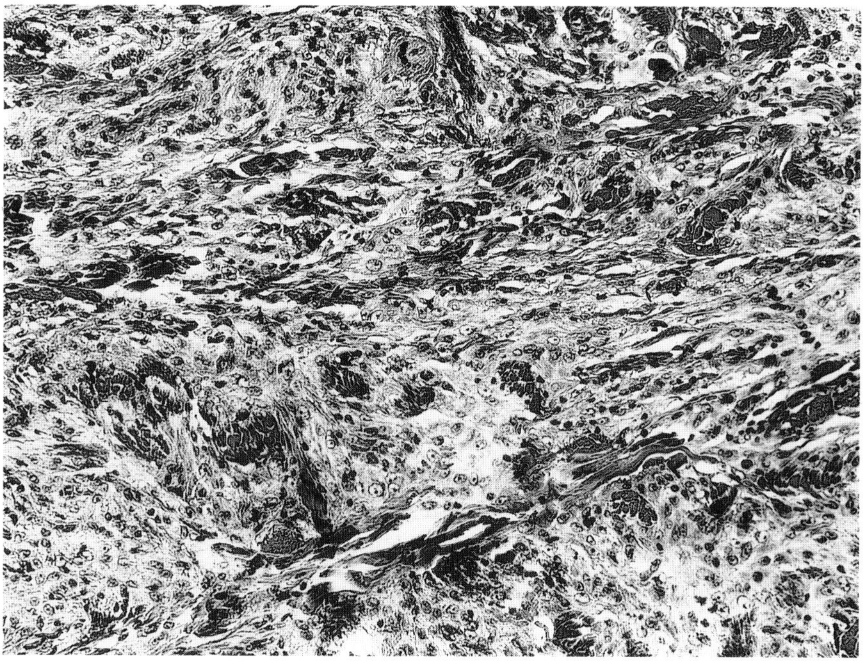

Fig. 382. Tracts of thick collagen bundles course between loose accumulations of histiocytes

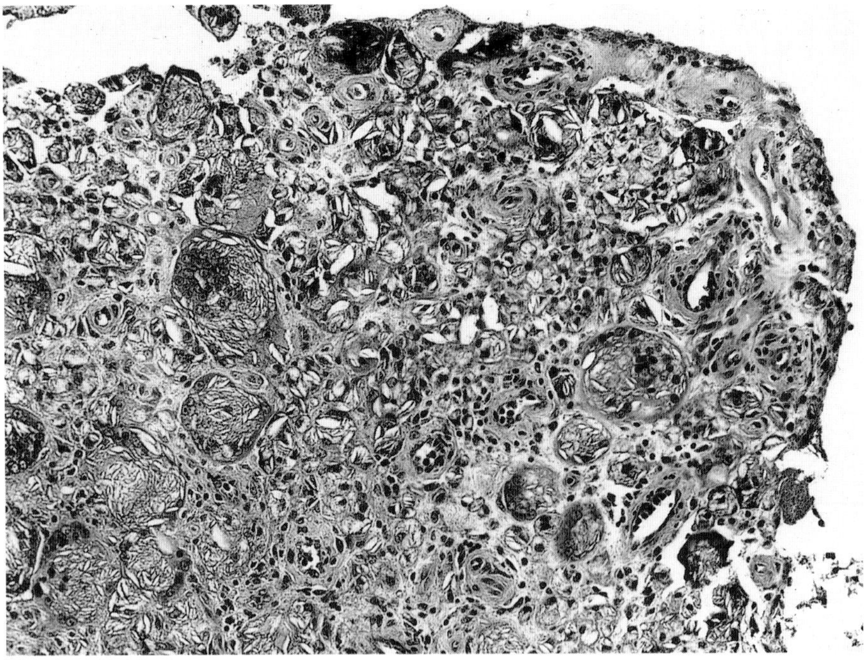

Fig. 383. The synovial membrane is very cellular by a marked increase in fibrocytes. Large multinucleated giant cells with a coarse trabecular cytoplasm are scattered among finely vacuolated histiocytes

eventually decreases. A larger number of fibrocytes amid increased bundles of collagen fibers takes the place of the giant cells. A progressive fibrosis eventually develops.

Electron-microscopic examinations [108, 915] disclose that the histiocytes contain a rough endoplasmic reticulum with many cisternae and a Golgi apparatus associated with vacuoles and inclusion bodies. Throughout the cytoplasm are scattered abundant electron-dense droplets and large vacuoles probably of lipidic origin. The giant cells additionally have nuclei with very irregular and condensed chromatinic material.

The articular cartilage is also an area of lipid deposition. Fine lipid droplets are loosely scattered in the upper zone, where empty lacunae of chondrocytes occur. However, more chondrocytes in the somewhat deeper zone are surrounded by broad halos of intensely stained ground substance (Fig. 384). The increase in ground substance is very conspicuous at the tide line, which is very broad and contains a large amount of lipid droplets. The reaction to lipid deposition is more pronounced in the subchondral subcortical marrow spaces (Fig. 385), which comprise loose connective tissue, surrounding cystic spaces, and containing granulomata, vacuolar histiocytes, and multinuclear giant cells.

The abnormal tissue elements have been studied histochemically for a possible explanation as to the etiology and pathogenesis of the condition. Orkin et al. [1206] noted that the histiocytes contained abundant material staining on periodic acid – Schiff which was removed by peptic digestion but not by lipid solvents, and which did not react with Alcian blue or toluidine blue. They concluded that the contained material was a glycoprotein. On the other hand, Barrow [77, 78], Davies [370], and Melton [1089] inferred that a part of the material in the histiocytes and giant cells was probably glycolipid, on the basis it stained black with Sudan IV. Barrow [77, 78], and Lyell [993] summarized that the material contained in the histiocytes and giant cells was composed of glycoprotein or mucoprotein, phospholipids, and other fat substances; thus it consisted of a glycol group, a lipid component, and some demonstrable protein.

Histopathological and histochemical examinations help to differentiate lipoid dermatoarthritis from rheumatoid arthritis, which also affects the peripheral joints in a symmetrical distribution and at gradual aggravation, and which is also associated with subcutaneous nodules. However, the latter are of harder consistency and nonregressing tendency and also lack foam cells and giant cells (Fig. 205). In addition, roentgenographs help to clarify the diagnosis because the alterations in rheumatoid arthritis leading to erosion of the articular cartilage are followed by narrowing (Fig. 189), not by widening of the joint space (Figs. 378, 379). The sharply punched-out areas in the bones (Figs. 378, 379) without periosteal reaction resemble those of eosinophilic granulomata, especially when occurring in the cervical spine, but these are not associated with nodules comprising numerous histiocytes.

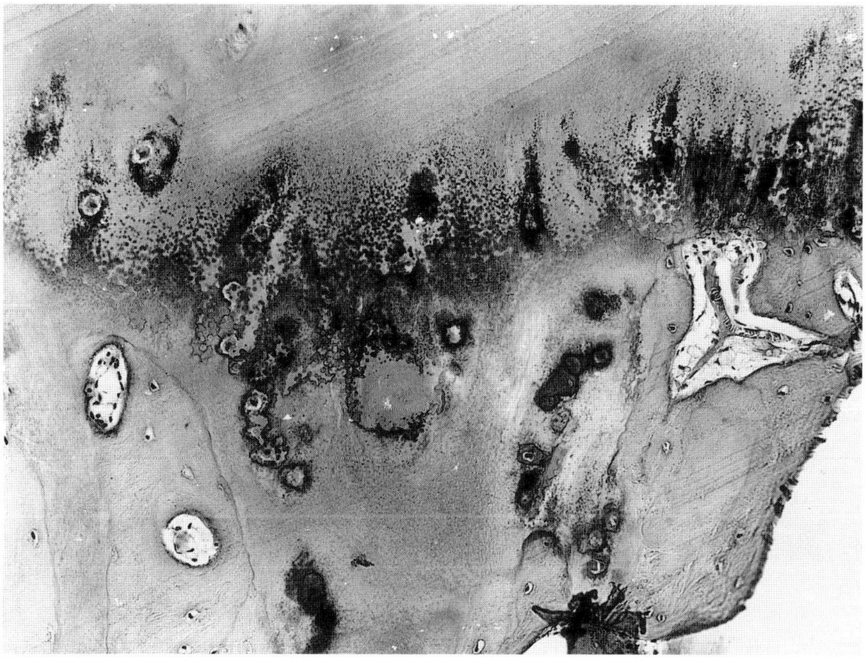

Fig. 384. The articular cartilage contains lacunae of chondrocytes, while other chondrocytes are surrounded by halos of increased ground substance. The tide line is intensely stained and broadened and contains numerous points of lucency due to deposition of lipid droplets

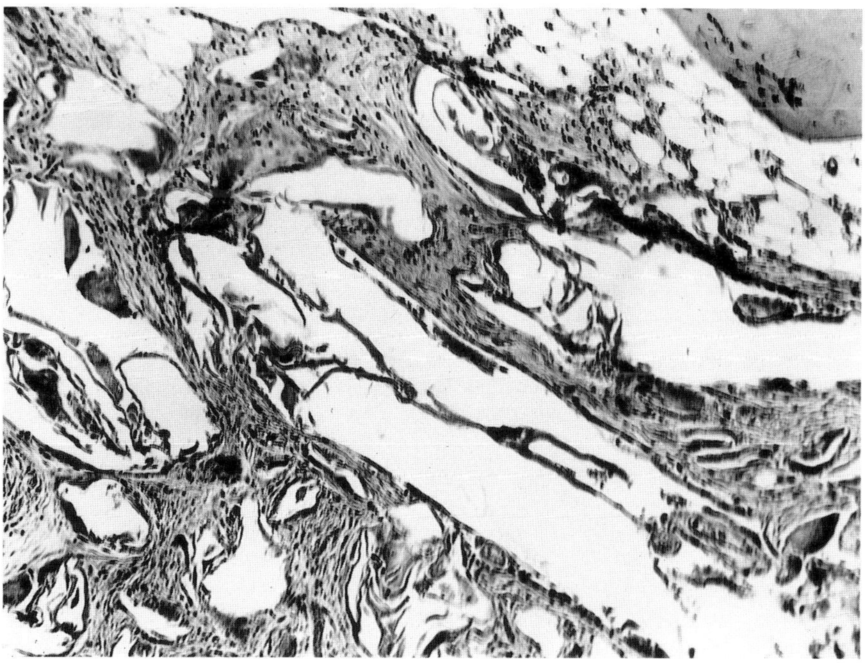

Fig. 385. The articular subcortical marrow spaces contain granulomata and organized connective tissue which comprises vacuolar histiocytes, multinuclear giant cells, and cystic spaces

The predominance of foamy histiocytes in several locations and various organs justifies the designation of systemic or multicentric reticulohistiocytosis [646]. The term lipoid dermatoarthritis, suggested by Warin et al. [1714], or rather lipid dermatoarthritis, also appears appropriate because it emphasizes the most significant clinical observations and their pathological relationship.

As long as the etiology of this condition has not been clarified, treatment remains symptomatic. Regular administration of salicylates and periodic application of shortwave diathermy help to relieve the aching joints. Restriction in the intake of fat-containing food is indicated, although so far no changes or improvement have been reported. Nonsteroidal antiinflammatory medications are of little help, and steroids in moderate doses may provide temporary benefits. Chloroquine and cytotoxic drugs (nitrogen mustard, phenambucin, chlorambucil, and cyclophosphamide) have been used

[719], but the results in a small number of patients and with a short follow-up do not permit a conclusive evaluation. The satisfactory experience [638] with clofibrate suggests the need for further trials with this medication. The intracutaneously or superficially located and cosmetically disturbing nodules may be excised, if they do not regress. Similarly, the subcutaneously located, larger nodes may be excised if conspicuously protruding or functionally impairing. In progressing deformations of peripheral joints (of fingers or wrist), individually molded plastic splints and passive mobilization exercises succeed in mitigating or correcting the deformations. If these modalities fail in the larger joints, tenotomies and capsulotomies are necessary, especially for flexion contracture of the elbow or knee joint. When advanced deformities of the articular epiphyses cause essential impairment in the function of the shoulder, hip, or knee joint, total arthroplasty as discussed in "Osteoarthritis" may represent the ultimate solution. On the other hand, arthrodesis supplemented with a reversed sliding bone graft (Figs. 209, 210, 213, 214, 215, 216, 217) is a stabilizing and reliable procedure on the long term [1549] for the wrist and ankle joint. However, before any surgical intervention is applied, all modalities of conservative treatment should be tried in view of the general systemic involvement. Beyond all therapeutic endeavors, the worrisome experience [612, 1206] remains that 20%–30% of these patients develop tuberculosis or malignancies in organs not related to the musculoskeletal system.

4. Joint Affections in Abnormal Deposition

a. Calcinosis of Joints

Deposition of amorphous calcium salts and calcium crystals can occur in articular and periarticular tissues; this has been termed calcium gout [1419], in analogy to such deposition of amorphous urates and urate crystals occurring in gout. However, in contrast to gout, no biochemical abnormality is noted in calcinosis. Calcium and phosphorus metabolism is normal. Thus, the term calcinosis refers to idiopathic, primary deposition of calcium salts in connective tissue [42]. On the other hand, Villiaumey et al. [1694] consider articular chondrocalcinosis among the metabolic disorders because anomalies in local metabolism lead to precipitation of calcium salts.

Besides idiopathic calcinosis, metastatic or secondary calcinosis of joints can occur in long-standing hypercalcemia such as associated with hypophosphatemia [1201] (Fig. 386), hyperparathyroidism [51, 1066, 1282], hypothyroidism, diabetes, gout, ochronosis, renal insufficiency [1292], tumorous bone

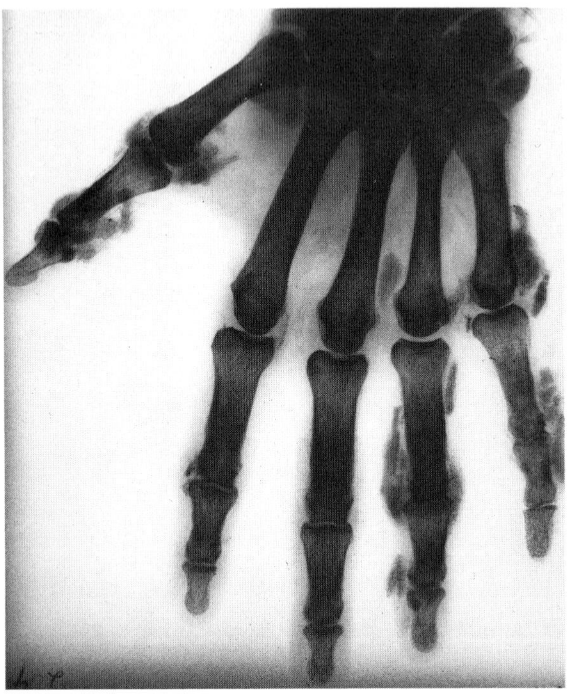

Fig. 386. Extensive calcification of joint capsules and periarticular tissues of the fingers in hypophosphatemia

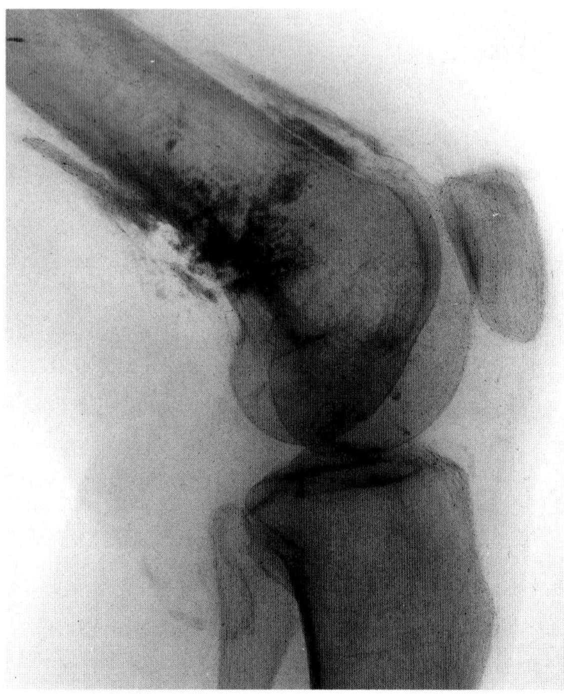

Fig. 387. Extensive calcification of paraarticular tissues of a knee took place secondary to an injury sustained 2 years ago

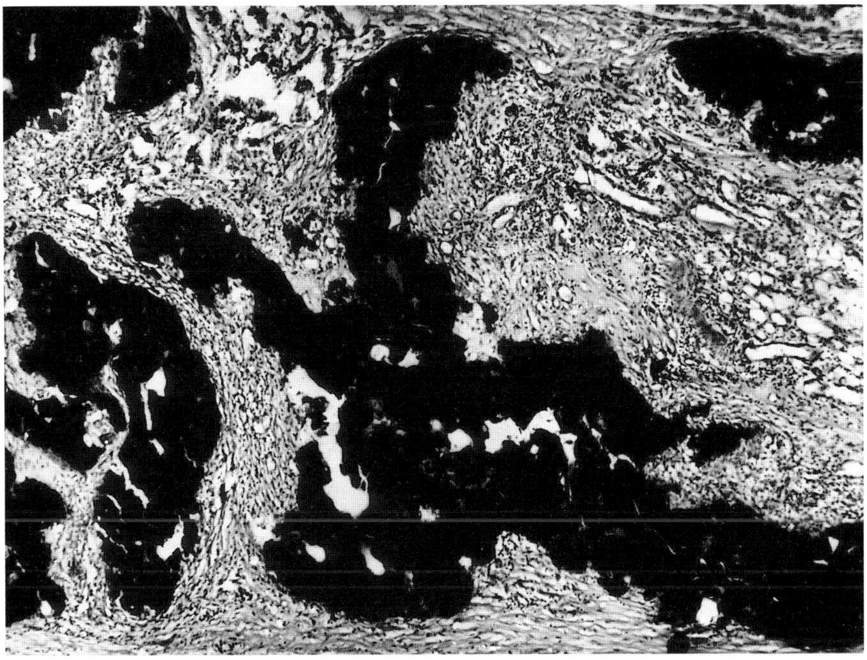

Fig. 388. Irregular and extensive calcium deposits lie in the paraarticular tissue and are surrounded by fibrosed tissue. The neighboring tissue is very cellular with fibrocytes and a small number of lymphocytes

destruction, or excessive intake of vitamin D. These types of calcinosis may be associated also with deposition of calcium salts in lungs, kidneys, and stomach, which have more alkalinity of the tissue ground substance due to their secretion of acids. On the other hand, dystrophic deposition of calcium salts is observed in localized regressive changes (Fig. 388) associated with degeneration and necrosis of cell complexes. Such changes develop secondary to intensive trauma (Fig. 387), specific and nonspecific inflammatory processes, marked impairment in local blood supply, or deposition of heterogenous material, as in dermatomyositis, neuropathic arthropathies, and lipid accumulation. The deposition of calcium salts in these areas is elicited by decrease or cessation of the local oxygen supply followed by increase of CO_2 concentration. The salts of the local tissue fluid are then no longer kept in solution, and precipitate. Dystrophic calcinosis therefore occurs principally in mesodermal tissues such as bursae (Figs. 544, 549), tendons, paraarticular ligaments (Fig. 388), articular cartilage, intervertebral disc and/or nucleus pulposus [1538], and subcutaneous tissue.

From these secondary types of calcification must be distinguished idiopathic primary calcinosis which is occasionally observed in the joint capsule (Figs. 393, 394), articular cartilage (Figs. 389, 396, 397), paraarticular structures (Figs. 554, 555), and intermuscular or subcutaneous connective tissue, and muscles. This presumably occurs without preceding inflammation, necrosis, or degenerative changes [407, 919, 1604]. Verse [1685] postulated here a constitutional defect of the mesoderm, similar to other collagen disease, and based on genetic mutations. The findings of Bjelle et al. [137, 138] support such a view, and indicate that the deposition of calcium crystals in cartilage may be a sequela to abnormal metabolism of chondrocytes from various causes [733]. On the other hand, Gatter et al. [578] and McCarty et al. [1052, 1054] explained the occurrence of calcium deposits by alteration in the ground substance (Figs. 394, 397) of connective tissue, in which phosphoric acid is readily liberated and combines with the available calcium to calcium salts. The same process occurs in articular cartilage following the release of phosphoric acid from dying chondrocytes and its combination with calcium [578, 1054]. Ryan et al. [1383] demonstrated that calcinosis occurs at reactive sites due to diminution or alteration in the proteoglycans which shield collagen fibers and block mineral nucleation. The calcium salts arrive (shedding of calcium salts) in the synovial fluid, from which they are deposited in the synovial membrane (Figs. 393, 394) and there provoke localized changes. Howell [781, 782] pointed out that the mere deposition of calcium salts is the cause of local or multilocal tissue changes, but it is not a systemic disease.

McCarty et al. [1052, 1054] identified calcium pyrophosphate dihydrate as the triggering agent of articular symptoms and described it as occurring in crystals (Fig. 28, a and b) of the monoclinic or triclinic morphism with characteristic weak or absent birefringence on polarized light. These crystals are deposited chiefly

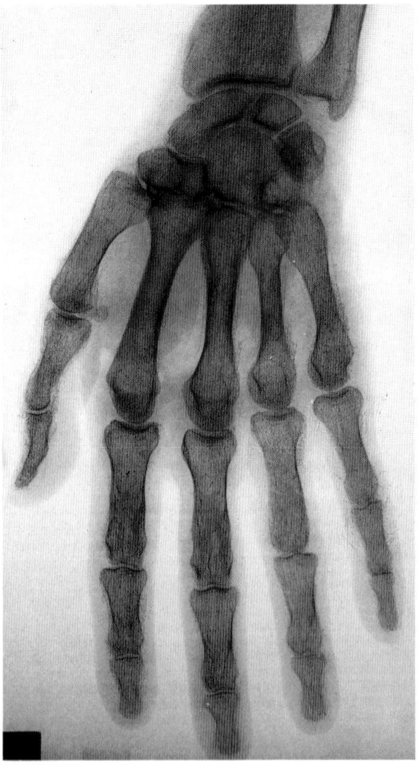

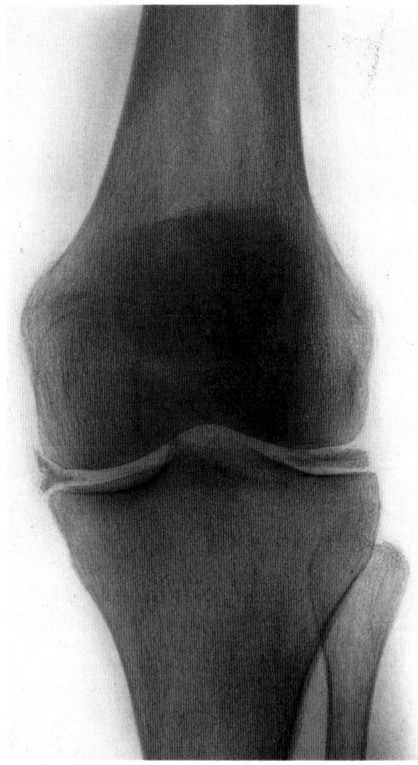

Fig. 389. The articular cartilages of the radiocarpal, intercarpal, and metacarpophalangeal joints are extensively calcified

Fig. 390. Both menisci are completely calcified

in the articular cartilage, synovial membrane, and intraarticular ligaments [716] and form punctate or linear small aggregates [716]. The joints affected by chondrocalcinosis are the knee, wrist (Fig. 389), metacarpophalangeal, interphalangeal, elbow, shoulder, ankle, and hip joints. Similarly, the fibrocartilages of the knees (Fig. 390), wrists, symphysis pubis, and intervertebral discs may be affected.

Zitnan et al. [1815] and Dieppe et al. [420, 422] identified hydroxyapatite (basic calcium phosphate or carbonate) as another crystal causing calcinosis. Nuki et al. [1196] conjectured that deposition of hydroxyapatite crystals follows changes in the composition of proteoglycan aggregates, leading to disintegration of the articular cartilage. These crystals have the shapes of straight or slightly curved rods or needles (Fig. 28 c) of the monoclinic system, but more often those of irregular rhomboid plates (Fig. 28 d) of the triclinic system, and are poorly or strongly birefringent on polarized light. Because of their small size (less than 1 μm) they can best be identified by electron microscopy [1442]. On light microscopy their aggregates are observed as shiny laminated cones [1383]. While hydroxyapatite is also deposited in articular cartilage and fibrocartilage, it is more frequently deposited in the joint capsule and its ligaments as well as in paraarticular organs such as the bursae (Fig. 544), tendons, and tendon sheaths (Figs. 383, 385). In these locations it tends to form plates or irregular clumps (Figs. 544, 549) of considerable size, up to a few centimeters in diameter.

Considering the fact that calcium deposition often follows osteoarthritis or rheumatoid arthritis [578, 716, 1308], Howell [782] inferred that this deposition is a consequence of disturbed cartilage metabolism. This view was supported by Schumacher et al. [1442], who noted calcium pyrophosphate dihydrate in 28%, hydroxyapatite in 30%, and both types of crystals in 43% of their cases of osteoarthritis or rheumatoid arthritis. The findings of Moskowitz et al. [1147, 1148] corroborated these reports.

Deposition of calcium salts [420, 421, 422, 1052, 1383] occurs in men more often than in women, chiefly those aged between 40 and 75 years. The knee joint (Figs. 390, 391, 392, 393) is most often affected, followed by the elbow, wrist (Fig. 389), finger, shoulder, ankle, and hip joint, and occasionally the spine [1259] (Fig. 293). Symptoms may be those of an acute attack, subacute arthritis, chronic arthritis, or chronic arthralgia [716, 1147, 1148]. The acute attack often follows stress or overexertion and is associated with intense pain usually localized in one joint. The attack may last 3–30 days and is manifested by swelling of the capsule of a diarthrodial joint, synovial effusion in a major joint, and locally elevated temperature. The acute attack may change after a short interval into subacute arthritis. In another type, the initial symptoms are per-

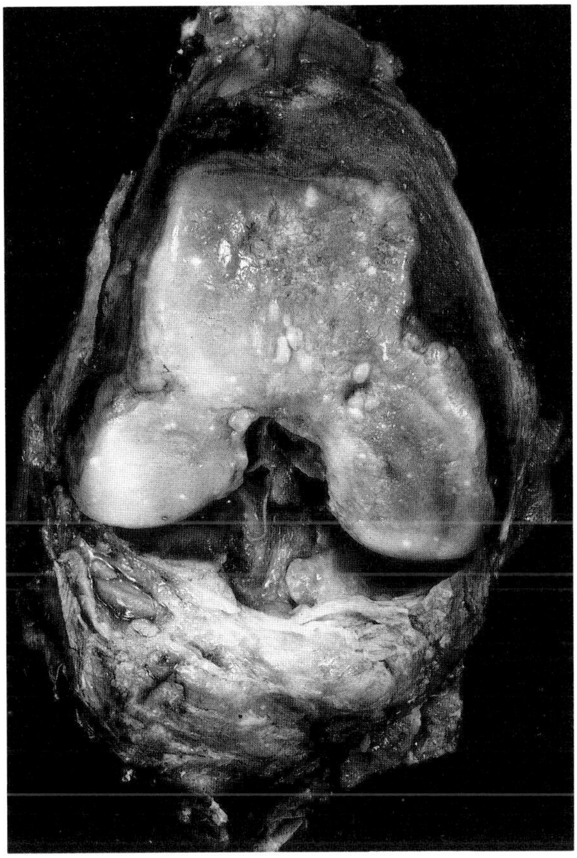

Fig. 391. The cartilaginous surfaces of the femoral condyles and the adjacent joint capsule contain several circumscribed and slightly elevated deposits of calcium

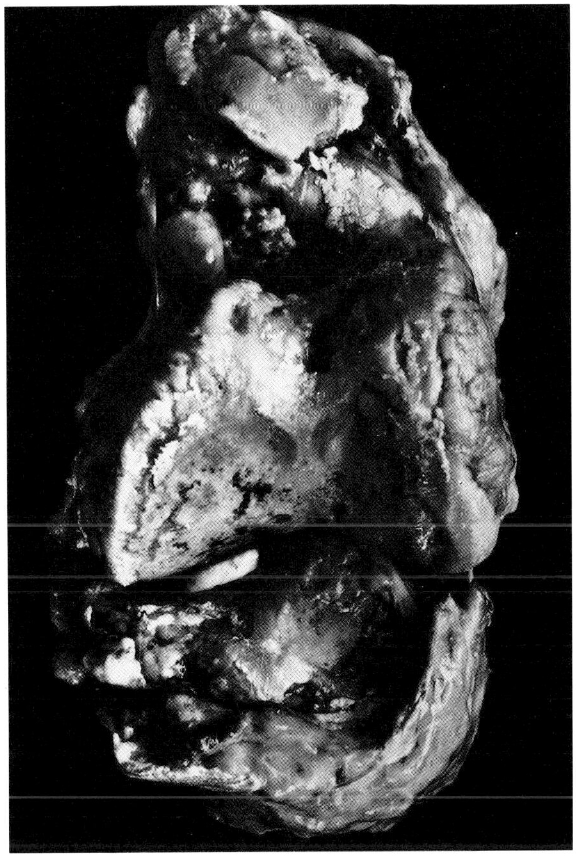

Fig. 392. The worn-off surfaces of the patella, femoral condyles, and tibial condyles comprise several irregular areas of white, crumbly material

sistent soreness in a few joints with moderate thickening and tenderness of the joint capsule, yet without locally elevated temperature or distinct bilaterality. The range of active motion is moderately limited, commensurate with the intensity of pain. This situation may last from a few to several weeks. The type of joint affection with episodes of reactivation simulates rheumatoid arthritis, especially when the sedimentation rate is significantly elevated, or the test result for rheumatoid factor is positive (in 6%–8% of patients). However, it does not become aggravated to deformity. Finally, in a course of slow aggravation and long duration the symptoms of osteoarthritis may develop [1323]. The latter type of calcinosis (Fig. 293) and osteoarthritis occurs principally in elderly individuals and involves mostly the joints of the lower extremities (Figs. 391, 392). It is manifested by thickening of the joint capsule and is often associated with limitation in the range of motion. On the other hand, calcinosis of the joint capsule and articular surfaces may sometimes be asymptomatic and may incidentally be detected as a coexistent feature in primary osteoarthritis of the elderly. In this sense, Villiaumey et al. [1694] emphasize the great frequency of calcinosis of joints and its diversified clinical picture. It thereby resembles several other joint affections and poses diagnostic problems. Such situations arise especially when chondrocalcinosis occurs as a secondary alteration in arthritic conditions of other etiology [1147, 1148, 1396] such as ochronosis (Fig. 361), diabetic arthropathy (Fig. 438), hemochromatosis, and gout.

In laboratory findings, the sedimentation rate may be elevated to 32–40 mm/h; the concentrations of calcium, phosphorus, alkaline phosphatase in serum are within normal limits. Calcium balance studies disclose normal results [200]. The latex fixation test yields false-positive results in 6%–8% of these cases; on the other hand, they may be true positive since interstitial calcinosis occurs in 3%–8% of patients with rheumatoid arthritis (Fig. 196). Microscopic examination of the synovial fluid [1051, 1146, 1148, 1254, 1439] discloses needles (Fig. 28, a and b) or plump sticks or rhomboid crystals (Fig. 28, c and d), with the former weakly positively birefringent and the latter strongly

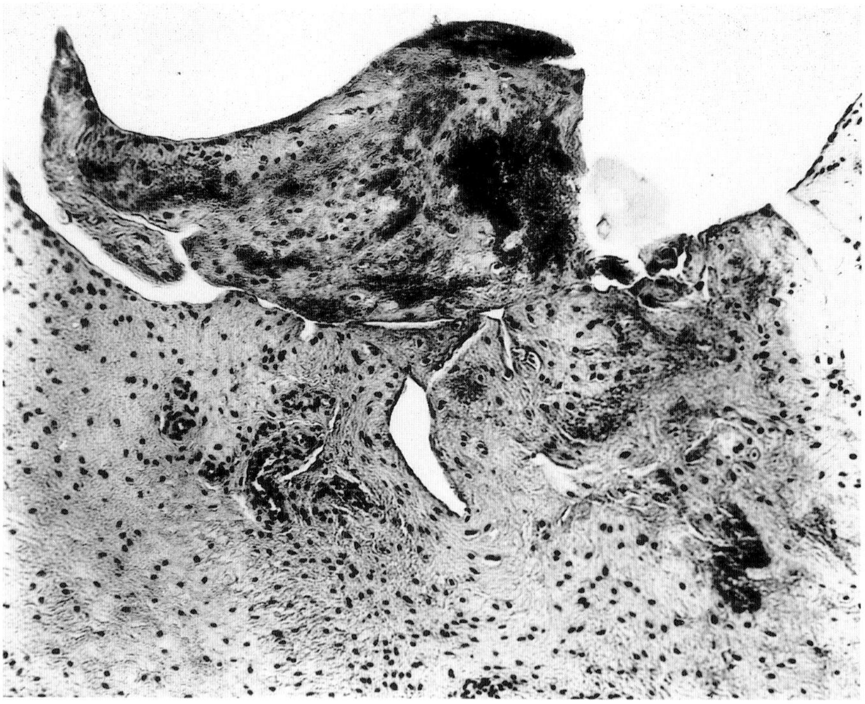

Fig. 393. The synovial membrane comprises a few irregular and dense deposits of calcium. The neighboring tissue is partly hypocellular and partly hypercellular with fibrocytes

positively birefringent on polarized light, in polymorphonuclear leukocytes and monocytes. Zitnan et al. [1815] demonstrated by electron microscopy apatite crystals in synovial fluid and in its leukocytes. Schumacher [1442] similarly identified apatite crystals by their slightly curved needle shape.

Roentgenographs (Figs. 386, 387) are very informative [6, 421, 591] when they reveal thin irregular shadows of small or larger extent in the joint capsule, periarticular tissues, and even adjoining musculature (Fig. 387). Calcification of the articular cartilage (Fig. 389) is noticeable as a sharply defined thick linear shadow which follows the outline of the subchondral bone in larger and smaller joints. Calcification of the intraarticular fibrocartilage (Fig. 390) is manifested in a few punctate or stippled shadows of varying density (as in the interpubic fibrocartilage or intervertebral disc); on larger spread it may assume the complete outline of this fibrocartilage, such as in the meniscus (Fig. 390) or intervertebral disc. However, the rather characteristic appearances of these calcifications are often overlapped in roentgenographs by coincident alterations in osteoarthritis and less often so by those of rheumatoid or other arthritis. Thus, additionally may be observed: densification of the joint capsule, narrowing of the cartilage space with irregular delimitation of the articular epiphyses, subchondral cysts, and varied formation of marginal osteophytes. Independently of these, the calcifications in the joint capsule are more extensive and completely irregular in outline [421, 1442]; those in calcinosis of the tendons resemble thick plates, and those in calcinosis of the bursae (Figs. 554, 555) appear like ovoid fluffy or denser shadows. The latter can appear either as single, rather well-circumscribed, or as a few, smaller shadows of various densities.

Gross-pathological examination [578, 1117] discloses in the subsynovial and periarticular tissue poorly vascularized areas which enclose white plaques or clumps of various sizes (Figs. 293, 392) as well as small clefts which contain (Fig. 293) lentil- to bean-sized clumps of white, crumbling material (Fig. 544). The uneven and fissured articular surfaces display areas of whitish stippling which may spread over rather large extents (Fig. 391). In the residual hyaline cartilage lie sharply defined white plaques [1118] (Figs. 391, 392) which due to their crumbling can be easily lifted, leaving behind irregular defects. Other areas of articular cartilage show whitish discoloration and loss of glistening.

Histopathological examination of the joint capsule discloses areas of swollen collagen bundles in the subsynoviocytic tissue, whereas in other areas this tissue contains accumulations of amorphous material (Fig. 393). The latter presents on light microscopy and on electron microscopy needle- or rodlike crystals of calcium pyrophosphate dihydrate or slightly curved needles, irregular rhomboid crystals, or clumps of hydroxyapatite in sparse accumulations. In rare situations the thickened synovial membrane is extensively impregnated with calcium salts, whereby its villi are completely filled with calcium salts (Fig. 394). In addi-

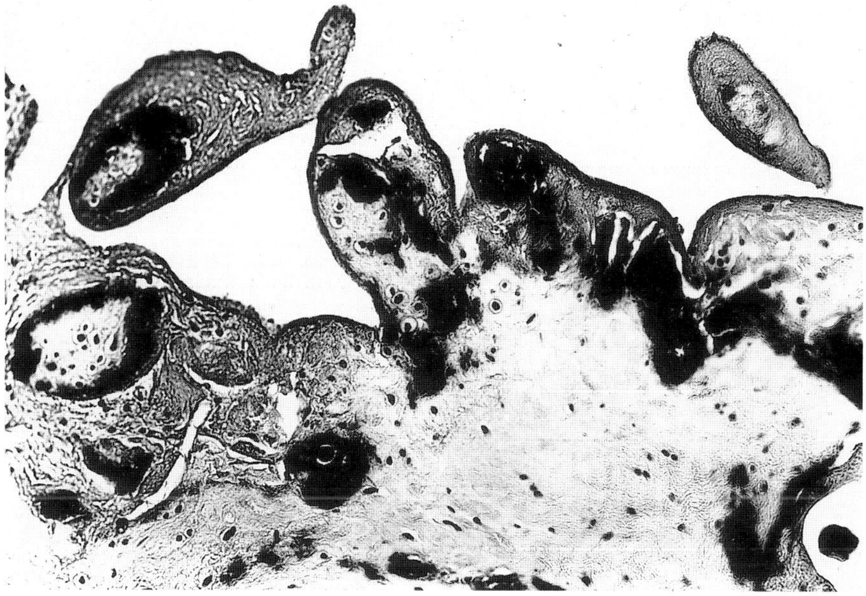

Fig. 394. The villi and the subsynoviocytic tissue comprise irregular deposits of calcium. The neighboring connective tissue is markedly hypocellular and is poor in fibers. Some of these cells have chondrocyte shape

tion to the usual changes in chronic inflammation, Moskowitz et al. [1146, 1147] observed in the calcium-containing synovial membrane also granulomatous inflammation with numerous giant cells and mononuclear cell infiltrates. Gaucher et al. [579] identified in the synovial membrane and articular cartilage large crystals in the shape of arrowheads and small crystals in the shape of prisms or rhomboids. Areas of calcium deposition are also present in the periarticular tissue, whose collagen bundles display hyaline degeneration and homogenization. On fusion of such areas calcific foci result, which are surrounded by a wall of large fibrocytes, lymphocytes, and solitary giant cells, and stain intensely blue with hematoxylin-eosin-phloxin-safran. The fibrocartilage of the meniscus (Fig. 395) contains extensive areas in which collagen bundles have lost their definition, being transformed into an almost homogeneous material which contains very few cells. Among these areas large accumulations of calcified material are interspersed. The articular cartilage contains in clefts and gaps small clumps of calcium salts (Fig. 396) directly neighbored by poorly stained

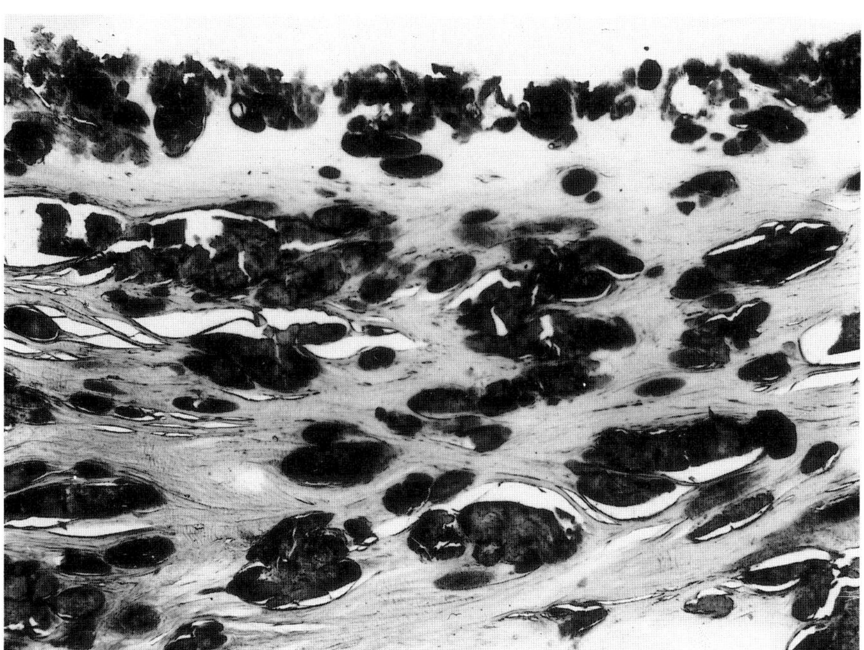

Fig. 395. The fibrocartilage of the meniscus is extensively hypocellular, and its staining ability is decreased. Many circumscribed calcium deposits lie in it

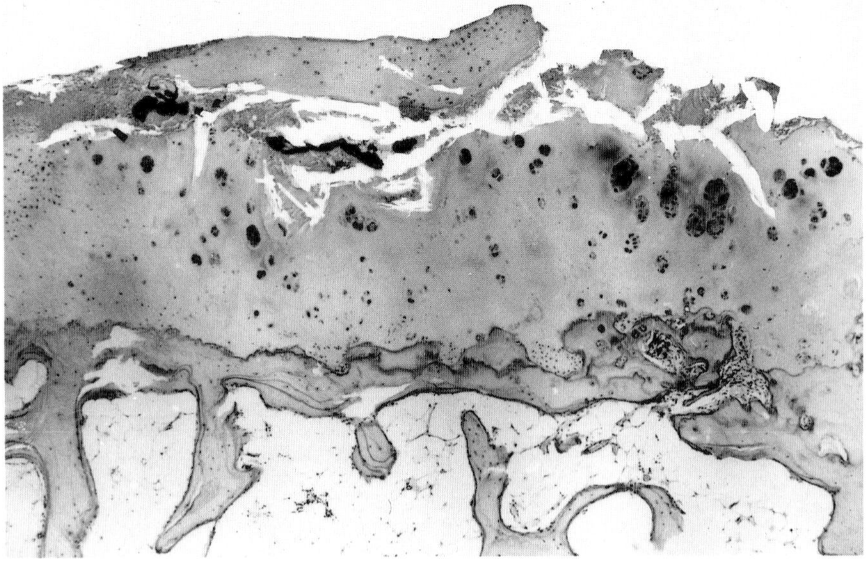

Fig. 396. The articular cartilage is disrupted on its surface by clefts. Close to these lie a few irregular deposits of calcium. Some of the chondrocytes in the deeper zone are hypertrophic and surrounded by large halos. The tide line is multiplied

chondrocytes with fragmented nuclei [23, 24]. Some halos or perilacunar zones are partly filled with calcium crystals. Somewhat distant chondrocytes are hypertrophic (Fig. 396) in clone formations and are surrounded by broad, intensely basophilically stained halos (Fig. 396). The presence of extensive disintegration in the intercellular matrix (Fig. 397) and the pronounced degenerative and necrotic changes of the chondrocytes in areas remote from the sites of deposition of calcium crumbs indicate, or at least strongly suggest, that regressive changes in the articular cartilage preceded the deposition of the calcium crumbs.

Electron-microscopic examinations [1442] revealed rhomboid or needlelike spaces in the synoviocytes and subsynoviocytic tissue, presumably the sites from which crystals have been dissolved by the water-based fixatives. Intact crystals or distinguishable remnants of crystals were observed only occasionally. Many crystals were distinctly membrane bound and appeared to be within phagosomes.

Differential diagnosis must consider inflammatory conditions of various nature [1147, 1148, 1396]. This consideration applies especially to the acute phase of calcinosis articularis, when its effusion and the tender-

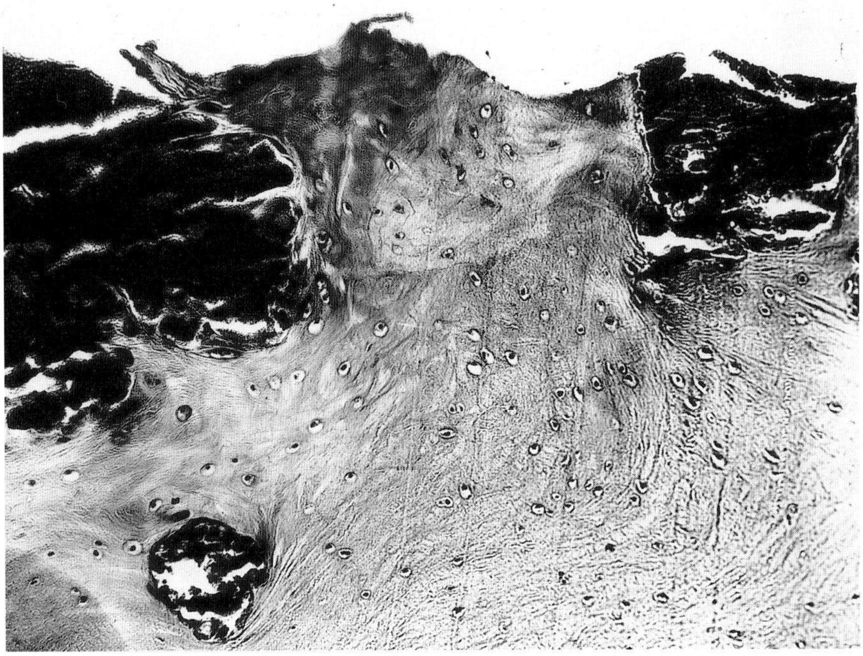

Fig. 397. The articular cartilage is distinctly hypocellular and contains lacunae. Unmasking of collagen fibers and extensive deposition of calcium occurs in this area

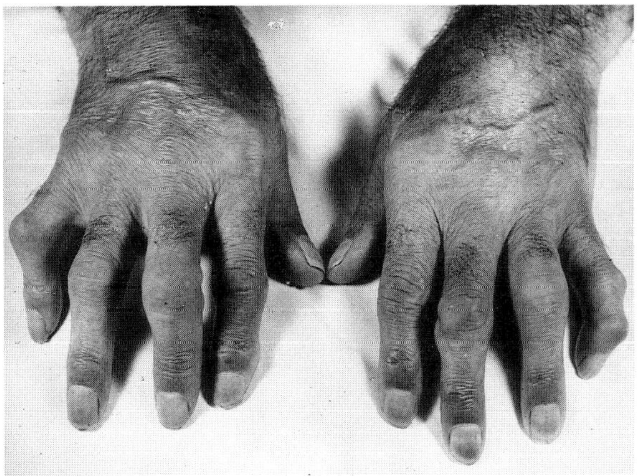

Fig. 398. The wrist joint, metacarpophalangeal joints, and proximal interphalangeal joints are thickened, and the latter are held in flexion contracture

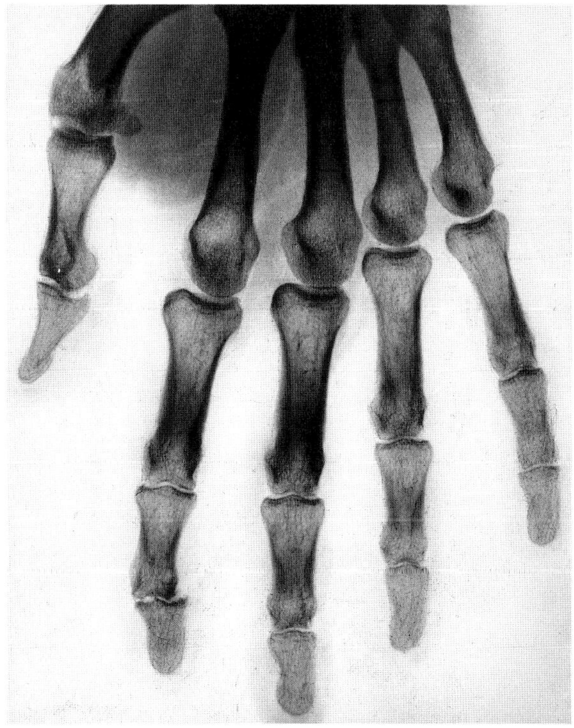

Fig. 399. The distal ends of the metacarpals as well as the proximal and distal ends of the first and second phalanges comprise extensive areas of radiolucency. Some metacarpophalangeal joints are uneven

ness of the joint capsule resemble those in any acute joint inflammation, whether of infectious, rheumatoid, or metabolic etiology. Examination of possibly increased joint fluid from all points of view, including microscopic examination, helps to clarify the nature of the joint affection. In those situations in which the roentgenographs reveal shadows of calcium deposits in the articular or periarticular tissues, they suggest the proper diagnostic direction. Finally, in the chronic phase with marked thickening of the joint capsule, coarse crepitation on motion of the joint, and possibly limitation of motion, osteoarthritis is very often suspected and may even be coexistent. Such situation is evidenced by roentgenographs with narrowing of the cartilage space, but with distinct calcium impregnation of the remnant articular cartilage and/or intraarticular fibrocartilage and possibly also of the joint capsule.

Treatment in the acute phase, after aspiration of the joint fluid, aims at reducing the inflammatory symptoms by rest, application of moist warm compresses, and administration of colchicine. The latter is given at 0.6 mg six to eight times daily for 1 week and then gradually descreasing for further 2 weeks. If colchicine does not fully suppress the crystal-induced soreness, nonsteroidal antiinflammatory medications are subsequently given as indicated in "Osteoarthritis". Similarly, compression of the acutely irritated joint by a firm strapping may provide beneficial rest. In chronic inflammations with marked thickening of the joint capsule, ultrasound at greater intensity (3.0–3.5 W/cm^2) in two series of eight sessions is able to reduce local symptoms such as tenderness and hardening of the tissue [687, 1541]. However, when extensive calcium deposits are present in larger clumps causing persistent pain and impediment of motion, excision of these masses is the practical solution (Fig. 544), especially in primary calcinosis. In the frequent cases of calcinosis associated with either primary or secondary pronounced osteoarthritis, regular administration of analgesics and/or nonsteroidal antiinflammatory medications combined with one or two series of eight sessions of shortwave diathermy and/or massage is necessary [944, 1613]. The application of hot mud packs in eight to ten sessions may provide long-lasting regression of symptoms. For the major joints, especially those of the lower extremities, supportive splints or braces are useful. In cases of very advanced joint alterations, representing rheumatoid arthritis or osteoarthritis followed by extensive calcinosis, arthroplastic procedures may be indicated. The here advisable procedures are discussed in "Rheumatoid Arthritis" and "Osteoarthritis".

b. Hemochromatosis of Joints

Hemochromatosis is the term used for a generalized disease characterized by deposition of protein-bound iron in organs and tissues of the body [349, 409]. It is most often the result of a disorder in iron metabolism [714] associated with increased absorption of the iron through the gastrointestinal tract. In these conditions it

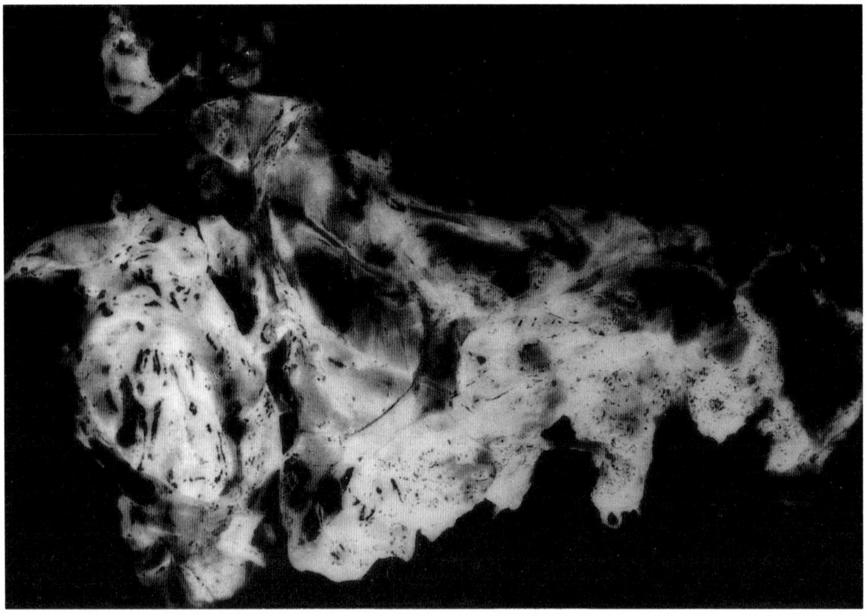

Fig. 400. The inner part of the joint capsule is uneven by several darkly discolored areas which are retracted secondary to shrinking

is the manifestation of a genetically transmitted, inborn failure as an autosomal recessive trait – therefore, the term primary hemochromatosis [455, 996]. In other conditions, hemochromatosis is secondary to iron overload resulting from numerous blood transfusions, disorders in erythropoesis, increased dietary intake of iron, or disorders of the liver either in alcoholism or hepatitis. The result is excessive hemolysis with elevation of the iron concentration in the blood. The substantially increased protein-bound iron, ferritin, in the circulating blood is subsequently deposited in parenchymatous organs and reticuloendothelial structures [85]. Therefrom results cirrhosis of the liver, pancreas, kidneys, parathyroid, and heart, and is associated with diabetes, hypercalcinosis, and myocardial failure.

In 20%–40% of patients iron is also deposited in the synovial membrane and hyaline cartilage, with resulting articular symptoms [1, 393, 409, 453, 1441]. These patients present gray discoloration of the skin of the face and trunk, and often the symptoms of diabetes, neuropathy, or heart failure. The affected joints [532, 1441] are primarily those of the fingers (Fig. 398), with special involvement of the metacarpophalangeal and interphalangeal joints of the second and third fingers; thereafter follow the wrist, elbow, shoulder, knee, hip, and ankle joints. In more advanced cases, especially in elderly individuals, the thoracic and lumbar spine is also affected. Initial symptoms are aching and moderate pain in these joints and are subsequently associated with the sensation of stiffness. Objectively observed limitation of motion eventually follows. The affected joints present distinct, although moderate thickening of the joint capsule. Flexion contractures of the metacarpophalangeal and first interphalangeal joints ensue particularly in the thumb and second and third fingers (Fig. 398); a rather characteristic deformity of the hand results. The wrist, ankle, and knee joints also become moderately thickened and limited in their movements. Eventually the shoulder and hip joints may become affected. An intraarticular effusion is sometimes seen in the knee joint.

Blood studies [532, 1518] disclose a distinct increase in the serum iron concentration from a normal maximum of 150 μg/dl to 275 μg/dl, a total ironbinding capacity of less than 320 μg/dl, and a ferritin saturation greater than 75%. The latter is elevated in most cases of primary and secondary hemochromatosis. The aspirated joint fluid contains a moderate number (600–1000/ml) of lymphocytes but no hemorrhage or increase of desquamated synoviocytes. The mucin forms a normal clot.

Roentgenographs [824] of the hands (Fig. 399) and elbows reveal moderate narrowing of the cartilage space, slight erosion with irregular delineation of the articular epiphyses, sometimes chondral sclerosis, and invariably subchondral cystic lesions. The joints of the fingers, wrist, knee, and/or ankle joint are sometimes contiguous with periarticular or paraarticular irregular shadows of calcified tissue. The destructive arthropathy of the metacarpophalangeal joints, the subchondral cyst formations, and the generalized osteopenia suggest an underlying iron disorder [6]. The shoulder and knee joints present slight narrowing of the cartilage space and irregular outlines of the articular epiphyses. Small osteophytes rise at the margins of the articular epiphyses, where the joint capsule is thickened and dense. In elderly patients with

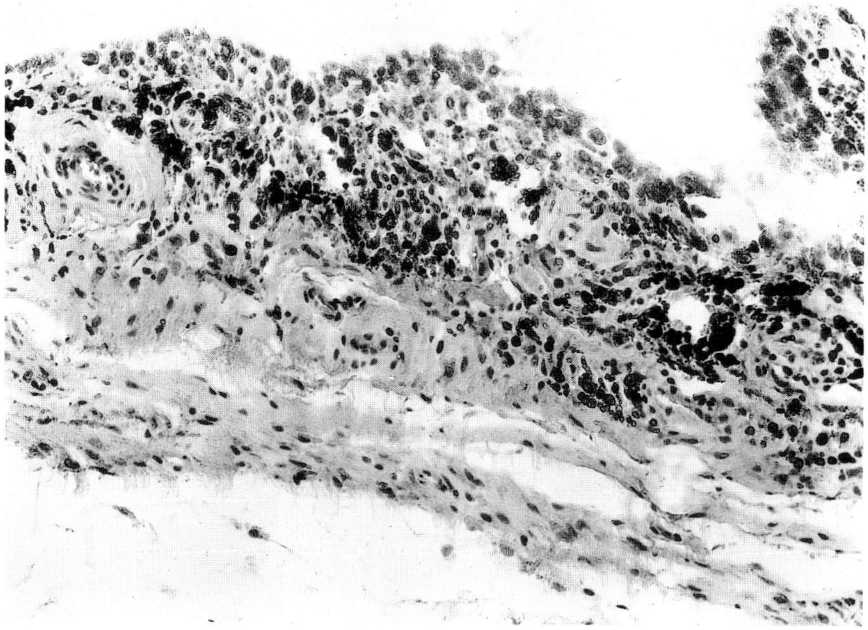

Fig. 401. The synovial membrane is delimited by hypertrophic synoviocytes and contains increased fibrocytes and numerous hemosiderin-laden histiocytes in the subsynoviocytic zone. Additional hemosiderin lies extracellularly and interstitially

hemochromatosis, calcinosis of the hyaline cartilage [733] may be noted in the finger joints, the major joints of the extremities, and the intervertebral discs [6, 714, 1713].

Gross-anatomical examination (Fig. 400) discloses that the inner part of the joint capsule is moderately uneven in several rather extensive areas. Some of these are slightly elevated, but most are shrunken and retracted below the level. All of the latter are discolored dark brown and are harder on palpation.

Histopathological examination of the joint capsule [1118, 1157, 1709] in the early phase discloses slight thickening of the synovial membrane by hypertrophy of the synoviocytes (Fig. 401). Golden brown granules in moderate amount are partly deposited in the synoviocytes and subsynoviocytic histiocytes and partly lie free in the interstitial tissue. Staining with potassium ferrocyanide discloses the presence of blue iron particles in these deposits. In the advanced phase the deeper subsynoviocytic tissue is thickened by rather extensive

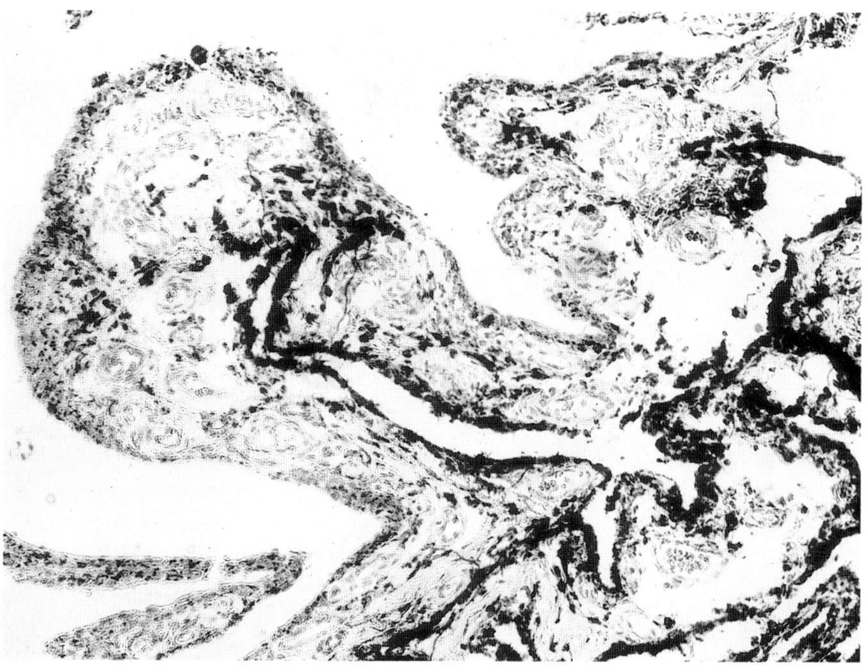

Fig. 402. The synovial membrane is elevated into many large villi whose synoviocytes are hypertrophic. Many of these synoviocytes are laden with hemosiderin granules; also subsynoviocytic histiocytes are laden with hemosiderin

proliferation of fibrocytes (Fig. 402). Similar iron-containing granules are noted in the chondrocytes and lacunae of the articular cartilage [1441, 1709]. On the other hand, numerous smaller and larger deposits of calcium salts, surrounded by disintegrating interstitial matrix, were observed [1118] in all zones of the articular cartilage.

On the basis of histopathological findings, other conditions with depositions of hemosiderin such as traumatic synovitis, hemosiderosis, pigmented villonodular synovitis (Fig. 65), and arthritis in hemophilia (Fig. 414) must be considered. Clinical and roentgenographic findings in hemochromatosis are more suggestive of primary osteoarthritis or chondrocalcinosis. Eventually the relevant laboratory studies contribute to establishing the diagnosis.

On more extensive deposition of iron particles in the joint capsule and articular cartilage, profound alteration in their interstitial tissue ensues as well as in their cellular metabolism. Disintegration continues here in the articular constituents, resulting in pronounced secondary osteoarthritic changes [54] and substantial impairment in the function of the joints.

Treatment [532, 714] endeavors primarily by regulation of the diet to restrict the intake of iron-containing food and secondarily to decrease periodically the iron-containing pool by phlebotomies. The iron load is periodically checked by determining the concentration of serum ferritin. Blood (500 ml) is withdrawn at intervals of 3–6 months until mild iron-deficiency anemia results, but with a hematocrit not below 34% and hemoglobin concentration not below 11 mm. The immediate benefits are noticeable in regression of a present heart congestion, improvement in liver function, and decrease in diabetes. As to the articular symptoms, regular application of moist hot packs and physical therapy with shortwave diathermy in one or two series of eight sessions provide a distinct benefit, which must nevertheless be supplemented with salicylates. On occasionally occurring more pronounced swelling of the joint capsule, antiinflammatory medications, especially phenylbutazone 100 mg twice daily for 8–10 days under control of the leukocyte count, are indicated. In rare situations, the deformation of the joints may become aggravated to such an extent that synovectomy (Fig. 400), surgical repair, or even total arthroplasty may be necessary.

5. Joint Affections in Blood Disorders

a. Arthropathy in Hemophilia

Of the joint affections in blood disorders, arthropathy in hemophilia is the most impairing condition, because of the eventually severe alterations of the articular structures [52, 399, 434, 609, 838, 1006, 1086, 1431, 1530]. Hemophilia is characterized by a tendency to frequent bleedings, with accumulation of hematomas in internal organs and extremities. These bleedings are the manifestations of disturbance in the physiological coagulation process of the blood due to a lack of the necessary clotting components. As such components have been identified factor VIII, whose deficiency accounts for the classic hemophilia, and factor IX, whose deficiency or lack accounts for so-called Christmas hemophilia. These two most frequent types of hemophilia are transmitted by asymptomatic female carriers through a sex-linked chromosome and therefore appear almost exclusively in males. Other types of bleeding disorders are caused by the lack of fibrinogen, prothrombin, or substances related to prothrombin. These deficiencies occur in both sexes without a precedence in the family history, thus suggesting a mutation of genes [207, 1006].

The disease often manifests itself as early as the age of 2–4 years and becomes more frequent and pronounced with adolescence. Besides bleeding in subcutaneous tissue, deep musculature, visceral cavities, internal organs, or skull, bleeding occurs also in joints. The first episode of the disease is usually elicited by a trauma, either a sharp wound or bruise, followed by prolonged bleeding, depending in its duration on the quantitative degree of deficiency in antihemophilic factor. In the mild form excessive bleeding may occur only in open wounds or at operations. In the moderate form bleeding occurs after any trauma, but this varies in intensity and duration with the severity of the inflicted injury. In the severe form bleeding may occur even with slight of unidentified injury. The moderate form is the most frequent. The first harm to a joint is caused by direct trauma, while subsequent harms to a joint may be elicited even by a moderate sprain or strain at routine activity.

The knee is the most often affected joint (Fig. 403), followed by the elbow, ankle, hip, wrist and shoulder joints. The symptoms vary according to the intensity, duration, and frequency of the joint affliction and justify the following classification of the clinical findings on the basis of the underlying changes. (a) Acute or very recent hemarthrosis, starting in childhood, with conspicuous swelling of the joint chiefly by intraarticular accumulation of blood. Other signs include moderate to marked tenderness of the joint capsule, slight tenseness of the regional musculature, and increased local warmth with occasional redness of the covering skin. The first few effusions may be absorbed spontaneously, and normalization of the joint capsule follows. (b) Repeated hemarthroses at shorter intervals, whereupon the joint capsule remains thickened, and the

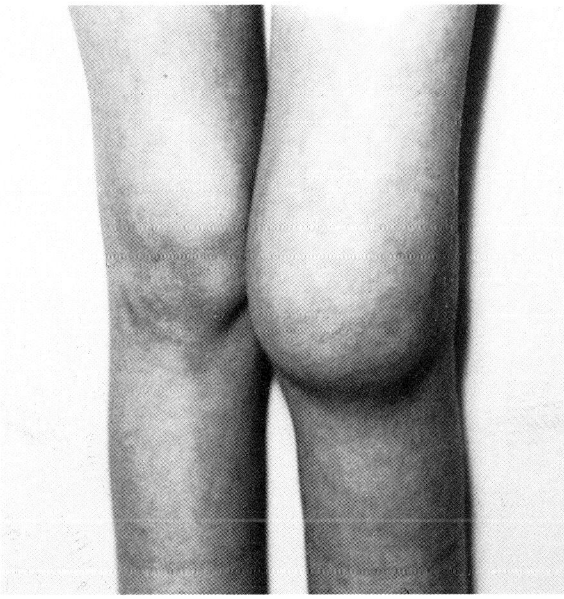

Fig. 403. The left knee is markedly enlarged by extensive and very pronounced thickening of the joint capsule

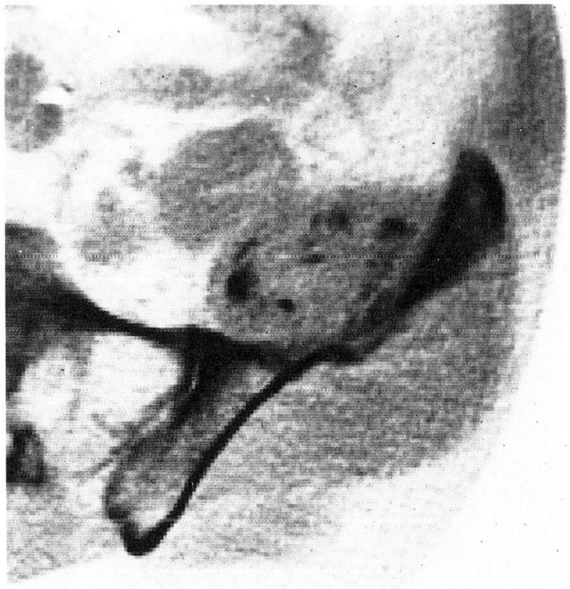

Fig. 404. CT scan evidences that the iliac bone is very thinned over a large extent, which is occupied by a circumscribed mass of soft tissue. The latter contains several osseous densities

regional musculature becomes tight. However, no inflammatory signs are noted, while the range of motion decreases, and a contracture of the joint may set in. (c) Advanced articular changes, occurring in adults several years after frequent and decreasingly absorbed hemorrhages. The joint capsule then becomes irregularly thickened (Fig. 403), and movements of the joint are limited by contracture or by concomitant advanced alterations of the articular epiphyses [1530]. The regional musculature is generally atrophic and weakened.

Besides the repeated hemorrhages into joints, hemorrhages often of greater extent occur in the musculature of the extremities and trunk, where they usually do not absorb but remain encapsulated. There they become organized under concurrent ossification of the musculature as well as under erosion of the adjacent cortical bone. The latter reacts subsequently with irregular proliferation. The resulting marked local enlargement in the upper or lower extremities, chest, or pelvis (Figs. 404, 408) has been termed hemophilic pseudotumor [434, 609, 771, 894, 1249].

Laboratory studies disclose the underlying anomalies in the blood. Due to deficiency in plasma factor VIII, thromboplastin – which in the presence of calcium ions activates prothrombin to the enzymatic clotting factor thrombin – is diminished. Consequently, the polymerization of fibrinogen to the insoluble fibrillar fibrin is delayed and diminished [755, 756]. Thus the clotting time, which physiologically is 4–14 min, depending on the laboratory method, is prolonged to 10–20 min. However, the physiological concentration of fibrinogen to 150–300 mg/dl is not changed in hemophilia. Bleeding time and prothrombin time are also not abnormal [191, 1767]. On the other hand, tests determining the clotting ability of the plasma in the coagulation of the blood yield abnormal findings [1767, 1777]. These are the partial thromboplastin time and the thromboplastin generation time. The former is more readily tested and normally amounts 60–85 s; it is prolonged to 160–400 s on decrease in factor VIII below 40% of the normal assay [1100]. The latter, normally measuring 10–32 s, is prolonged to 51–80 s on decrease of the factor VIII below 25% of the normal assay [1100]. In addition, studies for measuring the deficient clotting factor are of basic importance. Normal individuals have 50%–200% of 1 U factor VIII per 1 ml plasma [1006]. Individuals with this factor decreased below 30%–50% of the normal level are considered mild hemophiliacs, and those with this clotting factor below 5%–30% of the physiological level are considered moderate to severe hemophiliacs [1006]. Examination for the inhibitor antibody against factor VIII is of further essential importance. This antibody belongs to the IgG group. Its presence can be ascertained by incubating the patient's plasma with normal plasma, whereupon prolongation of the thromboplastin time follows. Such identification is of elementary importance in the management of extensive bleedings, because the inhibitor antibody frustrates the salutary effect of the transfusion with the concentrate of factor VIII and/or cryoprecipitate. Electromyo-

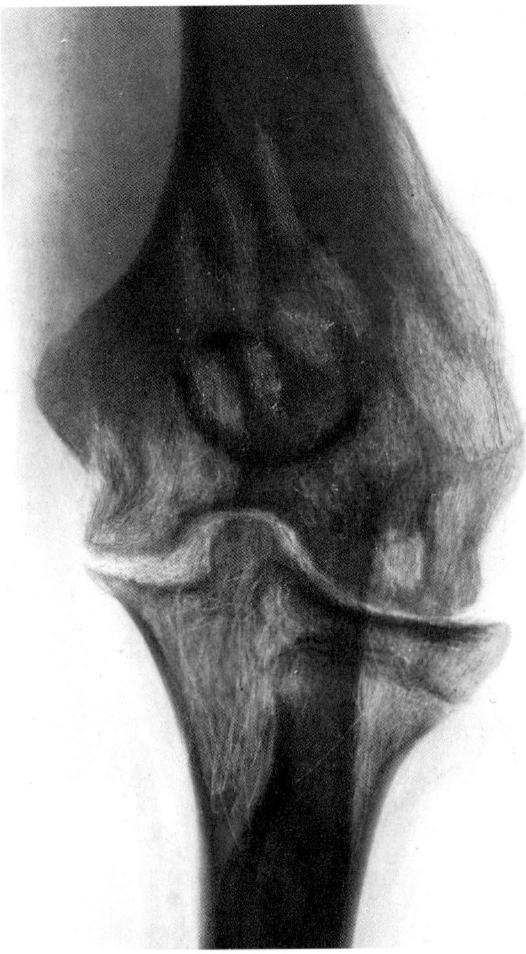

Fig. 405. The humeral condyles and the proximal epiphyses of the ulna and radius contain several delimited radiolucenct areas. The joint space is uneven and narrowed on the radial side, and the articular surfaces are sclerosed

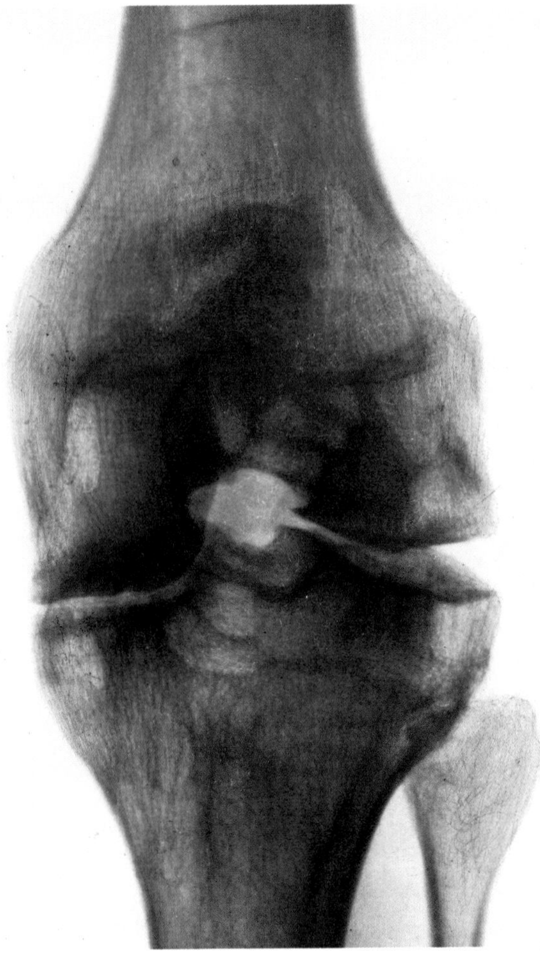

Fig. 406. The femoral and tibial epiphyses contain large areas of radiolucency. The joint space is uneven, medially narrowed, and laterally widened. The intercondylar space is bell-like widened

graphic studies disclose a decrease in the potential of motor units of the peripheral musculature.

Roentgenographs reveal no changes in the phase of brief hemorrhages. However, with repeated hemorrhages over a longer period of time a varying picture is manifested [399, 838, 1249, 1591]. This depends on the age of the individual and the frequency and duration of hemorrhages. Relating the clinical findings to the roentgenographs, Arnold et al. [52] and Hilgartner [755] drafted a five-grade scale. Moseley [1143] described in young individuals the sequelae of recurrent intraarticular hemorrhages as enlargement of the articular epiphyses due to overgrowth and accelerated maturation in the trabecular pattern. In adults with hemorrhages recurring over longer periods of time, the joint capsule is very densified while the articular epiphyses and adjoining metaphyses are irregularly osteoporotic. The cartilage space is substantially narrowed (Figs. 405, 406, 407) due to erosion of the articular cartilage, expanding from the margin to its center. In the subchondral and adjoining areas numerous spots of radiolucency (Figs. 405, 406, 407) delimited by densified trabecular rims appear as sequelae of hemorrhages. These cystic areas are greater in size and number, and also occur in other joints than in those usually observed in osteoarthritis. On further attrition, the cartilage space is unevenly narrowed, and large osteophytes rise at the margin of the articular surfaces (Fig. 407), thus contributing to the deformity of the articular epiphyses.

Additionally, specific local changes are observed roentgenographically in some joints [952]. In the shoulder joint, the osteoporotic humeral head is usually enlarged, comprises a few large cysts, and trespasses the rim of the glenoid cavity, which bears large marginal osteophytes. In the elbow joint (Fig. 405) the humeral condyles are very enlarged, and the radial head is flattened, while the trochlear groove of the ulna

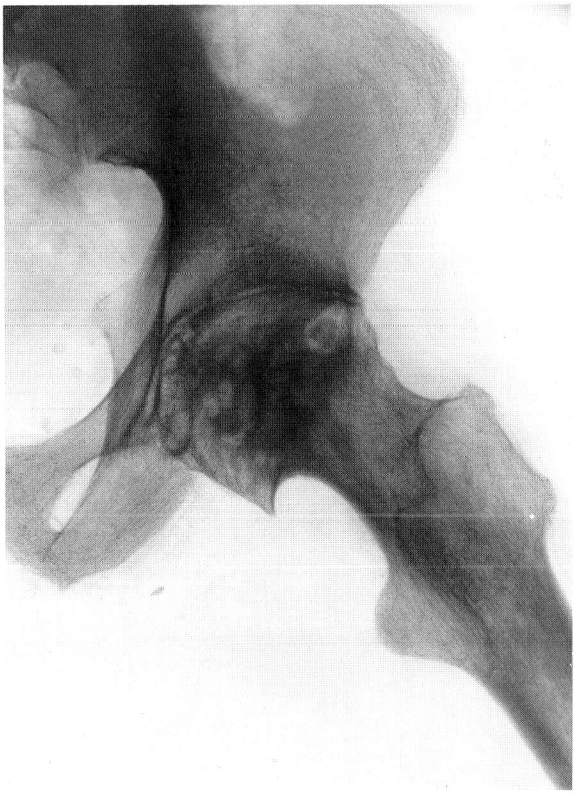

Fig. 407. The acetabular area contains a radiolucent area of moderate width, and the iliac bone contains a large radiolucent area. The femoral head contains many small radiolucent areas, most of them surrounded by sclerosis. The joint cleft is very narrowed

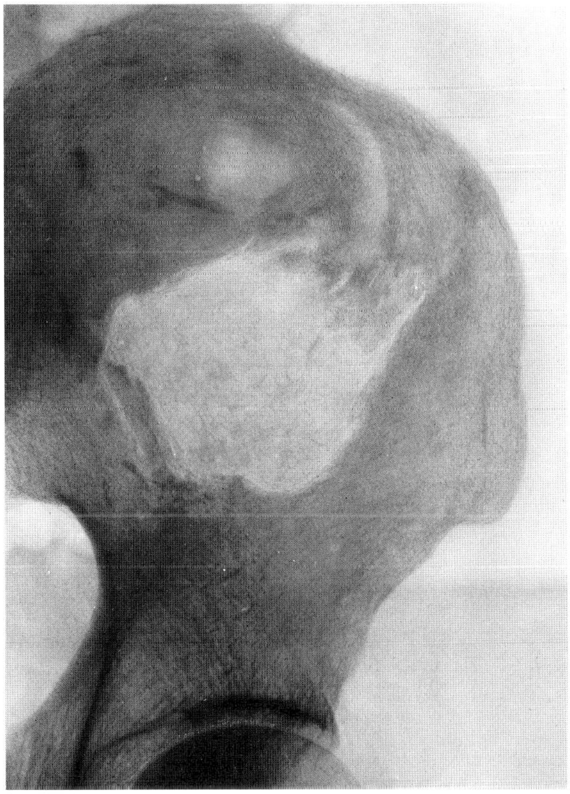

Fig. 408. The iliac bone comprises a very extensive and sharply, although irregularly delimited radiolucency

is widened, being dorsally delimited by an enlarged olecranon. In the wrist joint, the cartilage space is irregularly delimited by epiphyses which contain subchondral lucencies and densifications; the styloid processes are enlarged. In the hip joint (Fig. 407), the femoral head is flattened and bears marginal osteophytes at its upper contour; its subchondral area and the adjoining region of the femoral neck are partly osteoporotic and partly sclerotic. These changes are much more pronounced in the hip joints of children whose femoral head contains several large cystic lucencies which expand into the metaphyseal area. In the knee joint, the enlarged femoral condyles with rarefied trabecular structure delimit a conspicuously intercondylar groove widened like a bell (Fig. 406) while the tibial condyles are flattened. In the ankle joint, the mortise is widened, and its malleoli are enlarged; the cartilage space is very uneven. Roentgenographs of the hemophilic tumor [209, 434, 771] (Fig. 408) reveal extensive, irregular densification and ossification in the musculature, as well as extensive cavities and formation of new osseous areas in the adjacent bone. A mixed structural pattern develops here which is suggestive of myositis ossificans, osteitis fibrosa cystica, giant cell tumor, or osteogenic sarcoma. Additional studies as the tomogram, the computed tomography scan (Fig. 404), and the ultrasonogram aid in clarifying the diagnosis.

Gross-anatomical examination of joints affected over a longer range of time by repeated intraarticular hemorrhages reveals that the joint cavity is concentrically narrowed by a thickened joint capsule (Figs. 409, 410). Its inner part is discolored rusty brown to a large extent and is elevated in plump villi (Figs. 409, 410, 411). By the thickening of its superficial layer the resorptive capacity of the joint capsule had been diminished, whereupon the subsequent hemorrhagic effusions persist with increased pressure in the joint cavity. The subjacent tissue of the joint capsule contains a few organized hematomas, but is otherwise transformed into a dense fibrosed tissue. The cartilage of the articular ends has lost its glistening appearance and is discolored brownish gray (Fig. 412). It is only partly maintained (Fig. 412) and is mostly uneven and fibrillated or has the appearance of fibrocartilage. Another part of the articular surfaces is covered by connective tissue which stems from overgrowth and expansion of synovial pannus. In larger areas, however,

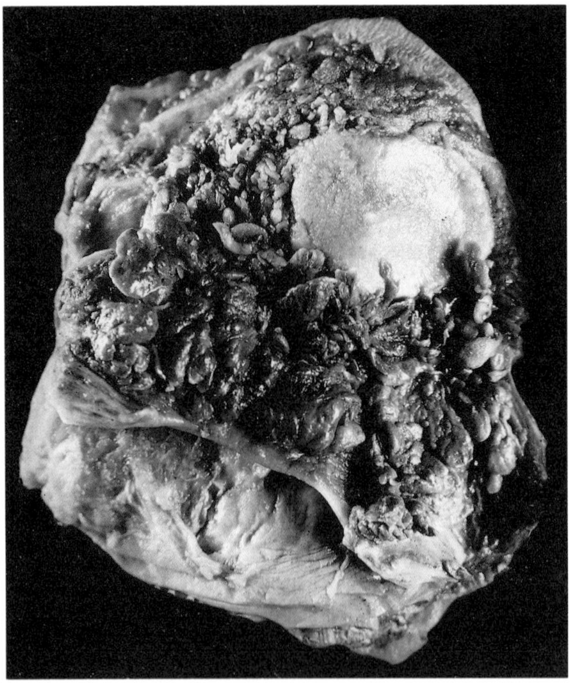

Fig. 409. The inner part of the joint capsule surrounding the patella is raised in many villi, most of which are discolored brownish or dark brown

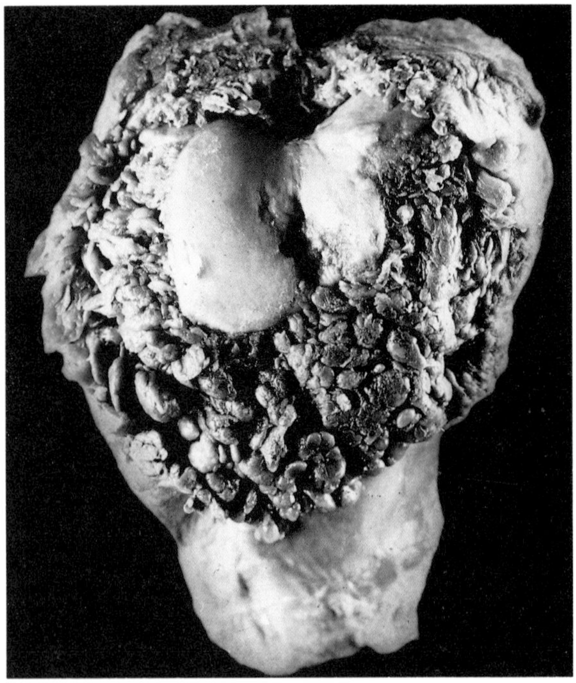

Fig. 410. The inner part of the joint capsule surrounding the femoral condyles is raised in many rather plump, brownish villi

the articular ends are bare of any cover (Fig. 413), which has been worn off. Wide areas of the denuded subchondral bones contain shallow and also rather deep indentations (Fig. 412), which account for the extensive irregularity of the articular surfaces. Intraarticular hematomata penetrate through the defects in the surface. The deeper bone is generally porotic and comprises cavities from lentil to hazelnut size. These cavities contain old organized hematomas (Fig. 413), bone spicules, or reddish brown loose connective tissue, and are delimited by densified osseous trabeculae. The edges of the articular epiphyses have become deformed and enlarged by the protrusion of marginal osteophytes, beneath which larger cavities, containing

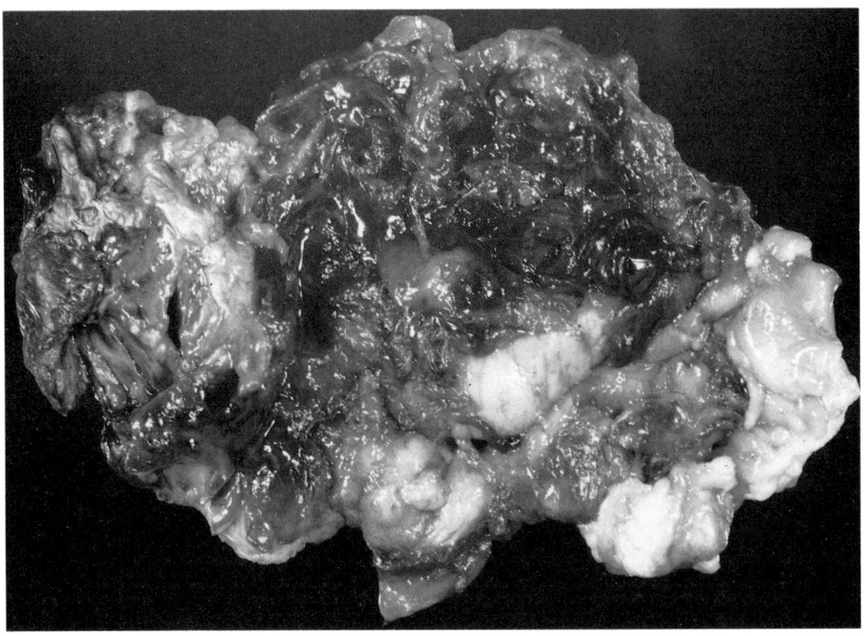

Fig. 411. The excised inner part of the joint capsule has normal appearance in a few areas. Otherwise, the surface is raised in many thick villi and plump nodes, most of which are discolored light brown or dark brown

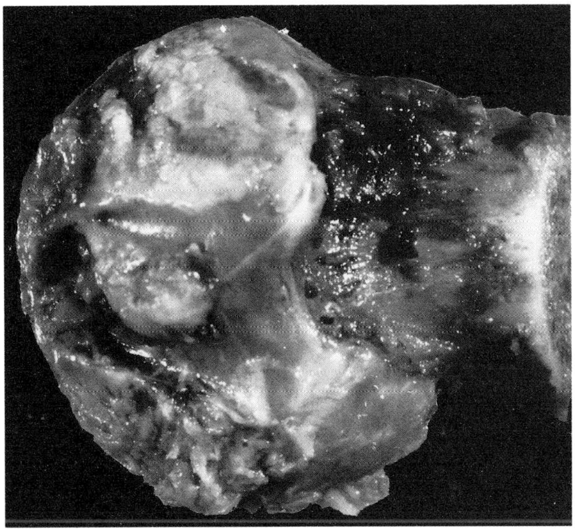

Fig. 412. The femoral head is very uneven and comprises several extensive indentations with thinned or lacking articular cartilage

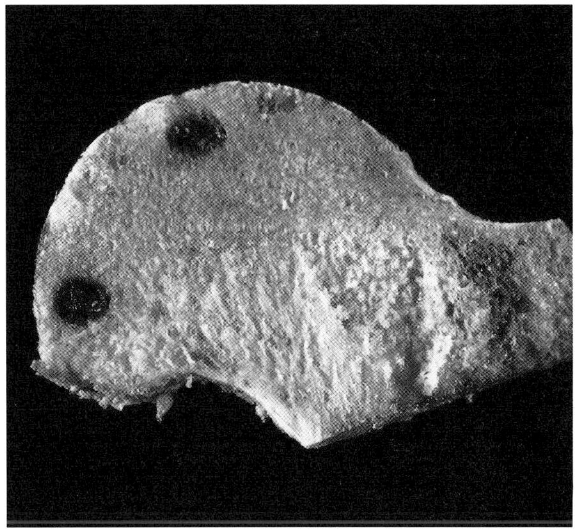

Fig. 413. The femoral head is mostly denuded of articular cartilage. The bone close to the surface is rather sclerosed and comprises two cavities filled with blood clots. A few smaller but empty cavities also lie close to the surface

organized hematomas sometimes lie. Concurrently, the thickened joint capsule has substantially shrunken, and the entire joint has become fibrotically contracted. Experimental studies by Puhl et al. [1287] confirmed the development of gross-anatomical and histopathological changes in the synovial membrane and articular cartilage, as are noted intraoperatively after repeated intraarticular hemorrhages.

Histopathological examination [1006] discloses the synovial membrane to be markedly thickened, partly by enlargement and multiplication of the synoviocytes which proliferate into short plump villi and partly by an increase in fibrocytes in the subsynoviocytic tissue (Fig. 414). Additional thickening is contributed here by extensive deposits of hemosiderin granules which have been engulfed by synoviocytes, fibroblasts, and histiocytes, but to a greater proportion lie extracellularly and interstitially (Figs. 414, 415). These granules stain golden brown with hematoxylin-eosin and dark blue with potassium ferrocyanide. Some blood vessels are

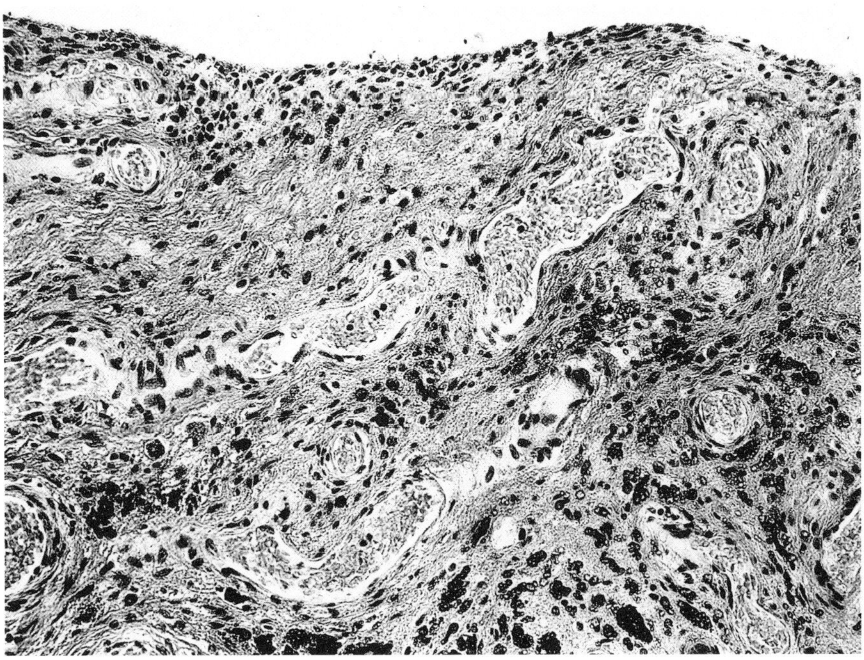

Fig. 414. The synovial membrane is very dense by an increase in fibrocytes and collagen fibers. Many fibrocytes and histiocytes are enlarged by hemosiderin granules. All blood vessels are dilated

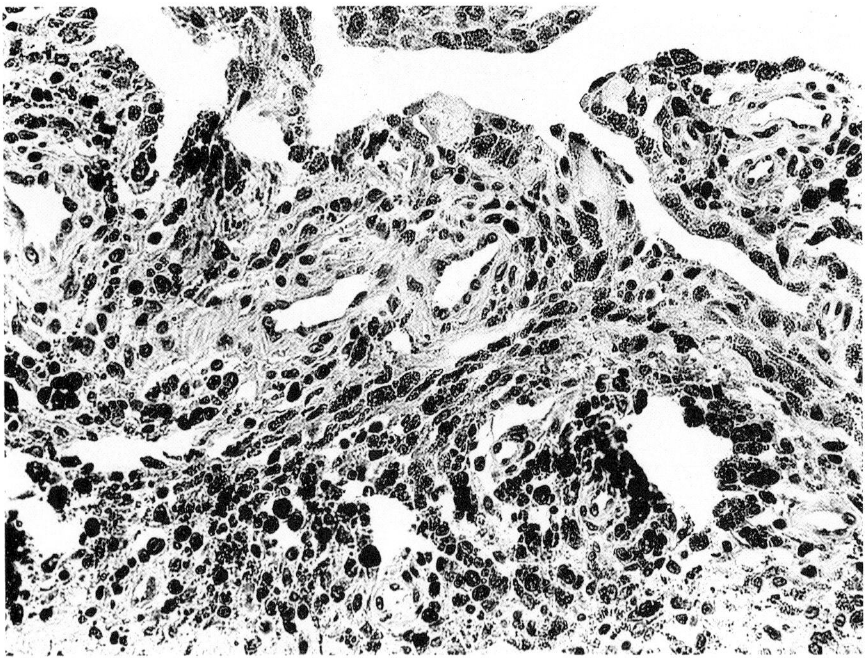

Fig. 415. The synovial membrane is elevated into broad villi. Many synoviocytes, fibrocytes, and histiocytes are enlarged by hemosiderin granules. A substantial amount of such granules lies extracellularly and interstitially

dilated and hyperemic, and others are disrupted. A few small agglomerates of lymphocytes are scattered. The intercellular matrix is extensively densified by an increase of collagen fibers from the subsynoviocytic zone to the peripheral layer (Fig. 414).

It appears that the ingestion of hemosiderin has changed the biology of the synoviocytes [603]. Roy et al. [1365] observed by electron-microscopic examination that the enlarged synovial cells contained erythrocytes or siderosomes resulting from their phagocytosis.

Culture and histochemical studies [1006] disclose that the hemosiderin laden synoviocytes and fibroblasts release protease and collagenolytic enzyme in sufficient quantity to cause degradation of the intercellular ground substance of the articular cartilage, leading to osteoarthritic changes. Accordingly, Schulitz [1431] emphasized the disintegration of chondrocytes on release of enzymes by synoviocytes after their phagocytosis of erythrocytes. Schulitz [1431] also demonstrated the loss of the lamina splendens of the articular cartilage, the resulting degradation of the matrix, and the structural changes in collagen fibers secondary to adherence of blood to the cartilage surface. The articular cartilage (Figs. 416, 417) is of uneven surface throughout. In several areas it displays a changed staining pattern, lack of ground substance, and unmasking of collagen fibers, which are placewise separated by thin vertical clefts. The interjacent chondrocytes [780] contain hemosiderin granules close to their nuclei. Most of these cells have pyknotic or fragmented nuclei, and large lacunae surround their small mass of cytoplasm. Several lacunae completely devoid of chondrocytes are interposed. In a few directly neighboring areas the chondrocytes are multiplied in pairs and clusters. These are surrounded by halos with increased concentration of ground substance, as revealed by intensified pericellular staining (Fig. 416). In other areas, the articular cartilage also displays unmasking of the collagen fibers (Fig. 416) but with maintained ground substance, whereby it assumes the appearance of fibrocartilage. In contrast hereto is the epiphyseal cover in places, where the cartilage is missing (Fig. 417) and has been replaced by organized granulation tissue with irregularly coursing collagen fibers and a few blood vessels. Hemosiderin granules are deposited intracellularly and intercellularly in the fibrocartilage as well as in the organized pannus [1574]. However, in several extensive areas the articular epiphysis is completely devoid of any cover, and the denuded subchondral bone is sclerosed; in other areas the bone is thinned and porotic. In the subjacent zone several cystic cavities occur; they are partly filled with loose connective tissue, old organized hematomas, or fragmented material and are delimited by bony trabeculae. Extensive rarefaction involves the regional bone.

Differential diagnosis must consider, at the initial occurrence, primary traumatic hemarthrosis occurring in children and adolescents by an identified injury. In adults with posttraumatic thickening of the joint capsule and histopathologically verified, extensive hemosiderin deposits but without advanced alterations in the articular epiphyses or impairment in the function of

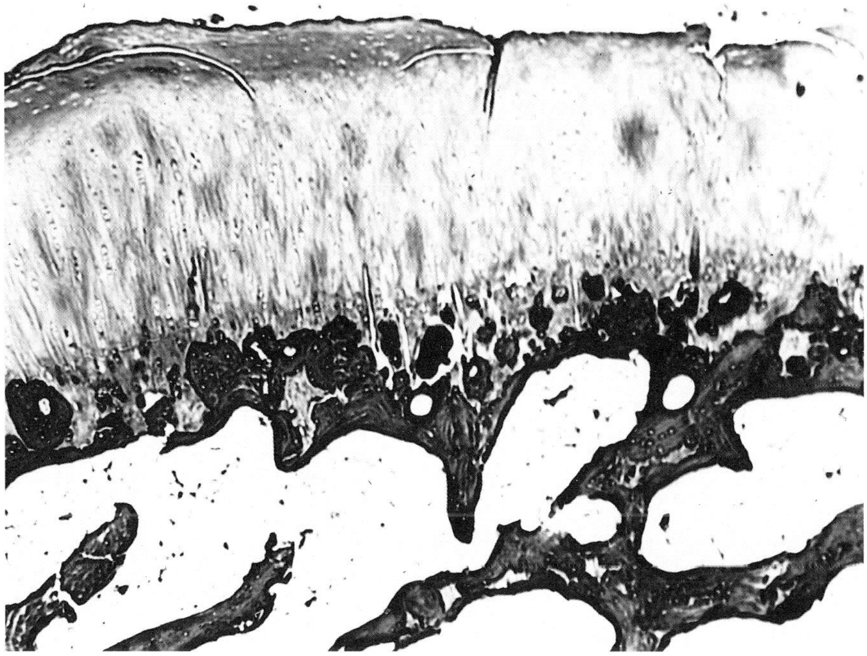

Fig. 416. The surface of the articular cartilage is slightly disrupted by fine clefts, and the subjacent collagen fibers are partly unmasked. Small ossifications lie in the zone of calcified cartilage

the joint, hemochromatosis (Fig. 401) and pigmented villonodular synovitis (Fig. 65) is also a probable diagnosis.

The treatment of fresh hemarthrosis endeavors to attain absorption of the hematoma by complete bedrest, with elevation of the affected extremity and regular application of cold wet compresses. In cases of a large and nonregressing hematoma, arthrocentesis using a syringe with a thin needle is indicated. Immediately thereafter the joint should be compressed by a firm strapping and the affected extremity should be elevated. The concurrent correction of the hemophilic disorder, as immediately ascertained by appropriate laboratory studies at the slightest suspicion of a clotting disorder, is followed by substitution of the absent clotting factor. This is the etiological treatment in an episode of protracted and laboratory-confirmed bleeding. Concentrates of the indicated clotting factor are transfused in plasma [52, 755] which also contains some fibrinogen, especially necessary in cases of coexisting

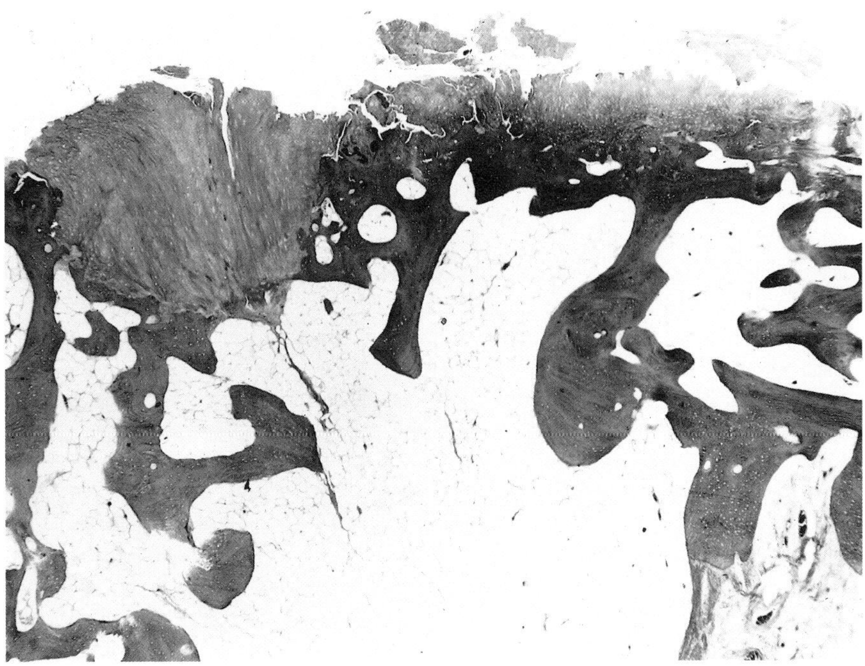

Fig. 417. The articular cartilage is uneven by small clefts and attrition. Several small fragments of cartilage are detached. A larger portion of articular cartilage is displaced into the depth through a gap in the cortical bone

fibrinogen deficiency. Determining the individual deficiency and the indicated type of plasma concentrate must be carried out in collaboration with a hematologist. In any extensive bleeding the clotting deficiency should be corrected by transfusion of an adequate amount of frozen plasma. The amount of clotting factor to be substituted is determined by the level of deficiency in the clotting factor, expressed in decreased percentage of the normal level of units per 1 ml plasma. The therapeutic material contains 1 U factor VIII in 1 ml pooled frozen plasma. Each unit of the infused factor per kilogram body weight yields a 2% rise in the factor level in the plasma [1006]. In moderate to severe hemophilia the amount of cryoprecipitate is doubled.

To minimize the amount of transfused plasma, supplements have been prepared from human and animal plasma which contain factor VIII in a much higher concentration than normal plasma. This consideration also applies to episodes of recurrent extensive bleeding in which the treatment for supervised chronic cases uses plasma administered at the home of the patient. Beyond this, frozen plasma is administered as a prophylactic measure in a hospital before any major surgical intervention on a joint, during this operation, and in immediately postoperative care as long as bleeding at the operative site is a potential complication. In view of the possibly frequent necessity of such plasma transfusion at any episode of extensive bleeding, a home care program has been instituted by the United States National Hemophilia Foundation. Relatives of the patient receive instruction here and are enabled, under the guidance of a physician in charge, to administer such transfusions. However, as a major complication after the transfusions some patients develop an inhibitor antibody against the factor VIII. This negates the effect of future transfusions.

In all articular conditions in which bleeding does not recur, the thickening of the joint capsule is a residual feature which limits motion; orally administered corticosteroids may provide a benefit. Nevertheless, a longer series (about 20–30 sessions) of physical therapy, consisting of muscle strengthening exercises and active/passive joint mobilizations, is an essential necessity. Understandably, vigorous activities, especially sportive exercises, should be avoided. As a further protection against disuse, supportive braces, either provided with hinges or completely stiff, are indispensable adjuncts for the joints of the lower extremities.

However, on further aggravation of the joint alterations and resulting deformities operative procedures can be applied [675]. These include: lengthening of the tendons of the contracted muscles, synovectomy, and in far-advanced cases osteotomy, total arthroplasty, and arthrodesis [52, 360, 451, 609, 625, 675, 755, 864, 990, 1032, 1056, 1226, 1274, 1526, 1596, 1675, 1745]. The lengthening of a tendon as the least invasive procedure is indicated in contracture of a joint not amenable to physical therapy; this must be followed by passive manipulations until an adequate range of mobility has been restored. In the cases of coexistent or independent, marked villous thickening of the joint capsule extensive synovectomy is able substantially to diminish the irritation of the joint as well as the tendency to bleeding; an even and fibrosed inner layer of the joint capsule is the result. Since invasion by the proliferating synovial membrane accounts for some of the alteration of the osteocartilaginous surfaces, prophylactic synovectomy has been applied by Melanotte [1086] and Montane et al. [1133] for the elbow, hip, knee, and ankle joints. Follow-up examinations and long-term roentgenographic controls by Esposito et al. [481] and Traldi et al. [1658] indicate that early synovectomy protects the joints from further deterioration. In pronounced axial deviation of a joint, metaphyseal osteotomy with inextensive exposure succeeds in correcting the deviation. This should not be combined with internal fixation by metallic devices because of the potential for recurrent bleedings and local resorption of bone with loosening of the internal fixation device. Stability at the site of osteotomy and the attainment of an adequate angle of correction should be entrusted to V-osteotomy, which protects the alignment of the fragments at any necessary angle. The operation is supplemented with a snug plaster cast until roentgenographically ascertained consolidation at the site of osteotomy. Mainly applied for the knee, osteotomy is performed according to the prevalent site of deviation either at the femoral supracondylar level or the tibial infracondylar level [1703] (Figs. 279, 280, 283, 284).

Total arthroplasty may be indicated for the knee [1721] and hip joints [278, 1152] in cases of very advanced deformity of the articular epiphyses and essential impairment in the function of these joints. While initial results appear promising in a satisfactory percentage of these operations [52, 990], a longer period of follow-up is necessary to ascertain the definite benefits. A modification of lesser extent for the hip joint is resurfacing arthroplasty [40, 1702]. The mobility of the elbow joint can be restored by economic resection of the radial head and extensive synovectomy of the joint capsule. The marked functional disorder caused by voluminous enlargment of a hemophilic pseudotumor requires prophylactic and/or early treatment. Doehring et al. [435] emphasized the necessity of supplementing the clotting factor for prevention of further bleeding, regular elevation of the affected part of the body, and local firm compression. If a pseudotumor nevertheless develops and causes symptoms, surgical treatment is indicated also for excluding a possibly malignant tumor and for preventing infection. Arthrodesis as primary choice appears indicated in advanced alterations of the wrist and ankle joint, but this should not be secured by compression devices for internal or external metallic fixation [279]. Internal fixation may be entrusted to a firmly impacted, arrow-shaped bone graft [1549] (Figs. 209, 210, 214, 215, 216, 217) and should be supplemented by immobilization by a well-molded plaster cast.

With the possibility of performing effective operative procedures, it is imperative before embarking on such procedures to ascertain hematologically a possible presence of inhibitors against the clotting factors. If such inhibitors are present, plasma replacement would not succeed in stopping the bleeding; therefore any surgical treatment is precluded.

b. Arthropathy in Lymphocytic Leukemia and Multiple Myeloma

Disorders of the blood manifested in excessive proliferation of some of its white cell types are rather often associated with arthritic symptoms. These are elicited either primarily by affection of the articular tissues through local accumulation of white cells emerging from the blood stream or secondarily by white cells spreading from the bone marrow of the epiphyses into the joint capsule and articular cartilage. These blood disorders causing symptoms of arthritis are lymphocytic leukemia and multiple myeloma [368, 618, 634].

According to its course, prevalent affection of patients as to age, hematological findings, and prognosis, lymphocytic leukemia may be of the acute or the chronic type.

Acute lymphocytic leukemia is a malignant expansion in B lymphocyte precursors [821] and occurs more frequently in children aged 3–10 years than in adults. Concurrently, the affection appears primarily in the joints in 20%–35%, and secondarily in the joints in 65%–80% of these patients. Nevertheless, the general symptoms in most patients with acute lymphocytic leukemia are similar and are manifested in elevation in temperature up to 40° C, sweating, pallor, pronounced malaise with prostration, weakness, and anorexia. Concurrently, intense pain is felt more often and of longer duration [1495] in the long bones than in the joints. The articular impairment is usually symmetrical in children but not in adults. On pauciarticular distribution in the extremities the fingers, wrist, elbow, shoulder, hip, knee, or ankle are affected, with the wrist, knee, and ankle being affected distinctly more often. These joints may be merely tender, but are usually also enlarged by swelling of the joint capsule. Joint fluid is sometimes increased in the elbow, knee, or ankle joint. The vertebral column is also tender along extensive areas, and its movements are avoided because of pain. The often associated peripheral neurological symptoms are caused by leukemic infiltrates in the marrow of the vertebral column. Even more worrisome are the leukemic infiltrates when accompanied by meningeal irritation and symptoms of the cranial nerves. Regional

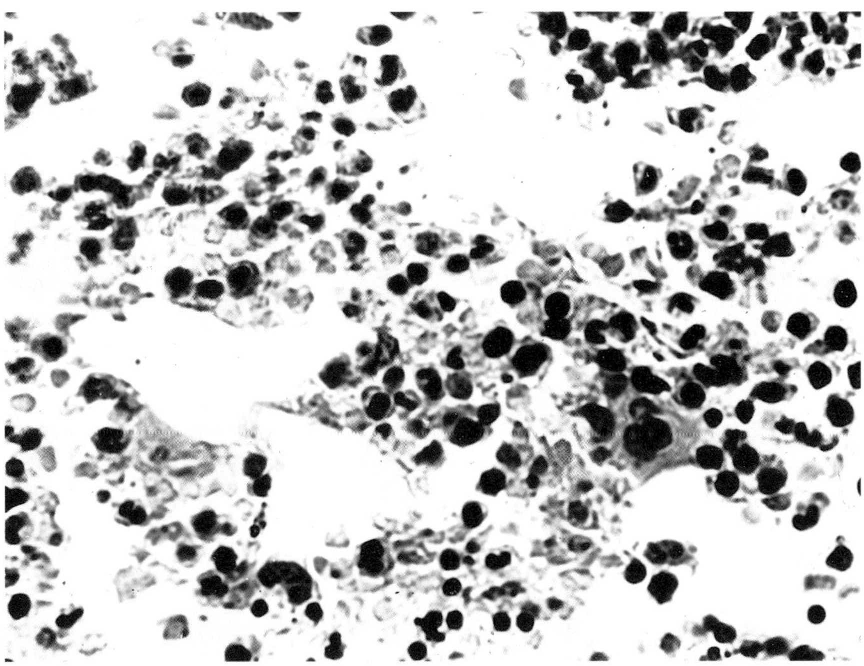

Fig. 418. Blood smear contains a distinct increase in mature lymphocytes and among them a large number of immature lymphocytes

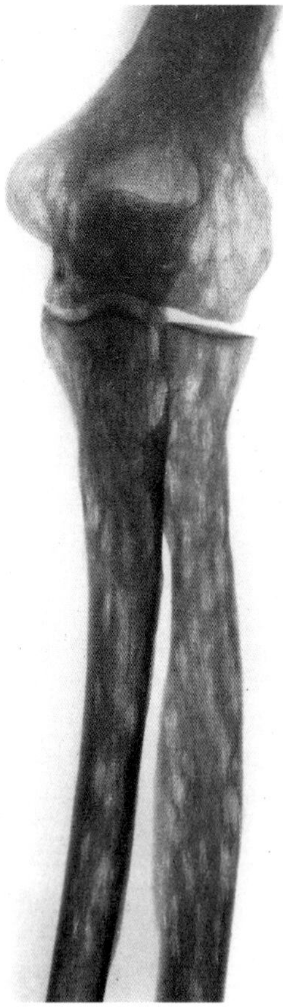

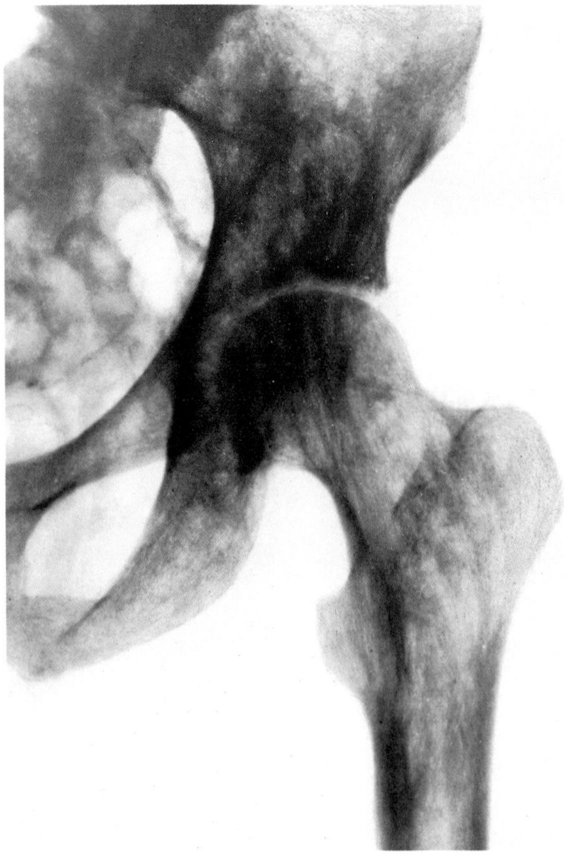

Fig. 419. The distal part of the humerus and the entire ulna and radius are penetrated by numerous areas of radiolucency bordered by sclerosed bone. The joint cleft between humeral condyle and radial head is uneven and slightly narrowed

Fig. 420. An area of the pelvic bone and the proximal part of the femur are extensively rarefied by radiolucenct areas. The joint space is unevenly delimited

lymph nodes are usually enlarged, and subcutaneous nodules can be palpated in the forearm and lower leg. Liver and spleen are enlarged in about 40% of cases, and the spleen may become very painful upon infarction.

In the laboratory studies, the sedimentation rate is elevated to 35–60 mm/h, especially in adults. The stained blood smear (Fig. 418) presents a predominance of immature lymphocytes and lymphoblasts [1100, 1767]. The latter are larger (15–22 μm) and have an abnormal cytoplasmic ratio and large nuclei of round, indented or lobulated outline. The nuclei contain fine chromatin particles and a few nucleoli [697]. The cell count discloses an increase of these cells up to 10000/ml in the majority of patients but between 10000 and 50000/ml in others [821]. Neutrophilic leukocytes and erythrocytes are distinctly decreased due to the substantial predominance of immature lymphocytes and lymphoblasts. The smear of aspirates from the bone marrow presents a greater percentage of lymphoblasts. Uric acid in the serum is often elevated to 10–12 mg% due to breakdown of an excessive quantity of nucleic acid; therefore, this condition has also been classified as secondary gout [1620]. The tests for rheumatoid factor yield positive results at a high titer in 20%–25%, especially in adults, and so are the tests for antinucleic antibodies. In the cases of joint effusion with an overwhelming proportion of abnormal lymphocytes (5000–50000/ml), a clue is offered to the pathological blood condition which affects the joints, provided that an active inflammation of other etiology (tuberculosis) can be disregarded.

Roentgenographs in acute lymphocytic leukemia [296, 1232, 1495, 1637] reveal, although less pronounced than in chronic lymphocytic leukemia (Figs. 419, 420), spots and slightly larger areas of radiolucency within the cancellous bone of the extremities. Thickening of the cortical bone sometimes also develops secondary to endosteal and periosteal detachment by lymphoblastic infiltration. Moseley [1143] emphasized transverse bands of radiolucency across the metaphyses as a characteristic, but not pathognomonic sign in children. This is a manifestation of lymphocyte-suppressed enchondral bone formation. In adults the areas of intense osteoporosis or radiolucency in the marrow spaces are wider. These occur in the bones of the extremities, with occasional irregular thickening of the cortex, as well as in the skull, vertebral bodies, and pelvis.

Punch biopsies or arthroscopies with removal of specimens from the affected joint capsule disclose (Fig. 421) extensive and dense agglomerations of im-

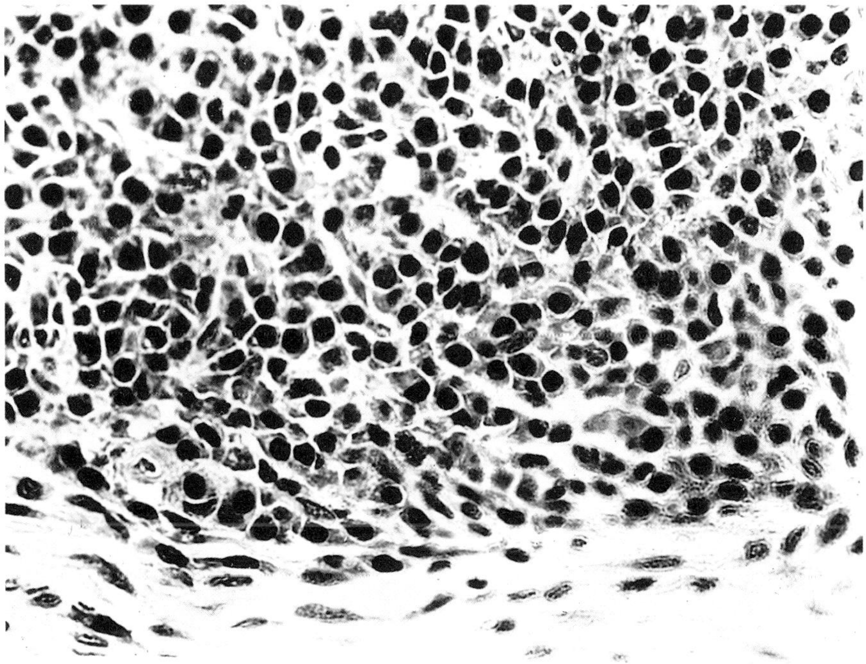

Fig. 421. The peripheral part of the joint capsule contains extensive dense accumulations of mature lymphocytes, among which larger lymphoblasts are scattered

mature lymphocytes in the subsynoviocytic tissue up to the fibrous capsule. However, in other cases no characteristic infiltrates of lymphocytes, but hyperemia and extensive edema, are observed in the joint capsule, an indication that the joint swelling in these cases has been elicited by an immunobiological reaction against the antigens of the lymphocytes in leukemia [1560, 1637]. On the other hand, biopsies of bone from areas of rarefaction invariably disclose widening of the marrow spaces which are extensively filled principally with blast cells. These spaces are bordered by thin trabeculae along which osteoclasts and small giant cells lie.

Differential diagnosis must consider acute arthritis of rheumatic fever and juvenile rheumatoid arthritis in children and rheumatoid arthritis in adults. However, the roentgenographically revealed multiple lytic areas in the bones and their histopathological examination provide a clue to the underlying lymphocytic leukemia.

At the start of treatment a thorough examination must ascertain whether the persistent fever is not caused by the coexistence of an infection. In this situation, administration of the indicated antibiotic and sufficient hydration are the necessary therapeutic measures [1777]. Subsequently a substantial benefit is obtained in 90% of children with acute lymphocytic leukemia by prednisone 30–40 mg daily during 4–6 weeks [1637]. For induction treatment cortisone is followed by or administered with vincristine 1.5–2.0 mg intravenously once weekly for 3 weeks, daunorubicin 30–60 mg daily for 3–5 days and repeated after 3–4 weeks, cytosine arabinose 100–200 mg in daily infusions for 1 week and repeated after 4 weeks, or asparaginase 1000 IU intravenously for 10 days [821, 1777]. These cytotoxic medications may also be used for maintenance of remission or may be alternated with methotrexate 4–6 mg daily for 2–3 weeks, chlorambucil 4–10 mg daily for 3 weeks, mercaptopurine 75–150 mg daily for 2–3 weeks, cyclophosphamide 50–100 mg for 1–2 weeks, or doxorubicin 60–75 mg once in 3 weeks [697]. The potential adverse effects of these cytotoxic and alkylating or antimetabolic medications are gastrointestinal disorders, inflammatory changes of the skin, aplastic anemia, renal failure, and disorders of the central nervous system. With leukemic areas in the skull or spine complicated by symptoms of the central nervous system or peripheral nerves, radiation treatment with 20 Gy is necessary. In adults with acute lymphocytic leukemia the chemotherapy is similarly implemented. The course of these medications is carried out until suppression of the lymphoblasts is ascertained.

Combination of the therapeutic modalities provides remission for up to 5 years, especially in children; even a lasting cure may be obtained in about 50% of children [821, 1777]. However, less encouraging results are obtained in adults. The prognosis is even more guarded in cases with a great number of immature lymphocytes and lymphoblasts prevailing in the blood at the initial examinations. Eventually the prognosis becomes hopeless in patients with extensive leukemic infiltrates in the lungs, heart, liver, and kidneys.

Chronic lymphocytic leukemia is characterized by a substantial increase in B-lymphocytes [821] in the blood and bone marrow. In contrast to acute lymphocytic leukemia, the chronic form rarely occurs in children but is increasingly frequent with advancing age. Symptoms are rather moderate and include weakness, headache, general malaise, and loss of appetite. Temperature is irregularly and moderately elevated to 39.2°–40.0°C but becomes regularly and more elevated with concurrent internal infection. Clinical examination discloses occasional macular, small vesicular or exfoliative dermatitis on the trunk and extremities, and regionally enlarged lymphnodes. Spleen and liver may also be enlarged. A few joints (elbow, hip, and knee) or diaphyseal areas of the extremities are enlarged and moderately tender, but not limited in their movements. The vertebrae may be moderately tender, and sometimes painful on extensive infiltrates. However, in contrast to acute lymphocytic leukemia, neurological symptoms originating from the skull or spine are very rare.

Blood studies disclose a lymphocyte count above 5000/ml and up to 100000/ml [821], with most of these cells being of the normal small size (9–10 μm). However, a moderate number of lymphocytes may be pleomorphic and larger than average; their nuclei are of irregular or indented outline (Fig. 418). Erythrocytes and platelets are diminished in numbers. The smear of bone marrow presents a distinct increase in lymphocytes and a larger number of immature lymphocytes. Thus it substantiates the diagnosis in cases in which the lymphocyte level in the blood does not present conclusive findings. Roentgenographs of the long bones (Figs. 419, 420) and vertebrae disclose irregularly delimited or diffuse osteoporosis and only occasionally small and sharply delimited areas of bone erosion. Histopathological examination of biopsies from thickened joint capsule (Fig. 421) discloses diffuse spread of small lymphocytes and somewhat larger lymphocytes with irregularly outlined nuclei in the subsynoviocytic zone and up to the fibrous capsule.

Before treatment all cases with elevated temperature should be evaluated to determine whether an infection is not the cause; this requires antibiotic treatment. Otherwise, prednisone 50–80 mg is daily given for 6–8 weeks, which results in a distinct alleviation of symptoms by the regression of infiltrates [1473]. However, in situations with persistent symptoms such as fever, loss of appetite and body weight, increase in enlarged lymph nodes, progressive enlargement of spleen and liver, anemia and thrombocytopenia, and aggravation of articular and osseous symptoms, chemotherapy by cytotoxic drugs must be instituted. In induction treatment, vincristine 2.0–4.0 g intravenously once weekly or chlorambucil 4–10 mg daily for 3 weeks is administered. If inadequate remission is obtained, cyclophosphamide 40–100 mg daily for 1 week, methotrexate 4–6 mg for 1 week, or mercaptopurine 75–150 mg is given daily for a week and then repeated after 3 weeks [697]. The effects of these cytotoxic medications and the necessity of switching from one to another are indicated by periodic counts of white blood cells. Treatment is continued until normalization of these counts and should be supplemented with administration of allopurinol 200–300 mg daily. This eliminates the excessive concentrations of uric acid resulting from the decomposition of the leukemic nuclei. Follow-up blood studies at 3- to 6-months intervals provide information on whether the treatments should be repeated [152]. In cases of excessive localized accumulation of lymphocytes and extensive enlargement of the affected organs (lymph nodes, spleen, liver, vertebrae), local radiation with 15–20 Gy is indicated. With more extensive or excessive leukocyte infiltrates, whole-body radiation with 30–40 Gy may provide significant improvement or complete remission.

Multiple myeloma is a disorder characterized by excessive proliferation of mature and immature plasmacytes as well as of myeloma cells and by concomitant excessive production of abnormal immunoglobulins. It occurs almost exclusively in adults aged between 50 and 65 years, many of whom have suffered or are suffering from chronic infection. General symptoms are pallor, weakness, loss of appetite and body weight, and frequent fatigue associated with irregular elevations in temperature. Multiple myeloma also often causes episodes of rather intense and localized pain in the long bones, ribs, and/or vertebrae elicited by osteolytic lesions in these bones. Pain becomes more aggravated with the occurrence of pathological fractures in the ribs or long bones, causing periods of disability. When affecting the skull or vertebral bodies, the myelomatous proliferations may compress the regional nerves and cause symptoms from the cranial nerves or intervertebral nerve roots. On expansion of the lytic lesions within bones and developing hypercalcemia, apathy, polydipsia, and polyuria become pronounced symptoms. By advanced proliferations, the spleen and liver become enlarged. Furthermore, in the late phase extensive depositions of abnormal globulins in the kidneys lead to obstruction and degeneration of renal tubules and thus to renal failure. Intercurrent infections are frequent complications.

In conjunction with the affection of the bone, multiple myelomata also occur in joints in about 15%–20% of these patients [258, 753, 1174] after they had appeared in the bones. The joints affected without symmetricality are those of the fingers, wrist, elbow, shoulder, hip, knee, and ankle. They are tender and

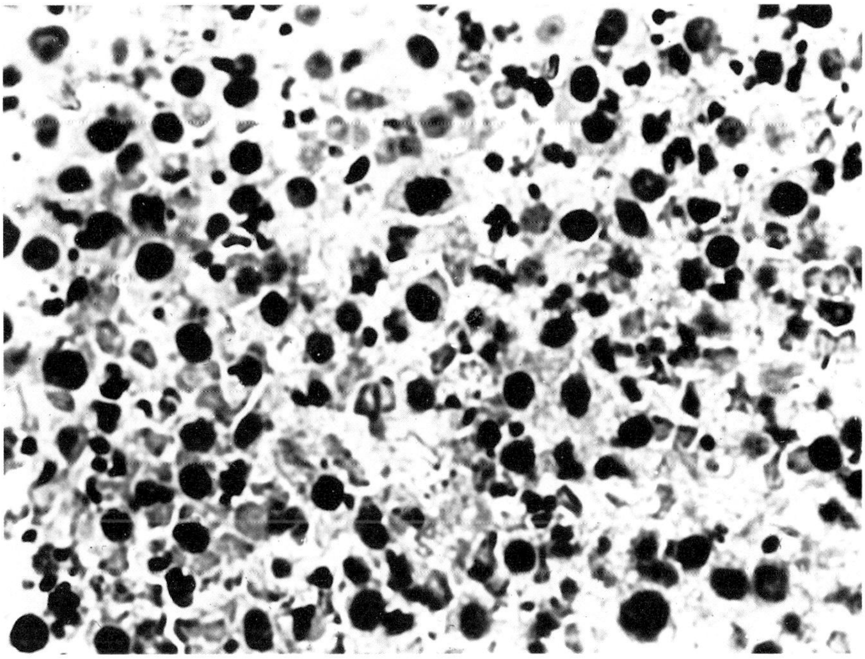

Fig. 422. The blood smear discloses the presence of a significant proportion of plasmacytes, among which myeloma cells occur

often present rather dense swelling of the joint capsule [651]. When these hard infiltrates are of larger extent, the range of motion becomes concentrically limited; eventually contractures of the finger, elbow, and knee joints develop. A carpal tunnel syndrome may occur due to compression in amyloid arthropathy of the wrist. Extensive infiltration of the glenohumeral joint capsule may produce a characteristic shoulder pad appearance [651].

Of the laboratory studies, the sedimentation rate is invariably elevated to 35–60 mm/h due to the increase in globulins to 3.9–5.0 g%; total proteins are 6.8–8.0 g%, and albumin is 3.0–3.4 g%. Accordingly, electrophoresis shows a large band in the gammaglobulin region, and immunoelectrophoresis discloses that these proteins correspond to the IgG, IgA, IgM, and IgI. On extensive osteoclasis and disintegration of large bone areas, calcium salts appear at an increased concentration of 11 mg/dl and higher in the serum. Consequently, calcium salts are deposited in the renal parenchyma. Examination of the blood smear discloses that the neutrophilic leukocytes are relatively decreased, but that plasmacytes and immature lymphocytes (Fig. 422) have appeared, with the former being distinctly increased [1100, 1767]. Examination of the bone marrow is more instructive, especially when obtained from the areas of radiolucency. This discloses a significant proportion of plasmacytes densely aggregated in sheets or heaps. Between them myeloma cells are scattered, which are 20- to 35-μm large, round or ovoid, and contain one or two nuclei 5–7 μm in size. The single nucleus is eccentrically located; its chromatin is not as dense as in the normal plasmacyte, nor is the wheelspoke arrangement present. The cytoplasm is basophilic and often contains spherules (Russel's bodies), which are immunoglobulin. In cases of malignant proliferation, one also observes a significant percentage of atypical myeloblasts and atypical plasmacytes, with large bizarre or multilobated nuclei [924]. Uric acid in the serum may be elevated to 16.8 mg% due to excessive breakdown of nucleic acid from the disintegrating plasmacytes, leading to secondary gout [1620]. Results of the test for Bence-Jones protein, representing amyloid derived from the light-chain IgG produced by the abnormal plasmacytes [362, 1524], are positive in the urine in 45%–60% of cases. This finding may be practically regarded as pathognomonic for multiple plasmacytoma. Elimination of paraproteins (amyloid) through the kidneys may lead to obstruction of nephrons and to marked impairment in the renal function. Joint fluid, when increased in amount, is cloudy and contains an increased concentration of mucin and a larger number (1200–5000 ml) of white blood cells. These are represented by a few polymorphonuclear leukocytes but particularly by lymphocytes and plasmacytes.

Roentgenographs reveal [737] sharply delimited, "punched-out" areas of homogeneous radiolucency in the skull (Fig. 423) and/or some long bones of the extremities (Fig. 424). With further duration such areas appear in the pelvis and other bones of the extremities (Fig. 424). Moseley [1143] reported that lesions occurring in the ribs and vertebrae may be of uneven radiolucency and unsharp outline and thus may be inter-

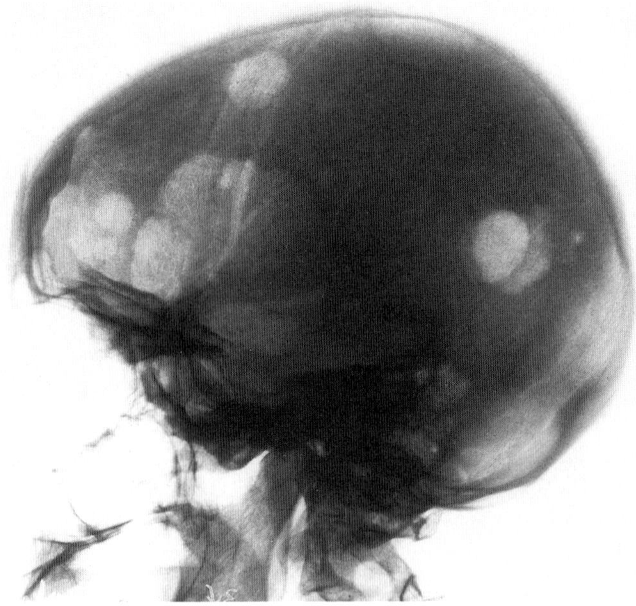

Fig. 423. The skull is penetrated by several areas of rather extensive, sharply demarcated radiolucency

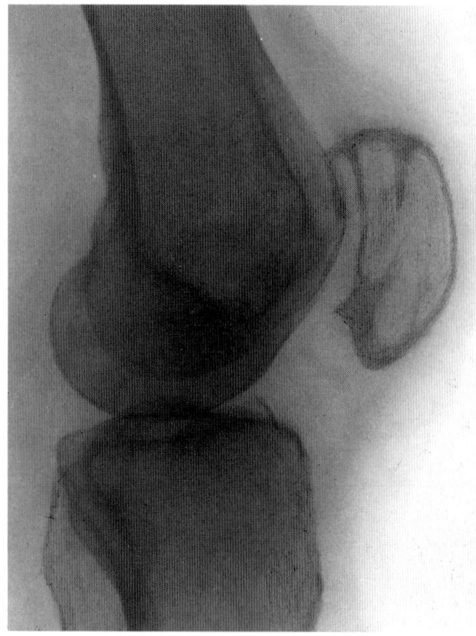

Fig. 424. The patella is extensively penetrated by an area of intense radiolucency which left only a thin cortical border

preted as metastases or inflammatory conditions. Other occasional changes are focal sclerotic lesions in intramedullar areas, fairly uniform sclerosis of the medullary cavity, and cortical thickening with perpendicular spicules. Pathological fractures may eventually occur in the ribs, long bones, and vertebrae, leading to their compression.

Gross-pathological examination [36, 1119] (Fig. 425) discloses that the femoral neck and trochanteric area, similarly to the humerus, are overlain by moderately soft bags. Their dissection discloses them to be filled with a white cheesy material. An identical material completely fills the trabecular meshes of the femoral head and trochanteric area (Fig. 426).

Histopathological examination of specimens removed from the punched-out areas of bone lesions disclose that these areas, similarly to the blood smears (Fig. 422), are filled with myeloblasts and a significant number of abnormal plasmacytes, and are bordered by a conspicuous number of osteoclastic giant cells. It appears that these myeloma cells and plasmacytes do not directly erode the bony trabeculae but exert a stimulating effect on the osteoclasts, provoking their enlargement and enhancing their bone eroding activity.

Histopathological examination of the joint capsule (Fig. 427) discloses hypertrophic synoviocytes and diffuse infiltrates of lymphocytes and/or plasmacytes in the subsynoviocytic tissue. Larger, irregularly delimited areas in this tissue are occupied by an eosinophilic amorphous material, which stains metachromatically with toluidine blue. Small deposits of similar material are observed in the wall of middle-sized arteries and veins. The material of these deposits is amyloid resulting from the action of proteolytic enzymes produced by the plasmacytoma [258], and it extends from the subsynoviocytic zone peripherally into the fibrous capsule [1119, 1753]. The material, appearing homogeneous on light microscopy [36], stains pinkish red with hematoxylin-eosin and is metachromatic on crystal violet or toluidine blue. It also stains specifically with Congo red, with which under polarized light it displays an apple-green birefringence [164, 258, 1579, 1592]. The enlarged synoviocytes stained with Congo red display a content of amyloid under polarized light. Similarly, most of the precipitated material from the joint fluid stains with Congo red. Gallo et al. [561] emphasized the usefulness of immunofluorescence microscopy for identification of amyloid deposits in tissue. The osteocartilaginous surface (Fig. 428) bears an intensely hematoxylin-stained articular cartilage in which the chondrocytes are diminished. Some of the chondrocytes are hypertrophic, and others are fragmented. The subchondral subcortical spaces are extensively and densely filled with a few lymphocytes and numerous plasmacytes. A few myeloma cells are scattered among the latter.

Franklin et al. [540] maintained that the initial concept, amyloid being deposited in situations in which the antigenic stimulus is excessive for the immune system, had to be revised. The reason for this was the finding that the biochemical make-up of amyloid varies

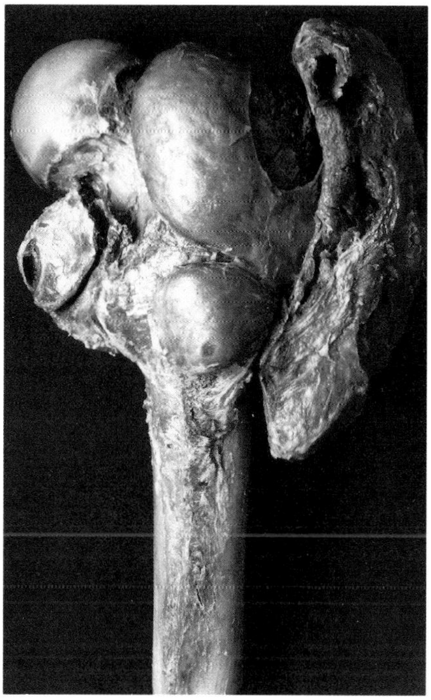

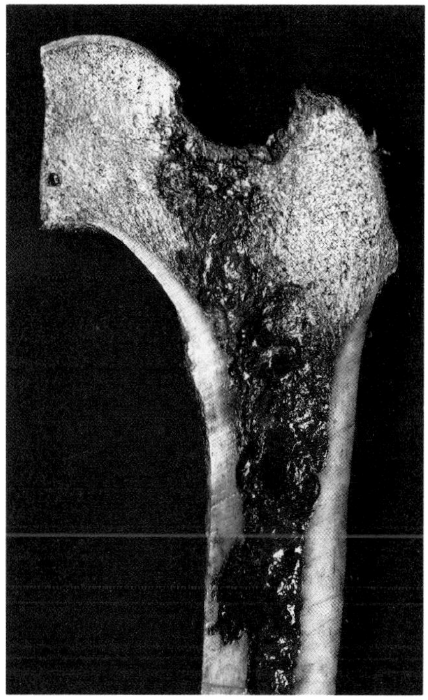

Fig. 425. The lateral area of the femoral neck and the intertrochanteric area are covered by baglike formations filled with amyloid

Fig. 426. The femoral head and the proximal part of the neck as well as the greater trochanter are filled in their cancellous bone with amyloid

in different conditions [966]. Primary amyloid, associated with multiple myeloma, consists of Ig light chains [619] while the secondary amyloid, which accompanies chronic inflammatory conditions such as rheumatoid arthritis, derives from serum amyloid A [619]. Immunochemical and sequence analyses of Bence-Jones protein by Prelli et al. [1279] revealed antigenic and structural features not previously described for the Ig light chains. Amyloid polymerizes to fibrils which were found [1277] by fractionation to be composed of three proteins as determined by their amino terminal sequence. Electron-microscopic studies [307] revealed that the amyloid consists of two distinctly formed elements: thin fibrillar components and a pentagonal unit.

Differential diagnosis of the articular changes must consider rheumatoid arthritis [1446] and arthropathy in

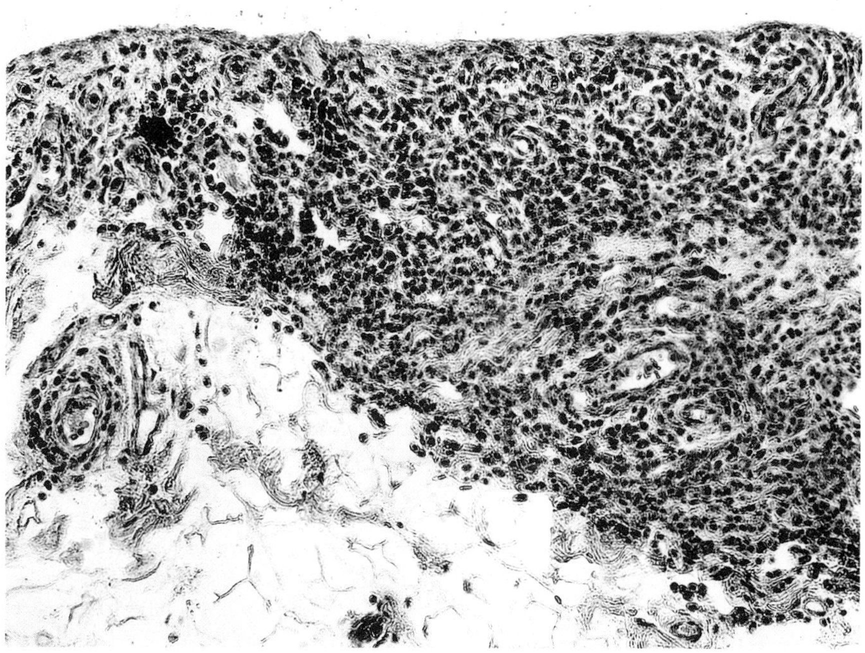

Fig. 427. The synovial membrane comprises in its superficial zone a broad accumulation of plasmacytes among which a few myeloma cells are scattered

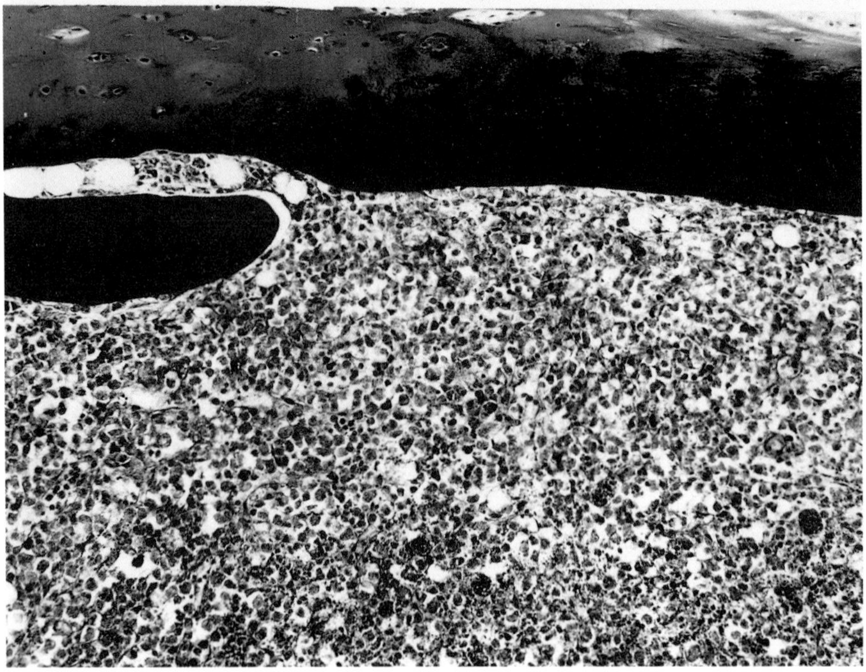

Fig. 428. The subchondral subcortical area comprises an extensive, rather dense accumulation of plasmacytes, among which typical and atypical myeloma cells are scattered

psoriasis [553], which in rare instances may contain amyloid deposits in the joint capsule. Goldberg et al. [624] pointed out that articular and paraarticular deposits of amyloid in multiple myeloma simulate the clinical picture of rheumatoid arthritis. Yet the multiple small and large lytic lesions in the skull, long bones, and pelvis may have been caused by metastases originating from a carcinoma of the lungs, breast, thyroid, or ovaries. Histopathological examination of lesions which contain a significant percentage of plasmacytes and myeloma cells, examination of a blood smear presenting a similar cell content, and abnormal globulins identified by immunoelectrophoresis assist in identifying the forelying lesions as caused by multiple myeloma.

In view of the extensive areas of osteoporosis, especially in the long bones and vertebrae, the patients should avoid very long periods of bedrest and be advised to be as active as possible. Braces or other orthopedic devices are often necessary for protection of the lower extremities and for prevention of pathologic fractures. Medicamentous treatment is started with prednisone 50 mg daily, given for 3–6 weeks. This reduces soreness and pain in the bone, but has little effect on the extensive bone lesions. Therefore, prednisone should be combined with an alkylating cytotoxic agent [697, 821, 924, 1777]. Mephalan 1.5–2.0 mg three times daily for 5–7 days and repeated after 3–4 weeks, cyclophosphamide 50–150 mg daily for 1–2 weeks and repeated after 3 weeks, or chlorambucil 4–10 mg daily for 3–4 weeks and repeated after 1–2 months is usually a very helpful addition to prednisone. However, if not effective, one of the following cytotoxic drugs should be administered: vincristine 2–4 mg daily for 3 weeks and repeated after 4 weeks, arabinoside 100–200 mg daily for 2 weeks and repeated after 4 weeks, cytosine 100–150 mg daily for 3 weeks and repeated after 4 weeks, mercaptopurine 100–200 mg daily for 2 weeks and repeated after 4 weeks, or methotrexate 5–10 mg daily for 1 week and repeated after 2–4 weeks [697]. The effect of these chemotherapeutic agents is periodically evaluated by blood counts and by examination of the smears from bone marrow. Accordingly, chemical treatment is continued as long as myeloma cells and immature plasmacytes are noticed. In addition, radiation treatment with 15–30 Gy is strongly recommended for expanded and very painful lesions of the peripheral skeleton or for solitary lesions of the skull and vertebrae. The latter lesions have the potential to encroach upon the central nervous system. Normalization of the count and percentage of the white cells in the blood and of the thrombocyte count indicates the beneficial effect of these treatments. Concurrently, the concentration of the monoclonal gammaglobulins decreases, and thus also the formation of amyloid, which is partly eliminated in the urine. Nevertheless, the frequent adverse effects of cytotoxic drugs and especially of the antimetabolites must not be disregarded; these include suppression of the bone marrow manifested by pancytopenia. Thus, regular examination of the blood is an indispensable safeguard in these treatments.

In the course of multiple and extensive plasmacytoma, decalcification of the bone is followed by a significant increase in the calcium concentration in blood and urine [924]. The great potential for nephrocalcinosis and renal failure requires abundant intake of fluids and the administration of sodium phosphate and allopurinol 300 mg twice daily. Colchicine 0.6 mg two or three times daily is beneficial for decreasing the painful attacks on the bones. Combination of these therapeutic modalities provides a satisfactory remission [821, 1777], approaching a cure, in about 50%–60% of the patients. In the other patients, the prognosis is very guarded due to the high potential for infections, hypercalcemia, and renal failure.

6. Joint Affections in Neuropathies

Anatomical and especially histological examinations of the joint capsule disclose that the synovial membrane, articular ligaments, and fibrous capsule contain myelinated and nonmyelinated nerve fibers. These have the shapes of free endings (Fig. 10), treelike ramifications (Fig. 10), or encapsulated endings as the Golgi-Mazzoni and Vater-Pacini corpuscles (Fig. 11) [386, 871, 1299 1794]. Other free endings enter the articular tissues by their location in the walls of the blood vessels (Fig. 10) which surround and intrude the joints.

Most of these nerve endings actually are the incepts of the emerging nerves which, in association with nerves originating from other deep organs and the skin, convey the sensations of proprioception, pain, and deep touch. The united afferent nerves enter the spinal cord via the spinal ganglion and posterior root. From the posterior horn these nerves emit association collaterals, which synapse with motor ganglion cells in the anterior horn. This establishes the pathway of the direct reflex (Fig. 429). However, the major part of the nerve fibers ascend in the dorsal column. The shorter of these fibers cross in the white commissure and synapse with secondary neurons which ascend anterolaterally in the spinothalamic tract (Fig. 429) and arrive in the contralateral thalamus opticus. From there tertiary neurons depart, terminating in the corona radiata, the sensory sphere of the cerebrum (Fig. 429). The longer nerve fibers ascend in the dorsal (Clarke) column, where they synapse with secondary neurons ascending in the tractus spinocerebellaris dorsalis, pass through the medulla oblongata, and enter the cerebellum through the corpus restiforme [653, 1623] (Fig. 429). Other secondary neurons from the dorsal column pass as the tractus spinocerebellaris ventralis through the medulla oblongata into the mesencephalon, from which they terminate retrogradely through the brachia conjunctiva in the cerebellum (Fig. 429). Thus the proprioceptive sensations are conveyed partly as conscious elements to the cerebrum and partly as unconscious elements to the cerebellum [653, 1623].

Resulting motor impulses are emitted from the cortex and subcortical nuclei of the cerebrum. The main motor tract is the lateral corticospinal or pyramidal tract, which originates from the cortical pyramidal cells. Their fibers converge to a compact bundle and enter the medulla oblongata. There they divide into a few bundles which cross and continue in the lateral corticospinal tract (Fig. 429). Another centrifugal tract, also crossing into the contralateral fascicle, is the rubrospinal tract, which runs to the end of the lumbar spinal cord. All these neurons carry motor impulses and synapse with ganglion cells in the anterior horn [653, 1623] (Fig. 429). Identical functions are fulfilled by the secondary neurons in the anterior corticospinal, tectospinal, and vestibulospinal tracts in the anterior fascicle. The ganglion cells in the anterior horn emit efferent nerve fibers which run in the anterior nerve roots and convey motor impulses to the voluntary musculature (Fig. 429). Along with the efferent nerve fibers also run sympathetic nerve fibers which originate from sympathetic preganglionic cells located in the lateral horn of the spinal cord (Fig. 429).

The rich supply of the joints throughout with nerve endings of various shapes and apparently of various functions in conveying different sensations indicates the elementary role of the nerves as regulatory organs in the trophic and function of the joints. Consequently, disruption in the role of the nerve fibers is invariably followed by a profound impact on the biology and function of the joints.

With clinically ascertained disorders in the central nervous system or peripheral nerves [1782] the function of the joints is basically impaired due to lack of sensory control and inadequate action of the regional musculature. Secondary to loss of proprioceptive reflexes, which protect the joints from uncoordinated or exaggerated movements, alterations in the constituent articular structures invariably set in, and spontaneous fractures may occur [830]. Substantially impaired use of the joints is the result. Permanent dysfunction eventually leads to conspicuous deformation and dysorganization of joints [102, 276, 470, 839, 912, 1529]. Such changes occur in congenital and acquired affections of the brain, spinal cord, peripheral nerves, or all of these in combination:

Alcoholic neuropathy and neuropathy in other circulatory impairment
Diabetic neuropathy

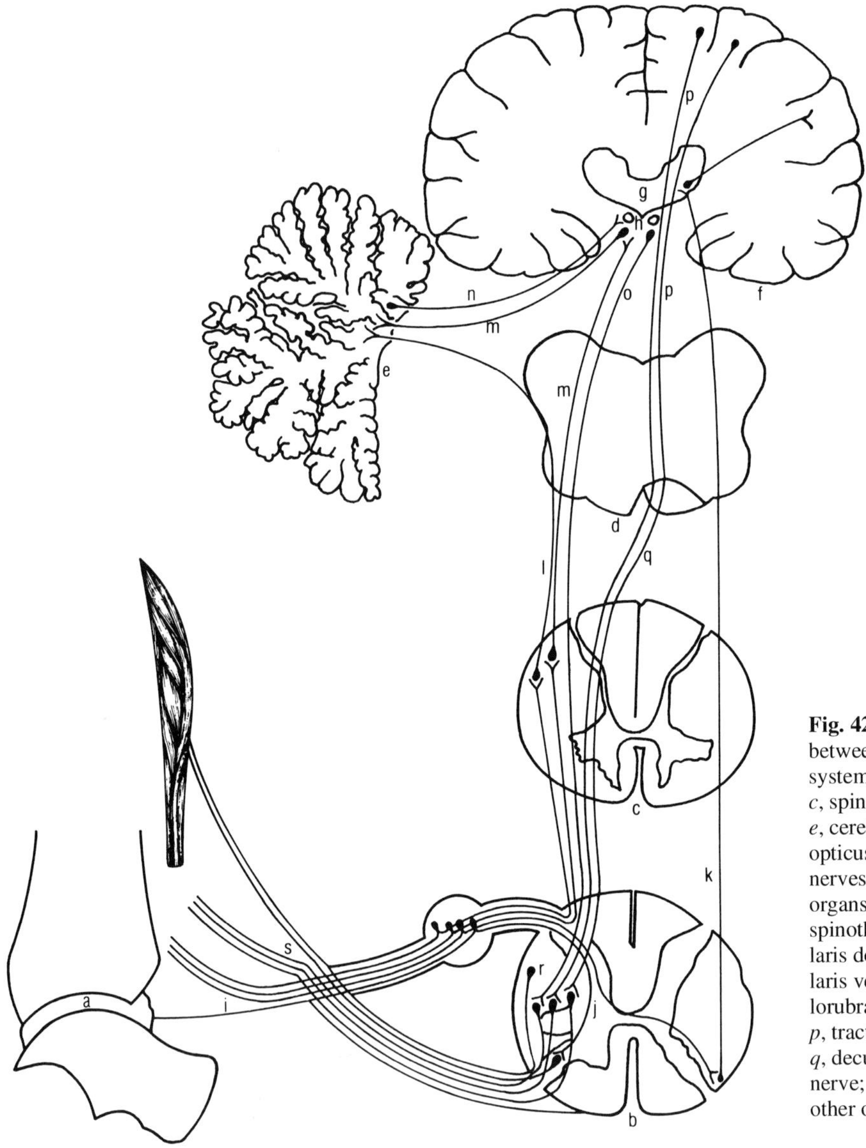

Fig. 429. The mutual relationship between the joints and the nervous system: *a*, ankle joint; *b*, spinal cord L4; *c*, spinal cord T1; *d*, medulla oblongata; *e*, cerebellum; *f*, cerebrum; *g*, thalamus opticus; *h*, nucleus ruber; *i*, efferent nerves from ankle joint and other organs; *j*, reflex collateral; *k*, tractus spinothalamicus; *l*, tractus spinocerebellaris dorsalis; *m*, tractus spinocerebellaris ventralis; *n*, tractus cerebellorubralis; *o*, tractus rubrospinalis; *p*, tractus corticospinalis lateralis; *q*, decussatio pyramidum; *r*, sympathic nerve; *s*, efferent nerves to muscles and other organs

Tabes
Syringomyelia
Multiple sclerosis
Paraplegia or hemiplegia
Meningitis or arachnoiditis
Gliomatosis of the spinal cord
Injuries to the spinal cord in fractures, stab wounds, or shot wounds
Myelodysplasia
Spina bifida with myelomeningocele
Pernicious anemia and degeneration of spinal cord
Injuries to peripheral nerves
Familial dysautonomia or other hereditary neuropathies
Congenital analgia
Leprosy

a. Arthropathy in Chronic Alcoholism and Other Aseptic Necrosis

In regard to the sequelae of chronic alcoholism, it has become evident that one of its noxious effects is necrosis of the femoral head and neck. This represents about 17%–29% of all cases of aseptic necrosis of the femoral head [789, 790, 814, 1227]. While the etiology of bone necrosis in alcoholism has not yet been fully clarified, it appears that obliteration of the regional blood vessels [406, 836] by fat embolism is one of the factors responsible for disruption of the local circulation. This is supported in part by the findings of a disorder of fat metabolism with hyperlipemia in 53% of patients with chronic alcoholism [309, 712]. Thus fat embolism probably also accounts for the analogous necrosis in the humeral head, distal end of the femur, and proximal part of the tibia in chronic alcoholism.

This view of the etiology is further substantiated by the finding of intravascular fat globules in some resected femoral heads [789, 790, 1227] and of fatty degeneration of the local bone marrow. Furthermore, Melanotte et al. [1088] emphasized that general organic, local, and functional pathogenetic factors may be responsible for the local interruption in the blood supply in many cases of aseptic necrosis of the femoral head. Another frequent cause is thrombosis of the terminal blood vessels occurring in sickle cell anemia. This leads to infarction and necrosis of bone in the femoral head and neck and sometimes in other bones of the extremities [955, 1464].

The expanding ischemic necrosis of the subchondral bone accounts for a substantial decrease in the resistance of the articular surface to any stress, which unavoidably initiates degenerative articular changes. These changes become conspicuously manifested in the area corresponding to the extent of the necrosis and where continued weight bearing is superimposed on the femoral head. Unlike in other causes (abnormal hemoglobinemia, hyperuricemia, or prolonged use of steroids), an additional and specific factor in alcoholism compounds the aggravating changes of the arthropathy. Victor [1688] and others [1581, 1743] emphasized the development of peripheral neuropathy in chronic alcoholism due to noninflammatory toxic changes of the peripheral nerves. These are manifested histopathologically in degeneration of the myelin sheath and axis cylinder. In advanced cases both the anterior and the posterior nerve roots are affected.

Such impairing features occur in about 9%–10% of patients with chronic alcoholism [814]. The prevailing symptoms are those of polyneuropathy involving principally the lower extremities and less often the upper extremities. In very severe cases the central nervous system (cerebellum) is also affected, as manifested by concurrent ataxia [1743]. The disuse particularly of the lower extremities which is associated with these neurological deficiencies, is invariably followed by substantial aggravation of the articular changes, initiated by ischemic osteonecrosis of the articular ends. The patients thus affected are predominantly men, aged between 35 and 55 years, who for 2–5 years have experienced sensations of tingling, pricking, heat, or burning in the extremities, more frequently in the lower than in the upper extremities. Also, weakness is experienced in the arms and legs and

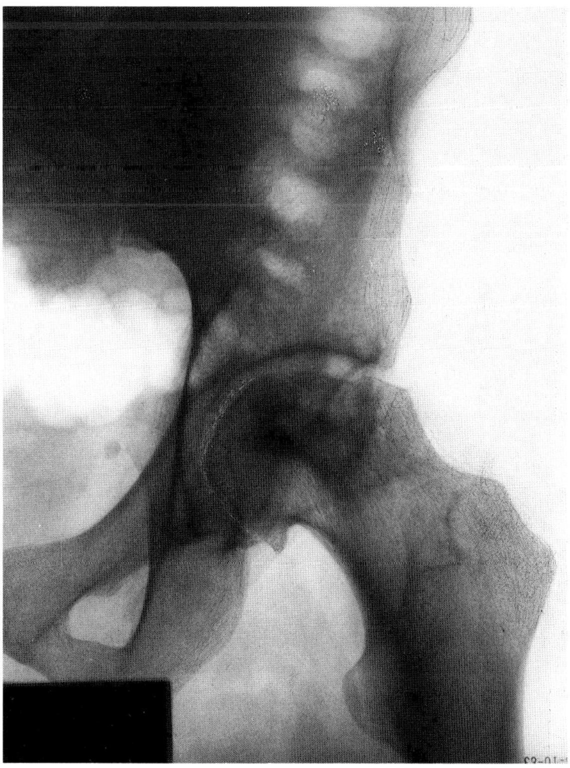

Fig. 430. The femoral head is depressed in its upper area, which also is sclerosed in wedge outline. The joint space is widened in this area and otherwise is uneven. Osteophytes protrude at the inferior margin of the joint space

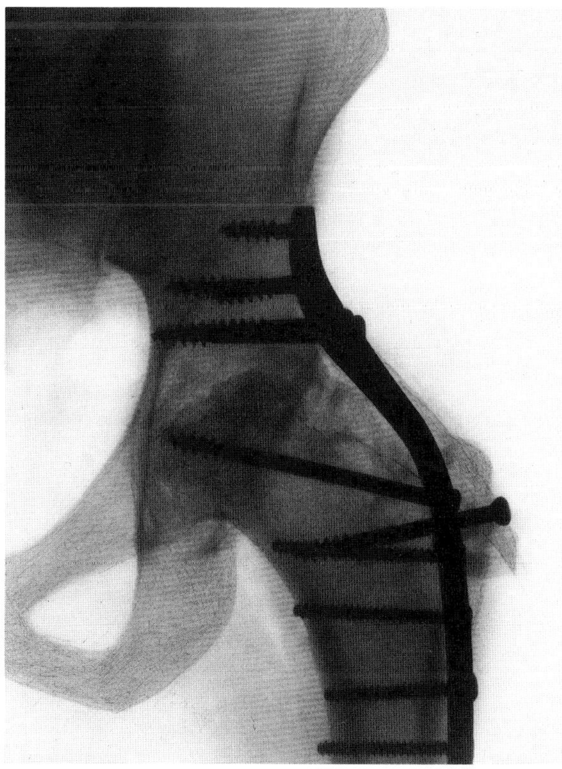

Fig. 431. Arthrodesis of the hip joint in Fig. 430 by insertion of a cobra plate and by apposition of a bone graft

subsequently increasing pain. Pain in the shoulders becomes manifest on extreme or forceful movements of the arms. Pain in the hips, thighs, and lower legs becomes aggravated on standing and walking, which leads to ambulation becoming minimized.

Examination of the usually emaciated patients, with a history of irregular and improper nutrition, shows a generally neglected condition with abnormal pigmentation of the reddish face, thickened skin on the nose and lips, shrunken and wrinkled skin over the entire body, and enlarged liver. Neurological examination discloses varying signs of affection of the sensory, motor, and/or autonomic nerves. The perception of touch, pressure, pinprick, temperature, and vibration is markedly diminished, especially in the lower extremities; anesthesia in a symmetrical, stockinglike pattern is very common. The musculature of the thigh or calf may be very sensitive, even painful, to pressure; it lacks the normal tonus, and its motor response is decreased. Concurrently with aggravation of the sensory symptoms, the anterior tibial, peroneal, and calf muscles have diminished or have lost their functions and become atrophic. The deep reflexes of the lower extremities are usually depressed or completely absent. The resulting foot drop and stomping gait worsen the attritional changes in the joints of the lower extremities. Plantar flexion contracture of the ankle joint sometimes ensues. Intense perspiration of the lower legs and feet indicates harm to the autonomic nerve fibers. On tenderness in the groin and its anterior aspect, the motion of the hip joint is usually limited in terms of internal rotation and abduction. The knee joint presents a distinct thickening of the joint capsule, sometimes associated with a flexion contracture and most often with coarse grating. Thus the mechanics of the major peripheral joints is distinctly impaired; added to this shortcoming is the unreliable function of the musculature.

Laboratory studies reveal anemia and decreased albumin with increased globulin and bilirubin. Some serum enzymes (alkaline phosphatase, glutamic-oxalacetic transaminase, and glutamic-piruvic transaminase) are invariably elevated [309, 1508], indicating the extent of the damage to the liver cells. The most sensitive test is that for bromosulfaleine retention, which is distinctly elevated in liver damage [712]. Except for the latter, all tests approach normalcy on discontinuation of alcohol intake and on resumption of normal nutrition [712]. Electromyographic examination discloses the presence of fibrillation potentials and random fasciculations in the muscles of the lower extremities. Conduction velocity in the major nerves of the lower extremities (anterior femoral, peroneal, tibial) is decreased, and motor unit potentials are larger.

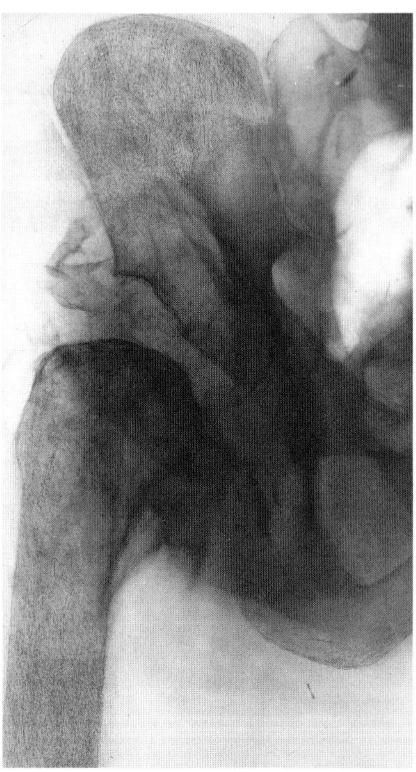

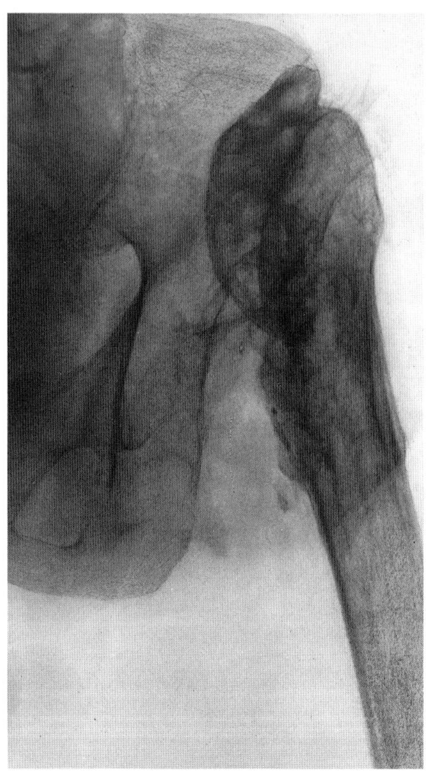

Fig. 432. The joint space is excessively widened due to extensive attrition of the acetabulum. The femoral head is partly worn off and sclerosed

Fig. 433. The roof of the acetabulum is completely worn off. The femoral head, excessively worn off and yet of roundish outline, is upward dislocated

Of important diagnostic value are the roentgenographs [1193], which in the initial stage reveal a wedgelike area of density (Fig. 430) directly beneath the articular surface of the femoral head. This area is bordered in the progressing phase by one of radiolucency and irregular structure. Peripherally and distally to this follows normally structured bone. These distinct differences change with longer duration of the condition. The dense area becomes mottled partly by deposition of osteoid along the necrotic bone and partly by hypercalcification of necrotic bony trabeculae (Figs. 432, 433). In the lucent area, new formation of bone sets in, and provides a fine trabecular structure. Thus, irregularly delimited areas of sclerosis and of osteoporosis alternate, indicative of genuinely weakened structure (Figs. 432, 433). The weight-bearing ability of the femoral head is substantially decreased. Consequently, it progressively loses its roundness in the central and cranial areas. Following this deformation, deformation also takes place in the contiguous acetabular surface. On expanding attrition of the acetabular roof the femoral head subluxates from the joint (Fig. 432) and eventually becomes completely dislocated (Fig. 433). The tomograph separates these alterations into planes and provides information on the extent of osseous changes in the depth, especially where density of the overlying soft tissues obscures the structural details of the bone. Important information of the evolving structural alterations is also provided by scintigraphy, which by scanning osseous tissue for absorbed radionuclides, phosphonates labeled with radioactive tritium, permits early identification of these changes before they become evident by radiography [361, 620, 677, 1816, 1817]. Scintigraphy indicates cold areas (Fig. 19) in the early phase due both to absent blood supply in the necrotic area and to diminished local uptake of radionuclides. In the increasing uptake of the radioinuclides (Fig. 20), it also reveals beginning of restructuring, secondary to revascularization and apposition of new bone, as the repair of bone progresses [361].

Pathological-anatomical examination [260, 1088, 1227] discloses areas of moderate unevenness and discoloration in the articular cartilage. With longer duration the cartilage presents wide clefts (Fig. 434) and is separated in places from the subjacent bone. On sagittal section (Fig. 435) three zones are evident here [1227]. Immediately beneath the hyaline cartilage and close to the surface lies a wedge-shaped zone of gray-white coloring and irregularly structured necrotic osseous tissues (Fig. 435). This is surrounded by a zone of whitish gray tissue of soft consistency. At the outer margin follows a zone of regular trabecular structure and of normal osseous consistency. Corresponding to the width of the necrotic zone, the femoral head is indented over a rather large extent and has lost its roundness as well as its congruency with the acetabulum. However, this clear structural delimitation becomes irregular and almost indistinct in later phases when restructuring changes of the osseous tissue take place.

Histopathological examination (Fig. 436) in the early phase of necrosis discloses that the articular cartilage is of normal structure on most of its extent. Hypertrophic chondrocytes are present in a few areas

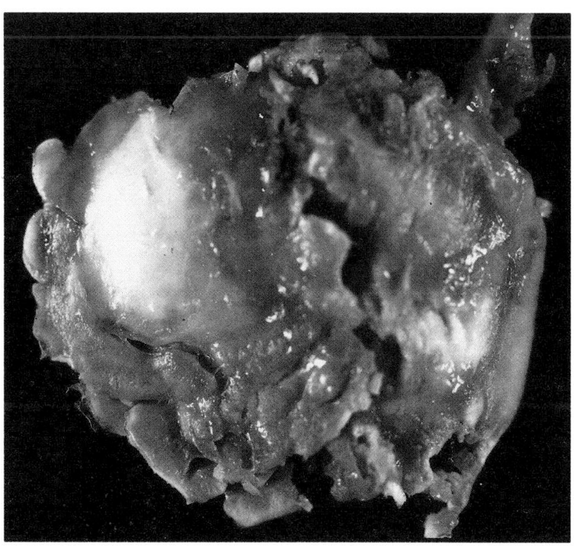

Fig. 434. The articular cartilage from a femoral head is very uneven by several extensive areas of attrition

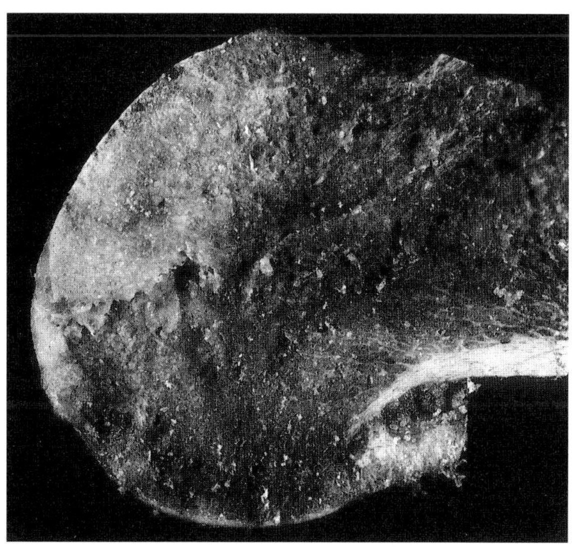

Fig. 435. A wedge-shaped whitish area in the femoral head indicates necrosis and local lack of circulation

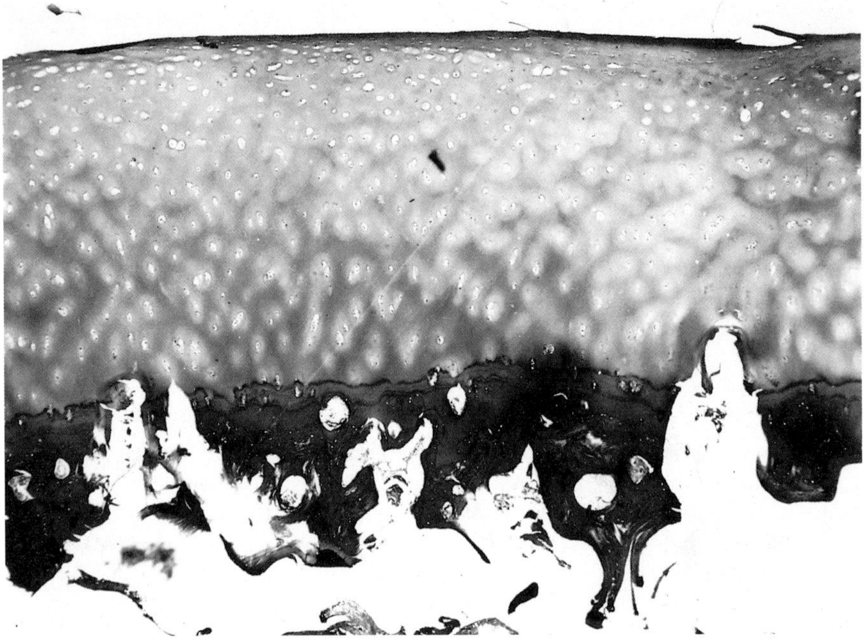

Fig. 436. The articular cartilage contains a few lacunae from chondrocytes in the superficial zone. The subchondral bone is necrotic over its entire extent

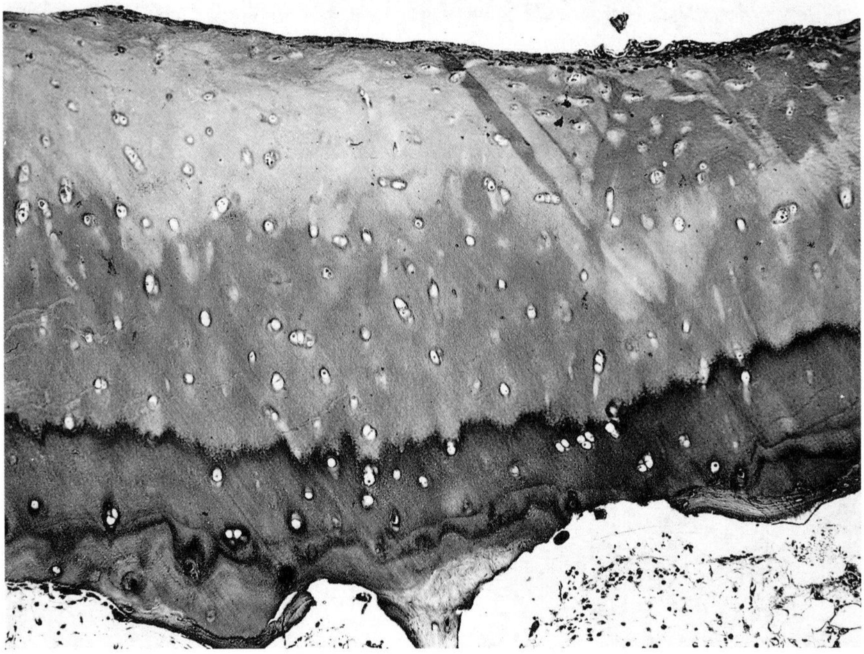

Fig. 437. The articular cartilage comprises empty lacunae from chondrocytes in all zones. The subchondral bone is necrotic all over, and the narrow spaces comprise granulation tissue and young connective tissue

[1088]. In the immediately subchondral and deeper zones, most bone trabeculae comprise lacunae left after osteocytes (Figs. 436, 437). Some of these trabeculae are very thin, and others are compact and irregularly arranged. Directly neighboring is a zone composed of loose connective tissue (Fig. 437) which contains hyperemic blood vessels. Peripheral to this is an adjacent zone in which vivid formation of new bone trabeculae takes place, partly by membranous and partly by enchondral ossification. In a later phase extensive resorption and thinning of bone trabeculae by osteoclasts takes place in the necrotic zone. The overlying articular cartilage comprises numerous lacunae and disintegrating ground substance (Fig. 437). Its interstitial fibers are unmasked, and extensive clefts are formed. Concurrently, vivid new ossification in the peripheral osseous zone expands into the fibrous zone and farther into the necrotic zone. In the latter, newly formed trabeculae of osteoid become ossified but do not have normal mechanical alignment. Concomitantly with these changes and the disintegration of the articular cartilage, the articular surface collapses.

In view of the breakdown of chronically alcoholic patients, psychological reeducation appears an elementary initial step in general treatment. For the cooperative patient systematic muscle training, massage, electrical stimulation of the weak musculature, and galvanization along the nerves are physiological and promising modalities. Higher doses of nonsteroidal antiinflammatory medications are indicated for the articular pain and should be combined with a few series of sessions of shortwave diathermy. The latter, by producing deep heat, may also have a beneficial effect on revascularization of necrotic areas in the articular epiphyses. On marked deformation of articular ends arthroplastic procedure may be considered only in those patients who manifest insight into the detriments of their former habits and a determination to alter these. Improvement in general condition then becomes evident in normalization of metabolism and most significant laboratory tests, except for that of bromosulfaleine retention. However, in view of the almost invariably associated neuropathy, restoration of the peripheral musculature is unlikely. A successful outcome of arthroplasty is here very questionable. Therefore, with severe impairment in the function of a joint (especially the hip joint) and its regional musculature, arthrodesis [73] by operative denudation of the articular surfaces and internal fixation of the epiphyses (Fig. 431) appears the more advisable treatment. This restores stability in a very unreliable extremity. However, where the symptoms of cerebellar ataxia are already manifest, an operative procedure cannot succeed and thus should not be embarked on.

b. Arthropathy in Diabetic Neuropathy

While diabetes is basically a metabolic disease, the incident arthropathy is not caused by any abnormal metabolites occurring in diabetes and possibly affecting the synovial membrane and hyaline cartilage. On the other hand, clinical examinations of patients with diabetes of longer duration (more than 3–5 years) disclose that most of them suffer from neuropathies. These are sequelae of impaired trophic of peripheral nerves secondary to alterations in the walls of blood vessels in diabetes. In the ensuing involvement of the peripheral nerves, chiefly their sensory and sympathetic fibers are affected. The pain sensation becomes lost mainly in the lower extremities, with maintenance of the motor capacity. Concurrently, the loss of or decrease in sympathetic tonus leads to regional vasodilatation associated with hyperemia and osteoporosis of bones. In agreement with Foster et al. [529], clinical observations point out that affections particularly of the sensory fibers of the peripheral nerves and of their posterior root ganglia are responsible for the disuse of the joints. At the same time, the motor nerve fibers and muscles often remain intact. In addition to the lack of proprioceptive reflexes, repeated minor injuries or intensive use, with frequently coincident overweight, account for the excessive attrition of joints.

Since the weight-bearing joints are more exposed to overuse, the tarsometatarsal, midtarsal, and ankle joints display more often than the other joints of the extremities the changes of diabetic arthropathy [48, 1706]. The joints of the lumbar spine are rarely affected. Thus the ankle and midtarsal joints have traditionally been regarded as the prototypes of manifestation of diabetic arthropathy. However, more recent publications [235, 467, 501, 1447] indicate that on longer duration of diabetes the joints of the upper extremities are also often affected. The patients are over middle age and mostly men. They sometimes experience pain in the upper or lower extremities, but more often they have become aware of the impaired use through clumsiness and inadequate control, rarely mixed with soreness, of the joints of the feet (Fig. 443). These patients often volunteer the information of suffering from diabetes for a period of several years. The affected joints display moderate to marked thickening of the joint capsule and of the surrounding soft tissue. The enlargement becomes more conspicuous when subluxation and deviation supervene, principally in the ankle, midtarsal and/or elbow joints. These subluxations are clinically discernible in the ankle joint by faulty alignment, with valgus deviation and lateral subluxation, in the foot by complete flattening of the longitudinal arch, and in the elbow joint by valgus deviation. The movements in these joints are free of pain, but they are carried out along new and false axes. Marked osteoarthritic changes characterize the affected joints during clinical examination (Figs. 442, 443).

The neurological examination discloses a varying picture of disorders [839] consisting of: (a) irritations of posterior nerve fibers and nerve roots, manifested by lancinating pain and tenderness of peripheral nerves along their course; (b) predominant but moderate affection of anterior nerve fibers, resulting in weakness and atrophy of muscles of the extremities; or (c) combined but unequal involvement of sensory, motor, and autonomic nerve fibers. The eventual effects are primarily lack of pain on pinprick, of temperature sensation and vibratory sense, muscle weakness and atrophy, and hyperemia and altered local temperature [199, 1720].

In the first type, with sole involvement of the sensory nerve fibers, symptoms start with lancinating pain or burning sensation in the extremities. These gradually change to numbness and anesthesia with symmetrical and extensive glove- or stockinglike distribution; eventually decreased proprioception, extensive paresthesia and anesthesia, and absence of regional reflexes ensue. The loss of sensitivity is followed by frequent traumatization even on pressure by tight shoes, propensity for local infection at the slightest harm, and tendency to very slowly healing trophic ulcers. The second type, with selective involvement of the motor fibers, is very rare and is associated with paresis of the major muscles of the lower extremities, such as quadriceps, anterior tibialis, and peronei. The regional deep tendon reflexes are often depressed or even absent. The last type, polyneuropathy, is most often observed and presents involvement of the different types of nerve fibers to a varying degree; the sensory fibers are predominantly affected, the motor fibers are less affected, and the autonomic fibers are sometimes almost as intensely affected as the sensory fibers.

Diagnostically characteristic for all these patients are the laboratory findings related to abnormal carbohydrate metabolism as manifested in the significantly increased fasting blood sugar and glucose tolerance test. Levels of fasting blood sugar above 120 mg/dl are suggestive of and levels above 150 mg/dl diagnostic of diabetes mellitus. The glucose tolerance test is carried out during an unrestricted diet containing at least 150 g carbohydrate daily for 3 days. If two or three consecutive blood specimens drawn at 2-h intervals contain a concentration of 200 mg/dl sugar in plasma, diabetes mellitus must be diagnosed [712]. Electromyographic examinations disclose early degenerative changes in nerve fibers by determining the sensory potential amplitudes and spinal somatosensory conduction [199]. The tests for nerve function disclose significantly impaired and slowed conduction velocity, especially in the median, tibial, sural, and peroneal nerves, indicative of loss of the large motor axons [199, 706].

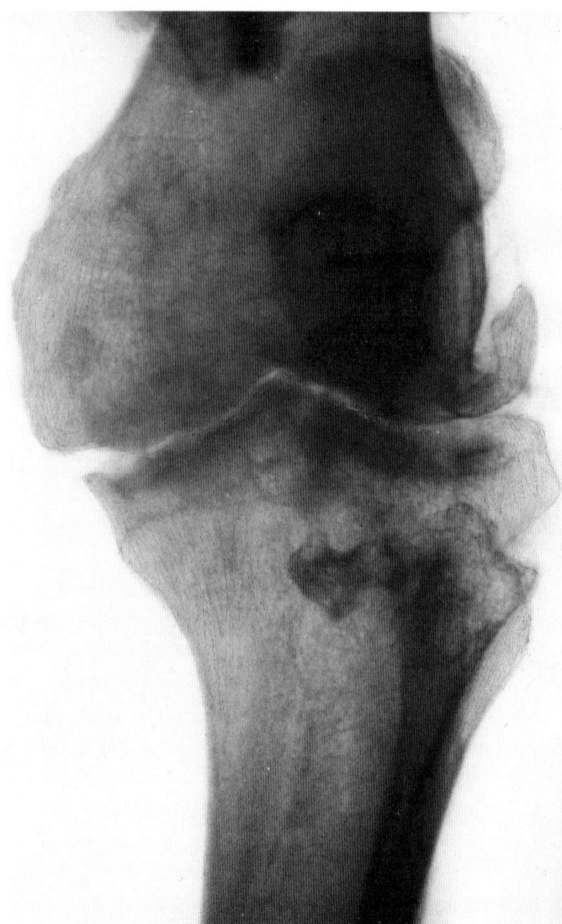

Fig. 438. The articular ends of the femur and tibia are sclerosed and worn off, and osteophytes rise from their margins. The joint space is narrow

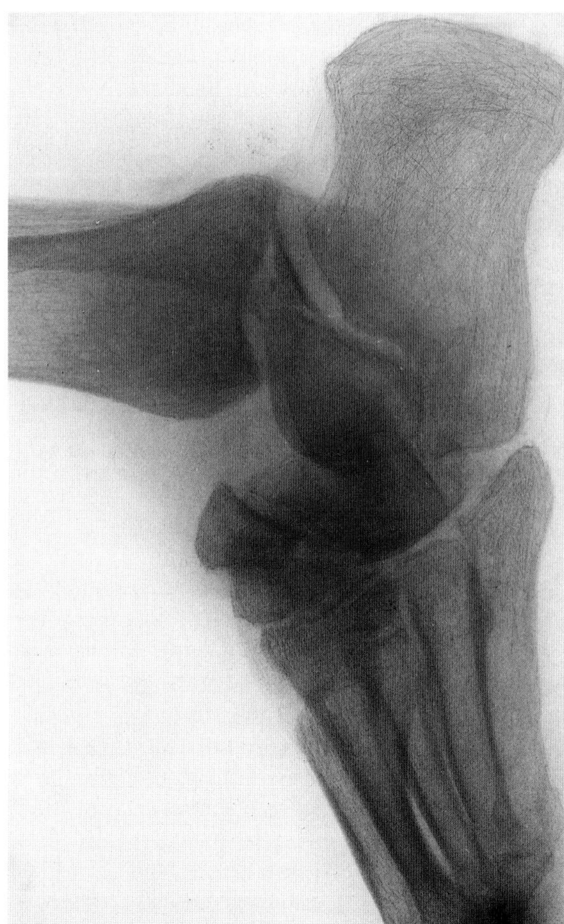

Fig. 439. The body of the talus is compressed, thinned, and subluxated. The joint space between talus and calcaneus is narrowed. The cuneiforms are dislocated dorsally

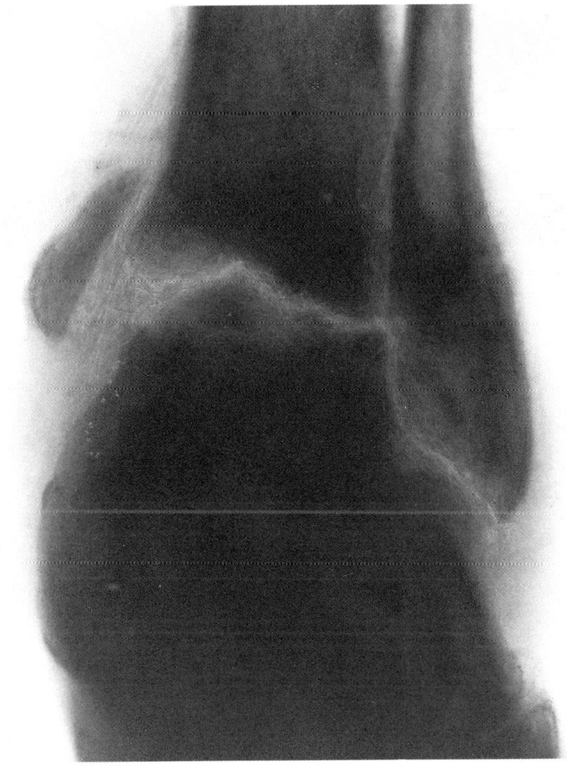

Fig. 440. The medial malleolus is widely separated from the tibia. The joint space between the tibia and talus is very uneven, and the contiguous epiphyses are sclerosed

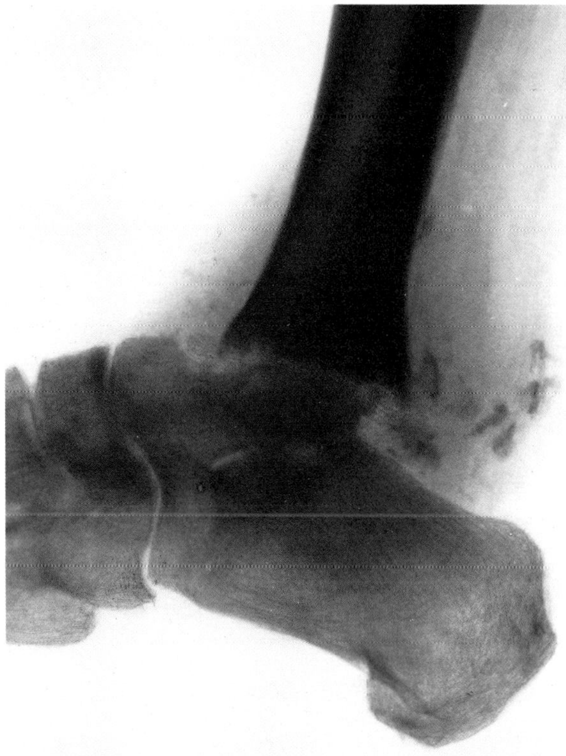

Fig. 441. The joint space between tibia and talus is very narrow and uneven. The tibial epiphysis is sclerosed, and the body of the talus is compressed. Bone fragments lie in the periarticular tissue

Roentgenographs [235, 303, 469, 501, 1193] are very informative as to the extent of alteration both in the articular epiphyses and within the joints. These generally reveal atrophy and osteoporosis, which with progression may lead to complete resorption and disappearance of bone (Figs. 439, 440) with the lack or scarcity of reactive new bone formation. The specific bone changes in the shoulder joint are deformation of the humeral head by subchondral bone resorption at irregular delimitation and widening of the glenoid cavity. In the elbow joint the lateral humeral condyle and/or, more commonly, the radial head become partly disintegrated, with deformation of their articular surfaces and lateral deviation of the forearm. In the fingers juxtarticular cortical erosions occur. The knee joint (Fig. 438) presents attrition of the tibial condyles with contiguous sclerotic bony changes and with substantial narrowing of the cartilage space or with subluxation. Similar changes may be noted in the hip joint. The ankle joint displays marked swelling of the joint capsule and extensive osteoporosis as well as fragmentation of the head of the talus (Figs. 439, 441); the latter is subluxated secondary to fracture of a malleolus (Figs. 440, 441). Similar extensive and almost pathognomonic resorption is noticeable in the tarsal bones, which may be fragmented into loose portions (Fig. 439), whereupon the longitudinal arch of the foot is completely abolished. The tarsometatarsal joints present fragmentation and osteoporosis alternating with sclerosis of their articulating bones, which are separated from each other with resultant subluxation (Fig. 439).

Gross-anatomical examination discloses marked thickening of the inner part of the joint capsule pertaining to any affected joint and more pronounced in the ankle and midfoot joints. This part has lost its pliability, is rather dense, and encapsulates a number of osteocartilaginous fragments obviously stemming from the articular epiphyses. The latter present in the ankle and knee joints extensive irregularity and disruption of their surfaces (Figs. 442, 443) by broad defects secondary to separation of fragments. More deeply extending fragmentation involves the cranial surface of the talus (Fig. 443), which has lost its alignment with the tibial articular epiphysis and is most often laterally subluxated secondary to displaced fracture of the fibular end. These alterations are more extensive and varied in the intertarsal and tarsometatarsal joints (Fig. 443), in

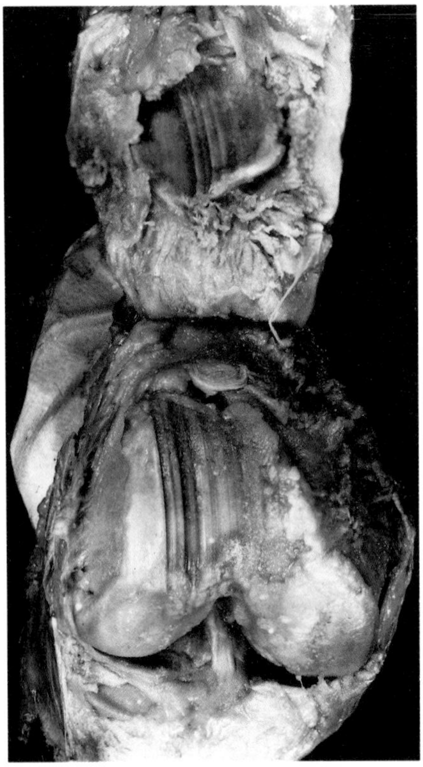

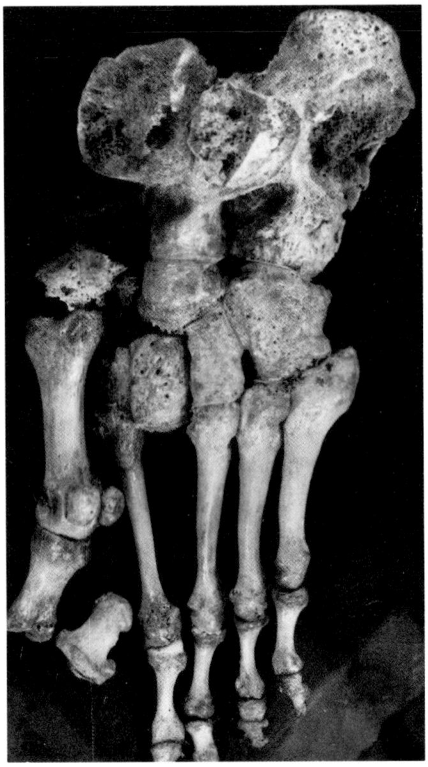

Fig. 442. The articular surfaces of the patella and femoral condyles are worn off and remain over small extents with their articular cartilage. Their central areas are deepened by cartwheel traces

Fig. 443. The articular surfaces of the talus, toward the tibia and the calcaneus are extensively worn off, as are the surfaces between the cuboid and metatarsals. The first cuneiform is worn off and subluxated

which the articulating bones are broken up into a number of fragments. Some of these are large and sclerosed, and others are small and soft from osteolysis [967, 1078].

Histopathological examination discloses that the articular cartilage (Fig. 444) is disrupted by vertical and horizontal clefts, with large fragments separated from the uneven surface. The remaining deeper zone of the cartilage contains fragmented nuclei and numerous lacunae empty of chondrocytes. Large free fragments from the articular epiphyses present sclerosis and partly necrosis of osseous tissue, while small fragments are osteoporotic. The synovial membrane is thickened and fibrosed up to the surface. This is disrupted in a few areas through which large fragments composed either of hyaline cartilage and subchondral bone or solely of cartilage have been dislodged into the depth (Fig. 445). No extensive inflammatory infiltrates are observed, but rhomboid calcium crystals sometimes lie in proximity to these intracapsular fragments.

The almost invariably present neurological signs concomitant with the pronounced disorganization of a joint point to a neuropathic alteration. Especially syringomyelia for the upper extremity and tabes for the lower extremity must be considered, in addition to all other possible etiologies of neuropathic joint disorganizations. However, the bony changes in the first two arthropathies are predominantly of the sclerosing type, whereas those in diabetes are more of the atrophic and rather catabolic type. Guided by a complete neurological examination and considering the pronounced deformities of the lower extremities, the laboratory studies regarding the carbohydrate metabolism succeed in elucidating the etiology.

In view of the sensory impairment and the poor healing tendency in diabetes, treatment of the arthropathies should preferably be conservative. It can be easily and routinely implemented for the elbow and knee by a brace with metal hinges and for the knee, ankle, or midtarsal joints by a plaster cast or stiff brace. Such immobilization is indicated especially when a fracture arises. In cases with excessive lateral subluxation in the ankle joint, osteotomy at the smallest extent through the fibula may be indicated to correct the deviation, and this should be supplemented with a plaster cast or a stiff brace. A similar treatment may suffice in disorganization of the midtarsal joints, where the longitudinal arch may be restored by osteotomy or arthrodesis through the midtarsal bones. After completion of the plaster cast immobilization, a supportive brace is invariably indicated. Arthrodesis of the ankle joint, even reinforced by a compression clamp, is not advisable because of the poor consolidation ability of the talus.

Equally, any operative procedure in or close to the knee joint, including supracondylar osteotomy of the femur or infracondylar osteotomy of the tibia, is not

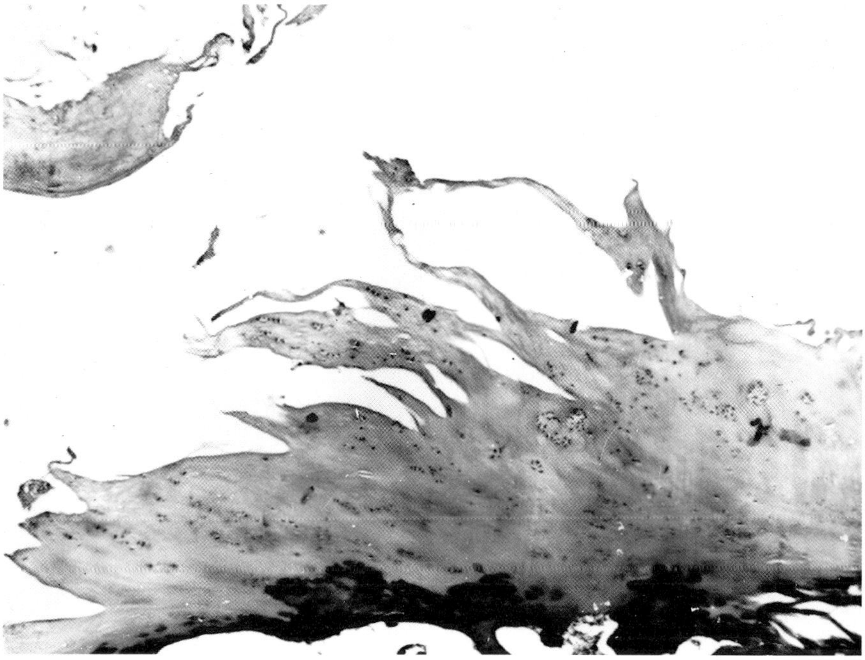

Fig. 444. The articular cartilage is thinned, and its surface is disrupted by several clefts. A large fragment is separated

advisable because of the impaired healing potential. In view of the probability of postoperative infection and poor consolidation tendency, the outcome may be very serious in such complications; amputation may present the final solution. Villiaumey et al. [1691] therefore pointed out the grave prognosis in diabetic neuropathy and advised early prophylactic measures especially concerning the lower extremities.

Nevertheless, Gerhart et al. [598], Skolnik et al. [1527], and Sprenger et al. [1562] performed arthroplasties in diabetic hip joints and reported satisfactory results. Long-term follow-up examinations are indicated in all operative cases to evaluate the duration of benefits provided by surgical modalities in the treatment of diabetic arthropathies.

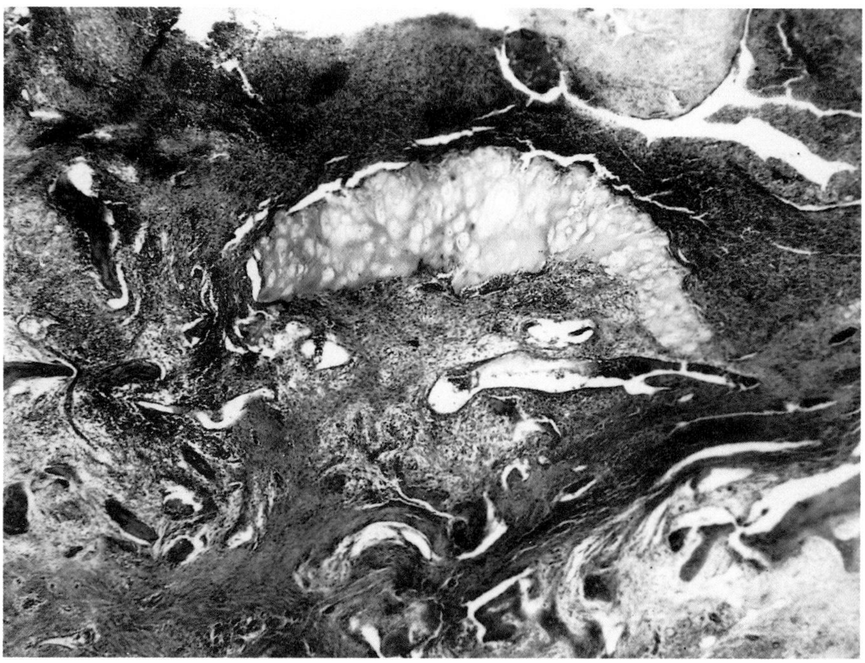

Fig. 445. The synovial membrane is very cellular and extensively thickened. It comprises a loose portion of articular cartilage and a denuded articular surface

c. Arthropathy in Tabes

The importance of innervation for the physiology of joints impressively emanates from the articular alterations in tabes [464, 470]. Charcot [276] explained these changes as the sequelae of innervational lack. Due to loss of function of the afferent and efferent nerve fibers following degeneration in the posterior and anterior tracts of the spinal cord (Fig. 429) in the late phase of syphilis, the function of the correlated organs is profoundly affected [391]. Nevertheless, the overall incidence of tabes and thus also the incidence of arthropathy in tabes have been substantially decreased [1337] by extensive public education and effective measures in the treatment of syphilis.

The pathogenesis of the conspicuous articular alterations occurring in tabes is partly the outcome of the changed trophic of osseous tissue [197]. The primary disorder of sensory innervation impairs the regulation of flow in the blood vessels and thereby the nutrition of the osseous tissue. A disproportion results between the organic and inorganic components of this tissue, with its mechanical capacity becoming diminished. Thus the bone in tabes is stigmatized by enhanced vulnerability, which in awkward movements or even with normal use permits occurrence of intrinsic discontinuities. In addition to the peripheral disturbance in vasomotor reflexes, a disorder of supraordinated trophic centers [391] situated in the gray substance of the spinal cord contributes to the ensuing disintegrating articular changes. While the diminished mechanical resistance of the osseous tissue is manifested in susceptibility to small pathological fractures, the performed ataxic movements intensify the harm to the bone due to absence of sensibility. Disruption of articular sensation precludes the reflex blockage of any excessive excursion and the appropriate comportment of a joint after a trauma. By the absence of the pain sensation all protective measures of the joints and the body are abolished – measures which could prevent the occurrence of injuries or could lead to the healing of injured structures.

The discussion of these factors indicates that the joint alterations do not necessarily require ataxia to produce at least the initial osseous and articular changes. Indeed, tabic arthropathy may appear at the preataxic stage; sometimes it is the first clinical sign suggesting the presence of tabes. When additional ataxia supervenes, any movement, by its uncontrolled range and uncoordinated course, can mean a traumatization of joints. Especially the joints of the vertebral column, hip, and knee are subjected to excessive disuse and attrition. By a stomping gait the cartilage or fibrocartilage of these joints is progressively worn away, the bone is beaten off, the ligaments are overstretched, and the joint capsule is distended.

About 30%–40% of tabic patients develop changes in the joints between the ages of 45 and 60 years. The knee joint (Fig. 446) is most often affected, followed in

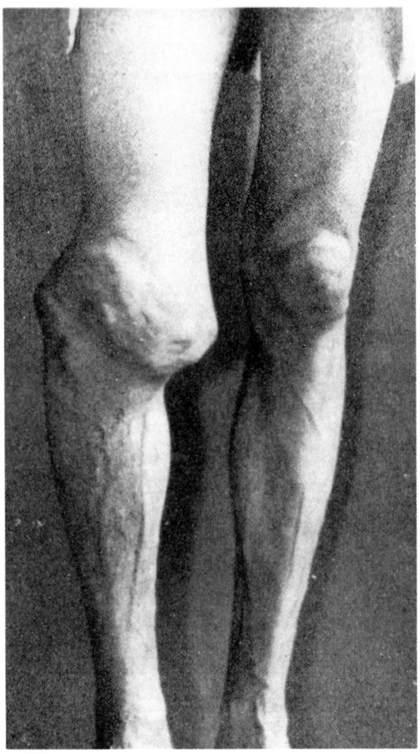

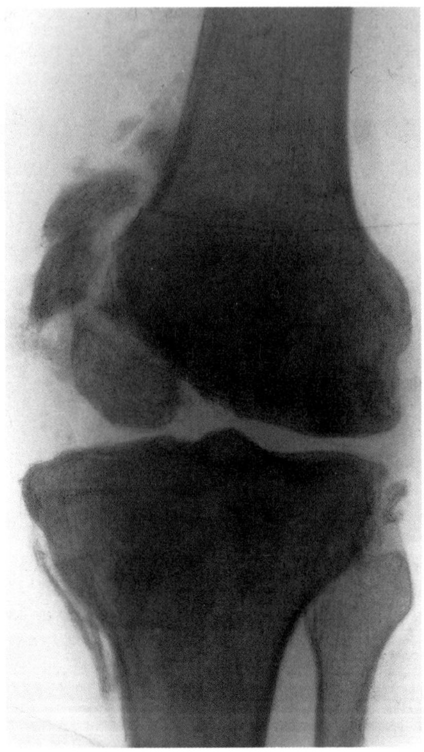

Fig. 446. The right knee is very deformed by the femoral condyles, dislocated medially and distally

Fig. 447. The medial femoral condyle is separated from the shaft, and a few fragments of it lie paraarticularly. The medial tibial condyle has periosteal apposition

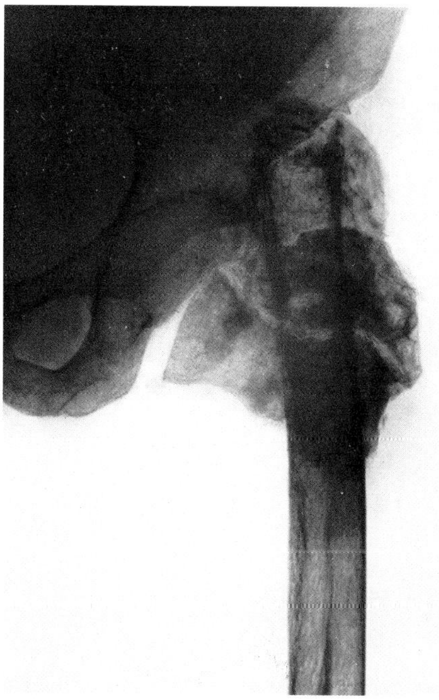

Fig. 448. The proximal femoral end is disrupted by fracture lines. The femoral head is dislocated to the iliac bone, and the femoral neck articulates in the acetabulum

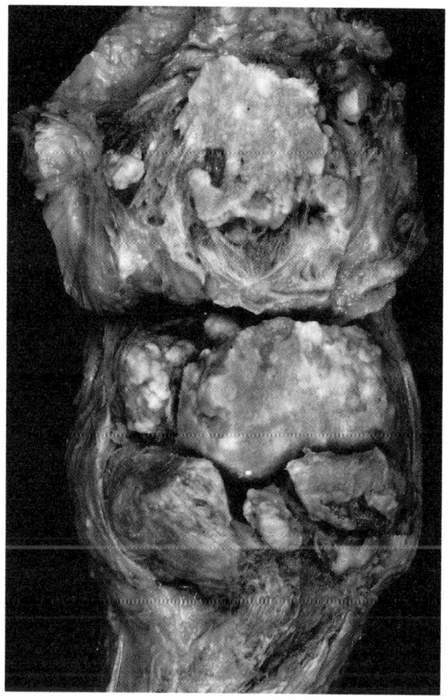

Fig. 449. The articular surface of the patella is partly denuded of its cartilage, and its outline is uneven. The femoral condyles and tibial condyles are disrupted by deep fractures, and their articular surfaces are covered with cartilage only to small extents. Fragments of cartilage and bone lie in their proximity

frequency by the joints of the hip, ankle, and vertebral column. The first sign of joint affection is limited use or distinct swelling which occurs spontaneously or after a minor trauma and partly regresses. Nevertheless, the swelling recurs and gradually progresses to enlargement of joints (Fig. 446). This is associated with discomfort caused by the instability of the joints, especially those of the lower extremities. The knee joint is occasionally sore. The use of these joints causes more pain to the observing physician than to the patient himself. The conspicuously minimal pain, disproportionate to the marked impairment in function, indicates the need for neurological examination. This discloses the lack of deep pain and temperature sensation and the absence of reflexes, especially those of the quadriceps and Achilles tendons. Due to decreased or absent pain sensation and the lack of protective muscle reflexes, the joints are abused beyond the ranges of physiological motions. The ligaments become overstretched, and the articular surfaces are moved at excessive ranges. The characteristic changes in this joint disease, conspicuous deformity with substantially impaired function and absence of pain, follow at varying intervals. Therefore benign and malignant tabic arthropathies have traditionally been distinguished. However, this distinction is not very justified because transitions very often exist between these two types. Apart from these variations, the progression of the joint affection is dictated not only by the individual severity of the neurological affection but also by the comportment of the patient. While the joints are abused due to painlessness, the loss of muscular tonus permits increasing distention of the joint capsule and overstretching of the articular ligaments. At each subsequent movement, the articular epiphyses are further worn off, with resulting pathological subluxations or fracture dislocations [830].

Examination discloses those joints which lie close beneath the skin to be conspicuously thickened and deformed. The hip protrudes, and its trochanteric area is close to the skin with concomitant shortening of the leg; the passive movements of this joint display an excessive range. However, the tabic arthropathy manifests itself most conspicuously in the knee joint, which on weight bearing deviates into valgus and recurvation (Fig. 446). On further attrition of the articular epiphyses, the lower leg is often laterally and posteriorly subluxated; the distal end of the femur then protrudes (Fig. 446). The knee joint is also enlarged by swelling of the joint capsule; inside the latter a number of hard, angularly edged free bodies can be palpated. The active movements of the knee are free, and the lower leg can be moved passively in abnormal directions. Similar abnormal passive excursions, although of lesser ranges, can be noticed in other joints such as the ankle joints. The vertebral column is very deformed and usually presents shortening and kyphoscoliosis of the dorsal and lumbar segment without local soreness. However, nerve root symptoms are sometimes observed here, but are inconclusive due to involvement of the central nervous system. Besides the conspicuous, sometimes even grotesque deformities of joints and their excessive ranges of motion in the advanced phase

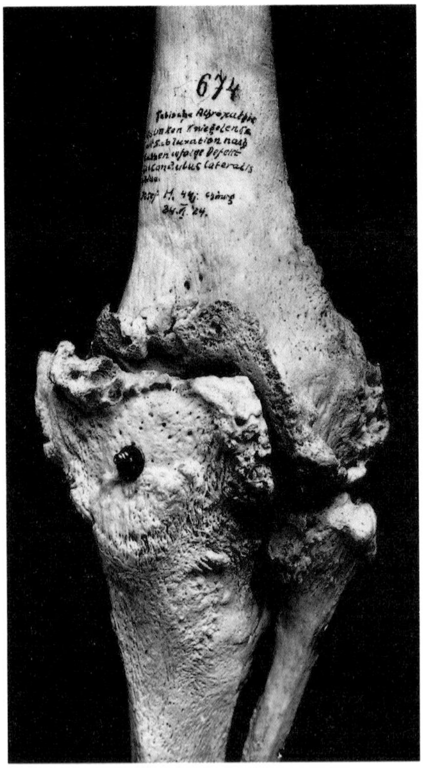

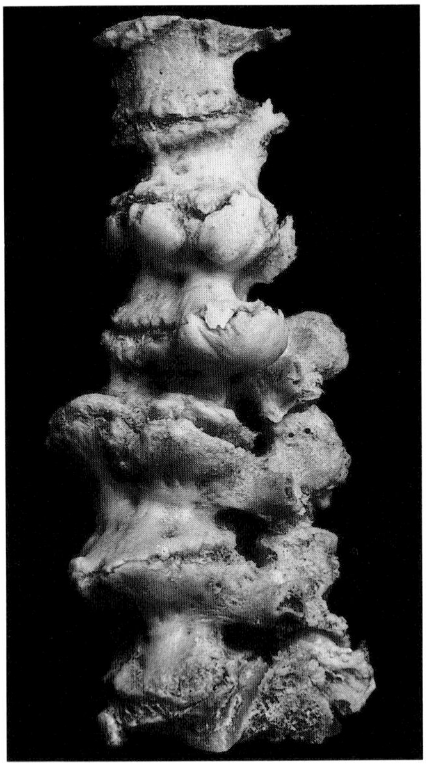

Fig. 450. The medial femoral condyle is completely missing, and its defect articulates with the tibia, while the dislocated lateral femoral condyle articulates with the fibula

Fig. 451. The lumbar vertebrae are very uneven at their intervertebral margins from which large osteophytes rise. The apophyseal joints are similarly uneven

of this disease, the obvious lack of pain with these motions provides a ready clue to the diagnosis.

Routine laboratory studies disclose no specific findings, and even the results of serological tests for syphilis are positive in no more than 10%–20% of cases. On the other hand, roentgenographs are quite characteristic as they reveal even in an early phase excessive attrition of the rather sclerosed articular surfaces and several loose bodies of osseous structure lying within the articular cavity (Fig. 447). The density of the subchondral bone often extends peripherally into the diaphysis. Each joint also presents its own rather typical changes. The lower thoracic and entire lumbar spine are deviated into scoliosis; all their vertebrae are worn off in a wedgelike manner, and their intervertebral spaces are substantially or even extremely narrowed, yet sharply delimited. In the hip joint (Fig. 448) spontaneous fractures divide the femoral neck or the femoral head, which are extensively sclerosed. The femoral head may be completely worn off, and the smoothened stump of the femoral neck is dislocated out of the acetabulum, whose roof is worn off. In the knee joint (Fig. 447) one of the tibial condyles, more frequently the lateral one, is separated or completely worn off from the tibial metaphysis. The tibia is then axially deviated and subluxated posteriorly with concomitant formation of congruent grooves and elevations on the contiguous epiphysis of the femur. The attempt at repair by formation of excessive callus is observable at the site of these fractures, while shadows of osseous density lie paraarticularly close to the articular epiphyses. In the ankle joint the medial and lateral malleolus is shorn off, and the talus is subluxated concurrently with subluxation and wearing off at the midtarsal joint. Lesser changes are observed in the elbow and wrist joints.

Gross-anatomical examination of most joints of the extremities discloses that the articular cartilage is missing over wide areas. Large parts of the articular surfaces, especially in the central regions, are denuded (Fig. 449). At their peripheries, the articular cartilage is uneven and rough. Discontinuities expand from the articular surfaces into the depth of the articular epiphyses, with wedgelike fragments of considerable sizes being partly separated (Fig. 449). Clefts in between have been filled with connective tissue. The extraarticular endings of these fracture lines are signified by massive periosteal callus formations which cause local hardness of the bone. Several loose bodies from lentil to walnut size, smoothly polished by articular function, lie in the joint cavity (Fig. 449). Other separated small fragments are displaced in outpouchings of the joint capsule; their residual defect is delimited by a sclerosed smooth surface which conveys the impression of having been ground off. The contact surfaces of the opposite articular epiphyses show an adaptation (Fig. 450) to this defect by steplike protrusions. The marginal areas of the articular surfaces are

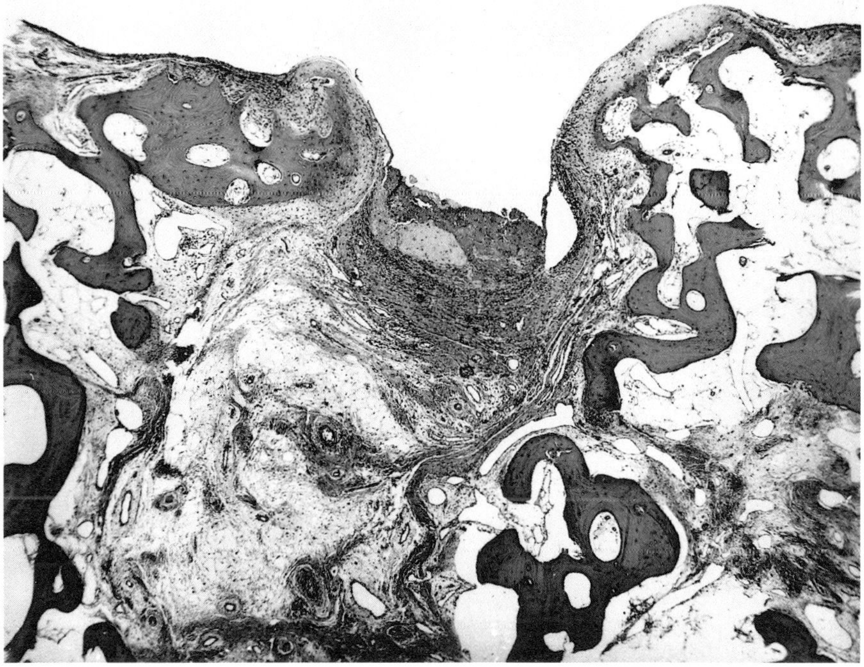

Fig. 452. The articular surface, covered partly with thinned articular cartilage and partly with connective tissue, is disrupted by a wide defect which is filled with loose and dense connective tissue. The latter comprises a fragment of articular cartilage

occupied by massive exostoses (Fig. 450) of bizarre shapes which are partly of cartilaginous and partly of membranous origin. The joint capsule is markedly thickened and widened. Its inner surface is very uneven; the synovial membrane is dense and bare of pliability. Several areas of the fibrous capsule are calcified or comprise cartilaginous-osseous fragments (Fig. 453) which are separated from the articular epiphyses. Individual changes characterize the major joints. In the hip joint (Fig. 448) the femoral head has been ground off; the femur is subluxated or completely displaced with its neck, depending on the remainder of the acetabular roof. In the knee joint (Figs. 449, 450) one of the tibial condyles, more frequently the lateral one, is completely worn off or separated from the metaphysis; the femoral condyles are also worn off at their posterior aspects, whereby the tibia is subluxated posteriorly. The articular constituents of the spine (Fig. 451) are completely worn off at their endplates and apophyseal joints; the substantially shortened vertebral bodies lie close to each other.

Histopathological examination discloses extensive necrosis and attrition of the articular cartilage and its partial substitution by fibrocartilage. In other places the cartilage defect is filled with vascular connective tissue which extends through the line of provisional calcification from the cancellous bone (Fig. 452). By these subchondral protrusions and by the expansion of synovial tissue from the surface, the hyaline cartilage has been progressively replaced (Fig. 452). Conspicuous exostotic formations and loose bodies rise at the articular margins (Fig. 453), while cystlike cavities in the subchondral bone are delimited by dense osseous borders and are filled with loose connective tissue. The synovial membrane is considerably thickened (Fig. 453) upon hyperplasia of the synoviocytes and by infiltrates with histiocytes and lymphocytes. The subsynoviocytic tissue is markedly hypercellular with fibrocytes, and it comprises organized hemorrhages, bone fragments, necrotic calcified tissue, and metaplastic new formations of osseous tissue. The wall of the blood vessels is thickened by proliferation of the intima, and the lumina are thus substantially narrowed.

Differential diagnosis may present difficulty in the rare cases of swollen painful joints when primary osteoarthritis or arthropathy in diabetes is being considered. However, on conspicuously progressing deformity of a joint with axial deviation or spontaneous nontraumatic subluxation, the excessive range of motion at freedom of pain provides a clue to the correct diagnosis, which is confirmed by the neurological examination.

Treatment is primarily prophylactic by the advice to abstain from excessive activities, even prolonged walking or standing. When the vertebral column becomes deviated, it may be straightened out by pelvic traction and may be held so by a high dorsolumbosacral brace or a dorsolumbosacral belt of firm canvas with metal stays (Fig. 51). Even in an already existing deviation of the vertebral column, such supports are of benefit by

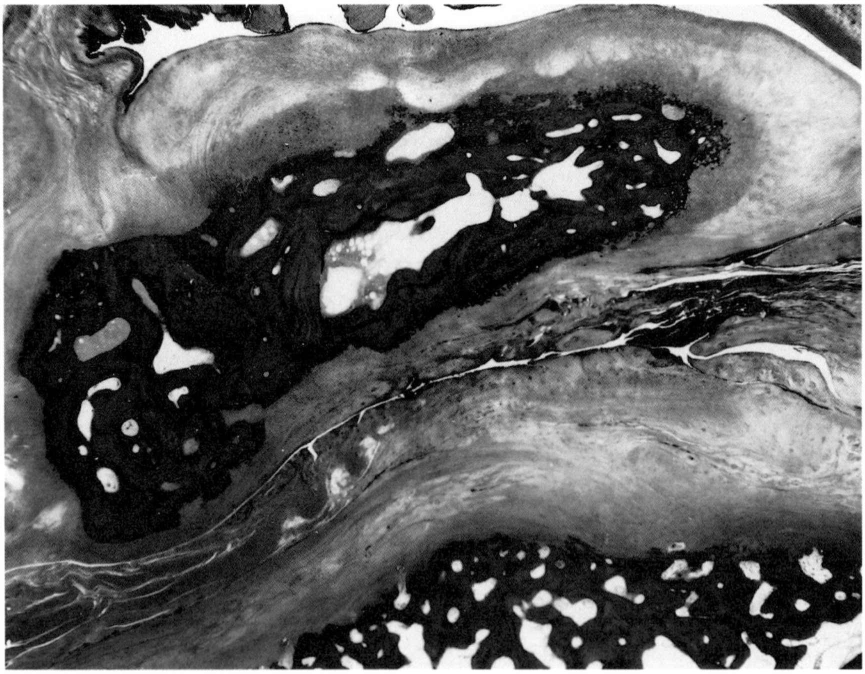

Fig. 453. Close to the articular surface lies a loose body of similar structures as the former, and it is partly connected with the joint capsule

preventing further deviation. The use of a supportive brace is also indicated for a beginning as well as an advanced stage of involvement of the knee or ankle joint in which further aggravation may be prevented. In this sense, immobilization of the hip, knee, or ankle joint by a plaster cast for an adequate period of time, followed by a brace with articulations, may be of substantial and enduring benefit. Overstretched ligaments have the possibility of shrinking, and paraarticular ossifications can consolidate without further expansion. This results in a firmer hold in the joint at the price of limitation of motion, but with the advantage of preventing deformation.

If further shearing of the articular surfaces and formation of free bodies nevertheless follow, with increasing thickness of the joint capsule, an operation is rarely followed by unequivocal success. The slow healing tendency of the operative wound is a serious shortcoming, and removal of the capsular ossifications decreases the stability of the joint. However, in cases with relentlessly progressing subluxation or dislocation in the knee joint, correction of the malalignment by resection of the articular epiphyses followed by internal fixation with a rod or compression clamp appears an advisable treatment [443, 555, 836]. This should invariably be supplemented by immobilization with a plaster cast in view of the stresses imposed upon the operated joint and the possibility of breakage of the metallic fixation device. Similarly, the dislocated ankle joint could be benefited by realignment osteotomy or triple arthrodesis [836]. However, ankle arthrodesis has little potential for healing because of the shattered talus and its poor healing tendency. On the other hand, it appears that the hip joint, even if subluxated or dislocated, does not require operation because the stump of the femoral neck meets sufficient support at the remainder of the hip socket (Fig. 448). An ischial weight-bearing brace may be of substantial benefit here. With increasing application of total arthroplasty, this procedure has also been used in tabic hip and knee joints [598, 1507, 1562]. Long-term follow-up examinations are necessary here to evaluate the lasting benefits and advisability of such procedure. In addition to the poor tendency for healing in the operated joint, the potential problem of difficult to be combated infection must not be disregarded. This should be an elementary factor in deciding between conservative and operative management of the joint affection. Disregarding the possibility of such complication may lead to amputation of the extremity.

d. Arthropathy in Syringomyelia

Schlesinger [1414] reported in 1901 the occurrence of joint alterations in syringomyelia and pointed out that these alterations often are the first symptoms indicating an affection of the central nervous system. Subsequent observations [142, 470, 606, 1434, 1529] revealed a similarity with tabic joint alterations regarding pathogenesis and clinical aspects. However, in contrast to the latter, which affects predominantly the joints of the lower extremities, the joint alterations in syringomyelia appear in the upper extremities and upper part of the

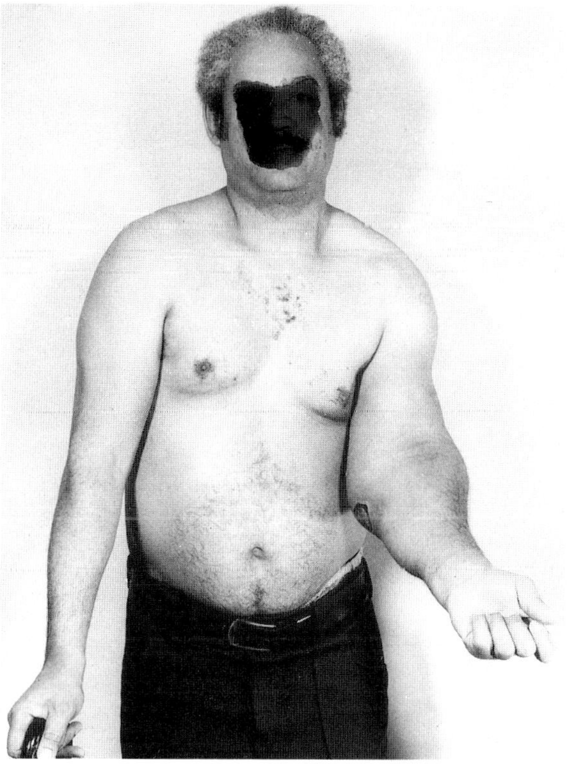

Fig. 454. The left elbow is extensively thickened and deformed and presents a large ulceration at its medial aspect

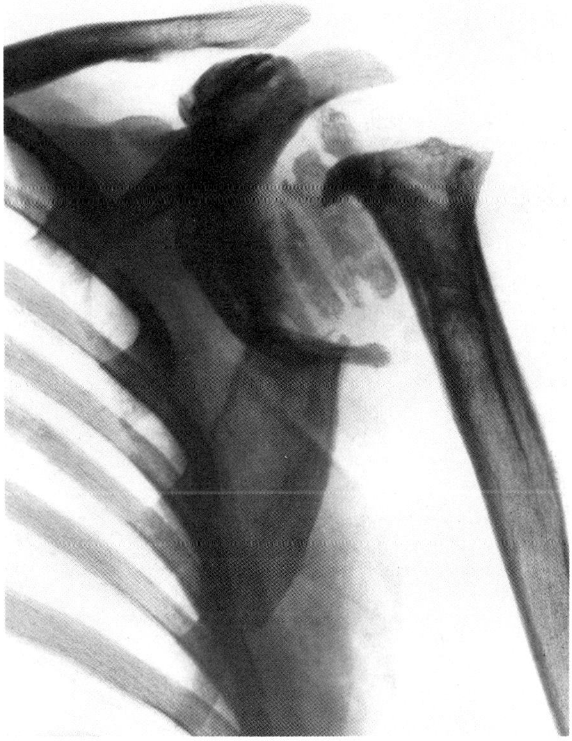

Fig. 455. The glenoid cavity is extremely widened but evenly delimited and contains a few large osseous densities. The humeral head is completely worn off, and its neck is smoothly delimited

vertebral column. The primary pathology resides in cystic widening of the central canal of the spinal cord, chiefly at the level of the lower cervical area. Syringomyelia affects the gray substance in the ependymal region and the posterior horns, specifically in the lower cervical and upper thoracic spinal cord. This is associated with alterations in the anterior white commissure in which the fibers of the secondary sensory neurons cross; the senses for pain and temperature are lost (Fig. 429). Concurrently, the corticospinal tract and its correlated cells of the anterior horn are affected (Fig. 429). This results in degeneration of the lower motor neuron, being associated with weakness or insufficiency of the musculature particularly of the upper extremity.

The neurological symptoms include analgesia, loss of temperature and position sense, impairment of proprioceptive reflexes, and associated regional trophic disorders. Brower [197] emphasized that the primary pathogenesis in trophic alterations of the joints is of neurovascular nature, leading by neurally elicited vascular disorders to active bone resorption and followed by inadequate bone repair. Corresponding to the main localization of the affection in the cervical spinal cord, chiefly the upper extremities are involved, and the sequelae of neurological deficits are manifested in their joints [1529]. Due to the lack both of sensibility and sense of statics, the joints are used improperly. These also are not protected due to lack of muscle reflexes and are thus subjected to traumatization even on normal function. Consequently, the articular ends become extensively disorganized in their hyaline cartilage and subchondral bone. Such disintegration becomes even more profound when a real trauma harmed these joints.

Syringomyelic arthropathy [1414, 1529] appears in the shoulder and elbow joints, also in the joints of the lower cervical and upper dorsal spine, but substantially less often in the wrist joint [1576]. Similarly as in tabic arthropathy, it begins insidiously with swelling of the joint capsule and frequent intraarticular effusion; these increase slowly while the disintegration of the articular ends advances extensively. Accordingly, the joints become enlarged by thickening of the joint capsule (Fig. 454) and/or increase of the joint fluid. Their active motion does not transgress the barriers of the normally stabilizing structures as in tabes unless the joint space is excessively widened. To the contrary, the active motion is very often limited, sometimes associated with soreness and coarse crepitation noises. The first

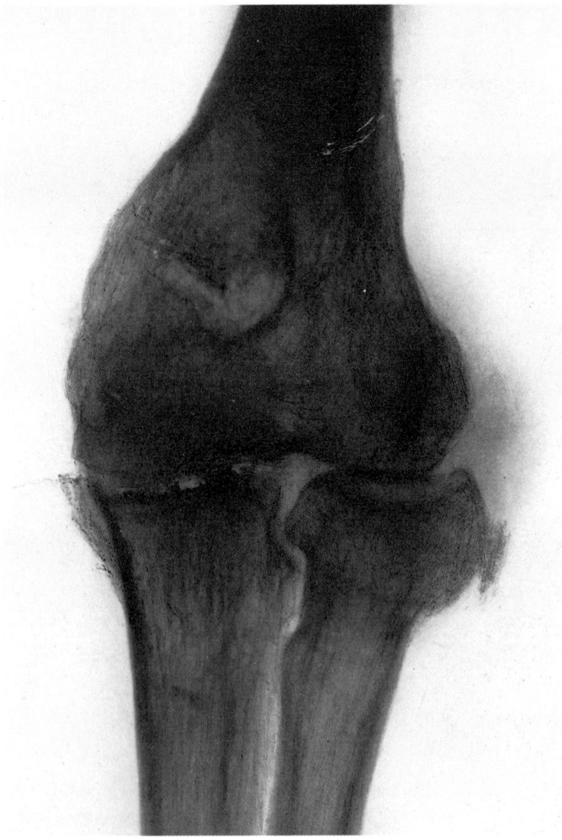

Fig. 456. The proximal end of the ulna is broader and sclerosed. The radial head is also broader and is laterally subluxated; its articular surface is wider. The joint capsule is thickened

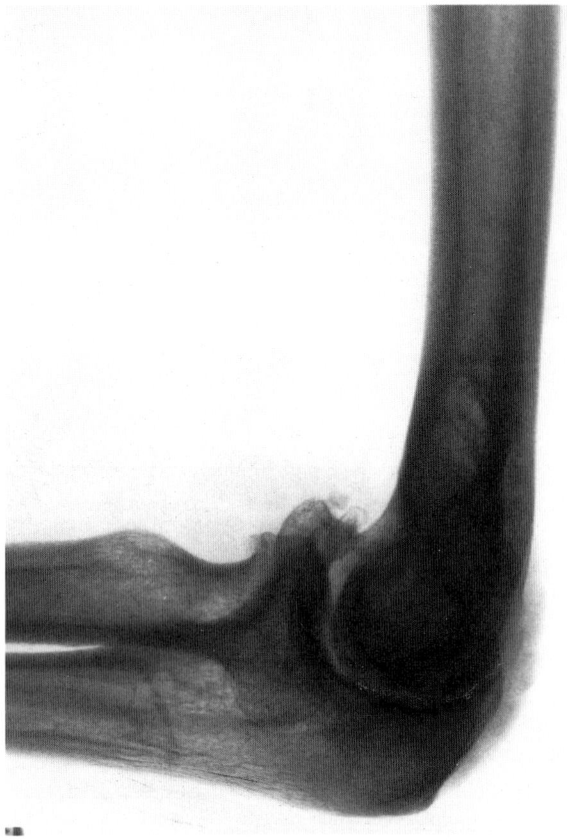

Fig. 457. The humeral condyles are worn off, as are the articular surfaces of the ulna and radius. A loose joint body lies close to the latter

neurological symptom characteristic for syringomyelia is dulling of the pain and temperature sense. Subsequently the tactile sensitivity becomes lost; superficial vasomotor disturbances and trophic alterations of the skin and subcutis follow. Eventually ulcerations of the skin develop, with very slow healing propensity (Fig. 454) and tendency to form draining sinuses with mixed infection.

Blood studies yield no significant findings. However, roentgenographs reveal extensive, rather characteristic homogeneous dissolution of the bone of the contiguous articular epiphyses of the shoulder joint, with broad separation of the sharply delimited remainders of the epiphyseal ends (Fig. 455). Due to lack of coherence by articular ligaments, an excessive widening of the shoulder joint space results, associated with enlargement of the entire joint; this is recognizable by the dense calcifications and numerous bone fragments located in the joint capsule (Fig. 455). Large marginal osteophytes arise from the extensively worn-off and sharply delimited articular epiphyses in the shoulder joint. Such conspicuous changes with extensive dissolution of the articular ends are not observed in the elbow joint. Nevertheless, the latter too undergoes substantial attrition of the articular ends and formation of very protruding marginal osteophytes, with irregular outlining of the joint space (Figs. 456, 457). The remaining stumps of the articular ends of the shoulder joint and the articular ends of the elbow joint present extensive sclerosis of the metaphyseal bone (Figs. 456, 457) in the advanced stage. This alteration is similar to that of arthropathy in tabes, but differs from that of arthropathy in diabetes. The disorganization of the articular epiphyses is less extensive, but more osteoporosis prevails in the residual articular epiphyses in diabetes. In the lower cervical and upper dorsal spine in syringomyelia the vertebral bodies comprise areas of osteoporosis alternating with areas of osteosclerosis. Their densified and irregularly delimited endplates border narrowed intervertebral spaces.

Gross-pathological examination discloses conspicuous thickening of the joint capsule, partly by villous proliferation and extensive fibrosis but especially by numerous deposits of smaller and larger fragments of bone, obviously separated from the articular epiphyses. The latter are worn off chiefly in the shoulder joint, are

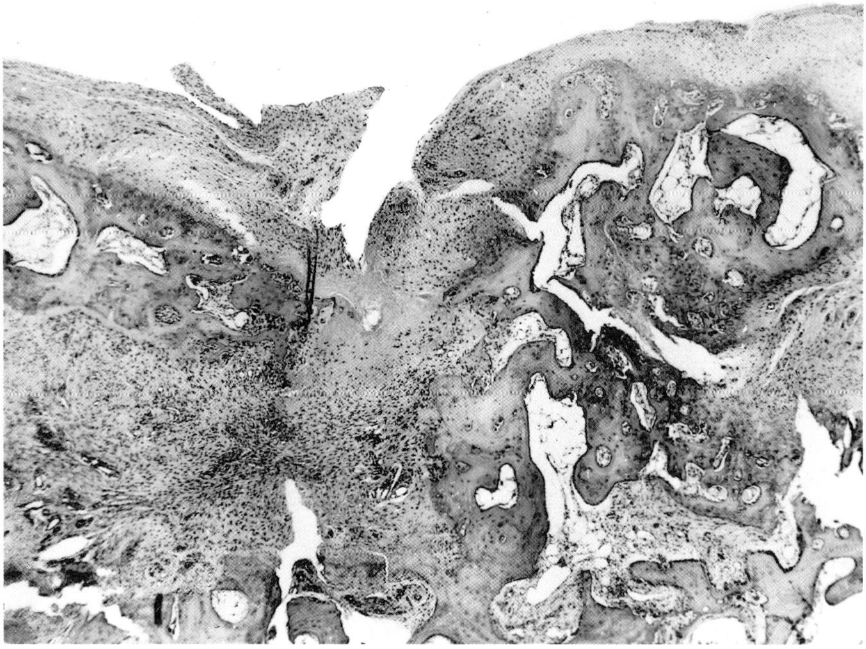

Fig. 458. The articular surface is partly covered with thinned cartilage and partly with connective tissue and is disrupted by a deep cleft filled with connective tissue

disintegrated, and entirely lack a cover of hyaline cartilage. The residual epiphyseal stumps are hardened and sclerosed. The joint fluid, as a sequela of the persistent articular irritation, is almost regularly increased in amount, is discolored dark yellow or sometimes brownish-hemorrhagic, and of dense viscosity.

Histopathological examination of the radial head discloses that its articular surface (Fig. 458) is covered partly with thinned articular cartilage and partly with fibrosed connective tissue. A broad cleft disrupts this surface; being filled with dense connective tissue, it expands deeply into the subchondral osseous tissue. The inner part of the joint capsule is very uneven, partly by villous proliferations but more so by deep disruptions and discontinuities of the synoviocyte cover. The subsynoviocytic and deeper tissues contain a few infiltrates of lymphocytes and are extensively densified by fibrocyte hypercellularity and fibrosis. Within the latter most blood vessels appear compressed (Fig. 459). This fibrosed tissue also contains numerous

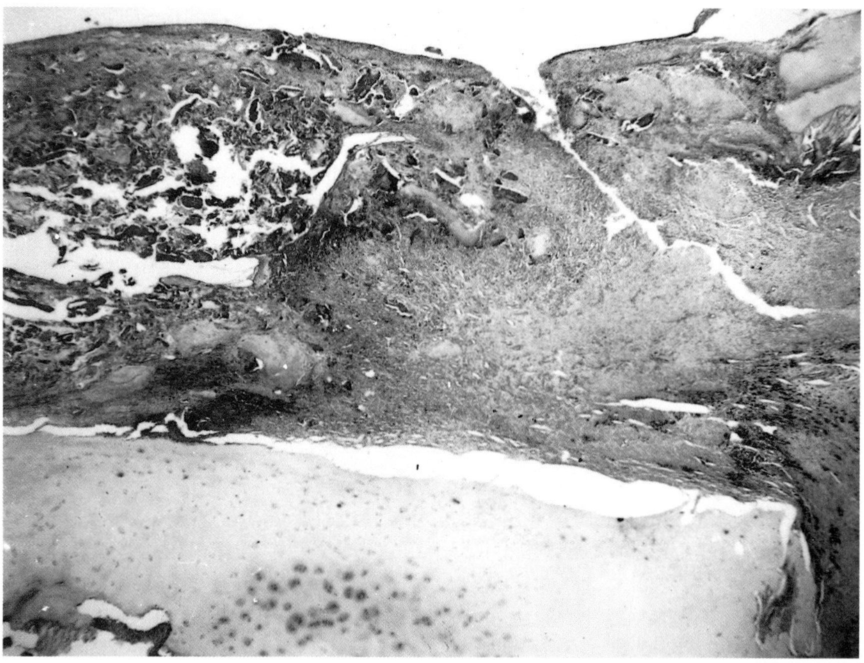

Fig. 459. The inner part of the joint capsule is very dense and thickened by substantial increase of the fibrocytes and collagen fibers. It is disrupted in a few areas and comprises several small fragments and one large fragment of articular cartilage

irregularly shaped fragments of articular cartilage and large fragments of sclerotic bone (Fig. 459).

Differential diagnosis presents little difficulty in cases of reported sensory disturbances, but a primarily traumatic alteration of the shoulder joint may come into consideration in the initial phase and without manifest sensory changes. In an advanced phase, the presence of conspicuous deformities of the articular epiphyses, excessive thickening of the joint capsule which comprises numerous fragments of bone, and possibly associated trophic ulcerations of the skin facilitate establishing the diagnosis. In this context Villiaumey et al. [1692] pointed out the morphological and roentgenographic similarity of alterations in the shoulder joint following an injury to the upper spine with those occurring in syringomyelia. The possibility of destruction by tumorous growth must also be considered, and, if indicated, the diagnosis should be supported by a biopsy.

Since arthropathy in syringomyelia involves chiefly the joints of the upper extremities, no weight-bearing support is needed. Similarly, no major operation may be performed, considering the contraindications presented by the distinct sensory disturbances and the poor healing capacity of the skin. On the other hand, a supportive brace with hinges is indicated for the elbow joint upon its tendency to axial deviation.

7. Joint Affections in Hormonal Disorders

a. Endocrine Arthropathies

With increasing insight into the etiology of joint diseases, dysfunctions of endocrine glands have come to be recognized as significant causes of some joint diseases [1066]. The difficulty in identifying the endocrine etiology and the actual role of any endocrine gland in a joint disease lies in the fact that most endocrine glands do not act independently but in concert with each other. Furthermore, their hormones often also affect other organs, and it is the dysfunction of these, when becoming manifest, which is likely to be considered the etiological factor in the joint alterations. Nevertheless, the participation of endocrine glands in the biology and pathology of joints is especially evident in some patients following the operative removal of a gland or in others after spontaneous hyperfunction of a gland. These observations have been confirmed in animal experiments either by excision of an endocrine gland or by its additional administration to an existing gland. Therapeutic results have corroborated that the hypophysis, thyroid, parathyroids, adrenals, ovaries, and testes – individually or in relationship with each other – have a direct influence on bone, articular cartilage, and joint capsule [348, 1068].

Silberberg et al. [1487–1491] demonstrated on the basis of in vivo and in vitro studies [150, 433, 1627] that cartilage cells proliferate and hypertrophy upon administration of hypophyseal extract. This effect is followed by exaggerated degeneration and calcification. Thus intensification of the growth process leads to an earlier incidence and increased severity of articular changes. Regarding growth hormones, Smith et al. [1520] differentiated the somatotropin produced by the hypophysis from the somatomedin produced by the liver. Somatotropin has a direct action on the articular cartilage by the synthesis of glucosaminoglycans, whereas somatomedin has a stimulating effect on cartilage replication and matrix synthesis [1510]. Similarly, on administration of thyroxin [708, 1487] the growth of cartilage cells is enhanced – but so is also their aging, associated with sclerosis and hyalinization of the ground substance. On the other hand, hypothyroidism inhibits the breakdown of cartilage cells [1487]. The parathyroid glands have a similar effect on the articular cartilage [1488] by promoting its hypertrophy and the subsequent disintegration and ossification. Sex hormones also play a role. Castration causes increased hyperplasia and hypertrophy of the articular cartilage, but once aging has set in, degeneration occurs more rapidly than otherwise [1461, 1490]. Furthermore, differences between sexes may be noticed under certain conditions. Accentuated hypertrophic changes in the articular cartilage are manifested in castrated female animals, whereas calcification and ossification outbalance proliferation in castrated male animals [892, 1490]. On the other hand, the administration of estrogen [1622] decreases the growth rate of cartilage and hastens its regressive changes.

Silberberg et al. [1489] assessed these findings by correlating the hormonal stimulation of cartilage cell function with the synthesis of mucopolysacharides and glycogen. Estrogen induces an arthrosis effect by increased deposition of cytoplasmic glycogen, increased collagenization, and hyalinization. Progesterone does not affect the growth in cartilage and maintains the youthful appearance of cartilage for a long period of time, but eventually the regressive changes in cartilage proceed more rapidly. The administration of testosterone inhibits proliferation of cartilage and accelerates its aging by promoting degeneration and hyalinization [1457]. Regarding the effect of steroids, Silberberg et al. [1489] noted diminution of chondrocyte size and underdevelopment of cytoplasmic organelles compounded by early cell death. Similarly, Mankin et al. [1018] observed a progressive decline in the concentration of hexosamine after administration of corticosteroids. Consequently, the production of chondroitin sulfate was impaired, and the fibrillation of the matrix was accelerated due to depletion of the ground

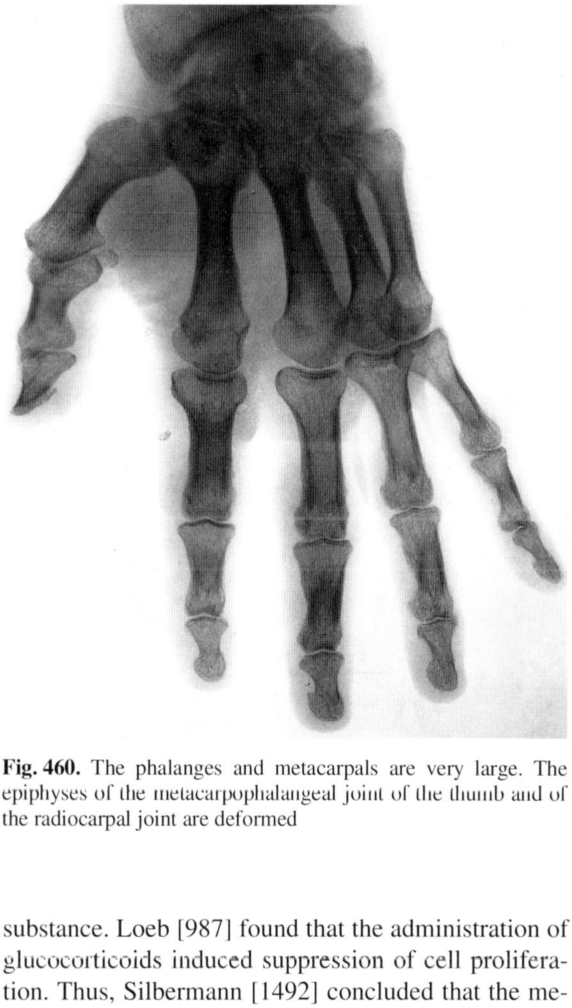

Fig. 460. The phalanges and metacarpals are very large. The epiphyses of the metacarpophalangeal joint of the thumb and of the radiocarpal joint are deformed

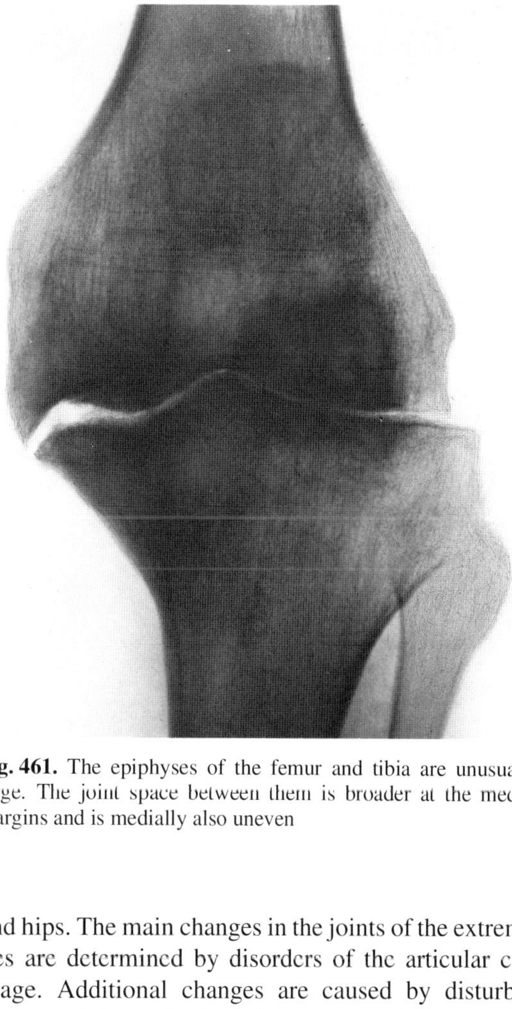

Fig. 461. The epiphyses of the femur and tibia are unusually large. The joint space between them is broader at the medial margins and is medially also uneven

substance. Loeb [987] found that the administration of glucocorticoids induced suppression of cell proliferation. Thus, Silbermann [1492] concluded that the metabolism of the articular cartilage is distinctly influenced by various endocrine agents.

Aside from these experimental findings, sufficient clinical observations have been reported [87, 438, 757, 776, 1039, 1068, 1384] indicating that disorders in the function of endocrine glands can cause significant alterations in the skeleton as well as in the articular cartilage and joint capsule. These changes are associated with distinct symptoms in the joints. In view of the interplay of the endocrine glands and their reactions to conditions of the body, such as anomalies in metabolism or electrolyte imbalance, Bland [139, 140] distinguished the following possibilities of dysfunction of the endocrine glands: primary hyperfunction, secondary hyperfunction, primary hypofunction, and secondary hypofunction.

Marie [1028] reported the occurrence of osteoarticular changes in acromegaly involving the vertebral column and extremities. Since then the disorders of the anterior lobe of the hypophysis have been recognized as leading to changes in axial and peripheral joints, especially those of the thoracolumbar spine (Fig. 462), fingers (Fig. 460), hands, shoulders, knees (Fig. 461), and hips. The main changes in the joints of the extremities are determined by disorders of the articular cartilage. Additional changes are caused by disturbed growth of the articular epiphyses and their resulting incongruence (Fig. 461) associated with disuse of the articular cartilage and joint capsule. The specific changes in the vertebral column and peripheral joints in acromegaly were described by Waine et al. [1705], who pointed out that the histopathological changes resemble those in severe degenerative joint disease. However, these changes are different in some features, and are unphysiological for the age of the patients. In conclusion, Bluestone et al. [147] emphasized the characteristic active proliferation of the cartilage cells, which resulted in thickening of the articular cartilage (Figs. 464, 465, 466), and was followed later by pronounced degenerative changes of the peripheral joints (Fig. 461) and hyperostosis of the vertebral bodies (Fig. 462).

Beyond stimulating the growth of osseous tissue and articular cartilage, the pituitary gland also causes growth and swelling [348] of the mesodermal soft structures. This is seen especially in the joint capsules, bursae, articular ligaments, and periarticular tendons. Fibrosis and ossification follow in the latter two structures. Similar enlargements and swellings of other

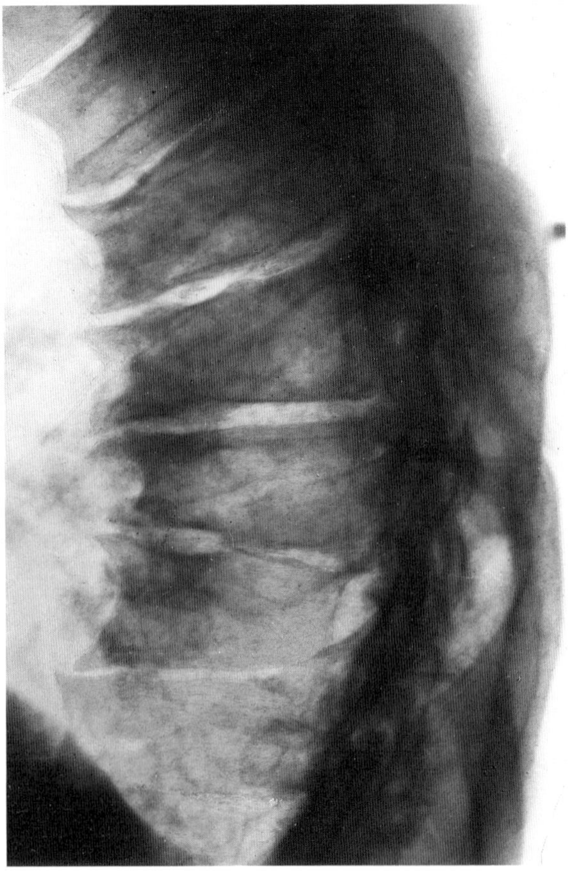

Fig. 462. All vertebrae are unusually large but shorter at their ventral height. They also are uneven at their ventral cortex and at the intervertebral plates. Concomitantly the intervertebral spaces are of unequal width

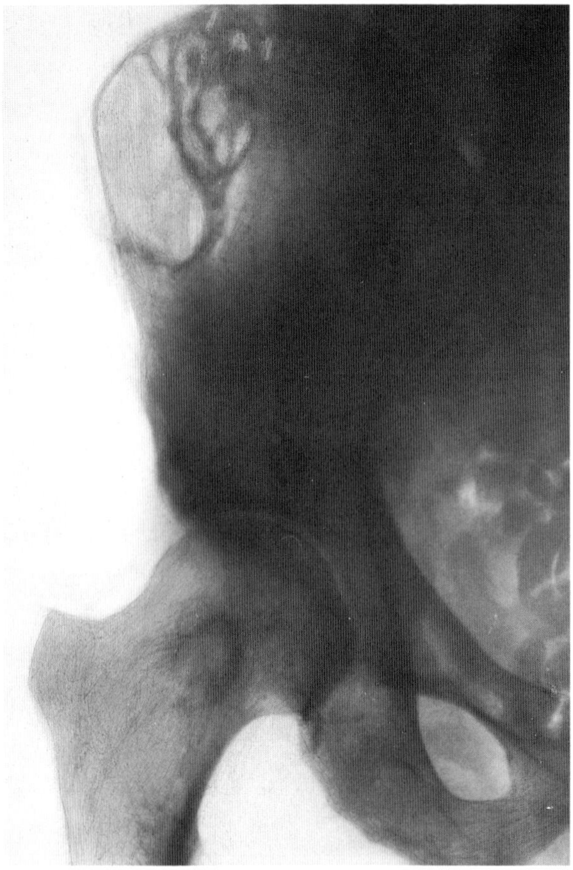

Fig. 463. The pelvic bone is sclerosed in its lower and medial region but otherwise presents a large area of osteoporosis and cystic radiolucency at its upper lateral zone

structures account for the coarsening of facial features and for the plumpness of the entire body. The symptoms are primarily related to the peripheral joints. The fingers, hands, shoulders, knees, and hips are often affected by aching or pain and the sensation of stiffness. The usual findings in the majority of these patients are deformities of the hands by enlargement of the end and middle phalanges and thickening of the interphalangeal and metacarpophalangeal joints. The knee joints too are deformed, partly by broadening of the articular epiphyses and partly by thickening of the joint capsules. The elbow and ankle joints are less often affected. All these joints are slightly to moderately tender, and the knee joints occasionally present slight effusions. The ranges of the movements vary with the duration of the joint affection [873]. In the initial stage, mobility has a greater range than normal, especially in the vertebral column [776]. However, as alterations advance in the joints, their movements are substantially decreased and are associated with coarse crepitation. The shoulder joints are eventually limited in elevation and external rotation. On the other hand, the vertebral column, although painful at its thoracic and lumbar portion, is mobile [147]. The subdeltoid, olecranon, prepatellar bursa, or all three may be enlarged.

Roentgenographs of the skull reveal widening of the sella turcica due to pituitary adenoma and enlargement noticeable chiefly in the frontal and occipital bones and mandible due to overgrowth of bone. The cartilage spaces in the joints of the fingers, hands, and knees are initially widened upon enlargement of their articular epiphyses (Fig. 460). Their joint capsules occasionally contain areas of ossification. More frequent and more extensive ossifications occur in the areas of attachment of the articular ligaments and paraarticular tendons at the larger peripheral joints. Squaring of the epiphyses results at hooklike protruding marginal osteophytes (Fig. 461). Their cartilage spaces are eventually narrowed, and the bordering subchondral bones are uneven and very sclerosed (Fig. 461). On the other hand, the deeper cancellous bone appears osteoporotic due to widening of the trabecular spaces despite increased thickness of the trabeculae. In the advanced stage the contiguous articular epiphyses are flattened at very nar-

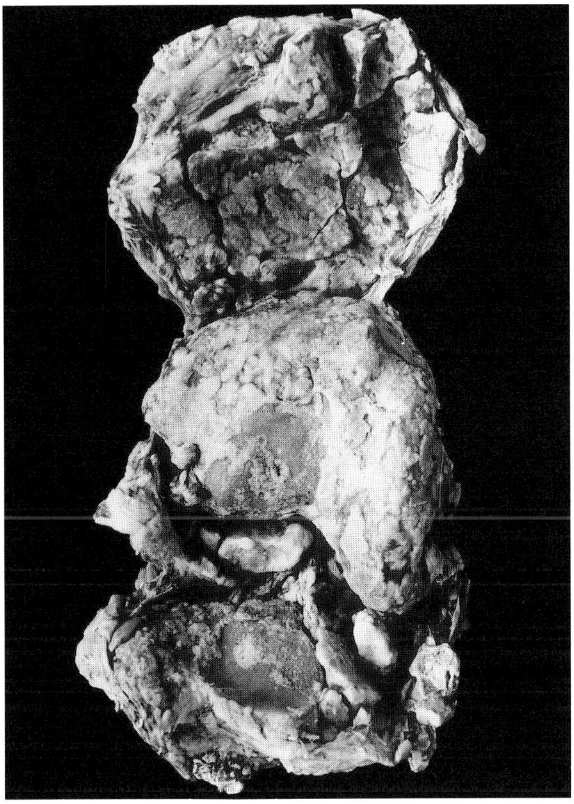

Fig. 464. The articular cartilage is thickened in several areas of the patella and femoral condyles. Otherwise, the articular surfaces especially those of the tibial condyles present deep defects

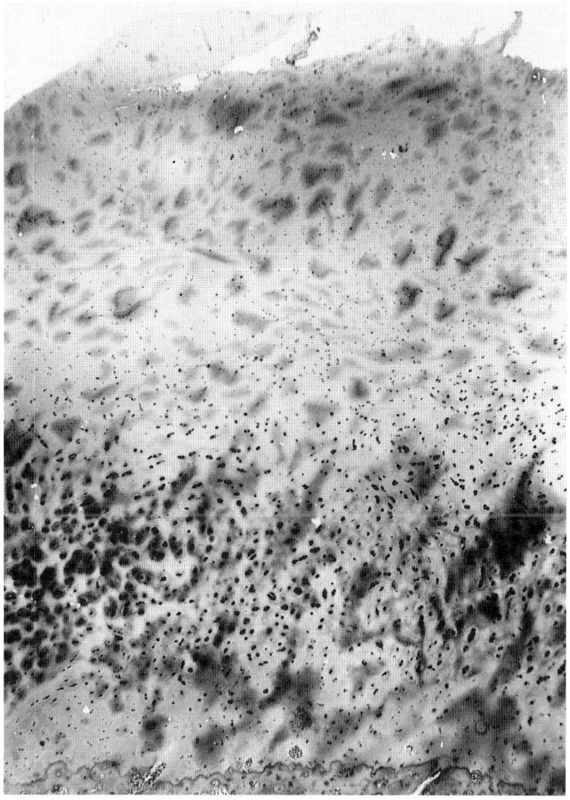

Fig. 465. The articular cartilage is substantially thickened by hyperplasia of chondrocytes in the deeper zone and by marked hypertrophy of chondrocytes in the superficial zone

rowed joint space, and their peripheral zones carry numerous marginal osteophytes as in a wreath. These contribute to mushrooming of the humeral and femoral heads [413, 873]. The vertebral column presents increased kyphosis of its dorsal part. Pronounced marginal osteophytes arise on the entire spine (Fig. 462). In the lateral view, the vertebral bodies have a concave contour and a longer anteroposterior diameter secondary to bone overgrowth at their anterior aspects (Fig. 462). The intervertebral spaces are partly widened and are irregularly delimited by sclerosed vertebral plates (Fig. 462). Sometimes calcifications and ossifications of the intervertebral discs occur in advanced phase.

These findings are explained by the gross-anatomical examinations. Bluestone et al. [147] noted regeneration and advanced degenerative changes in abnormally growth-stimulated articular cartilage as well as very active remodeling of bone. The interphalangeal joints of the fingers had thickened, uneven articular cartilage with fibrocartilaginous changes and marked marginal osteophytes. The femoral head contained an area of ragged ulceration with undermined edges. The knee joint displayed fibrillation of cartilage and deep defects in some places, and thickening of the cartilage (Fig. 464) and eburnation in other places. The lower thoracic vertebrae presented disruptions of the endplates and considerable formations of osteophytes with moderate degeneration of the discs. The lumbar spine had hypertrophic cartilage covers at its endplates and discs of greater than normal height.

Histopathologically [147, 873], the inner part of the joint capsule displays noninflammatory fibrous thickening as well as thickening of its adipose tissue. Alteration in the articular cartilage was initially described by Erdheim [477] who identified degeneration of the articular cartilage with cleft formation. The resulting deep-reaching and undermined ulcers are characteristic of the cartilage defects in acromegaly. The articular cartilage of most joints is considerably thickened by irregular cellular overgrowth and substantial increase in the matrix, which expands beyond the calcification line deeply into the subchondral bone (Fig. 465). The latter area of the cartilage is intensely metachromatic. In other specimens of articular cartilage, excised from younger individuals, the chondrocytes of the upper zones are hypertrophic and broadly surrounded by basophilic ground substance (Fig. 466). Here the articular

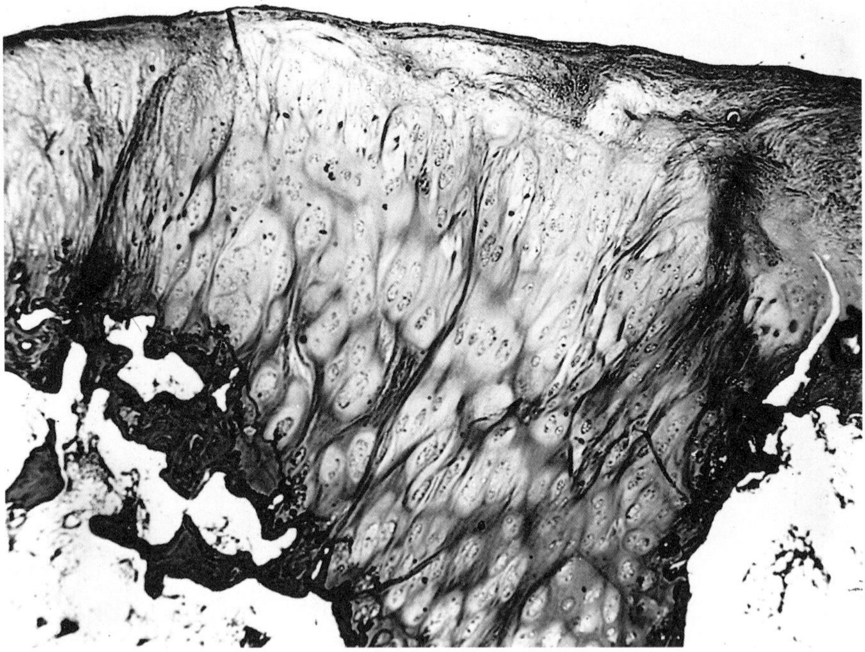

Fig. 466. The articular cartilage is thickend by extensive hypercellularity of the chondrocytes and locally expands deeply into the subcortical space

cartilage is substantially thicker. Nevertheless, fissures and clefts disrupt the articular cartilage in a few areas.

The pronounced degenerative articular alterations in acromegaly necessitate treatment because of the significant symptoms and functional impairment. While in most cases primary treatment of the enlarged hypophysis by radiation or operative resection is embarked on, the articular symptoms require specific treatment following the guidelines described in "Osteoarthritis". Detenbeck et al. [413] emphasized the potentially concurrent other endocrine disorders (diabetes and/or hyperthyroidism) which also require treatment.

Articular changes have been described in hyperfunction of the thyroid gland [87, 708, 888, 1636]. Payr [1230] reported regression of arthritic symptoms after excision of a hyperthyreotic struma. Besides the alterations in the joints, trophic changes in the skin, hair, and nails are observed in hyperthyroidism. Articular symptoms in hyperthyroidism start insidiously and are usually expressed either in arthralgias of short duration or bothersome dragging and radiating pain associated with thickenings of the joint capsules. The hands, elbows, shoulders, knees, and ankles are most commonly affected. Pronounced weakness of the musculature of the back and extremities, often concurs. Further examinations disclose clubbing of the fingers and toes and swelling of the hands, forearms, and ankles due to local edema. Joint capsules present moderate doughy thickening and slight tenderness. The range of mobility is increased due to laxity of the articular ligaments. The knee joint is often enlarged by an increase in the joint fluid. Body temperature is slightly and irregularly elevated. Blood studies reveal an abnormally high level of thyroxin and protein-bound iodine, above the physiological level of 3.5–8.5 μg/dl thyroxin and 4–8 μg/dl protein-bound iodine [424]. Concurrently, the thyroidal uptake of radioactive iodine is significantly increased. Increased immunoglobulins are also detected, probably as antibodies to thyroid-stimulating hormone [1698]. Roentgenographs of patients with pronounced swelling of the fingers and toes [888, 1636] reveal thickening of the phalanges, metacarpals, and metatarsals by periosteal apposition of new bone. However, in other patients with very active hyperthyroidism osteoporosis of the hands, feet, and vertebral column is noted, as related to the concurrent negative calcium and phosphorus balance.

In primary hypothyroidism in adults, the changes affect the hands and feet but in more pronounced way the wrist, knee, and ankle joints. All ailing joints are moderately tender, but are fully moveable. Laxity prevails in the knee joint. Myalgias are common, sometimes associated with cramps; neuralgias are scattered irregularly in the extremities. These symptoms account for the frequent weakness in the use of the extremities. The knee joint often contains increased joint fluid which is hyperviscous due to an increased concentration of hyaluronic acid and forms a firm mucin clot. Joint fluid also sometimes contains calcium crystals [438]. Roentgenographs reveal irregular densifications in the tibial plateau similar to chondrocalcinosis [438]. On histopathological examination the joint capsule and periarticular tissues present myxedematous swelling by increased accumulation of hyaluronic acid and other proteoglycans [138, 438]. The articular cartilage is very actively invaded at the calcified zone by blood vessels from the subchondral marrow spaces [828].

Treatment depends on the functional status of the thyroid gland. In most cases effectively treated for hyperthyroidism, a subsequent low level of thyroid hormone requires supplementation with thyroid hormone for a longer period of time until regression of the symptoms. As an alternative, the administration of prednisolone 20–30 mg daily for 3–4 weeks provides more rapid resolution of the symptoms, but a longer follow-up is indicated in view of the possibility of recurrence of the symptoms. Swelling of the joints and the associated symptoms may regress fully by hormonal and/or surgical treatments of the under- or over-functioning thyroid gland. Subsequent physical therapy is beneficial with shortwave diathermy and massage in one series of eight to ten sessions. Articular symptoms following excision of a hyperthyreotic struma respond satisfactorily to the administration of thyroidin. Judging by this success, the thyreogenic etiology of the incident joint alterations may be reasonably inferred.

Hyperparathyroidism [828], as primarily caused by adenomatous enlargement of the parathyroid gland, has a stimulating effect on osteoclasts, which by increased dissolution of bone release calcium and phosphate. Further effects of hyperparathyroidism are stimulation of the intestine in absorption of calcium ions and influence on the renal tubules with resulting increase in the reabsorption of calcium ions and decrease in the reabsorption of phosphate ions. General symptoms in hyperparathyroidism are caused by the hypercalcemia and are manifested in nausea, polydipsia, constipation, weakness, and depression. The complaints of aching or intense pain are chiefly confined to the joints of the fingers, hands, shoulders, hips and knees and less often to the diaphyseal areas of the contingent bones [409, 1824]. Most joints present laxity of their ligaments due to increased collagenase activity in hyperparathyroidism. The thickenings of the joints are caused principally by deformation of the articular epiphyses and less by swelling of the joint capsule. These joints are tender but not stiff.

Laboratory studies on serum disclose increased parathyroid hormone, increased calcium to 12.4–14.1 mg%, frequently decreased phosphorus to 3.0–3.2 mg%, and concomitantly increased alkaline phosphatase to more than 100 IU. These findings indicate that calcium salts have been released from physiological sites. Laboratory findings of abnormal levels of calcium and phosphorus in serum point to the underlying endocrine disorder. High levels of serum calcium may occur and then may cause life-threatening cardiac arhythmias. Serum uric acid is elevated in about 30% of patients with long-standing hyperparathyroidism due to renal damage by hypercalcemia. Roentgenographs reveal deformities in the articular epiphyses of the fingers, hands, knees, sternoclavicular, and acromioclavicular joints. Their articular surfaces are uneven and collapsed secondary to the subchondral erosions. Concomitantly, the cartilage spaces are irregularly delimited and partly widened. Pronounced sharply delineated cortical and/or endosteal erosive defects are noted also in the diaphyses of the phalanges, metacarpal, and carpal bones as well as in the humerus, clavicle, femur, and iliac bone (Fig. 463). Punctate and linear calcifications may be seen in the articular cartilage of the fingers, wrist, and knee. More extensive calcifications are dispersed in the intervertebral discs and soft tissues of the hands in about 25%–33% of these patients [211, 826, 1319]. The thinner deposits consist of calcium pyrophosphate dihydrate crystals while the more extensive deposits consist predominantly of calcium hydroxyapatite [433, 438, 1282]. Roentgenographic studies show that changes in hyperparathyroidism are very similar secondary to renal failure but more extensive in calcification of soft tissues and blood vessels. The resulting changes in areas of bones close to joints are associated with collapses of articular surfaces. Infractions in the mechanically inferior articular epiphyses contribute to their deformation and to the development of osteoarthritis. Differential diagnosis must consider in view of the elevated calcium level and bone resorption areas a multiple myeloma, and in view of the increased alkaline phosphatase a damage to the liver.

Treatment seeks to correct the hyperparathyroidism. Excision, resection, or radiation of the parathyroid adenoma is necessary in cases of increased serum calcium. Oral and intravenous overhydration with addition of sodium phosphate is indicated to enhance elimination of calcium ions and restore the phosphate balance. Concurrently, the function of the kidneys should be checked regularly. Salicylates are of benefit for relief of articular symptoms and may be supplemented in more pronounced symptoms with nonsteroidal antiinflammatory medications. In addition, local treatment with shortwave diathermy in two or three series of eight sessions, application of moist warm packs, and supportive splints or braces are of benefit.

Underfunction of the parathyroid gland also causes a disorder in the metabolism. Low serum calcium levels of 7.3–8.2 mg% result from decreased intestinal absorption of calcium ions and are occasionally accompanied by high phosphate levels of 4.1–5.0 mg%. This is associated with paresthesias in the extremities and episodes of convulsion or tetany. Additionally, arthralgias are experienced in the joints of the fingers and/or in larger joints (shoulder, hip, or knee). Examination discloses moderate thickening of the periarticular tis-

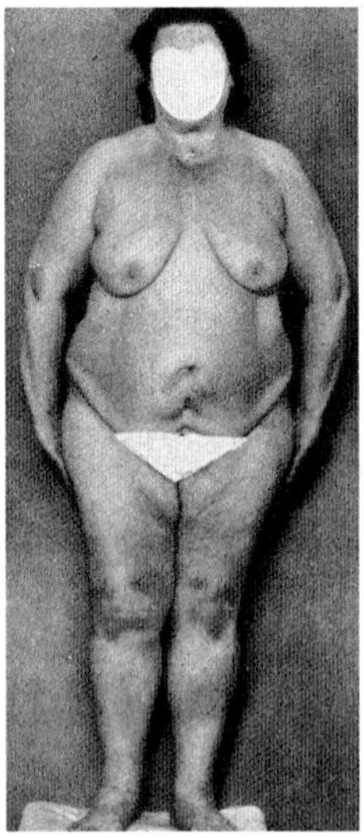

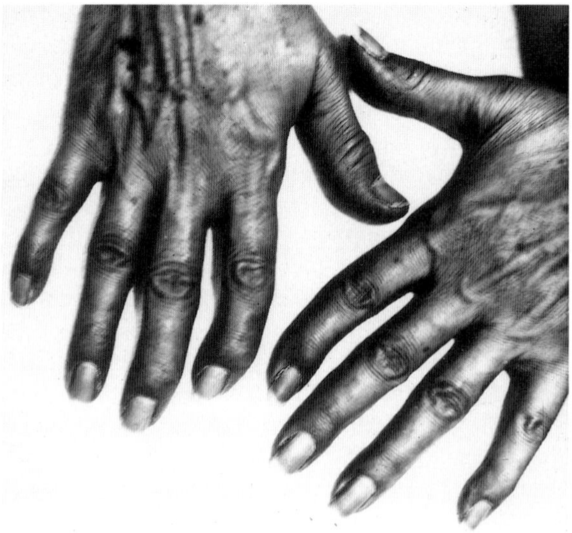

Fig. 467. Secondary to ovarectomy, the body and especially the extremities have become edematous, and the joints have become swollen

Fig. 468. The interphalangeal joints are moderately thickened and are ulnarward deviated in the distal joints of the indices and middle fingers

sues, circumscribed moderate tenderness of the joint, but no essential limitation of motion. Roentgenographs reveal calcifications in the soft tissues close to joints (Fig. 386) and vertebral column, large areas of densification within bones, and parosteal new bone formation close to large bones. Treatment aims at normalizing the level of calcium ions by administering calcium carbonate and vitamin D and at decreasing the absorption of phosphate ions by administering antacids. Prior to these, carefully determined substitution of parathormone is the most indicated modality.

The research of Hench et al. [741], Kyriazis et al. [925], Loeb [987], Mankin et al. [1018], Selye [1462, 1463] among others indicates that the hormones of the adrenal gland have an important bearing on the immune defense of the organism. Hence the probability that lack of or inadequate production of these hormones changes the resistance of the mesodermal organs and facilitates the occurrence of abnormal processes in the articular structures. The results reported by Hench et al. [741] after having administered adrenal hormone or adrenocorticotropic hormone of the hypophysis demonstrate that these hormones distinctly affect the inflammatory changes of the joint capsule. The endogenous hyperproduction of these hormones also has a pronounced effect on the metabolism of the osseous tissue by increasing its catabolism. An extensive osteoporosis of the axial and peripheral skeleton results. The diminished weight-bearing capacity of the skeleton expresses itself in frequent fatigue aggravated by generalized weakness of the musculature. This condition is often complicated by pathological fractures. The thoracic and lumbar vertebrae undergo wedge deformation; femoral head and tibial plateau collapse. Treatment attempts to correct the hyperfunction of the pituitary or adrenal gland either by radiation with 10–15 Gy or by surgical resection. These modalities are combined with a high protein diet supplemented with vitamins C 1000 mg and D 250 IU daily.

The most frequently observed articular affection caused by endocrine dysfunction occurs in women of the postmenopausal age. Actually, the symptoms, although of minor degree, start with the onset of menopause due to the substantial decrease in the major steroids estrogen and progesterone secreted by the ovaries. In this phase, diffuse arthralgias begin in the lumbar spine and major peripheral joints. Instability and fatigue are experienced in the lower extremities, but no objective findings are noted. However, the clinical picture changes in the advancing postmenopausal phase. Patients often present obvious changes in endocrine disorder such as swollen face, hyperpigmentation of the skin on the face and extremities, loss of hair on the scalp, laxity of the skin due to looseness of the subcutaneous tissues, edematous swelling of the forearms, lower legs, and knees (Fig. 467), and increasing body weight despite normal intake of food. It may be inferred from the young women of nutritional overweight but with normal ovarian function and without articular changes that the greater body weight as such is not alone the cause of this arthritis, which involves the extremities and the vertebral column [140]. Indeed, a great number of women of normal weight or even underweight but in the postmenopausal phase present attritional and deforming changes of the joints of the fingers, hands, knees, ankles, and vertebral column. The past histories in the overwhelming majority of these women indicate that the affected joints were not subjected to excessive or unphysiological mechanical

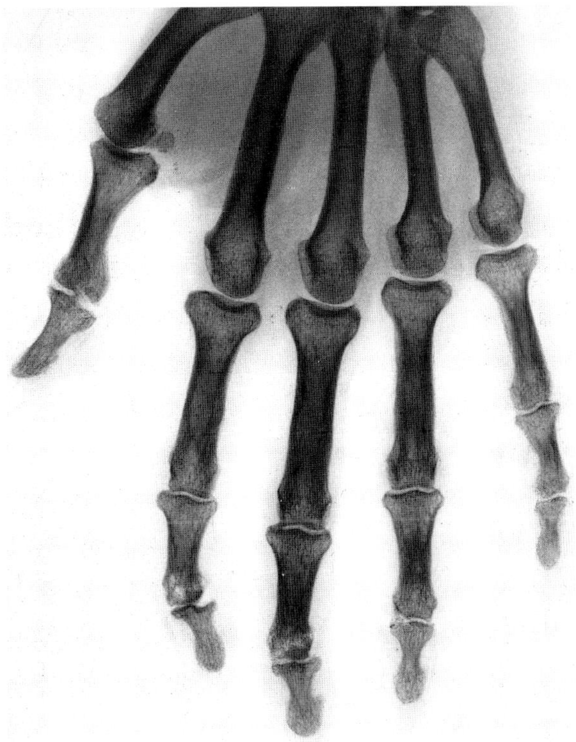

Fig. 469. The distal interphalangeal joints of the index and middle finger are partly eroded and are ulnarward deviated

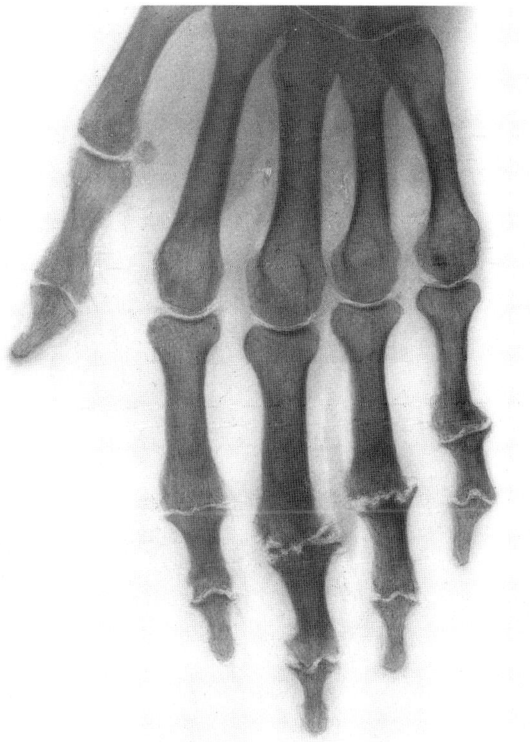

Fig. 470. The distal and proximal interphalangeal joints of four fingers are very uneven and are widened by extensive erosion of their articular surfaces

activities, either in private or in professional life. Menge [1092] reported similar articular attritions after intensive X-ray irradiation of the ovaries and therefore termed these changes arthritis ovaripriva. Also Cecil et al. [262] emphasized in cases after excision of the ovaries, that the lack of or disorder in ovarian function is the principal etiological factor in the ensuing articular symptoms. On the other hand, the beneficial effect of the ovarian function on active joint alterations may be inferred in rheumatoid arthritis, which distinctly regresses during pregnancy due to concurrent hyperfunction of the ovaries and increased production of estrogen and progesterone [266].

Patients in the postmenopausal age complain of stiffness and rigidity in the hands, knees, and cervical and lumbar spine [872]. Symptoms are pronounced in the morning at the start of activities and regress or become more pronounced during day. A sensation of numbness and stiffness often persists in the hands and fingers. Similarly, nerve root symptoms, emanating from the lumbar spine into the lower extremities, are often experienced. Local findings are characterized by swelling of the joint capsule predominantly involving the distal and proximal interphalangeal joints and the metacarpophalangeal joints (Fig. 468). Distinct swelling of the joint capsule is also observed at the ankles and knees (Fig. 467). On palpation the joint capsule of affected joints of the extremities present a doughy consistency and slight to moderate tenderness which becomes intensified by moving these joints to extreme ranges. The finger, wrist, and knee joints are often slightly warmer than the neighboring areas [458]. Nodular enlargements and protrusions can be palpated at the bases of the endphalanges [734] and sometimes at those of the middle phalanges. With long-standing disease, the swollen joint capsules become denser and tighter, resulting in their rigidity. In this stage the entire joints are tender and their movements limited. Eventually ulnar deviation in the finger joints (Fig. 468) and valgus deviation in the knee joints (Fig. 467) may ensue. Other joints of the extremities are also moderately tender and are slightly limited in their active movements. However, after longer duration of the joint condition, the joints particularly of the lower extremities become more painful, more thickened, and more limited in their active movements. Even more pronounced symptoms are then noticed in the lumbar spine, which very often is painful, persistently tender, and moderately to markedly limited in its movements. This situation is often compounded by irritation of the nerve roots in the

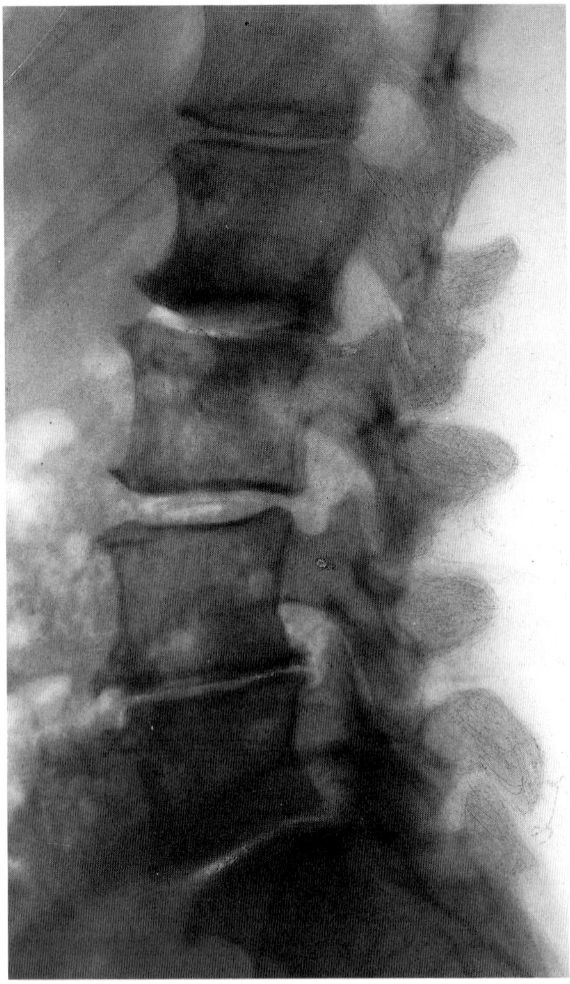

Fig. 471. The intervertebral spaces of the lumbar spine are uneven by erosion of the intervertebral plates and are very narrowed between the lower vertebrae. Marginal osteophytes rise from the vertebrae, and cavitation is noticed in the intervertebral spaces L2-3 and L5-S1

lumbar spine and manifested by radiating pain and/or paresthesias in the gluteal areas and lower extremities (Figs. 300, 301).

Johanson [828] indicated that chondrocyte proliferation is diminished due to the lack of estrogen in the postmenopausal age. Changes follow in the chondrocyte metabolism, regional concentration of proteoglycans, and enchondral ossification. Johanson [828] also pointed out that, with the concurrent deregulation of the calcium metabolism and associated changes in the strength of the osseous tissue, the subchondral bone has a diminished weight-bearing capacity. This results in deformations of the osteocartilaginous surfaces. Seidel [1460] emphasized the concurrent atrophy of the regional musculature which is associated in this phase with a typical appearance of the hands. Their skin displays roughness, cracking, and thickening.

Blood studies disclose no abnormality except for very low levels of ovarian hormones; total estrogen produced in 24 h is less than 0.1 mg/l, and total progesterone in 24 h is 0.2–0.1 mg/l [424]. The sedimentation rate is elevated in about 25% of patients above 30 mm/h and in some to 50–60 mm/h.

Roentgenographs reveal thickenings of the joint capsules of the fingers, wrists, knees, and ankles; these thickenings increase with the duration of the joint ailment. Narrowing of the cartilage space and irregular delimitation of the subchondral bone are the concomitant changes. A rather frequent and characteristic finding is the deepening into the articular epiphyseal cortex of the end and middle phalanges of the fingers (Heberden's and Bouchard's nodes; Figs. 469, 470). This often results in angular deviation in the interphalangeal joints. Eventually more pronounced changes are observed in the hip joints, with marked narrowing of the cartilage space, sclerosis of the articular epiphyses, and marginal osteophyte formation. Brandt [174, 175] demonstrated that the marginal osteophytes have a molten-wax, softer appearance rather than the usual sharp tapering. The middle and lower parts of the cervical spine sometimes bear moderate marginal osteophytes at the vertebral bodies. The lumbar spine (Fig. 471) often presents osteoporosis of the vertebral bodies, narrowing of the intervertebral spaces with occasional vacuum phenomenon (Fig. 471), sclerosis of the adjacent vertebral plates, and marginal attritions and/or osteophyte formation. Slight to moderate osteoporosis is often observed over the entire extent of the spine.

Gross-anatomical examination of the peripheral joints discloses thickening of the joint capsule by swelling and villous proliferation of the synovial membrane. This swelling is more pronounced in the interphalangeal joints of the fingers, where it expands into the joint cleft, and deeply ingresses into the cartilaginous surfaces of the adjacent phalanges. Here the articular cartilage has been substantially thinned or completely eroded, and the subchondral bone has been denuded on great extent. Concurrent deepening follows in part of the articular surfaces. Histopathological examination of the inner part of the interphalangeal joint capsule discloses proliferation of slender villi and moderate fibrocytic hypercellularity, as well as occasional lymphocyte agglomerations in the subsynoviocytic tissue (Fig. 472). In the latter, small cavities appear by separation of fibrocytes and collagen fibers from each other, but without any degeneration or necrosis of cells or disintegration of fibers (Fig. 472). These cavities are from the very incept well delimited, have a rather roundish outline, and remain so under progressive widening. Eventually they attain very large extent with concurrent thickening of the surrounding tissue. They then become cysts which are delimited by a synovio-

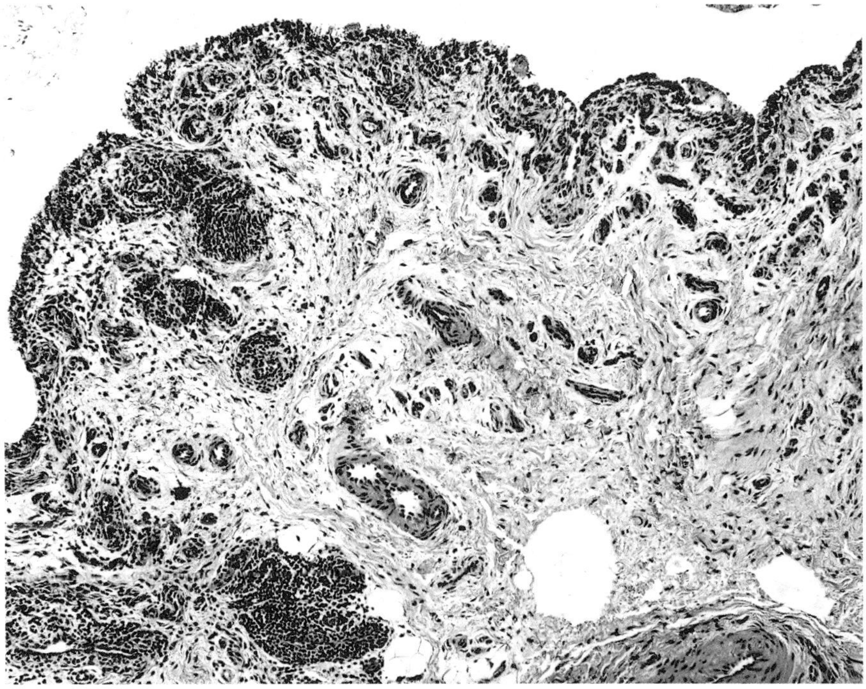

Fig. 472. The synovial membrane is hyperplastic at the synoviocyte cover and comprises a few circumscribed agglomerations of lymphocytes. Two small cystic cavities are present in the deeper subsynoviocytic tissue. No necrosis or degenerative changes are noticed in the neighboring tissue

cyte lining. Such cystic formations are not observed in the inner part of the joint capsule removed from the hip, knee, or ankle joint of patients in the postmenopausal phase. Eventually these synovial cysts deeply erode into the articular cartilage of the adjacent phalangeal epiphyses (Fig. 473). The surfaces of the phalangeal articular epiphyses bear substantially thinned cartilage in some areas and are devoid of articular cartilage in most others where the subchondral bone is eburnated (Fig. 473).

On the basis of clinical findings, Umber [1668] designated this type of joint alteration as periarthritis, implying that the tissues around the joints are inflamed. However, gross-anatomical and histopathological examinations do not support such a concept; they clearly indicate that the joint capsules and the articular

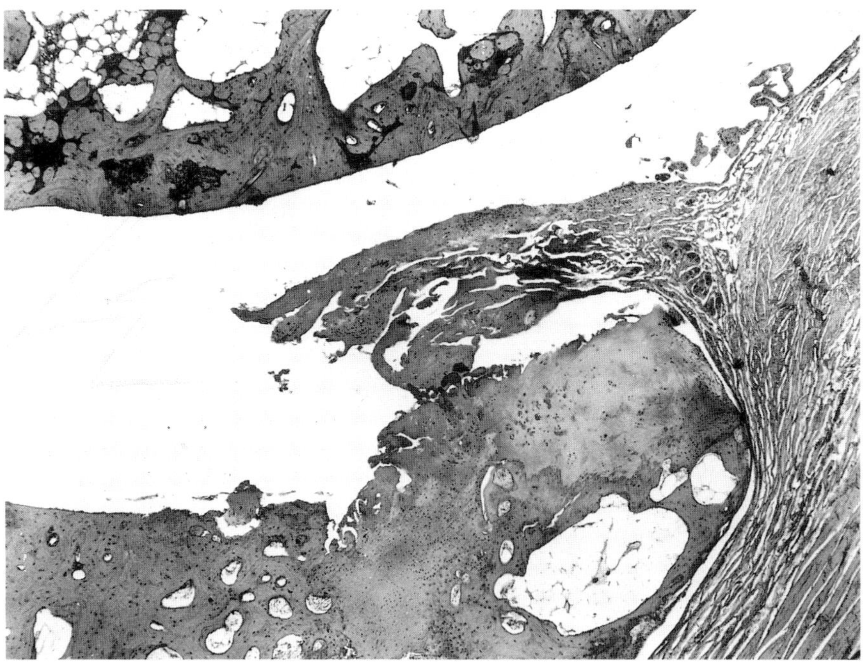

Fig. 473. Processes of synovial membrane comprising cystic spaces intrude into the joint cavity and penetrate into the articular cartilage

epiphyses are the prime and main tissues involved in the joint affection. The roentgenographically visualized marginal deepenings at the articular epiphyses of the end and middle phalanges of the fingers are distinct pertinent manifestations. These deepenings point to the underlying alterations. The causative synovial cystic erosions represent rather characteristic changes, which are especially observed in the postmenopausal phase and may thus be specifically related to the ovarian insufficiency. Such cystic erosions are not observed in elderly men who, occasionally, present osteoarthritic attritions and marginal exostoses in the interphalangeal joints secondary to overuse of the fingers. No overuse or injury of the fingers can be ascertained in the histories of most female patients. Stecher et al. [1565, 1566] reported that 72 of 74 patients with Heberden's nodes were postmenopausal women. This ratio can be verified in any larger number of patients with Heberden's or Bouchard's nodes.

Differential diagnosis must distinguish generalized arthritis developing secondary to metabolic disorders and infection. A history considering all diseases sustained by the patient in the past usually succeeds in clarifying this question. However, the differentiation versus primary osteoarthritis unrelated to any hormonal insufficiency is more difficult. This manifests itself in women aged over 60 years and chiefly in those who repeatedly strained their axial and peripheral joints in their work or private lives. On the other hand, arthropathy secondary to hormonal insufficiency manifests itself in women over the age of 45 years and independently whether they used their axial and peripheral joints intensely. Actually, most of these women report no strenuous prolonged activities of their hands. Additional informative criteria are the characteristic appearance of the fingers with nodes in their interphalangeal joints (Fig. 468, 469, 470) and the laboratory studies, which disclose a decreased production of estrogen and progesterone.

Treatment aims at correcting the lack of estrogen which is principally responsible for the articular symptoms. Daily administration of 0.6–1.2 mg estrogen in tablets for 3 weeks followed by 1 week without estrogen appears a physiological modality advisable throughout the postmenopausal age [560]. Local applications of moist warm packs to the painful joints and shortwave diathermy in distant series of eight to ten sessions provide symptomatic relief [944]. The episodic administration of androgens may be advisable less for a possible effect on the articular cartilage than for their effect on the general metabolism and thereby on the osteoporosis of the vertebral column. However, these patients must be watched for possible masculinizing effects, which would require immediate discontinuation of the androgens. Finally, a proper diet, low in carbohydrates and fat but high in proteins, fruit, and vegetables, is very necessary.

In men the testosterone and the androstenedione are the hormones (androgens) produced by the testes. The major sex hormone is testosterone, present in the serum at a concentration of 300–1200 mg/100 dl [424]. With advancing age the androgen levels decrease only slightly in most men and thus without untoward effect. However, those few men who suffer a substantial decrease in androgens go through a phase in their life in terms of articular symptoms similar to the climacterium in women. Clinical findings in the joints are similar to those in postmenopausal women, as is the treatment by administering testosterone on a regular basis.

VIII. Acquired Dysfunctions and Deformities of Joints

1. Laxity and Instability of Joints

The articular ends are invested by a joint capsule, and together with this form a joint. The outer fibrous part of the joint capsule keeps the articular ends together by virtue of its reinforcements, the ligaments. These secure the proper contact of the articular ends at all angles of excursion. That these ends, despite their incomplete congruence, do not come apart even at the extreme ranges of motion attests to the mechanical reliability of the ligaments.

However, under abnormal circumstances the articular ends are not held reliably together, and can deviate from each other even with normal function. Such disorder is termed laxity or instability of a joint. The cause of instability of a joint may lie in excessive changes in the joint capsule and its ligaments or those in the articular ends.

a. Constitutional weakness of the entire connective tissue system [1072] accounts for the idiopathic instability of any joint. Rotes-Querol et al. [1358] stress the composition of the ligaments by elastic fibers and collagen fibers. The elastic fibers are coiled and distensible but promptly reattain their original length once the distracting force has ceased. On the other hand, the collagen fibers, arranged in bundles, have a great resistance to distension but do not reattain their original length after being overdistended. Rotes-Querol et al. [1358] explain constitutional laxity of the ligaments by abnormal distensibility due to a basic disorder in their amino acids which are the interlacing molecules of the collagen fibers. Thus all joints of the body are involved in this disorder and can be moved to abnormal ranges of excursion which sometimes lend these joints a grotesque appearance. Such extreme mobility of individual joints (hand, vertebral column) may be beneficial for certain aptitudes or activities such as in musical performance, sports, or acrobatics [659, 660]. Otherwise, the instability of joints, especially those of the lower extremities, may be an impairing disability in daily needs.

b. If by injury a ligament is detached from its site of insertion, or its fibers are torn within their course and do not heal together, the result is insufficiency of the ligament. If a joint capsule is distended by chronic swelling and/or intraarticular effusion for a longer period of time, the ligaments remain overstretched. If in the treatment of fracture a traction device is applied with heavy weights, the pull is exerted not only at the site of the fracture but also on the joint capsule and its ligaments. Elderly persons or patients with poor muscle tone may then remain with overstretched ligaments. Similarly, in generalized or regional paralysis, the lack of muscle tone permits overstretching of ligaments, especially by prolonged weight bearing on an unprotected lower extremity.

c. Changes in the configuration of the articular ends often occur by intraarticular fractures which, if not adequately reduced, are followed by deformation and diminished height. A relatively excessive length of ligaments is associated with this, and their insufficiency is the outcome because proper tension is essential for the fixative role of the ligaments. Similarly, disturbances in the development of articular ends, such as those caused by bone diseases during the years of growth or an inflammatory destructive bone process, may result in incongruence of articular ends. In these situations, the points of attachment of the ligaments are brought more closely together; a relatively excessive length and decreased tension of ligaments are the sequelae.

Insufficiency of the ligaments or of the entire joint capsule and the associated instability of the joint cause symptoms which depend not only on the degree of the laxity but particularly on the involved joint [527, 659, 660]. In the vertebral column abnormal laxity of joints permits movements of abnormal ranges and unusual distortions of the body which may be useful in acrobatics or circus activities. In the shoulder joint laxity of the joint capsule due to inadequately healed tears of ligaments and/or tendons may be followed by unreliable retention of the humeral head in its glenoid cavity; thus the tendency of the humeral head to slip out of its joint may result, and a recurrent subluxation or dislocation is the outcome. In the elbow joint laxity is not very hindersome, and in the wrist and hand increased mobility may occasionally be beneficial in the practice of music or for manual skills. In contrast, laxity of joints of the lower extremity may be very disabling. When standing and especially when walking, each step with weight bearing on the ailing hip is associated with the sensation of instability and is manifested by a tilt of the pelvis to the affected side. In the knee joint [55, 1513] frequent buckling and the sensation of giving way, sometimes even the loss of control over the lower leg, cause a constant feeling of insecurity. The concomitant strains of the knee joint result in frequent pain and/or recurrent swelling. At higher degree of instability in the knee joint, the lower leg deviates from the thigh at each movement. In the ankle joint the tendency to trip over the foot or to twist the ankle joint at the slightest unevenness of the ground causes persistent soreness and chronic swelling of the ankle.

On physical examination the unstable joint or joints are not characterized by deformity unless a malunited fracture or a bone disease has resulted in a misshapen

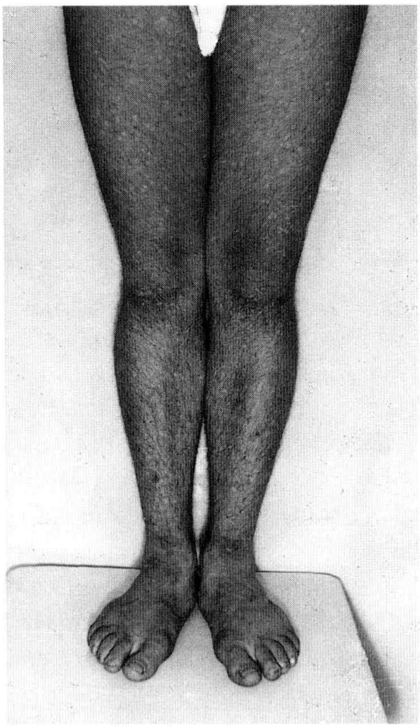

Fig. 474. Both knees are in straight alignment on upright standing and less weight bearing on the left leg

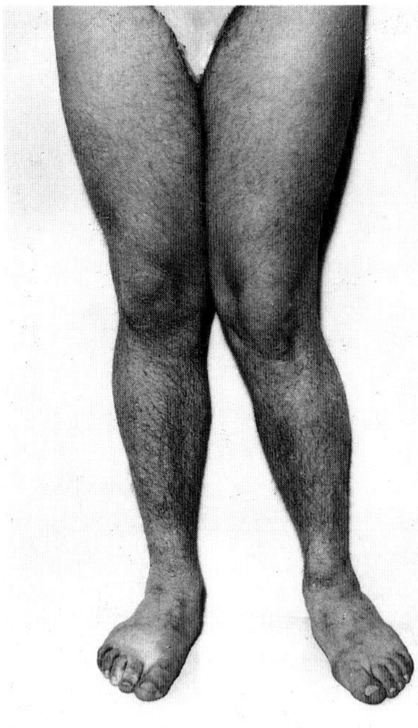

Fig. 475. The left knee deviates into valgus position on equal weight bearing on both legs

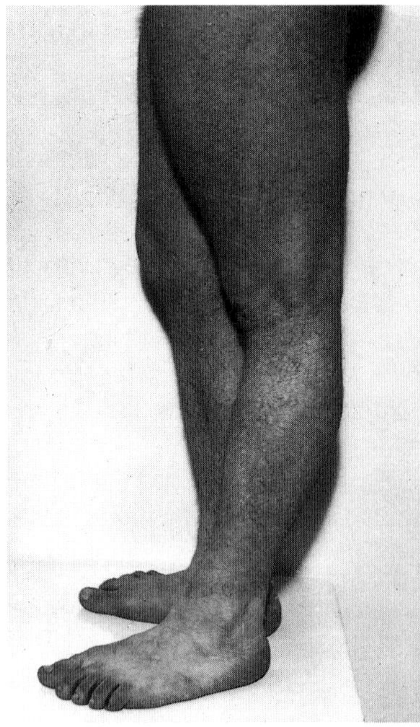

Fig. 476. The left knee deviates into recurvation on equal weight bearing on both legs

articular end. This becomes the cause of ligamentous insufficiency; permanent swelling is often an associated symptom. In the joints of the lower extremity instability is readily manifested on full weight bearing and standing without an external support (Figs. 474, 475, 476), and especially on walking. Additionally, the instability of any joint of an extremity is detected by examination for passive mobility. The proximal articular end is steadied with one hand of the examiner, and the distal end is grasped with the other hand, which attempts to tilt that part of the extremity into abnormal directions. It is necessary here that the regional musculature be completely relaxed because reflectory tightness of the musculature may preclude such kinking of a part of the extremity. Another and conclusive test is roentgenographic examination. Here especially in fresh posttraumatic cases, the tender area should be locally anesthetized to eliminate any muscle defense. The joint is then forced into abnormal deviations, while roentgenographs are taken (stress films; Figs. 46, 47). These permit precise determination of the angle of deviation and the one-sided gaping of the joint space. In longstanding injuries of the ligaments (Fig. 45) as well as in cases of late posttraumatic or postinflammatory alteration of the articular epiphyses the specific stress roentgenographs reveal the degree of ligamentous insufficiency and the one-sided widening of the articular cartilage space. In addition, in most cases with articular instability of longer duration, attritional changes with uneven narrowing of the cartilage space, subchondral sclerosis, and slight formation of marginal osteophytes may be noted.

Treatment of instability of joints, except for that caused by constitutional weakness of connective tissue, should be prophylactic. This means preventing or correcting those situations which could lead to instability. Any sprain with injury to ligaments should be treated as soon as feasible and preferably by immobilization so that healing of the damage may result. In cases with obvious and extensive disruption of the soft tissues, surgical repair of the damage is indicated [1200]. Any injury to the articular epiphyses should be treated with the aim of correcting an angulation, restoring the normal height of the epiphyses, and preventing relative insufficiency of ligaments. All bone injuries treated by traction should be managed by keeping in mind the possibility of distracting ligaments. All bone diseases should be treated with the concomitant endeavor to prevent, if possible, deformities of the articular ends.

For the instability of joints which occurs primarily in conjunction with constitutional weakness of the connective tissue of the body systematic strengthening of the entire musculature by regular exercises (isometric and isotonic contractions) and swimming may help to compensate for this weakness. In addition, strengthening of regional muscle groups for particular joints can be accomplished by faradic stimulation in two or three series of eight to ten sessions. Regular intake of vitamin

C 500 mg two to three times a day is of benefit because this vitamin participates in the build-up of proteins for the connective tissue.

In localized ligamentous disorder treatment should aim at correcting the underlying defect, especially in view of the otherwise developing secondary osteoarthritic changes. In laxity of the shoulder joint with propensity to recurrent subluxations or dislocations, surgical repair by plicating or reefing the joint capsule and by overlapping it with the tightened subscapularis tendon, the Putti-Platt procedure [1209], is indicated. The other joints of the upper extremity do not need surgical repairs and can be secured effectively by elastic or semirigid splints or hinge braces.

The unstable hip can be stabilized by a brace extending from above the iliac crest to the knee joint, with specially designed articulations to prevent any excessive motion. For those patients desiring surgical repair, the correction must be according to the direction or directions of excessive mobility. Plication of the joint capsule and iliofemoral ligament, possibly with reinforcement by flaps of the tendons of the iliopsoas muscle or the gluteal muscles, may prove adequate. The unstable knee joint [787, 1185] is a frequent object of surgical reconstruction for repairing insufficient ligaments. This is performed either by reinforcing them with neighboring dense connective tissue or more frequently by replacing them with transposed grafts from the sartorius or semitendinosus tendons, fascia lata, or patellar ligament. More than in any other joint, a thorough preoperative examination of the knee joint is necessary to determine precisely which of the ligaments, medial or lateral collateral, anterior or posterior cruciate, or possibly a combination of them, is deficient. Additionally, a concurrent injury to one of the menisci may complicate the clinical picture; this possibility must be kept in mind and the treatment adjusted accordingly. In less severe cases and commensurately with the degree of instability, or where surgery is not feasible, external support by an elastic knee cap reinforced with metal stays should be used. In more difficult cases and according to the degree of instability, a knee brace with articulations is indicated. This can be either a conventional long leg brace or a free knee brace with excentric joints. In cases of defectively healed fractures of the condyles of the knee, a reconstructive operation of the bones is necessary to restore the normal height of the condyles and the full tension of the ligaments. The ankle joint is a very frequent site of instability particularly in women, due partly to constitutional laxity but especially due to neglected or inadequately healed sprains of the ankle joint (Fig. 48). In most of these situations the ligaments at the lateral aspect of the ankle are affected. Frequently coexisting overweight contributes to the increased stresses upon the ankle and should be corrected first. Regular strapping of the ankle with a firm elastic bandage or application of an anklet with lateral hinges usually suffices. Otherwise, plication of the ligaments or their substitution by grafts from the peroneal tendons may be indicated.

2. Snapping of Joints

The undisturbed course of motion in a joint depends primarily on the congruent configuration and the even surface of its articular ends as well as on the full patency of the articular space. These prerequisites permit the articular ends, kept together by ligaments, to glide smoothly along one another when they are pulled by the tendons of contracting muscles. A pliable joint capsule invests them in all excursions. If one of these components presents gross-anatomical alterations, its contribution to normal joint functioning is diminished or lost, and the movement of the entire joint is disturbed or put in jeopardy. However, if the gross-anatomical changes involve only a portion of such articular component, the impediment arises at a certain angle of excursion, and the movement is momentarily blocked. This is followed by an intensified contraction of the regional muscles by which the articular ends overcome the obstacle and continue the remaining range of articular excursion at an accelerated speed. This disturbance in the function of a joint, manifested in a brief arrest of movement followed by its acceleration, is referred to as snapping.

Such snapping may involve any joint of the body, but it is most common in the knee, hip, metacarpophalangeal, and rarely in the shoulder and ankle joints. The snapping is elicited by different changes of the various articular constituents in the case of each joint.

The patients presenting a snapping phenomenon are aged from 6 to 65 years and are of either sex. Their histories are similar in that they report a dysfunction of the joint described as jumping. This disorder is often blamed on a strain, sprain, or misstep, but in other cases no such cause can be identified. In cases following an inflammation the snapping becomes manifest on resumption of full function. Although the examinations of younger patients suggest that the alterations leading to snapping are of congenital nature, the functional disturbance starting years later can be explained by adaptation in the changing shape of the intra- and extracapsular components during the years of growth. The patients are often able to point to the site where the snapping occurs. When a joint of the lower extremity is involved, the functional disturbance is much more pro-

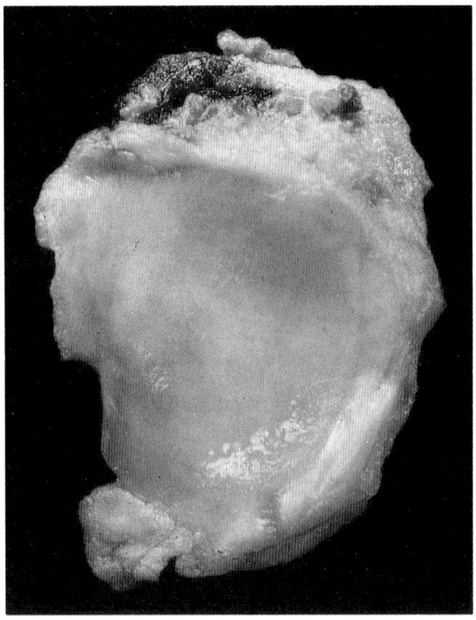

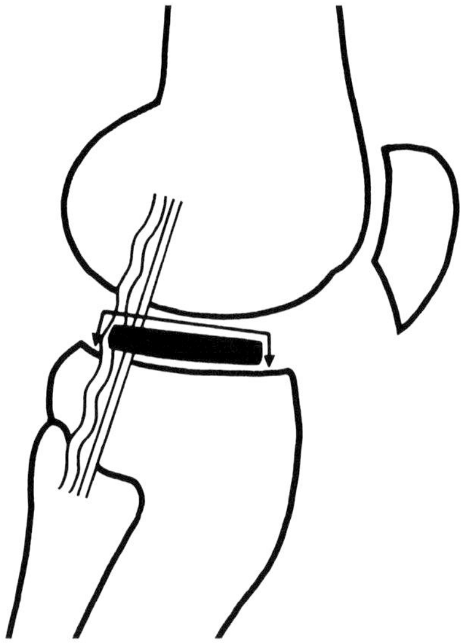

Fig. 477. The meniscus presents a congenital malformation by being a discoid plate with an extensive central indentation

Fig. 478. The misshapen meniscus is an impediment on any movement of the knee. It is overcome by enforced muscle contraction, whereupon at flexion the femoral condyles come down behind the meniscus

nounced because a feeling of insecurity or of falling often prevails, especially when fast motion is attempted.

Inspection occasionally discloses atrophy of the regional musculature. Palpation often reveals a protruding thickening or diffuse swelling involving a paraarticular organ or intraarticular structure and tenderness localized to the tissue accounting for the snapping. With the hand applied on the joint in motion, one can perceive roughness or friction in the paraarticular tendons, circumscribed thickening in the joint capsule or a ligament, prominent bulging from the joint cavity, or coarse crepitation between the articular ends. Sometimes a smacking noise is heard on motion. Nevertheless, the most instructive examination is the observation of the snapping phenomenon. This can occur at any angle of articular excursion, but most characteristically it occurs shortly after the start of flexion, before the termination of extension, or on combining these movements with a certain degree of rotation. The motion is suddenly arrested on attainment of the critical angle and is then resumed with acceleration until completion of the excursion. The snapping phenomenon can be mitigated by applying longitudinal traction to the extremity while the patient carries out the impaired motion. Roentgenographic examination generally reveals no significant findings since alterations of the soft structures usually account for the snapping phenomenon. However, in the case of osteochondritis dissecans, a migrating free body is detected between the articular epiphyses. In other cases, temporarily interposed calcified villi of the joint capsule are the cause.

The knee joint is affected more often than any other joint by the snapping phenomenon, and also presents the greatest variety of pathoanatomical alterations accounting for the phenomenon. Depending on the site [1555], the extraarticularly located alterations are uneven thickenings of the distal portion of the quadriceps tendon, patellar ligament, anserine bursa and contiguous tendons, or tractus iliotibialis. The intraarticularly located alterations causing a snapping phenomenon are villonodular synovitis, synovial chondromatosis, osteochondritis dissecans, chondropathia patellae, uneven thickening of the cruciate or collateral ligament, or congenital malformation of the meniscus [832]. The latter alteration, presented by a platelike or discoid misshaped meniscus (Fig. 477), accounts for the most characteristic snapping phenomenon [98]. This is elicited in the following way. When the collateral ligaments become tense on transition from extension to flexion at the angle of 155°–160°, the normally unnoticed switching in the knee joint from rocking to gliding or vice-versa encounters an impediment in the thickness of the malformed meniscus. The latter causes a substantial narrowing of the joint cleft. The movement is suddenly stopped, but thereafter continues with accelerated speed due to the intensified energy and enforced contraction of the regional muscles. On the way to flexion, the meniscus plate slips forward and is overridden backward (Fig. 478) by the femoral condyle which comes down with an audible pop on the tibial condyle. On the way to extension, the meniscus plate is squeezed backward (Fig. 478) and outward with a noisy snap. Roentgenographs sometimes reveal a loose intraarticular body or conspicuous widening of the joint cleft by lodging of a malformed meniscus. Since this dysfunction of the knee joint impairs basic stability and security during walking, correction of the disorder is imperative. The indicated operation resects or excises the interfering articular component, nodular thickening of the joint capsule, interposed free body, irregular thickening of the intraarticular ligaments, or usually malformed meniscus (Fig. 477). On the other hand, when alterations in the extraarticular structures are the cause, one or a few topical injections of hydrocortisone induce a distinct regression of the symptoms. Otherwise, resection or excision of the interfering tissue portion from the affected tendon is indicated.

In the hip joint the trochanteric bursa is often the seat of chronic inflammatory changes associated with thickening and roughness of the bursal wall. When the fascia lata is tensed in extended position of the hip joint, it encounters an impediment at the elevated, uneven trochanteric area on internal or external rotation of the femur. This impediment is shortly afterward overcome, and the remaining range of motion is completed with a visible and audible snapping. In flexed position of the hip joint the fascia lata is relaxed and does not rub against the thickened bursal wall; hence no snapping occurs. Such snapping may be very disturbing because of the functional impediment and the insecurity during walking manifest on each internal and external rotation of the leg. Avoidance of long walks and of rotation at each step may decrease the intensity and frequency of snapping. However, to reduce the thickening of the bursal wall moist hot packs should be applied to the trochanteric area once daily for one hour, and ultrasound with 2.5–3.0 W/cm^2 should be administered in eight to ten sessions. The next therapeutic step is topical injections with hydrocortisone solution. If this treatment also fails, the final procedure is an oblique division of the fascia lata by subcutaneous discission or an open lengthening combined with excision of the thickened bursa. This minimizes the apposition of the fascia lata to the greater trochanter and the friction by the interposed bursa. Another cause of snapping of the hip joint may lie in posttraumatic thickening of the iliofemoral ligament. This snapping manifests itself in the attempt at active full extension when the shortness and unevenness of the ventral ligament are overcome by intensified contraction of the gluteal musculature. A precipitated extension and external rotation of the hip joint then follow. Two or three topical injections of hydrocortisone usually succeed in softening the densified tissue and providing relief from the symptoms.

The snapping shoulder joint is caused by similar conditions – chronic inflammation of the subdeltoid bursa with thickening of its capsule. This interferes with the gliding of the deltoid muscle over the humeral head and blocks the elevation of the shoulder joint particularly in internal rotation. Another alteration causing snapping of the shoulder joint is bicipital tenosynovitis which by its protruding thickening interferes with the final flexion or final extension of the shoulder joint, especially on internal rotation. The impediment is overcome by intensified contraction of the deltoid and supraspinatus muscles, on the one hand, and the teres major muscle on the other, whereupon the movements complete their ranges at accelerated speed. The snapping shoulder blade is manifested in frequent snapping sensations associated with palpable and audible cracking produced on movements between a scarified subscapularis muscle and an uneven surface at the superoposterior wall of the chest cage. The symptoms in the shoulder joint are less disturbing and are remedied by application of moist hot packs and topical injections of hydrocortisone in the first few of the above conditions. The snapping shoulder blade requires prolonged treatment: it responds best to application of moist hot mud packs and diathermy in two series of eight sessions.

Snapping or trigger finger refers to a disturbance in the function of a finger characterized by obstruction on extension with transient locking at an angle of 100°–120° flexion. Thereafter on effort, either by active vigorous contraction of the extensor muscles or by passive manipulation, the finger snaps suddenly to full extension as if a trigger were released. Although the impediment to full extension is experienced in the metacarpophalangeal joint, the underlying pathological changes are extraarticular and involve the flexor tendons of the finger and their sheath. When this surrounding sheath becomes swollen secondary to mechanical irritation or any inflammation, it loses the smoothness of its inner surface by inflammatory ridges. Similar elevations develop on the surface of the flexor tendon. Thus irregularities are facing each other mainly at the site where the tendon sheath is relatively too narrow. This is the site where the superficial flexor tendon broadens by dividing into two slips to permit the exit of the deep flexor tendon to its insertion into the end phalanx. Triggering of the finger is then caused by the opposing ridges of the tendons and tendon sheaths which interlock with each other. This site on the volar aspect of the metacarpophalangeal joint is manifested clinically in nodular thickening (Fig. 535) of the tendon sheath and moderate tenderness. Since these irregularities are generally of inflammatory nature (Fig. 535), they may regress. Therefore, moist hot packs should be applied once or twice daily for 30 min. At that time gentle passive exercises by the other hand should also be carried out to stretch adhesions or shortened fibers. However, no active forced extension exercises may be undertaken as these aggravate the irritation of the tendon sheath. Should these modalities not provide essential improvement within 6–8 weeks, intrathecal (into the tendon sheath) and perithecal injections of hydrocortisone solution are routinely administered. These injections are commonly followed by regression of the inflammatory changes and subsidence of the symptoms. However, the tendinous tissue may become so disorganized by the topical hydrocortisone

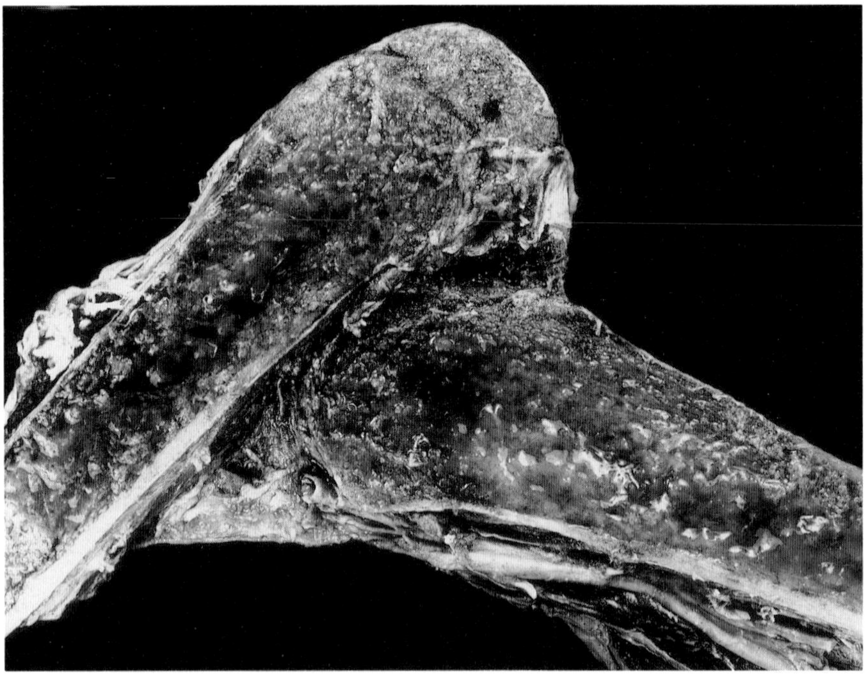

Fig. 479. The condyles of the tibia are eroded and are dorsally and proximally dislocated. The inner part of the joint capsule is thickened and uneven by large villi

injection that the flexor tendons may tear on any forceful extension. Thus an operation is more advisable. The tendon sheath is exposed and split, combined with excision of its thickened portion; the flexor tendon is then freed from its dentate constriction.

The ankle joint is often subjected to sprains in daily activities or sports and sustains injuries of the ligaments chiefly on its lateral aspect, the fibulotalar and fibulocalcaneal ligaments. If these ligaments do not heal adequately, they remain the cause of instability in the ankle joint. The tendons of peroneus longus and brevis can then slip forward and backward even in normal activity. The surrounding fascia and sheaths become distended. A frequent snapping in the ankle joint and subtalar joint results. These episodes are associated with a very disturbing feeling of insecurity which requires stabilization of the ankle joint and subtalar joints, at least by an anklet reinforced by plastic or metallic stays. Should this device not suffice, operative plication of the ligaments at the lateral aspect and reinforcement of the tendon sheaths are indicated to stabilize the tendons.

3. Contracture of Joints

The changes in a joint occurring in any disease often show that alteration of one articular component substantially affects the organic condition and/or function of other articular components. The sequential changes indicate the close interrelationship not only among the various tissues of a particular joint but also among this joint and all other organs participating in the functioning of the joint. This interconnection makes all ostensibly independent tissues and organs appear as a single functional unit, whose individual parts when harmed exert a reciprocal aftereffect upon one another; these are able to disrupt the functioning of the whole unit. Therefore, the term kinetic chain can be used to describe the assembly to a joint, indicating that harm to one part entails secondary impairment of the other parts.

If a joint capsule becomes inflamed or mechanically irritated, the articular ends may be drawn or tightened into a faulty position (Fig. 479) initially by the swelling of the joint capsule, and later by shrinking of the joint capsule as well as by concomitant reflectory muscle contraction at one side of the joint (Fig. 479). While the points of insertion of the contracted muscle group are brought closer together on this side, the antagonist muscles are overstretched and become atrophic on the opposite side. The equilibrium of the regional muscles is disturbed. Concurrently, the ligaments and periarticular tissues on the former side of the joint shrink; the deviation initiated by one tissue is followed in the same direction by the other structures of the joint. The elastic fixation of a joint at a certain angle within the physiological range of motion is associated with limitation of the active and passive movements of the joint in a specific direction. This is referred to as contracture [700]. Since the fixation is caused by shrunken soft tissues on one side [1788], the possibility of movement still exists in the direction of increasing the faulty position but not in the opposite direction with correction of

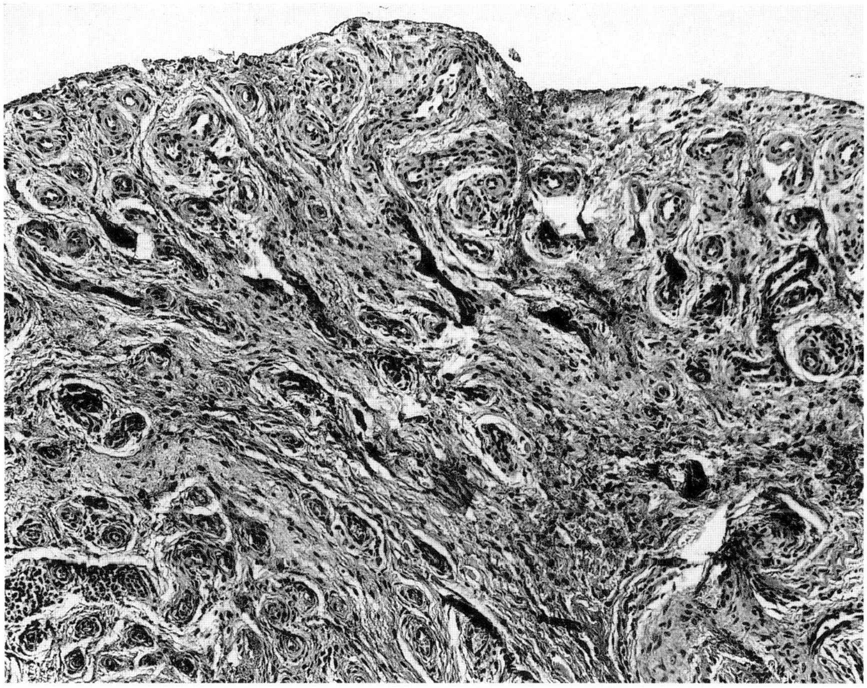

Fig. 480. The inner part of the joint capsule is very dense by a substantial increase in fibrocytes and by marked thickening of the collagen fibers

the deformity. Nevertheless, the indispensable prerequisite for moving the articular ends into any of the remaining directions is a maintained patency of the joint space (Fig. 479).

With an intact joint capsule, the cause for a contracture may reside in the regional musculature. If secondary to paralysis a muscle group atrophies, the antagonist muscles become overly dominant; they contract and remain contracted. Subsequently, the joint capsule shrinks at the side of the contracted muscles. The joint cannot be moved even passively toward the side of the paralytic muscles. Similarly, a contracture of a joint may develop if its musculature shortens after injuries or inflammations or in spastic conditions. Since the periarticular and articular tissues one-sidedly shrink in these conditions, the joint is held contracted in one direction of motion. According to the primarily affected tissue or organ, the contracture is designated as arthrogenic, myogenic, neurogenic, or desmogenic.

Gross-anatomical examination discloses alterations chiefly related to the affection of the organ which initiated the contracture. Thus in primary arthrogenic contracture the joint capsule invariably is thickened, and its inner surface is uneven by villi and folds (Fig. 479). The joint cavity is irregularly narrowed. The thickening expands into the fibrous capsule, while the articular ligaments are substantially shortened. Otherwise, in contractures originating from the surrounding organs, the inner surface of the joint capsule is even, and the joint cavity entirely extends. Of the surrounding structures, especially the regional musculature manifests its participation in the pathogenesis of the contracture by some of its groups being tight and densified while their antagonists are flaccid and soft.

Histopathological examination of the joint capsule in cases of primary arthrogenic contracture discloses conspicuous uneveness of the synovial membrane by plump villous elevations and a substantial increase in fibrocytes in the subsynoviocytic zone (Fig. 480). Infiltrates of inflammatory cells are of small extent. Whether of primary arthrogenic or extraarthrogenic origin, a dense fibrosis expands through the subsynoviocytic zone (Fig. 480) and involves peripherally the fibrous capsule.

Since the shortening and shrinking, initiated by different organs pertaining to any one joint, have the same outcome – an elastic rebounding contracture in a faulty position – the treatment is directed more at the deviation in contracture of any individual joint than at the tissue or organ which originated the contracture.

Contracture of the shoulder joint [445] generally develops secondary to a sprain of the shoulder, fracture of the humerus, clavicle, or scapula, inflammation such as bursitis or bicipital tenosynovitis, or any other painful regional condition, especially arthritis, which prevented the shoulder joint from being normally used. Indeed, it suffices to keep the shoulder joint immobile for 3–4 weeks to develop a contracture. Since during the period of rest the arm is kept close to the body, the unused inferior part of the joint capsule, the recessus infraglenoidalis, shrinks and becomes obliterated. The periarticular tissues, ligaments, tendons, and muscles

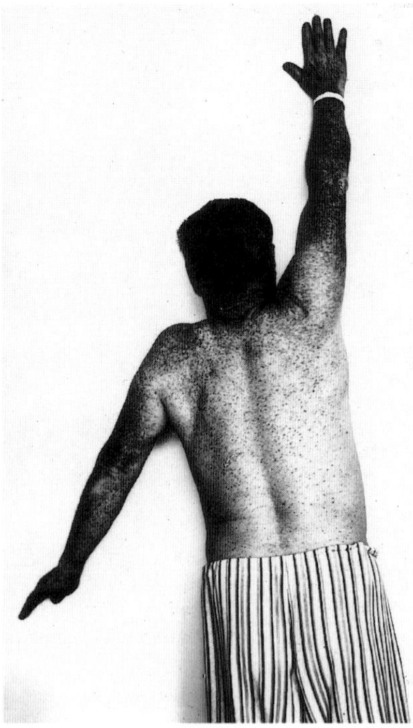

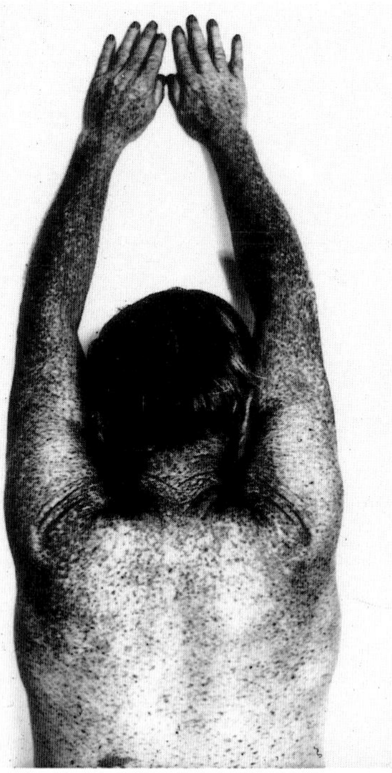

Fig. 481. The left arm can not be abducted beyond 40° either actively or passively

Fig. 482. The left arm of the patient in Fig. 481 can be raised to full elevation following manipulation under general anesthesia and subsequent active exercises

then become shortened. The tissues in the axilla and in front of the shoulder hold the arm close to the chest cage; an adduction contracture of the shoulder joint is present. The arm can be abducted away from the trunk maximally to about 45°–50° (Fig. 481) but cannot be raised to horizontal level or higher. The still available range of active motion does not provide exact information on the extent of limitation within the humeroscapular articulation, because part of the motion of the shoulder girdle is being carried out between the shoulder blade and the chest wall. The attempt at passive motion does not essentially increase the range of abduction and external rotation. Secondarily to inadequate use of the shoulder joint on longer duration, the musculature atrophies, and the configuration of the shoulder changes; it loses its roundness (Fig. 481). Contracture of the shoulder joint represents not only an impediment to the use of the arm but also a painful condition due to compression of the nerve fibers passing from the cervical spine to the arm by the shrunken tissues around the shoulder joint. Symptoms may include pain along the nerve fibers and occasionally numbness extending to the wrist and fingers. Unless advanced inflammatory or posttraumatic changes in the humeroscapular articulation are present, roentgenographs rarely reveal significant changes except for calcified bursae and inactivity osteoporosis of the articular epiphyses.

Once the diagnosis has been established, mobilization of the joint should be started without delay. Most important is to position the arm in maximally attainable abduction and for periods as long as feasible. During the day the arm is positioned on a table on which heavy books in increasing number are placed, and during the night a few pillows are placed between the chest and arm. In view of the increased pain and muscle tenseness caused by the corrective modalities, stronger analgesics and muscle relaxants are necessary. Additionally, regular application of moist hot packs are very beneficial; their mode of use and effects are discussed in "Osteoarthritis". However, the effective stretching of the shortened tissues of the shoulder joint can be accomplished only by energetic exercises. In upright standing, a cane is grasped with both hands and lifted as far as possible upward and backward. By raising the cane with both hands, the healthy arm serves as a guide to the ailing arm. When following these exercises the arm can be elevated above the horizontal level, rotating exercises are added. The elevated arm is grasped by the healthy hand and pulled behind the head toward the ear on the healthy side. Subsequently, the ailing arm is placed along the body and is pulled by the healthy hand behind the lower back toward the opposite hip. As a routine two other mobilization exercises are generally used. (a) The pendulum exercise: the upper body is bent forward, and the ailing arm is swung like a pendulum in all directions. However, this exercise does not provide a range beyond 90° abduction and is therefore not able completely to stretch the shrunken tissue. (b) The climbing exercise: the arm is raised above the horizontal level by climbing with the fingers along a wall as high as possible. This exercise, however, is

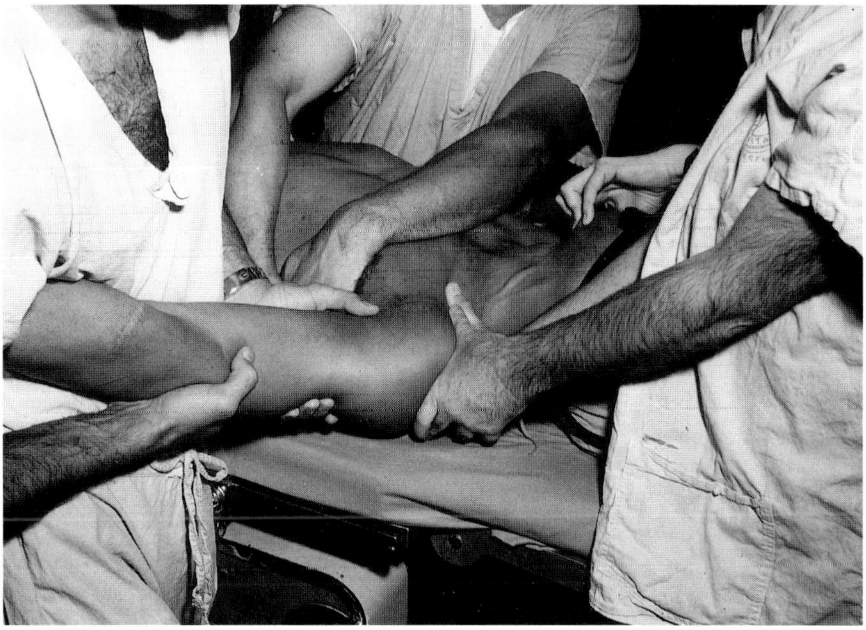

Fig. 483. With the patient under general anesthesia, the chest and shoulders are steadied, while traction and gradual abduction is exerted on the arm

effective only when carried out with the body in a position lateral to the wall, not facing the wall. If the active exercises by the patient do not provide an essential increase in the range of motion, they should be supplemented by passive exercises with the assistance of a physical therapist. Shortwave diathermy in two series of eight sessions for deep heating and ultrasound of similar frequency at 3–4 W/cm^2 intensity for softening the tissue are often beneficial. One to three periarticular injections of hydrocortisone, combined with a local anesthetic, sometimes succeed in suppressing persistent soreness confined to circumscribed areas and helping to expedite reattainment of the motion.

However, if these modalities do not succeed in restoring the ability to elevate the arm beyond the horizontal level, manipulation of the shoulder joint under general anesthesia is indicated. The shoulder blade and the shoulder are steadied by assistants, and the arm is distracted from the shoulder blade by the physician's maximal force (Fig. 483). This lengthens the shrunken tissues, joint capsule with its ligaments, and the surrounding tendons. The manipulations act principally upon the soft tissues, and the potential danger of fracture of the humerus is minimized. The arm is progressively brought by the physician's stretching maneuvers into increasing abduction (Fig. 483), subsequent elevation, and final external rotation. The benefit of such manipulation is usually a substantial increase in the range of motion (Fig. 482); this must be perpetuated by regular active elevation exercises with a cane for a few more months. Despite its impressive benefits, manipulation of the shoulder joint under general anesthesia should not be embarked on as the first modality but only after all conservative methods have failed. Complications of such manipulation may be a fracture of the osteoporotic humerus or overstretching of nerve fibers in the axilla with resulting, albeit transient, numbness and motor impairment in the arm and hand. Only rarely does such a manipulation not provide satisfactory improvement. In these cases operation may be necessary to dissect and lengthen the shortened soft structures (tendons, ligaments, and joint capsule) at the anterior and axillary aspect of the shoulder. Nevertheless, diligent mobilization exercises are then indispensable for maintaining the result obtained by surgery.

The elbow joint is often prone to contracture not only after inflammatory processes of long duration but also after such shorter periods of immobilization as are necessary in the treatment of fractures and other injuries to the elbow. The elbow joint then becomes usually contracted in a position between 90° and 110° from which neither further flexion nor further extension is possible; pronation or supination are also not possible to their full ranges. In some cases extension can be carried out to an adequate range, but flexion does not succeed to less than the right angle. Therefore the elbow should be mobilized as soon as possible after healing of the injury or regression of the inflammation. With the chest apposed to a table, the ailing arm rests firmly on the top of table. In contracture of the elbow joint the forearm usually rises to erect position. This forearm is grasped by the patient's other hand and is slowly but firmly pressed backward in the direction of flexion. Then the forearm is progressively turned more inward, then more outward, and is finally stretched in the direction of extension. Each of these exercises

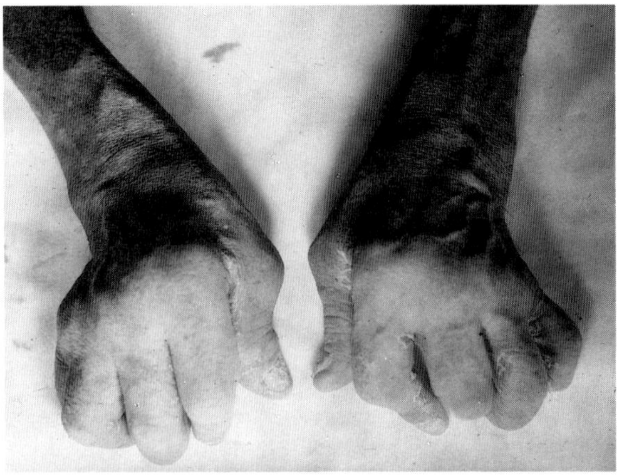

Fig. 484. The wrist joints are contracted in extension, while the metacarpophalangeal and interphalangeal joints are contracted in flexion secondary to arthritis in psoriasis. Ulcerations affect the left fingers

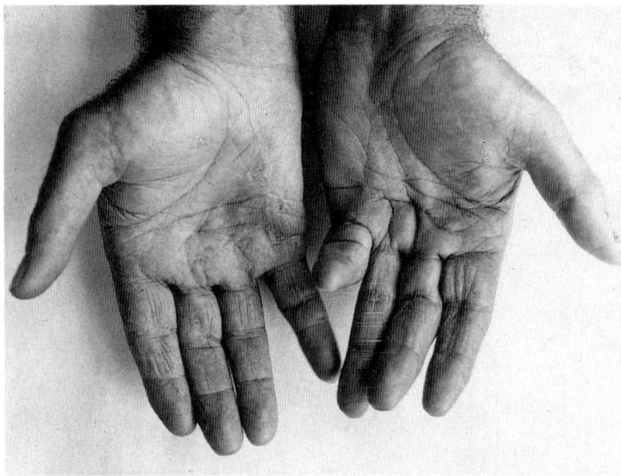

Fig. 485. The skin in the left palm is shrunken and deepened by two vertical folds. The third and fifth fingers are contracted in flexion

should be carried out three times daily, and analgesics should be taken in advance. It is also advisable to apply moist warm packs before the exercises in order to soften the tight tissues. These exercises require a firm grip by the manipulating hand and rarely are adequately carried out by the patient himself. Therefore they should be performed by another person or by a physiotherapist who steadies with one of his hands the patient's arm and forces with the other hand the patient's forearm into further flexion, pronation, supination, and finally extension. In cases of persistent contracture, manipulation under general anesthesia is necessary. Here too, long aftercare with regular mobilization exercises in all physiological directions is indispensable.

The wrist joint develops contracture secondary to intraarticular inflammation (Figs. 187, 484) or fracture at the distal end of the radius. Similarly, proliferative inflammations of the tendon sheaths be on the dorsal or volar aspect of the wrist or paralyses of the forearm musculature are followed by contracture of the wrist joint. Depending on the site of the shrunken tissues, the wrist joint becomes contracted in neutral position or more often in volar flexion. Occurrence of the latter can be prevented by timely immobilization of the wrist with a splint in cocked position. However, once a deviation developed, it should be corrected without delay. In whatever position the wrist joint became contracted, it must be mobilized by exercises. The forearm is placed on a table in such a way that the wrist joint extends closely beyond the edge of the table. The wrist is grasped by the other hand and is manipulated in dorsal and volar, radial and ulnar directions and is finally rotated in all directions. These exercises should be carried out daily. It is also necessary to apply moist warm packs each day to soften the shrunken tissues. When volar flexion contracture exists, manipulation exercises particularly in the direction of dorsal extension should be supplemented with a cocked splint as long as the volar flexion contracture has not been fully corrected. When the exercises by the patient or his relatives are not sufficient, the additional services of a physiotherapist are necessary. Because of swelling recurring with the exercises, application of an elastic bandage during the day and elevation of the arm on pillows during the night are advisable.

The finger joints often become contracted in conjunction with a contracture of the wrist joint (Figs. 187, 188) or alone secondary to intrinsic affections, injuries, or inflammations usually of their tendon sheaths (Fig. 484). The contracture usually develops in the direction of flexion, unless the flexor tendon has become insufficient secondary to injury, whereupon contracture in extension position follows. With the more frequent flexion contracture (Figs. 186, 187, 188) the extension ability is limited or absent, and mobilization exercises should concentrate on this direction. With the second and third fingers of the patient's nonaffected hand pressing the adjacent phalanges from the volar aspect, the thumb of his nonaffected hand presses the interphalangeal joint from its dorsal aspect in the volar direction. This manipulation is performed on all interphalangeal joints as well as on the metacarpophalangeal joint since all joints of a finger or of the fingers are generally affected. These exercises should be daily carried out in a sink with warm water to soften the tight tissue. In view of the tendency of these small joints to persist in deviation, overnight immobilization of the finger in fully corrected position by metal or plastic splint is very useful.

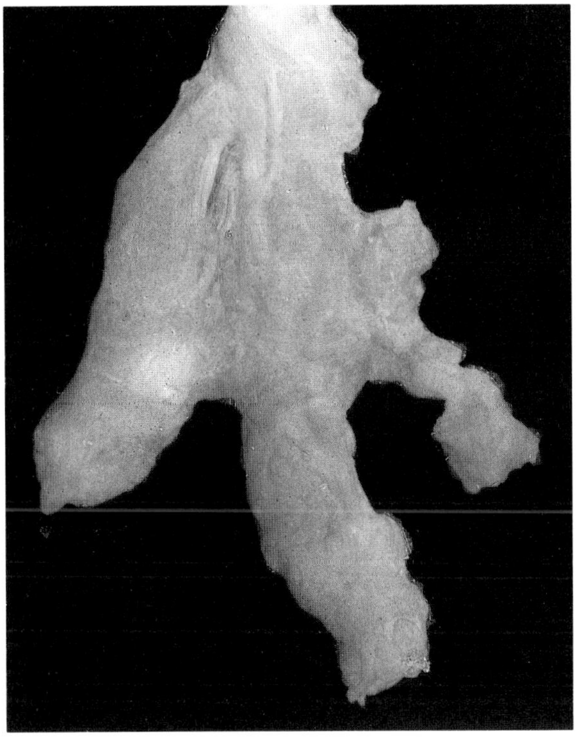

Fig. 486. The in toto excised palmar fascia consists of very dense greyish white connective tissue

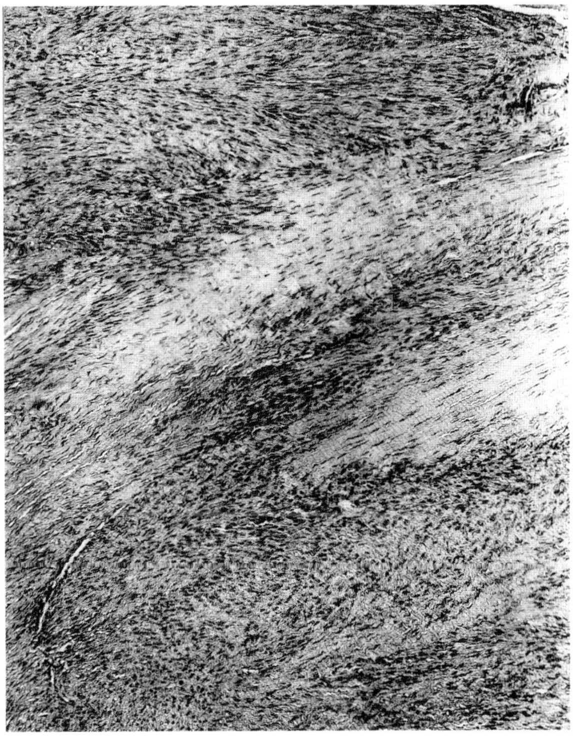

Fig. 487. The connective tissue from the excised palmar fascia is very dense by a marked increase in fibrocytes and collagen fibers

Dupuytren's contracture [449] is an intrinsic alteration of the hand associated with flexion contractures of the fingers (Fig. 485). This contracture proceeds from the palmar fascia which overlies the flexor tendon sheaths of the hand and becomes increasingly thickened due to proliferation of its fibroblasts and fibrocytes. In the late phase collagen fibers predominate in lamellar and nodular arrangements. Here the tissue (Fig. 487) resembles histopathologically a fibroma or even a fibrosarcoma. The cause of the benign tumorlike proliferation of fibrocytes is explained [785] as the reaction to intensive activities of the hand, possibly connected with the patient's type of work. However, it also occurs in individuals who do not perform manual work, and in some in combination with tumorous thickening of the plantar fascia, an indication that constitutional predisposition may be here the cause. Secondary to dense formation of collagen fibers, the fibrosed fascia shrinks and by its distal expansions draws the metacarpophalangeal and interphalangeal joints into flexion (Fig. 485). Due to persistence of this position the volar capsule and ligaments of these joints eventually shrink, and the desmogenically initiated deformity becomes arthrogenically perpetuated. The thickening of the palmar fascia becomes obvious by its nodular elevations and by the creasing of the overlying skin (Fig. 485) due to fibers extending into the skin. In the initial phase passive stretching exercises of the involved fingers should be carried out, and these should be followed by splinting in extended position; hereby shrinking of the fascia and its pull on the fingers may be minimized. If such deformity has already developed, two or three topical injections with hydrocortisone may succeed in softening the palmar fascia and making the contracture of the fingers more amenable to corrective exercises. In more advanced contracture the fibers of the fascia can be divided by subcutaneous discission under local anesthesia; this procedure is indicated chiefly in diabetics or elderly persons. However, if the flexion contracture of the fingers is so firm that no passive extension manipulations can effectively be carried out, the fascia should be excised in toto (Fig. 486) together with its fibers extending into the tendon sheaths and interphalangeal joints. Partial fasciectomy does not succeed because remaining scattered fibrocyte nodules (Fig. 487) subsequently proliferate and cause another contracture [1231]. The incision follows the palmar distal crease with proximal and distal undermining of the skin; in the case of very shrunken skin, a Z-plasty is indicated. Usually the fibrous joint capsules of the metacarpophalangeal and interphalangeal joints are so shrunken and thickened that they must be divided to allow extension of the joints. Immediately after surgery the fingers should be held in flexion to permit proper closure of the wound and adaptation of the circulation. After healing of the wound diligent passive extension exercises are instituted, supplemented with temporary immobilization of the fingers on a straight volar splint until an adequate range of extension of all finger joints has been obtained.

The hip joint becomes contracted mostly in inflammatory or degenerative conditions which involve the joint capsule and articular ends, but it may also occur in posttraumatic shrinking of the surrounding tendons and muscles, and in cases of muscle imbalance secondary to neurological disorders. Due to the predominance of the iliopsoas and the adductor muscles, the affected hip joint usually assumes a flexion-adduction position which is recognizable by the bent-forward position and relative shortening of the leg. This type of shortening can be ascertained by measuring the length of the supposed shorter leg and that of the normal leg. Apart from the stress upon the hip joint, each step in upright attitude causes a strain on the lumbar spine which is held overstretched to maintain the trunk erect. The ipsilateral knee joint is held in flexed position to permit downward vertical thrust of the lower leg. Such a hip joint represents a restriction in many activities and also an impediment for women because of the limitation in spreading the thighs apart. Thus both components of the contracture, adduction and flexion, of the hip joint must be corrected. For the adduction, regular abduction exercises are essential; in supine position on a firm mattress or on the floor, the legs are spread as widely as possible with the hands being used additionally to pull the hips apart. For the flexion deformity, resting or sleeping regularly in prone position on a firm mattress is of elementary necessity. A sandbag of increasing weight from 3 to 15 lb, placed on the buttocks, helps to stretch the shortened tissue at the anterior aspect of the hip joint. Moist warm packs should be applied at least once daily to make the shrunken tissues more amenable to the corrective exercises. If these are not performed strongly enough by the patient and relatives, passive exercises by a physiotherapist should be added to obtain more stretching of the shortened tissues. However, if these do not yield adequately, a traction device can be applied around the ankle to pull the leg into abducted position. At the same time, a sandbag is placed under the buttocks with the patient in supine position to bring the hip joint into extension. If these modalities fail to obtain adequate yielding of the shortened soft tissues, these must be lengthened by an operation. The tendons of the iliopsoas and adductor muscles and the ligaments at the anterior aspect of the hip joint are exposed and divided. The hip joint is then manipulated into the correct positions, and a plaster cast or firm brace is applied for 4–6 weeks to secure healing of the dissected tissues in satisfactory alignment with the hip joint. Subsequent mobilization exercises of the hip joint are performed for 3–4 months. Since this procedure corrects only the shortened soft tissues, any underlying disease of the articular epiphyses may require special treatment.

The knee joint is often involved by contracture; depending on the persistent position, as determined by the affected main structures, this is termed extension contracture or flexion contracture. Extension contracture [1635, 1704] usually develops as a sequela of immobilization of the knee joint for periarticular inflammations or for injuries to the ligaments, tendons, or bones. The first change noted here is atrophy of the quadriceps muscle, caused by inactivity and trophic disorders secondary to irritation of vasomotor nerve fibers. Atrophy of the muscle fibers is followed by vicarious proliferation of the interstitial connective tissue, which by its subsequent fibrotic shrinking leads to hardening and shortening of the quadriceps muscle. If the joint capsule is also affected, its response alterations may cause it to become adherent to the articular ends and may substantially limit motion by the narrowing of the joint cavity. A knee joint stiffened in extended position, although free of pain and fully capable of weight bearing, interferes with many activities of daily life and work. When sitting, such a leg is held straight, and when walking or running, it prevents fast locomotion due to longer duration in getting started. For those wishing to take part in sports activities, a nonyielding, straight knee joint is a permanent impediment. Roentgenographic examination reveals the presence of a patent although sometimes narrowed or uneven joint space and a thickening of the articular or periarticular soft structures. The most important factor in the treatment of an extension contracture [1300] is its prevention. Immobilization of an injured knee joint with a plaster cast or a stiff brace or by traction should be carried out only for the minimum necessary period of time. Similar considerations apply to all inflammations of the knee joint or its periarticular structures. Upon completion of the rest period, mobilization of the knee joint must be started without delay by forcing the lower leg backward with both hands into flexion position three times daily in a warm bath. Another modality is to lie across the bed with the knee joint on the edge of the bed and with a sandbag, starting with 3 lbs and increasing to 15 lb, attached around the ankle. The sandbag pulls the lower leg downward and backward, forcing the knee into progressive flexion. Additionally, various splints and braces have been designed for use by the patient in supine or prone position; these are based on the principle of pulling or pressing the lower leg into flexion. Further help in increasing the range of flexion can be provided by energetic flexion manipulations carried

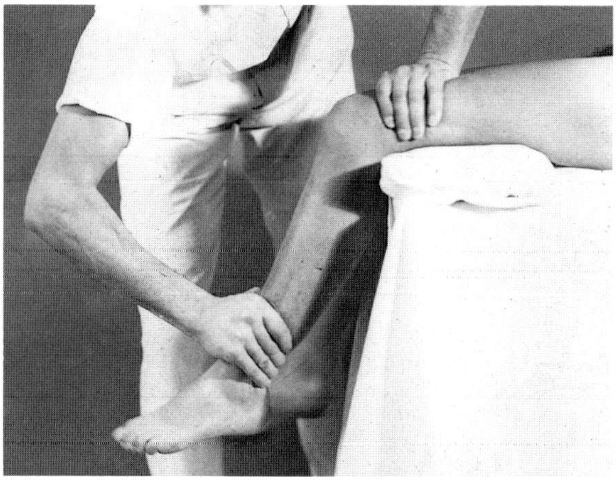

Fig. 488. With the thigh resting on a table and a folded sheet beneath its distal part, the lower leg is gently manipulated into progressing flexion

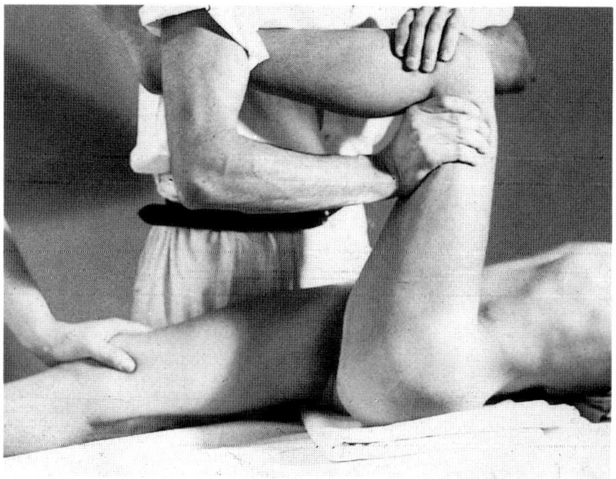

Fig. 489. If sufficient flexion can not be attained by positioning in Fig. 487, the hip joint is flexed to 90°, and the knee joint is gradually manipulated at least to a right angle

out by a physiotherapist. The combination of regular active and passive exercises eventually results in a physiological range of motion.

However, if the exercises are hampered by nonyielding tissue and tense pain in and around the knee joint, manipulation of the knee joint under general anesthesia is indicated. Such manipulation is rejected by some physicians because it may cause tears of articular tissues, hemorrhages followed by renewed shrinking, and serious fractures; however, this nonsurgical procedure should be attempted since it offers the greatest probability for reattaining mobility. Nevertheless, the manipulation must not be carried out as a forced brisement with tearing of the shortened fibers but as a gentle redressment with gradual stretching of all scars. With the patient in the supine position, first the patella must be mobilized from the femur because an adherent patella may be the main obstacle in regaining the flexion. Forcing the knee into flexion may cause either a fracture of the patella or a tear of the quadriceps tendon. Therefore, the patella is grasped and moved against the femur medially and laterally, upward and downward. After the mobility of the patella has been restored, the leg is shifted distally on the table so that the joint cleft of the knee comes to lie directly on the edge of the table (Fig. 488). A folded sheet is placed beneath the distal part of the thigh, which is steadied by the left hand of the surgeon, while the lower leg is grasped by the right hand, which elastically and gradually presses the lower leg downward and backward (Fig. 488). Here the crepitation of the stretched fibers is perceived; the range of motion progressively increases until it stops at a nonyielding hold. Continuation of the manipulation beyond this stop may lead to tears and fractures. One rarely succeeds by forced manipulation to attain the full range of flexion in one stage, but one should endeaver to attain a flexion range to the right angle (Fig. 489). With less than 90° flexion attained, the knee joint loses the newly gained flexion. After completion of the manipulation, the knee is surrounded by wet cold compresses. Flexion exercises are started a day later by dangling the lower leg over the edge of the bed and suspending a sandbag with increasing weight from 3 to 15 lb on the ankle. Once an angle of flexion of about 75°–80° (taking the straight knee as being in 180° extension) has been attained, kneeling exercises are practised daily on a pillow either on the floor or in a tub with warm water, which soothes the soreness and softens the tissues; the weight of the body presses the knee into increasing flexion. If the full range of flexion has not yet been attained, but a good excursion range has been accomplished, a further manipulation may be applied 3–4 weeks later (Fig. 489). At any rate, full weight bearing on the manipulated leg should not be started before the possibly final angle of flexion is reached.

For those cases in which the manipulation of the knee joint was rejected or was unsuccessful, exploration and repair of the structures and organs thought to be the obstacles to flexion is carried out by an open operation. If the scar and adhesions are in the quadriceps tendon, this should be freed from the femur and lengthened [114] to the distance which permits flexion beyond the right angle. If the obstacle to mobilization of the knee joint lies in obliteration of the patellofemoral space, these adhesions must be divided to permit free gliding of the patella; interposition of a flap of synovial tissue between the patella and femur, such as in chondropathia patellae (Fig. 244), is indicated to provide frictionless gliding in this space.

Flexion contracture of the knee joint [1163, 1291] develops as a sequela after intensive inflammation as-

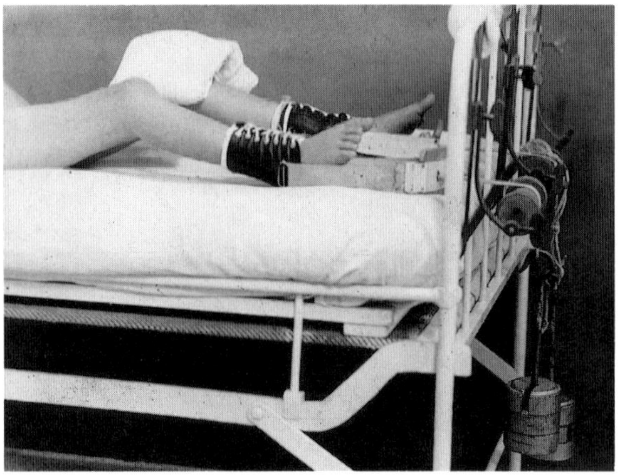

Fig. 490. Cuff traction with attached adequate weight and a sandbag placed on top of the knee joint often correct a flexion contracture

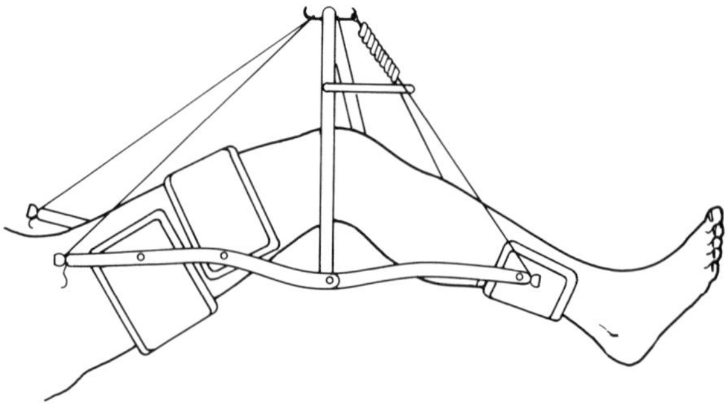

Fig. 491. The turnbuckle brace exerts greater vigor and thus is able to straighten out a tenacious flexion contracture

sociated with marked swelling of the joint capsule. An increase in joint fluid and/or the reflectory muscle spasm causes the joint automatically to assume the middle position of about 120°–130° (full extension being 180°), in which all portions of the joint capsule are equally relaxed. By persistence of the flexion position the flexor muscles shorten and the posterior joint capsule shrinks. The ligaments also participate in this shrinking. The shortened collateral ligaments pull the tibia backward away from the femur; this is also the case with the cruciate ligaments, which together with the hamstring tendons initiate a posterior subluxation of the tibia (Fig. 186). Thus the changes leading to flexion contracture reside primarily inside the knee joint. Beyond these, injuries or inflammations of the regional muscles and/or affections of the central nervous system or peripheral nerves also lead by disturbance of the muscular equilibrium to persistent contraction of the flexor muscles and hence to flexion contracture of the joint. Similarly, inflammations or burn scars of the skin and subcutaneous tissue in the popliteal area with secondary shrinking may also be followed by flexion contracture. This deviation becomes especially obvious in the upright position, when weight bearing on this leg is possible only with the hip joint flexed, the lumbar spine hyperlordosed, and the foot in equinus attitude to touch the ground. With more advanced flexion contracture, walking is possible only supported by crutches, but without weight bearing on the affected leg and with the lower leg deviated backward. Accordingly, the flexion may have a larger or smaller range, but no extension is feasible.

A flexion contracture of the knee joint can be prevented [396, 1298] in many cases by immobilizing the knee joint – in cases of soft tissue injuries, inflammatory processes, or nerve disorders – with a lateral plaster cast splint or a dorsal metal splint in fully extended position until these disorders regress. A very effective method to correct a beginning flexion contracture is the Buck's traction or a cuff attached to the ankle, pulled by a rope and weight via a pulley (Fig. 490). The initial weight of 5 lb may be gradually increased to 10–15 lb, provided that the skin beneath the traction device is checked regularly for pressure sores. Even a fully developed flexion contracture may yield after 3–4 weeks of such traction. The latter can be made more effective by sandbags, starting with 2 lb and increased to 10 lb and placed on top of the knee joint (Fig. 490). Once the fully extended position of the knee joint has been attained, it should be maintained by a long leg brace with joint locks. If the traction device is not effective, various apparatuses or braces can be used which are constructed on the same principle: longitudinal and ventral pull on the lower leg and dorsalward pressure on the distal area of the femur. However, due to shrinking of the cruciate and collateral ligaments, such ventral pull may result in concomitant dorsal subluxation of the lower leg by a lever effect unless this apparatus also exerts distraction within the knee joint and stretches the ligaments. Because of similar considerations a manipulation is not advisable for correction of a flexion contracture since it may aggravate a beginning dorsal subluxation of the lower leg. In consideration of this complication, apparatuses similar to the turnbuckle plaster cast (Fig. 491) have been designed which exert distraction of the knee joint under concurrent lengthening of the cruciate and collateral ligaments. Another effective correcting method is that of skeletal traction; here a Kirschner wire is drilled through the tibial tubercle and is attached to a traction clamp which pulls the lower leg distally and distracts the shortened ligaments. This prevents dorsal subluxation of the tibia and corrects the flexion position of the knee joint.

However, in flexion contracture of long duration, the posterior joint capsule, periarticular structures, and all tendons crossing the popliteal space are so shortened that no traction is able to effect a lengthening of the shrunken tissues. The only solution in this situation is the surgical exposure of the popliteal space with identification of each local organ (particularly nerves and blood vessels), lengthening of all shortened connective tissue structures (deep fascia and medial and lateral hamstring tendons), and stripping off the posterior joint capsule from femur and tibia. Additionally , the tensor fasciae latae and the lateral intermuscular septum should be divided because their shrinking aggravates the contracture. After correcting all impediments, the knee joint is extended only as far as the circulation permits and is placed on a splint with a traction device on the ankle. The circulation of the lower leg must be watched hourly for the following 2 days; should this be compromised, the corrected position must be decreased to the angle, at which satisfactory circulation of the lower leg is restored. Immobilization by traction of the knee at the maximum obtainable extension is then carried out for about 2 weeks under regular observation of the peripheral circulation until the operative wound has healed. Thereafter, the knee is systematically mobilized in the directions of extension and flexion by daily active and passive exercises with the help of a physiotherapist until the movement of extension has been secured. During that time it is necessary to wear a long leg brace with locks to maintain the maximal possible range of extension. This range may be increased by long-term continuation of forced mobilization treatment. On the other hand, when dissection of the popliteal space is not feasible or not advisable because of extensive and dense scar formation, supracondylar osteotomy of the femur and infracondylar osteotomies of the tibia and fibula succeed in straightening the leg, although at the price of shortness and unimproved range of motion.

The ankle joint becomes contracted in the course of arthritis of various etiologies or in severe injuries with intraarticular fracture. The often unavoidable shrinking of the joint capsule and ligaments may become aggravated if tendons have also shrunk. This occurs principally when the ankle was immobilized for a longer period of time to maintain proper reduction of a comminuted fracture or the ankle joint was held in persistently faulty attitude due to muscular imbalance in neurological disorders. Shortening of the Achilles tendon then generally leaves the ankle joint contracted in pronounced plantar flexion. The contracture can be minimized if treatment is started once the inflammation subsides, or the injury of the ankle heals. The ankle joint is mobilized actively by flexing the foot in the dorsal and plantar directions and by rotating it to all sides at least twice daily. For passive mobilization the foot is grasped with one hand, and the lower leg is firmly held above the ankle with the other hand; the foot is forced in dorsal and plantar directions and in a circle twice daily. Concurrent soaking of the foot in warm water softens the tissue, thus making the exercises more effective. While mobilization in the direction of plantar flexion usually progresses satisfactorily, reattaining an adequate angle of dorsal flexion encounters difficulty due to persistent shortening of the Achilles tendon. Stretching of the Achilles tendon can be effectively carried out by placing a folded sheet around the middle of the foot, grasping each end of the sheet with a hand, and pulling on these ends with maximal force. If these exercises do not succeed in restoring the normal range of dorsal flexion, lengthening of the Achilles tendon and division of the posterior joint capsule is a necessary operation. To secure the corrected position, a lower leg brace with an ankle stop at the right angle is indispensable for 6–12 months in the aftercare. During this time dorsal flexion exercises in the ankle joint are regularly carried out. The much less frequent contracture of the ankle joint in dorsal flexion is usually the sequela of a malunited fracture involving the talus and/or the calcaneus or the sequela of disproportionate action of the lower leg musculature in a flaccid or spastic paralysis. Initial treatment consists in diligent passive elongation exercises of the shortened tendons on the anterior aspect of the lower leg and in forced manipulations to lengthen the joint capsule on the anterior aspect of the ankle joint. Beyond this , the primary etiological condition must be corrected either by osteotomy and open reduction of the malunited fracture, concluding with internal fixation, or by transposition of tendons such as the anterior tibialis or peronei into the tuber calcanei. Achilles tenodesis may also help to correct the muscle imbalance.

4. Ankylosis of Joints

Stiffness of a joint associated with absolute lack of mobility in any direction is referred to as ankylosis. It is characterized by obliteration of the entire joint space concomitant with fusion of the contiguous articular epiphyses. This is the outcome of conditions in which the articular cartilage has been widely destroyed, with the articular epiphyses becoming denuded and fused with each other. In addition, the joint capsule, being intensely irritated, initiated or participated in the destruction of the articular cartilage and subsequently contributed to the welding of the articular epiphyses.

Such extensive damage to the articular cartilage often occurs in comminuted intraarticular fractures. If exact reduction of the fragments could not be accomplished, the contiguous articular surfaces, deprived in large areas of their cartilage, merge due to the outgrowth of the exposed subchondral bone. The capsular

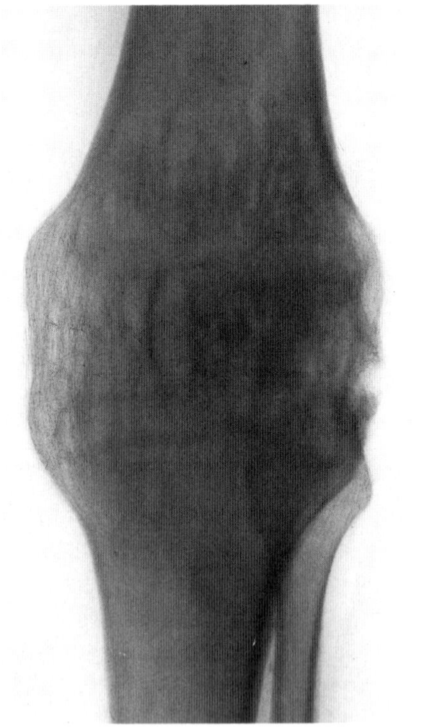

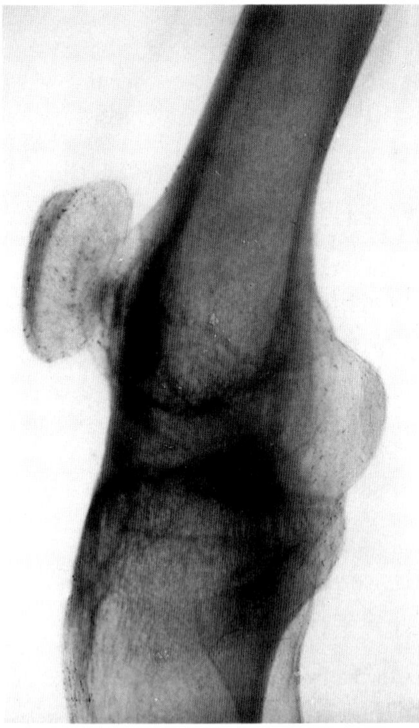

Fig. 492. Osseous ankylosis developed secondary to suppurative arthritis. Areas of osteoporosis and osteosclerosis expand in the femoral and tibial condyles

Fig. 493. Osseous ankylosis developed secondary to gonorrhoic arthritis. Dense trabeculae pass continuously from one to the other epiphysis

and periarticular tissues shrink secondarily to the trauma and participate in the fusion of all damaged tissues into a single block. Extensive damage is more commonly inflicted in severe inflammations, when the articular cartilage becomes necrotic and disintegrates due to toxic harm by microorganisms and/or enzymatic digestion by the inflamed synovial membrane. The latter expands as a pannus from the margins over the articular epiphyses (Fig. 86) and intrudes with granulation tissue into the resulting cartilage defects (Fig. 87) as well as into the joint cleft. By the following obliteration of all capsular recessuses (outpouchings, reserve spaces) and of the articular space (Figs. 87, 101), the entire joint cavity becomes filled with soft, inflamed tissue and finally with dense, fibrosed tissue. When the bone of the denuded articular ends is concomitantly stimulated, osteoid and osseous tissue grows out into the obliterated joint cavity and leads to ossification of the fibrosed tissue. Stresses such as vertical pressure by weight bearing upon the subchondral bone are especially apt to stimulate the outgrowth of osteoid tissue. The fibrous union of the articular ends eventually becomes transformed into an osseous fusion.

The symptoms and findings in the two conditions, fibrous or osseous fusion, are identical. Neither active nor passive movements can be carried out in such a joint due to lack of yielding in the obliterated joint space. The periarticular tissues are thickened, and the regional musculature is atrophic due to lack of action. The thickening and deformity of the joint thereby become more conspicuous. The joint is sometimes stiffened in full extension or, more often, in a degree of middle flexion. No local signs of inflammation are noted, nor are areas of tenderness detectable. Body temperature is normal. Blood studies, including sedimentation rate, do not disclose any specific anomaly because the traumatic and/or local inflammatory reactions have subsided by the time that the ankylosis is completed.

Roentgenographs reveal the type of ankylosis. In fibrous ankylosis the joint space is partly discernible, although most often significantly narrowed and irregularly delimited due to erosion of the osteocartilaginous borders. In osseous ankylosis the previous joint space is filled with bone which sometimes leaves the outline of the former articular ends still discernible (Figs. 492, 493). Roentgenographs further help to identify the changes in the bones leading to ankylosis, whether comminuted intraarticular fracture, inflammation of the epiphyseal bone as in osteomyelitis (Figs. 492, 498, 504), or severe inflammation or suppuration within the joint cleft (Figs. 192, 492). The articular epiphyses have lost their normal outline secondary to profound traumatic alterations or inflammatory destructive processes (Figs. 498, 504). The trabeculae pass continuously from one articular epiphysis to the adjacent articular epiphysis in osseous ankylosis (Fig. 492) and display a characteristic arrangement. More pronounced endosteal bone growth is observed in the areas of greater mechanical stress and pressure, while osteoporosis

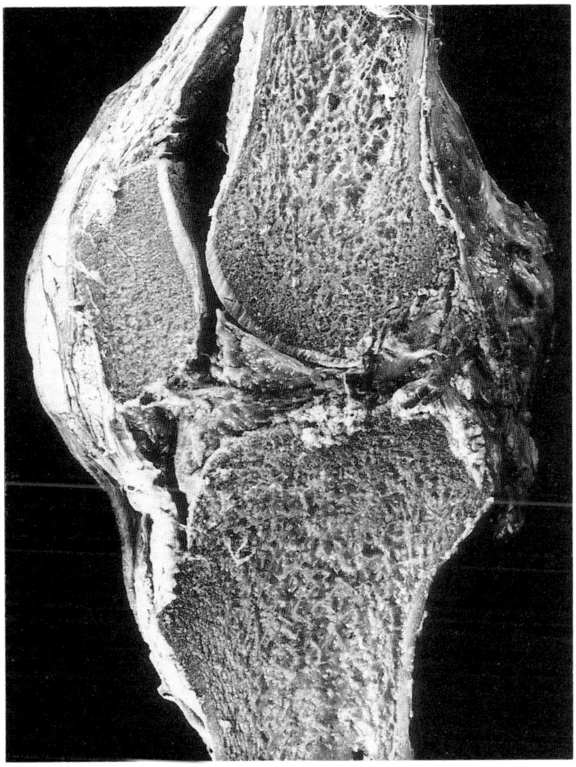

Fig. 494. Incomplete fibrous ankylosis secondary to suppurative arthritis. The dorsal part of the articular surfaces is fused by dense fibrous tissue. In the ventral part the tibia is fused with the patella, but the femoral condyle partly maintains the articular cartilage

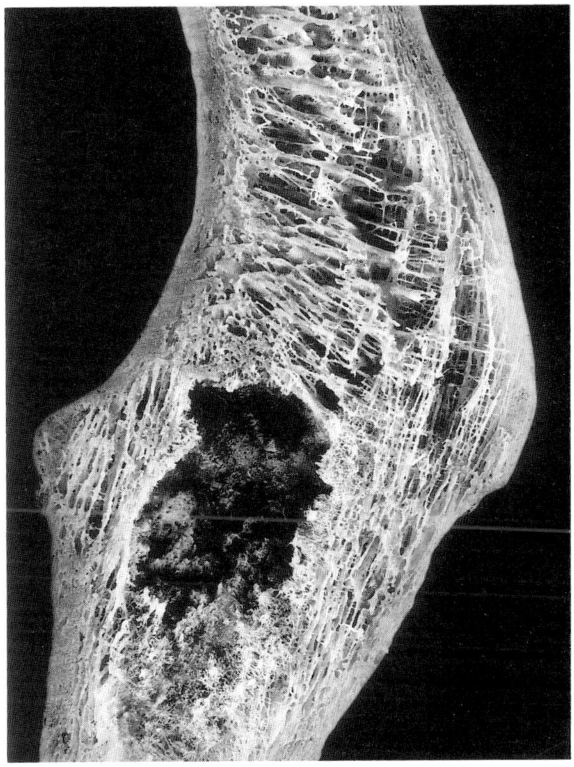

Fig. 495. Complete osseous ankylosis has occurred secondary to staphylococcal osteomyelitis. A large abscess cavity occupies the posterior parts of the epiphyses. In the other parts trabecula pass in continuity from one to the other epiphysis

with rarefaction of the trabeculae has set in in the areas spared of pressure (Fig. 492). Finally, roentgenographs permit the distinction between fibrous ankylosis and contracture with very tight musculature which clinically simulates such ankylosis; in the latter condition the joint space maintains its width, and the outlines of the articular epiphyses are slightly or not at all altered.

Gross-anatomical examination discloses that a proximal and a distal articular epiphysis are extensively united (Fig. 494) and the joint capsule adheres firmly. The latter is transformed into a dense fibrosed tissue which can be separated from the articular epiphyses only by dissection. Opening a fibrotically ankylosed joint (Figs. 197, 494) exposes uneven articular surfaces which in places maintain a cover of defective cartilage but otherwise and mostly are covered by dense connective tissue. The latter completely fills the articular space (Fig. 494). In cases of osseous ankylosis no articular surface can generally be identified because bony tissue expands as a bridge from one articular end to the contiguous articular end, thus establishing a nonyielding firm bony unit (Fig. 495).

Histopathological examination discloses that the articular cartilage of the epiphysis has been destroyed to a large extent and has been substituted by fibrosed connective tissue (Fig. 496). This emerges in some cases from the subchondral spaces and in others penetrates from the articular surfaces into the depth, but it fills the cartilage space in all cases. The dense connective tissue connects the extensively disrupted or destroyed osteocartilaginous borders of the adjacent articular epiphyses. This establishes a fibrosed overall union of two adjacent articular epiphyses (Fig. 496). In osseous ankylosis (Fig. 497) the previous cartilage space and the joint cleft are extensively obliterated by trabeculae (Fig. 497) which have established a continuous connection of the articular epiphyses by merging in both of them with the trabeculae of the subchondral bone. In the majority of these cases the pattern of osseous trabeculae passing from one epiphysis to the other one and merging in each of them with the local trabeculae is disrupted by intervening areas of sclerosis and irregular osseous structure as the sequelae of initial inflammation and/or destruction.

Differential diagnosis must consider a very tight contracture, especially when associated with reflectory tenseness of regional musculature. In this situation elimination of the muscle spasm by an intravenously

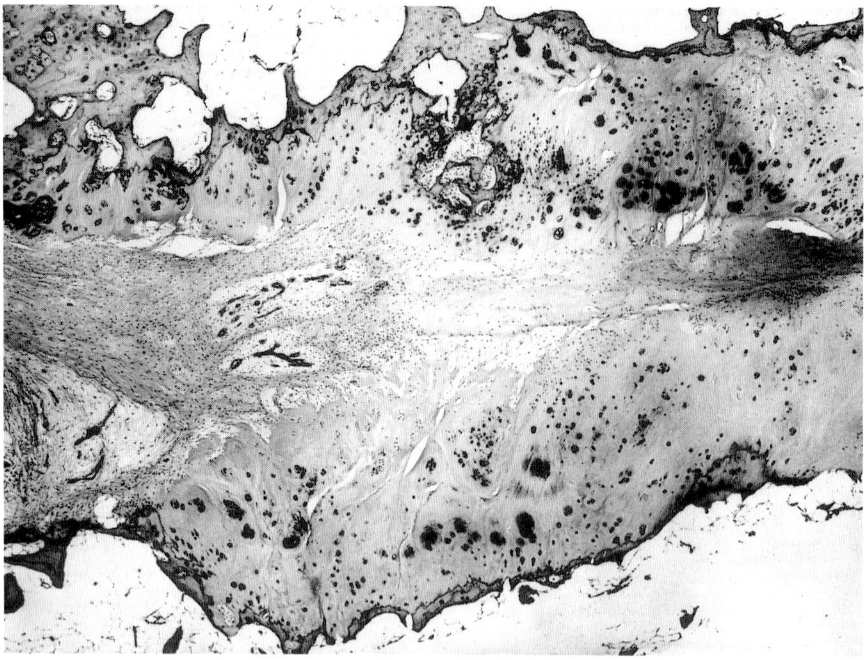

Fig. 496. The joint space is completely occupied by dense connective tissue which also connects the adjacent articular epiphyses. However, articular cartilage has partly remained on the epiphyses in this fibrous ankylosis

administered muscle relaxant helps to ascertain whether the hindrance to joint motion lies in obliteration of the joint cavity or in tightness of the regional musculature. In the situation of osseous ankylosis ascertaining the etiology plays an important role in determinating the necessity for antibiotic treatment or surgical treatment. Roentgenographic evaluation here is of great use. In infectious arthritides and especially gonococcal arthritis leading rapidly to ankylosis, the contours of the articular epiphyses remain rather unaltered (Fig. 493). In primary suppurative arthritis or that expanding secondarily from osteomyelitis the articular epiphyses have deep erosions and a structure with osseous rarefactions and densifications (Fig. 492). In tuberculous ankylosis, the articular epiphyses also have an irregular contour but a rather homogeneous osseous rarefaction and no areas of sclerosis.

The best treatment for ankylosis is the prophylaxis because fusion of a joint can be prevented in many instances. In intraarticular fractures with displacement,

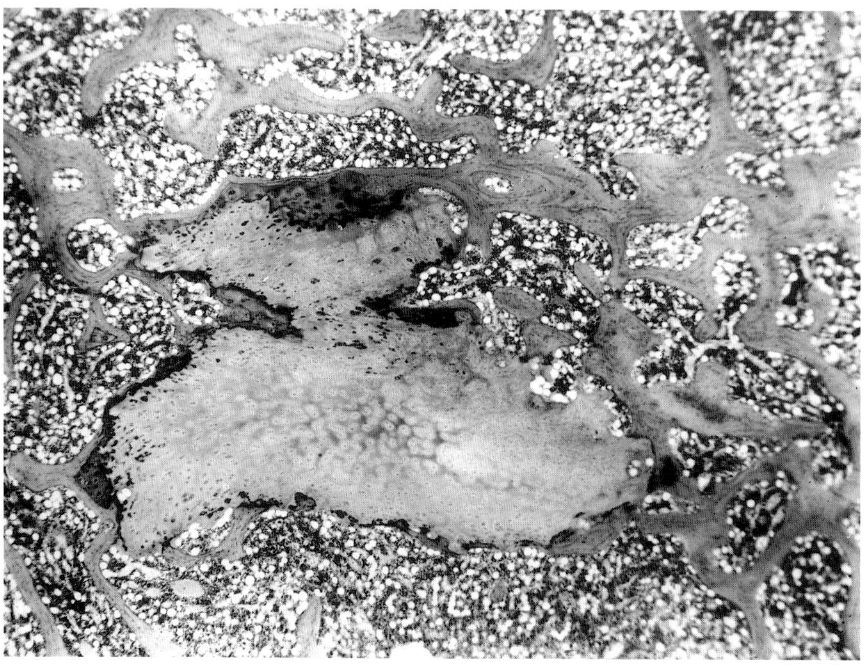

Fig. 497. A large island of articular cartilage, partly contiguous with bone, indicates the site of a previous joint space which is completely occupied by cancellous bone in this osseous ankylosis

skeletal traction may succeed in obtaining proper reduction of the fragments, restoration of the joint space, and prevention of soft tissue shrinking. Immediately after consolidation of the fracture mobilization of the joint is started by regular active and passive exercises, and these are continued until a satisfactory range of motion is attained. In all suspected infections of a joint, high doses of multivalent antibiotics are instantly administered and continued. If, nevertheless, the inflammation does not regress, aspiration of joint fluid and irrigations of the joint with solutions of the antibiotic, determined by culture and sensitivity tests of the pathogenic microorganism, are of elementary necessity, as is oral or parenteral administration of this antibiotic. Concurrently, the extremity should be kept in traction with large weights to prevent shrinking of the joint capsule and periarticular tissues. Once the acute inflammation and the presence of microorganisms subsides, and while the traction is continued, mobilization of the joint is started by gentle active exercises; passive exercises are added subsequently. In inflammatory conditions of granulomatous nature, while the indicated medications are administered, and the extremity is kept in traction, the joint is similarly mobilized after regression of the acute inflammatory phase.

Ankylosis is a state which, in view of the freedom from pain, does not cause discomfort. Nor does it cause a conspicuous deformity unless the joint is fused in a faulty position. Nevertheless, the lack of motion represents such an impairment in many situations that correction is desired by most patients. Treatment is determined individually according to the age, sex, and occupation of the patient as well as the specific joint involved and the type of its affection.

The shoulder joint rarely fuses because of the small contact surfaces, unless it was severely injured and sustained comminuted fractures of the humeral head and glenoid cavity, such as occur in explosions or gunshot wounds, and complicated by extensive injuries of the soft tissues. A similar condition results after long-lasting suppuration. If this joint is ankylosed in a good functional position (about 70° abduction, 30° flexion before the frontal plane, and 15° external rotation) it can be used for most functions of daily life and in many occupations. Of substantial benefit is here the available mobility between the shoulder blade and the chest cage, which permits movements of 25°–30° in terms of adduction and elevation, and of 10°–15° ventral flexion. However, if the ankylosis occurs in a non-functional position, such a shoulder joint represents a constant impediment in the use of the arm. Then, according to the individual desires and needs, this malposition and dysfunction may be corrected surgically by the following techniques: (a) osteotomy through the surgical neck of the humerus, combined with internal or external immobilization, which improves the malalignment of the arm but leaves the ankylosis unchanged; (b) excision of the humeral head a procedure which restores the mobility of the shoulder joint but does not restore the balance of the shoulder musculature and therefore also not the stability of the shoulder joint; or (c) total arthroplasty with metallic and/or polymeric inserts, which restore the mobility of the joint and the balance of the shoulder musculature. Regarding the types of replacement inserts, unconstrained [1179] (Fig. 212), the semiconstrained [1275], and the constrained [683] total arthroplasties are in general use. After healing of the operative wound, the patient is instructed in active mobilization exercises to be carried out for 4–6 months. However, as in any total arthroplasty, this arthroplasty is also fraught with complications such as loosening of the stem, dislocation or subluxation of the endoprosthesis, and postoperative infection. Thus, when infection was the cause of the ankylosis, an intraarticular operation should not be undertaken unless the complete subsidence of the infection is ascertained by blood culture, gallium scan, and aspiration of local tissue fluid subjected to bacteriological tests. Even then the probability of a reinfection cannot be excluded. Details of total arthroplasty of the shoulder joint are discussed in "Rheumatoid Arthritis" and "Osteoarthritis".

The ankylosed elbow joint (Fig. 498), even when stiff in a position of 90°–110° flexion, represents an impairment in daily life and manual occupations; an essential motion, the inward and outward rotation of the forearm and wrist, is lacking. Using the rotation in the shoulder joint for such needs cannot compensate the missing rotation in the elbow joint. Another elementary function for activities of daily life is the ability to flex the elbow. Thus, when rotation as well as a range of flexion in the elbow joint are necessary, arthroplasty (Fig. 499) is indicated. The currently most used method is excision of the fused articular ends in one block and the insertion of metallic and/or polymeric substitutes. In total arthroplasty of the elbow joint, three types of arthroplastic implants are used. These are: the unconstrained prosthesis [484, 917, 988], the semiconstrained prosthesis [804, 1412] (Fig. 499), and the totally constrained prosthesis [387, 690]. These are described in "Rheumatoid Arthritis". Long-term follow-up examinations are needed to evaluate the results. Apart from the potential complications as in any total arthroplasty, the arthroplastic inserts, while permitting full flexion and extension, often do not provide sufficient rotation. Therefore, less extensive natural arthroplasty has been used; a procedure excising the interposed bony bridges and reshaping the economically resected articular ends succeeds in producing a more naturally shaped elbow joint. This type

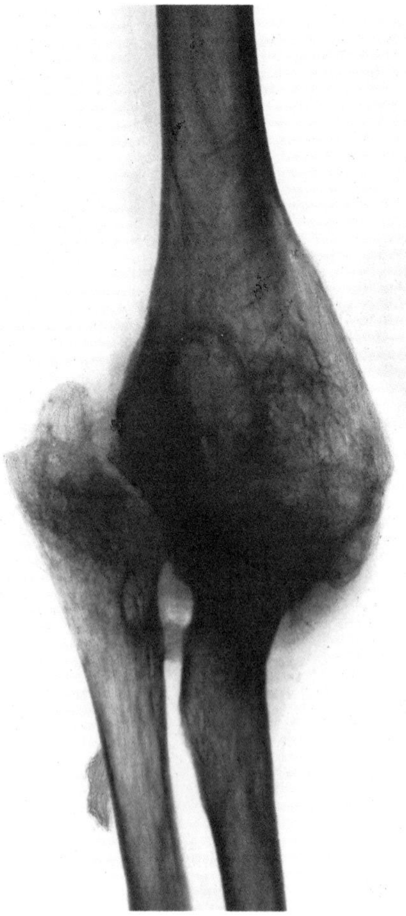

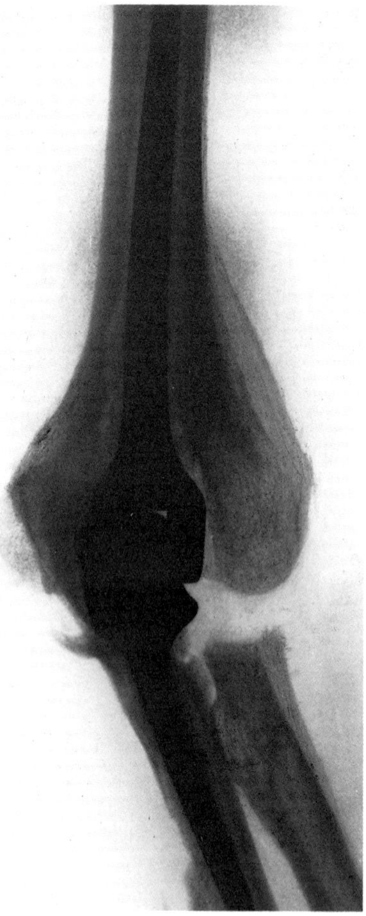

Fig. 498. Osseous ankylosis between the lateral humeral condyle, which comprises large areas of osteosclerosis, and the radial head. The proximal end of the ulna is subluxated and also comprises areas of osteoporosis and osteosclerosis

Fig. 499. The radial head and neck have been resected. Components of total semiconstrained arthroplasty have been inserted into the medial humeral condyle and the proximal end of the ulna

of organic arthroplasty requires: (a) interposition of a flap of fascia lata together with its adipose tissue to prevent fusion of the resected articular ends and (b) overnight traction of the forearm for several weeks to months to keep the articular ends separated from each other and to forestall shrinking of the soft structures. A satisfactory range of motion is obtained in the majority of these patients [903, 1672]. However, the resulting instability associated with pain in some patients is a considerable shortcoming of this procedure, as is the heterotopic bone formation associated with decreased mobility. Independently of the type of operation, any arthroplasty of the elbow joint is fraught with a frequent complication specific for this joint: operative damage to the ulnar, median, and/or radial nerves.

Ankylosis of the wrist joint follows severe injuries or inflammations. When occurring in middle position or slight dorsal extension at the radiocarpal junction, it permits the hand to be used to a good range. The wrist, being composed of three rows of articulations, retains adequate function owing to the combined range of motion in some of its small joints, which are left moveable. However, if ankylosis occurs in a faulty position, this has to be corrected by osteotomy through the wrist. The remaining motion in some of the small joints does not suffice to compensate a pronounced misalignment.

Ankylosis of the metacarpophalangeal and interphalangeal joints of the fingers follows after severe crush injuries or infection and is usually associated with stiffness in pronounced flexion. This limits the normal use of the fingers and interferes with the use of the hand. As treatment, arthroplasty appears indicated which restores the motion and corrects the malposition. Arthroplasty by excision of the articular ends and their substitution by polymeric inserts (Fig. 208) is a widely used procedure, as described in "Rheumatoid Arthritis". However, due to impaired blood circulation the operative wound does not always heal well; a wound infection may follow which requires removal of the arthroplastic inserts. Even with a well-healed wound, intense movements may cause the pins of the arthroplastic inserts to become loose after a period of time. This adverse effect requires removal of the arthroplastic inserts, followed by implantation of more tightly fitting inserts. An alternative is arthroplastic resection of the articular ends with the convex articular ends in a

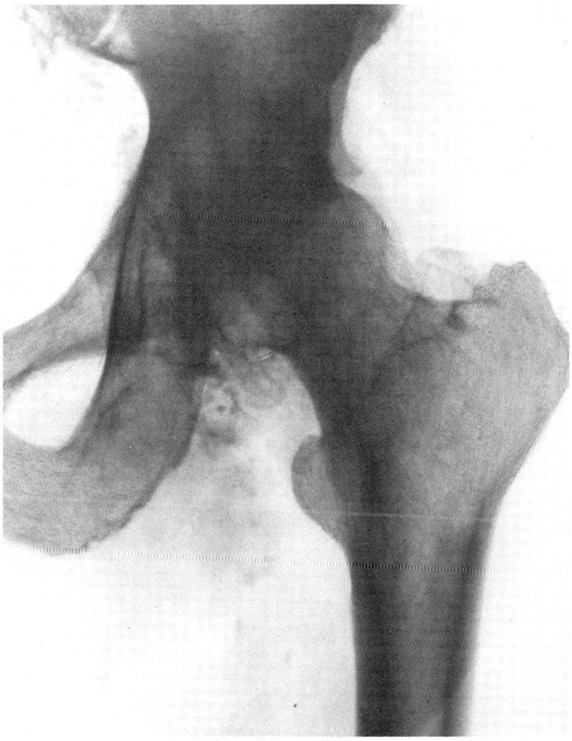

Fig. 500. The articular surfaces of the acetabulum and femoral head are fused together. Osseous trabecula pass in continuity from one to the other epiphysis.

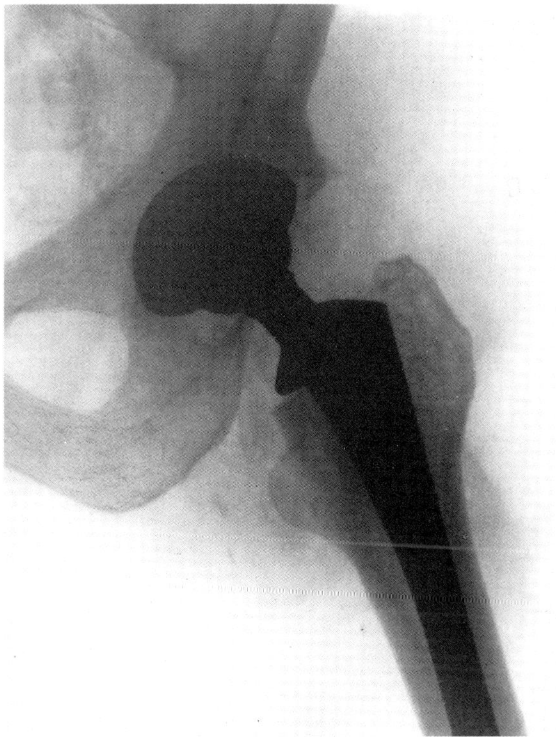

Fig. 501. A total arthroplasty of the noncemented type was performed. Both components, the femoral one with a long stem, are centrally inserted

wedgelike manner. Shortly after the operative wound has healed, mobilization of the operated joint is instituted by regular active and passive exercises, and this is continued until it is evident that the motion is definitely secured.

Ankylosis of the hip joint develops after extensive harm to the articular ends and joint capsule, as caused by deep comminuted fractures, gunshot wounds, severe inflammation or suppuration (Fig. 500). Ankylosis of the hip joint is sometimes an associated complication in ankylosing spondylitis (Fig. 227), Reiter's syndrome, and arthritis in ulcerative colitis (Fig. 340). Ankylosis of the hip joint may be noticeable by faulty posture of the body depending on the alignment of the thigh. It is more conspicuous in the flexion-adduction position of the hip, when the leg is apparently shorter, and the lumbar spine is overstretched. It is less conspicuous in the extension-abduction position of the hip, when the leg is apparently longer. Independently of the alignment, a completely stiff hip joint represents an essential impediment in daily life, especially for women. Thus the desire for restoration of motion is well motivated and can be implemented by total arthroplasty (Fig. 501). Its modalities and technique are described in "Rheumatoid Arthritis" and "Osteoarthritis" assuming that no general medical contraindication exists, and that no active inflammation of the hip can be detected by any method, especially in the cases with infection in the past as the cause of the ankylosis. Since the latter condition is essential for embarking on hip surgery, three deep shortwave diathermy sessions are administered as provocations to ascertain by clinical signs and laboratory tests whether a dormant infection is present and has been activated. In the case of doubt, regular arthroplasty must not be carried out because of the probability of a reinfection. Nevertheless, the motion of such a hip joint can be restored by resection of the femoral head, such as in the Girdlestone's procedure [613]. However, following the removal of a larger portion from the proximal end of the femur the action of the iliofemoral musculature is dynamically impaired, and the hip joint is unstable on upright standing and weight bearing. This instability of the hip joint can be partly corrected by pelvic support osteotomy at the intertrochanteric level of the femur [1546]. When indicated without previous infection, the performed total arthroplasty of the hip joint is followed in 3%–7% of cases by infection [203, 300, 1811]. This cannot be prevented despite all precautions due to the magnitude of the operation, and may necessitate removal of all arthroplastic inserts in the majority of the patients with this complication, as indicated in "Rheumatoid Ar-

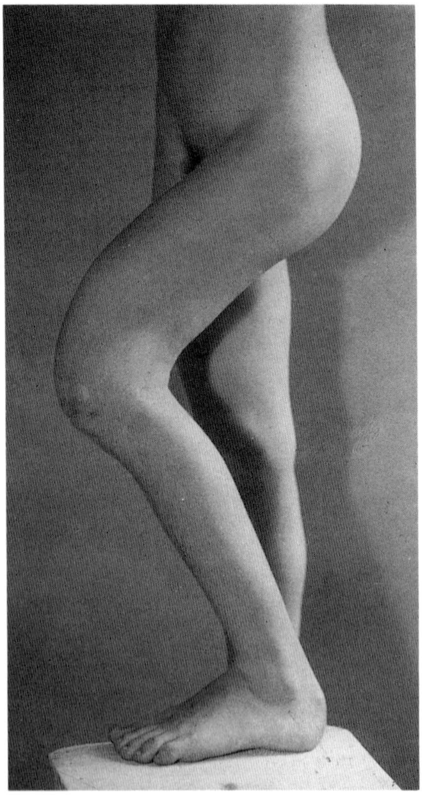

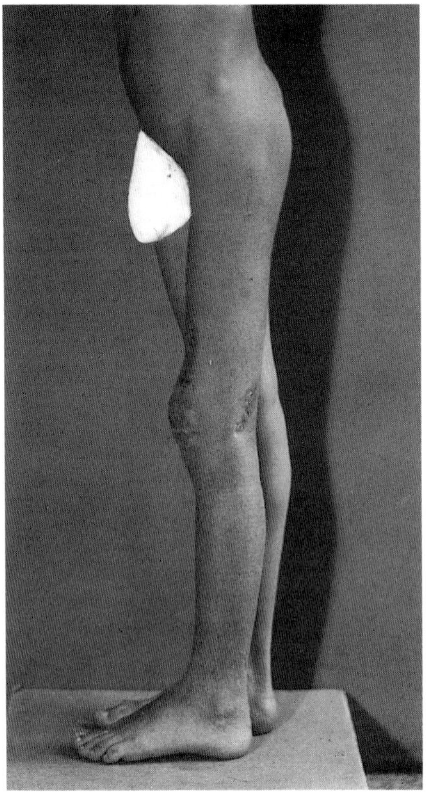

Fig. 502. The left knee ist stiff in flexion at 120°, and the left leg appears much shorter

Fig. 503. The left knee of Fig. 502 has been brought to straight alignment by a femoral osteotomy, and the length of the left leg has been almost fully restored

thritis" and "Osteoarthritis". Herefrom a mechanically insufficient hip joint would result. Therefore, one should not embark lightly on radical operation for restoring the mobility of an ankylosed hip joint.

Ankylosis of the knee joint may occur in a position of flexion (Figs. 495, 502, 504) or of extension (Figs. 493, 494). Since the former represents a conspicuous deformity (Fig. 502), associated with either apparent or real shortening, correction is highly necessary. After establishing the indication by evaluating the individual etiology of the ankylosis, the sex, age and occupation of the patient, this can be achieved either by total arthroplasty or by osteotomy. Total arthroplasty restores the mobility and proper alignment in the knee joint; its details are discussed in "Rheumatoid Arthritis" and "Osteoarthritis" (Figs. 287, 288). On the other hand, osteotomy restores only the straight alignment of the leg (Figs. 503, 505) but not the mobility of the knee joint. Thus it is indicated in those cases in which arthroplasty of the knee is not advisable because of the possibility of an existing local inflammatory process (Fig. 504) or is precluded because of extremely dense scarification in the popliteal space. Osteotomy can be performed as a dome-shaped or a V osteotomy (Fig. 297) through the distal part of the femoral shaft (Figs. 503, 505). Excision of an adequate additional wedge portion of bone is necessary in cases of pronounced flexion deformity. Otherwise, on straightening the operated part of the femur into extended position, the blood vessels and nerves in the popliteal space are liable to become overstretched. The circulation of the lower leg and foot may be disrupted, and neurological symptoms appear. Therefore, the circulation of the foot must be checked at the completion of osteotomy and at hourly intervals for the following 48 h. Any signs of obliteration of the circulation or of neurological dysfunction require decreasing instantly the attempted full extension in order to restore the normal circulation. The extension may subsequently be increased gradually at further concurrent examination of the circulation and innervation. Disregard for these warning signs may lead to gangrene of the lower leg. On the uncomplicated completion of the operation, the leg is immobilized by traction or by a plaster splint with the provision that both these modalities decrease the extension position if the circulation of the foot requires so. It is not necessary to use metallic devices for internal fixation at the site of osteotomy since the bones have here broad contact. It is also not advisable to do so as the need may arise to change the alignment of the bones to accommodate the blood vessels, and internal fixation device would preclude such correction. With these potential complications in mind, osteotomy for correction of a flexion deformity may be undertaken when a straight, although stiff knee joint would represent a distinct advantage in private life or

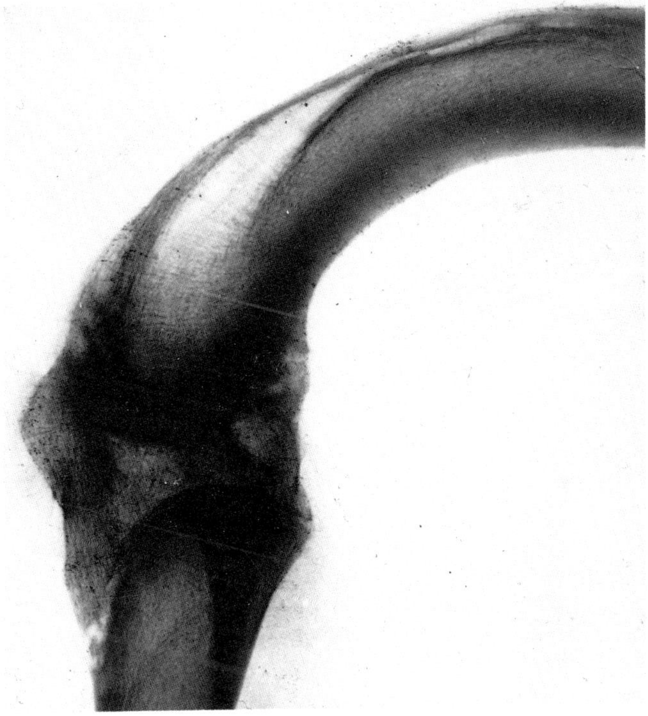

Fig. 504. Osseous ankylosis with extensive areas of osteoporosis, suggesting incomplete healing of a suppurative process, in the knee joint of an adolescent. The femoral shaft is curved to 120° at its distal part

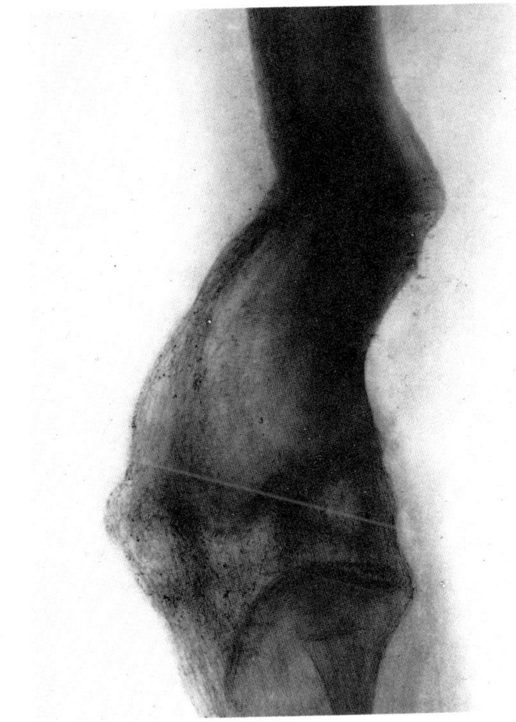

Fig. 505. The femoral shaft in Fig. 504 has been brought to straight alignment by an osteotomy which is consolidated. The extensive areas of osteoporosis are still noticeable

work. However, in certain occupations carried out in sitting attitude, such as cobblers, cab drivers, tractor drivers, a knee joint ankylosed in flexion position is functionally, although not morphologically, of advantage compared with a knee joint ankylosed in extension.

On the other hand, with the knee joint ankylosed in full extension (Figs. 493, 494), the difficulty with stockings and shoes, and the hindrance in sitting and in social life compel many patients to desire an operation to restore the ability of bending the knee joint. Total arthroplasty carries the promise of such satisfactory result, but only with the fulfillment of certain requirements. These factors must be taken into consideration, before establishing the indication for arthroplasty. The evaluations applied to the knee joint may serve as a paradigm for all other ankylosed joints of the extremities. The basic considerations apply to the organic condition of the ankylosed joint and the individual situation and psychological attitude of the patient. In the fulfillment of these requirements lies the chance of satisfactory outcome of arthroplasty.

Regarding the organic condition, it is advisable to permit an interval of at least 2–3 years from the subsidence of inflammation which led to the ankylosis. This interval makes it probable that all inflammatory foci have healed and been transformed into scars. If palpation does not disclose areas of tenderness or elevated local temperature, roentgenographs reveal no lesions of active destruction or recent periosteal apposition, and the sedimentation rate is within normal limits, further investigations should be carried out for latent inflammation or encapsulated foci of inflammation. On three alternating days, the knee joint is subjected to quartz lamp irradiations of 15-min duration and at decreasing distances, or to short wave diathermy. If these provocations do not result in an increase in general and local temperature, leukocytosis, elevation of sedimentation rate, local swelling, tenderness, and redness, blood culture and gallium scan are carried out. Furthermore, other local organic factors must be considered. Those forms of ankylosis are best amenable for arthroplasty which are not associated with excessive scarification of the joint capsule and periarticular soft structures. Therefore, posttraumatic and postgonorrhoic ankyloses are especially suited. Ankyloses secondary to suppurative processes offer fair chances, if the joint capsule and articular cartilage were mainly affected but not also the periarticular tissues surrounding the blood vessels and nerves. Similarly undetected foci in the depth of the bone marrow may be followed by infection of the new artificial joint.

In the individual indication, the patient's occupation plays an important role because an artificial joint is not fully stable and is sometimes also painful. Thus heavy laborers, farmers, and craftsmen are better served with a stable and pain-free, although stiff knee joint. On the other hand, office employees, intellectuals, and most women prefer a movable, although less reliable joint. In addition to the proper technique in the operation and an immediately postoperative course free of complications, the success of the operation depends on continuing postoperative rehabilitation management and the conscientious cooperation of the patient. Only those individuals should be accepted for arthroplasty who understand the risks of this operation, have the endurance to tolerate the pain afterwards, and also have the willpower to carry out the mobilization extercises and muscle training until the immediate goals and subsequently the final goals of the operation have been secured. Children and debilitated or mentally incompetent patients should be excluded from arthroplasty. Since attaining and maintaining mobility in the newly created joint depend also on the functional condition of the regional musculature and the ability to use it, preoperative conditioning of this musculature by massage, faradic stimulation, and isometric contraction exercises are valuable adjuncts.

After evaluation of these factors and ascertaining that no contraindication is present, arthroplasty can be performed as an entirely organic procedure or as an operation supplemented with anorganic (metallic and polymeric) inserts.

In organic arthroplasty the adherent joint capsule is stripped off the bones under preservation of the collateral ligaments. The patella is freed from the femur, and the latter is severed from the tibia by an osteotome which also molds the bony ends. The articulating end of the femur is shaped like a blunt wedge, while a shallow transversal furrow is molded into the proximal end of the tibia. The patella is shaped convexely on its posterior surface. Thereupon a thick flap of the fascia lata is excised and inserted into the newly created joint cavity. After closure of the soft tissues, the lower leg is placed on skeletal or cuff traction, and systemic high doses of antibiotics are administered. Mobilization of the joint is started by assisted active and passive exercises on the 8th–10th days after the operation. Weight bearing on the operated leg is started when flexion of 90° has been attained. Organic arthroplasty by modeling resection of the articular ends and interposition of fascia lata was improved by Albee [19], Campbell [234], and Putti [1290] among others. Following this method, Miller et al [1110] reported good results in 30% of their patients and mediocre or poor results in the others. Lacheretz [927] similarly reviewed arthroplasties of ankylosed knee joints; 50% presented good results, but the other 50% presented mediocre or poor results. In view of the good results reported in only 30%–50% of patients, organic arthroplasty has been replaced by total arthroplasty using implants of metal and polymeric material. This is discussed in "Rheumatoid Arthritis" and "Osteoarthritis".

Ankylosis of the ankle joint may occur as a sequela to extensive intraarticular fractures or to wounds with long-lasting suppuration. If such ankylosis develops in a functional position, which is between 90° and 100° plantar flexion, and the subtalar as well as the midtarsal joints have been spared, the patient is able to walk with moderate impairment in the deployment of the foot. He compensatorily uses the movements in the latter joints especially when wearing a shoe with a heel of normal height. On the other hand, arthroplasty by means of metal and polymeric material provides adequate mobility but with the disadvantage that these inserts become loose after 4–5 years [1723]. Since painless stability in the ankle joint is an essential requirement for adequate locomotion, and total arthroplasty with polymeric and metallic inserts does not fully guarantee such stability on long duration, arthroplasty should be undertaken primarily when the ankylosis occurred in a deforming position. Under the same organic conditions in the ankylosed ankle joint the individual consideration plays an important role in the indication for arthroplasty. The latter and its technique are discussed in "Rheumatoid Arthritis" and "Osteoarthritis". For men with office work and for women generally, an ankle joint made moveable again is the preferable organic condition (Figs. 273, 274). On the other hand, for most men, especially heavy laborers, a stiff ankle joint provides a reliable support in all situations. In ankylosis of the subtalar joints in proper alignment and with mobility left in the neighboring smaller joints and chiefly in the ankle joint, no surgical correction is indicated.

IX. Tumors of Joints

1. Benign Tumors of Joints

While joints are often affected by inflammations and attrition, they are rather rarely the sites of tumors [308, 1408]. It is peculiar that the connective tissue, which in other areas of the body is rather often involved by excessive proliferation, so rarely displays neoplastic growth in joints. No satisfactory explanation has yet been offered for this fact. It appears that this feature may be related to the biology of the joints, whose function is performed in a different way than that of the other organs of the body.

The possibility of developing articular tumors of various cellular compositions derives from the common matrix for all constituents of the joints. At the early ontogenetic stage, the joints are represented by an assembly of mesodermal formative cells (Fig. 506) from which the various component tissues of the joints individually develop. By absent or incomplete differentiation, rudiments of tissue remain behind until they are activated and develop in an exaggerated or aberrant mode. New formations appear, reaching a range from mucinous to osseous tissue. Publications [160] and clinical observations indicate that connections exist between traumata and tumorous formations in joints in some cases. However, in other cases the histories and examinations are not able to disclose the causative factors in the development of tumors in joints. The most frequently affected joint is that of the knee; with lower frequency follow the shoulder, hip, elbow, and ankle joints. Depending on the predominant tissue component in the benign tumors, the following six types are distinguished.

1. The fibroma originates from the subsynoviocytic tissue; with increasing size it impairs the movements of a joint and may even block movements. When protruding outward (Fig. 507), it may cause pain by pressure on nerves. It can be palpated as a thickening which is movable within its ground. On gross-anatomical examination it is a circumscribed tumor (Fig. 508) from hazelnut to plumsize which protrudes above the inner surface and becomes covered on longer existence by a chronically inflamed, swollen synovial membrane. The tumor is composed partly of whitish gray shiny bundles of dense fibers and partly of loosely textured, edematously swollen fibers [1598]. Depending on the predominance of one or the other of these components, the fibroma may be of hard or soft consistency. Microscopic examination discloses slender cells having long nuclei and long cytoplasmic processes, which lie in a more or less densely woven network of fibers. These enclose ground substance. Differential diagnosis must consider a myxoma or a tightly filled fibrosed cyst. Treatment is arthrotomy with a direct approach which permits complete excision of the tumor and circumspective examination of the inner joint capsule for other, clinically undetected fibromata.

2. The pure myxoma [1769] is a very rare tumor and is not associated with other connective tissue variations. Its symptoms somewhat resemble those of a fibroma, but it arises from the synovial surface or from the immediately subsynoviocytic tissue, where it dif-

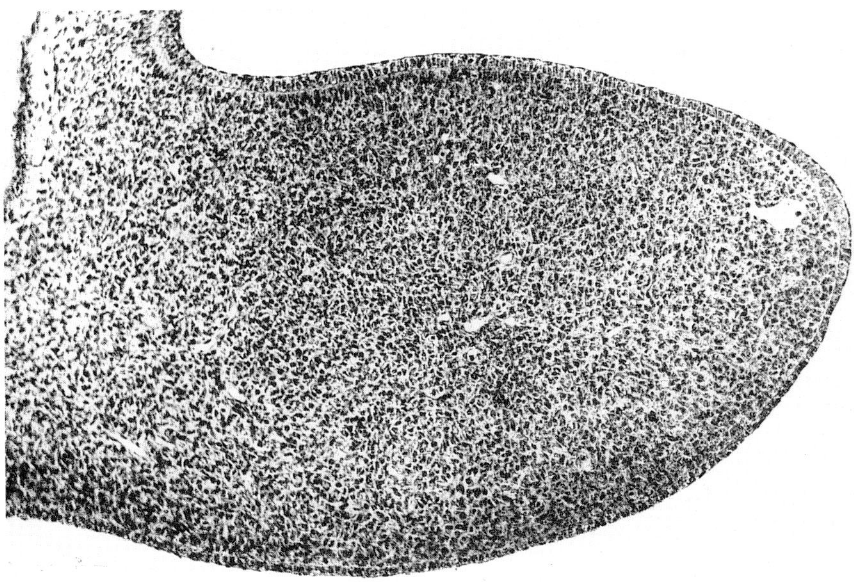

Fig. 506. The lower extremity of an embryo 7 mm in size is filled with mesodermal blastema cells

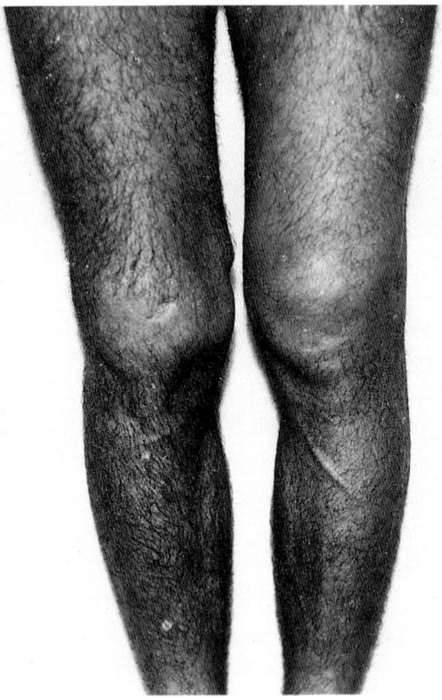

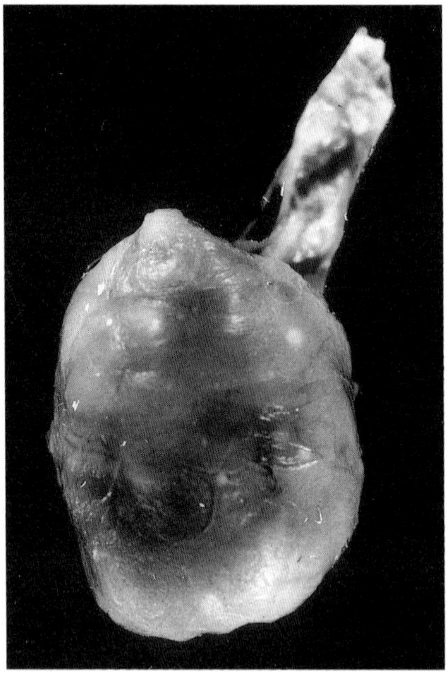

Fig. 507. The left suprapatellar area presents a circumscribed protrusion by an intracapsular thickening

Fig. 508. A circumscribed ovoid fibroma has a stalk by which it was attached to the inner surface of the joint capsule

fusely expands. Thus it is poorly delineated and does not rise above the level of the neighboring tissue. The myxoma forms an irregular or ovoid, whitish gray mass with very viscous, translucent mucinous content on cross-section. It can be differentiated by its shiny surface and on palpation by its elastic compressibility, like that of a rubber ball from the fibroma. Both of these characteristics are due to an excessive amount of mucopolysaccharides, which are partly interstitially and partly intracellularly accumulated. The increased and rather clear joint fluid is very viscous (Fig. 26). Histopathological examination discloses in a strongly basophilic ground substance the constituent cells to be large and to appear as ovoid or spindle-shaped fibroblasts (Fig. 509). They may be loosely separated or lie closely together as in a mesenchyma [1597]. Thin

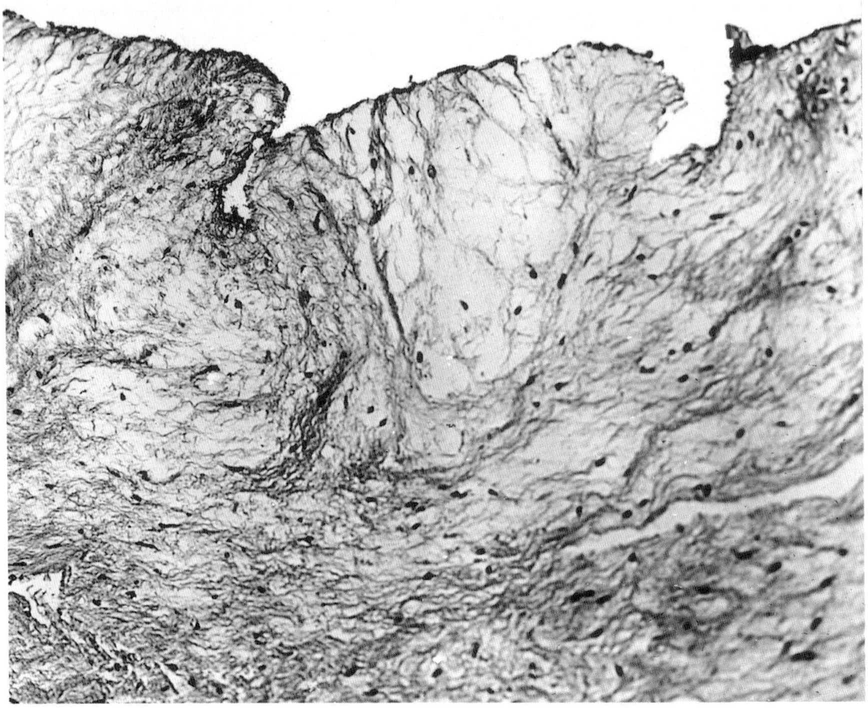

Fig. 509. The synovial membrane is extensively loosened by accumulation of a large amount of interstitial mucinous ground substance. The slender cells and collagen fibers are widely separated

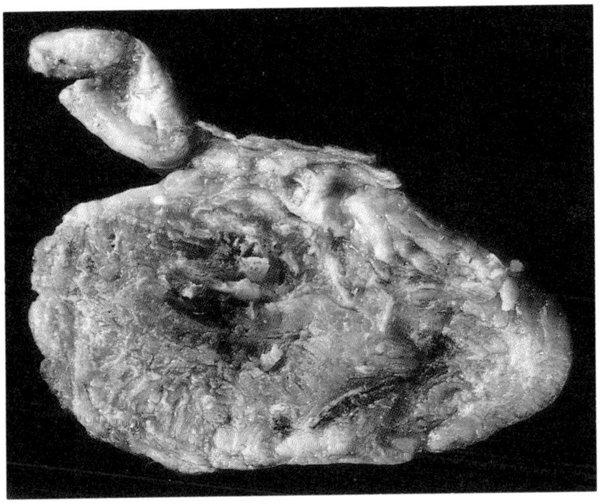

Fig. 510. An ovoid lipoma has a stalk and presents on dissection two cavities which contain small bone formations

fibers course and cross through the areas of wide cellular separation. Treatment consists of radical excision extending into normal tissue. Otherwise, the myxoma may form again, but it does not metastasize [1000, 1769].

3. The lipoma is a tumorous formation of the joint capsule [333], and should be differentiated from both lipoma arborescens and liposynovitis infrapatellaris which develop as proliferative responses to chronic stimuli. The tissue of origin is the subsynoviocytic adipose layer with which this tumor remains connected by a stalk. On increasing size, the lipoma protrudes into the joint cavity and impairs the movements of the joint. If long-stalked, the lipoma may cause the symptoms of incarceration by torsion of its stalk. On inspection, the lipoma is a protruding circumscribed swelling (Fig. 510). Palpation discloses a soft, well-delineated, and easily moveable thickening which can be differentiated by its consistency from the fibroma and by its lobulated surface from the myxoma. The lipoma can sometimes attain the size and weight of a small potato (Fig. 510) and is composed of yellow, roundish or ovoid nodes. On cross-section it may contain, besides normal adipose tissue traversed by bundles of collagen fibers, areas of disintegrating tissue with deposition of calcium salts or areas of combination with other types of tumors such as fibroma, myxoma, or osteoma (Fig. 510). Microscopic examination discloses broad agglomerations of large adipose cells and multinucleated lipoblasts held together by thin septa of connective tissue; trabeculae of osteoid or cancellous bone are sometimes interspersed. The tumor may be excised in toto.

4. The hemangioma is frequent [401, 1408] among the benign tumors of joints and usually manifests itself as early as childhood or early adolesence. This fact indicates that the hemangioma is a congenital malformation, a hamartoma, rather than a new formation. It undergoes rapid enlargement during the growth years and then provokes symptoms. Being mostly a regional malformation of the synovial blood vessels, the hemangioma is in continuity with the autochthonous blood vessels and is thus difficult to separate from the latter.

The presence of a larger hemangiomatous tumor is suggested by pain which characteristically regresses or recurs on decrease or increase of congestion of the local blood vessels. The diagnosis of hemangioma of the joint capsule is also sometimes suggested by conspicuous enlargement of the blood vessels in the regional skin. This indicates a wide communication of the intracapsular blood vessels with the blood vessels of the surrounding region of the extremity. In involvement of the knee, the lower leg may be longer secondary to accelerated growth in the distal epiphysis of the femur [622]. On palpation the abnormal joint capsule presents a spongy consistency which changes to almost normal by elevation of the extremity or by manual squeezing out of the blood unless the joint cavity contains an increased amount of fluid [731]. On the other hand, the swelling of the joint capsule increases on prolonged lowering of the extremity or after application of a tourniquet. The range of active motion of the affected joint may be decreased, whereupon a contracture may develop with longer persistence of this situation. Atrophy of the regional musculature accompanies this.

Arthrocentesis at joint effusion yields hemorrhagic fluid which requires differential diagnosis against primary traumatic effusion, effusion in hemophilic arthropathy, and effusion in pigmented villonodular synovitis. Roentgenographs [526, 1317] sometimes reveal small roundish shadows of calcified density due to formation of phleboliths or thickening of the joint capsule in extensive hemangioma. In the latter, arteriovenography is indicated [707] to ascertain the possible presence of an arteriovenous shunt and to determine precisely the extent of the hemangioma.

Gross-anatomical examination reveals the therapeutically and prognostically important factors, whether the hemangioma is of the localized circumscribed or the extensive diffuse type. The more frequent circumscribed type is a grapelike [897], bluish red or dusky red discolored formation already often with macroscopically noticeable, enlarged blood vessels. The circumscribed hemangioma protrudes only slightly beyond the level of the thickened synovial membrane, but manifests its presence by a spongy surface and discoloration. The neighboring areas of the synovial membrane are rustlike brownish discolored and are often thickened by villous proliferation. The diffuse heman-

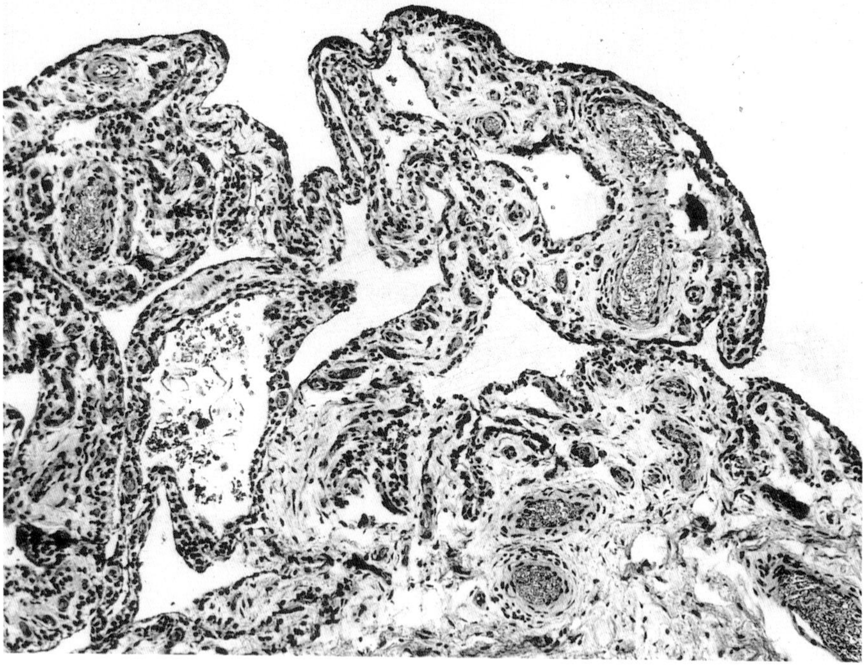

Fig. 511. The synovial membrane is elevated in several villi which comprise numerous wide capillaries

gioma displays either small, berrylike nodules over a large extent of the inner surface of the joint capsule or a bluish, elevated surface with an underlying convolute of serpentine blood vessels. The neighboring reddish brown inner part of the joint capsule resembles, by its thickening and unevenness, pigmented villonodular synovitis. The adjoining articular cartilage is often also brownish in color.

Principally by microscopic examination [1344] one can determine the predominant type of blood vessels. Histopathologically the following types of hemangioma may be distinguished (a) the capillary, (b) the venous, (c) the cavernous, and (d) the mixed type. In the capillary hemangioma (Fig. 511) the number and diameter of the capillaries are substantially increased. Numerous capillaries are widened to three- – fivefold

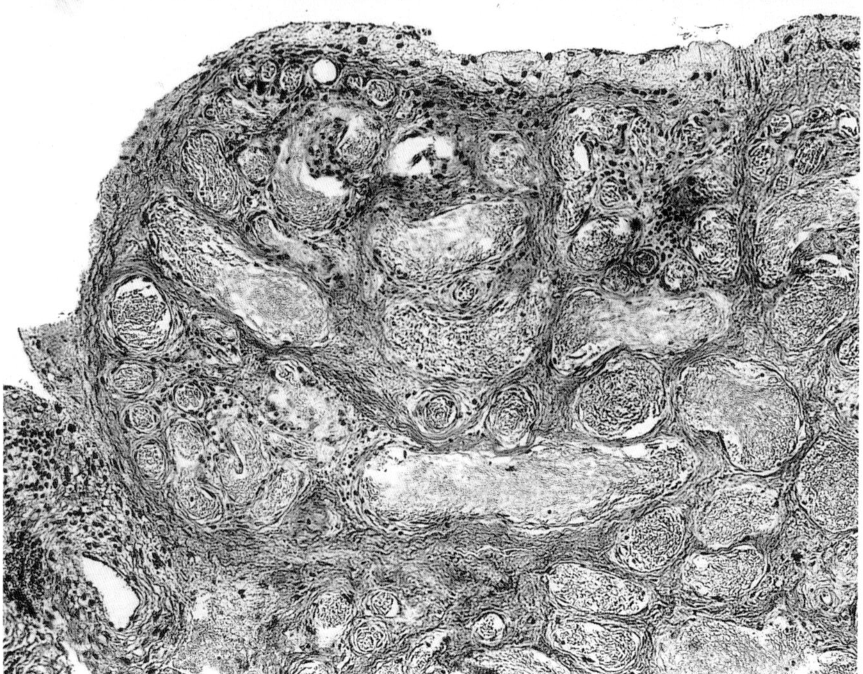

Fig. 512. The synovial membrane comprises a multitude of veins of various width and which lie close to each other

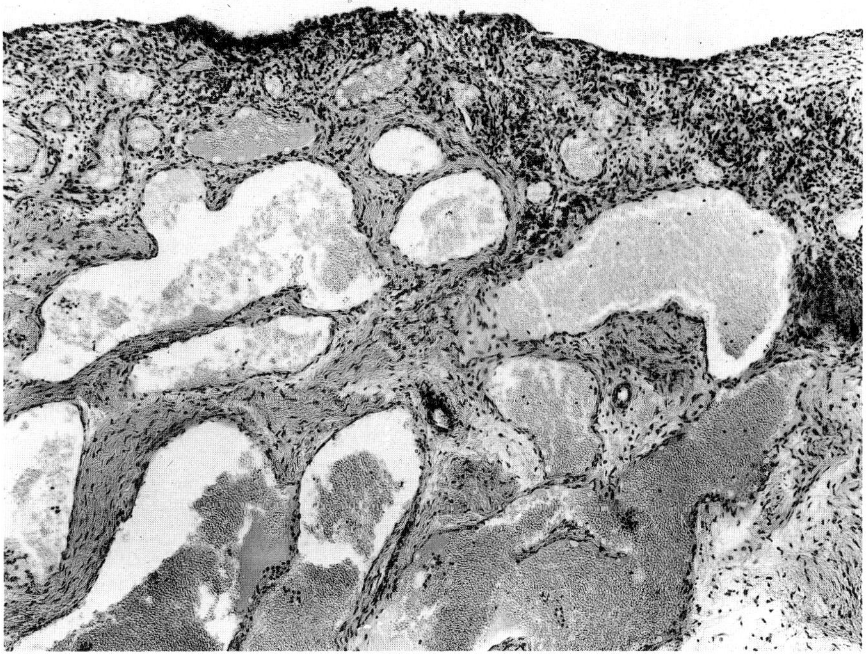

Fig. 513. The synovial membrane is occupied by numerous thin-walled cavernous blood vessels which are extensively filled with blood

their physiological diameter and are conspicuously evident. The dilatation of the capillaries resembles the widening in acute intense inflammation but without the otherwise perivascular cell infiltration. The venous hemangioma is the most frequent type and is characterized by numerous large blood vessels (Fig. 512) having a winding course and sometimes intertwining branches. Their thick walls, in places protruding into the lumina, are composed of fibrocytes irregularly scattered between a subendothelial elastic net and thick collagen bundles. The interstitial connective tissue contains numerous hemosiderin-laden histiocytes. Similar but much lesser inclusions of hemosiderin are contained in the hypertrophic synoviocytes which cover the villous surface. The cavernous hemangioma (Fig. 513) is composed of blood vessels with walls of endothelium, collagen fibers, and pericytes. These blood vessels are maximally distended to lakelike spaces and often communicate with each other by ramifications. A labyrinth is thus formed which contains more blood than the venous hemangioma. It also may be distinguished by its completely irregular course and arrangement, indicating that it is not an ectasia but a local dysplasia of blood vessels. Beyond this, by combined ectasia and dysplasia, all types of malformation of blood vessels may be observed together in the mixed diffuse hemangioma, which expands from the synovial layer into the fibrous capsule.

A special type of angiomatous formation in the joint capsule, albeit very rare, is the angiomyoneuroma, or the glomus tumor [1047]. It is characterized by numerous medium-sized vascular spaces lined by large endothelial cells and surrounded by a stroma of fine fibers among which glomus cells are loosely scattered.

The treatment, consisting of electrosurgical excision, suffices fully in the localized hemangioma, but it may not succeed in the extensive hemangioma despite the attempt at radical exstirpation. Therefore, cobalt irradiation should follow in the latter cases [35, 1632], but this must be carefully considered in children and adolescents in view of potential harm to the epiphyseal cartilage.

5. The osteochondroma or, more correctly, chondroosteoma arises by metaplastic propensity from the synovial membrane due to its development from a common embryonal layer. The transformation into cartilage cells may be explained by colloidal changes inside the subsynoviocytic fibrocytes, leading to accumulation of proteoglycan substances. These cells then become enlarged, and assume roundish shapes (Fig. 518). Clinical observations in a substantial number of cases suggest that trauma is probably an eliciting factor in the chondromatous metaplasia, which by embryogenetic determination is followed by partial ossification.

Symptoms depend on the size, number, and extent of the chondroosteomata in the joint capsule and their mobility within the joint cavity. With lesser size of the chondroosteomata and lesser involvement of the joint capsule, only vague discomfort and occasional effusion develop after strenuous use of the joint. However, when the joint capsule becomes progressively more plump and rigid by the intracapsularly spreading development of firm bodies, pain often arises even on

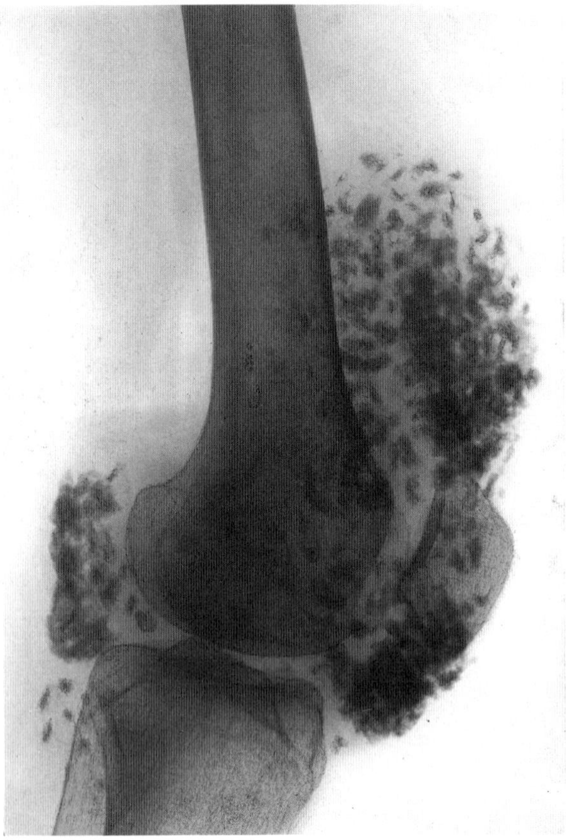

Fig. 514. Numerous shadows of osseous density resembling a swarm of bees widely surround the epiphyses

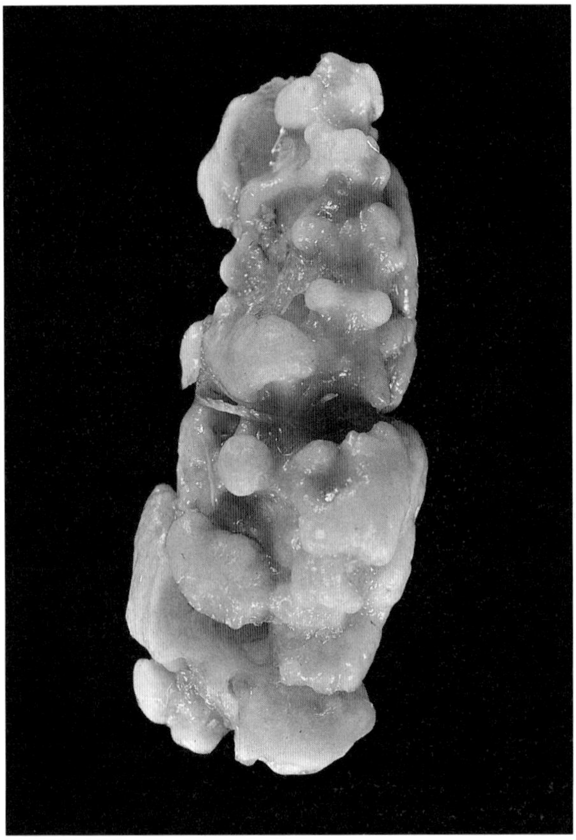

Fig. 515. The solitary chondroosteoma is of rather large size and characteristically has a very uneven surface

normal movements which are concentrically limited. In these situations the joint is enlarged and deformed, and its movements are limited and associated with coarse crepitation and cracking. When some of these chondroosteomata are fully detached, they migrate in the joint cavity and may become entrapped between the articular epiphyses (Fig. 322). Thereby the symptoms of locking of the joint are elicited. Some of these bodies may be moved around by digital pressure.

Roentgenographs are very instructive especially in the cases of multiple chondroosteomata when they reveal numerous roundish or ovoid shadows of osseous density lying close together like grapes or a swarm of bees (Fig. 514). The solitary chondroosteoma is much longer and irregularly delimited, having several roundish indentations and protrusions.

Gross-anatomical examination discloses that the solitary chondroosteoma (Fig. 515) may attain a length of up to 8–9 cm and contains a mixture of myxomatous, cartilaginous, and osseous tissue. Multiple chondroosteomata (Figs. 516, 517) are much smaller, measuring 0.6–1.5 cm in diameter, and present upon arthrotomy a very interesting picture. They loosely cover like white cobblestones (Fig. 516) the inner surface of the joint capsule and adhere like glistening pieces of mother-of-pearl to it. Other chondroosteomata are palpable closely beneath the synovial membranes or behind inner folds of the joint capsule. In their totality (Figs. 516, 517) they may number up to 100 or more. They are cartilage hard and present on transversal section softer and harder areas originating from myxomatous degeneration to osseous transformation. On their longer existence and free migration in the joint cavity, the cartilage cover of the articular surfaces may become worn off.

Microscopic examination [817, 1106] of the inner part of the joint capsule discloses that in some areas the synoviocytes as well as the subsynoviocytic fibrocytes have lost their cytoplasmic processes and have assumed a globular shape (Fig. 518). Especially the fibrocytes are larger in diameter by an increase of their intracellular material, chiefly proteoglycans, as ascertained by metachromatic stain and safranin stain; their nuclei lie centrally. These cells are surrounded by halos of more intensely staining basophilic material or by empty lacunae and thus appear to have become cartilage cells. On their multiplication the cartilage cells come to lie in clusters, while the entire area is divided

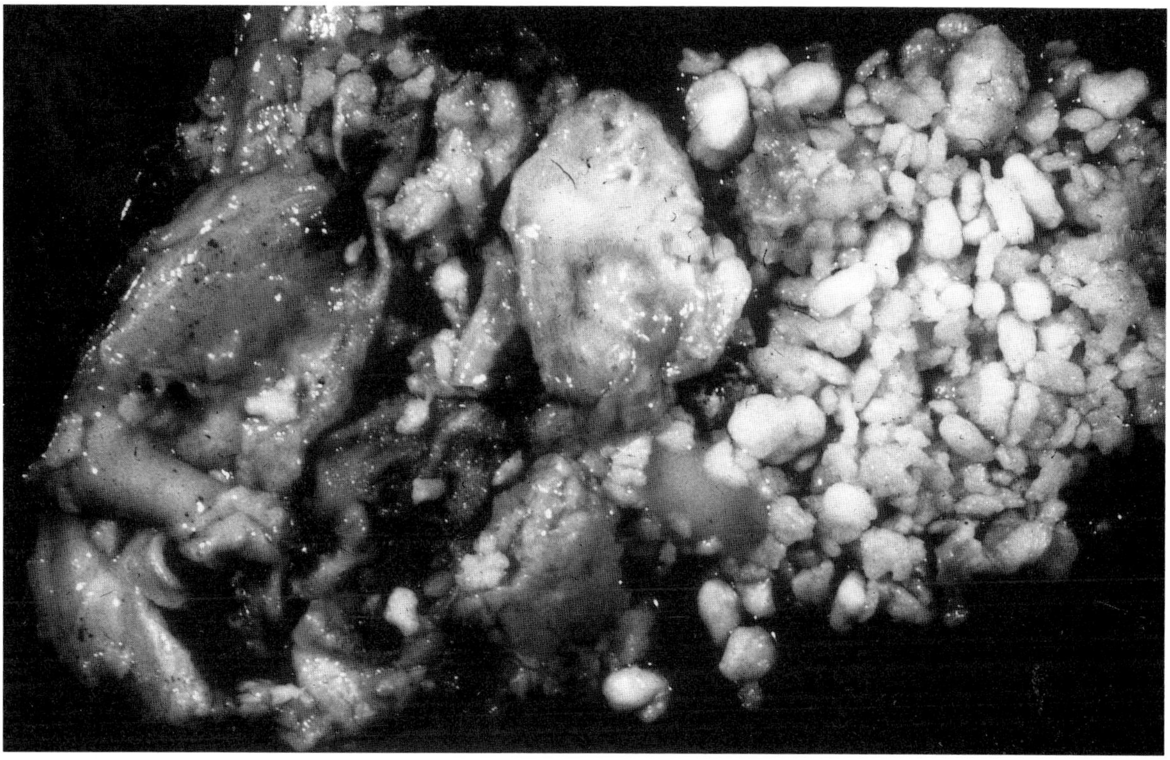

Fig. 516. On opening a joint with multiple chondroosteomata, the latter lie like cobblestones or pieces of mother-of-pearl on the articular epiphyses and the inner surface of the joint capsule

into lobules by a markedly densified intercellular material and strands of fibrocartilage (Fig. 519). Some of these lobules manifest regressive changes by decreased staining of cell bodies, disintegration of nuclei, and the presence of large vacuoles. By increased softening and rarefaction of the intercellular material, mucoid transformation occurs, and cavities develop. In other lobules necrosis of cartilage cells, impregnation of the ground substance with calcium salts, formation of osteoid, and fully matured osseous tissue are observed. The latter encloses spaces with adipose marrow. On the other hand, chondroosteomata sometimes contain irregularly shaped cartilage cells of various sizes with plump hyperchromatic nuclei, suggesting a turn to malignancy. However, being clinically confirmed as benign, these changes may be interpreted as signs of active growth [1160].

Despite the roentgenographically rather characteristic appearance, differential diagnosis must consider traumatically detached fragments from the articular epiphyses and free bodies representing separated cartilage-bone pieces in osteochondritis dissecans or osteoarthritis. In the first two situations, the areas from which the free bodies have been detached are identifiable, while in the third situation the significant narrowing of the cartilage space and the protrusion of marginal spurs provide a clue to the primary joint disease. Arthrotomy helps to establish the diagnosis by providing a survey of the inner aspect of the joint and permits the removal of the solitary or multiple chondroosteomata. In the latter situation, total synovectomy must complete the operation. Otherwise, since the inner part of the joint capsule is likely to develop further chondroosteomata, the previous symptoms would repeat themselves and would require another operation.

6. The xanthoma [562, 1793] was considered a benign giant cell tumor by Albertini [21, 22] and Hellner [739], while Wegelin [1726] and Stedtfeld [1567] interpreted the observed tissue changes merely as posttraumatic inflammatory responses. The symptoms – affecting mostly the knee joint and less often the hip, shoulder, or ankle joint – consist of vague but frequent discomfort and impaired motion of the joint. Episodes of locking of the joint sometimes occur, and a circumscribed thickening of the joint capsule can be palpated in these cases. Laboratory studies, including those pertaining to the fat metabolism, do not disclose abnormal findings. Roentgenographs may reveal irregular areas of moderate thickening within the joint capsule.

Gross-anatomical examination discloses protruding globular tumors of cherry to walnut size which are broadly based in the inner surface of the joint capsule or, more rarely, are slightly elevated above and exten-

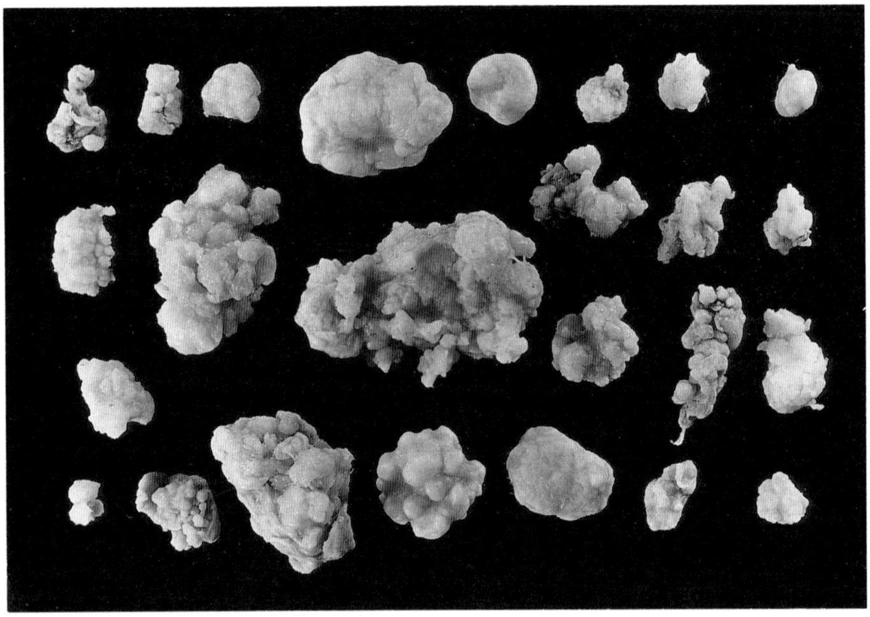

Fig. 517. The multiple chondroosteomata are much smaller than the solitary chondroosteoma (Fig. 516), but many of them also have very uneven surfaces

sively spread in the synovial membrane. They are distinct by their brownish yellow hue and softer consistency from the neighboring swollen and hyperemic synovial membrane. Microscopic examination of the latter provides a clue to the nature of these formations, showing connective tissue with fibrocytes, fibroblasts, and numerous thin-walled blood vessels situated between loose collagen bundles. Among these, agglomerations of large histiocytes (Fig. 520) are extensively interspersed; most of them are lipid-laden and contain fat acids and cholesterol, as identified by special stains, histochemical examination, and birefringence in polarized light. Rhomboid cholesterol crystals may also be detected in occasional joint effusions [482]. In other cases cholesterol clefts [333], identified by their sharply pointed ends and alignment in rosette patterns (Fig. 521), penetrate the loose connective tissue. In the latter multinucleated giant cells are occasionally scattered; these have a diameter of 40–65 μm and contain from three to seven eccentrically located chromatin-rich nuclei lying in lipid-laden, eosinophilic cytoplasm. Deposits of hemosiderin and agglomerations of inflammatory cells are occasionally observed.

The insignificant to moderate participation of inflammatory infiltrates among the observed tissue changes makes inflammation unlikely as the patho-

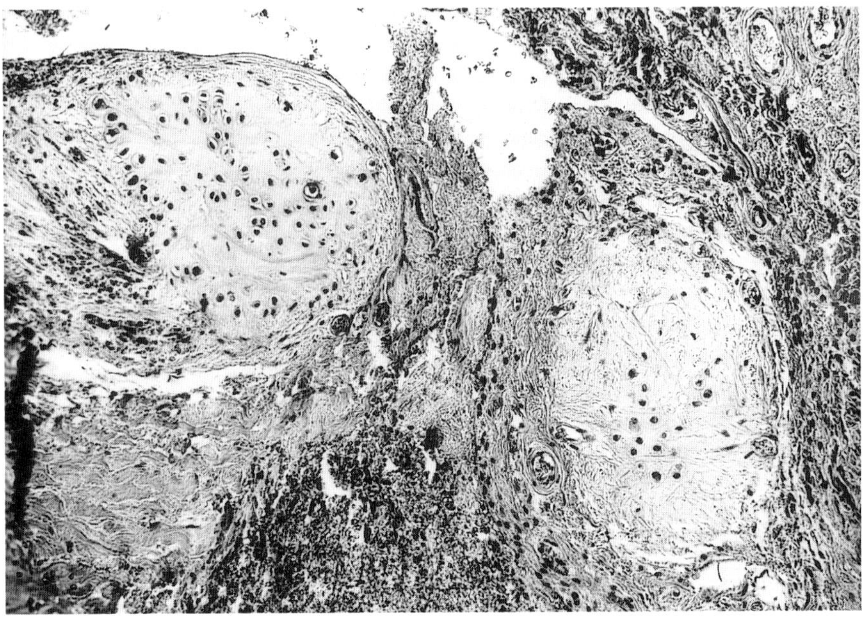

Fig. 518. The start of chondroma formation may be observed in a conspicuous increase in ground substance and a change of fibrocytes to larger sizes and round shapes

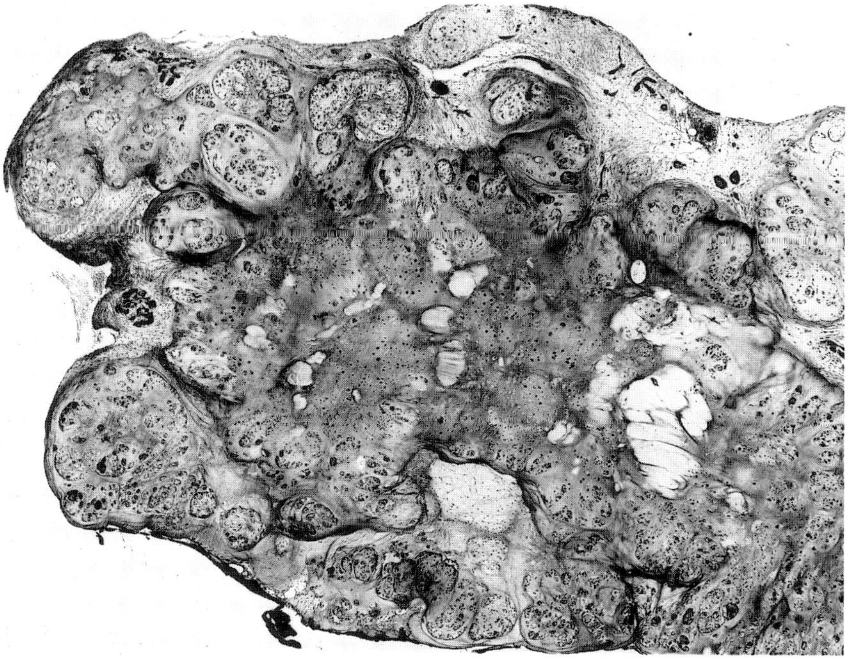

Fig. 519. The early chondroosteoma is composed chiefly of numerous circumscribed agglomerations of chondrocytes surrounded by dense ground substance and interspersed accumulations of mucinous substance

genetic factor in the formation of the xanthoma. On the other hand, the invariably present lipid-laden cells with their content of cholesterol and fat acids led to the initial concept [1260] that a generalized disorder in fat metabolism elicited these tumorlike formations. However, the almost regularly normal findings in blood pertaining to fat metabolism make it more likely that local factors, such as traumata, caused dense hemorrhages with following disintegration of erythrocytes and liberation of cholesterol. The latter was ingested by the ubiquitous histiocytes of the joint capsule. The lower incidence of multinucleated giant cells points to the possibility of tumorous proliferation, at least as a participating factor in the formation of these joint alterations. Thus Chiari [283] in contrast to Albertini [21, 22] does not regard the xanthoma as a truly neoplastic formation and concludes that its true etiology is still controversial. Similarly, Minear [1114] emphasizes that the true nature of the xanthoma has not yet been clarified.

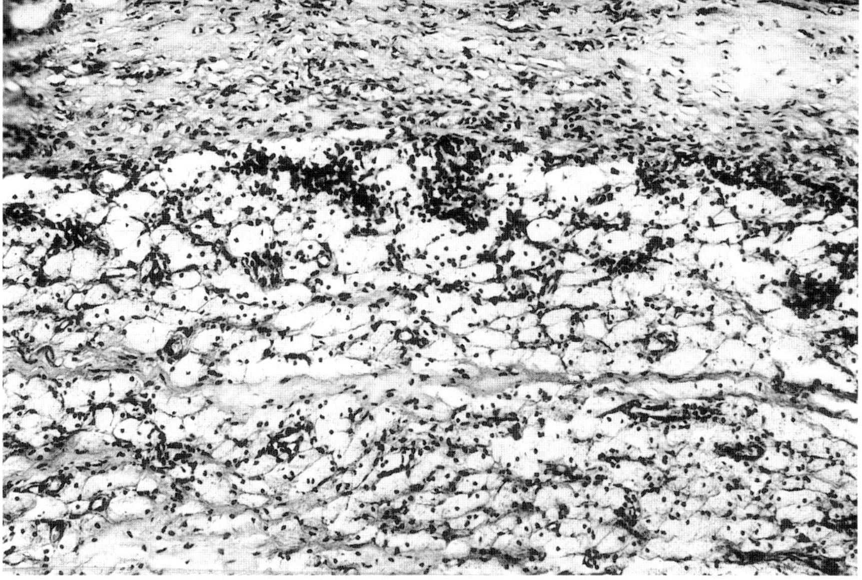

Fig. 520. The subsynoviocytic tissue is extensively composed of lipid-laden histiocytes, among which inflammatory cells are scattered

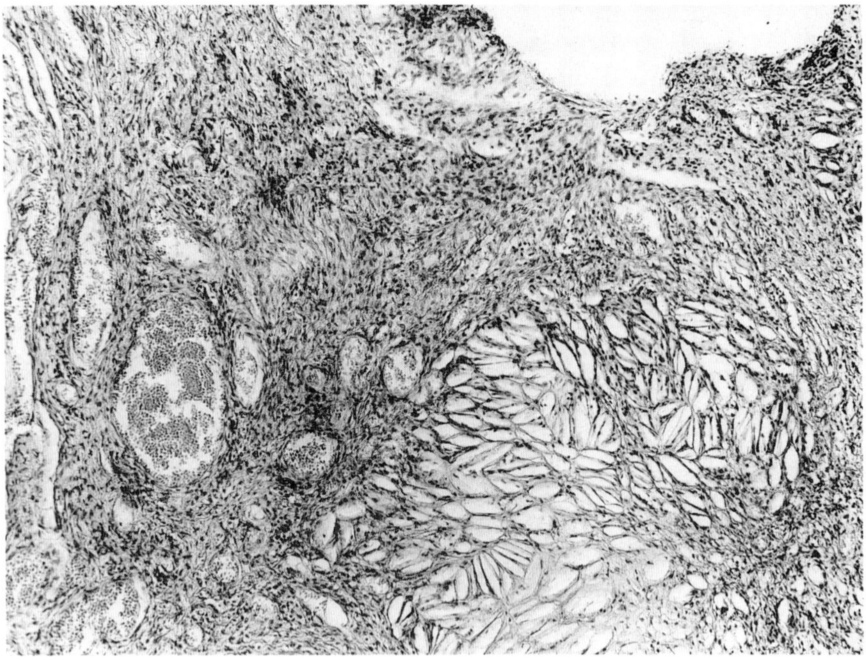

Fig. 521. The subsynoviocytic fibrocyte-dense tissue comprises pointed spaces in a rosette pattern, representing cholesterol clefts

Nevertheless, arthrotomy is indicated, using the most direct approach to the site of the palpable thickening. This generally discloses a circumscribed tumor which, when bulging, can be excised in toto [333]. However, in the case of a diffusely spread and broad-based tumor, the excision should be carried out extensively into healthy tissue. Otherwise, with persistence of local disturbance of metabolism, retention of lipids and recurrent formation of an expanding xanthoma may follow. Nonetheless, despite the possibility of local recurrence, the lack of unlimited infiltrative growth and the absence of metastases confirm the benign character of the xanthoma.

2. Malignant Tumors of Joints

Among the malignant tumors affecting joints [1306] (about 13.8 % of all malignant tumors of the soft tissues [621]) those originating from the inner part of the joint capsule assume major importance because of their greater incidence. Their rather characteristic structure [388] points to this part of the joint as the site of origin [308, 1408]. Nevertheless, Lejars et al. [957], acknowledging these origins and structures, applied the term endothelioma to them. However, due to the emphasis placed by Lubarsch [989], Smith [1516] used the term synovioma. In view of the malignant features, Franceschini [534] and Sabrazes et al. [1386] considered the designation synovial sarcoma more descriptive, and this has met with general acceptance. Other terms such as synovialoma, sarcomesothelioma, and synovial sarcomesothelioma are still occasionally used for these tumors [1306]. On the basis of similar structure, King [886] and Zwahlen [1825] pointed to the related origin of malignant tumors developed from tendon sheaths [125] or intermuscular septa. Thus the term synovial sarcoma is also applied to them. Of equal considera-

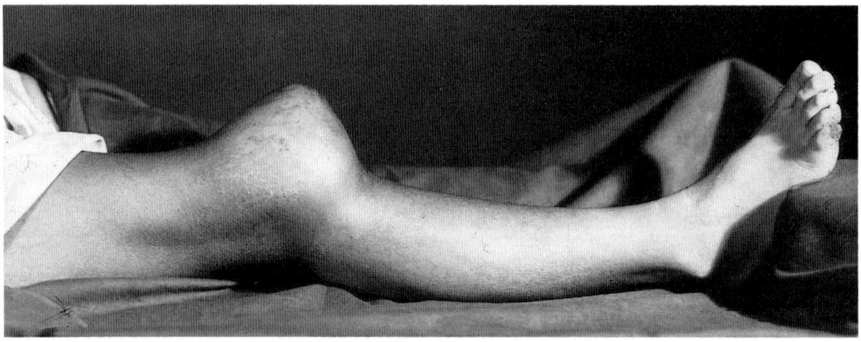

Fig. 522. Excessive enlargement of the knee by synovial sarcoma

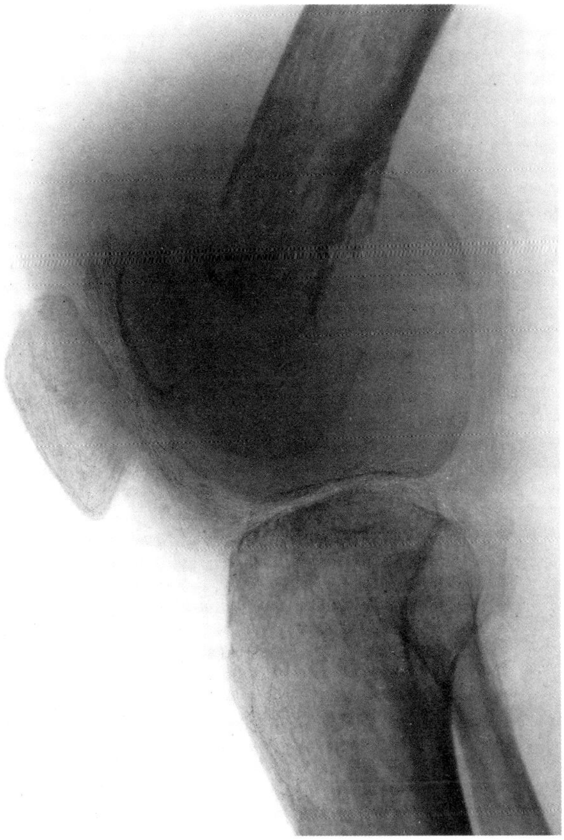

Fig. 523. The dorsal area of the femoral condyles is very porotic at blurred structure, and the adjacent soft tissue is globularly densified by a synovial sarcoma in the early phase

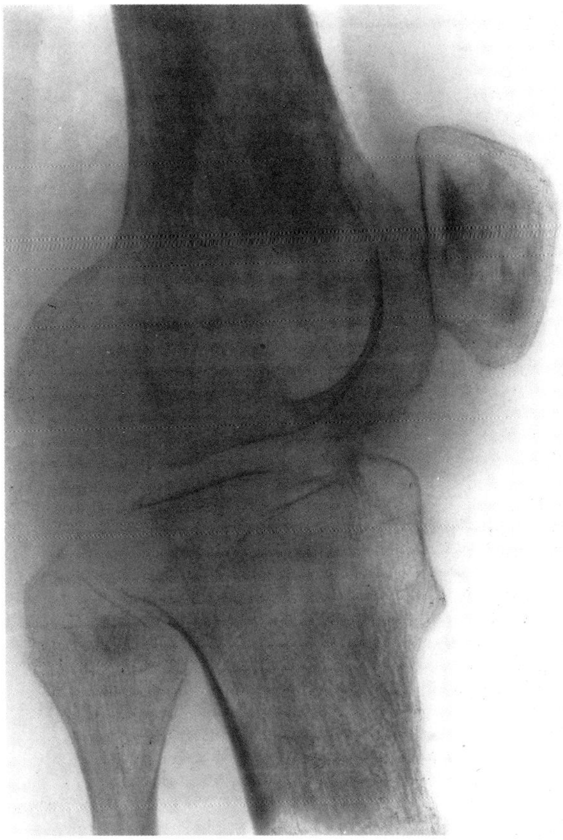

Fig. 524. The dorsal areas of the femoral and tibial condyles are extensively eroded by an advanced synovial sarcoma, and the neighboring areas are osteoporotic. The surrounding soft tissues are extensively densified

tion, Berger [125] applied the term synovial sarcoma to the malignant tumors originating from the paraarticular bursae.

The synovial sarcoma arises in the joint capsule and spreads within the joint capsule. Its origin may also be paraarticular [125], and it represents, at least in the initial stage, an extracapsular node or lump; eventually it often and diffusely invades the joint capsule. With regard to its etiology, direct blunt traumata have often been implicated yet without detectable external signs of injury. This explanation seems to apply principally in the case of men, who are in a slight majority here over women. Young adults aged between 20 and 30 years are most commonly affected by these tumors, and the incidence decreases with progressing age. The knee is by far the most frequent location, followed by the elbow, hip. ankle, hand, and forearm. Other regions (neck, back, buttock, chest wall) may also be the primary sites of synovial sarcoma, yet at much lower incidence [204, 222, 308, 705, 1521].

Patients present a rather slowly enlarging swelling of the involved joint or of its neighboring region. In the initial stage this swelling is generally free of pain, but with progressing growth the tumor becomes sore and distinctly impairs the use of the limb. Palpation discloses: (a) a rather broadly pedunculated intracapsular tumor which occasionally interferes with or blocks movements: (b) a circumscribed node of walnut to plum size within the joint capsule or close to the joint, having developed in the latter location from a paraarticular bursa or tendon sheath and without impediment to the function of the joint; (c) a diffuse thickening of the joint capsule which causes marked enlargement (Fig. 522) of the joint and deformation of the region and is associated with persistent pain, distinct limitation in the function of the joint, and frequent local elevation in temperature; or (d) an excessive growth originating either from the joint capsule or from the paraarticular structures, infiltratingly invading the neighboring organs and finally leading to local ulceration. The latter two situations are associated in about 60% of the cases with enlargement of the regional lymph nodes and/or pulmonary metastases.

Laboratory studies show the sedimentation rate to be elevated in the latter two situations. Arthrocentesis sometimes yields a hemorrhagic exudate which con-

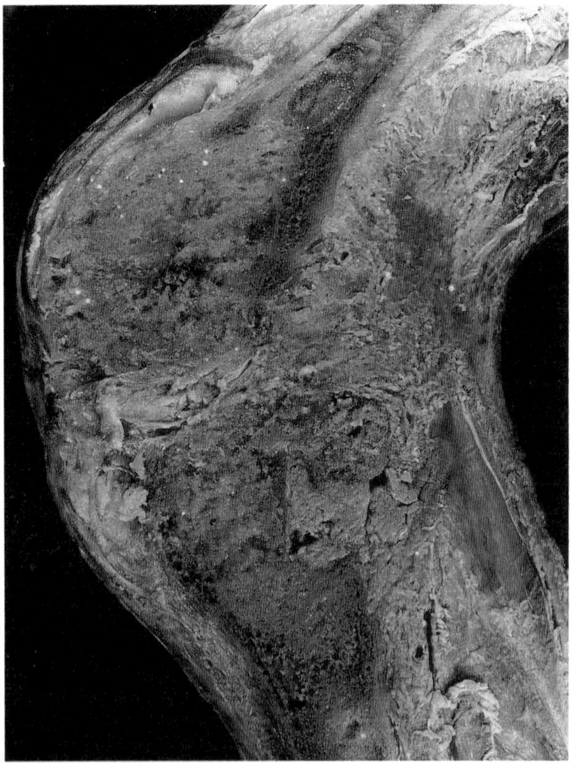

Fig. 525. Sarcoma of the joint capsule diffusely invaded the femoral and tibial condyles

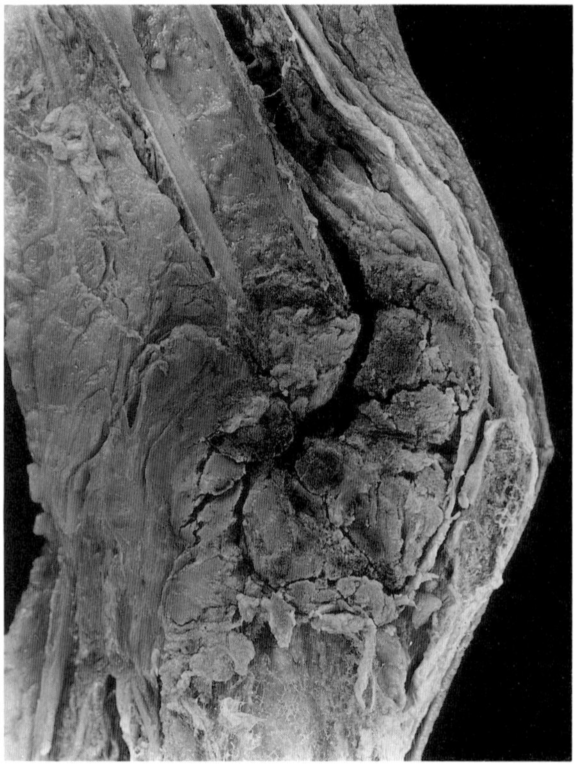

Fig. 526. Sarcoma, emanating from a tendon sheath close to the femoral condyles, invaded the knee joint

tains hypertrophic synoviocytes with hyperchromatic nuclei, as well as fibrocytes of irregular sizes and with hyperchromatic nuclei.

Roentgenographs, taken by soft tissue technique, reveal either localized or more extensive, irregularly delimited densifications of the joint capsule (Fig. 523) and/or of the neighboring soft tissues (Fig. 524). However, the initial osteoporosis of the directly adjoining articular epiphyses (Fig. 523) [13] becomes more pronounced and is followed by extensive erosion of the epiphyses (Fig. 524). This indicates the complete destruction of the bone. Computed tomography [639] is helpful in outlining the invasive tissue, while the increased uptake of radioactive nuclides indicates the size and active growth of the tumor as well as its metastases. Spots of calcifications are occasionally noticeable within the areas of densified soft tissue or bone destruction, making a calcified lipoma or a chondrosarcoma possibilities to be considered in the differential diagnosis.

Gross-anatomical examination discloses: (a) a completely intracapsular large node, distinguishable by its consistency and structure; (b) uneven lobulated nodes (Fig. 527) of walnut to potato size measuring sometimes up to 10 cm in diameter; they are extracapsularly located but are sometimes adherent to the joint capsule and then infiltrate and diffusely expand into the interstitial spaces of the adjacent tendons and muscles; (c) an inseparable diffuse mass within the joint capsule causing capsular enlargement beyond the physiological confines and protruding into the joint cavity, invading in a funguslike manner the articular epiphyses (Figs. 525, 526). Regardless of location, these foreign masses differ from the neighboring tissue by their mesenchymatous consistency and pinkish gray color, or more often by their elastic compressibility, grayish yellow or salmon pink color, and shiny cut surface (Fig. 527).

Histopathological examination discloses, as indicated by Amouroux [35] and Klein et al. [896], extreme polymorphism of the constituent cells, a very characteristic feature of the malignant synovial tumors. Accordingly, the following arrangements and structural compositions may be distinguished among the synovial sarcomata. (a) The mesothelial synoviocytic type is represented by formations resembling villi of various shapes (Fig. 528), some of them ramified and all of them covered by hypertrophic cuboidal, roundish, or polygonal synoviocytes with large pale or chromatin-containing nuclei. The core of the villi is a substrate of sparse bundles of thin collagen and reticulin fibers. Because of its great similarity with villous synovitis,

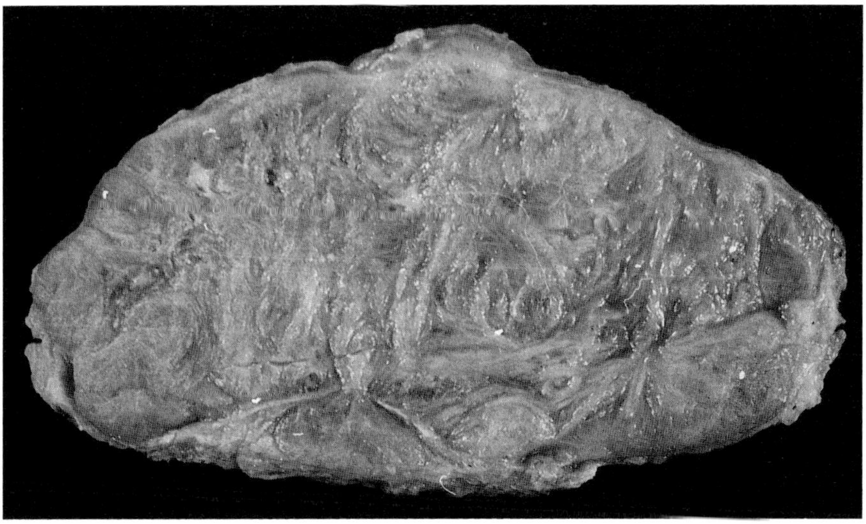

Fig. 527. Synovial sarcoma originating from a bursa is initially circumscribed, and presents on cross-section dense bundles of connective tissue, between which glandular spaces with mucinous content are interspersed

the use of the term synovioma appears understandable. (b) The mesothelial sarcomatous type is composed of elongated glandular or irregular alveolar (Fig. 529) spaces, all lined by one layer of hypertrophic cuboidal, roundish, or polygonal synoviocytes with large ovoid or round hyperchromatic nuclei. Some glandular spaces contain desquamated synoviocytes with vacuoles of mucinous material, and others contain a homogeneous substance which stains with mucicarmin, Alcian blue, and periodic acid–Schiff, an indication of its mucinous composition. All glandular spaces are surrounded and delimited from each other by an interposed broad stroma of whorled collagen bundles, between which lie numerous fibrocytes. Most of the fibrocytes are elongated and contain a thin nucleus and scant cytoplasm, while other fibrocytes are distinctly larger and contain larger irregularly shaped nuclei with occasional mitotic figures. Separate agglomerations of synoviocytes form compact cords of roundish nests, and are distinct by their plump size from the surrounding spindle-shaped fibrocytes. (c) The differentiated mesothelial fibrosarcoma (Fig. 530) is composed principally of a stroma of broad collagen bundles among which spindle-shaped fibrocytes with large, hyperchromatic, irregularly shaped nuclei are interspersed. Some of these cells are polymorphic with atypical sizes and shapes, and some contain mitoses. Within this stroma lie small, roundish, cystic spaces

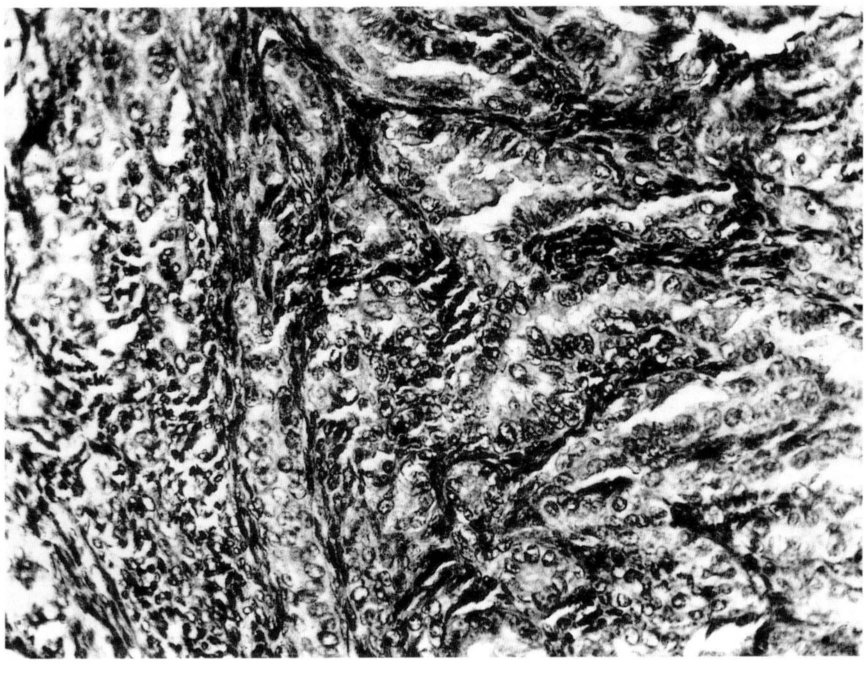

Fig. 528. The mesothelial synoviocytic type is composed of elongated glandular spaces lined by hypertrophic cuboidal or polygonal synoviocytes

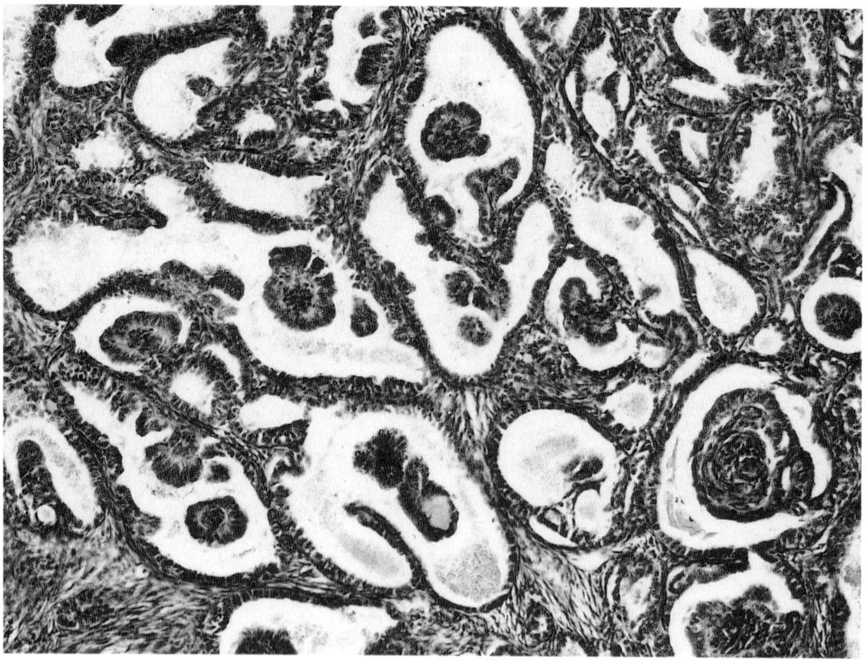

Fig. 529. The mesothelial sarcomatous type is composed of numerous alveoli lined by one row of hypertrophic cells with large nuclei. The interstitial tissue is composed of similar cells and very scarce interstitial fibers

(Fig. 530) lined by one row of either flat spindle-shaped or, more often, of prismatic hypertrophic cells with hyperchromatic nuclei. (d) The undifferentiated mesothelial fibrosarcoma is composed principally of polymorphic and anaplastic fibrocytes (Fig. 531); some of these are of ovoid or spindle shape, and among them lie rarefied collagen bundles. Accumulations of cells occur focally and are separated from each other by intervening mucinous material. In some cases, the fibrocytes and collagen bundles comprise amorphous areas of myxoid or hyaline material in which fragmented fibrocytes occasionally lie. A few larger irregular spaces resembling glandular spaces (Fig. 531) also occur here, and their linings of larger angular cells identify them as synoviocyte-delimited formations.

Between these four main types of malignant tumors, intermediate forms occur [1785] which comprise features of one or the other type in varying proportions. Nevertheless, the prime origin of these tumors may be inferred from their composition and structure. The first two types originate chiefly from the inner part of the joint capsule, whereas the third and fourth types derive

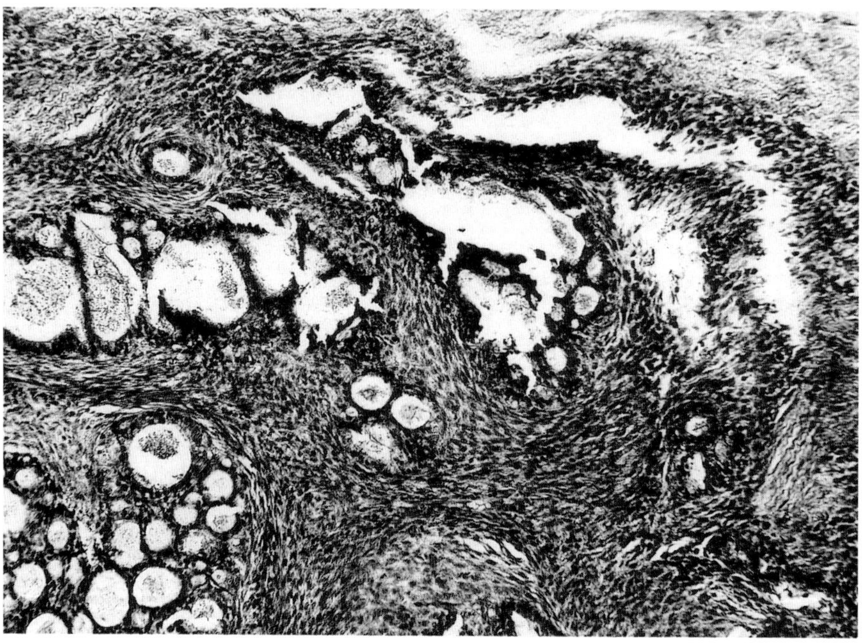

Fig. 530. A few villi-like elevations of multiangular fibrocytes rise from a substratum, densely composed of similar cells between which thin collagen fibers course

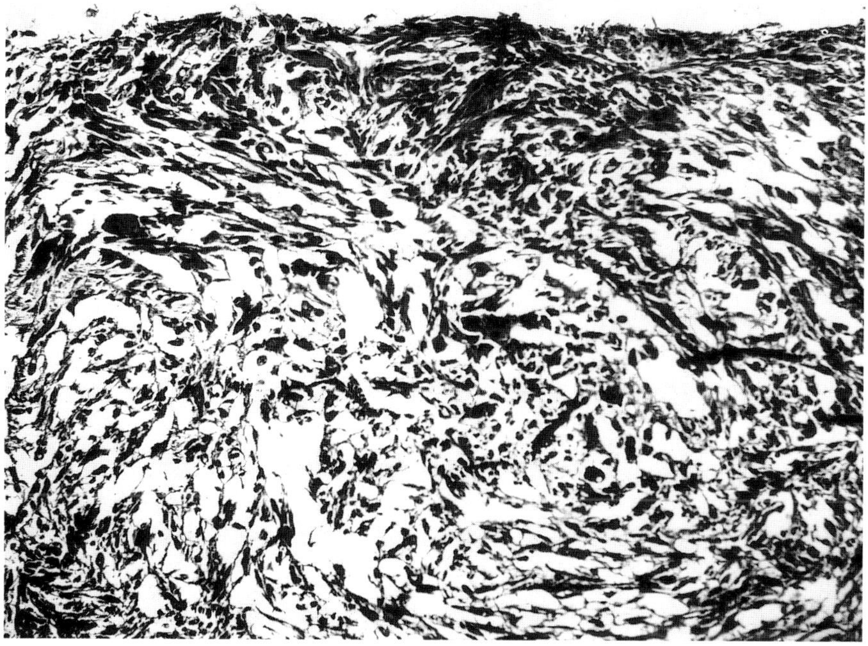

Fig. 531. Thin collagen fibers course between a multitude of large pleomorphic fibrocytes. A few large empty or mucin-containing spaces, lined by similar pleomorphic cells, are interspersed

particularly from the bursae, tendon sheaths, and intermuscular septa.

Treatment of these tumors should be based on the experiences published in the past and obtained from treatments and follow-up examinations. Pack et al. [1218, 1219] reported an overall survival rate of 19% after 5 years in patients treated solely with radiation. Goidanich et al. [621] and Pack et al. [1218, 1219] considered the specification of the histopathologically ascertained type of tumorous growth to be of essential significance for determining the prognosis; according to their experiences [621, 1218], a distinct relationship exists between the histopathological aspect and the survival rate following various modalities of treatment. The mesothelial synoviocytic type had a zero survival rate after 5 years, even after 3 years, due to pulmonary metastases despite radical excision and intensive radiation or high amputation. In the mesothelial sarcomatous type, the prognosis was less pessimistic but still guarded, as no survival after 5 years was expectable.

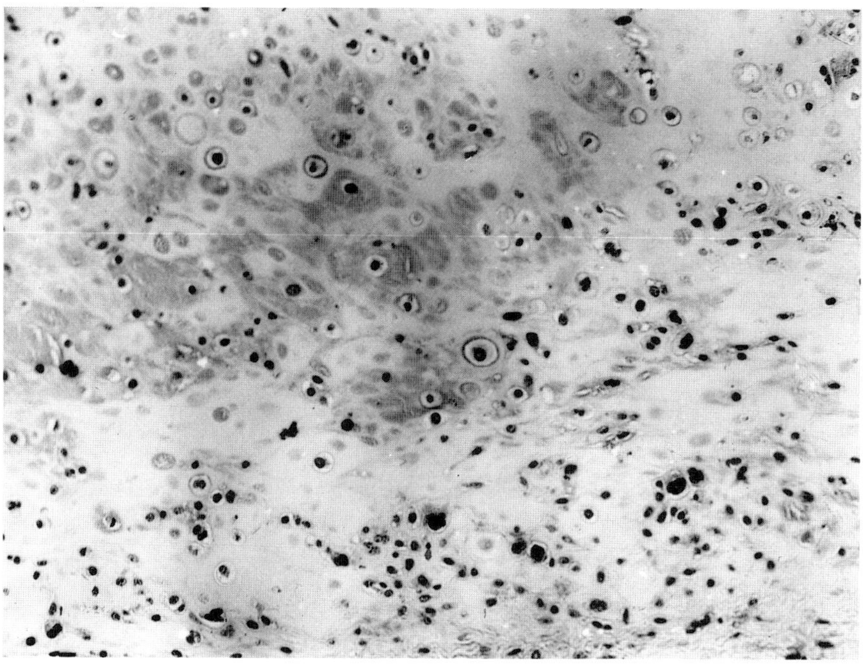

Fig. 532. An area of rather homogeneous ground substance of hyaline cartilage comprises round chondrocytes with dense nuclei. Among them, chondrocytes with small nuclei and other chondrocytes with very large, irregularly shaped and very dense nuclei are scattered

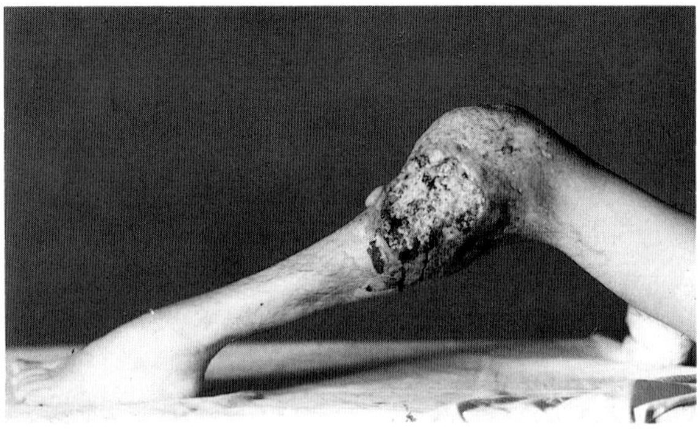

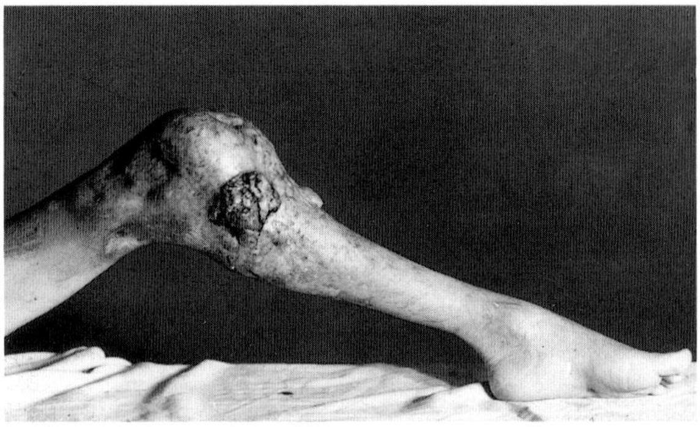

Fig. 533 and 534. The knee joint is stiff in flexion position and presents a few deep scars at the supracondylar area of the thigh. Extensive exulcerations persist on the lateral and medical aspects of the tibial condyles secondary to tuberculous fistulae with more than 20 years drainage

On the other hand, in the differentiated mesothelial fibrosarcoma the prognosis was essentially more favorable, attaining a survival between 3 and 17 years, either by radical excision and intensive radiation or by high amputation. The tumors of the undifferentiated mesothelial fibrosarcomatous type had a less favorable prognosis but a better than the mesothelial synoviocytic and mesothelial sarcomatous types. DeLutio et al. [397] underlined these prognostic considerations and emphasized the necessity of histopathological specification of the tumor, besides the knowledge of its duration and location, as the basic factors for establishing the prognosis and for determining the treatment. The exhaustive statistics of DeLutio et al. [397] show the average postoperative survival rate to be 3.3 years, wherefore the synovial sarcoma must be regarded as a very malignant tumor. Moberger et al. [1120] confirmed these evaluations and indicated that among the synovial sarcomata those with a predominantly fibrosarcomatous structure had a better 5-year survival rate than those with a predominantly mesothelial glandular structure.

Thus, in any case of rapid growth in articular or paraarticular structures, an expeditious biopsy and histopathological verification followed by radical excision extensively in healthy-appearing tissue and intensive radiation treatment are necessary. A trial with concurrent chemotherapy is advisable. At the slightest sign of metastatically enlarged regional lymph nodes, a high amputation is necessary, primarily in synovial sarcoma of the hand and foot. These drastic treatments also appear justified in the light of more recent statistics [599, 705, 1359, 1785]. The latter indicate that, despite the application of all therapeutic modalities, the overall survival rate after 5 years is 36%–58% and that after 10 years 27%–48%. The eventual outcome is that of widespread metastases in the lymph nodes, lungs, and brain. Recent surveys [980, 1480, 1481, 1603] indicate that regional recurrence and general metastases can be reduced by preoperative and postoperative radiation therapy at a widely resected extremity.

With the potential for chondromatous metaplasia in the inner part of the joint capsule, the possibility of chondrosarcomatous malignancy also exists in the joint capsule. However, it is rare and definitely rarer than that of synovial sarcoma, as reported by Dunn et al. [446], Goldman et al. [642] and King et al. [887]. The pathogenesis, case history, and clinical findings differ from that of synovial sarcoma because the chondrosarcoma takes its origin solely from the joint capsule, develops insidiously, and causes a pronounced uneven thickening of the joint capsule. Thus the joint is enlarged, and its outlines are distorted. The motion of the affected joint becomes gradually and substantially limited, leading to a marked impairment in its use, but without significant pain. Laboratory studies of the blood show normal results, but roentgenographs reveal a conspicuous densification of the joint capsule, with diffusely scattered and irregularly delimited (some of them lobular) shadows of calcifications.

Gross-pathological examination discloses conspicuous thickening and areas of firmness or hardness in the joint capsule. Its uneven, plump-villous surface is studded in one or a few places with whitish, rather hard bodies of pea size. Numerous other hard bodies lie closely beneath the surface, contributing to its unevenness, and can be palpated through the synovial membrane. Histopathological examination discloses markedly fibrocytic synovial tissue which comprises roundish portions of hyaline cartilage, divided by thin collagen bundles into lobules. These contain groups of roundish chondrocytes of similar size (Fig. 532), whose hyperchromatic nuclei lie in lacunae. In their vicinity, other chondrocytes of conspicuous pleomorphism (Fig. 532) are scattered; their nuclei are much larger, of irregular bizarre shape or duplicated, and all of them are markedly hyperchromatic. Some areas contain only a few chondrocytes, of which most are necrotic, as identified by their fragmentation or lack of nuclei. The ground substance in their vicinity is focally impregnated with calcium salts.

Despite its slow growth the synovial chondrosarcoma is very malignant and has the tendency to metastasize rapidly. Therefore, once the diagnosis has been established histopathologically, radical resection followed by intensive radiation appears as the least aggressive and an effective treatment. However, in cases with operatively ascertained invasion by the joint capsule into the neighboring bones, a high amputation appears the only modality to carry a probability of salvaging the situation.

Beyond the malignant tumors which originate in the joint capsule or paraarticular synovial organs, the joint may also be invaded by malignant tumors originating in the articular epiphyses and their metaphyses. Such tumors start with the picture of an enchondroma, osteitis fibrosa, giant cell tumor, or reticulum cell sarcoma and thereafter manifest their malignant character by unlimited destruction of the regional bone and expansion into the joint (Fig. 526). Eventually the clinical picture of a primary joint tumor is simulated. The diagnosis is corroborated by biopsy and histopathological examination, which usually discloses a spindle cell sarcoma and less often an osteogenic sarcoma with scant sclerosis. The reasonable treatment is high amputation, which should be followed by radiation treatment 30–40 Gy to the area of operation and to the regional lymph nodes.

A similar picture may be caused by a pathogenetically completely different tumor, the carcinoma. The past histories of these patients invariably disclose that they have suffered for 12–16 years from articular epiphyseal tuberculosis or chronic osteomyelitis associated with ulcerations of the skin and draining sinuses (Figs. 533, 534). Roentgenographs reveal diffuse destruction of the articular epiphyses and densification of the joint capsule. Histopathological examination of the tissue obtained by biopsy discloses a squamous cell carcinoma of the ulcerated skin, in the fistular tracts, and in the joint. These findings pose the question as to the origin of this tumor, since a carcinoma is improbable as a tumor originating from the mesodermal articular tissue. Indeed, the skin, irritated by chronic suppuration, eventually developed malignant proliferation which expanded as a carcinoma along the fistulous tracts into the joints, where it invaded the joint capsule and the articular epiphyses. Treatment consists of high amputation and subsequent regional and lymph node radiation in two series of 30–40 Gy. Grosspathological examination discloses a dense, reddish gray mass expanding diffusely into the joint capsule and completely occupying the joint.

Besides the malignant tumors originating from the articular and paraarticular structures, and thus representing primary regional tumors, the joint capsule is very rarely the site of secondary tumors, such as metastases emanating from a carcinoma of the lung, colon, kidney, uterus, or ovary [116, 491, 629, 856, 1164, 1501]. Caroit et al. [247] reported metastases simulating a primary tumor in the joint capsule of the shoulder, ankle, or hip and originating from a cancer of the rectum, skin, or unidentified location. Treatment of these secondary tumors is not able to provide substantial improvement, even by excision of the primary tumor. As palliative treatment, local radiations with 30–40 Gy are advisable.

X. Related Affections

1. Tenosynovitis and Hygroma

The tendons, endportions of muscles, are invested by sheaths; here they are exposed to intensive use by contiguous epiphyseal protrusions or by tightness of the surrounding connective tissue. The sheaths ensure smooth gliding for the tendons by their inner lining with synoviocytes.

When the tendon sheaths are exposed to repeated stresses, especially those of friction, their synoviocyte linings respond to these irritations; they also respond to other noxious agents. Their reactions are manifested in inflammatory changes of various sorts. According to the etiology and concomitant changes, the following types of tenosynovitis may be discerned:

a. The most frequent type is traumatic tenosynovitis, caused by mechanical irritations in strenuous activities at work, sport, or pastime more often than by direct trauma. The reactions to these insults are similar; after a brief period of pain the area of the tendon sheath becomes swollen and tender. Active movement of the joint involving this tendon or these tendons is limited, and passive movement in the opposite direction of the tendon action elicits intense pain along the tendon sheath by distraction. On continued disuse, the tendon sheath swells, partly by augmented production of intrathecal synovial fluid but more by gradual thickening and unevenness of its inner lining. This impairs the gliding of the encased tendon. Treatment should be directed at avoiding the harmful activities. Inflammation of the sheaths is also mitigated by regular application of moist warm packs, and by protection of the involved joints and extremity from excessive activities by an elastic bandage, firm strapping, or plastic splint. On protracted course of these symptoms, additional shortwave diathermy in one or two series of eight sessions and antiinflammatory medications provide substantial improvement if carried out over a period of a few months. If satisfactory recovery is not obtained, an injection of hydrocortisone into the tendon sheath may provide dramatic relief, but this should be used judiciously. Local administration of corticosteroids impairs the biology of the local fibrocytes and thereby the composition of the local collagen fibers; spontaneous tears of the treated tendon (especially long biceps head or Achilles tendon) may occur thereafter even in normal activities. This potential complication urges careful evaluation of each case before injecting hydrocortisone into the peritendineum. In certain tendon sheaths (flexor tendon sheaths of the fingers), operative splitting with partial excision of the thickened portions may be indicated especially in the case of a "snapping finger". The latter condition is discussed in "Snapping of joints". Histopathological examination of the excised portion of the tendon sheath (Fig. 535) discloses chronic inflammatory changes with considerable increase of fibrocytes, extensive fibrosis, and interspersed giant cells.

b. Rheumatoid tenosynovitis is a concomitant paraarticular manifestation and occurs in 20%–28% of

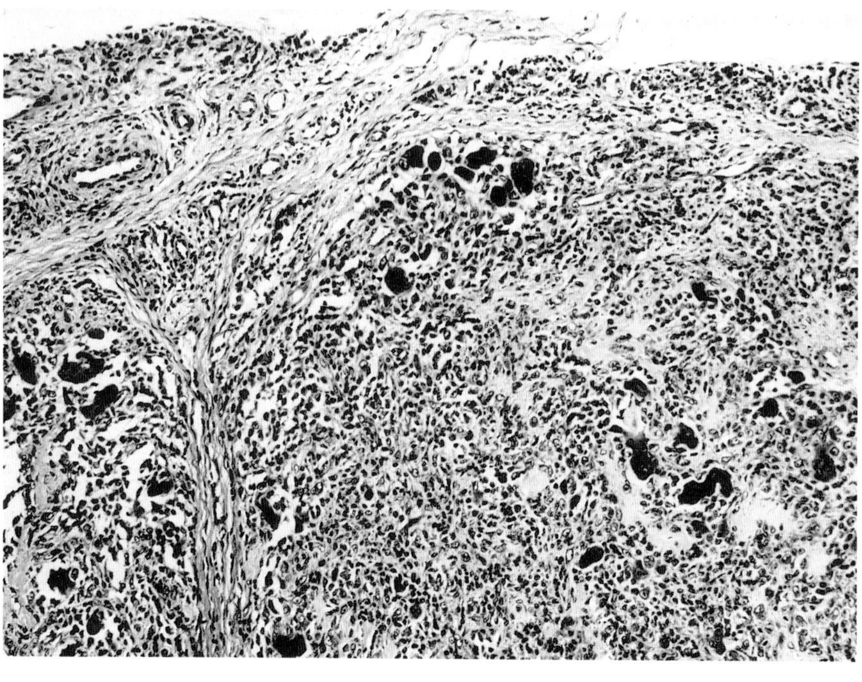

Fig. 535. Connective tissue delimited by synoviocytes is very cellular in fibrocytes. Middle-sized giant cells are scattered in between

patients suffering from rheumatoid arthritis. It starts with moderate swelling which progresses slowly to marked enlargement, more by thickening of the synovial lining and less by increase of the synovial fluid. The result is a local protrusion and deformation of this region (Fig. 536) and substantial limitation in the function of the encased tendons. The most affected sheaths are those of the extensors of the wrist and fingers (Fig. 536) and those of the extensors of the ankle and toes. The active motion of the adjacent joints is limited, but their passive motion has almost normal range. Treatment of rheumatoid tenosynovitis follows the principles outlined in "Rheumatoid Arthritis". Nonsteroidal antiinflammatory medications are indicated. Parenteral administration of gold salts may be of similar benefit, but should respect the adverse effects indicated in "Rheumatoid Arthritis". However, if all these modalities fail, and chronic swelling of the tendon sheaths persists with substantial limitation of motion of the local joints, excision of the tendons sheaths (Fig. 537) is indicated down to their attachment to the bone and joint capsule. Concurrent opening of the subjacent joint capsule reveals that the alterations in the latter are far less advanced than those of the tendon sheaths. Gross-anatomical examination discloses substantial thickening of the tendon sheaths and unevenness in their inner lining. Histopathological examination discloses, besides villosities on the surface, extensive lymphocytic infiltration and fibrocytic hypercellularity of the subsynoviocytic layers.

c. Tenosynovitis may occur in gout. Tendon sheaths as well as the neighboring tissues are often the sites of urate precipitations which cause painful episodes in the acute phase. Lobulated tophi are formed on the inner surface of the tendon sheaths. Microscopic examination discloses deposits of amorphous material and needlelike crystals in the tendon sheaths, and corroborates the clinical diagnosis. Laboratory studies disclose a significant increase in uric acid in the serum; the normal average levels of uric acid in the serum are 7–8 mg/100 ml in men and 6–7 mg/100 ml in women. The general treatment is outlined in "Arthritis in Gout". Beyond this, nonregressing large nodules within the tendon sheaths which mechanically interfere with the tendon action should be excised. The operation is indicated especially when the nodules are close to eruption through the sheaths. Active and passive mobilization exercises restore the gliding of these tendons, provided that no additional urate deposits in the joint capsule limit the motion of the joint.

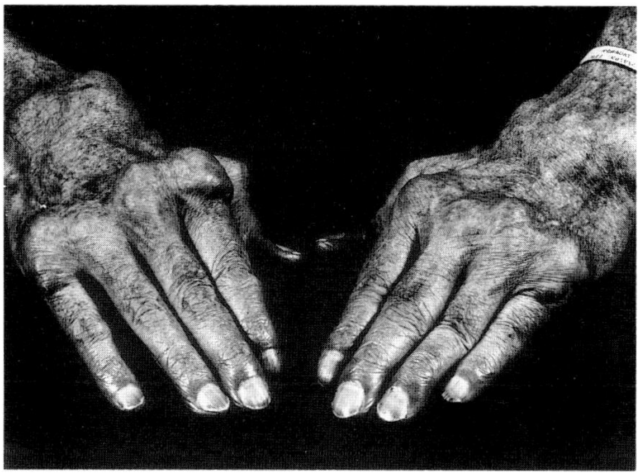

Fig. 536. Both hands, particularly the right one, present circumscribed thickenings on their dorsal aspects. The fingers are deformed

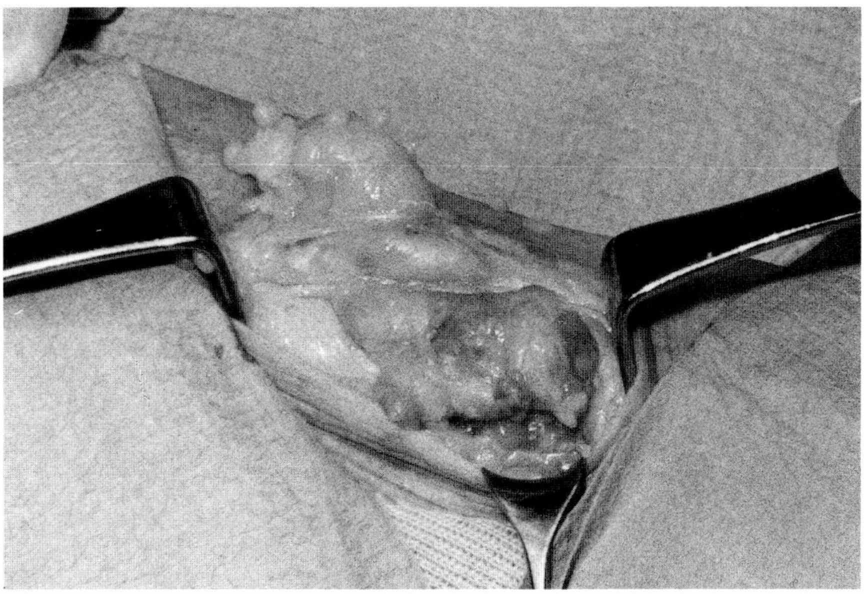

Fig. 537. At operation of the hands in Fig. 536, unevenly thickened soft tissue surrounds the tendons on the dorsal aspect of the hand

d. Tenosynovitis in gonorrhea results in the tendon sheaths, especially around the ankle or in the sole of the foot, being affected by the spread of gonococcal toxins via the bloodstream. The relationship between gonorrhea and affection of the tendon sheath must be supposed because no other causative factor can be ascertained in these situations. On the other hand, since no bacteria can be identified in the washings aspirated from the site of the tendinous inflammation, a direct bacterial infection must be excluded and a bacterioantigenic inflammation has to be assumed. This inflammation is very painful from its inception and is associated with moderate swelling but marked impairment in the use of the tendons. Reflexive tightness of the regional muscles causes the joint to assume an intermediate position unless an intraarticular inflammation coexists which also has an effect on the position of the joint. The etiology, suggested by concurrent and similar involvement of joints and/or bursae, can be clarified by the case history, genital examination, and stained smear of the urethral secretion. Once the etiology is ascertained, treatment follows the guidelines in "Arthritis in Gonorrhea". In addition, diligent application of moist hot packs, protection of the tendon sheaths, prevention of malposition of the joint by immobilization with a splint, and deep diathermy in two series of eight sessions are very beneficial. These modalities help to restore the function of the tendons unless intrinsic contracture or ankylosis of the adjacent joint supervenes.

e. Suppurative tenosynovitis [521] derives from a wound of the covering skin or an infection of the neighboring structures. It is usually caused by staphylococci and less often by streptococci or other bacteria. The rapid development of swelling, redness, and local warmth as well as the severe pain point to the septic character of this inflammation. Immediate treatment is required by immobilization of the extremity with a splint, application of mild warm compresses, and administration of a generally effective antibiotic against staphylococci. This medication is continued until the causative microorganism is identified by smear with Gram stain and culture and the proper antibiotic ascertained by sensitivity tests. If the symptoms continue unabated, and aspiration reveals the presence of pus, the tendon sheath or sheaths should be opened widely to permit free drainage. The indicated specific antibiotic should be regularly administered orally or intravenously as well as in bidaily wound irrigations until the suppuration stops and the operative wound is healing. The time between the onset of infection and instituting the antibiotic administration, on the one hand, and that between the appearance of frank pus and evacuation of the pus, on the other, greatly influence the outcome with respect to irreversible tissue damage, adhesions, necrosis of tendons, and corresponding functional impairment.

f. Tuberculous tenosynovitis [132] is a manifestation of the generalized disease caused by the mycobacterium tuberculosis. This can be identified in the wall of the tendon sheaths by specific staining with carbolfuchsin in the characteristic greenish, turbid intrathecal fluid by smear with Ziehl-Neelsen stain and by culture on Löwenstein-Jensen medium. With the overall decrease in pulmonary and generalized tuberculosis [132], tuberculous tenosynovitis has become rare. The insidious development of a doughy diffuse swelling without significant pain but with impaired function of the tendons suggests the specific etiology. This is confirmed by general examination, roentgenographs of the chest, skin tests, and biopsy of the tendon sheaths (Fig. 538), which discloses the presence of granulomata and Langhans' giant cells. Administration of streptomycin, isoniazid, and ethanbutol, as outlined in "Tuberculosis of Joints" effects regression of the swelling and healing of the tuberculous process. Residual adhesions and stiffness may mar the outcome.

g. Mycotic tenosynovitis, as an aspect of systemic coccidioidomycosis, sporotrichosis, or histoplasmosis [389, 1708], is rare and is observed mostly in southern regions of the United States. It is of insidious onset and is manifested by diffuse, indurated swelling of the tendon sheaths of the shoulder, hand, hip, knee, or ankle but without an increase in intrathecal fluid. The functional impairment is very pronounced. Biopsies of the tendon sheaths reveal the presence of the causative fungus, both histopathologically and by specific culture on Sabouraud's agar. Frequent draining sinuses in the proximity of tendon sheaths or a joint permit identification of the causative fungus in the fistular fluid by smear and culture. The treatment, outlined in "Mycotic Arthritis", consists of administration of amphothericin and excision of the indurated tendon sheaths [389].

While various possibilities exist in the etiology of inflammation of each tendon sheath, it also appears that the tendon sheaths of various regions are affected predominantly by inflammations of different specific etiologies. In conjunction with such inflammations, the functional symptoms differ from one region to the other and also necessitate different treatments.

The tendon sheath of the long head of the biceps muscle becomes inflamed chiefly after repeated strenuous activities entailing forward flexion of the shoulder joint combined with flexion of the elbow joint, as carried out in some sports and occupational activities. It is characterized by pain and circumscribed tenderness along the bicipital groove and by increased pain on passive hyperextension of the shoulder joint. This condition responds well to discontinuation of the offending activities, application of moist hot packs and shortwave

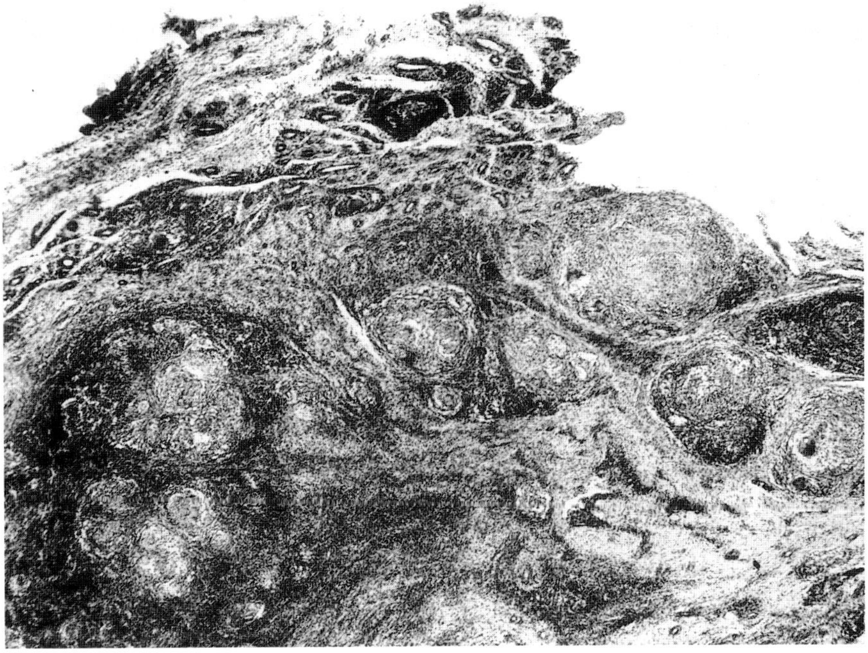

Fig. 538. Connective tissue, delimited by synoviocytes, is elevated into a few villi. The subjacent tissue is very cellular by fibrocytes and comprises several large granulomata; a few of these contain Langhans' giant cells

diathermy, and administration of antiinflammatory medications. Subsequent mobilization exercises prevent contracture of the shoulder joint. Topical injection of hydrocortisone is contraindicated because of the possibility of a subsequent tear of the tendon.

The sheaths of the tendons activating the wrist and fingers are often affected due to intensive and frequent use of the hand in activities in private and occupational life [1762]. While this consideration applies to the flexor tendons as well as to the extensor tendons, the latter tendon sheaths may also be affected by gout, tuberculosis (Fig. 538), mycosis, and rather often in rheumatoid arthritis (Fig. 187). Each of these types of inflammation has a slow, protracted course and is manifested by swelling associated with limitation in the flexion of the wrist and finger joints. Gout affecting the tendon sheaths generally causes uneven nodular thickenings expanding principally toward the skin (Fig. 349). Tuberculosis and especially rheumatoid arthritis expand into the depth and often cause adhesions of the tendon sheaths to the joint capsule, limiting the motion of the wrist joint. The proliferating granulations of the tendon sheaths may sometimes erode into the tendons, thus leading to their spontaneous rupture. The tendon sheaths of the extensor carpi radialis and extensor carpi ulnaris, although separated from the extensor digitorum communis, are affected by inflammation of the same etiology. Whereas antiinflammatory medications may provide a temporary regression of the swelling, most of these inflammations, except for those elicited by occasional strenuous activities, show a protracted course. Regular application of moist warm packs, and protection of the wrist by an elastic bandage are effective modalities. Intrathecal injections with hydrocortisone provide substantial regression of the swelling, but are contraindicated in cases of specific infectious inflammation and because of the potential for disorganization of tendinous tissue and subsequent tear of tendons. Thus thorough excision of these tendon sheaths (Fig. 537) is an effective treatment in all situations, especially rheumatoid arthritis, with extensive chronic swelling of the tendon sheaths and concomitant essential limitation of motion of the wrist and finger joints, and where administration of antiinflammatory medications do not provide a distinct benefit. When followed by prolonged physical rehabilitation, this is able to restore the motion of the wrist and fingers. The prognosis is good because concurrent inspection of the wrist joint through its opened joint capsule, at the operation of the tendon sheaths, discloses that its articular cartilage and synovial membrane are only moderately affected.

The tendon sheaths of the extensor pollicis brevis and abductor pollicis longus are affected by frequent, intense use in various occupations, musical practice, and handcraft. Thus the dominant etiology is recurrent mechanical irritation followed by circumscribed dense thickening of the tendon sheaths and surrounding ligamentous compartment. The distal part of the radius is also thickened and very tender. Pain in the thumb is intensified by forced active abduction or extension or by forced passive adduction and opposition. The gliding of the tendons inside the sheaths is mechanically and substantially impaired – thus the term tenosynovitis stenosans [404]. This condition may be confused [110] with osteoarthritic changes of the first carpometacarpal joint, peritendinitis of the extensor carpi radialis, and carpal tunnel syndrome. The treatment consists of restriction of those activities which impose stress on the thumb and protection of the thumb by a plastic splint or elastic bandage. Regular applications of moist hot packs are very helpful and should be supplemented with antiinflammatory medications. Patients, who do not respond to these modalities, need an operation which should be carried out upon precise identification of the compartment through which these tendons run. Resection of the constricting, rather hard portion of the tendon sheath and its surrounding ligament should be carried out economically to preclude subluxation of the tendons.

Of great frequency is also affection of the tendon sheaths of the flexors, which usually involves the second or third finger and most commonly the thumb. The symptoms are very characteristic and are manifested in the affected finger being "locked" in pronounced flexion of all its joints. From this position, the finger can be brought to extension either passively by manipulation with the other hand or actively by forceful contraction of the extensor muscles. Thereupon the finger attains full extension with a jerking phenomenon ("snapping"). The examination discloses a circumscribed nodular thickening involving the flexor tendon sheath and its fibrous reinforcements at the level of the metacarpophalangeal joint. The treatment, consisting of avoidance of vigorous activities, application of moist hot packs, and gentle passive extension mobilizations over a period of a few months, usually restores full active extension. Otherwise, persistence of the locking episodes and shrinking of the joint capsule may lead to flexion contracture of the metacarpophalangeal joint which is more difficult to correct. Hydrocortisone injection is not advisable because it structurally weakens the tendinous tissue and may subsequently facilitate a tear in the flexor tendon on attempted forceful active extension. Therefore, the tendon sheath should be longitudinally divided and its firm nodular portion excised. Histopathological examination of this portion (Fig. 535) discloses beneath the synoviocyte cover fibrosed connective tissue with marked hypercellularity of fibrocytes, among which giant cells are interspersed in considerable number. Surgical inspection and excision may also be necessary when extensive thickening of the tendon sheaths on the volar aspect of the wrist compresses the median nerve and causes a carpal tunnel syndrome.

In the lower extremity the tendons of the knee have no surrounding sheaths, but synovial bags or cysts are interposed between the popliteal tendons. Their inflammatory alterations are discussed in "Hygroma".

The tendon sheaths of the extensors of the toes and the anterior tibialis develop frequent inflammations secondary to strains of the foot or excessive activities in sport, long-distance routine walking, or walking with a deformed foot. Diffuse swelling on the dorsum of the foot, tenderness along these tendons, and increased pain on passive forced plantar flexion of the toes characterize this condition. As primary care, all strenuous activities of the foot and toes should be curtailed; an elastic bandage or foot strap should be applied regularly as well as moist warm packs. On longer duration of the symptoms, a firm compression strapping for 4–6 weeks puts the irritated tissue at rest. On the other hand, in the frequently observed deformity of the mid- or forefoot the deformity of the metatarsal arch should be corrected by forced passive exercises of the toes, well molded arch supports with metatarsal pads, and/or metatarsal bars on the soles of the shoes. In rigid deformities not correctible by manipulations angulation osteotomy, a midtarsal wedge resection, or triple arthrodesis may provide the necessary correction. The primary cause of peritendinous swelling may be gout, which accounts for extensive, uneven local urate deposits. However, more frequent and rather uniform thickening occurs in rheumatoid arthritis, in which the affection of the tendon sheaths presents a conspicuous swelling extending from the distal part of the lower leg along the anterior aspect of the ankle down to the dorsum of the foot. The movements of the ankle joint and toes are substantially limited. In view of the usually insufficient response to physical therapy and treatment by antiinflammatory medications, excision of the tendon sheaths adherent to the joint capsule remains the ultimate solution. Concurrent opening of the joint capsule reveals that the inner part of the joint capsule is distinctly less altered than the tendon sheaths. The postoperative course supplemented by elastic bandaging and mobilization exercises substantiates these findings by the reattainment of a fair range of motion in the ankle joint as well as by increased active motion of the toes.

Conservative modalities can be used in tenosynovitis of the peroneal tendons which develops secondary to a sprain and presents a posttraumatic inflammation, generally associated with marked swelling and increase of synovial fluid. This causes a conspicuous protrusion at the lateral aspect of the ankle. If the swelling does not regress after complete bedrest with elevated leg and application of moist warm compresses, aspiration of the synovial fluid is indicated. A firm compression strapping must be applied for a longer period of time and should be followed by regular application of an elastic bandage for several months.

The tendon sheaths of the short foot musculature on the sole and the peritenon of the Achilles tendon are

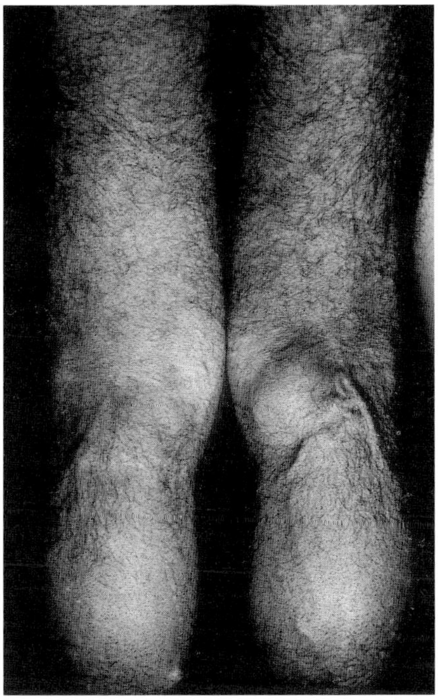

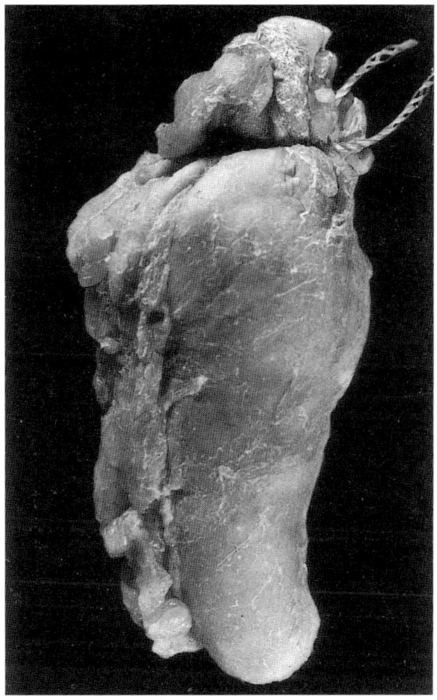

Fig. 539. The popliteal area of the right knee has a large egglike protrusion at its medial aspect. The neighboring veins are very enlarged

Fig. 540. The excised cystic formation partly has a smooth outer wall and partly merges with the adjacent connective and adipose tissue. It is compressible

often irritated by persistent strain in deformities of the foot, faulty footwear, or mechanical strains imposed by intensive activities in sport or at work. Correction of the foot deformity or of the footwear or discontinuation of these activities, supplemented with application of moist warm packs and elastic bandages, usually succeeds in bringing these irritations to regression. Additional physical therapy may be necessary with shortwave diathermy or ultrasound in six to eight sessions. However, no topical hydrocortisone injection may be administered because a spontaneous tear in these tendons may then follow especially any strenuous activity. These tendon sheaths as well as the tendon sheaths on the anterior and medial aspects of the ankle are also often affected in gonorrhea and respond satisfactorily to shortwave diathermy and moist, intensely hot applications.

Besides the inflamed tendon sheaths, synovial cysts as independent formations or by fusion of adjacent tendon sheaths may occur between tendinous ends. These are located chiefly between the tendons on the popliteal aspect of the knee [63] and rarely between the tendons on the dorsal and lateral aspects of the ankle. The baglike preformed or resultant synovial cyst (Fig. 539) is termed hygroma [1367]. The popliteal cyst is sometimes subdivided into two cysts, whereby the caudally located cyst often communicates with the capsule of the knee joint. This cyst may become affected by any strain or ailment involving the capsule of the knee joint as well as by any injury or stress imposed upon the directly adjacent tendons and muscles. Baker [63] regarded the communicating type of cyst as an outpouching of the synovial capsule which protrudes between muscle and tendon and concurrently contains more synovial fluid when the knee joint becomes irritated. Upon its excessive enlargement by accumulation of fluid, the outpouchings often become strangulated between the adjacent muscles and tendons and have no possibility of emptying their fluid content.

Even without communication with the knee joint cavity, this cystic tumor causes discomfort and impairment in the function of the knee. At maximally extended knee joint, it protrudes into the popliteal space (Fig. 539) and is easily discernible from the adjacent tendons and muscles. At flexed knee joint, it is drawn into the depth and disappears between these structures. It presents a fluctuation, and its content can be squeezed out into the knee joint if the cyst communicates with the knee joint. The propagation of the fluid into the knee joint can be ascertained by the immediately subsequent enlargement of the knee joint and the ballotement of the patella. On the other hand, in a hygroma without communication, a varicosity, aneurysma, cold abscess, and lipoma must be considered in the differential diagnosis.

Aspiration of the cystic fluid is diagnostically and therapeutically of great benefit and should be followed in cases without communication with the joint by intracystic injection of a hydrocortisone solution or at least by a firm compression strapping. However, sometimes even repeated aspirations do not succeed in bringing lasting relief from reaccumulation of fluid, especially in a cyst communicating with the joint. The only chance of permanent success lies in the excision

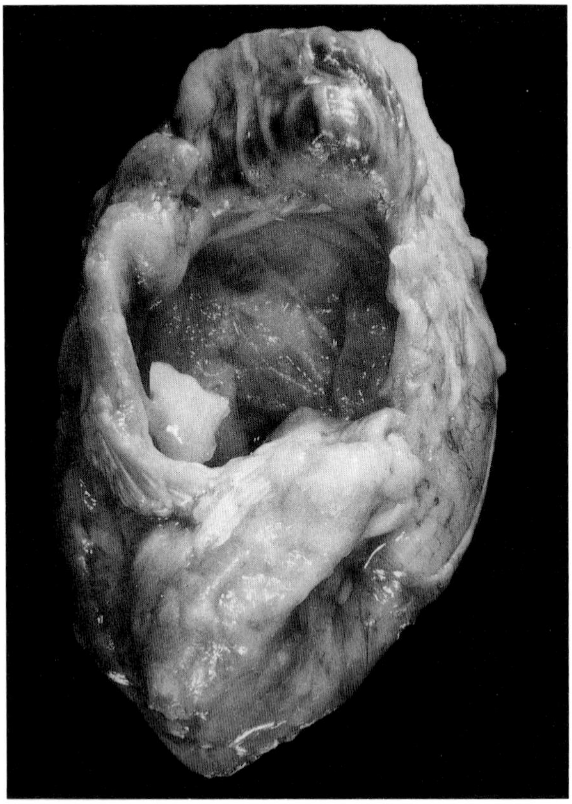

Fig. 541. On opening a cyst, its shiny inner surface becomes evident. It contains serous fluid and sometimes a small cartilaginous or osseous formation

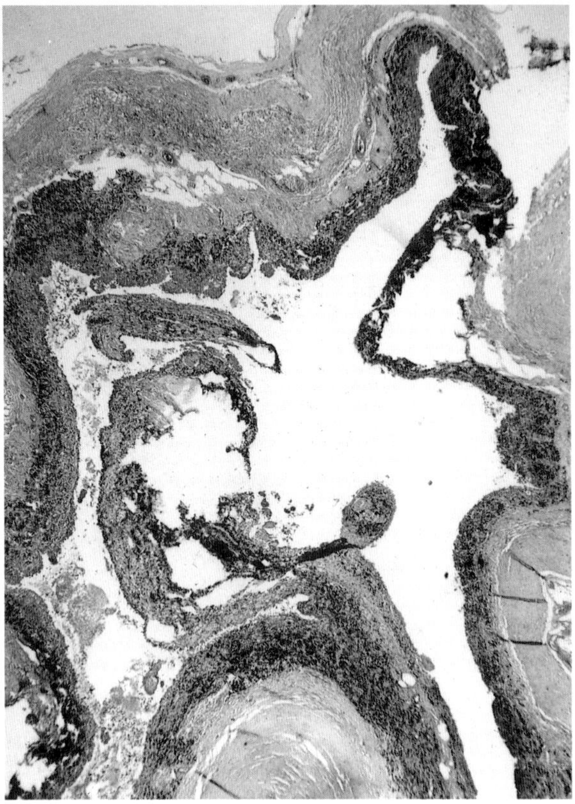

Fig. 542. The inner wall of the cyst is rather well delimited, consists of cellular connective tissue, and has a few protrusions into the cavity

of this cyst by a surgical approach which uses a broad anatomical exposure and permits radical excision of the cyst (Fig. 540) together with its occasional stalk communicating with the joint capsule. Since the wall of the cyst merges in places with the superficial tissue of the adjacent tendon and muscle head, it may become disrupted even on careful dissection. The remnants of the cyst wall should then be thoroughly excised together with the directly merging neighboring tissue. Otherwise, leaving fragments of the cyst wall may lead to recurrent formation of a synovial cyst and recurrence of a hygroma. This discussion of the gastrocnemio-semimembranosus hygroma applies gross-anatomically, histopathologically, and therapeutically to all other hygromata which may occur in other regions of the body.

Gross-anatomical examination discloses that the excised long-lasting cyst (Fig. 541) has a wall of rather dense connective tissue and an uneven inner surface with numerous folds and shallow deepenings. It contains a large amount of dense, dark yellow fluid and sometimes irregularly shaped loose bodies of cartilaginous or osseous consistency. The histopathologically ascertained alterations (Fig. 542) are initially slight hypertrophy of the synoviocytes, and marked edema of the subsynoviocytic tissue. With continued inflammation, hyperemia of the subsynoviocytic blood vessels persists, and serous exudation into the cystic cavity follows. Fibrinous exudation occurs from the areas with desquamation of synoviocytes and ulcerations, which merge in the depth with areas of hyaline degeneration of collagen fibers and necrosis. In the vicinity of these areas, fibroblasts proliferate and transform into fibrocytes under concurrent deposition of collagen fibers. Eventually, extensive hypercellularity and fibrosis (Fig. 542) produces a thickening of the wall of this synovial cyst.

Examination of the fluid from the cyst discloses increased viscosity up to 270 units as determined by the viscometer and a solid mucin clot; the cell count is 320–1500 cells/mm^3 with 87%–90% of these being mononuclear cells. The majority of these cells, desquamated synoviocytes, have a larger cystoplasmic body which contains a few vacuoles and an ovoid nucleus with several chromatin particles.

2. Bursitis

The ligaments within joint capsules and tendons close to joints are subjected to local friction where they are

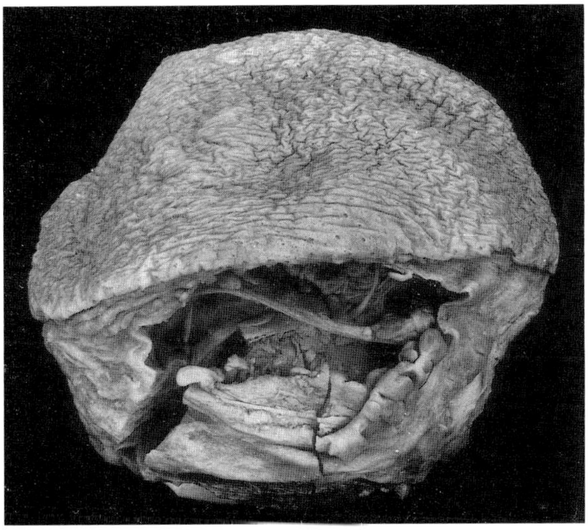

Fig. 543. The inner surface of a bursa is very uneven by large villous protrusions. Long, thin organized fibrin formations traverse the bursal cavity

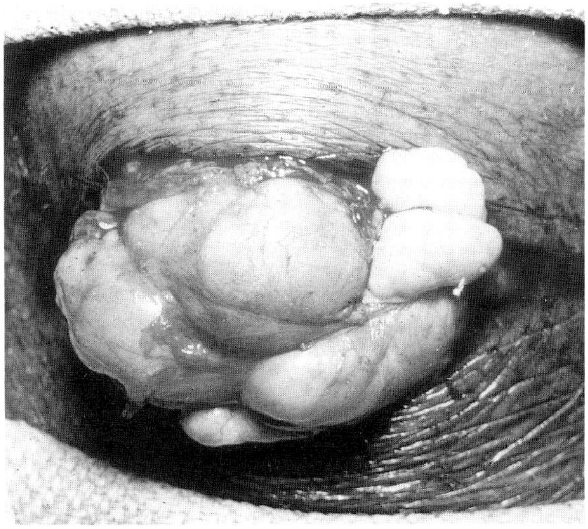

Fig. 544. Large egglike formations of white anorganic material lie in a bursal cavity

attached to or pass by protruding configurations of bone. In these areas, bursae are interposed and transform the friction into tangential gliding. This protects the ligaments and tendons from mechanical overuse. Similarly to joints, the bursae have an inner lining which produces synovial fluid; therefore they are referred to as arthroms [520]. The bursae also develop by cleft formation within mesodermal tissue during the fetal stage. While in most locations the bursae are completely separated from joints, in some cases (shoulder, hip, knee), the bursae communicate through narrow channels with the joint cavities. In addition to the preformed bursae of known locations, accessory bursae may develop at incidental sites of constant overuse of tendons.

Due to the structural similarity with the joint capsule, the bursae are affected by the same noxious agents: (a) mechanical disuse or repeated injuries lead in most cases to acute and/or recurrent irritation [237]; (b) rheumatoid arthritis affecting several joints involves the regional bursae [637]; (c) any infection [525, 764, 1025, 1638] by microorganisms, such as staphylococcus aureus, streptococcus hemolyticus, hemophilus influenzae, gonococci, pneumococci, mycobacterium tuberculosis, or other mycobacteria [1606, 1775] or fungi such as coccidioides (Fig. 163) or sporothrix [389, 1775] may affect bursae primarily or on expansion from adjacent organs; (d) chemical substances as abnormal products in generalized or local disorders of metabolism (urates, calcium salts) may be deposited in bursae [238, 375, 601, 1259].

According to the predominant changes elicited, the inflammation of the bursae may be of serous, purulent, necrotizing, or proliferative character. Transitions between these types occur, and the bursae then present a mixed gross-pathological picture. When traumatization or acute inflammation elicited by noxious agents affects a bursa, moderate effusion develops, either yellowish-serous by transudation or tenifluous-hemorrhagic by injuries to blood vessels. If the harm ceases, and this fluid is absorbed, complete healing may follow. On repeated irritations, however, recurrence of the exudation and precipitation of fibrin follow with proliferative reaction of the inner bursal wall. In other situations of more intensive harm to the bursal wall, some of its areas undergo mucoid degeneration and disintegration while others respond with proliferation. Hereby a chronic reaction and repeated thickening is perpetuated [151]. Eventually the inner wall of the bursa bears numerous and large villi (Fig. 543), some of which become detached under further mucoid degeneration and lie as free bodies in the bursal cavity. Formation of rice bodies (Fig. 150) secondary to such detachments and fibrin precipitates is observed especially in tuberculosis of bursae. In other cases the inner wall is transformed into a calcified whitish, uneven, and fragmented tissue. Egglike formations of calcified material (Fig. 544) then fill the bursal cavity.

Histopathological examination in the acute phase discloses edematous rarefaction of the bursal wall composed principally of fibrous connective tissue. Its inner surface is delimited by a single row of flat mesothelial cells. On continuation of the inflammation, collagen bundles in the subjacent tissue lose their sharp delineation and become thicker or fragmented. In other areas interstitial amorphous substance accumulates beneath the surface, an indication of mucoid degeneration. On intensification of the harm by microorganisms, cells

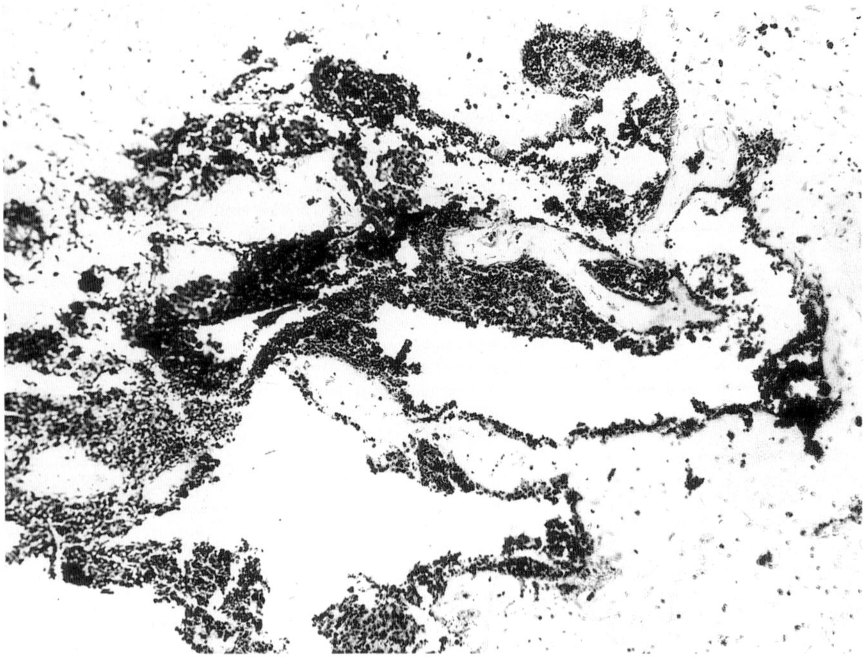

Fig. 545. Spaces of a bursal cavity contain many extensive agglomerations chiefly of polymorphonuclear leukocytes and, less so of lymphocytes

forming the lining of the bursal wall become necrotic and desquamated. The bursal spaces are filled with polymorphonuclear leukocytes and microorganisms (Fig. 545) and eventually become narrowed by fibrosis. In situations with continued inflammation but without necrosis fibroblasts proliferate throughout and, followed by proliferating capillaries, produce ramified villi (Fig. 546). However, the subsequent fibrosis accounts for most of the thickening of the bursal wall. In some cases, ulcerations occur on the inner surface of the bursa, and fibrinogen exudes into the bursal cavity. Fibrin becomes deposited on the inner surface, and fibrin clots fill the bursal cavity (Fig. 547). These fibrin masses become organized by intruding fibroblasts and capillaries (Fig. 547). Eventually, with regressing inflammation, as manifested in dense fibrosis of the bursal wall, calcium salts or cholesterol crystals (Fig. 548) are deposited in the bursal cavity. In other frequent

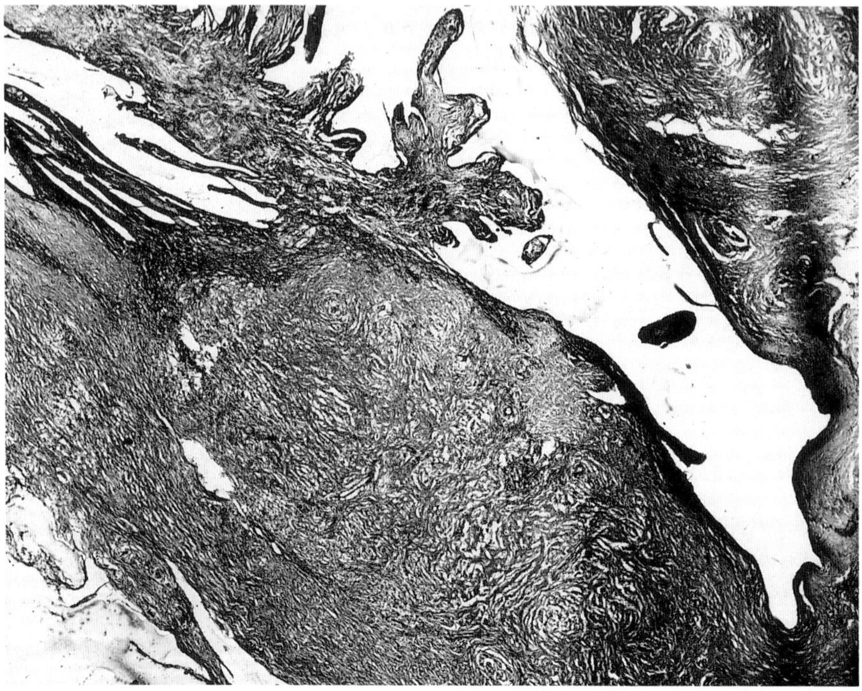

Fig. 546. The inner wall of a bursal cavity is uneven by villous elevations and is thickened by fibrocytic hypercellularity and an increase in collagen fibers

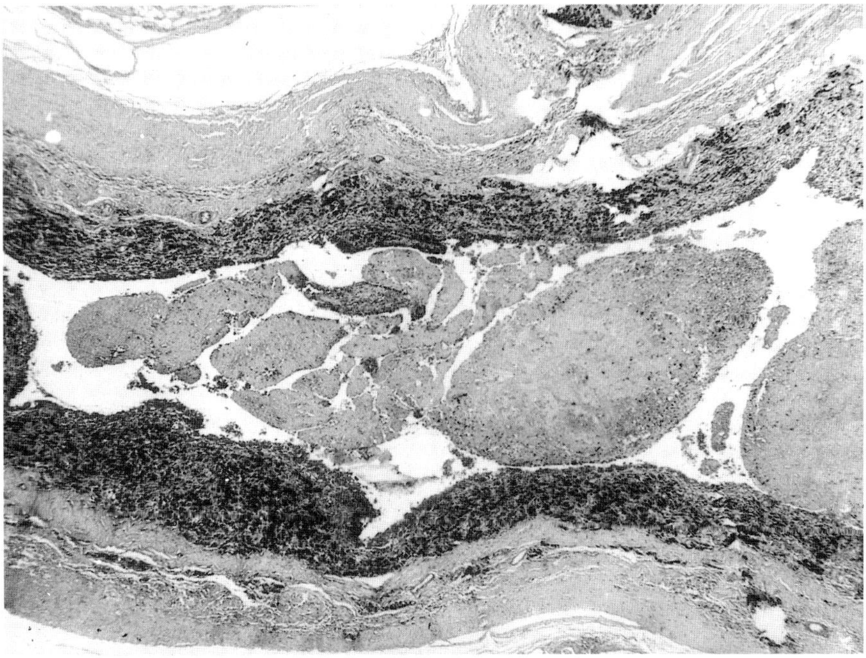

Fig. 547. The inner layer of a bursal wall is thickened and densified by marked increase of fibrocytes. The bursal cavity contains many large clumps of clotted and partly organized fibrin

instances, the proliferation of the fibroblasts is of slight degree and limited to small areas, whereas degeneration and especially necrosis involve more of the connective tissue. The latter becomes inspissated with calcium salts (Fig. 549), identified more often as hydroxyapatite and less so as calcium pyrodiphosphate by chemical examination, X-ray diffraction, and polarization microscopy for birefringence. Areas of the necrotic tissue are disrupted by deep clefts, and larger portions of it lie detached; the inner surface of the bursa is completely irregular and devoid of inner lining.

While any bursa in the body may potentially become the seat of inflammation, clinical experience indicates that certain bursae are predominantly affected by inflammatory processes. Those on the anterior aspect of the body (Fig. 550) are the (a) subacromial bursa, (b)

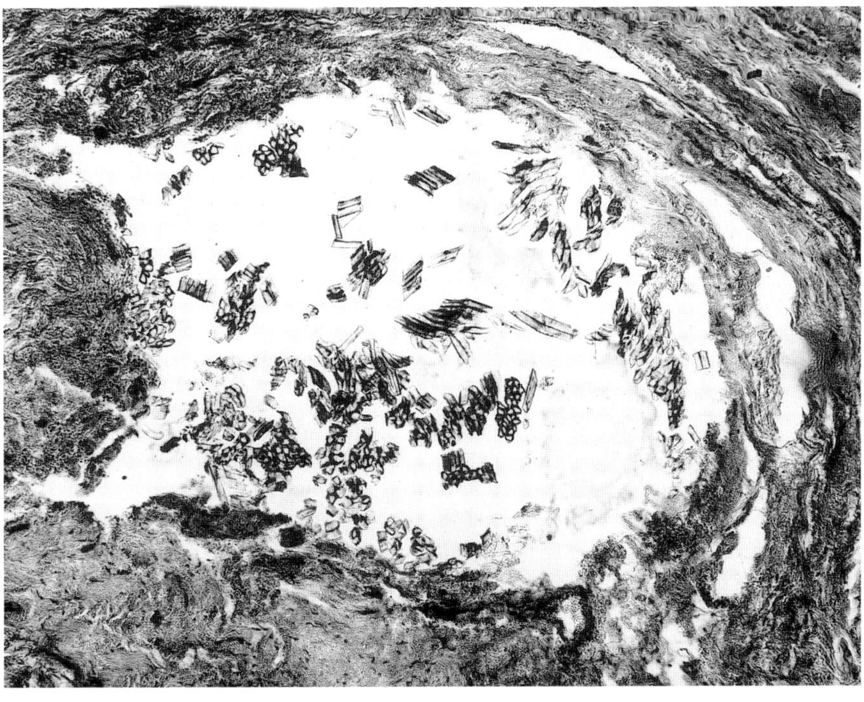

Fig. 548. The bursal wall is uneven and very densified by a marked increase in fibrocytes and collagen fibers. The bursal cavity contains many rhomboid crystals of cholesterol

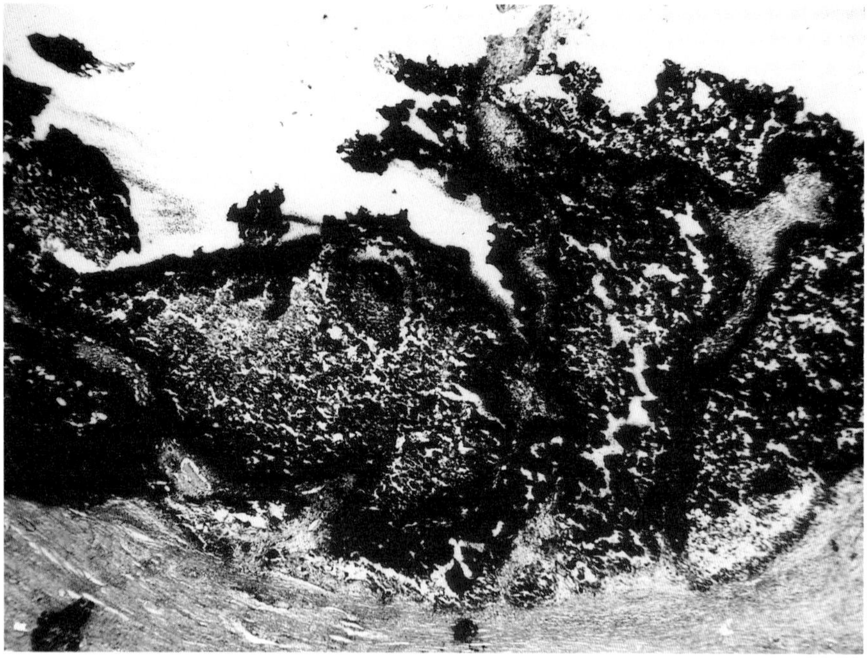

Fig. 549. The bursal wall is densified by fibrosis, and its cavity is extensively filled with calcium salts

subdeltoid bursa, (c) preglenoidal bursa, (d) iliopsoas bursa, (e) trochanteric bursa, (f) prepatellar bursa, (g) bursa at the fibular head, (h) anserine bursa, (i) bursa between medial collateral ligament and neighboring tendons, (j) bursa between lateral collateral ligament and neighboring tendons, and (k) infrapatellarpretibial bursa. The predominantly affected bursae on the posterior aspect of the body (Fig. 551) are the: (a) olecranon bursa, (b) ischiogluteal bursa, (c) bursa at insertion of the lateral hamstring tendons, (d) bursa at insertion of the medial hamstring tendons, (e) bursa at insertion of the Achilles tendon, and (f) bursa at origin of plantar tendons.

The cause of most of these bursitides may be found in repeated strenuous activities performed in sports, work, or household, in which the extremities or certain regions of the body are repeatedly subjected to intensive friction, pressure, or other mechanical irritations. A thorough case history helps substantially to elucidate the etiology. In the presence of rheumatoid arthritis an identical etiology is highly likely; with a history of infection of any nature the possibility is strong that it is a bacterial or bacteriotoxic affection. Such an etiology is also suggested by the presence of an inflammation or a wound of the regional skin. Prevalence of certain etiologies of inflammations may be noticed in the bursae at various regions of the body. The bursae in the shoulder are affected principally by strenuous activities or gout, those in the elbow [237, 375, 601] by trauma or inflammation in the proximity or by rheumatoid arthritis, those in the hip by strenuous activities or tuberculosis, those in the knee [1733] by injuries, strenuous activities, rheumatoid arthritis, or any septic inflammation in the neighboring area, and those in the ankle and foot by strenuous activities or urethral inflammations, especially in gonorrhea.

The onset of the bursitis is usually insidious, but it may also be rather sudden, when it develops within 1–3 days to a very painful condition. Physical examination discloses intensive circumscribed tenderness and a slight to moderate swelling of the deeper lying local soft tissues. When the bursa is affected by a septic infection or is located superficially such as the olecranon bursa or prepatellar bursa, the inflammation may produce a prominent enlargement (Figs. 552, 553) with distinct fluctuation by accumulation of a considerable amount of intrabursal fluid. The general temperature is usually not elevated, but the temperature in the painful area becomes elevated in proportion to the extent of the inflamed bursa or the intensity of its inflammation (Fig. 163). This sign of intensive underlying inflammation may be elicited by a septic infection and must not be neglected. However, without the presence of such infection acute bursitis in gout simulates the same symptoms. Upon localized intense pain, the regional musculature becomes tense, and active movements of the contiguous joint are limited. The attempt at increased passive movement is countered by reflex tenseness of the regional musculature.

The leukocyte count may be increased with an elevated percentage of polymorphonuclear neutrophilic leukocytes in cases of longer duration and with greater extent. The sedimentation rate may also be moderately increased. However, examination of the increased bur-

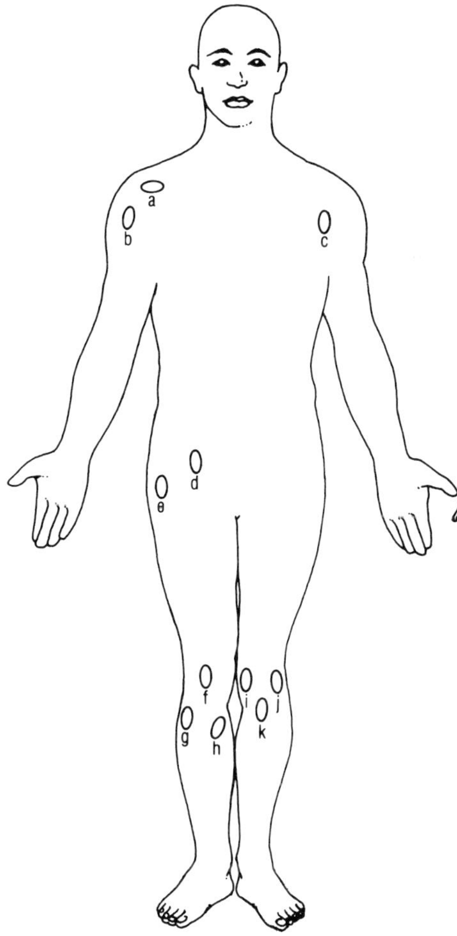

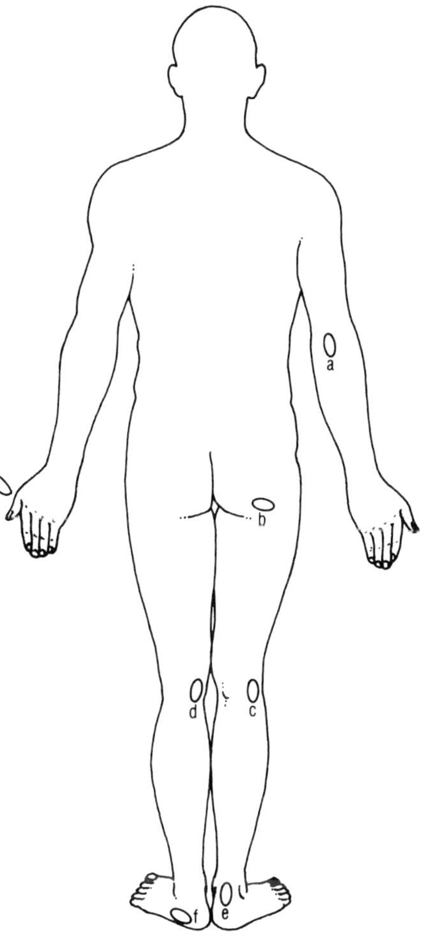

Fig. 550. Occurrences of bursitis at the anterior aspect of the body

Fig. 551. Occurrences of bursitis at the posterior aspect of the body

sal fluid is much more informative. In traumatic bursitis the fluid is clear to slightly hemorrhagic, with decreased viscosity and poor mucin clot; the number of erythrocytes is increased to 5000–150000, and that of white blood cells may be increased to 1000–3000. In these cases, a substantial number of mononuclear cells with large ovoid nuclei containing chromatin particles is also observed; these are desquamated cells from the inner bursal surface. On the other hand, in septic bursitis the bursal fluid is yellowish-turbid to thin purulent, with a leukocyte count of 5000–80000 comprising 65%–85% polymorphonuclear neutrophilic leukocytes, and positive bacterial findings in the stained smear. Staphylococcus aureus is the most frequent causative microorganism, less so streptococcus hemolyticus and rarely hemophilus influenzae [525, 764, 1025, 1638]. However, any other microorganism (Fig. 163) may cause bursitis [389, 1606, 1775, 1776], and therefore all differential culture methods should be applied. Furthermore, in the presence of a white smeary bursal content the chemical and optical examinations should be carried out for the presence of calcium salts or urates.

Roentgenographs usually yield negative results, at least in cases of shorter duration. In a few cases even of recent onset of symptoms and without preceding history, roentgenographs especially of the shoulder (Fig. 554) and trochanteric area may reveal calcification at the site of the bursa, an indication of longer, yet symptom-free existence of this bursitis. Otherwise, in most bursitides of longer duration, roentgenographs more likely reveal extensive calcification and even periosteal apposition, again, more often in the area of the shoulder, elbow, hip, and knee (Fig. 555).

Differential diagnosis must consider tenosynovitis or peritendinitis of the neighboring tendons.

In the treatment of acute bursitis, the extremity should be rested in a position which facilitates backflow of fluid, permits relaxation of the regional musculature, and prevents contracture of the joint. Thus the shoulder or the hip joint should be placed in abduction and the knee joint in extension or slight flexion with leg elevated. In addition to analgesics and muscle relaxants, nonsteroidal antiinflammatory medications, as discussed in "Rheumatoid Arthritis" are indicated. Regularly applied moist warm packs provide substan-

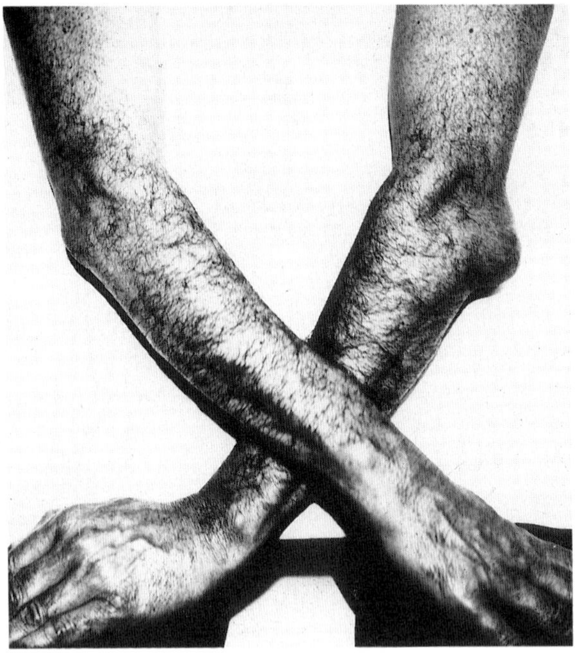

Fig. 552. The left elbow is conspicuously deformed at its posterior aspect by enlargement of the olecranon bursa

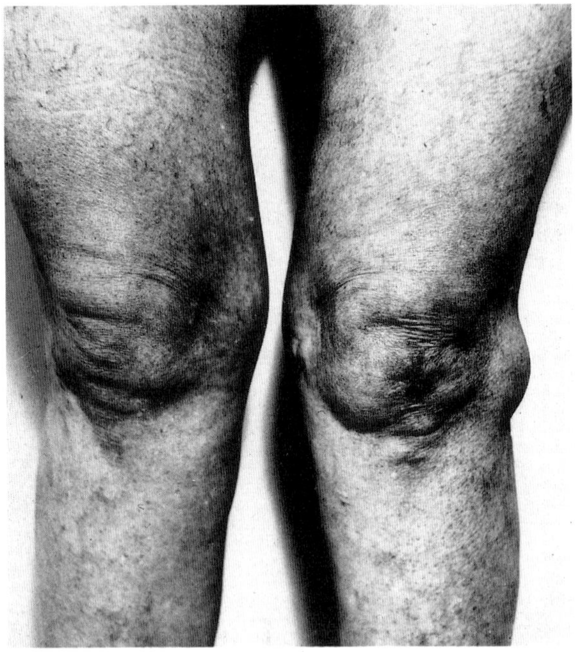

Fig. 553. The left knee is deformed by enlargement of both the prepatellar bursa and the bursa at the fibular head

tial relief. If local swelling develops by intrabursal effusion, the fluid should be aspirated and completely examined, as discussed in "Examination of Synovial Fluid", especially from the bacteriological point of view. According to these findings, the indicated antibiotics should be administered. Such treatment should be instituted from the very onset of bursitis in cases of a generalized bacterial infection or one localized elsewhere [765, 1638].

If bursal effusion nevertheless develops in these situations (Fig. 163) and becomes or remains purulent despite antibiotics, a broad incision (Fig. 164) is necessary for evacuation of the purulent material. Under concurrent general administration and local irrigation with the indicated antibiotics, healing of the suppurative process can usually be attained (Fig. 164). Rehabilitation treatment by active and passive mobilization exercises, as discussed in "Contracture of Joint", should immediately afterward be instituted to prevent contracture of the contiguous joint and to restore the function of the involved extremity. Operative treatment may also be necessary in extensive calcified bursitis (Fig. 544), chiefly at subdeltoid or prepatellar location. Otherwise, disruption of the bursal capsule and dispersion of the calcified material into the neighboring area elicit episodes of pain. Broad excision of the grossly evident abnormal tissue (Figs. 543, 544) provides abatement of symptoms. Similar treatment may be indicated with excessive tophaceous deposits in the bursae to prevent eruption of the urate masses into the subcutaneous tissue and the formation of a draining sinus. On the other hand, in situations of chronic nonseptic bursitis with repeated episodes of intense pain refractory to oral medications and physical therapy by ultrasound and with confirmed absence of bacterial infection, one to three topical injections with hydrocortisone are able to provide a long period of freedom from pain [1600]. However, such treatment should not be considered in cases of acute nonseptic bursitis; here nonsteroidal antiinflammatory medications, analgesics, moist warm packs applied two or three times daily, and shortwave diathermy in six to eight sessions are very effective.

3. Ganglion

The ganglion – a term used by Hippocrates [759] to designate a knot of tissue filled with mucin – is a cystic formation in the proximity of joints or tendon sheaths. In view of this location, it was formerly considered [1697] to be a prolapse of synovial tissue which continued to produce synovial fluid and gradually enlarged because of its impaired outflow. However, Carp et al. [248], King [885], and Mayer [1050] subsequently arrived at the conclusion that a degenerative myxomatous process of paraarticular connective tissue under-

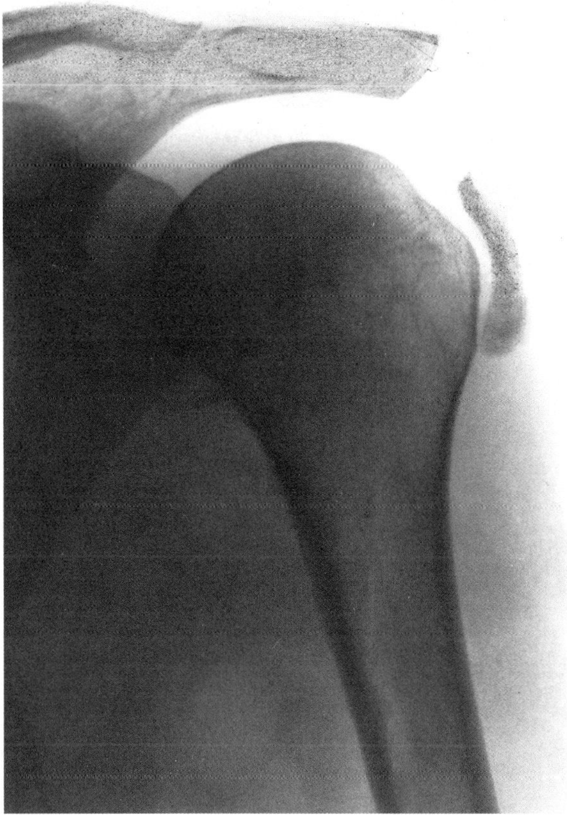

Fig. 554. The shadow of a calcified bursa is close to the greater tuberosity

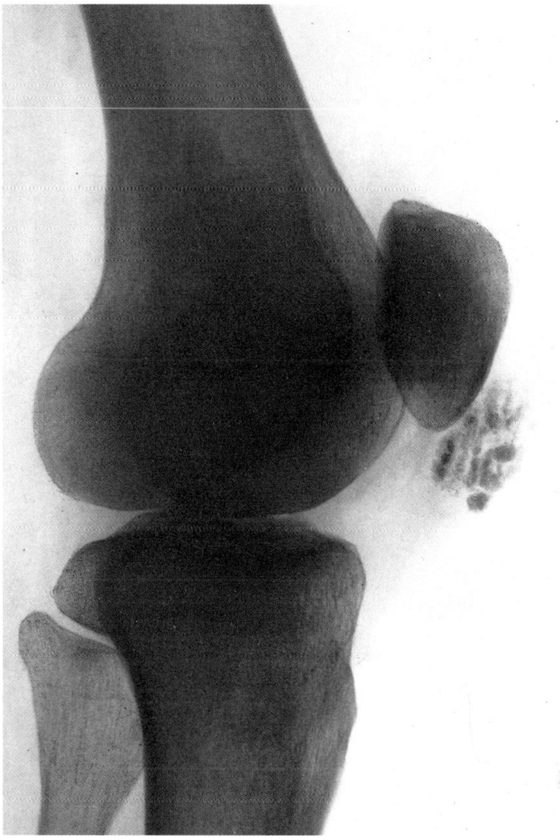

Fig. 555. A few small shadows of calcified material lie in the prepatellarinfrapatellar bursa

lies the formation of the ganglion. The primary cause for this formation has not yet been fully elucidated, but it appears that frequent strains occurring at work, sports, or other intense activities are associated with overuse of the regional connective tissue. This then undergoes regressive changes [520]. The predominant occurrence of the ganglion in the proximity of joints may be explained by the loose texture of the paraarticular tissue, which physiologically contains a great amount of interstitial ground substance. Moreover, a constitutional inferiority of the connective tissue system must be assumed in the etiology; otherwise, it could not be explained why some individuals develop a ganglion or even a few ganglia in various locations, while others with identical activities continue these without ganglia.

The ganglion comes into evidence as a circumscribed swelling, since it most often occurs in distinctly shaped regions and is well delimited from the neighboring organs. Its most frequent location is the dorsum of the wrist between the extensor tendons of the fingers (Figs. 556, 559). Less frequent locations are the volar aspect of the wrist between the transverse carpal ligament and the flexor tendons of the wrist and fingers, the medial aspect of the knee between the collateral ligament and the semimembranosus tendon, the lateral aspect of the knee in front of the fibular head (Fig. 560), and the dorsum of the foot between the tendon of tibialis anterior and the extensor tendons of the toes. Symptoms elicited by the ganglion are usually slight. The local discomfort or ache after intensive use of the adjacent joint is moderate, and no functional disturbance is experienced. However, when the ganglion is adherent to the tendon sheaths of the hand (Fig. 559), the gliding of these tendons and active motion of the fingers are impaired. A ganglion on the volar aspect of the wrist may elicit paresthesias and motor deficits by pressure on branches of the median nerve or the ulnar nerve. A ganglion located close to the fibular head (Fig. 560) may cause compression symptoms in the distribution area of the peroneal nerve. On palpation, the ganglion appears as an elastic or dense tumor which usually displays cystic composition by its compressibility. When its capsule is thick, no differentiation as to unilocular or multilocular can be ascertained. However, a conclusion may be

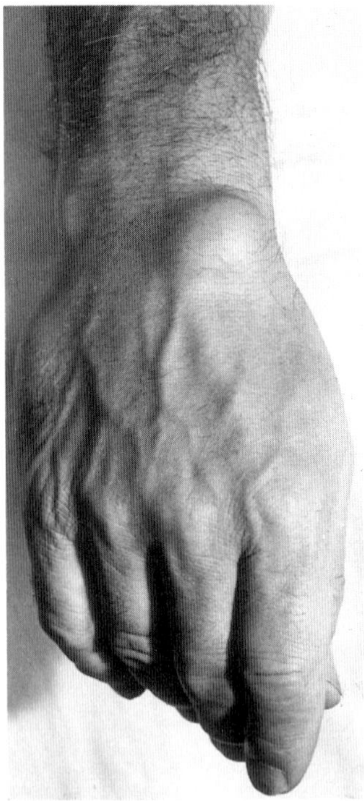

Fig. 556. A circumscribed thickening protrudes distinctly on the dorsal aspect of the wrist

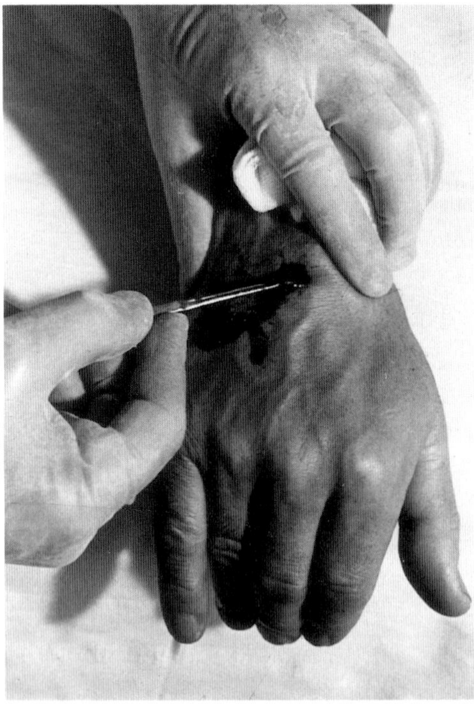

Fig. 557. The ganglion is treated by subcutaneous discission with a tenotome

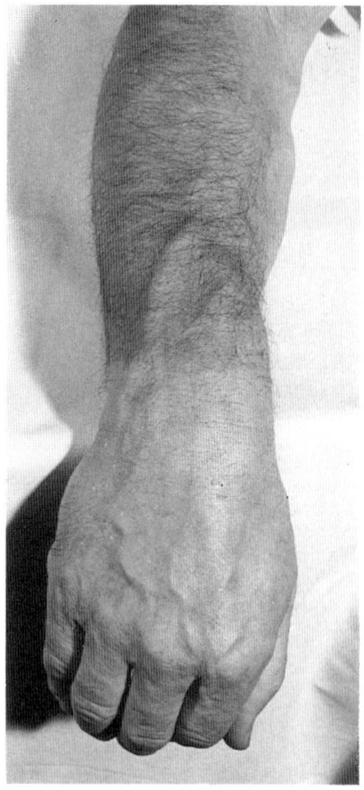

Fig. 558. The thickening on the dorsum of the wrist has completely regressed secondary to subcutaneous discission. No scar is noticeable in the skin

drawn from its consistency regarding its duration and its prevalent composition of liquid content or capsular connective tissue.

Roentgenographs do not reveal the presence of the ganglion unless its composition of soft tissue is sufficiently dense.

Gross-anatomical examination [1550] on transversal section (Fig. 561) discloses the cystic character of the ganglion and its formation by a capsule of dense connective tissue. This tissue commonly encloses a larger central cavity surrounded by a few smaller cavities. Sometimes a few larger cavities are interspersed between the smaller cavities. The individual cavities are separated from each other by septa which have a shiny lining and are soft in younger ganglia but denser and thick in ganglia of longer duration. Accordingly, the ganglion has a spongy consistency varying from elastic to dense. Due to increasing fibrosis, delimitation of the ganglion from the neighboring loose tissue becomes more distinct. The contained thin, jellylike, mucinous fluid has a viscosity of 140–300 units as determined by viscometer owing to its high content of proteoglycans (96–245 mg per 100 ml), among them much hyaluronic acid. Addition of alcohol or acetic acid causes precipitation of a white clumpy or ropy sediment, whereupon the viscosity of the supernatant fluid decreases to 38–75. The fluid also contains 2.8–3.2 g albumin and 1.2–1.9 g globulin per 100 ml.

Histopathological examination [1550] discloses not only in several ganglia of varying duration but often also in a single ganglion the various tissue changes leading to its formation. In the initial phase many collagen fibers in loose connective tissue are swollen, without sharp outlines, and indistinctly structured. Other fibers are separated from each other and form a network comprising increased ground substance by the admixture of decomposing fibers (Fig. 562). In this process of disintegration also participate fibrocytes, which swell, contain vacuoles with fluid and fragmented or indistinct nuclei in their cytoplasm, and are eventually incorporated into the liquefaction. Homogeneous, intensely hematoxylin-staining areas appear which are separated from each other by septa of collagen bundles. On further disintegration of some of these, larger cavities are formed containing mucoid substance (Fig. 563) manifesting metachromasia upon toluidine blue or acridin orange staining. When the decomposition process apparently comes to an end, the surrounding capsule assumes a dense texture due to additional formation of collagen fibers in the course of fibrosis.

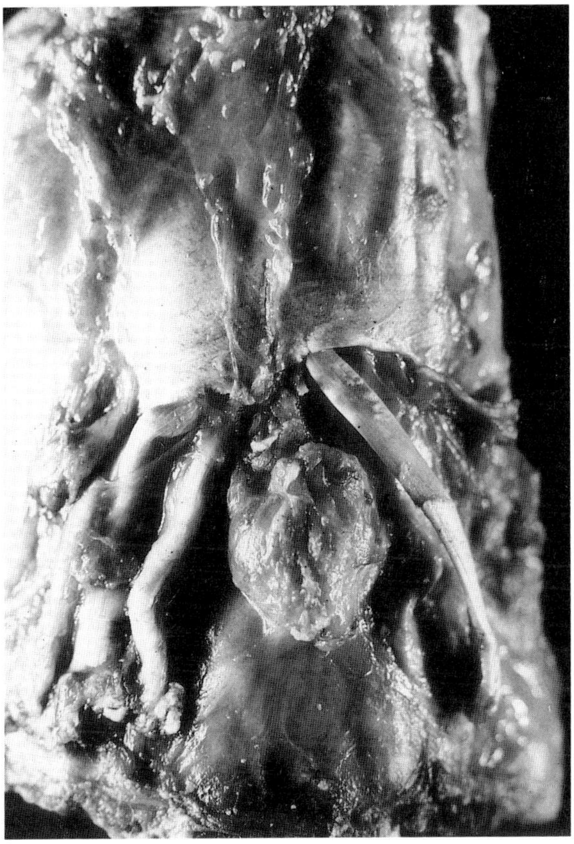

Fig. 559. The ganglion is an egglike, well-delimited cystic formation which lies between tendons on the dorsum of the hand

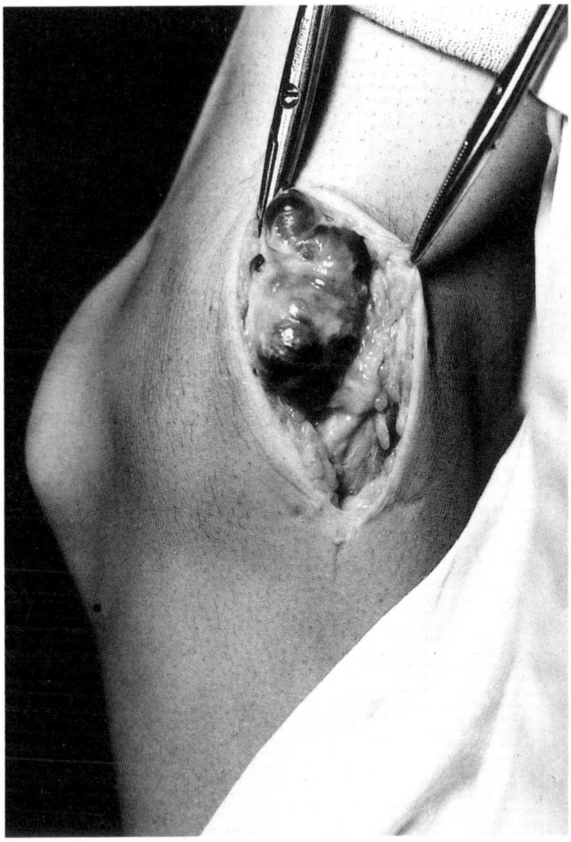

Fig. 560. The ganglion is a multicystic, well-delimited formation which lies close to the peroneal tendons

This phase is suggested by the increased number of plump and slender fibrocytes which lie between and along the collagen bundles. Other fibrocytes lie with their longitudinal diameter along the cavities on the surface of the septa of collagen bundles and form a more or less coherent lining (Fig. 564). Nevertheless, a few marginal areas still display various phases of disintegration of thin collagen septa, whereupon they are incorporated into the larger cavity. By its cavities filled with mucinous fluid and a surrounding capsule of dense connective tissue, the ganglion presents structural similarity with a bursa, but the former does not exist as a preformed organ, and its development is initiated by degeneration of connective tissue.

The desire to remove this primarily cosmetically disturbing deformity leads the patient to seek medical care which depends on the duration of the ganglion. When of shorter duration (1–3 months), the ganglion may be brought to bursting by firm compression with the tip of the thumb. In the aftercare a firm object, a padded big button or a padded big coin, is applied tightly onto this area for the following 3–4 weeks to prevent reaccumulation of mucoid substance. Such a ganglion may sometimes recur, especially if adjacent areas undergo disintegration and liquefaction. A further compression is then necessay and may be effective as long as the capsule is soft. However, if the capsule of the ganglion and its septa have already developed a denser structure, the compression fails. The removal of the mucinous content can be accom-

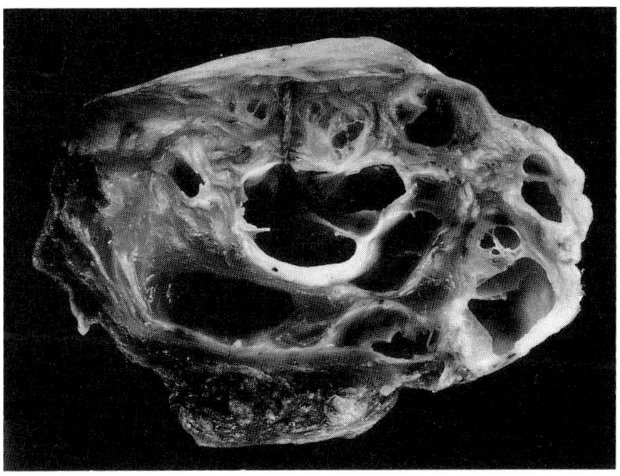

Fig. 561. Transversal section discloses that the ganglion comprises a few cystic spaces filled with a dense mucinous liquid

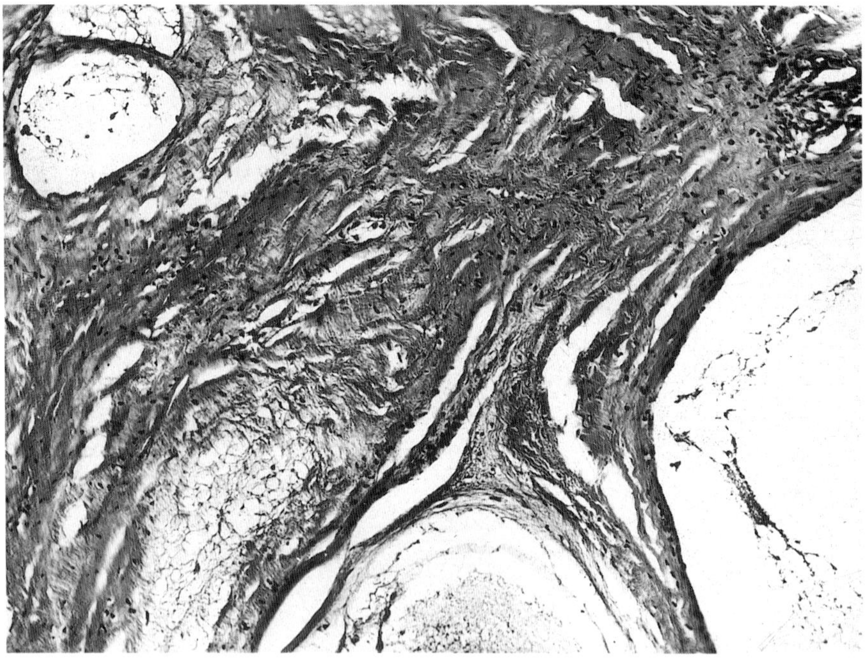

Fig. 562. A few areas of connective tissue undergo progressing degeneration and disintegration of their collagen bundles. Phases of liquefaction and formations of fluid-filled cavities follow

plished by aspiration with a large bore needle which, attached to a syringe, is inserted under local anesthesia in a few directions in order to penetrate into all cystic cavities. The entire mucinous content can be extracted; a hydrocortisone solution is then injected, followed by application of a firm compression dressing. Since this procedure does not remove the capsule and septa of the ganglion, residual thickening continues. Therefore, primary excision of the ganglion is generally practiced. However, Hand et al. [720], Hvid-Hansen [798], and McEvedy [1061] reported recurrence of the ganglion in 15%–40% of operated cases despite radical excision. This failure rate can be explained by the fact that even with broad exposure not all tissue involved in degeneration is perceived and removed at the operation. The remnants of such tissue progress to degenerate and to liquefy and to form another ganglion.

As an alternative, subcutaneous discission (Fig. 557) has been recommended [1550] which, with a recurrence rate of 18%, avoids the risks of an open operation

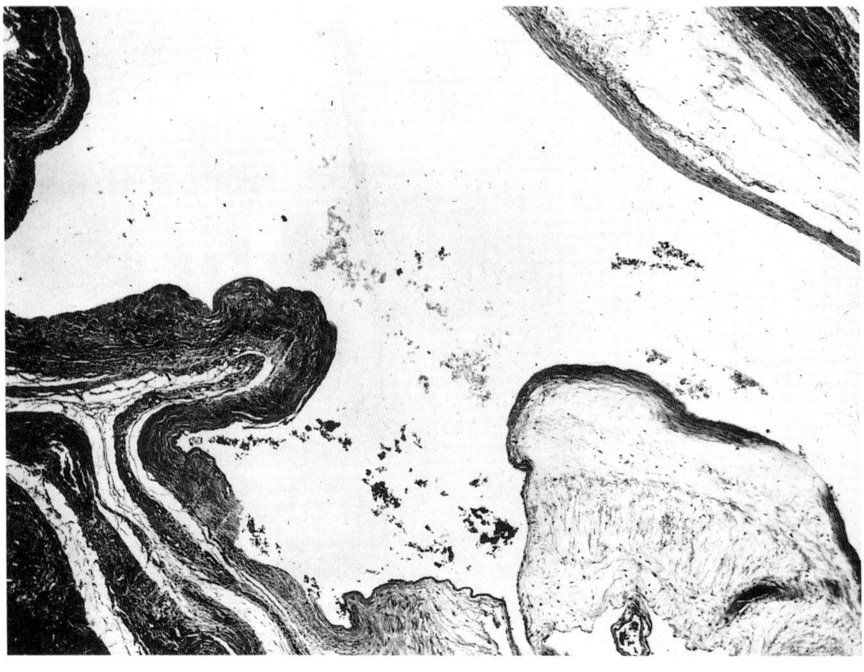

Fig. 563. Extensive cystic cavities have formed. Some of their delimiting connective tissue protrusions are still in disintegration

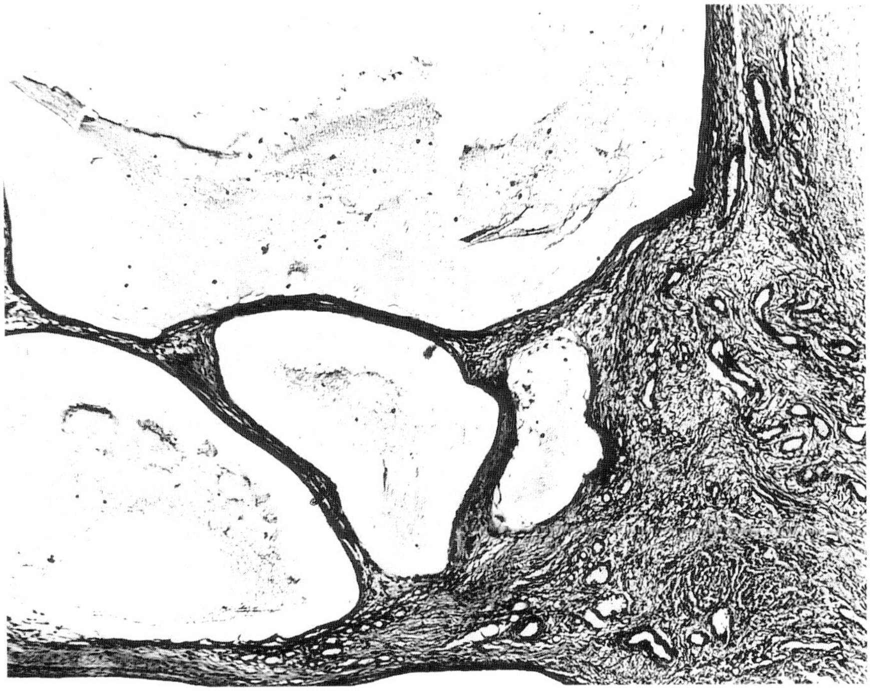

Fig. 564. The process of collagen liquefaction is no longer active. All cystic cavities are well delimited by dense connective tissue

and is free of the disadvantage of a resulting scar (Fig. 558) on the most often affected, uncovered regions of the extremities. The discission is performed with a tenotome (Fig. 557) which under local anesthesia is inserted through the skin and is so directed that it divides the ganglion circularly and in a number of planes [1550]. Thereby all cysts of the ganglion are opened and their viscid content is pressed out. A compression strapping is applied for 2 weeks. After its removal, no scar is noticeable (Fig. 558); only a subcutaneous thickening is palpable, which gradually decreases and eventually is no more palpable. However, this technique must not be applied on a ganglion located on the volar aspect of the wrist because of its proximity to the radial artery. The same limitations apply to ganglia located in other areas in proximity to blood vessels and/or nerves.

4. Fibrositis

The muscles, acting by their tendinous ends on the joints of the trunk and extremities, originate from and insert into bones. These areas of the bones, invested with periost, are exposed to irritations of various nature. Consequently, painful episodes develop locally which are considered the expression of inflammation. The term fibrositis [67, 656] or fibrosis [994] is used for the alterations and symptoms confined to the fibrous tissue of the tendinous ends, the areas of attachment of these ends or of fasciae onto bone [1499].

The etiology of primary fibrositis commonly lies in repeated, not necessarily very intense, local traumatizations, such as those caused by athletics or work in which larger parts of the body or the extremities are used strenuously. Other causes are stereotype movements in such activities as hobbies (practice of music, handcraft, etc.). In addition, some generalized inflammations of the body may secondarily affect the tendinous attachments. These are influenza or other viral infections, nonspecific inflammations of the intestine such as in regional ileitis or ulcerative colitis, urethral infections such as in gonorrhea or Reiters disease, rheumatoid arthritis and its variants such as ankylosing spondylitis, and beginning osteoarthritis of the spine. However, in some women aged between 20 and 50 years the symptoms occur without previous mechanical or inflammatory factors but are elicited psychogenically as stress reactions [67, 1522, 1523].

Symptoms include spontaneous aching localized in specific areas corresponding to the attachment of tendons, ligaments, or fasciae and/or pain following the performance of certain strenuous activities. The pain may remain confined to these specific areas for a longer period of time. A sensation of stiffness or limitation of motion is associated with these symptoms and is experienced especially in the lower cervical spine, upper thoracic spine, or lower lumbar spine. Smythe [1522, 1523] reported that regional aching and stiffness combined with localized numbness or burning sensation can arise either during the night, disrupting sleep, or in the morning after a sleepless night. Symptoms

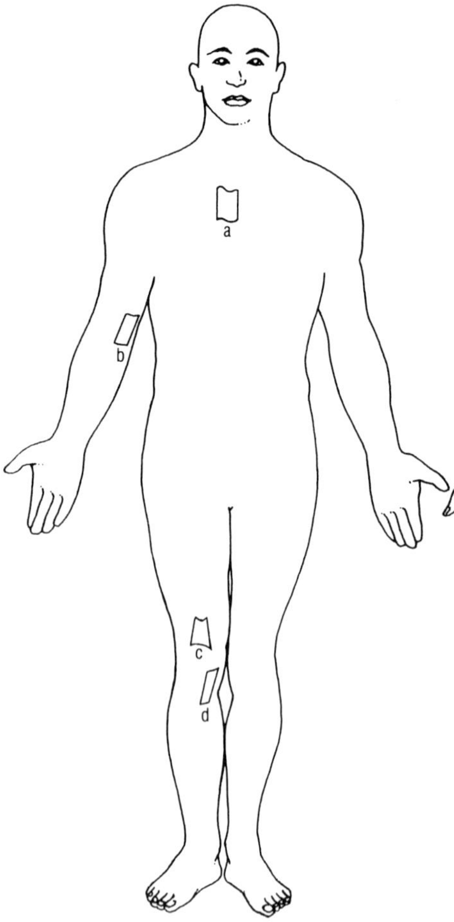

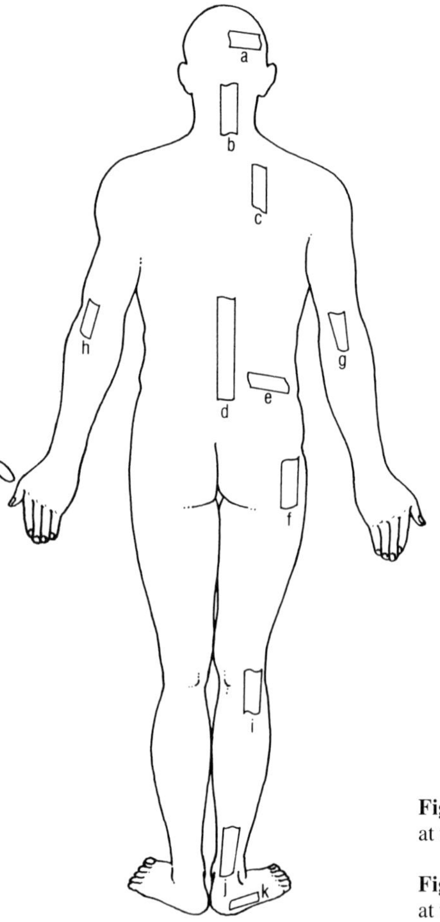

Fig. 565. Localization of fibrositis at the anterior aspect of the body

Fig. 566. Localization of fibrositis at the posterior aspect of the body

become aggravated by tension, headache, fatigue, exhaustion, or chill as well as by stress, grief, or fear. Similarly, Yunus et al. [1805] described a fibromyalgia with diffuse musculoskeletal aches and stiffness influenced by inclement weather, insomnia, and anxiety. However, after psychologically testing such female patients and a group of control patients, Clark et al. [294] arrived at the conclusion that no significant differences existed in the majority of these cases; the presence of a psychological condition accounted for the persistence of this condition in only some patients with fibrositis.

The areas most frequently affected by fibrositis on the anterior aspect of the body (Fig. 565) are at insertion of the (a) pectoralis tendons to the upper sternocostal joints, (b) flexor tendons to the medial humeral epicondyle, (c) quadriceps tendon to the upper border of the patella, and (d) medial collateral ligament and anserine tendons to the medial tibial condyle. Those most commonly affected areas on the posterior aspect of the body (Fig. 566) are at insertion of the (a) semispinal and splenius tendons to the occipital bone, (b) interspinous ligaments and semispinal tendons to the middle and lower cervical spine, (c) levator scapulae, supraspinatus, and rhomboidei tendons to the scapula, (d) interspinous ligaments and interspinal and semispinal tendons to the lumbar spine, (e) gluteal tendons to the iliac crest, (f) gluteal tendons to the greater trochanter, (g) triceps tendon to the olecranon, (h) extensor tendons to the lateral humeral epicondyle, (i) iliotibial band and biceps tendon to the lateral tibial condyle, (j) Achilles tendon to the calcaneus, and (k) plantar fascia to the calcaneus.

Palpation into depth sometimes discloses thickening or hardness of the terminal portion of a tendon or a ligament or in a fascia, and persistent circumscribed tenderness at the site of its attachment to bone. The localized pain increases on activation of the relevant muscles and with pull on tendons and ligaments. Correspondingly, the range of active movements of the involved joint or the body area is limited. The attempt passively to increase the range of movements intensifies the pain and is associated with reflex tenseness of the regional musculature. Blood studies disclose no specific changes except those related to a possibly primarily etiological disease. However, roentgenographs

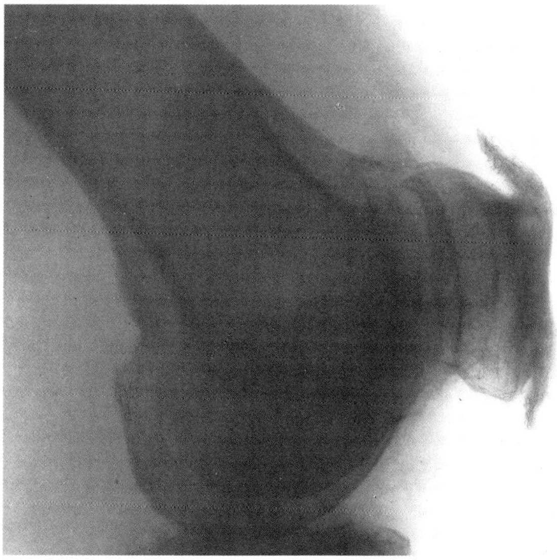

Fig. 567. Pointed exostoses rise cranially and caudally from the anterior aspect of the patella corresponding to the insertion sites of tendons

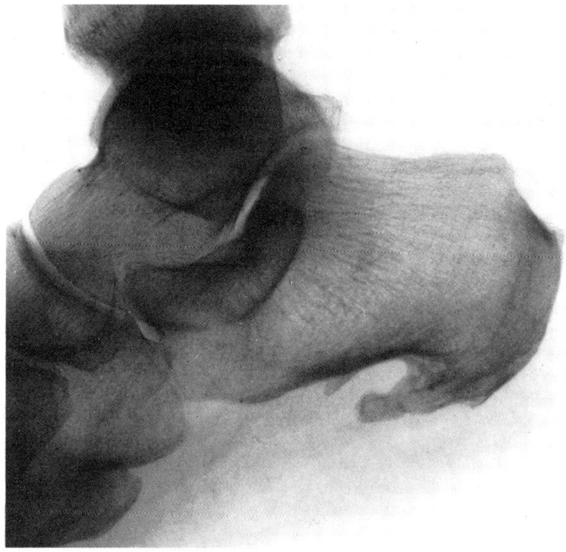

Fig. 568. A broad exostosis expands from the plantar aspect of the calcaneus into the insertion of the plantar fascia

(Figs. 567, 568) reveal in a small percentage of these patients irregular shadows of osseous density located in the terminal portion of the tendon, ligament, or fascia adjacent to bone. These densities are sometimes observed at the posterior aspect of the occipital bone, at the superior aspect of the scapula or humerus, at the superior aspect of the pelvic bone, and are relatively more common in the extremities at the medial or lateral epicondyle of the elbow, the medial or lateral condyle of the knee, at the base of the patella (Fig. 567), and the superior or plantar aspect of the tuber calcanei (Fig. 568).

Gross-pathological examination (Fig. 569) generally discloses no conspicuous changes in the inserting ends of connective tissue; however, after splitting these areas, hyperemia becomes evident. An exostotic thickening occasionally protrudes from the cortex at a length of 1.0–3.5 cm into the abutting tendon, ligament, or fascia [1554]. Such protrusion is observed chiefly in the lower extremities. Histopathological examination [1554] (Fig. 570) discloses occasional dilatation and hyperemia of the small and middle-size blood vessels and rather broad perivascular infiltration by lymphocytes in the areas of loose connective tissue. Extensive and very dense agglomerations of normal and larger fibrocytes are interspersed within the connective tissue, an indication of very active proliferation (Fig. 571). In other areas fibroblasts are surrounded by halos of light ground substance and resemble chondrocytes; osteoblasts containing large dense nuclei also occur here. These changes are accompanied by calcification of the ground substance. In contiguity, membranous bone is formed, and cavities appear in it through dissolution by intruding osteoclasts and blood vessels (Fig. 572). Peripherally hereto osteoblasts depose osteoid shells which assume a lamellar arrangement and become calcified to osseous tissue [1554]. Thurner et al. [1643] pointed out that the insertional area of this connective tissue into bone presents degeneration and necrosis of its cells as the first changes from imposed stresses. Proliferation of fibrocytes and blood vessels sets in as a reparative process and is followed by meta-

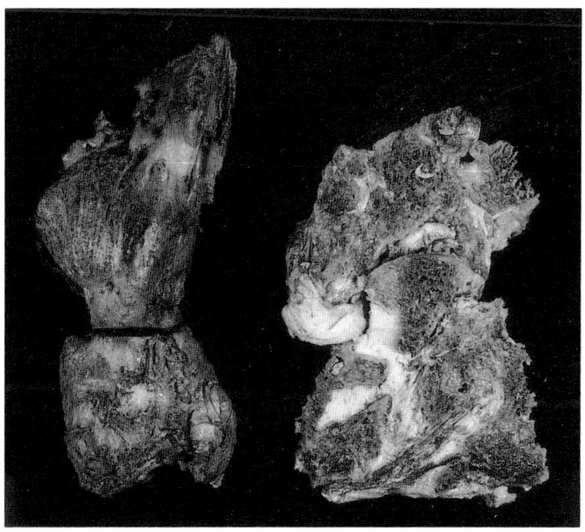

Fig. 569. Formations of osseous tissue lie within dense connective tissue

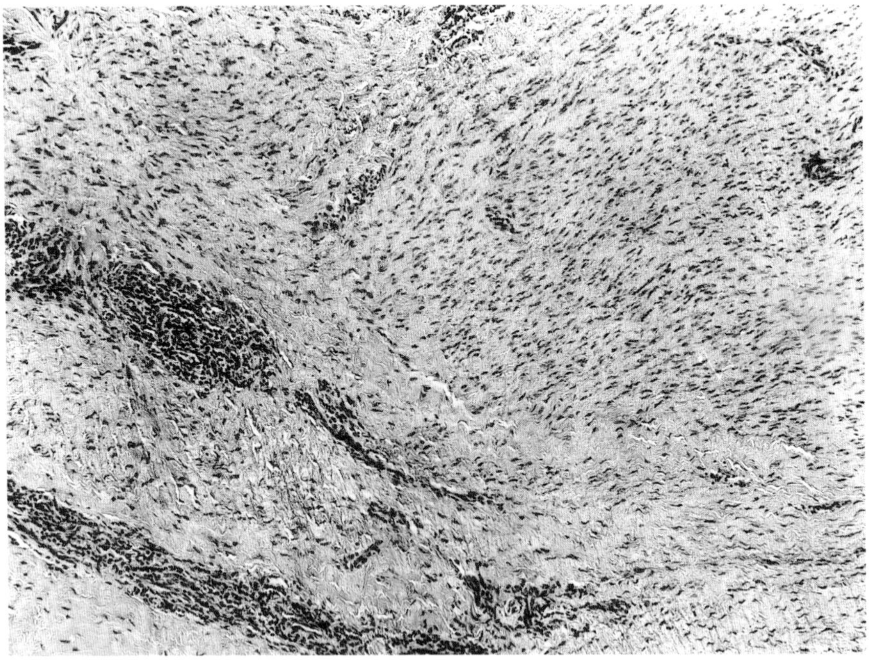

Fig. 570. Hypercellular and fibrosed connective tissue comprises a few small and two more extensive, dense infiltrates of inflammatory cells

plasia into chondrocytes and osteocytes. With the local formation of osseous tissue, the reparative process attains its completion [1643].

Differential diagnosis must consider all inflammatory conditions which may be associated secondarily with inflammatory changes of the periarticular structures. Especially bursitis and myositis should be here included; roentgenographs may reveal calcifications of varying extents. Furthermore, psychological evaluation appears indicated in all situations in which no distinct mechanical, traumatic, or inflammatory influence can be ascertained as etiological factor.

Treatment should address any primary general disease which may elicit fibrositis. Treatment is also designed to discontinue or decrease these activities associated with excessive strain to certain muscle groups or joints. Causative activities in the place of work and which are indispensable to the patient's employment should be

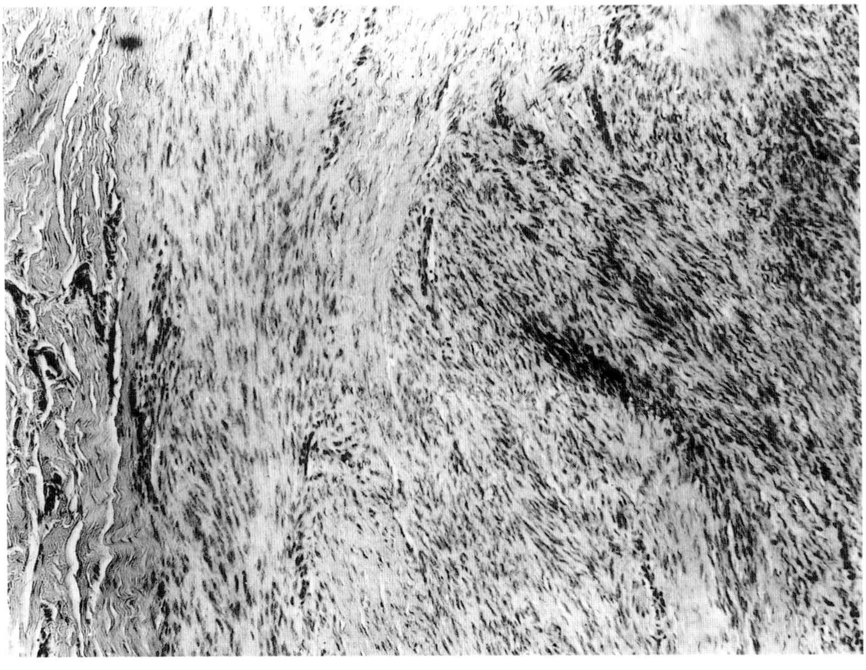

Fig. 571. Rather dense connective tissue comprises an area of conspicuously increased fibrocytes at concomitant increase of ground substance

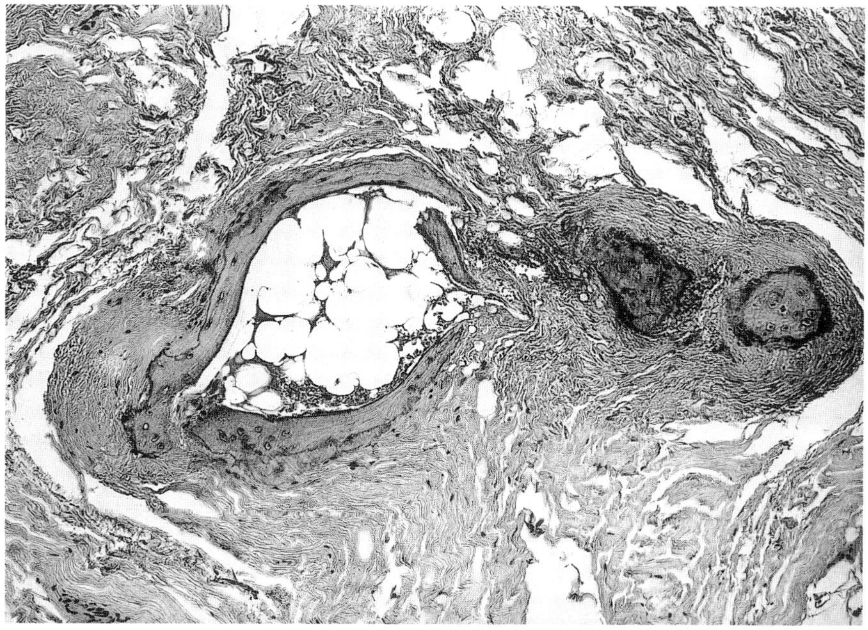

Fig. 572. Chondrification in two small areas and membranous ossification in a larger area took place in dense connective tissue

altered so that the harm they exert is mitigated, by changing the position of the body or of the participating joints or by restricting the vigor of movements by means of molded plastic splints, braces, straps, or belts. In addition, local treatment by regular application of moist hot packs and ultrasound of higher intensity (3–4 W/cm^2) proves very effective. If necessary, nonsteroidal antiinflammatory medications may be used. Where these modalities fail, two or three topical infiltrations with an anesthetic combined with hydrocortisone provide subsidence of the symptoms. In view of the fact that the fibrositis symptoms occur in some, albeit few, patients due solely to a psychological disorder involving a tension, it is understandable that medicamentous and physical therapy is not always followed by satisfactory regression of symptoms. In these situations, education and reassurance of the patients are necessary and of benefit. In cases of excessive extent of tissue densifications and/or ossifications causing mechanical interference in the function of the adjacent joint, excision of the impairing changes is the ultimate solution.

In view of its frequency, fibrositis localized at the epicondyles of the elbow – and therefore the term epicondylitis – deserves special attention. It commonly affects the lateral epicondyle (Fig. 566) at the origin of the caput commune of the extensor muscles for the wrist and fingers [636] and less often the medial epicondyle (Fig. 565) at the site of the conjoined tendons of the flexor muscles for the wrist and fingers. While generally termed "tennis elbow" because of its principal incidence among tennis players, this condition may also occur in other sports or occupational activities (typing, practice of music) in which intense strain is imposed on the elbow and wrist [319, 851]. Circumscribed tenderness at the epicondyle is associated with tenderness along the inserting muscle group. Substantial limitation in the use of these muscles often occurs and sometimes also neuralgia of the ulnar nerve or of the deep interosseal branch of the radial nerve. Roentgenographs sometimes reveal a paracondylar density or ossification in cases of longer duration.

Treatment [221] minimizes strains of the elbow by a reinforced strap applied around the elbow and proximal part of the forearm. The ailing arm is utilized with the elbow and wrist in positions which limit the strain of the involved muscle group. In addition, all the above local modalities are used. If necessary, topical infiltrations with an anesthetic and hydrocortisone should be applied. The results of hydrocortisone injection are very satisfactory and usually yield full subsidence of the symptoms. However, in 4%–10% of cases [129, 169] all local procedures fail, and surgical treatment is resorted to [1192]. The operation [166, 169] consists of exposure of the origin of the extensor muscles, sharp detachment of their tendons from the epicondyle, partial incision of the annular ligament, removal of the tip of the lateral epicondyle, excision of a fold of the joint capsule, and reattachment of the common head of the extensors. Gardner [575] totally excises the lateral epicondyle, whereas Bornhang [129] only curettes it thoroughly. The outcomes of these procedures were satisfactory according to the follow-up reports [129, 166, 169, 575, 1362].

Bibliography

1. Abbott DF, Gresham GA (1972) Arthropathy in transfusional siderosis. Br Med J 1: 418
2. Abernathy PJ, Townsend DR, Rose RN et al. (1976) Is chon dromalacia patellae a separate clinical entity. J Bone Joint Surg [Br] 60: 205
3. Abramson S, Korchak A, Ludwig R et al. (1985) Modes of action of aspirin-like drugs. Proc Nat Acad Sci USA 82: 7227
4. Ackermann R, Runne N, Klenk W et al. (1980) Erythema chronicum migrans mit Arthritis. Dtsch Med Wochenschr 105: 1779
5. Adams P, Muir H (1976) Qualitative changes with age of proteoglycans of lumbar discs. Ann Rheum Dis 35: 289
6. Adamson TC, Resnik CS, Guerra J et al. (1983) Hand and wrist arthropathies in hemochromatosis and calcium pyrophosphate deposition disease. Radiology 147: 377
7. Adlersberg AD, Parets D (1949) Genetic studies of 201 persons with hereditary hypercholesterolemia. J Clin Invest 28: 767
8. Afzelius A (1921) Erythema chronicum migrans. Acta Derm Venereol (Stockh) 2: 126
9. Agarwala BN, Peters JR, Levy HB (1981) Meningococcal septic arthritis in an infant. NY State J Med 81: 1512
9b. Agus B (1979) Hyperuricemia – when to start therapy. Curr Prescribing 5: 55
9c. Agus B, Nelson J, Kramer N et al. (1990) Acute central nervous system symptoms caused by ibuprofen in connective tissue disease. J Rheumatol 17: 1094
10. Ahuja SC, Bullough PG (1978) Osteonecrosis of the knee: a clinico-pathological study. J Bone Joint Surg [Am] 60: 191
11. Aichroth PM (1971) Osteochondritis dissecans of the knee: a clinical survey. J Bone Joint Surg [Br] 53: 440
12. Aidem HP (1968) Intraarticular amphotericin B in the treatment of coccidioidal synovitis of the knee. J Bone Joint Surg [Am] 50: 1663
13. Aitken AP (1941) Roentgenographic recognition of synovioma. J Bone Joint Surg 23: 950
14. Alarcon-Segovia D (1976) Symptomatic Sjoegren's syndrome in mixed connective tissue. J Rheumatol 3: 181
15. Alarcon-Segovia D (1983) Antibodies to nuclear and other intracellular antigens in the connective tissue disease. Clin Rheum Dis 9: 161
16. Alarcon-Segovia D, Ward LE (1965) Charcot-like arthropathy in rheumatoid. Consequence of overuse of a joint repeatedly injected with hydrocortisone. JAMA 193: 1052
17. Alarcon-Segovia D, Trujeque M, Tovar E et al. (1967) Scintillation scanning of joints with technetium 99m. Arthritis Rheum 10: 262
18. Alarcon GS, Koopman WJ, Acton RT et al. (1982) Seronegative rheumatoid arthritis. Arthritis Rheum 25: 502
19. Albee FH (1928) Original features in arthroplasty of the knee with improved prognosis. Surg Gynecol Obstet 47: 312
20. Albert J, Bruce W, Allen AC et al. (1960) Lipoid dermatoarthritis. Reticulohistiocytoma of the skin and joint. Am J Med 28: 661
21. Albertini VA (1929) Sehnenverknöcherung. In: Henke F, Lubarsch R (eds) Handbuch der pathologischen Anatomie. Springer, Berlin
22. Albertini VA (1934) Spezielle Pathologie der Sehnen, Sehnenscheiden und Schleimbeutel. In: Henke F, Lubarsch O (eds) Handbuch der speziellen pathologischen Anatomie und Histologie, vol 9/2. Springer, Berlin
23. Ali SY (1964) The degradation of cartilage matrix by an intracellular process. Biochem J 93: 611
24. Ali SY, Griffiths S (1981) New types of calcium phosphate crystals in arthritic cartilage. Semin Arthritis Rheum 11: 124
25. Alpert E, Iselbucher KJ, Schur PH (1971) The pathogenesis of arthritis associated with viral hepatitis. N Engl J Med 285: 185
26. Alspaugh MA, Fan EM (1976) Serum antibody in rheumatoid arthritis reactive with a cell associated antigen. Demonstrations by precipitation and immunofluorescence. Arthritis Rheum 19: 711
27. Alspaugh MA, Talal N, Tan EM (1976) Differentiation and characterization of autoantibodies and their antigens in Sjoegren's syndrome. Arthritis Rheum 19: 216
28. Alspaugh MA, Miller JJ (1977) A study of specificities of antinuclear antibodies in juvenile rheumatoid arthritis. J Pediatr 90: 391
29. Alspaugh MA, Henle G, Lennette ET et al. (1981) Elevated levels of antibodies to Epstein-Barr virus in sera and synovial fluid of patients with rheumatoid arthritis. J Clin Invest 67: 1134
30. Altman RD (1984) Osteoarthritis. Pathogenesis, differential diagnosis and treatment. Orthop Rev 13: 256
31. Altman RD, Rita JC, Howell DS (1973) Degradation of proteoglycans in human osteoarthritic cartilage. Arthritis Rheum 16: 179
32. Altman RD, Gray R (1985) Inflammation in osteoarthritis. Clin Rheum Dis 11: 353
33. Amor B, Coste F, Delbarre F (1965) Sur l'origine virale possible du syndrome oculo-urethro-synovial. Presse Med 73: 1825
34. Amouroux J (1971) La synovite villonodulaire hemopigmentee. Rheumatologie (Aix-le-Bains) 23: 81
35. Amouroux J (1971) Les tumeurs de la synoviale. Cah Med 12: 265
36. Amouroux J, Kemeny F (1977) Les arthropathies amyloides. Arch Anat Cytol Pathol 25: 439
37. Amouroux J, Arlet J, Durroux R (1981) Anatomie pathologique des osteoarthrites infectieuses. Rev Rhum Mal Osteoartic 48: 33
38. Amstutz HC (1973) Trapezoidal 28 total hip replacement. Clin Orthop 95: 158
39. Amstutz HC, Carey EJ (1966) Skeletal manifestations and treatment of Gaucher's disease; review of twenty cases. J Bone Joint Surg [Am] 48: 670
40. Amstutz HC, Graff-Radford A, Mai LZ et al. (1981) Surface replacement of the hip with the Tharies system. J Bone Joint Surg [Am] 63: 1069

41. Anadere I, Chmiel H, Laschner W (1979) Viscoelasticity of normal and pathological synovia. Biorheology 16: 179
42. Anderson HC (1983) Calcific diseases – a concept. Arch Pathol Lab Med 107: 341
43. Andrew R, Baldassare A, Weiss TD et al. (1981) Immunoprotein disposition in synovial tissue in Reiter's syndrome. Ann Rheum Dis 40: 281
44. Andrews CH (1950) Adventures among viruses; epidemic influenza. N Engl J Med 242: 161
45. Andriopoulos NA, Mestecky J, Miller EJ et al. (1976) Antibodies to native and degenerated collagens in sera of patients with rheumatoid arthritis. Arthritis Rheum 19: 613
46. Ansell BM (1977) Juvenile rheumatoid arthritis. Series 3. Arthritis Rheum 20: 176
47. Ansell BM (1981) Rehabilitation in juvenile chronic arthritis. Clin Rheum Dis 7: 469
48. Arcangelli P, Toccafondi R (1970) Les osteopathies du diabete. Etude clinique et pathologique. Rev Rhum Mal Osteoartic 37: 147
49. Argen RJ, St John Dixon A (1963) Clutton's joints with keratitis and periostitis. Arthritis Rheum 6: 341
50. Arkin AM, Schein A (1948) Aseptic necrosis in Gaucher's disease. J Bone Joint Surg [Am] 30: 65
51. Arnold W (1947) Epithelkörperchentumor mit allgemeiner Calcinose. Arch Pathol Anat 306: 427
52. Arnold WD, Hilgartner HL (1977) Hemophilic arthropathy, current concepts of pathogenesis and management. J Bone Joint Surg [Am] 59: 287
53. Aschoff L (1904) Zur Myocarditisfrage. Verh Dtsch Pathol Ges 8: 46
54. Atkins CJ, McIvor J, Smith PM et al. (1970) Chondrocalcinosis and arthropathy; studies in hemochromatosis and in idiopathic chondrocalcinosis. Q J Med 39: 71
55. Augustine RW (1956) The unstable knee. Am J Surg 92: 380
56. Axhausen G (1923) Die Arthritis deformans, ihre Abarten und Behandlung. Arch Klin Chir 126: 573
57. Axhausen G (1925) Zur Histologie und Pathogenese der Gelenkmausbildung im Kniegelenk. Beitr Klin Chir 133: 89

58. Babior BM (1978) Oxygen-dependent microbial killing by phagocytes. N Engl J Med 298: 659
59. Bach JF, Jacob L (1984) Prospects of the immunological treatment of rheumatoid arthritis. Clin Rheum Dis 10: 219
60. Bach TF (1940) Focal infection and arthritis. Med Clin North Am 24: 1673
61. Badalamente MA, Dee R, Propper M (1980) Ultrastructural study of joint innervation. Orthop Rev 13: 212
62. Bailey HL, Sister MG, Hodgson AR et al. (1972) Tuberculosis of the spine in children. Operative findings and results in one hundred consecutive patients. J Bone Joint Surg [Am] 54: 1633
63. Baker WM (1877) On the formation of synovial cysts in the leg in connection with disease of the knee joint. St. Bartholomews Hosp Rep 13: 245
64. Baldassare AR, Weiss TD, Tsai CC et al. (1981) Immunoprotein deposition in synovial tissue in Reiter's syndrome. Ann Rheum Dis 40: 281
65. Ballard A, Burkhalter WE, Mayfield GW et al. (1975) The functional treatment of pyogenic arthritis of the adult knee. J Bone Joint Surg [Am] 57: 1119
66. Ballmer PM, Jakob RP (1988) The non-operative treatment of isolated complete tears of the medial collateral ligament of the knee. Arch Orthop Trauma Surg 107: 273
67. Bankhurst AD (1983) The fibrositis syndrome: a common cause of soft tissue pain. In: Mediguide to inflammatory disease, vol 2. (p 8) Pfizer, New York
68. Banks BM, Korelitz BJ, Zetzel L (1957) The course of nonspecific colitis. Gastroenterology 32: 983
69. Barbour AG (1985) Lyme disease. Clin Microbiol Newslett 7: 39
70. Bargen JA (1929) Complications and sequelae of chronic ulcerative colitis. Ann Intern Med 5: 335
71. Barland P, Novikoff AB, Hammerman D (1962) Electron microscopy of the human synovial membrane. J Cell Biol 14: 207
72. Barland P, Novikoff AB, Hammerman D (1964) Fine structure and cytochemistry of the rheumatoid synovial membrane with special references to lysosomes. Am J Pathol 44: 853
73. Barmada R, Abraham A, Ray RD (1976) Hip fusion utilizing the cobra head plate. J Bone Joint Surg [Am] 58: 541
74. Barnert AL, Jerry EE, Persellin RH (1975) Acute rheumatic fever in adults. JAMA 232: 925
75. Barnett CH (1958) Measurement and interpretation of synovial fluid viscosities. Ann Rheum Dis 17: 229
76. Barrett AJ (1981) Which proteases degrade cartilage matrix. Semin Arthritis Rheum 11: 52
77. Barrow MV, Sunderman FW, Hachett RL et al. (1967) Identification of tissue lipids in lipoid dermatoarthritis (multicentric reticulohistiocytosis). Am J Clin Pathol 47: 312
78. Barrow MV, Holubar K (1969) Multicentric reticulohistiocytosis, a review of 33 patients. Medicine (Baltimore) 48: 287
79. Barry DW (1984) Influenza viruses. In: Joklik WK, Willot HP, Amos DB (eds) Zinsser Microbiology. Appleton and Lange, Norwalk
80. Bartfeld H (1967) Distribution of rheumatoid factor in nonrheumatoid states. Ann NY Acad Sci 168: 30
81. Bartfeld H (1975) Cell mediated immunity; its modulation by x-rays. Effect of X-irradiation on T-lymphocyte numbers and function. Ann NY Acad Sci 256: 342
82. Barth A (1919) Über die Entstehung der freien Gelenkkörper. Arch Klin Chir 112: 369
83. Bartholomew LE (1965) Isolation and characterization of mycoplasmas (PPLO) from patients with rheumatoid arthritis, systemic lupus erythematosus, and Reiter's syndrome. Arthritis Rheum 8: 376
84. Bassett A, LeBrigand H (1942) Lipome arborescente du genou. Mem Acad Chir 68: 210
85. Bassett ML, Halloday JW, Powell LW (1982) Ferritin synthesis in peripheral blood monocytes in idiopathic hemochromatosis. J Lab Clin Med 100: 137
86. Bateman JE (1974) Single assembly total hip prosthesis: preliminary report. Orthop Dig 2: 15
87. Bauer J (1929) Der sogenannte Rheumatismus. Steinkopf, Dresden
88. Baum C, Kennedy DL, Forbes MB (1985) Utilization of nonsteroidal antiinflammatory drugs. Arthritis Rheum 28: 686
89. Baum J (1977) Epidemiology of juvenile rheumatoid arthritis (JRA). Arthritis Rheum 20: 158
90. Baum J, Hurd B, Lewis H et al. (1973) Treatment of psoriatic arthritis with mercaptopurine. Arthritis Rheum 16: 139
91. Baum J, Ziff M (1989) Laboratory findings in rheumatoid arthritis. In: McCarty DJ (ed) Arthritis and allied conditions. Lea and Febiger, Philadelphia
92. Bayer AS, Yashikawa TT, Galpin JE et al. (1976) Unusual syndromes of coccidioidomycosis. Diagnostic and therapeutic considerations. Medicine (Baltimore) 55: 131
93. Bayer AS, Chaw AW, Louie JS et al. (1977) Gram-negative bacillary septic arthritis: clinical, radiographic, therapeutic and prognostic features. Semin Arthritis Rheum 7: 123
94. Bayer AS, Guze LB (1979) Fungal arthritis: II. Coccidioidal synovitis. Clinical, diagnostic, therapeutic and prognostic considerations. Semin Arthritis Rheum 9: 200
95. Bayer AS, Scott VJ, Guze LB (1979) Fungal arthritis: IV. Blastomycotic arthritis. Semin Arthritis Rheum 9: 145
96. Bayer AS, Choi C, Tillman DB et al. (1980) Fungal arthritis: V. Cryptococcal and histoplasmal arthritis. Semin Arthritis Rheum 9: 218

97. Bayliss MT, Ali SY (1978) Age related changes in the composition and structure of human articular cartilage proteoglycans. Biochem J 176: 683
98. Beals RK (1978) The snapping knee of infancy. J Bone Joint Surg [Am] 60: 679
99. Bechterew von W (1893) Steifigkeit der Wirbelsäule und ihre Verkrümmung als besondere Erkrankungsform. Neurol Centralbl 12: 426
100. Beckenbaugh RD, Tressler HA, Johnson EB (1977) Results after hemiarthroplasty of the hip using a cemented femoral prosthesis. Mayo Clin Proc 52: 349
101. Beckenbaugh RD, Ilstrup DM (1978) Total hip arthroplasty. J Bone Joint Surg [Am] 60: 306
102. Becker MH, Geniesser MB (1986) Congenital disorders with impaired pain sensation. In: Taveras TM, Ferrucci JT (eds) Radiology: diagnosis, imaging, intervention. Lippincott, Philadelphia
103. Becker WS, Obermayer BME (1947) Modern dermatology and syphililogy. Lippincott, Philadelphia
104. Bedendo A, Glorioso S, Venturi Pasini C et al. (1984) A family study of ankylosing spondylitis. Rheumatol Int 5: 29
105. Behrens F, Shepard N, Mitchell N (1975) Alteration of rabbit articular cartilage by intraarticular injection of corticosteroids. J Bone Joint Surg [Am] 57: 70
106. Behrman RE, Vaughan VC, Nelson WE (1983) Nelson textbook of pediatrics. Saunders Philadelphia
107. Beitzke H (1934) Syphilis der Gelenke. In: Henke H, Lubarsch O (eds) Handbuch der pathologischen Anatomie, vol 9. Springer, Berlin
108. Belaich S (1980) Multicentric reticulohistiocytosis. G Ital Dermatol Venerol 110: 77
109. Bell C, Talal N, Schur PH (1975) Antibodies to DNA in patients with rheumatoid arthritis and juvenile rheumatoid arthritis. Arthritis Rheum 18: 535
110. Belsole RJ (1981) DeQuervain's tenosynovitis: diagnostic and operative complications. Orthopedics 4: 899
111. Benassi E (1952) Spondiliti e sacro-ileiti brucellosi. Chir Organi Mov 37: 165
112. Benassi E (1956) Lesioni ossee ed articolare da infezioni tifo- paratifiche. Chir Organi Mov 41: 206
113. Benjamin JD, Ludwig JJ, Andersen CE (1969) Glucosamine and galactosamine distribution in human articular cartilage; relationship to age and degenerative joint disease. Clin Biochem 2: 461
114. Bennett G (1922) Lengthening of the quadriceps tendon. J Bone Joint Surg 4: 279
115. Bennett JC (1989) The etiology of rheumatoid arthritis. In: Kelley WN, Harris ED, Ruddy S, Sledge CB (eds) Textbook of rheumatology. Saunders, Philadelphia
116. Bennett RM, Ginsberg MH, Thomsen S (1976) Carcinomatous polyarthritis: the presenting symptom of an ovarian tumor and association with a platelet activating factor. Arthritis Rheum 19: 953
117. Bennett RM (1989) Psoriatic arthritis. In: McCarty DJ (ed) Arthritis and allied conditions. Lea and Febiger, Philadelphia
118. Benninghoff A (1925) Form und Bau der Gelenkknorpel in ihren Beziehungen zur Funktion. Z Anat 76: 43
119. Bentley G (1978) The surgical treatment of chondromalacia patellae. J Bone Joint Surg [Br] 60: 74
120. Bentley G (1985) Articular cartilage changes in chondromalacia patellae. J Bone Joint Surg [Br] 67: 769
121. Bentley G, Goodfellow JW (1969) Disorganization of the knees following intraarticular hydrocortisone injection. J Bone Joint Surg [Br] 51: 489
122. Berg E, Wainwright R, Barton B et al. (1977) On the nature of rheumatoid rice bodies; an immunological, histochemical and electron microscopic study. Arthritis Rheum 20: 1343
123. Berger BW, Clemmenson OJ, Ackerman AB (1983) Lyme disease is a spirochetosis. Am J Dermatopathol 5: 111
124. Berger H (1931) Intermittent hydroarthrosis with allergic basis. JAMA 112: 83
125. Berger L (1965) Synovial sarcomata in serous bursae and tendon sheaths. Am J Cancer 34: 501
126. Berger M, Gaither TA, Frank MM (1981) Complement receptors. Clin Immunol Rev 1: 471
127. Bernbeck R (1950) Intertrochantere Drehosteotomy zur Korrektur der Antetorsion and Coxa valga. Zentralbl Chir 75: 1559
128. Berney S, Goldstein M, Bishko F (1972) Clinical and diagnostic features of tuberculosis arthritis. Am J Med 53: 36
129. Bernhang AM (1979) The many causes of tennis elbow. NY State J Med 79: 1363
130. Bernstein HN (1982) Ophthalomologic considerations and testing in patients receiving long-term antimalarial therapy. Am J Med 75 (Symp IA): 25
131. Besredka A (1920) Anaphylaxis and antianaphylaxis and their experimental foundations. Mosby, St Louis
132. Bickel WH, Kimbrough RF, Dahlin D (1953) Tuberculous tenosynovitis. JAMA 151: 31
133. Bierbaum BE (1982) Acetabular revision arthroplasty. In: Turner RH, Scheller AD (eds) Revision total hip arthroplasty. Grune and Stratton, New York
134. Binette JR, Schmid K (1965) The proteins of synovial fluid: a study of the globulin ratio. Arthritis Rheum 8: 14
135. Bisno AL, Ofek I (1976) Serologic diagnosis of streptococcal infection. Comparison of a rapid hemaglutination technique with conventional antibody tests. Am J Dis Child 127: 676
136. Bittar ES, Petty W (1982) Girdlestone arthroplasty for infected total hip arthroplasty. Clin Orthop 170: 83
137. Bjelle A (1972) Morphological study of articular cartilage in pyrophosphate arthropathy. Ann Rheum Dis 31: 449
138. Bjelle A, Sunden G (1974) Pyrophosphate arthropathy; a clinical study of fifty cases. J Bone Joint Surg [Br] 56: 246
139. Bland JH,, Frymoyer JW (1970) Rheumatic syndromes of myxedema. N Engl J Med 282: 171
140. Bland JH, Frymoyer JW, Newberg AH et al (1979) Rheumatic syndromes in endocrine disease. Semin Arthritis Rheum 9: 23
141. Blau S (1979) Rheumatoid variants. Orthop Rev 8: 49
142. Blenke A (1933) Arthritis deformans and neuropathische Arthropathie. Z Orthop 59: 209
143. Bliznak J, Ramsey J (1976) Emphysematous septic arthritis due to Escherichia coli. J Bone Joint Surg [Am] 58: 138
144. Bloch KJ, Buchanan WW, Wohl MJ, et al. (1965) Sjoegren's syndrome. A clinical, pathological and serological study of 62 cases. Medicine (Baltimore) 44: 187
145. Blount WP (1964) Osteotomy in the treatment of osteoarthritis of the hip. J Bone Joint Surg [Am] 46: 1297
146. Bluestone R (1985) Ankylosing spondylitis. In: McCarty DJ (ed) Arthritis and allied conditions. Lea and Febiger, Philadelphia
147. Bluestone R, Bywaters EGL, Hartog M et al. (1971) Acromegalic arthropathy. Ann Rheum Dis 30: 243
148. Boardman PL, Hart FA (1967) Clinical measurement of the antiinflammatory effect of salicylates in rheumatoid arthritis. Br Med J 4: 264
149. Boddicker JH, Fong D, Walsh TE et al. (1980) Bone and gallium scanning in the evaluation of disseminated coccidioidomycosis. Am Rev Respir Dis 122: 279
150. Boehmig R (1928) Über die metaplastischen Veränderungen am Rippenknorpel. Beitr Pathol Anat 81: 172
151. Boehmig R (1954) Zur Pathogenese der unspezifischen und rheumatischen Schleimbeutelentzündungen. Zentrabl All Pathol 91: 252
152. Boggs DR, Sufferman SA, Wintrobe MM et al. (1966)

Factors influencing the duration of survival of patients with chronic lymphocytic leukemia. Am J Med 40: 243
153. Bollet AJ (1956) The intrinsic viscosity of synovial fluid hyaluronic acid. J Lab Clin Med 48: 721
154. Bollet AJ (1967) Connective tissue polysaccharide metabolism and the pathogenesis of osteoarthritis. Adv Intern Med 13: 33
155. Bollet AJ (1969) An essay on the biology of osteoarthritis. Arthritis Rheum 12: 152
156. Bollet AJ, Turner RA (1958) Psoriatic arthritis. Ann NY Acad Sci 73: 1013
157. Bollet AJ, Nance LJ (1966) Biochemical findings in normal and osteoarthritis articular cartilage: II. Chondroitin sulfate in concentration and chain length, water and ash content. J Clin Invest 45: 1172
158. Bombardieri S, Cattani P, Ciabattoni G et al. (1981) The synovial prostaglandin system in chronic inflammatory arthritis: differential effect of steroidal and nonsteroidal antiinflammatory drugs. Br J Pharmacol 73: 893
159. Bombelli R, Santore RF, Ross R (1984) Mechanics of the normal and osteoarthritic hip. Clin Orthop 182: 69
160. Bonacorsi A (1938) Le neoformazione benigne del ginocchio in raporto al trauma. Policlin Chir 45: 105
161. Boquien Y, Herrouet D, Hilleriteau F (1949) Resultat du traitement par la chloromycetin de soixante fievres typhoides. Bull Soc Med Paris 32: 1396
162. Bordet J (1904) Les propriétés des antisensibilitrices et les theories de l'immunité. Ann Inst Pasteur 18: 593
163. Bordet J, Gengou P (1903) Les sensibilitrices du bacille tuberculeux. C R Acad Sci Paris 87: 351
164. Bordin GM (1976) Natural green birefringence of amyloid. Am J Clin Pathol 65: 417
165. Borenstein DG, Gibbs CA, Jacobs RP (1982) Gas liquid chromatographic analysis of synovial fluid. Arthritis Rheum 25: 947
166. Bosworth DM (1965) Surgical treatment of tennis elbow. A follow up study. J Bone Joint Surg [Am] 47: 1533
167. Bouillaud J (1870) Traité clinique du rhumatisme articulaire et la loi de coincidence des inflammations du coeur. Bailliere, Paris
168. Bourdillon C (1888) Psoriasis et arthropathies. Thesis, Faculty of medicine, Paris
169. Boyd HB, McLeod AC (1973) Tennis elbow. J Bone Joint Surg [Am] 55: 1183
170. Bozzolan F, Cozzi F, Lazzarin P, Todesco S (1988) Il trattamento termale della coxartrosi nel bacino euganeo. Apparato Locom 2: 17
171. Brackertz D, Mitchell GF, Mackay IR (1977) Antigen-induced arthritis in mice. Arthritis Rheum 20: 841
172. Brady RO (1978) Glycosyl ceramide lipidosis: Gaucher's disease. In: Steinberg JB, Wyngaarden JB, Fredrickson WS (eds) The metabolic basis of inherited disease. McGraw Hill, New York
173. Branciforti S, Franz A (1952) Contributo allo studio radiologico delle artriti tifiche e paratifiche. Chir Organi Mov 37: 194
174. Brandt KD (1985) Osteoarthritis; clinical patterns and pathology. In: Kelley WN, Harris ED, Ruddy S, Sledge CB (eds) Textbook of rheumatology. Saunders, Philadelphia
175. Brandt KD (1989) Treatment of osteoarthritis. In: McCarty DJ (ed) Arthritis and allied conditions. Lea and Febiger, Philadelphia
176. Brandt KD, Cathcart ES, Cohen AS (1968) Studies of immune deposits in synovial membrane and corresponding synovial fluid. J Lab Clin Med 72: 631
177. Brandt KD, Cathcart ES, Cohen AS (1974) Gonococcal arthritis: clinical features correlated with blood, synovial fluid and genitourinary cultures. Arthritis Rheum 17: 502
178. Brandt KD, Palmoski M (1976) Organization of ground substance proteoglycans in normal and osteoarthritic knee cartilage. Arthritis Rheum 19: 209
179. Brauman A, Gilboa Y (1987) Recurrent pulmonary atelectasis a manifestation of familial Mediterranean fever. Arch Intern Med 147: 378
180. Braun DG, Holm SE (1970) Streptococcal anti-group A precipitins in sera from patients with rheumatic arthritis and acute glomerulonephritis. Int Arch Allergy Appl Immunol 37: 216
181. Braunstein EM, Martel W, Martel R (1982) Ankylosing spondylitis in men and women: a clinical and radiographic comparison. Radiology 144: 91
182. Bregeon C, Renier IC, Bontoux L (1981) Conduite generale du traitement des infections osteo-articulaires non-tuberculeuses en dehors de l-antibiotherapie. Rev Rhum Mal Osteoartic 48: 191
183. Brewer EJ (1977) Nonsteroidal anti-inflammatory agents. Arthritis Rheum 20: 513
184. Brewer EJ, Giannini EH, Parson DA (1982) Juvenile rheumatoid arthritis. Saunders, Philadelphia
185. Brewer EJ, Giannini EH, Barkley E (1986) Gold therapy in the management of juvenile rheumatoid arthritis. Arthritis Rheum 23: 404
186. Brewerton DA (1976) HLA-B27 and the inheritance of susceptibility to rheumatic disease. Arthritis Rheum 19: 656
187. Brewerton DA, Caffrey M, Hart FD et al. (1973) Ankylosing spondylitis and HLA-27. Lancet 1: 904
188. Brewerton DA, Caffrey M, Nicholls A et al. (1973) Reiter's disease and HLA-27. Lancet 2: 996
189. Brewerton DA, James DCO (1975) The histocompatibility antigen (HLA-27) and disease. Semin Arthritis Rheum 4: 191
190. Briggs J, Elings VB, Nicoli DF (1981) Homogeneous fluorescent immunoassay. Science 212: 1266
191. Brinkhous KM (1939) A study of the clotting defect in hemophilia; the delayed formation of thrombin. Am J Med Sci 198: 509
192. Broberg K (1983) On the mechanical behavior of the intervertebral disc. Spine 8: 151
193. Broderick PA, Corvese N, Pierik NG et al. (1976) Exfoliative cytology of synovial fluid of joint disease. J Bone Joint Surg [Am] 58: 396
194. Brodersen MP, Fitzgerald RH, Petersen LFA et al. (1979) Arthrodesis of the knee following failed total knee arthroplasty. J Bone Joint Surg [Am] 61: 181
195. Brook I, Reza MJ, Brickner KS et al. (1980) Abnormalities of synovial fluid of normal joints. Ann Rheum Dis 39: 168
196. Brooks BN (1954) Ulcerative colitis and its treatment. Livingstone, Edinburgh
197. Brower AC, Allman RM (1981) Pathogenesis of the neuropathic joint; neurotraumatic vs neurovascular. Radiology 139: 349
198. Brown IW, Ring PA (1985) Osteolytic changes in the upper femoral shaft following porous coated hip replacement. J Bone Joint Surg [Br] 67: 218
199. Brown MJ, Asburg AK (1984) Diabetic neuropathy. Ann Neurol 15: 2
200. Brown WE, Gregory TM (1976) Calcium pyrophosphate crystal chemistry. Arthritis Rheum 19: 446
201. Brumbaugh HL (1932) Tendinitis ossificans traumatica. J Bone Joint Surg 14: 953
202. Buchanan TM (1974) Brucellosis in the United States 1960–1972. Medicine (Baltimore) 53: 403
203. Buchholz HW, Gartmann HD (1972) Infektionsprophylaxe und operative Behandlung der schleichenden tiefen Infektion bei der totalen Endoprosthese. Chirurg 43: 466
204. Buck P, Nickelson MR, Bonfiglio M (1981) Synovial sarcoma, a review of 33 cases. Clin Orthop 156: 211
205. Buckingham RB (1977) Interactions involving antirheumatic agents. Bull Rheum Dis 28: 960

206. Buckingham RB, Rodnan PG (1985) Arthritis associated with hematologic disorders, storage disease, disorders of lipid metabolism, and dysproteinemias. In: McCarty DJ (ed) Arthritis and allied conditions. Lea and Febiger, Philadelphia

207. Buckingham RB, Rodnan PG (1985) Hemophilic arthritis. In: McCarty DJ (ed) Arthritis and allied conditions. Lea and Febiger, Philadelphia

208. Bucknall RC, Dixon AStJ, Glick EN (1975) Myasthenia gravis associated with penicillamine treatment for rheumatoid arthritis. Br Med J 1: 600

209. Buecheler E, Klammer HL (1974) Ossaere haemophile Pseudotumoren. Fortschr Roentgenstrahlther 120: 468

210. Buedinger R (1908) Über traumatische Knorpelnekrose im Kniegelenk. Dtsch Z Chir 92: 510

211. Bunch TW, Hunder GG (1973) Ankylosing spondylitis and primary hyperparathyroidism. JAMA 225: 1108

212. Bunch TW, Hunder GG, McDuffie FC et al. (1974) Synovial fluid complement determination as a diagnostic aid in inflammatory joint disease. Proc Mayo Clin 49: 715

213. Bunim JJ, Buchanan WW, Wertlake PT et al. (1964) Clinical pathologic and serologic studies in Sjoegren's syndrome. Ann Intern Med 61: 509

214. Burckhardt H (1929) Über Entstehung der freien Gelenkkörper. Beitr Klin Chir 130: 163

215. Burgan DW (1971) Lipoma arborescens of the knee. Another cause of filling defects on a knee arthrogram. Radiology 101: 583

216. Burgdorfer W, Barbour AG, Hayes SF et al. (1982) Lyme disease – a tick borne spirochetosis. Science 216: 1317

217. Busey JF (1972) Blastomycosis: III. A comparative study of 2-OH stilbamidine and amphotericin B therapy. Am Rev Respir Dis 105: 812

218. Butler MJ, Russel AS, Percy JS et al. (1979) A follow-up study of 48 patients with Reiter's syndrome. Am J Med 67: 808

219. Byeff PN, Suskiewicz L (1976) Meningococcal arthritis. JAMA 235: 2752

220. Byers PD, Cotten RE, Deacon AE et al. (1968) The diagnosis and treatment of pigmented villonodular synovitis. J Bone Joint Surg [Br] 50: 290

221. Cabot A (1987) Tennis elbow, a curable affliction. Orthop Rev 16: 322

222. Cadman NL, Soule EH, Kelly DJ (1965) Synovial sarcoma: an analysis of 134 tumors. Cancer 18: 613

223. Calabro JJ (1989) Juvenile rheumatoid arthritis. In: McCarty DJ (ed) Arthritis and allied conditions. Lea and Febiger, Philadelphia

224. Calabro JJ, Mody R (1966) Management of ankylosing spondylitis. Bull Rheum Dis 16: 408

225. Calabro JJ, Parrino GR, Atchoo PL et al. (1970) Chronic iridocyclitis in juvenile rheumatoid arthritis. Arthritis Rheum 13: 406

226. Calandriello B (1955) La sinovectomia nell idrartro cronico recidivante di ginocchio. Arch Putti Chir Organi Mov 6: 257

227. Calandruccio RA (1987) Arthroplasty of the hip. In: Crenshaw AM (ed) Campbell's operative orthopaedics. Mosby, St Louis

228. Calder MA, McHardy VU, Schonell ME (1970) Importance of pneumococcal typing in pneumonia. Lancet 1: 5

229. Calderon E (1938) Zur Kenntnis der als Lipoma arborescens bezeichneten Kapselveränderungen. Beitr Klin Chir 168: 364

230. Calin A (1980) HLA-B27: to type or not to type. Ann Intern Med 92: 208

231. Calin A (1989) Reiter's syndrome. In: Kelley WN, Harris ED, Ruddy S, Sledge CB (eds) Textbook of rheumatology. Saunders, Philadelphia

232. Calin A (1989) Ankylosing spondylitis. In: Kelley WN, Harris ED, Ruddy S, Sledge CB (eds) Textbook of rheumatology. Saunders, Philadelphia

233. Calin A, Fried JF (1975) The striking prevalence of ankylosing spondylitis in healthy W27 positive males and females. A control study. N Engl J Med 293: 835

234. Campbell WC (1921) Arthroplasty of the knee. J Orthop Surg 3: 430

235. Campbell WL, Feldman F (1975) Bone and soft tissue abnormalities in diabetes mellitus. Am J Roentgenol 124: 7

236. Campesi G, Patania S (1964) Evoluzione istologica e modificazione istochemiche in corso di sinoviti acute e croniche di causa non bacterica. Ortop Traum 12: 241

237. Canoso JJ (1977) Idiopathic or traumatic olecranon bursitis. Clinical features and bursal fluid analyses. Arthritis Rheum 20: 1213

238. Canoso JJ, Yood RA (1979) Acute gouty bursitis: report of 15 cases. Ann Rheum Dis 38: 326

239. Capello WN, Ireland PH, Trammel TR et al. (1978) Conservative total hip arthroplasty, a procedure to conserve bone stock. Clin Orthop 134: 59

240. Capener N (1950) The approach to the hip joint. J Bone Joint Surg [Br] 32: 147

241. Capener N (1964) Lateral rhachotomy. J Bone Joint Surg [Br] 36: 173

242. Cardell BS, Gurling KS (1954) Observations on pathology of Sjoegren's syndrome. J Pathol Bacteriol 68: 137

243. Carette S, Graham D, Little H et al. (1983) The natural disease course of ankylosing spondylitis. Arthritis Rheum 26: 186

244. Caroit M, DePerignon M, Levernieux J et al. (1975) Contribution au diagnostic etiologique des spondylodiscites. Rev Rhum Mal Osteoartic 40: 153

245. Caroit M, Forette B, Hubault A et al. (1976) Double blind study of ketoprofen against a placebo in osteoarthritis of the hip. Scand J Rheumatol 16: 123

246. Caroit M, Darbon L, Villiaumey J (1980) Pelvispondylite rhumatismale. Rev Rhum Mal Osteoartic 47: 61

247. Caroit M, Alia-Lerner C, Dubost JJ et al. (1983) Metastases synoviales des cancers. Practicien 1: 359

248. Carp L. Stout AP (1928) A study of ganglion. Surg Gynecol Obstet 47: 460

249. Carr WR (1983) Acute phase proteins. Clin Rheum Dis 9: 227

250. Carrera GF (1985) Computed tomography in the evaluation of low back pain. In: McCarty DJ (ed) Arthritis and allied conditions. Lea and Febiger, Philadelphia

251. Carson DS (1989) Rheumatoid factor. In: Kelley WN, Harris ED, Ruddy S, Sledge CB (eds) Textbook of rheumatology. Saunders, Philadelphia

252. Casscells SW (1980) The place of arthroscopy in the diagnosis and treatment of internal derangement of the knee. An analysis of 1000 cases. Clin Orthop 151: 135

253. Cassidy JT (1989) Juvenile rheumatoid arthritis. In: Kelley WN, Harris ED, Ruddy S, Sledge CB (eds) Textbook of rheumatology. Saunders, Philadelphia

254. Cassidy JT, Sullivan DB, Petty RE (1977) Clinical patterns of chronic iridocyclitis in children with juvenile rheumatoid arthritis. Arthritis Rheum 20: 224

255. Castor CW (1960) The microscopic study of normal human synovial tissue. Arthritis Rheum 3: 140

256. Castor CW (1972) Connective tissue activation: IV. Regulatory effects of antirheumatic drugs. Arthritis Rheum 15: 504

257. Catanzaro A, Einstein H, Levin B et al. (1982) Ketokonazole for treatment of disseminated coccidioidomycosis. Ann Intern Med 96: 436

258. Cathcart ES, Ignaczak TF (1985) Amyloidosis. In: Kelley WN, Harris ED, Ruddy S, Sledge CB (eds) Textbook of rheumatology. Saunders, Philadelphia

259. Catterall RD (1960) Uveitis, arthritis, and non-specific genital infection. Br J Vener Dis 36: 27
260. Catto M (1976) Pathology of aseptic bone necrosis. In: Davidson T (ed) Aseptic necrosis of bone. Excerpta Medica, Amsterdam
261. Cecchi E, Bisogno EM, Rocca-Rossetti G (1958) Ein weiterer Beitrag zur Untersuchung arthrotischer Knorpel unter dem Elektronenmikroskop. Z. Rheumaforsch 17: 197
262. Cecil RL, Archer BH (1925) Arthritis of the menopause. JAMA 89: 75
263. Cecil RL, Nicholls EE, Stainsby WJ (1929) Bacteriology of blood and joints in rheumatic fever. J Exp Med 50: 617
264. Cecil RL, Nicholls EE, Stainsby WJ (1931) The etiology of rheumatoid arthritis. Am J Med Sci 181: 12
265. Cecil RL, Algevine DM (1938) Clinical and experimental observations on focal infection with analysis of 200 cases of rheumatoid arthritis. Ann Intern Med 12: 577
266. Cecere FA, Persellin RH (1984) The interaction of pregnancy and the rheumatic disease. Clin. Rheum Dis 7: 747
267. Chafetz NI, Genant HK, Moon KL et al. (1983) Recognition of lumbar disk herniation with NMR. Am J Roentgenol 141: 1153
268. Claflin K, Milbauer J, Sullivan B (1983) Ketoconazole and blastomycotic osteomyelitis. Ann Intern Med 98: 260
269. Chandler GN, Jones DT, Wright V et al. (1959) Charcot arthropathy following intraarticular hydrocortisone. Br Med J 1: 952
270. Chandler HP, Reineck FT, Wizson L et al. (1981) Total hip replacement in patients younger than thirty years old. J Bone Joint Surg [Am] 63: 1426
271. Chandler RW, Robinson H, Masi AT (1971) Serological investigation for evidence of an infectious etiology of rheumatoid arthritis. Ann Rheum Dis 30: 274
272. Chang MJ, Controni G, Rodriguez WJ (1981) Ampicillin resistant hemophilus influenzae O type B in septic arthritis in children. Clin Pediatr (Phila) 20: 139
273. Chang YH (1975) Mechanism of action of colchicine. Arthritis Rheum 18: 493
274. Chaouat Y, Faures B, Ginet C et al. (1979) Les therapeutiques du rhumatisme psoriasique. Rev Rhum Mal Osteoartic 46: 561
275. Chapman M, Murray RD, Stoker DJ (1979) Tuberculosis of bones and joints. Semin Roentgenol 14: 266
276. Charcot JM (1868) Sur quelques arthropathies qui paraissent dépendre d'une lesion du cerveau ou de la moelle épinière. Arch Physiol Norm Pathol 1: 161
277. Charmot G, Radhaim R, Perez C (1982) Un cas d'arthrite de Lyme observé en France. Nouv Presse Med 11: 207
278. Charnley J (1950) Total hip replacement by low friction arthroplasty. Clin. Orthop 72: 7
279. Charnley J (1951) Compression arthrodesis of the ankle and shoulder. J Bone Joint Surg [Br] 33: 180
280. Charnley J (1972) The long term results of low friction arthroplasty of the hip performed as a primary intervention. J Bone Joint Surg [Br] 54: 61
281. Cheadle W (1889) The various manifestations of the rheumatic state exemplified in childhood and early life. Smith, London
282. Cheung HS, Ryan L, Kozin F et al. (1980) Synovial origins of rice bodies in joint fluid. Arthritis Rheum 23: 72
283. Chiari H (1934) Die Geschwülste der Gelenke. In: Henke F, Lubarsch O (eds) Handbuch der pathologischen Anatomie und Histologie, vol 9/2. Springer, Berlin
284. Chiroff RT, Cooke CP (1975) Osteochondritis dissecans. A histologic and microradiographic analysis of surgically excised lesions. J Trauma 15: 689
285. Chisholm DM, Mason DK (1968) Labial salivary gland-biopsy in Sjoegren's disease. J Clin Pathol 21: 656
286. Chisholm TS, Osterman K, Vankka E (1981) Osteochondritis dissecans of the elbow, ankle and hip. Clin Orthop 148: 245
287. Chrisman OD (1969) Biochemical aspects of degenerative joint disease. Clin Orthop 64: 77
288. Chrisman OD, Snook GA, Wilson FC (1972) The protective effect of aspirin against degeneration of articular cartilage. Clin Orthop 84: 193
289. Christie AB (1986) Infectious diseases. Epidemiology and clinical practice. Churchill Livingstone, Edinburgh
290. Chusid MJ, Sty JR (1975) Pneumococcal arthritis and osteomyelitis in children. Clin Pediatr (Phila) 20: 105
291. Chylak LT (1977) The ocular manifestations of juvenile rheumatoid arthritis. Arthritis Rheum 20: 217
292. Clanton TO, Delee JC (1982) Osteochondritis dissecans. History, pathophysiology, and current treatment concepts. Clin Orthop 167: 50
293. Clague RB, Shaw MJ, Halt PJL (1981) Incidence and correlation between serum IgG and IgM antibodies to native type II collagen in patients with chronic inflammatory arthritis. Ann Rheum Dis 40: 6
294. Clark S, Campbell SM, Forehand ME et al. (1985) Clinical characteristics of fibrositis. Arthritis Rheum 28: 132
295. Class RN, Cascio FS (1972) Histoplasmosis presenting as acute polyarthritis. N Engl J Med 287: 1133
296. Clausen N, Goetze H, Pedersen A et al. (1983) Skeletal scintigraphy and radiography at onset of acute lymphocytic leukemia in children. Med Pediatr Oncol 11: 292
297. Claus G, McEwen C, Brummer T et al. (1964) Microbiological studies of Reiter's disease. Br J Vener Dis 40: 170
298. Clayton ML (1989) Correction of arthritic deformities of the hip. In: McCarty DJ (ed) Arthritis and allied conditions. Lea and Febiger, Philadelphia
299. Clayton ML (1989) Correction of arthritic deformities of the foot and ankle. In: McCarty DJ (ed) Arthritis and allied conditions. Lea and Febiger, Philadelphia
300. Clegg J (1977) The results of the pseudarthrosis after removal of an infected total hip. J Bone Joint Surg [Br] 59: 298
301. Clemmensen I, Holund B, Andersen RB (1983) Fibrin and fibronectin in rheumatoid synovial fluid. Arthritis Rheum 26: 479
302. Cliff JM (1971) Spinal bony bridging and carditis in Reiter's disease. Ann Rheum Dis 30: 171
303. Clouse ME (1974) Diabetic osteoarthropathy. Clinical and roentgenographic observations in 90 cases. Am J Roentgenol 121: 22
304. Cobb S, Lawrence J (1957) Towards a geography of rheumatoid arthritis. Bull Rheum Dis 7: 133
305. Coburn A, Pauli R (1935) Studies on immune response of the rheumatic subject and its relationship to activity of the rheumatic process. J Exp Med 62: 129
306. Cohen AS (1975) Normal synovial membrane and fluid. In: Cohen AS (ed) Laboratory diagnostic procedures in the rheumatic diseases. Little and Brown, Boston
307. Cohen AS (1989) Amyloidosis. In: McCarty DJ (ed) Arthritis and allied conditions. Lea and Febiger, Philadelphia
308. Cohen AS, Canoso JJ (1985) Tumors joints and related structures. In: McCarty DJ (ed) Arthritis and allied conditions. Lea and Febiger, Philadelphia
309. Cohen JA, Kaplan MM (1979) The SGOT/SGPT ratio: an indication of alcoholic liver disease. Dig Dis Sci 24: 835
310. Collert S, Gillstrom P (1979) Osteotomy in osteoarthritis of the hip: a prospective study. Acta Orthop Scand 50: 555
311. Collins WRF (1939) Bacteriology of rheumatic fever. Lancet 2: 817
312. Compere CL, Hill JA, Lewinnex GE et al. (1979) A new method of patellectomy for patellofemoral arthritis. J Bone Joint Surg [Am] 61: 714
313. Comper WD, Laurent TC (1978) Physiological function of connective tissue polysaccharides. Physiol Rev 58: 255

314. Comroe B (1942) Arthritis and allied conditions. Lea and Febiger, Philadelphia

315. Cone RO, Resnick D (1985) Radiographic evaluation of articular diseases. In: Kelley WN, Harris ED, Ruddy S, Sledge CB (eds) Textbook of rheumatology. Saunders, Philadelphia

316. Convery FR, Minteer-Convery M, Malcolm LL (1980) The spherocentric knee: a re-evaluation and modification. J Bone Joint Surg [Am] 62: 320

317. Cooke CL, Owen DS Jr, Irby R et al. (1972) Gonococcal arthritis. JAMA 217: 204

318. Cooke TD, Jasin HE (1972) The pathogenesis of chronic inflammation in experimental antigen-induced arthritis. Arthritis Rheum 15: 327

319. Coonrad RW, Hooper WR (1973) Tennis elbow. Its course, natural history, conservative and surgical treatment. J Bone Joint Surg [Am] 55: 1177

320. Coonrad RW, Bryan RS (1974) Technique of Coonrad Elbow Arthroplasty. Zimmer, Warsaw

321. Coons AH, Creech HJ, Jones RW et al. (1942) The demonstration of pneumococcal antigen in tissue by the use of fluorescence antibody. J Immunol 45: 159

322. Cooper NS, Soren A, McEwen C et al. (1981) Diagnostic specificity of synovial lesions. Hum Pathol 12: 314

323. Cooper NS, Soren A. Statistical evaluation and diagnostic correlation of histopathological changes in articular cartilage. (in preparation)

324. Cooperating Clinics Committee of the American Rheumatism Association (1970) A controlled trial of cyclophosphamide in rheumatoid arthritis. N Engl J Med 283: 883

325. Cooperating Clinics Committee of the American Rheumatism Association (1973) A controlled gold salt therapy in rheumatoid arthritis. Arthritis Rheum 16: 353

326. Coste E (1958) La polyarthrite psoriasique. Z. Rheumaforsch 17: 90

327. Cotta H (1962) Elektronenoptische Untersuchungen an der Gelenkkapsel und ihre Bedeutung für die morphologisch-funktionelle Einheit des Gelenkes. Arch Orthop Unfall Chir 54: 443

328. Cotta H (1980) Chondropathia patellae. Fragen aus der Praxis. Dtsch Med Wochenschr 105: 1142

329. Cotta H, Puhl W, Niethard FU (1978) Knorpelschaden, Ursachen und Entstehung. Dtsch Ärztebl 75: 1889

330. Cotta H, Puhl W, Niethard FU (1982) Der Einfluß des Haemarthros auf den Knorpel der Gelenke. Unfallchirurgie 8: 145

331. Cotta H, Niethard FU (1983) Rücken- und Kreuzschmerz. Entstehung und Behandlung. Radiologie 23: 151

332. Court-Brown WM, Doll R (1965) Mortality from cancer and other causes after radiotherapy for ankylosing spondylitis. Br Med J 2: 1327

333. Coventry MB, Harrison EG, Martin JF (1966) Benign synovial tumors of the knee: a diagnostic problem. J Bone Joint Surg [Am] 48: 1350

334. Coventry MB, Tinerman GA, Robly LH et al. (1972) A new geometric knee for total knee arthroplasty. Clin Orthop 83: 157

335. Coventry MB (1973) Osteotomy about the knee for degenerative and rheumatoid arthritis. Indications, operative technique and results. J Bone Joint Surg [Am] 55: 23

336. Cowling P, Ebinger R, Cawdell D (1980) C-reactive protein, ESR and Klebsiella in ankylosing spondylitis. Ann Rheum Dis 39: 45

337. Coy JT, Wolf CR, Bronner DT et al. (1976) Pyogenic arthritis of the sacroiliac joint. J Bone Joint Surg [Am] 58: 845

338. Cozzi F, Tenon R, Todesco S (1985) Die Fangotherapie in der chronischen Polyarthritis (CP). Phys Med Baln Med Klin 14: 313

339. Cozzolino A (1955) Sul morbo di Hoffa Arch Ortop 68: 961

340. Craft JE, Grodziski RL, Steere AC. (1984) The antibody response in Lyme disease. Evaluation of diagnostic test. J Infect Dis 149: 789

341. Craun GG, Riley LA (1982) Evaluation of neck and associated arm pains. Surg Pract News 2: 13

342. Crellin RQ, Macabe JJ, Hamilton FBD (1970) Severe subluxation of the cervical spine in rheumatoid arthritis. J Bone Joint Surg [Br] 52: 244

343. Crenshaw AH (1980) Surgical approaches. In: Edmonsen AS, Crenshaw AH (eds) Campbell's operative orthopaedics. Mosby, St. Louis

344. Crespi M (1961) Nuove vedute etiopatogenetiche nell' idrartro intermittente. Arch Ortop 74: 327

345. Criep LH (1946) Allergy of joints. J Bone Joint Surg 28: 276

346. Crohn BB, Yarnis H (1958) Regional ileitis. Grune and Stratton, New York

347. Cromartie WJ, Craddock JG, Schwab JH et al. (1977) Arthritis in rats after systemic injection of streptococcal cells or cell walls. J Exp Med 146: 1585

348. Cronin ME (1989) Rheumatic aspects of endocrinopathies. In: McCarty DJ (ed) Arthritis and allied conditions. Lea and Febiger, Philadelphia

349. Crosby WH (1977) Hemochromatosis. The unsolved problems. Semin Hematol 14: 135

350. Cruickshank B (1960) Pathology of ankylosing spondylitis. Bull Rheum Dis 10: 211

351. Csonka GW (1960) Recurrent attacks in Reiter's disease. Arthritis Rheum 3: 164

352. Cummings NA, Schall GL, Asofsky R et al. (1971) Sjoegren's syndrome – newer aspects of research, diagnosis and therapy. Ann Intern Med 75: 937

353. Currey HLF, Harris J, Mason RM et al. (1974) Comparison of azathioprine, cyclophosphamide and gold in treatment of rheumatoid arthritis. Br Med J 3: 763

354. Currey HLF, Vernon-Robert B (1976) Examination of synovial fluid. Clin Rheum Dis 2: 149

355. Curtiss PH Jr (1973) The pathophysiology of joint inflammation. Clin Orthop 96: 129

356. Cush R, Light RK, George DB (1976) Clinical and roentgenographic manifestations of acute and chronic blastomycosis. Chest 69: 345

357. Cushing EH, Stout AP (1926) Gaucher's disease. Arch Surg 12: 539

358. Dalinka MK, Turner ML (1980) Knee arthrography. Contemp Orthop 2: 509

359. Dalldorf FG, Cromartie WG, Anderle SK et al. (1980) The relation of experimental arthritis to the distribution of cell wall fragments. Am J Pathol 100: 383

360. D'Ambrosia RD, Neiman KMW, O'Grady L et al. (1974) Total hip replacement for patients with hemophilia and hemorrhagic diathesis. Surg Gynecol Obstet 139: 381

361. D'Ambrosia RD, Shoji H, Riggins R et al. (1978) Scintigraphy in the diagnosis of osteonecrosis. Clin Orthop 130: 139

362. Dameshek W, Gunz F (1983) Leukemia. Grune and Stratton, New York

363. Dandy DJ (1984) Arthroscopic surgery. J Bone Joint Surg [Br] 66: 627

364. Danielopoulo D (1943) Die Klassifizierung des infektiösen Rheumatismus. Z Rheumaforsch 6: 209

365. Dans P, Rothenberg R, Holmes KK (1977) Gonococcal serology. How soon, how useful, and how much. J Infect Dis 135: 330

366. Datta SC, Radin NS (1988) Normalization of liver glucosylceramide levels in the "Gaucher" mouse by phosphatidyl serine injection. Biochem Biophys Res Commun 152: 155

367. David JR, Black RL (1960) Salmonella arthritis. Medicine (Baltimore) 39: 385

368. Davis JS, Wober FC, Bartfeld H (1957) Conditions involving the hemopoietic system resulting in pseudorheumatoid arthritis. Ann Intern Med 47: 10

369. Davidson PT, Horowitz I (1970) Skeletal tuberculosis – a review with patient presentations and discussion. Am J Med 48: 77

370. Davies NEJ, Roenigh, HH, Hawk WA et al. (1968) Multicentric reticulohistiocytosis. Arch Dermatol 97: 543

371. Davies PDO, Humphries MJ, Byfield SP et al. (1984) Bone and joint tuberculosis. J Bone Joint Surg [Br] 66: 326

372. Davis D, Ritvo M (1948) Osteoarthritis of the cervicodorsal spine (radiculitis) simulating coronary artery disease. N Engl J Med 238: 857

373. Davies SF, Khan M, Sarosi GA (1978) Disseminated histoplasmosis in immunologically suppressed patients. Am J Med 64: 94

374. Davis UH, Lee SL, Sokoloff L (1978) Boundary lubricating ability of synovial fluid in degenerative joint disease. Arthritis Rheum 21: 754

375. Dawes PT, Raman D, Haslock I (1983) Olecranon bursitis related to calcium pyrophosphate dihydrate crystal deposition. Ann Rheum Dis 26: 695

376. Dawes PT, Ghosh SK (1985) Tissue typing in Brucellosis. Ann Rheum Dis 44: 526

377. Dawson MH, Boots R (1930) Subcutaneous nodules in rheumatoid arthritis. JAMA 95: 1894

378. Dawson MH, Tysen JL (1938) Observations on certain features common to psoriasis and rheumatoid arthritis. Trans Assoc Am Physicians 53: 303

379. Day RO, Graham GG, Champion GD et al. (1984) Antirheumatic drug interactions. Clin Rheum Dis 10: 251

380. Dayer E, Gerster JC, Aguado MT et al. (1983) Capacity to solubilize immune complexes in sera and synovial fluids from patients with rheumatoid arthritis. Arthritis Rheum 27: 156

381. Dayer E, Lambert PH (1985) Immune complexes. In: Kelley WN, Harris ED, Ruddy S, Sledge CB (eds) Textbook of rheumatology. Lea and Febiger, Philadelphia

382. Deacon WE, Peacock ML, Freeman E et al. (1960) Fluorescent antibody tests for detection of the gonococcus in women. Public Health Rep 75: 125

383. Deburge A (1976) Guepar hinge prosthesis complications and results with two years follow-up. Clin Orthop 120: 47

384. Decker JL, Steinberg AR (1985) Immunoregulatory drugs. In: McCarty DJ (ed) Arthritis and allied conditions. Lea and Febiger, Philadelphia

385. Decker JL, Plotz PH (1985) Extraarticular rheumatoid disease. In: McCarty DJ (ed) Arthritis and allied conditions. Lea and Febiger, Philadelphia

386. Dee R (1978) The innervations of joints. In: Sokoloff L (ed) The joints and synovial fluid. Academic, New York

387. Dee R (1982) Reconstructive surgery following total elbow endoprosthesis. Clin Orthop 170: 196

388. DeGrailly R, Leger H (1952) Les tumeurs articulaires malignes. Masson, Paris

389. DeHaven KE, Wilde AH, O'Duffy JD (1972) Sporotrichosis arthritis and tenosynovitis. J Bone Joint Surg [Am] 54: 874

390. Dekker-Saeys BJ, Meuwissen JGM, VandeBorg Loon EM et al. (1978) Clinical characteristics and results of histocompatibility typing (HLA-B27) in patients with ankylosing spondylitis and inflammatory bowel disease. Ann Rheum Dis 37: 36

391. DeLano PJ (1946) The pathogenesis of Charcot's joint. Am J Roentgenol 56: 189

392. DeLauche MC, Kahn MF, Ryckewaert A (1981) Arthritis gonococciques. Rev Rhum Mal Osteoartic 48: 127

393. Delbarre F (1969) Les manifestations intra-articulaires de l'hemochromatose. Presse Med 72: 973

394. Delbarre F, Menkes CJ, Aignan M et al. (1973) La synovioorthese par le radioisotopes. Rev Rhum Mal Osteoartic 40: 205

395. Delbarre F, Rondier J, Delrieu F et al. (1975) Pyogenic infection of the sacroiliac joint: report of thirteen cases. J Bone Joint Surg [Am] 57: 819

396. Del Monte A, Teodorana G (1955) Trattamento del ginocchio flesso poliomyelitico. Chir Organi Mov 41: 325

397. DeLutio O, Pisani G (1961) Il sinovialsarcoma. Chir Organi Mov 47: 1

398. Deodhar SD, Michener WM, Farmer RG (1969) A study of the immunologic aspects of chronic ulcerative colitis and transmural colitis. Am J Clin Pathol 51: 591

399. DePalma AF (1967) Hemophilic arthropathy. Clin Orthop 52: 145

400. DePalma AF, Flynn JJ (1958) Joint changes following experimental partial and total patellectomy. J Bone Joint Surg [Am] 49: 395

401. DePalma AF, Mauler GG (1964) Hemangioma of the synovial membrane. Clin Orthop 32: 93

402. DePalma AF, Fenlin JM (1966) Arthrodesis of the hip with intramedullary fixation. Clin Orthop 48: 19

403. DePalma AF, McKeever DC, Subin DK (1966) Process of repair of articular cartilage demonstrated by histology and autoradiography with tritiated thymidine. Clin Orthop 48: 229

404. DeQuervain M (1912) Über das Wesen und die Behandlung der stenosierenden Tendovaginitis am Processus styloideus radii. Münch Med Wochenschr 59: 5

405. Disciascio G, Taranta A (1980) Rheumatic disease in children. Am Heart J 99: 635

406. DeSeze S, Welfling J, Lequesne M (1960) L'osteonecrose primitive de la tête femorale chez l'adulte; étude de 30 cas. Rev Rhum Mal Osteoartic 27: 117

407. DeSeze S, Ryckewaert A, Hubault A et al. (1966) Les chondrocalcinoses articulaires. Semin Hosp 42: 2461

408. DeSeze S, Ryckewaert A, Kahn MF et al. (1966) Sur quelques aspects particuliers du rhumatisme psoriasique. Rev Rhum Mal Osteoartic 33: 617

409. DeSeze S, Solnica J, Mitrovic D et al. (1972) Joint and bone disorders in hyperparathyroidism in hemochromatosis. Semin Arthritis Rheum 2: 71

410. Deshayes P, Houdent C, Heckketsweiler R (1976) Les manifestations rhumatismales de la maladie de Crohn. Rev Rhum Mal Osteoartic 43: 541

411. Detenbeck LC, Young HH, Underdahl LA (1970) Ochronotic arthropathy. Arch Surg 100: 215

412. Detenbeck LC, Coventry MD, Kelly RJ (1972) Intertrochanteric osteotomy for degenerative arthritis of the hip. Clin Orthop 86: 73

413. Detenbeck LC, Tressler HA, O'Duffy JD et al. (1973) Peripheral joint manifestation of acromegaly. Clin Orthop 91: 119

414. Devas MB (1960) Chondromalacia of the patella. Clin Orthop 18: 54

415. Dewar PJ (1983) HLA antigens. Clin Rheum Dis 9: 93

416. Diamant-Berger L, Siccard A (1931) La lipoarthrite traumatique du genou. Rev Orthop 18: 5

417. Diamond HS, Lazarus R, Kaplan D et al. (1973) Effect of urine flow rate on uric acid excretion in man. Arthritis Rheum 16: 539

418. Dick WC, Deodhar SD, Provan CJ et al. (1971) Isotope studies in normal and diseased knee joints: 99 m Tc uptake related to clinical assessment and to synovial perfusion measured by the 133 Xe clearance technique. Clin Sci Mol Med 40: 327

419. Dienes L (1947) Controversial aspects of the morphology of PPLO. Ann N Y Acad Sci 79: 356

420. Dieppe PA, Doyle DV, Huskisson EC et al. (1978) Mixed crystal deposition disease in osteoarthritis. Br Med J 1: 150

421. Dieppe PA, Alexander GJM, Jones AE et al. (1982) Pyrophosphate arthropathy; a clinical and radiological study of 105 cases. Ann Rheum Dis 41: 371
422. Dieppe PA, Doherty M, McFarlane DG et al. (1984) Apatite associated destructive arthritis. Br J Rheumatol 23: 84
423. Dietzman DE, Schaller JG, Ray CG et al. (1976) Acute myositis associated with influenza B infections. Pediatrics 57: 255
424. Dillon RS (1980) Handbook of endocrinology. Lea and Febiger, Philadelphia
425. DiMaggio C, Cavallo A, Pescarini L et al. (1979) La radiologia della mano con tecnica a basso tensione. Radiol Med (Torino) 65: 571
426. Dingle JT (1978) Articular damage in arthritis and its control. Ann Intern Med 88: 821
427. Dintenfass L (1963) Lubrication in synovial joints; a theoretical analysis. J Bone Joint Surg [Am] 45: 1241
428. Dirheimer Y (1977) The cranio-vertebral region in chronic inflammatory rheumatoid diseases. Springer, Berlin Heidelberg New York
429. Dismukes WE, Stamm AM, Graybill JR et al. (1983) Treatment of systemic mycosis with ketoconazole. Emphasis of toxicity and clinical response in 52 patients. Ann Intern Med 98: 13
430. Dixon JS, Bird HA, Litton NG et al. (1984) C-reactive protein in the serial assessment of disease activity in rheumatoid arthritis. Scand J Rheum 13: 39
431. Docken WP (1979) Pigmented villonodular synovitis; a review with illustrative case reports. Semin Arthritis Rheum 9: 1
432. Dodds GS (1939) Row formation and other types of arrangement of cartilage cells in enchondral ossification. Anat Rec 46: 383
433. Dodds WJ, Steinbach HL (1968) Primary hyperparathyroidism and articular cartilage calcification. Am J Roentgenol 104: 884
434. Doehring S (1985) Über die Haemophilie und deren Skelettveränderungen. Beitr Orthop Traumatol 32: 73
435. Doehring S, Hofman P (1985) Hemophilic pseudotumors. In: Doehring S, Schulitz KP (eds) Orthopaedic problems in hemophilia. Zuckschwerdt, Munich
436. Dolan CT (1971) A practical approach to identification of yeast like microorganisms. Am J Clin Pathol 55: 580
437. Dorff GJ, Ziolkowski JS, Rytel MW (1975) Detection by counter immunoelectrophoresis of pneumococcal antigen in synovial fluid from septic arthritis. Arthritis Rheum 18: 613
438. Dorwart BB, Schumacher HR (1975) Joint effusion, chondrocalcinosis, and other rheumatic manifestations in hypothyroidism. Am J Med 59: 780
439. Dorwart BB, Gall E, Schumacher HR et al. (1978) Chrysotherapy in psoriatic arthritis. Efficacy and toxicity compared to rheumatoid. Arthritis Rheum 21: 513
440. Doughty RA, Giesecke L, Athreya B (1980) Salicylate therapy in juvenile rheumatoid arthritis. Dose, serum level, and toxicity. Am J Dis Child 134: 461
441. Doyle DV (1982) Tissue calcification and inflammation in osteoarthritis. J Pathol 136: 199
442. Doyle DV, Lanham JG (1984) Routine drug treatment of osteoarthritis. Clin Rheum Dis 10: 277
443. Drennan DB, Fahey JJ, Maylahn DJ (1971) Important factor in achieving arthrodesis of the Charcot knee. J Bone Joint Surg [Am] 53: 1180
444. Dumonde DC, Glynn LE (1962) The production of arthritis in rabbits by an immunological reaction to fibrin. Br J Exp Pathol 43: 373
445. Duncan BF (1983) The frozen shoulder syndrome. Contemp Orthop 6: 69
446. Dunn EJ, McGavran MH, Nelson P et al. (1974) Synovial chondrosarcoma. J Bone Joint Surg [Am] 56: 811
447. Dunne JV, Carson DA, Spiegelberg HL et al. (1979) IgA rheumatoid factor in the sera and saliva of patients with rheumatoid arthritis and Sjoegren's syndrome. Ann Rheum Dis 38: 161
448. Dupuis PV, Watillon M, Despontin J et al. (1959) Ochronose et arthrite alcaptonurique. Rev Rhum Mal Osteoartic 26: 473
449. Dupuytren G (1832) Leçons orales de clinique chirurgicale. Balliere, Paris
450. Dustmann HD, Puhl W (1973) Die Reaktion des Gelenkknorpels nach chondralen und osteochondralen Verletzungen. Arch Orthop Chir [Suppl] 65: 334
451. Duthie RB, Mattews JM, Broza CK et al. (1972) The management of musculo-skeletal problems in hemophilias. Blackwell, Oxford
452. DuVivier A, Munro DD, Verbow J (1974) Treatment of psoriasis with azathioprine. Br Med J 1: 49
453. Dymock IW, Hamilton EBD, Laws JW et al. (1970) Arthropathy of hemochromatosis. Ann Rheum Dis 29: 469

454. Edelman J, Russel AS (1983) A comparison of patients with seropositive and seronegative rheumatoid arthritis. Rheumatol Int 3: 47
455. Edwards CQ, Carrol M, Bray P et al. (1977) Hereditary hemochromatosis; diagnosis in siblings and children. N Engl J Med 297: 1922
456. Egeland T, Munthe E (1986) Rheumatoid factor. Clin Rheum Dis 9: 135
457. Ehrlich GE (1973) Familial Mediterranean Fever (FMF). Bull Rheum Dis 24: 746
458. Ehrlich GE (1975) Osteoarthritis beginning with inflammation: definitions and correlations. JAMA 232: 157
459. Ehrlich GE (1977) Guidelines for antiinflammatory drug research. J Clin Pharmacol 17: 697
460. Ehrlich GE (1979) Pathogenesis and treatment of osteoarthritis. Compr Ther 58: 36
461. Ehrlich GE (1989) Intermittent and periodic arthritic symptoms. In: McCarty DJ (ed) Arthritis and allied conditions. Lea and Febiger, Philadelphia
462. Ehrlich GE, Young I, Mosheny SZ et al. (1972) Multicentric reticulohistiocytosis (lipoid dermatoarthritis) a multisystem disorder. Am J Med 52: 830
463. Eichenblat M, Hass P, Kessler I (1982) Synovectomy of the elbow in rheumatoid arthritis. J Bone Joint Surg [Am] 64: 1074
464. Eichenholtz SN (1966) Charcot joints. Thomas, Springfield
465. Eisenberg JM, Schumacher RH, Davidson PL et al. (1980) Usefulness of synovial fluid analysis in the evaluation of joint effusions. Arch Intern Med 144: 715
466. Eisenstein BI, Masi T (1981) Disseminated gonococcal infection (DGI) and gonococcal arthritis (GCA): I. Bacteriology, epidemiology, host factors, pathogen factors and pathology. Semin Arthritis Rheum 10: 155
467. Ellenberg M (1968) Diabetic neuropathy of upper extremities. J Mt Sinai Hosp NY 35: 134
468. Ellis HA, Felix-Davies D (1959) Serum complement, rheumatoid factor, and other serum proteins in rheumatoid disease and systemic lupus erythematosus. Ann Rheum Dis 18: 215
469. El-Khouri GY, Kathol MH (1980) Neuropathic fractures in patients with arthritis in diabetes mellitus. Radiology 134: 313
470. Eloesser L (1917) On the nature of neuropathic affections of joints. Ann Surg 66: 201
471. Ellsasser JC, Reynolds FC, Omohundro JR (1974) The nonoperative treatment of collateral ligament injuries of the knee in professional football plagues. J Bone Joint Surg [Am] 56: 1185
472. Emerson RH, Potter J (1985) The use of the McKeever metallic hemiarthroplasty for unicompartmental arthritis. J Bone Joint Surg [Am] 67: 208
473. Emkey RD, Mills J (1975) Aspirin and analgesic nephropathy. JAMA 247: 55

474. Enarson DA, Fuji M, Nakielna E et al. (1979) Bone and joint tuberculosis. A continuing problem. Can Med Assoc J 120: 139
475. England JM, Bain BJ (1976) Total and differential leukocyte count. Br J Haematol 33: 1
476. Enzinger FM, Weiss SK (1988) Soft tissue tumors. Mosby, St Louis
477. Erdheim J (1931) Die Lebensvorgänge im normalen Knorpel und seine Wucherung bei Akromegalie. Springer, Berlin
478. Eriksson E, Pitman NJ (1984) Arthroscopy and arthroscopic surgery of joints other than the knee. In: Shariaree H (ed) O'Connor's textbook of arthroscopic surgery. Lippincott, Philadelphia
479. Escobar MR, Dalton HP, Allison MJ (1976) Fluorescent antibody tests for syphilis using cerebrospinal fluid. Clinical correlation in 150 cases. Am J Clin Pathol 53: 886
480. Espinoza LR, Vasey FB, Oh JH et al. (1978) Association between HLA-BW38 and peripheral psoriatic arthritis. Arthritis Rheum 21: 72
481. Esposito C, Melanotte PL, Olmeda A et al. (1982) La sinovectomia precoce nell' emofilia. Ital J Orthop Traumatol 8: 311
482. Ettlinger RE, Hunder GG (1979) Synovial effusions containing cholesterol crystals. Mayo Clin Proc 54: 366
483. Evanski PM, Waugh TR, Orofino CF et al. (1976) UCI knee replacement. Clin Orthop 120: 33
484. Ewald FC, Jacobs MA (1984) Total elbow arthroplasty. Clin Orthop 182: 137
485. Exner G (1951) Beitrag zur Pathogenese der Osteochondritis dissecans. Z Orthop 81: 386
486. Eyring EJ (1969) The biochemistry and physiology of intervertebral disc. Clin Orthop 67: 16
487. Eyring EJ, Longert A, Bass JD (1971) Synovectomy in juvenile rheumatoid arthritis. J Bone Joint Surg [Am] 53: 638
488. Fahey JJ (1949) Surgical approaches to bones and joints. Surg Clin North Am 29: 65
489. Fallahi S, Halla JT, Hardin JG (1982) The influence of B-27 antigen in the clinical and radiographic picture of definite and classical rheumatoid arthritis. J Rheumatol 9: 13
490. Fam AG, Tenenbaum J, Stein JL (1977) Clinical forms of meningococcal arthritis: a study of five cases. J Rheumatol 6: 567
491. Fam AG, Kolin A, Lewis AJ (1980) Metastatic carcinomatous arthritis and carcinoma of lung. J Rheumatol 7: 98
492. Fanelli GM Jr (1975) Uricosuric agents. Arthritis Rheum 18: 853
493. Farber GA, Forshner JG, O'Quinn SE (1967) Reiter's syndrome treatment with methotrexate. JAMA 200: 171
494. Fassbender HG (1975) Pathology of rheumatic diseases. Springer, Berlin Heidelberg New York
495. Fassbender HG, Gay S (1988) Synovial processes in rheumatoid arthritis. Scand J Rheumatol Suppl 76: 1
496. Fehr K, Boeni A (1973) Rheumafaktor. Nachweis durch einfachen Haemagglutinations Tropfentest. Praxis 61: 1086
497. Fehr K (1976) Rheumaserologie bei juveniler rheumatischer Arthritis. Dtsch Med Wochenschr 101: 516
498. Fehr K (1982) Autoimmune reactions and rheumatoid arthritis. Eur J Rheumatol Inflamm 5: 439
499. Feinstein AR, Spagnuolo M (1962) Sore throats, streptococcal infection and prevention of rheumatic fever. J Chronic Dis 15: 623
500. Feinstein AR, Spagnuolo M (1962) The clinical patterns of acute rheumatic fever: a reappraisal. Medicine (Baltimore) 41: 279
501. Feldman F, Johnson AM, Walter JF (1974) Diabetes and axial neuropathy. Radiology 111: 1
502. Fenelon GCC, Foerster G, von Engelbrecht L (1980) Disarticulation of the hip as a result of failed arthroplasty. J Bone Joint Surg [Br] 62: 441
503. Ferguson RH (1985) Enteropathic arthritis. In: McCarty DJ (ed) Arthritis and allied conditions. Lea and Febiger, Philadelphia
504. Ferguson RH, Dowair WW (1968) Gastrointestinal amyloidosis in psoriatic arthritis. Ann Rheum Dis 27: 245
505. Fernandez-Herlihy L (1959) The articular manifestations of chronic ulcerative colitis. N Engl J Med 261: 259
506. Fetto JF (1986) Knee lesions. In: Jenkins DJR (ed) Ligament injuries and their treatment. Chapman and Hill, London
507. Fialk MA, Moravec RC, Armstrong D (1986) Cryptococcal bone. A manifestation of disseminated cryptococcosis. Clin Orthop 158: 219
508. Ficat RP, Philippe J, Hungerford DL (1979) Chondromalacia patellae. A system of classifications. Clin Orthop 144: 55
509. Fielding WJ (1980) Rheumatoid arthritis of the cervical spine. Instr Course Lect Am Acad Orthop Surg 29: 114
510. Fiessinger N, Leroy E (1916) Contribution a l'étude d'une epidemie de dysenterie dans la Somme. Bull Soc Med Hosp Paris 40: 2030
511. Fink CW (1977) Patients with JRA: a clinical study. Arthritis Rheum 20: 183
512. Firooznia H (1986) Newer radiographic modalities in diagnoses of disease of the spine. Bull NY Acad Med 62: 149
513. Firooznia H (1988) Clinical applications of magnetic resonance imaging of the spine. Proc NY Acad Med 64: 741
514. Firooznia H, Golimbu C, Rafii M (1983) Application of computed tomography in detection of disorders of the joints, intraarticular and periarticular structures. Orthop Rev 12: 69
515. Fischbach M, Char D, Christensen M et al. (1980) Immunocomplexes in Sjoegren's syndrome. Arthritis Rheum 23: 791
516. Fischer W (1988) Das Roentgenbild der Knochen in der Diagnose des Morbus Gaucher. Fortschr Roentgenstrahlther 37: 158
517. Fitzgerald RH, Rosenblatt JE, Tenney JH et al. (1982) Anaerobic septic arthritis. Clin Orthop 164: 141
518. Fearon DT, Austin KF (1980) The alternative pathway of complement – a system of host resistance to microbial infection. N Engl J Med 303: 259
519. Flatt AE (1989) Correction of arthritic deformities of the hand. In: McCarty DJ (ed) Arthritis and allied conditions. Lea and Febiger, Philadelphia
520. Fluderus B (1915) Studien in der Biologie der Skelettgewebe mit besonderer Berücksichtigung der Pathogenese der histoiden Gelenkgewebegeschwülste. Friedländer, Berlin
521. Flynn JE (1950) Acute suppurative tenosynovitis of the hand. N Engl J Med 242: 241
522. Ford DK (1963) Rheumatoid arthritis – an infection. Arthritis Rheum 6: 159
523. Ford DK (1986) Reactive arthritis; a view point rather than a review. Clin Rheum Dis 12: 389
524. Ford DK, Vallis DG (1959) The clinical course of arthritis associated with ulcerative colitis and regional ileitis. Arthritis Rheum 2: 526
525. Forouzesh S, Fan PT, Bluestone R (1981) Septic bursitis, a neglected diagnosis. Orthop Rev 10: 111
526. Forrest J, Staple TW (1971) Synovial hemangioma of the knee; demonstration by arthrography and arteriography. Am J Roentgenol 112: 512
527. Forrest JE, Owen DS, Sagar KB (1980) The benign hypermobile joint syndrome. Arthritis Rheum 23: 1053
528. Forrester DM, Brown JC (1983) The radiographic assessment of arthritis. The plain film. Clin Rheum Dis 9: 291
529. Foster DB, Basset RC (1947) Neurogenic arthropathy (Charcot joint) associated with diabetic neuropathy. Arch Neurol Psychiatry 57: 173
530. Fountain FF (1973) Acute blastomycotic arthritis. Arch Intern Med 132: 684

531. Fowler PD, Woolf D, Alexander S (1975) Phenylbutazone and hepatitis. Rheumatol Rehabil 14: 71
532. Fox IH (1985) Arthropathy with iron storage disease. In: Kelley WN, Harris KJ, Ruddy S, Sledge CB (eds) Textbook of rheumatology. Saunders, Philadelphia
533. Fox R, Calin A, Gerber PC et al. (1979) The chronicity of symptoms and disability in Reiter's syndrome. Ann Intern Med 91: 190
534. Franceschini P (1956) Il sistemo istiocitario. Salpietra, Firenze
535. Franco AE, Schur PH (1971) Hypocomplementemia in rheumatoid arthritis. Arthritis Rheum 14: 231
536. Frangione B (1975) Structure of human immunoglobulins and their variants. In: Benacerraf B (ed) Immunodeficiency and immunogenetics. Medical and Technical Lancaster, UK
537. Frangione B, Milstein C, Franklin EC (1969) Clinical typing of immunoglobulins. Nature 221: 149
538. Frangione B, Buxbaum JN (1985) Immunoglobulins and their genes. In: Kelley WN, Harris ED, Ruddy S, Sledge CB (eds) Textbook of rheumatology. Saunders, Philadelphia
539. Franklin EC (1979) Plasma cell dyscrasias. In: Parker (ed) Clinical immunology. Saunders, Philadelphia
540. Franklin EC, Zucker-Franklin D (1972) Current concepts of amyloid. Adv Immunol 15: 249
541. Fraser GL (1981) Treatment of nongonococcal bacterial septic arthritis. Drug Clin Pharm 15: 531
542. Fredrickson DS, Hoffman AF (1960) Gaucher's disease. In: Stanbury JB, Wyngaarden JB, Fredrickson DS (eds) The metabolic basis of inherited disorders. McGraw-Hill, New York
543. Fredrickson DS, Levy RI, Lees RS (1967) Fat transport and lipoproteins – an integrated approach to mechanisms and disorders. N Engl J Med 276: 215
544. Fredrickson DS, Levy RI (1970) Familial hyperlipoproteinema. In: Stanbury JB, Wyngaarden JB, Fredrickson DS (eds) The metabolic basis of inherited disorders. McGraw-Hill, New York
545. Freeman MAR (1980) ICLH arthroplasty of the knee. Contemp Orthop 2: 38
546. Freeman MAR, Meachim G (1970) Ageing and degeneration. In: Freeman MAR (ed) Adult articular cartilage. Pitman Medical, Kent
547. Freeman R, Janes MR (1983) Microbiology. Clin Rheum Dis 9: 3
548. Fremont AJ, Jones CIP, Denton J (1983) The synovium and synovial fluid in multicentric reticulohistiocytosis; a light macroscopic, electron microscopic, and cytochemical analysis of one case. J Clin Pathol 36: 860
549. Freyberg RH (1950) Present status of gold therapy for rheumatoid arthritis. JAMA 143: 418
550. Friberg S, Hirsch C (1949) Anatomical and clinical studies on lumbar disc degeneration. Acta Orthop Scand 19: 222
551. Friedman B, Kapur VN (1973) Newer knowledge of chemotherapy in the treatment of tuberculosis of bones and joints. Clin Orthop 97: 5
552. Friedman DM, Moore ME (1980) The efficacy of intraarticular corticosteroid for osteoarthritis of the knee. J Rheumatol 7: 850
553. Friedman R, Agus B, Ames E (1981) Amyloid arthropathy in a patient with psoriasis. Arthritis Rheum 24: 1320
554. Fritz P, Müller J, Wegner G et al. (1981) Beitrag zur Verteilung der Immunglobulin-Klassen in Gelenkkapseln bei Osteoarthritis (Arthrose) und chronischer Polyarthritis. Z Rheumatol 40: 187
555. Frymoyer JW, Hooglund FF (1974) The role of arthrodesis in reconstruction of the knee. Clin Orthop 101: 82
556. Funk FJ (1971) Surgery of the foot in rheumatoid arthritis. Semin Arthritis Rheum 1: 25
557. Furcolow ML, Balows A, Menges RW et al (1966) Blastomycosis. JAMA 198: 529
558. Gaafar HA, D'Arcangelis DC (1975) Fluorescent antibody test for the serological diagnosis of gonorrhea. J Clin Microbiol 3: 438
559. Gaines JJ (1989) The pathology of alkaptonuric ochronsosis. Hum Pathol 20: 40
560. Gallagher JC, Riggs BL, DeLuce AF (1980) Effect of estrogen on calcium absorption and serum metabolites in postmenopausal osteoporosis. J Clin Endocrinol Metab 51: 1359
561. Gallo GR, Feiner HD, Chuba JV et al. (1986) Characterization of tissue amyloid by immunofluorescence microscopy. Clin Immunol Immunopathol 39: 479
562. Galloway JDB, Broders CC, Ghormley RK (1940) Xanthoma of the tendon sheaths and synovial membranes. Arch Surg 40: 485
563. Gambari PT, Marson P, Cavallo G et al. (1985) Effetti tossici della D-penicillinamine nel trattamento del' artrite reumatoide. Reumatismo 37: 283
564. Gambari RF, Volante D, Stone GC et al. (1981) Complemento nel liquido sinoviale. Recenti Prog Med 71: 69
565. Gamboa ET, Eastwood AB, Hays AP et al. (1979) Isolation of influenza virus in myoglobinuric polymyositis. Neurology 29: 1323
566. Gardner DL (1962) Amyloidosis in rheumatoid arthritis treated with hormones. Ann Rheum Dis 21: 298
567. Gardner DL (1972) The influence of microscopic technology on knowledge of cartilage surface structure. Ann Rheum Dis 31: 235
568. Gardner DL (1980) General pathology of joints. In: Sokoloff L (ed) The joints and synovial fluid. Academic, New York
569. Gardner DL (1983) The nature and causes of osteoarthrosis. Br Med J 186: 418
570. Gardner DL (1986) Pathology of rheumatoid arthritis. In: Scott JD (ed) Copeman's textbook of rheumatic diseases. Churchill Livingstone, Edinburgh
571. Gardner ED (1954) Physiology of blood and nerve supply of joints. Bull Hosp Jt Dis 15: 35
572. Gardner ED (1963) Physiology of joints. J Bone Joint Surg [Am] 45: 1061
573. Gardner FH, Nathan DG (1961) Secondary gout. Med Clin North Am 45: 1273
574. Gardner RC (1973) A simple, rapid, and esthetic exposure of the shoulder joint. Surg Gynecol Obstet 137: 99
575. Gardner RC (1974) Surgery for tennis elbow. Orthop Rev 3: 45
576. Garrod, AB (1859) A treatise on gout and rheumatic gout. Walton and Maberly, London
577. Gatenby PA, Engleman EG (1981) Immunoregulation in the synovium of rheumatoid arthritis. Lancet 2: 1348
578. Gatter, RA, McCarty DJ (1967) Pathological tissue calcifications in man. Arch Pathol 84: 346
579. Gaucher A, Faure G, Netter P et al. (1977) Identification des cristaux observés dans les arthropathies destructives de la chondrocalcinose. Rev. Rhum Mal Osteoartic 44: 505
580. Gaucher OC (1882) De l'epithelioma primitive de la rate, hypertrophic sans leucemie. Thesis, Faculty of medicine, Paris
581. Gay RE, Palmoski MJ, Brandt KD et al. (1983) Aspirin causes in vivo synthesis of type I collagen by atrophic articular cartilage. Arthritis Rheum 26: 1231
582. Gay S, Mueller PK, Lemmen C et al (1976) Immunohistological study on collagen in cartilage-bone metamorphosis and degenerative osteoarthritis. Klin Wochenschr 54: 969
583. Gay S, Gay RE, Miller EJ (1980) The collagen of the joint. Arthritis Rheum 23: 937
584. Gehlbach SH, Hamilton JD, Canant WF (1973) Coccidioidomycosis. Arch Intern Med 131: 254

585. Gehweiler JA, Capp MP, Chick EK (1970) Observations on the roentgen patterns in blastomycosis of bone. Am J Roentgenol 108: 497
586. Geiler G (1971) The antibody synthesis of the synovial membrane in rheumatoid arthritis. In: Mueller W, Horworth HG, Fehr K (eds) Rheumatoid arthritis. Academic London
587. Geiler G (1977) Die Pathologie der Systeme und Systemgrenzen am Beispiel der Gelenkerkrankungen. Nova Acta Leopold 47: 250
588. Geiler G (1985) Common and contradictory aspects of inflammation and the pathogenic immune reactions. Zbl Allg Pathol 130: 307
589. Geiler G, Stiehl P (1974) Zur Bedeutung der Begriffe Basisaktivität und aktuelle Aktivität der Synovialmembran bei der morphologischen Beurteilung der Synovialmembran bei Rheumatoid Arthritis. Z Rheumatol 33: 73
590. Geiler G, Riedel R (1985) Detection by the PAP technique of lysosome containing synoviocytes, and their quantity in rheumatoid arthritis and osteoarthrosis. Histochem J 17: 562
591. Genant HK (1970) Roentgenographic aspects of calcium pyrophosphate dihydrate crystal deposition disease (pseudogout). Arthritis Rheum 19: 307
592. Genant HK (1985) Radiology of rheumatic diseases. In: McCarty DJ (ed) Arthritis and allied conditions. Lea and Febiger, Philadelphia
593. Genant HK, Doi K, Mall JC et al. (1977) Direct radiographic magnification for skeletal arthrography, an assessment of image quality and clinical application. Radiology 123: 47
594. George AL, Taylor Hayes JT, Graham BS (1985) Blastomycosis as monoarticular arthritis. Arthritis Rheum 28: 516
595. George DL, Glass DN (1983) Quantitation of complement proteins in rheumatic diseases. Clin Rheum Dis 9: 177
596. George RC, Chrisman OD (1968) The role of cartilage polysaccharide in osteoarthritis. Clin Orthop 57: 259
597. Gerber N, Ambrosini GC, Boeni A et al (1977) Spondylitis ankylosans (Bechterew) und Gewebsantigen HLA-B27. Z Rheumatol 36: 219
598. Gerhart TN, Scott RD (1983) Hip arthroplasty in patients with tabetic Charcot joints. Orthopedics 6: 179
599. Gerner RE, Moore GE (1975) Synovial sarcoma. Ann Surg 181: 22
600. Gerster JC, Guggy J, Perroud H et al. (1981) Lyme arthritis affecting outside the United States. A case report from Switzerland. Br Med J 283: 951
601. Gerster JC, Lagier R, Boivin G (1982) Olecranon bursitis related to calcium pyrophosphate dihydrate crystal deposition disease. Arthritis Rheum 25: 989
602. Gewuerz H, Mold C, Siegel J et al. (1982) C-reactive protein and the acute phase response. Adv Intern Med 27: 345
603. Ghadially FN (1978) Fine structure of joints. In: Sokoloff L (ed) Joints and synovial fluid. Academic, New York
604. Ghadially FN (1981) Structure and function of articular cartilage. Clin Rheum Dis 7: 1
605. Ghadially FN, Roy S (1967) Ultrastructure of synovial membrane in rheumatoid arthritis. Ann Rheum Dis 26: 421
606. Ghormley R (1926) Charcot joints in a case of syringomyelia. Surg Gynecol Obstet 43: 695
607. Giannini EH, Brewer EJ, Person DA (1983) Anaurofin in the treatment of juvenile rheumatoid arthritis. J Pediat 102: 138
608. Gibson T, Grahame R (1981) Rehabilitation of the elderly arthritic patient. Clin Rheum Dis 7: 485
609. Gilbert MS (1977) Musculoskeletal manifestations of hemophilia. Mt Sinai J Med 44: 339
610. Gilchrist TC (1984) Protozoan dermatitis. J Cut Gen Urin Dis 12: 496
611. Giliberty RP (1985) Bipolar endoprosthesis minimizes protrusio acetabuli. Orthop Rev 14: 27
612. Ginsburg NW, O'Duffy JD (1985) Multicentric reticulohistiocytosis. In: Kelley WN, Harris ED, Ruddy S, Sledge CB (eds) Textbook of rheumatology. Saunders, Philadelphia
613. Girdlestone GR (1943) Acute pyogenic arthritis of the hip. An operation giving free access and effective drainage. Lancet 1: 419
614. Gitelis S, Heligman D, Morton T (1989) The treatment of pigmented villonodular synovitis. Clin Orthop 239: 154
615. Glasgow MM (1976) Brucellosis of the spine. Br J Surg 63: 283
616. Glasser L (1980) Body fluids: II. Reading the signs in synovia. Diagn Med 3: 35
617. Glassroth J, Robins AG, Snider DEJ (1980) Tuberculosis in the 1980's. N Engl J Med 302: 1441
618. Glenchur H, Zinneman H, Hall W (1959) A review of fifty-one cases of multiple myeloma. Arch Intern Med 103: 173
619. Glenner GG, Terry W, Harada M et al. (1971) Amyloid fibrin proteins, proof of homology with immunoglobulin light chains by sequence. Science 172: 1150
620. Glimcher MJ, Kenzora JE (1979) The biology of osteonecrosis of the human femoral head and its clinical implications: II. The pathological changes in the femoral head as an organ and in the hip joint. Clin Orthop 139: 283
621. Goidanich IF, Battaglia L (1957) I Sarcomi de origine sinoviale. Chir Organi Mov 44: 335
622. Goidanich IF, Companacci M, Beodgni C (1963) Amartomi vascolari intraarticolari. Chir Organi Mov 52: 351
623. Gold RH, Metzger AL, Mirra JM et al (1975) Multicentric reticulohistiocytosis (lipoid dermatoarthritis). An erosive polyarthritis with distinctive clinical, roentgenographic and pathologic features. Am J Roentgenol 124: 610
624. Goldberg A, Brodsky I, McCarty DJ (1964) Multiple myeloma with paraamyloidosis presenting as rheumatoid disease. Am J Med 37: 653
625. Goldberg VM, Heiple KG, Ratnoff OA et al. (1981) Total knee arthroplasty in classic hemophilia. J Bone Joint Surg [Am] 63: 695
626. Goldberg VM, Norby DP, Sachs BL et al. (1984) Correlation of histopathology and sulfated proteoglycans in human osteoarthritic hip. J Orthop Res 1: 302
627. Goldenberg DL (1989) Gonococcal arthritis. In: McCarty DJ (ed) Arthritis and allied conditions. Lea and Febiger, Philadelphia
628. Goldenberg DL, Brandt KD, Cohen AS et al. (1975) Treatment of septic arthritis. Comparison of needle aspiration and surgery as initial modes of joint drainage. Arthritis Rheum 18: 83
629. Goldenberg DL, Kelley W, Gibbons RG (1975) Metastatic adenocarcinoma of synovium presenting as an acute arthritis. Arthritis Rheum 18: 107
630. Goldenberg DL, Cohen AS (1978) Synovial membrane histopathology in the differential diagnosis of rheumatoid arthritis, gout, pseudogout, systemic lupus erythematosus, infectious arthritis, and degenerative joint disease. Medicine (Baltimore) 57: 239
631. Goldenberg DL, Cohen AS (1978) Arthritis due to Gram negative bacilli. Clin Rheum Dis 4: 197
632. Goldenberg DL, Cohen AS (1978) Arthritis due to tuberculous and fungal microorganisms. Clin Rheum Dis 4: 211
633. Goldenberg DL, Egan MS, Cohen AS (1982) Inflammatory synovitis in degenerative joint disease. J Rheumatol 9: 204
634. Goldenberg GJ, Paraskevas F, Israels LG (1969) The association of rheumatoid arthritis with plasma cells and lymphocytic neoplasm. Arthritis Rheum 12: 569
635. Goldfinger WG (1972) Colchicine for familial Mediterranean fever. N Engl J Med 287: 1302
636. Goldie I (1965) Epicondylitis lateralis humeri. Acta Chir Scand Suppl 339

637. Goldin DS, Stangler DA, Canoso JJ (1981) Rheumatoid subcutaneous bursitis. J Rheumatol 8: 974
638. Golding DN (1968) Clofibrate in the management of a case of lipoid dermatoarthritis; a clinical and metabolic study. Ann Rheum Dis 27: 475
639. Golding SJ, Husband JE (1982) The role of computed tomography in the management of soft tissue carcinoma. Br J Radiol 55: 740
640. Goldings EA, Jericho J (1986) Lyme disease. Clin Rheum Dis 12: 343
641. Goldman JA, Glueck CJ, Abrams NR et al. (1972) Musculoskeletal disorders associated with type IV hyperlipoproteinemia. Lancet 2: 449
642. Goldman RL, Lichtenstein L (1964) Syovial chondrosarcoma. Cancer 17: 1233
643. Goldsand G (1989) Actinomycosis. In: Hoeprich PD (ed) Infectious diseases. Harper & Row, Philadelphia
644. Goldstein RC, Schwabe AD (1974) Prophylactic colchicine therapy in familial Mediterranean fever. A controlled double blind study. Ann Intern Med 81: 792
645. Golimbu C, Firooznia H, Rafii M (1986) The intervertebral vacuum sign. Spine 11: 1040
646. Goltz RW, Laymon CW (1954) Multicentric reticulohistiocytosis of the skin and synovia. Arch Dermatol Syphilol 69: 717
647. Good AE, Schultz JS (1977) Reiter's syndrome following Shigella Flexneri. Arthritis Rheum 20: 100
648. Goodfellow J, Hungerford AL, Woods L (1976) Patellofemoral joint mechanics and pathology. Chondromalacia patellae. J Bone Joint Surg [Br] 58: 291
649. Goodwin JS, Cluppens JL (1983) Effect of nonsteroidal antiinflammatory medications on immune function. Semin Arthritis Rheum 13: 134
650. Goodwin RA, DesPrez RM (1918) Histoplasmosis. Am Rev Respir Dis 117: 929
651. Gordon DA, Pinzanski W, Ogryzlo NA et al. (1974) Amyloid arthritis simulating rheumatoid disease in five patients with multiple myeloma. Am J Med 55: 142
652. Gordon G, Kabins SA (1980) Pyogenic sacroileitis. Am J Med 69: 50
653. Goss CM (1959) Anatomy of the human body by Henry Gray. Lea and Febiger, Philadelphia
654. Gotazzo E, Alarcon GS, Bocanegra TS et al. (1982) Articular involvement in human brucellosis. A retrospective analysis of 304 cases. Semin Arthritis Rheum 12: 245
655. Gottlieb NL, Riskin WG (1980) Complications of local corticosteroid injections. JAMA 243: 1547
656. Gowers WRA (1904) A lecture on lumbago, its lessons and analogues. Br Med J 1: 117
657. Grady GF, Kensch GT (1971) Pathogenesis of bacterial diarrhea. N Engl J Med 285: 831
658. Graham GG, Day KO, Champion DG (1984) Aspects of clinical pharmacology of nonsteroidal antiinflammatory drugs. Clin Rheum Dis 10: 229
659. Grahame R (1971) Joint hypermobility – clinical aspects. Proc R Soc Med 64: 32
660. Grahame R, Jenkins JM (1972) Joint hypermobility – asset or liability. Ann Rheum Dis 31: 109
661. Granberry GM (1977) Soft tissue release in children with juvenile rheumatoid arthritis. Arthritis Rheum 20: 565
662. Granowitz SP, D'Antonio J, Mankin HJ (1976) The pathogenesis and long term end results of pigmented villonodular synovitis. Clin Orthop 114: 335
663. Gray RG, Gottlieb NL (1983) Intraarticular corticosteroids: an updated assessment. Clin Orthop 177: 235
664. Grayzel AI, Liddle L, Seegmiller JE (1961) Diagnostic significance of hyperuricemia in arthritis. N Engl J Med 265: 763
665. Green CA (1939) Research into the etiology of acute rheumatism: rheumatic carditis, post-mortem examinations of nine consecutive cases. Ann Rheum Dis 1: 86
666. Green DP, Parkes JC, Stinchfield FE (1967) Arthrodesis of the knee. J Bone Joint Surg [Am] 49: 1065
667. Green HN (1950) Suggested mode of action of corticotrophin in rheumatoid arthritis and its allergic state. Br Med J 1: 1165
668. Green L, Meyers OL, Gordon W et al. (1987) Arthritis in psoriasis. Ann Rheum Dis 40: 366
669. Green WT (1940) Mono-articular and pauci-articular arthritis in children. JAMA 115: 2023
670. Greenblatt JJ, Hunter N, Schwab JH (1980) Antibody response to streptococcal cell wall antigen-associated experimental arthritis in rats. Clin Exp Immunol 42: 450
671. Greenman R, Becker J, Campbell C et al. (1975) Coccidioidal synovitis of the knee. Arch Intern Med 135: 526
672. Greenstein AJ, Janowitz HD, Sachar DB (1976) The extraintestinal complications of Crohn's disease and ulcerative colitis. A study of 700 patients. Medicine (Baltimore) 55: 401
673. Greenwald AS, Haynes DW (1969) A pathway for nutrients from the medullary cavity to the articular cartilage of the human femoral head. J Bone Joint Surg [Br] 51: 747
674. Greenwood BM, Whittle HC, Bryceson A (1973) Allergic complications of meningeal disease. Br Med J 2: 737
675. Greer RB (1980) Operative management of hemophilic arthropathy – an overview. Orthopedics 3: 135
676. Greiling H, Herberta J, Schuler B et al. (1962) Biochemische Untersuchungen über die Ursachen der Harnsäureablagerung im Bindegewebe der Gicht. Z Rheumaforsch 21: 50
677. Greyson ND (1980) Radionuclide bone and joint imaging in rheumatology. Bull Rheum Dis 30: 1034
678. Gribble M deG (1955) Rheumatoid arthritis and psoriasis. Ann Rheum Dis 14: 198
679. Griffith GC, Huntington RW (1946) Sudden death in rheumatic fever. Ann Intern Med 25: 283
680. Gristina AG (1987) Biomaterial centered infection: microbial adhesion versus tissue integration. Science 237: 1588
681. Gristina AG, Marchetti PG (1961) Arthrodesis of the knee. Bull Hosp Spec Surg 4: 81
682. Gristina AG, Rovere GD, Shoji H (1974) Spontaneous septic arthritis complicating rheumatoid arthritis. J Bone Joint Surg [Am] 56: 1180
683. Gristina AG, Webb L (1982) Proximal humeral and monospherical glenoid replacement surgical technique. Howmedica, Rutherford
684. Grobois B, Pawlotsky Y, Oger J et al. (1979) Secrétion intrasynoviale d'anticorps antibrucelliens. Nouv Presse Med 8: 3752
685. Gross D (1963) Chemische Synovektomie mit Senfgas bei primär chronischer Polyarthritis. Z Rheumaforsch 22: 456
686. Gross L, Ehrlich JC (1934) Studies on the myocardial Aschoff body. Descriptive characteristics of the lesions. Am J Pathol 10: 467
687. Grynbaum BB (1954) An evaluation of the clinical use of ultrasonics. J Phys Med 33: 75
688. Gschwend N (1980) Surgical treatment of rheumatoid arthritis. Thieme, Stuttgart
689. Gschwend N (1989) Synovectomy. In: Kelley WN, Harris ED, Ruddy S, Sledge CB (eds) Textbook of rheumatology. Saunders, Philadelphia
690. Gschwend N, Scheier H (1974) Elbow arthroplasty with the new GSB-prosthesis. Scand J Rheumatol 3: 177
691. Gschwend N, Winer J, Boeni A et al. (1976) Die operative Synovektomie. Z Rheumatol 35: 32
692. Gschwend N, Boeni A, Fehr K (1982) Rheumatische Arthritis, rheumatischer Formenkreis. In: Witt AN, Rettig H,

Schlegel KF (eds) Orthopädie in Praxis und Klinik, vol 4. Thieme, Stuttgart
693. Guhl JF (1982) Arthroscopic treatment of osteochondritis dissecans. Clin Orthop 167: 65
694. Gumpel JM, Hibbs JR (1970) Serum immunoglobulins in Sjoegren's syndrome. Ann Rheum Dis 29: 681
695. Gundel M (1942) Ansteckende Krankheiten. Thieme, Leipzig
696. Gunston FH (1973) Polycentric knee arthroplasty prosthetic simulation of normal knee movement. Clin Orthop 94: 128
697. Gunz F, Baikie AG (1983) William Dameshek and Frederick Gunz's Leukemia. Grune and Stratton, New York
698. Gutman AB (1973) The past four decades of progress in the knowledge of gout with an assessment of the present status. Arthritis Rheum 16: 431
699. Gutman AB, Yu TF (1968) Uric acid nephrolithiasis. Am J Med 45: 756

700. Hackenbroch M (1946) Kontrakturen and Gelenksteifen. Z Orthop 76: 97
701. Hackenbroch MHJr (1982) Degenerative Gelenkerkrankungen. In: Witt AN, Rettig H, Schlegel KF et al. (eds) Orthopädie in Praxis und Klinik, vol 4. Thieme, Stuttgart
702. Hackenbroch MHJr (1982) Koxarthrose. In: Witt AN, Rettig H, Schlegel KF et al. (eds) Orthopädie in Praxis und Klinik, vol 8. Thieme, Stuttgart
703. Hadler NM (1976) A pathogenetic model for erosive synovitis. Lessons from erosive synovitis. Arthritis Rheum 19: 256
704. Hadler NM, Gronovetter DA (1978) Phlogistic properties of bacterial debris. Semin Arthritis Rheum 8: 1
705. Hajdu SI, Shiu NA, Fortner JG (1977) Tendosynovial sarcoma; a clinicopathologic study of 136 cases. Cancer 39: 1201
706. Halar EM, Graf RJ, Halter JB et al. (1982) Diabetic neuropathy. A clinical, laboratory, and electro-diagnostic study. Arch Phys Med Rehabil 63: 298
707. Halborg A, Hansen H, Sneppen HO (1968) Haemangioma of the knee joint. Acta Orthop Scand 39: 209
708. Hall FC, Monroe RT (1933) Thyroid gland deficiency in chronic arthritis. J Lab Clin Med 18: 439
709. Hall GH, Jones BJM, Head AC et al. (1978) Intraarticular methotrexate; clinical and laboratory studies in rheumatoid and psoriatic arthritis. Ann Rheum Dis 37: 351
710. Halla JT, Volanakis JE, Schrohenloher RE (1977) Immune complexes in rheumatoid arthritis sera and synovial fluids. Arthritis Rheum 22: 440
711. Halla JT, Volanakis JE, Schrohenloher RE (1979) Circulating immune complexes in mixed connective tissue disease. Arthritis Rheum 22: 484
712. Halsted JA, Halsted CH (1981) The laboratory in clinical medicine: interpretation and application. Saunders, Philadelphia
713. Hamdy H, McKendry RJ, Mierins E et al. (1987) Low dose methotrexate compared with azathioprine in the treatment of rheumatoid arthritis. Arthritis Rheum 30: 361
714. Hamilton EBD (1986) Arthritis in ochronosis, hemochromatosis, and Wilson's disease. In: Scott JD (eds) Copeman's textbook of the rheumatic diseases. Churchill Livingstone, Edinburgh
715. Hamilton PJ (1983) The hematology laboratory and the rheumatologist. Clin Rheum Dis 9: 69
716. Hamilton EBD (1976) Diseases associated with CPPD deposition disease. Arthritis Rheum 19: 353
717. Hamerman D, Sandson J, Schubert M (1963) Biochemical events in joint diseases. J Chronic Dis 16: 835
718. Hamerman D, Rosenberg L, Schubert M (1970) Diarthrodial joints revisited. J Bone Joint Surg [Am] 57: 725
719. Hanauer LB (1972) Reticulohistiocytosis; remission after cyclophosphamid therapy. Arthritis Rheum 15: 636
720. Hand BH, Patey DH (1952) The treatment of ganglion of the wrist. Practitioner 169: 195
721. Handsfield HH, Wiesner PJ, Holmes KR (1976) Treatment of the gonococcal arthritis-dermatitis syndrome. Ann Intern Med 84: 661
722. Hanson V, Kornreich H, Bernstein B et al. (1977) Prognosis of juvenile rheumatoid arthritis. Arthritis Rheum 20: 279
723. Hardy AV (1937) Arthritis in Brucella Melitensis infections. Med Clin North Am 21: 1747
724. Harris EDJr (1985) Biology of the joint. In: Kelley WN, Harris EJ, Ruddy S, Sledge CB (eds) Textbook of rheumatology. Saunders, Philadelphia
725. Harris EDJr (1985) Diagnosis of rheumatoid arthritis. In: Kelley WN, Harris ED, Ruddy S, Sledge CB (eds) Textbook of rheumatology. Saunders, Philadelphia
726. Harris EDJr (1989) Pathogenesis of rheumatoid arthritis. In: Kelley WN, Harris ED, Ruddy S, Sledge CB (eds) Textbook of rheumatology. Saunders, Philadelphia
727. Harris TN, Harris S (1949) Studies in the relation of the hemolytic streptococcus to rheumatic fever. Am J Med Sci 217: 174
728. Haslock I (1979) Clinical features of the seronegative spondylarthritides. Rheumatol Rehabil 18: 214
729. Haslock I, Wright V (1973) The musculoskeletal complications of Crohn's disease. Medicine (Baltimore) 52: 217
730. Hatcher VB, Borg JP, Levitt MA et al. (1981) Enhanced neutral protease activity in proliferating rheumatoid synovial cells. Arthritis Rheum 24: 919
731. Hawley WL, Ansell BM (1981) Synovial hemangioma presenting as monoarticular arthritis of the knee. Arch Dis Child 56: 558
732. Head WC (1981) Wagner surface replacement arthroplasty of the hip. J Bone Joint Surg [Am] 63: 420
733. Hearn PR, Russell RGG, Eliott JC (1978) Formation product of calcium pyrophosphate crystals in vitro and the effect of iron salts. Clin Sci Mol Med 54: 29
734. Heberden W (1803) Commentaries on the history and cure of diseases. Payne, London
735. Hedberg H (1967) Studies on synovial fluid: I. The total complement activity. Acta Med Scand Suppl 479. 1
736. Heine J (1926) Über die Arthritis deformans. Arch Pathol Anat 260: 521
737. Heiser S, Schwartzman JJ (1952) Variations in the roentgen appearance of the skeletal system in myeloma. Radiology 58: 179
738. Heller H, Gafni J, Michaeli D et al. (1966) The arthritis of familial Mediterranean fever. Arthritis Rheum 9: 1
739. Hellner H (1950) Die Knochengeschwülste. Springer, Berlin Göttingen Heidelberg
740. Helms CA, Vogler JB (1983) Computed tomography on spinal stenosis and arthroses. Clin Rheum Dis 9: 417
741. Hench P, Kendall E, Slocumb C et al. (1949) The effect of a hormone of the adrenal cortex and of pituitary adrenocorticotropic hormone in rheumatoid arthritis. Ann Rheum Dis 8: 97
742. Henkind P, Rothfield NE (1963) Ocular abnormalities in patients treated with systemic antimalarial drugs. N Engl J Med 269: 433
743. Henry JB (1984) Todd-Sanford-Davidson: clinical diagnosis and management by laboratory methods. Saunders, Philadelphia
744. Herd JK, Morris RL, Metzger AL et al. (1974) HAL-W27 spondylitis and enteritis. N Engl J Med 291: 680
745. Hermann G, Alvarez E, Lavine LS (1977) Value of knee arthrography in nonmeniscal damage. NYState J Med 77: 916
746. Hermann G, Hedberg F (1980) Lipoma arborescens: arthrographic findings. Orthopedics 3: 19
747. Hermann G, Wagner LD, Gendal ES (1989) Spinal cord compression in type I Gaucher disease. Radiology 170: 147

748. Hermans PE, Keys FF (1983) Antifungal agents used for deep mycotic infections. Mayo Clin Proc 58: 223
749. Herness D, Makin M (1975) Articular damage in familial Mediterranean fever. J Bone Joint Surg [Am] 57: 265
750. Herrell WE, Barber TE (1952) Treatment of brucellosis with aureomycin or ferramycin combined with dihydrostreptomycin. Postgrad Med 11: 476
751. Hess EV, Hunter DK, Ziff M (1965) Gonococcal antibodies in acute arthritis. JAMA 191: 531
752. Heyderman E (1979) Immunoperoxydase technique in histopathology: application method and controls. J Clin Pathol 32: 971
753. Hickling P, Wilkins M, Newman GA (1981) A study of arthropathy in multiple myeloma. Q J Med 50: 417
754. Highton GS, Panayi GS, Shepherd P et al. (1981) Fall in immune complex levels during gold treatment of rheumatoid arthritis. Ann Rheum Dis 40: 575
755. Hilgartner MW (1975) Hemophilic arthropathy. Acta Pediatr Scand 21: 139
756. Hilgartner MW, McMillan CW (1989) Coagulation disorders. In: Miller DR, Parson HA, Baehner RL, McMillan CW (eds) Smith's blood diseases of infance and childhood. Mosby, St. Louis
757. Hill DJ (1979) Stimulation of cartilage zones of the calf costochondral growth plate in vitro by growth hormone dependent; rat plasma somatomedin activity. J Endocrinol 83: 219
758. Hill JA, Compere CL (1981) Comparative study of patellectomy. Orthop Rev 10: 41
759. Hippokrates. Translation by Withington ET (1927) On joints. Heineman, London
760. Hirsch C (1944) The pathogenesis of chondromalacia patellae. Acta Chir Scand Suppl 90: 83
761. Hirsch C, Ingelmark BE, Miller M (1963) The anatomical basis for low back syndrome. Acta Orthop Scand 33: 1
762. Hirsch C, Goldie I, Ryla W (1972) Intertrochanteric osteotomy for osteoarthritis of the hip: a radiological evaluation. Clin Orthop 86: 63
763. Hirschkorn K, Wilkinson CF (1959) The mode of inheritance in essential familial hypercholesterolemia. Am J Med 26: 60
764. Ho GJr, Tice AD (1979) Comparison of nonspecific and septic bursitis. Arch Intern Med 139: 1289
765. Ho GJr, Su EY (1989) Antibiotic therapy of septic bursitis. Its application in the treatment of septic arthritis. Arthritis Rheum 24: 905
766. Ho GJr, Gadbow JJ, Glickstein SL (1983) Hemophilus influenzae septic arthritis in adults. Semin Arthritis Rheum 12: 314
767. Hoaglund FT, Lord GP (1967) Hemophilus influenzae septic arthritis in adults. Arch Intern Med 119: 648
768. Hoffa A (1904) The influence of the adipose tissue with regard to the pathology of the knee joint. JAMA 43: 795
769. Hoffman GS (1985) Mycobacterial and fungal infections of bones and joints. In: Kelley WN, Harris ED, Ruddy S, Sledge CB (eds) Textbook of rheumatology. Saunders, Philadelphia
770. Hoffman WL, Goldberg ML, Smiley JD (1982) Immunoglobulin P subclass production by rheumatoid synovial tissue cultures. J Clin Invest 69: 136
771. Hofmann P, Doehring S, Schumpe G et al. (1982) Haemophile Pseudotumoren. Z Orthop 120: 125
772. Hogan DB, Pritzker KPH (1985) Synovial fluid analysis. Another look at the mucin clot test. J Rheumatol 12: 242
773. Hollander JL (1979) Arthrocentesis and intrasynovial corticosteroid therapy. In: McCarty DJ (ed) Arthritis and allied conditions. Lea and Febiger, Philadelphia
774. Hollander JL, Reginato A, Torralba TN (1966) Examination of synovial fluid as a diagnostic aid in arthritis. Med Clin North Am 50: 1281
775. Hollister JR, Mannik M (1974) Antigen retention in joint tissues in antigeninduced synovitis. Clin Exp Immunol 16: 615
776. Holt PJL (1986) Endocrine disorders in metabolic bone diseases. In: Scott JT (ed) Copeman's textbook of the rheumatic diseases. Churchill Livingstone, Edinburgh
777. Holzman RS, Florman AL, Lyman M (1980) Gentamycin resistant and sensitive strains of s. aureus. Am J Epidemiol 112: 352
778. Hong CZ, Lee S, Lum P (1986) Cervical radiculopathy. Clinical, radiographic and EMG findings. Orthop Rev 15: 433
779. Hood RW, Varmi M, Insall JN (1981) The correction of knee alignment in 225 consecutive total condylar replacements. Clin Orthop 160: 94
780. Hough AJ, Banfield WG, Sokoloff L (1976) Cartilage in hemophilic arthropathy. Arch Pathol Lab Med 100: 91
781. Howell DS (1985) Osteoarthritis. Biochemical studies. In: McCarty DJ (ed) Arthritis and allied conditions. Lea and Febiger, Philadelphia
782. Howell DS (1985) Diseases due to deposition of calcium pyrophosphate and hydrooxyapatite. In: Kelley WN, Harris ED, Ruddy S, Sledge CB (ed) Textbook of rheumatology. Saunders, Philadelphia
783. Howell FA, Chamberlain MA, Perry RA et al. (1972) IgG antiglobulin levels in patients with psoriatic arthropathy, ankylosing spondylitis, and gout. Ann Rheum Dis 31: 129
784. Howie S, Feldman M (1978) Cellular interactions in antibody production. Clin Rheum Dis 4: 481
785. Hueston JT (1984) Dupuytren contracture. Livingstone, London
786. Hughes JG, Griffith JF (1984) Synopsis of pediatrics. Mosby, St. Louis
787. Hughston JC, Andrews JR, Cross MJ et al. (1976) Classification of knee ligament instability. J Bone Joint Surg [Am] 58: 159
788. Hunder GG, McDuffie FC, Muller BJ (1977) Activation of C3 and fraction B in synovial fluid. J Lab Clin Med 89: 160
789. Hungerford DS (1981) Pathogenetic considerations in ischemic necrosis of bone. Can J Surg 24: 583
790. Hungerford DS, Zizic TM (1978) Alcoholism associated ischemic necrosis of the femoral head. Clin Orthop 130: 144
791. Hunter G, Dandy D (1977) The natural history of the patient with an infected total hip replacement. J Bone Joint Surg [Br] 59: 293
792. Hunter J, Gordon DA, Ogryzlo MA (1974) The ground pepper sign of synovial fluid: a new diagnostic feature of ochronosis. J Rheumatol 1: 45
793. Hurd ER (1979) Extra-articular manifestations of rheumatoid arthritis. Semin Arthritis Rheum 8: 151
794. Huskisson EC (1984) How to choose a nonsteroidal antiinflammatory drug. Clin Rheum Dis 10: 313
795. Huskisson EC, Doyle DV, Lanham JG (1985) Drug treatment in osteoarthritis. Clin Rheum Dis 11: 421
796. Huth F, Soren A, Klein W (1972) Structure of synovial membrane in rheumatoid arthritis. Curr Top Pathol 56: 55
797. Huth F, Soren A, Rosenbauer A et al. (1973) Fine-structural changes of the synovial membrane in arthrosis deformans. Arch Pathol Anat 359: 201
798. Hvid-Hansen O (1978) On the treatment of ganglion. Acta Chir Scand 136: 471
799. Hyla JF, Frank WA, Chavis JS (1976) Lack of association of HLA-B27 with radiographic sacroileitis in inflammatory bowel disease. J Rheumatol 3: 196

800. Ilousz G, Hewitt J (1981) A propos de l'arthrite de Lyme. Polyarthrite inflammatoire après un erythema annulaire migrant. Rev Rheum Mal Osteoartic 48: 813
801. Indelicato PA (1983) Non-operative treatment of complete

tears of the medial collateral ligament of the knee. J Bone Joint Surg [Am] 65: 323
802. Inerot S, Heinegard D, Andell L et al. (1978) Articular cartilage proteoglycans in aging and osteoarthritis. Biochem J 169: 143
803. Inglis AE (1989) Correction of arthritic deformities of the shoulder and elbow. In: McCarty DJ (ed) Arthritis and allied conditions. Lea and Febiger, Philadelphia
804. Inglis AE, Pellicci PM (1980) Total elbow replacement. J Bone Joint Surg [Am] 62: 1252
805. Insall JN (1985) Correction of arthritic deformities of the knee. In: McCarty DJ (ed) Arthritis and allied conditions. Lea and Febiger, Philadelphia
806. Insall JN, Tria AJ, Aglietti SP (1979) Resurfacing of the patella. J Bone Joint Surg [Am] 62: 933
807. Insall JN, Binazzi R, Soudry M et al. (1985) Total knee arthroplasty. Clin Orthop 192: 13
808. Ishikawa H, Ohno A, Hirohata K (1986) Long term results of synovectomy in rheumatoid arthritis. J Bone Joint Surg [Am] 68: 198

809. Jackson R (1977) The cervical spine. Thomas, Springfield
810. Jackson R (1985) Syndrome of cervical nerve root compression. In: McCarty DJ (ed) Arthritis and allied conditions. Lea and Febiger, Philadelphia
811. Jackson RW, Dandy DJ (1976) Arthroscopy of the knee. Grune and Stratton, New York
812. Jackson RW (1983) Current concepts review; arthroscopic surgery. J Bone Joint Surg [Am] 65: 416
813. Jacobs MR, Koornhof HJ, Robins-Brown RM et al. (1978) Emergence of multiple resistant pneumococci. N Engl J Med 299: 735
814. Jacobs B (1978) Epidemiology of traumatic and nontraumatic osteonecrosis. Clin Orthop 130: 51
815. Jacobsen ST, Levinson JE, Crawford AH (1985) Late results of synovectomy of juvenile rheumatoid arthritis. J Bone Joint Surg [Am] 67: 8
816. Jacoby RK, Jayson MIV (1974) HL-A27 in Crohn's disease. Ann Rheum Dis 33: 422
817. Jaffe HL (1958) Tumors and tumorous conditions of the bones and joints. Lea and Febiger, Philadelphia
818. Jaffe HW (1975) The laboratory diagnosis of syphilis. New concepts. Ann Intern Med 83: 846
819. Jaffe IA (1989) Penicillamine. In: McCarty DJ (ed) Arthritis and allied conditions. Lea and Febiger, Philadelphia
820. Jajic I (1968) Radiological changes in the sacroiliac joints and spine of patients with psoriatic arthritis. Ann Rheum Dis 27: 1
821. Jandl JH (1985) Blood. Textbook of hematology. Grune and Stratton, Orlando
822. Jasin HE (1985) Autoantibody specifics of immune complexes sequestered in articular cartilage of patients with rheumatoid arthritis and osteoarthritis. Arthritis Rheum 28: 241
823. Jayson MIV, Barks JS (1973) Structural changes in the intervertebral disc. Ann Rheum Dis 32: 10
824. Jensen PS (1976) Hemochromatosis: a disease often silent, but not invisible. Am J Roentgenol 126: 343
825. Jergesen HE, Mankin HJ, Schiller AL (1978) Diffuse pigmented villonodular synovitis mimicking primary bone neoplasm. J Bone Joint Surg [Am] 60: 825
826. Jimenea CV, Frame B, Chaykin LB et al. (1971) Spondylitis of hyperparathyroidism. Clin Orthop 74: 84
827. Johansen PE, Sylvest O (1961) Synovial fluid changes in degenerative joint disease, rheumatoid arthritis, and traumatic arthritis. Acta Rheumatol Scand 7: 240
828. Johanson NA (1985) Endocrine arthropathies. Clin Rheum Dis 11: 297
829. John JT, Haugh RJ, Sergent JS (1979) Pericardial disease in rheumatoid arthritis. Am J Med 66: 385
830. Johnson JT (1967) Neuropathic fractures and joint injuries. J Bone Joint Surg [Am] 49: 1
831. Johnson LL (1986) Diagnostic and surgical arthroscopy. Mosby, St. Louis
832. Johnson RG, Simmons EH (1982) Discoid medial meniscus. Clin Orthop 167: 176
833. Johnson RP, Brower B (1985) Chondromalacia patellae. In: McCarty DJ (ed) Arthritis and allied conditions. Lea and Febiger, Philadelphia
834. Johnston RB (1978) Oxygen metabolism and the microbicidal activity of macrophages. Fed Proc 37: 2759
835. Johnston YE, Duray PH, Steere AC et al. (1985) Lyme arthritis spirochetes found in synovial microangiopathic lesions. Am J Pathol 118: 26
836. Jones JRJr (1971) Alcoholism, hypercorticism, fat embolism, and osseous avascular necrosis. In: Zinn WN (ed) Idiopathic ischemic necrosis of the femoral head in adults. Thieme, Stuttgart
837. Jones VE, Jacoby RH, Wallington T et al. (1981) Immune complexes in early arthritis. Clin Exp Pathol 44: 512
838. Jordan HH (1958) Hemophilic arthropathies. Thomas, Springfield
839. Jordan WR (1936) Neuritic manifestations in diabetes mellitus. Arch Intern Med 57: 307
840. Josefsson PO, Genta CF, Johnell O et al. (1987) Surgical versus nonsurgical treatment of ligamentous injuries following dislocation of the elbow joint. J Bone Joint Surg [Am] 69: 605

841. Kahn MF, Baillet F, Amouroux J et al. (1972) Le rhumatisme inflammatoire subaigu de la syphilis secondaire. Rev Rhum Mal Osteoartic 37: 431
842. Kahn RL, McDermott EB (1948) Studies on cardiolipin antigen. J Lab Clin Med 33: 1220
843. Kalbak K (1947) Agglutination of hemolytic streptococci (group A) in serum from patients with rheumatoid arthritis. Ann Rheum Dis 6: 230
844. Kalliomaki JL, Halonen P, Salmi A (1975) Virus antibodies in serum and synovial fluid of patients with rheumatoid arthritis and other connective tissue diseases. Ann Rheum Dis 34: 43
845. Kammer GM, Soto AN, Gibson DJ et al. (1979) Psoriatic arthritis: a clinical immunologic and HLA study of 100 patients. Semin Arthritis Rheum 9: 75
846. Kantor TG (1976) Antiinflammatory drugs. In: Miescher PA, Mueller-Eberhard HJ (eds) Textbook of immunopathology. Grune and Stratton, New York
847. Kantor TG (1984) Peripherally acting analgesics. In: Kuhar M, Pasternak G (eds) Analgesics: neurochemical, behavioral and clinical perspectives. Raven, New York
848. Kantor TG (1987) Current modalities in arthritic diseases. Am J Med 83 (suppl 4 B): 2
849. Kantor TG (1988) New strategies for the use of antiinflammatory agents. In: Dubner R, Gebhart SF, Bond MR (eds) Proceedings of the 5th world congress on pain. Elsevier, Amsterdam
850. Kaplan D, Meyer K (1959) Aging of human cartilage. Nature 183: 1267
851. Kaplan EB (1968) The etiology and treatment of epicondylitis. Bull Hosp Jt Dis 29: 77
852. Kaplan EL, Top FH, Dudding BA et al. (1971) Diagnosis of streptococcal pharyngitis. Differentiation of active infection from the carrier state in the symptomatic child. J Infect Dis 123: 490
853. Kappis M (1920) Über Bau, Wachstum und Ursprung der Gelenkmäuse. Dtsch Z Chir 157: 214
854. Karlson L (1940) Chondromalacia patellae. Acta Chir Scand 83: 847
855. Karr RW, Rodey GL, Lee T et al. (1980) Association of

HLA-D2 with rheumatoid arthritis in black and white patients. Arthritis Rheum 23: 1241
856. Karten I, Bartfeld H (1972) Bronchogenic carcinoma simulating early rheumatoid arthritis. JAMA 179: 162
857. Kassan SS, Gardy M (1978) Sjoegren's syndrome: an update and overview. Am J Med 64: 1037
858. Kastert J (1957) Die Spondylitis Tuberculosa und ihre Behandlung. Hippokrates, Stuttgart
859. Kaufer H (1979) Patellar biomechanics. Clin Orthop 144: 51
860. Kaufer H, Mathews LS (1985) Spherocentric arthroplasty of the knee. J Bone Joint Surg [Am] 63: 545
861. Kauffman CA, Watanakunakorn C, Phaer JP (1976) Pneumococcal arthritis. J Rheumatol 3: 409
862. Kaufman L, Kaplan W (1961) Preparation of a fluorescent antibody specific for the yeast phase of histoplasma capsulatum. J Bacteriol 82: 729
863. Kawamura A (1977) Fluorescent antibody techniques and their applications. University Park Press, Baltimore
864. Kay L, Stainsby D, Buzzard B et al. (1981) The role of synovectomy in the management of recurrent hemarthrosis in hemophilia. Br J Haematol 49: 53
865. Keenan JD, Matz CW (1982) Brucella spondylitis. Clin Orthop 82: 87
866. Keil H (1938) The rheumatic erythemas: a critical survey. Ann Intern Med 11: 2223
867. Keiser H, Ruben EL, Wolinski E et al. (1968) Clinical forms of gonococcal arthritis. N Engl J Med 279: 234
868. Kelley WN, Greene ML, Rosenbloom JF et al. (1969) Hypoxanthine-guanine phosphoribosyl transferase deficiency in gout. Ann Intern Med 70: 155
869. Kelley WN, Wyngaarden JB (1983) Clinical syndromes associated with hypoxanthine-guanine phosphoribosyl transferase deficiency. In: Steinberg JB, Wyngaarden JB, Fredrickson WS (eds) The metabolic basis of inherited diseases. McGraw Hill, New York
870. Kelley WN, Fox IH (1985) Gout and related disorders of purine metabolism. In: Kelley WN, Harris ED, Ruddy S, Sledge CB (eds) Textbook of rheumatology. Saunders, Philadelphia
871. Kellgren JH, Samuel EP (1950) The sensitivity and innervation of the articular capsule. J Bone Joint Surg [Br] 32: 84
872. Kellgren JH, Moore R (1952) Generalized osteoarthritis and Heberden's nodes. Br Med J 1: 181
873. Kellgren JH, Ball J, Tutton GR (1952) The articular and other limb changes in acromegaly. Q J Med 21: 405
874. Kellner G, Klein G (1976) Richtlinien zur Synovialzytologie. Z Rheumatol 35: 141
875. Kelly PJ, Marton WJ, Scheriger A et al. (1960) Brucellosis of the bones and joints: experience with thirty-six patients. JAMA 174: 347
876. Kelly R (1971) Cultivation of Borrelia hermsii. Science 173: 443
877. Kendall MJ, Lawrence DS, Shuttleworth GR (1973) Haematology and biochemistry of ankylosing spondylitis. Br Med J 2: 235
878. Kennedy JF (1976) Chemical and biochemical aspects of the glycosaminoglycans and proteoglycans in health and disease. Adv Clin Chem 18: 1
879. Kerr WR, Bryne DJH, Robertson L et al. (1967) Immunoglobulin class of brucella antibodies in human sera. Immunology 13: 223
880. Kersley G (1950) Rheumatic diseases. Heineman, London
881. Kettunen KO (1959) Cartilaginous metaplasia of connective tissue in clinical skin arthroplasty. Acta Orthop Scand 28: 190
882. Key JA (1925) The reformation of synovial membrane in the knees of rabbits after synovectomy. J Bone Joint Surg 7: 793
883. Key JA, Large AM (1942) Histoplasmosis of the knee. J Bone Joint Surg 24: 281
884. Khan MA, Khan MK (1982) Diagnostic value of HLA-B27 testing in ankylosing spondylitis and Reiter's syndrome. Ann Intern Med 96: 70
885. King ES (1937) The pathology of ganglion. Aust N Z J Surg 1: 637
886. King ESJ (1952) Tissue differentiation in malignant synovial tumors. J Bone Joint Surg [Br] 34: 97
887. King JW, Spjut HG, Fechner RE et al. (1967) Synovial chondrosarcoma of the knee joint. J Bone Joint Surg [Am] 49: 1389
888. Kinsella RA, Beck DF (1968) Thyroid acropathy. Med Clin North Am 52: 395
889. Kinsella TD, Norton WL, Ziff M (1968) Complement fixing antibodies to bedsonia organisms in Reiter's syndrome and ankylosing spondylitis. Ann Rheum Dis 27: 240
890. Kinsella TD, Bauer J, Ziff M (1969) Immunofluorescent demonstration of IgG-BIC complex in synovial lining cells of rheumatoid synovial membrane. Clin Exp Immunol 4: 265
891. Kinsella TD, Baum J, Ziff M (1970) Studies of isolated synovial lining cells of rheumatoid and non-rheumatoid synovial membrane. Arthritis Rheum 13: 734
892. Kippen AA, Loeb L (1930) The effect of gonadectomy on the thyroid gland in the guinea pig. Endocrinology 20: 201
893. Kirkaldy-Willis WH (1958) Arthrodesis of the hip with staple fixation. J Bone Joint Surg [Am] 40: 114
894. Kitchens CS (1982) Computed tomography in two cases of hemophilic pseudotumor. Am J Hematol 12: 277
895. Klein G, Rainer F (1977) Herzmanifestationen bei rheumatischen Erkrankungen. Wien. Med Wochenschr 4: 132
896. Klein W, Huth F (1974) The ultrastructure of malignant synovioma. Beitr Pathol Anat All Pathol 153: 194
897. Klein W, Steinhaus M (1979) Angiomaehnliche Dysplasie der Synovialmembran. Z Orthop 116: 394
898. Klein W, Schulitz KP (1981) Outpatient arthroscopy under local anesthesia. Arch Orthop Surg 96: 131
899. Klestov AC, Webb J, Latt D et al. (1981) Treatment of xerostomia: a double blind trial in 108 patients with Sjoegren's syndrome. Oral Surg Oral Med Oral Pathol 51: 594
900. Klinenberg JR (1984) Current concepts in rheumatoid arthritis. Orthop Rev 13: 245
901. Klinge F (1933) Der Rheumatismus. Bergman, Munich
902. Kluge R, Schmidt M, Barth WF (1973) Pneumococcal arthritis. Ann Rheum Dis 32: 21
903. Knight RA, Van Zandl IL (1952) Arthroplasty of the elbow: an end result study. J Bone Joint Surg [Am] 34: 610
904. Knox WE (1958) Sir Archibald Garrod's inborn errors of metabolism: II. Alkaptonuria. Am J Hum Genet 10: 95
905. Kobayashi I, Ziff M (1975) Electron microscopic studies of the cartilagepannus junction in rheumatoid arthritis. Arthritis Rheum 18: 475
906. König F (1887) Über freie Körper in Gelenken. Dtsch Z Chir 20: 97
907. König F (1923) Reaktive Vorgänge am Knorpel nach verschiedenen Schädigungen. Arch Klin Chir 124: 1
908. Koenigsberg M, Freeman L (1976) Radionuclide bone imaging. Curr Probl Diagn Radiol 6: 1
909. Koopman WJ (1985) Genetic control of immune responses, in: Kelley WN, Harris ED, Ruddy S, Sledge CB (eds) Textbook of rheumatology. Saunders, Philadelphia
910. Koopman WJ, Schrohenloher RE (1985) Rheumatoid factor. In: Utsinger PD, Zvaifler NJ, Ehrlich GE (eds) Rheumatoid arthritis. Lippincott, Philadelphia
911. Koopman WJ, Schrohenloher RE, Crago SS et al. (1985) IgA rheumatoid factor synthesis by dissociated synovial cells. Arthritis Rheum 28: 1219
912. Kornberg M (1983) Neuropathic arthropathy. Orthop Rev 12: 45

913. Krane SM (1975) Collagenase production by human synovial tissues. Ann N Y Acad Sci 256: 289
914. Kremer D, Deodhar SD, Dick WC (1973) A function of the synovial membrane of normal and diseased humans in relation to the movement of small molecular weight ions. Clin Sci Mol Med 44: 611
915. Krey PR, Comerford FR, Cohen AS (1974) Multicentric reticulohistiocytosis. Fine structural analysis of the synovium and synovial fluid cells. Arthritis Rheum 17: 615
916. Krey PR, Bailen DA (1979) Synovial fluid leukocytes. A study of extremes. Am J Med 67: 436
917. Kudo H, Iwano K, Watanabe S (1980) Total replacement of the rheumatoid elbow with a hingeless prosthesis. J Bone Joint Surg [Am] 62: 277
918. Kudoh T, Wenger DA (1982) Diagnosis of metachromatic leukodystrophy, Krabbe disease and Farber's disease after uptake of fatty acid labeled cerebroside sulfate into cultured skin fibroblasts. J Clin Invest 70: 89
919. Kuehne W (1965) Beitrag zur Klinik der Calcinosis interstitialis universalis. Z Orthop 99: 473
920. Kummerle F, Wessinghage D, Schweikert CH (1971) Risks of alloplastic replacements in degenerative and inflammatory diseases of joints. Acta Orthop Belg 37: 541
921. Kushi Y, Rokakawa C, Handa S (1988) Direct analysis of glycolipids in glycolipid storage disorders. Anal Biochem 175: 167
922. Kushner I (1985) Acute phase reactants. In: Kelley WN, Harris ED, Ruddy S, Sledge CB (eds) Textbook of rheumatology. Saunders, Philadelphia
923. Kutty MK, Iqbal QM (1973) Ochronotic arthropathy. A comparative study of light microscopic and ultrastructural features. Arch Pathol 96: 100
924. Kyle AR (1982) Plasma cell disorders. In: Newcom SR, Kadin ME (eds) Hematologic malignancies in the adult. Addison-Wesley, Menlo Park
925. Kyriazis AP, Tsaltas TT (1971) Changes in the chemical composition of ear cartilage matrix after administration of various hormones. Am J Pathol 63: 149

926. Lacey A (1980) Lacey total knee. Data Sheet L095-0009. Dow Corning Wright
927. Lacheretz M (1953) Traitement des ankyloses. Rev Chir Orthop 39, 495, 1953
928. Lachiewicz PF, Lane TM, Wilson PD (1981) Total hip replacement in Gaucher's disease. J Bone Joint Dis [Am] 63: 602
929. Ladd JR, Cassidy JT, Martel W (1971) Juvenile ankylosing spondylitis. Arthritis Rheum 14: 579
930. LaDu BN (1960) Alkaptonuria. In: by Stanbury JB, Wyngaarden JB, Fredrickson DS, (eds) The metabolic bases of inherited disease. McGraw-Hill, New York
931. LaDu BN, Zannoni VG, Laster L et al. (1958) The nature of the defect in thyrosine metabolism in alkaptonuria. J Biol Chem 230: 251
932. Laewen A (1925) Knorpelresektion bei fissuraler Knorpeldegeneration der Patella – eine Frühoperation der Arthritis deformans. Beitr Klin Chir 134: 265
933. Laewen A (1928) Zur Behandlung chronischer und rezidivierender Kniegelenkergüsse. Ref Zentralorg Chir 37: 829
934. Lakha S (1983) Immune complexes. Clin Rheum Dis 9: 199
935. Lambert JR, Wright V (1977) Psoriatic spondylosis: a clinical and radio logical description of the spine in psoriatic arthritis. Q J Med 46: 411
936. Lancefield RC (1928) The antigenic complex of streptococcus hemolyticus: II. Chemical and immunological properties of the protein fractions. J Exp Med 47: 469
937. Land MA, Bisno AL (1983) Acute rheumatic fever: a vanishing disease in suburbia. JAMA 249: 895
938. Landells JW (1957) The reactions of injured human articular cartilage. J Bone Joint Surg [Br] 39: 548
939. Lane ME (1984) Recent developments in the electrodiagnosis of radiculopathies. Bull Hosp Jt Dis 44: 56
940. Langness U, Banavsky D, Akropoulos J et al. (1971) Differentiation of inflammation and ossification in spondylarthritis ankylopoetica. Acta Rheum Scand 17: 15
941. Lannigan R, Zaki SA (1967) Ultrastructure of lesions of rheumatic carditis. J Pathol Bacteriol 93: 449
942. Lansbury J, Crosby W, Bello C (1950) Precipitation reaction of serum from rheumatoid arthritis with homologous connective tissue extract. Am J Med Sci 22: 414
943. Lunseth PA, Herple KG (1979) Prognosis in septic arthritis of the hips in children. Clin Orthop 139: 81
944. Lanyi VF (1988) Rehabilitation management in arthritis and related disorders. In: Goodgold J (ed). Rehabilitation medicine. Mosby, St. Louis
945. Larmon WA (1965) Pigmented villonodular synovitis. Med Clin North Am 49: 141
946. Larmon WA, Kurtz JF (1958) The surgical management of chronic tophaceous gout. J Bone Joint Surg [Am] 40: 743
947. Larson HE, Nicholson KG, Loewi G et al. (1977) Arthritis after meningococcal meningitis. Br Med J 1: 618
948. Laurent MR, Panayi GS, Sheppard O (1981) Circulating immune complexes serum in immunoglobulins, and acute phase proteins in psoriasis and psoriatic arthritis. Ann Rheum Dis 40: 66
949. Laurin CA, Desmarchais J, Dariano L et al. (1974) Long term results of synovectomy of the knee in rheumatoid patients. J Bone Joint Surg [Am] 56: 521
950. Lawrence HS (1973) Mediators of cellular immunity. Transplant Proc 5: 49
951. Lawrence JS (1974) Family survey of Reiter's disease. Brit J Vener Dis 50: 140
952. Layani F, May V, Pelisson J et al. (1959) Arthropathies hemophiliques. Rev Rhum Mal Osteoartic 26: 463
953. Leczinsky CG (1948) The incidence of arthropathy in a ten year survey of psoriasis cases. Acta Derm Venereol Scand 28: 483
954. Lee P, Roonig PJ, Sturrock RD et al. (1974) The etiology and pathogenesis of osteoarthritis. Semin Arthritis Rheum 3: 189
955. Lee REJ, Golding JSR, Serjeant GR (1981) The radiological features of avascular necrosis of the femoral head in homozygous sickle cell disease. Clin Radiol 32: 205
956. Leirisalo M, Skylo G, Kousa M et al. (1982) Follow-up studies on patients with Reiter's disease and reactive arthritis with special reference to HLA-B27. Arthritis Rheum 25: 249
957. Lejars F, Rubens-Duval H (1910) Les sarcomes primitives des sinoviales articulaires. Rev Chir 13: 290
958. Lemaire V, Peltier A, Jouvent C et al. (1981) Resultats de l'examen cytologique du liquide synoviale dans diverses arthropathies. Rev Rhum Mal Osteoartic 48: 229
959. Lemaire V, Ryckewaert A (1981) Monoarthrites Brucelliennes chroniques des membres en dehors de la coxite. Rev Rhum Mal Osteoartic 48: 149
960 Lennhoff C (1948) Spirochaetes in aetiologically obscure diseases. Acta Derm Venerol 28: 295
961. Lepow ML, Gold R (1977) Further conquest of the meningococcus. N Engl J Med 297: 721
962. Leppelman HJ (1959) Der Mukopolysaccharidgehalt des Knorpels in Abhängigkeit von Lebensalter. Z Rheumaforsch 18: 348
963. Leriche R (1931) A propos des osteomes metatraumatiques paracondyliens internes du femur. Bull Soc Chir Paris 57: 737
964. Lever JD, Ford EHR (1958) Histological, histochemical and electron microscopical observations on synovial membrane. Anat Rec 132: 523

965. Levin B (1961) Gaucher's disease. Clinical and roentgenological manifestations. Am J Roentgenol 85: 685
966. Levin M, Pras M, Franklin EC (1973) Immunologic studies of the major nonimmunoglobulins of amyloid. J Exp Med 138: 373
967. Levin ME, Borisseau VC, Avioli LV (1976) Diabetes mellitus and bone mass in juvenile and adult onset diabetes. N Engl J Med 294: 241
968. Levine DB (1989) The painful back. In: McCarty DJ (ed) Arthritis and Allied conditions. Lea and Febiger, Philadelphia
969. Levinsky WJ (1972) Sporotrichial arthritis. Arch Intern Med 129: 118
970. Levinson DJ, Silcox DC, Rippon JW et al. (1974) Septic arthritis due to non-encapsulated cryptococcus neoformans with coexisting sarcoidosis. Arthritis Rheum 17: 1037
971. Levinson JE (1981) Gold salts in the rheumatic disease. In: Moore JD (ed) Arthritis in childhood. Ross Laboratories, Columbus
972. Levy M, Ehrenfels M, Levy J et al. (1980) Circulating immune complexes in recurrent polyserositis (familial Mediterranean fever). J Rheumatol 7: 886
973. Lewis G, Holstein A (1960) End results study in patellectomy. Bull Hosp Jt Dis 21: 71
974. Lewis JL, Rabinovich S (1972) The wide spectrum of cryptococcal infections. Am J Med 53: 315
975. Lewis RB (1982) The absence of reactive arthritis after Shigella Sonnei infection. Arthritis Rheum 25: 1267
976. Lewison M, Jackson H (1914) A case of systemic blastomycosis. Arch Intern Med 13: 575
977. Lichtenstein L, Kaplan L (1954) Hereditary ochronosis. Pathologic changes observed in two necropsied cases. Am J Pathol 30: 99
978. Lifeso RM, Harder E, McCorkell SJ (1985) Spinal Brucellosis. J Bone Joint Surg [Br] 67: 345
979. Lightfoot LW (1989) Treatment of rheumatoid arthritis. In McCarty DJ (ed) Arthritis and allied conditions. Lea and Febiger, Philadelphia
980. Lindberg RD, Martin RG, Romsdahl MM et al. (1981) Conservative surgery and postoperative radiation therapy in 300 adults with soft tissue sarcoma. Cancer 47: 2391
980 b. Lindblad S, Hedfors E (1987) Arthroscopic and immunohistologic characterization of knee joint synovitis in osteoarthritis. Arthritis Rheum 30: 1081
980 c. Lindblad S, Wredmark T (1990) Traumatic synovitis analyzed by arthroscopy and immunohistopathology Br J Rheumatol 29: 422
981. Linden B (1977) Osteochondritis dissecans of the femoral condyles. J Bone Joint Surg [Am] 59: 769
982. Lindholm S, Pylkaenen P (1977) Recurrent effusions in the synovectomized knee joint. Scand J Rheumatol 6: 11
983. Lindholm TS, Osterman K, Vankka E (1981) Osteochondritis dissecans of the elbow, ankle and hip. Clin Orthop 148: 245
984. Lindner J, Grasedyck K, Bartelheimer H (1979) Der Stellenwert der Morphologie in der Diagnostik der chronischen Polyarthritis. Z Rheumatol 38: 189
985. Lindsley CB (1981) Pharmacotherapy of juvenile rheumatoid arthritis. Pediatr Clin North Am 28: 161
986. Ling CM, Overby LR (1972) Prevalence of hepatitis B virus antigen as revealed by direct radioimmune assay with I-antibody. J Immunol 109: 834
987. Loeb JN (1976) Corticosteroids and growth. N Engl J Med 295: 547
988. Lowe LW, Miller AJ, Allum RL et al. (1984) The development of an unconstrained elbow arthroplasty. J Bone Joint Surg [Br] 66: 243
989. Lubarsch O (1950) Quoted in Pack, GT, Ariel, IM (1950) Synovial sarcoma. Surgery 28: 1047
990. Luck JV Jr (1985) Surgical management of advanced hemophilic arthropathy. In: Doehring S, Schulitz KP (eds) Orthopaedic problems in hemophilia. Zuckschwerdt, München
991. Lustberg FJ, Schulman JD, Seegmiller JE (1970) Decreased binding of C-homogentisic acid induced by ascorbic acid in connective tissue of rats with experimental alcaptonuria. Nature 228: 770
992. Lutzker LG, Alave R (1976) Bone and marrow imaging in sickle cell disease. Diagnosis of infarction. Semin Nucl Med 6: 83
993. Lyell A, Carr AJ (1959) Lipoid dermatoarthritis (reticulohistiocytosis). Br J Dermatol 71: 12
994. Lynch M, Jayson ML (1979) Fasciitis and fibrosis. Clin Rheum Dis 5: 833

995. Ma SM, Kabo JM, Amstutz HC (1983) Frictional torque in surface and conventional hip replacement. J Bone Joint Surg [Am] 65: 366
996. MacDonald RA (1964) Hemochromatosis and hemosiderosis. Thomas, Springfield
997. Mach RS, Bruegger Y, Della Santa R, et al. (1950) L'hormone hypophysaire corticotrope. Schweiz Med Wochenschr 80: 5
998. MacIntosh DL (1971) Arthroplasty of the knee in rheumatoid arthritis using the hemiarthroplasty prosthesis. In: Cruess RS, Mitchell NS (eds) Surgery of rheumatoid arthritis, Lippincott, Philadelphia
999. MacIntosh DL, Hunter G (1972) The use of the hemi-arthroplasty prosthesis for the knee. J Bone Joint Surg [Br] 54: 244
1000. Mackenzie DH (1981) The myxoid tumors of somatic soft tissues. Am J Surg Pathol 5: 443
1001. Macrae I, Wright V (1973) A family study of ulcerative colitis and particular reference to ankylosing spondylitis and sacroileitis. Ann Rheum Dis 32: 16
1002. Maggio ET, Nakamura RM (1981) Immunology: current and future technology assessment. Clin Lab Med 1: 77
1003. Magnuson PB (1941) Joint debridement; surgical treatment of degenerative arthritis. Surg Gynecol Obstet 73: 1
1004. Maibach E (1953) Histochemische Untersuchungen an der Synovialmembran als Beitrag zum Problem der Herkunft der Synovia. Acta Anat (Basel) 17: 175
1005. Mainardi CL, Levine PH, Werb Z et al. (1978) Proliferative synovitis in hemophilia. Biochemical and morphologic observations. Arthritis Rheum 21: 137
1006. Mainardi CL, Levine PH (1985) Hemophilia and arthritis. In: Kelley WN, Harris ED, Ruddy S, Sledge CB (eds) Textbook of rheumatology. Saunders, Philadelphia
1007. Makin M, Robin GC (1964) Chronic synovial effusion treated with intraarticular radioactive gold. JAMA 188: 725
1008. Makin M, Levin S (1965) The articular manifestations of periodic disease (familial Mediterranean fever). J Bone Joint Surg [Am] 47: 1615
1009. Malcolm AJ (1983) Diagnostic pathology in rheumatology. Clin Rheum Dis 9: 27
1010. Malek J, Brodkin R (1973) Multicentric reticulohistiocytosis with extensive bone and joint destruction. NY State J Med 73: 2487
1011. Malemud CJ, Moskowitz RW (1981) Physiology of articular cartilage. Clin Rheum Dis 7: 29
1012. Mallinger R, Geleff S, Boeck P (1985) Histochemistry of glycosaminoglycans in cartilage ground substance. Histochemistry 85: 121
1013. Mallinger R, Stockinger L (1987) Histochemistry of the extracellular matrix of aging hyaline cartilage. Folia Histochemcytobiol 25: 129
1014. Manicourt DH, Orloff S (1982) Gonococcal arthritis-dermatitis syndrome. Arthritis Rheum 25: 574

1015. Mandell GL, Douglas RG, Bennett JE (1990) Principles and practices of infectious diseases. Churchill-Livingstone, New York
1016. Mankin HJ (1974) The reaction of articular cartilage to injury and osteoarthritis. N Engl J Med 291: 1285
1017. Mankin HJ (1981) Symposium – can cartilage heal. Contemp Orthop 3: 138
1018. Mankin HJ, Zarins A, Jaffe NL (1972) The effect of systemic corticosteroids in rabbit articular cartilage. Arthritis Rheum 15: 593
1019. Mankin HJ, Trasher AL (1975) Water content and binding in normal and osteoarthritic human cartilage. J Bone Joint Surg [Am] 57: 76
1020. Mankin HJ, Johnson ME, Lipiello L (1981) Biochemical and metabolic abnormalities in articular cartilage from osteoarthritic human hips. J Bone Joint Surg [Am] 63: 131
1021. Mannik M (1989) Characteristics of immune complexes and principles of immune complex diseases. In: McCarty DJ (ed) Arthritis and allied conditions. Lea and Febiger, Philadelphia
1022. Mansat C, Mansat M, Duroubean L et al. (1978) Osteochondrite dissequante du genou. Rev Rhum Mal Osteoartic 45: 177
1023. Manthorpe R, Frost-Larsen K, Isager H et al (1981) Sjoegren's syndrome. A review with emphasis on immunological features. Allergy 36: 139
1024. Maquet P (1979) Mechanics and osteoarthritis of the patellofemoral joint. Clin Orthop 144: 70
1025. Marchildon A, Slonim RR, Brown HW et al. (1963) Primary septic bursitis. J Fla Med Assoc 50: 139
1026. Margolis HM (1941) Diagnosis and treatment of arthritis and allied disorders. Hoeber, New York
1027. Margolis HM, Caplan R (1951) Effect of pituitary adrenocorticotropic hormone ACTH in rheumatoid arthritis. JAMA 145: 381
1028. Marie P (1886) Sur deux cas d'acromegalie. Rev Med 6: 29
1029. Marks MI (1985) Pediatric infectious diseases. Springer, Berlin Heidelberg New York
1030. Marmor L (1968) Surgery for rheumatoid arthritis. Am J Surg 115: 630
1031. Marmor L (1976) The modular (Marmor) knee. Case report with a minimum follow-up of two years. Clin Orthop 120: 86
1032. Marmor L (1977) Total knee replacement in hemophilia. Clin Orthop 125: 192
1033. Marmor L, Chan KP, Ho KC et al. (1967) Surgical treatment of tuberculosis of the hip in children. Clin Orthop 67: 133
1034. Maroudas A (1976) Balance between swelling, pressure and collagen tension in normal and degenerated cartilage. Nature 260: 808
1035. Maroudas A (1979) Physiochemical properties of articular cartilage. In: Freeman MAR (ed) Adult articular cartilage. Pitman Medical, Kent
1036. Maroudas A, Bayliss MT, Venn MF (1980) Further studies on the composition of human femoral head cartilage. Ann Rheum Dis 39: 514
1037. Martel W, Braunstein E, Barbara G et al. (1979) Radiologic features of Reiter's disease. Radiology 132: 1
1038. Martel W, Holt JF, Cassidy JT (1982) Roentgenologic manifestations in juvenile rheumatoid arthritis. Am J Roentgenol 88: 400
1039. Martin E (1961) Les arthropathies endocriniennes. Med Hyg 19: 1023
1040. Marti GE, Ryan MM, Papadopoulos NM et al. (1988) Polyclonal B-lymphocytes and hypergammaglobulinemia in patients with Gaucher disease. Am J Hematol 29: 189
1041. Marzouk JB (1986) Lyme disease and arthritis. J Musculoskel Med 3: 12
1042. Masi AT, Eisenstein BI (1981) Disseminated gonococcal infection (DGI) and gonococcal arthritis (GCA): II. Clinical manifestations, diagnosis, complications, treatment, and prevention. Semin Arthritis Rheum 10: 173
1043. Mason AMS, Gumpel JM, Golding RL (1973) Sjoegren's syndrome – a clinical review. Semin Arthritis Rheum 2: 301
1044. Mason RM (1986) Ankylosing spondylitis. In: Scott, JW (ed) Copeman's textbook of rheumatic diseases. Churchill Livingstone, Edinburgh
1045. Mason RM, Murray RS, Oates JK et al. (1959) A comparative radiological study of Reiter's disease, rheumatoid arthritis and ankylosing spondylitis. J Bone Joint Surg [Br] 41: 137
1046. Massias P, Letournel E, Evrard J et al. (1981) Place de la chirurgie dans le traitement des infections pyogenes. Rev Rhum Mal Osteoartic 48: 213
1047. Masson P (1927) Le glomus neuromyo-arteriel des regions tactiles et ses tumeurs. Lyon Chir 21: 257
1048. Matzner Y (1987) Complement in the pathophysiology of human disease. Engl J Med 317: 1542
1049. Mayer L, Burman M (1939) Arthroscopy in the diagnosis of meniscal lesions of the knee joint. Am J Surg 43: 501
1050. Mayer M (1950) Über das Ganglion. Helv Chir Acta 17: 155
1051. McCarty DJ (1989) Synovial fluid. In: McCarty DJ (ed) Arthritis and allied conditions. Lea and Febiger, Philadelphia
1052. McCarty DJ, Silcox DL, Jacobelli S et al. (1974) Diseases associated with calcium pyrophosphate dihydrate crystal deposition: a controlled study. Am J Med 56: 704
1053. McCarty DJ, Carrero GT (1982) Treatment of intractable rheumatoid arthritis with combined cyclophosphamide, azathioprine and hydrooxychloroquine. JAMA 248: 1718
1054. McCarty DJ, Halverson P (1985) Basic calcium phosphate (apatite orthocalcium phosphate, tricalcium phosphate) crystal deposition diseases. In: McCarty DJ (ed) Arthritis and allied conditions. Lea and Febiger, Philadelphia
1055. McClure J, Smith OS, Gramp AA (1983) Calcium pyrophosphate dihydrate (CPPD) in ochronotic arthropathy. J Clin Pathol 36: 894
1056. McCollough NC, Enis JE, Loot J et al. (1979) Synovectomy or total replacement of knee in hemophilia. J Bone Joint Surg [Am] 61: 69
1057. McCutchen CW (1981) Joint lubrication. Clin Rheum Dis 7: 241
1058. McDevitt HO (1985) Genetic structure and functions of the major histocompatibility complex. In: McCarty DJ (ed) Arthritis and allied conditions. Lea and Febiger, Philadelphia
1059. McDanald EC, Weisman MH (1978) Articular manifestations of rheumatic fever in adults. Ann Intern Med 89: 917
1060. McDuffie FC, Bunch TW (1976) Immunologic tests in the diagnosis of rheumatic diseases. Bull Rheum Dis 27: 900
1061. McEvedy BV (1954) The simple ganglion: a review of modes of treatment and an explanation of the frequent failures of surgery. Lancet 266: 135
1062. McEwen C (1968) Arthritis accompanying ulcerative colitis. Clin Orthop 57: 9
1063. McEwen C, Ziff M, Carmel P et al. (1958) The relationship to rheumatoid arthritis of its so-called variants. Arthritis Rheum 1: 481
1064. McEwen C, DiTata D, Lingg C et al. (1971) Ankylosing spondylitis and spondylitis accompanying ulcerative colitis, regional ileitis, psoriasis and Reiter's disease. Arthritis Rheum 14: 291
1065. McGahan JP, Graves DS, Palmer PES et al. (1981) Classic and contemporary imaging of coccidioidomycosis. Am J Roentgenol 136: 393
1066. McGill PE, Grange AJ, Royston CSM (1984) Chondrocalcinosis in primary hyperparathyroidism. Scand J Rheumatol 13: 56

1067. McGinty JB (1979) Arthroscopy of the knee: update and review. Orthop Dig 7: 17
1068. McGuire JL (1989) Arthropathies associated with endocrine disorders. In: Kelley WN, Harris ED, Ruddy S, Sledge CB (eds) Textbook of rheumatology. Saunders, Philadelphia
1069. McKee GK (1957) Arthrodesis of the hip with a lagscrew. J Bone Joint Surg [Br] 39: 477
1070. McKee GK, Watson-Farrar J (1966) Replacement of arthritic hips by the McKee-Farrar prosthesis. J Bone Joint Surg [Br] 48: 245
1071. McKeever DC (1960) Tibial plateau prosthesis. Clin Orthop 18: 86
1072. McKusick VA (1972) Heritable disorders of connective tissue. Mosby, St. Louis
1073. McMaster MJ, Coventry MD (1973) Spinal osteotomy in ankylosing spondylitis. Technique, complications and long-term results. Mayo Clin Proc 48: 476
1074. McMaster PE, Gilfillan C (1939) Coccidioidal osteomyelitis. JAMA 112: 1233
1075. McMaster PE (1960) Pigmented villonodular synovitis with invasion of bone. J Bone Joint Surg [Am] 42: 1170
1076. McMichael AJ, Sasazubi T, McDevitt HO et al. (1977) Increased frequency of HLA-3C and HLA-DW4 in rheumatoid arthritis. Arthritis Rheum 20: 1037
1077. McMurray TP (1935) Osteoarthritis of the hip joint. Br J Surg 22: 716
1078. McNair P, Christiansen C, Christiansen MS et al. (1981) Development of bone mineral loss in insulin treated diabetes. Eur J Clin Invest 11: 55
1079. Meachim G (1969) Age changes in articular cartilage. Clin Orthop 54: 33
1080. Meachim G, Ghadially FN, Collins DH (1965) Regressive changes in the superficial layer of human articular cartilage. Ann Rheum Dis 24: 23
1081. Meachim G, Roberts C (1971) Repair of the joint surface from subarticular tissue in the rabbit knee. J Anat 109: 3
1082. Meachim G, Stockwell R (1979) The matrix. In: Freeman MAR (ed) Adult articular cartilage. Pitman Medical, Kent
1083. Meak G (1946) Rheumatische Erkrankungen und die Frage der Herde. Z Stomatol 43: 148
1084. Mejlszenkier JD, Safran AP, Healy JJ et al. (1973) Severe myositis of influenza. Arch Neurol 29: 441
1085. Melanotte PL (1964) Fiziopatologia del cartilagine articolare. 49th congress of the Società Italiana di Ortopedia e Traumatologia, Padua, 1964
1086. Melanotte PL (1978) Le sinovectomie nella emofilia. G It Ortop Traum 4: 171
1087. Melanotte PL, Ferracini B, Operti F (1956) Aspetti clinicopatologici di una forme di sinovite iperplastica nodosa. Riv Anat Pat Onc 11: 306
1088. Melanotte PL, Agostini S (1966) Necrosi idiopatica della testa femorale del' adulto. Clin Ortop 18: 131
1089. Melton JW, Irby R (1972) Multicentric reticulohistiocytosis. Arthritis Rheum 15: 221
1090. Meltzer M, Franklin EC, Elias K et al. (1966) Cryoglobulinemia – a clinical and laboratory study. Am J Med 40: 837
1091. Menezes AH, VanGilder JC, Graf CJ et al. (1980) Craniocervical abnormalities. A comprehensive surgical approach. J Neurosurg 53: 444
1092. Menge F (1924) Über Arthropathia ovaripriva. Zentralbl Gynokol 30: 1617
1093. Menninger H, Lambusch M, Mohr W et al. (1983) Immunkomplexe, Mediatoren für die Bildung von entzündlichem Granulationsgewebe. Z Rheumatol 42: 7
1094. Messner, RP (1985) Tuberculosis of joints. In: McCarty DJ (ed) Arthritis and allied conditions. Lea and Febiger, Philadelphia
1095. Metzger AL, Morris RI, Bluestone R et al. (1975) HLA-W27 in psoriatic arthropathy. Arthritis Rheum 18: 111
1096. Meyer GA (1985) Correction of arthritic deformities of the spine. In: McCarty DJ (ed) Arthritis and allied conditions. Lea and Febiger, Philadelphia
1097. Meyer K (1969) Biochemistry and biology of mucopolysaccharides. Am J Med 47: 664
1098. Meijers KAE, VanBueskon GT, Luyendigk W et al. (1974) Dislocation of the cervical spine with cord compression in rheumatoid arthritis. J Bone Joint Surg [Br] 56: 668
1099. Meynadier J, Guilhou JJ, Clot J et al. (1979) Pathogenie du psoriasis. Rev Rhum Mal Osteoartic 46: 529
1100. Miale JB (1977) Laboratory medicine, hematoloy. Mosby, St. Louis
1101. Michotte L, Herrard E (1955) La pathologie de la bourse sereuse sousrotulienne. Rev Rhum Mal Osteoartic 22: 665
1102. Middleton PJ, Alexander RM, Szymanski MJ (1970) Severe myositis during recovery from influenza. Lancet 2: 533
1103. Mielants H, Dhondt E, Goethals L et al. (1982) Long term functional results of the non-surgical treatment of common bacterial infection of joints. Scand J Rheumatol 11: 101
1104. Mikulicz J (1937/1938) Concerning peculiar symmetrical disease of lacrimal and salivary glands. Med Classics 2: 165
1105. Milgram JE (1947) Shoulder anatomy. American Academy of Orthopedic Surgery Instructional Course Lections vol 4. Edwards, Ann Arbor
1106. Milgram JW (1977) Synovial osteochondromatosis. A histologic study of 30 cases. J Bone Joint Surg [Am] 59: 792
1107. Milgram JW (1978) Radiological and pathological manifestations of osteochondritis dissecans of the distal femur. Radiology 126: 305
1108. Milgram JW (1983) Morphologic alterations of the subchondral bone in advanced degenerative arthritis. Clin Orthop 173: 293
1109. Millender LH, Nalebuff EA (1975) Reconstructive surgery in the rheumatoid hand. Orthop Clin North Am 6: 709
1110. Miller A, Friedman B (1952) Fascial arthroplasty of the knee. J Bone Joint Surg [Am] 34: 55
1111. Miller JJ, Freud JM (1977) Myocarditis in juvenile rheumatoid arthritis. Am J Dis Child 131: 205
1112. Miller JJ, Olds-Arroyo J, Akasaka T (1977) Antiglobulins in juvenile rheumatoid arthritis. Arthritis Rheum 20: 729
1113. Miller JL, Lewin P (1927) Evidence of the anaphylactic character of intermittent hydraarthrosis. JAMA 82: 1177
1114. Minear WL (1951) Xanthomatous joint tumors. J Bone Joint Surg [Am] 33: 451
1115. Mital MA, Willington PF (1970) Osseous pathway of nutrition to the articular cartilage of the human femoral head. Lancet 1: 842
1116. Mitchell DM, Tries JF (1982) An analysis of The American Rheumatism Association criteria for rheumatoid arthritis. Arthritis Rheum 85: 481
1117. Mitrovic DR (1983) Pathology of articular deposition of calcium salts and their relationship to osteoarthritis. Ann Rheum Dis 42: 19
1118. Mitrovic DR, Mazaroud D, Joffres R et al. (1966) Etude histologique et histochimique des lesions articulaires de la chondrocalcinose survenant au cours d'une hemochromatose. Arch Anat Pathol 14: 264
1119. Mitrovic DR, Stankovic A, Quintero M et al. (1985) Amyloid deposits in human knee and hip joints. Rheumatol Int 5: 83
1120. Moberger G, Nilsonne H, Friberg S (1968) Synovial sarcoma. Acta Orthop Scand Suppl 11:
1121. Moccia G (1937) La fenestrazione della capsule nel'idrartro cronico del ginocchio. Chir Organi Mov 22: 464
1122. Modic MT, Weinstein M, Pavlicek W et al. (1983) Nuclear magnetic resonance of the spine. Radiology 148: 757
1123. Mohing W (1960) Die Osteochondrosis dissecans des Kniegelenkes. Z Orthop 92: 543

1124. Mohing W (1969) Die Stellung der Synovektomie in der Behandlung chronisch entzündlicher und degenerativer Gelenkveränderungen. Z Orthop 104: 82
1125. Mohr W (1984) Gelenkkrankheiten, Diagnostik und Pathogenese makroskopischer und histologischer Struckturveränderungen. Thieme, Stuttgart
1126. Mohr W, Wessinghage D, Lendshau E (1980) Die Ultrastruktur in hyalinem Knorpel und Gelenkkapselgewebe bei der alkaptonurischen Ochronose. Z Rheumatol 39: 55
1127. Mohr W, Wessinghage D, Putzier R et al. (1980) Corpora oryzoidea (Reiskörperchen). Acta Rheumatol 5: 207
1128. Mohr W, Westerhellweg H, Wessinghage D (1981) Polymorphonuclear granulocytes in rheumatic tissue destruction: III. An electron microscopic study of polymorphonuclears at the pannus cartilage junction in rheumatoid arthritis. Ann Rheum Dis 40: 396
1129. Moll JMH (1979) The clinical spectrum of psoriatic arthritis. Clin Orthop 143: 66
1130. Moll JMH, Wright V (1973) New York clinical criteria for ankylosing spondylitis. Ann Rheum Dis 32: 354
1131. Moncada S, Vane JR (1979) Mode of actions of aspirin-like drugs. Adv Intern Med 24: 1
1132. Monghal JP, Dorfman H, Caroit M et al. (1981) Contribution à l'étude de la synovite villonodulaire du genou. Rev Rhum Mal Osteoartic 48: 397
1133. Montane I, McCullough NC, Chun-Yet Lian E (1986) Synovectomy of the knee for hemophilic arthropathy. J Bone Joint Surg [Am] 68: 210
1134. Moon KL, Genant HK, Helms CA et al. (1983) Musculoskeletal application of NMR. Radiology 147: 161
1135. Moore AT (1957) The self locking metal hip prosthesis. J Bone Joint Surg [Am] 39: 811
1136. Moore TL, Sheridan RW, Traycoff PP et al. (1982) Immune complexes in juvenile rheumatoid arthritis. J Rheumatol 9: 395
1137. Morcacci G (1951) Ginocchio a scatto extraarticulare. Minerva Ortop 11: 379
1138. Morgan CJ, Hendee WR (1984) Introduction to magnetic resonance imaging. Multi Media, Denver
1139. Morgan WS, Castleman B (1953) A clinicopathologic study of "Mikulicz's disease." Am J Pathol 29: 471
1140. Morrey BF, Bianco AJ, Rhodes KH (1975) Septic arthritis in children. Orthop Clin North Am 6: 923
1141. Morrey BF, Bryan RS, Dobyns JH et al. (1981) Total elbow arthroplasty: a five-year experience at the Mayo Clinic. J Bone Joint Surg [Am] 63: 1050
1142. Morton NE (1979) Genetics of hyperuricemia in families with gout. Am J Med Genet 4: 103
1143. Moseley JE (1963) Bone changes in hematologic disorders. Roentgen aspects. Grune and Stratton, New York
1144. Moskowitz RW (1979) Treatment of osteoarthritis. In: McCarty DJ (ed). Arthritis and allied conditions. Lea and Febiger, Philadelphia
1145. Moskowitz RW (1981) Management of ankylosing spondylitis. Bull Rheum Dis 31: 35
1146. Moskowitz RW (1989) Clinical and laboratory findings in osteoarthritis. In: McCarty DJ (ed). Arthritis and allied conditions. Lea and Febiger, Philadelphia
1147. Moskowitz RW, Harris BK, Schwartz A et al. (1971) Chronic synovitis as a manifestation of calcium crystal deposition disease. Arthritis Rheum 14: 109
1148. Moskowitz RW, Garcia F (1973) Chondrocalcinosis articularis (pseudogout syndrome). Arch Intern Med 132: 87
1149. Moskowitz RW, Goldberg VM, Schwab W et al. (1975) Effects of intraarticular corticosteroids and exercise in experimental models of inflammatory and degenerative arthritis. Arthritis Rheum 18: 417
1150. Mudge P (1974) Epidemic polyarthritis in South Australia. Med J Aust 2: 823
1151. Mueller F (1912) Differenzierung der chronischen Gelenkerkrankungen. Trans Int Congr Med (Lond) 17: 501
1152. Mueller ME (1970) Total hip prostheses. Clin Orthop 72: 46
1153. Mueller MN, Sorensen LB, Strandjord N et al. (1965) Alkaptonuria and ochronotic arthropathy. Med Clin North Am 49: 101
1154. Mueller W (1919) Die Pirquet Reaktion in Influenza Patienten. Dtsch Med Wochenschr 455: 853
1155. Muir H (1977) Heberden oration: molecular approach to the understanding of osteoarthrosis. Ann Rheum Dis 36: 199
1156. Muir H, Bullough P, Maroudas A (1970) The distribution of collagen in human articular cartilage with some of its physiological implications. J Bone Joint Surg [Br] 52: 554
1157. Muirden KD, Senator GB (1968) Iron in the synovial membrane in rheumatoid arthritis and other joint diseases. Ann Rheum Dis 27: 38
1158. Muller-Eberhard HJ (1975) Complement. Annu Rev Biochem 44: 697
1159. Munoz AJ (1978) Gonococcal and meningococcal arthritis. Clin Rheum Dis 4: 169
1160. Murphy FP, Dahlin VC, Sullivan CR (1962) Articular synovial chondromatosis. J Bone Joint Surg [Am] 44: 77
1161. Murphy GE (1963) The characteristic rheumatic lesions of striated and of nonstriated or smooth muscle cells of the heart. Medicine (Baltimore) 42: 73
1162. Murphy TF, Senterfit LB, Christian CL (1980) Arthralgia associated with acute urinary retention. A syndrome of probable viral etiology. Am J Med 68: 386
1163. Murray DC (1976) Some thoughts on flexion deformity and how to correct it. Orthop Rev 5: 15
1164. Murray GC, Perselin RH (1980) Metastatic carcinoma presenting as monoarticular arthritis. Arthritis Rheum 23: 95
1165. Myers AR (1985) Septic arthritis. In: Kelley WN, Harris ED, Ruddy S, Sledge CB (eds) Textbook of rheumatology. Saunders, Philadelphia.
1166. Myers BW, Masi AT, Feigenbaum SL (1980) Pigmented villonodular synovitis and tenosynovitis; a clinical epidemiologic study of 166 cases and literature review. Medicine (Baltimore) 59: 223

1167. Nachemson A (1976) The lumbar spine an orthopaedic challenge. Spine 1: 59
1168. Nachlas IW (1934) Pseudo-angina pectoris originating in the cervical spine. JAMA 103: 323
1169. Nachlas IW, Olpp JJ (1945) Para-articular calcification (Pellegrini Stieda) in affections of the knee. Surg Gynecol Obstet 81: 206
1170. Nagant de Deuxchaisnes C, Huaux JP, Friasse P et al. (1974) Ankylosing spondylitis, sacroilitis, regional enteritis and HLA-27. Lancet 1: 1239
1171. Nakane PK (1975) Recent progress in the peroxidase-labelled antibody method. Ann N Y Acad Sci 254: 203
1172. Nakayama DA, Barthelemy C, Carrere G et al. (1984) Tophaceous gout; a clinical and radiographic assessment. Arthritis Rheum 27: 468
1173. Namey TC (1985) Nuclear medicine and special radiologic imaging. In: Kelley WN, Harris ED, Ruddy S, Sledge CB (eds) Textbook of rheumatology. Saunders, Philadelphia
1174. Nashel DJ, Widerlitz LW, Pekin JT (1973) IgD myeloma with amyloid arthropathy. Am J Med 55: 426
1175. Nathan CF, Silverstein SC, Bruckner LH et al. (1979) Extracellular cytolysis by activated macrophages and granulocytes: II. Hydrogenperoxide as a mediator of cytotoxicity. J Exp Med 149: 100

1176. Natvig JB, Kunkel HG (1973) Human immunoglobulins. Classes, subclasses, genetic variants and idiotypes. Adv Immunol 16: 1
1177. Natvig JB, Froland SL, Wisloff F et al. (1975) Different lymphocyte populations in rheumatoid arthritis and their relationship to anti-Ig activities. Ann Clin Res 7: 146
1178. Neer CS (1972) Anterior acromioplasty for the chronic impingement syndromes of the shoulder. A preliminary report. J Bone Joint Surg [Am] 54: 41
1179. Neer CS, Watson KC, Stanton FK (1982) Recent experiences in total shoulder replacement. J Bone Joint Surg [Am] 64: 319
1180. Nelson JP (1971) Antibiotic concentrations in septic joint effusions. N Engl J Med 284: 394
1181. Nelson JP (1977) Deep infection following total hip arthroplasty. J Bone Joint Surg [Am] 59: 1042
1182. Neustadt DH (1977) HL-A antigens in rheumatic diseases. Orthop Rev 6: 19
1183. Newton P, Sharpe J, Barnes KL (1982) Bone and joint tuberculosis in Greater Manchester 1969–1979. Ann Rheum Dis 41:1
1184. Newton SE (1982) Total ankle arthroplasty: clinical study of fifty cases. J Bone Joint Surg [Am] 64: 104
1185. Nicholas JA (1973) The five-one reconstruction for anteromedial instability of the knee. J Bone Joint Surg [Am] 55: 899
1186. Nicholas JA, Freiberger RH, Killoran PJ (1970) Double contrast arthrography of the knee. Its value in the management of 225 knee derangements. J Bone Joint Surg [Am] 52: 203
1187. Nielsen H, Svehag SE (1976) Detection and differentiation of immune complexes and IgG aggregates by a complement consumption assay. Acta Pathol Microbiol Scand 84: 261
1188. Niethard FU (1981) Therapie degenerativer Gelenkerkrankungen. Dtsch Med Wochenschr 106: 478
1189. Niethard FU (1983) Die klinische Bedeutung von lumbosakralen Übergangstörungen. Z Orthop 121: 333
1190. Niethard FU, Puhl W (1978) Mikroverletzungen der Gelenkfläche als Präarthrose. Z Orthop 116: 438
1191. Niethard FU, Cotta H (1985) Die Pathogenese und konservative Behandlung der posttraumatischen Arthrose. Ber Unfallmed 51: 227
1192. Nirschl RP, Pettrone FA (1979) The treatment of lateral epicondylitis. J Bone Joint Surg [Am] 61: 832
1193. Norman A, Robbins H, Milgram JE (1968) Acute neuropathic arthropathy; severely disorganizing form of arthritis. Radiology 90: 1159
1194. Norton WL, Lewis D, Ziff M (1966) Light and electron microscopic observations on the synovitis in Reiter's disease. Arthritis Rheum 6: 747
1195. Norton WL, Ziff M (1966) Electron microscopic observations in the rheumatoid synovial membrane. Arthritis Rheum 9: 589
1196. Nuki G, Ferguson J (1971) Studies on the nature and significance of macromolecular complexes in the rheology of synovial fluid from normal and diseased human joints. Rheol Acta 10: 2

1197. Oates JK, Young AC (1959) Sacroiliitis in Reiter's disease. Br Med J 1: 1013
1198. O'Brien WM, LaDu BN, Bunim JJ (1963) Biochemical, pathologic and clinical aspects of alkaptonuria and ochronotic arthropathy. Am J Med 34: 813
1199. Odensten M, Hamberg P, Norden M et al. (1985) Surgical or conservative treatment of the acutely torn anterior cruciate ligament. Clin Orthop 198: 87
1200. O'Donoghue DH (1950) Surgical treatment of fresh injuries to the major ligaments of the knee. J Bone Joint Surg [Am] 32: 721
1201. O'Duffy JD (1970) Hypophosphatasia associated with calcium pyrophosphate dihydrate deposits in cartilage. Arthritis Rheum 13: 381
1202. Oldstone MBA, Dixon FJ (1971) Immune complexes in chronic viral infections. J Exp Med 134: 32
1203. O'Leary PA (1941) What proportion of cases with psoriasis have arthritis? J Invest Dermatol 4: 425
1204. Olhagen B, Manson I (1974) Fecal clostridium perfringens and rheumatoid arthritis. J Infect Dis 130: 444
1205. Opitz JC (1979) Isolated acute meningococcal arthritis. Clin Pediatr (Phila) 18: 444
1206. Orkin M, Goltz RW, Good RA et al. (1964) A study of multicentric reticulohistiocytosis. Arch Dermatol 89: 640
1207. Oronsky AL, Porper RJ (1975) Connective tissue degrading enzymes of human leukocytes. Ann N Y Acad Sci 256: 233
1208. Ortega OA, Larrea PR, Calderon JN (1955) Erythromycin in human brucellosis. Antibiot Med 1: 513
1209. Osmond-Clarke H (1948) Habitual dislocation of the shoulder. The Putti-Platt operation. J Bone Joint Surg [Br] 30: 19
1210. Ostuni PA, Cavasin F, Marson P et al. (1968) Elbow involvement in rheumatoid arthritis: a clinical and radiological study: V. Symposium EULAR. Rev Rhum Mal Osteoartic 868:
1211. Ott VR (1956) Roentgenologische Beobachtungen bei Ochronose. Z Rheumaforsch 15: 65
1212. Ott VR, Schmidt KL (1980) Bases experimentales de la thermotherapie des inflammations. Acta Rheumatol 4: 28
1213. Otte P (1958) Die Regenerationsunfähigkeit des Gelenkknorpels. Z Orthop 90: 299
1214. Ottoson L (1978) Lateral instability of the ankle treated by a modified Evans procedure. Acta Orthop Scand 49: 302
1215. Ozdemir AI, Sotzmen C (1969) Familial Mediterranean fever among the Turkish people. Am J Gastroenterol 51: 311

1216. Pace N, Kantor T, McEwen C (1964) Evaluation of an intraarticularly injected alkylating agent in arthritis. Arthritis Rheum 7: 337
1217. Pachman LM, Baldwin SM (1977) Assays of complement in polyarticular juvenile rheumatoid arthritis. Arthritis Rheum 20: 467
1218. Pack GT (1954) End results in the treatment of sarcoma of the soft somatic tissues. J Bone Joint Surg [Am] 36: 241
1219. Pack GT, Ariel IM (1950) Synovial sarcoma. Surgery 28: 1047
1220. Pageaut G, Guidet M, Corbillet JP et al. (1971) Anatomie pathologique de l'ochronose. Rev Rhum Mal Osteoartic 38: 277
1221. Palmoski MJ, Brandt KD (1980) Effects of some nonsteroidal antiinflammatory drugs on proteoglycan metabolism and organization in canine articular cartilage. Arthritis Rheum 23: 1010
1222. Pancoast SJ, New JC (1980) Antibiotic levels in human bone and synovial fluid. Orthop Rev 9: 49
1223. Pappas AM (1981) Osteochondritis dissecans. Clin Orthop 158: 59
1224. Parker LP, Seward CW, Osterland CK (1974) Occurrences of antigammaglobulins in effusion fluids of diverse etiology. Ann Rheum Dis 33: 262
1225. Parker RH, Schmid FR (1971) Antibacterial activity of synovial fluid during therapy of septic arthritis. Arthritis Rheum 14: 96
1226. Patel MR, Pearlman HS, Lavnic LS (1972) Arthrodesis in hemophilia. Clin Orthop 86: 168
1227. Patterson RJ, Bickel WH, Dahlin AD (1964) Idiopathic avascular necrosis of the head of the femur. A study of fifty-two cases. J Bone Joint Surg [Am] 46: 267
1228. Paul H, Reginato AJ, Schumacher HR (1983) Alizarin red staining as a screening test to detect calcium compounds in synovial fluid. Arthritis Rheum 26: 191

1229. Pauwels F (1940) Neue Richtlinien für die operative Behandlung der Koxarthrose. Verh Dtsch Orthop Ges 48: 152
1230. Payr E (1926) Behandlung der primären und sekundären Arthritis. Beitr Klin Chir 136: 260
1231. Peacock EE (1976) Dupuytren disease: controversial aspects of management. Clin Plast Surg 3: 29
1232. Pear BL (1974) Skeletal manifestation of the lymphomas and leukemias. Semin Roentgenol 9: 229
1233. Pekin TJ, Zvaifler NJ (1964) Hemolytic complement in synovial fluid. J Clin Invest 43: 1372
1234. Pekin TJ, Malinin TT, Zvaifler NJ (1967) Unusual synovial fluid findings in Reiter's syndrome. Ann Intern Med 66: 677
1235. Pellegrini A (1905) Sulla ossificazione paraarticulare del ginocchio. Clin Med 12: 433
1236. Pelletier JP, Martel-Pelletier J, Howell DS et al. (1983) Collagenase and collagenolytic activity in human osteoarthritic cartilage. Arthritis Rheum 26: 63
1237. Peltier AR, Cyna L, Dryll A et al (1973) Immunofluorescence de la membrane synoviale. Rev Rheum Mal Osteoartic 40: 619
1238. Pemberton R (1926) The etiology and pathology of arthritis. JAMA 87: 1253
1239. Pennelli M (1983) Diagnosi oncologica al microscopo elettronica applicata alla biopsia aspiratorie con ago sottile. V Congr Naz Soc It Anat Pat 5: 284
1240. Pepys MB, Baltz MI (1983) Acute phase proteins with special reference to C-reactive protein and related proteins and serum amyloid A protein. Adv Immunol 34: 141
1241. Pere C, Jegou D, Obaid M et al. (1976) Spondylodiscite à pyogenes de l'adulte. Rev Chir Orthop 62: 703
1242. Perry BA (1937) Erythema marginatum (rheumaticum). Arch Dis Child 12: 233
1243. Persellin ST, Ramirez G, Moatamed F (1982) Immunopathology of rheumatic pericarditis. Arthritis Rheum 25: 1054
1244. Person DA, Sharp JT, Rawls WE (1973) A search for viruses and mycoplasma in connective tissue disease. Arthritis Rheum 16: 677
1245. Person DA, Sharp JT (1976) The etiology of rheumatoid arthritis. Bull Rheum Dis 27: 888
1246. Peter G, Smith AL (1977) Group A streptococcal infection of the skin and pharynx. N Engl J Med 297: 311, 365
1247. Peters SP, Lee RE, Glew RH (1977) Gaucher's disease. Medicine (Baltimore) 56: 425
1248. Petersen BH, Lee TJ, Snyderman R et al. (1979) Neisseria meningitidis and Neisseria gonorrheae associated with C6, C7 or C8 deficiency. Ann Intern Med 90: 917
1249. Pettersson H, Kentro T, Gilbert MS (1985) Radiologic diagnosis of musculoskeletal complications in hemophilia. In: Doehring S, Schulitz KP (eds) Orthopaedic problems in hemophilia. Zuckschwerdt, München
1250. Petty RE, Cassidy JT, Sullivan DB (1977) Serologic studies in juvenile rheumatoid arthritis. A review. Arthritis Rheum 20: 260
1251. Petty W, Goldsmith I (1980) Resection arthroplasty following total hip arthroplasty. J Bone Joint Surg [Am] 62: 889
1252. Peyron J (1972) Revue des apports récents en physiopathologie du cartilage articulaire. Rev Rhum Mal Osteoartic 39: 157
1253. Peyron J (1972) Le cartilage et l'arthrose. Les traits du cartilage arthrosique. Rev Rhum Mal Osteoartic 39: 313
1254. Phelip X, Verdier JM, Gras JR et al. (1978) Les hemarthroses de la chondrocalcinose. Rev Rhum Mal Osteoartic 43: 259
1255. Phillips PE, Waxman J, Hirshaut Y et al. (1976) Virus antibody levels and delayed hypersensitivity in rheumatoid arthritis. Ann Rheum Dis 35: 152
1256. Piatier D, LeGo A, Brouilhet H et al. (1976) Immunofluorescence of synovial membrane – multifactorial analysis of the results. Biomedicine 24: 359
1257. Pick L (1933) Classification of the diseases of lipoid metabolism and Gaucher's disease. Am J Med Sci 185: 453
1258. Pinals RS (1977) Meningococcemia presenting as acute polyarthritis. J Rheumatol 4: 420
1259. Pinals RS, Short CL (1960) Calcific arthritis involving multiple sites. Arthritis Rheum 9: 566
1260. Pinkus S, Pick L (1908) Zur Struktur und Genese der symptomatologischen Xanthome. Dtsch Med Wochenschr 43: 1426
1261. Pirquet CE (1911) Allergy Arch Intern Med 7: 259
1262. Pirquet CF, Schick B (1951) Serum sickness. Williams and Wilkins, Baltimore
1263. Pisani G (1961) Gonalgia e pseudoblocco in estensione del ginocchio da malformazione del ligamento adiposo. Chir Organi Mov 50: 427
1264. Placeo F, Tassi D (1953) Considerazioni cliniche su 62 osservazioni di lipoma arborescente posttraumatico del ginocchio come entita pathologica a se stante ed associata a lesione meniscale. Minerva Chir 8: 316
1265. Platzgummer H (1954) Die Osteochondritis dissecans (Koenig). Arch Orthop Chir 46: 650
1266. Platt PN (1983) Examination of synovial fluid. Clin Rheum Dis 9: 51
1267. Polacek B (1964) Receptors of joints. Acta Fac Med Univ Brun
1268. Pollard AC, Carey WT, Nelson PV et al. (1980) Enzymological diagnosis of a group of lysosomal storage diseases. Med J Aust 2: 549
1269. Polley HF, Bickel WH (1951) Punch biopsy of synovial membrane. Ann Rheum Dis 10: 277
1270. Pommer G (1927) Über die mikroskopischen Kennzeichen und die Entstehungsbedingungen der Arthritis deformans. Arch Pathol Anat 213: 434
1271. Pope RM, Rutstein JE, Straus DC (1982) Detection of antibodies to streptococcal mucopeptide in patients with rheumatic disorders and normal controls. Int Arch Allergy Appl Immunol 67: 267
1272. Porter JL, Lonergan RC (1932) Intermittent hydrarthrosis. J Bone Joint Surg 14: 631
1273. Portnoy J, Julian AJ, Smith J et al. (1963) Fractionation studies of antibodies detected in serological tests for syphilis. Br J Vener Dis 39: 33
1274. Post M, Telfer MC (1975) Surgery in hemophilic patients. J Bone Joint Surg [Am] 57: 1136
1275. Post M, Haskell SS, Jablon M (1980) Total shoulder replacement with a constrained prosthesis. J Bone Joint Surg [Am] 62: 327
1276. Prager RJ, Mall JC (1976) Arthrographic diagnosis of synovial chondromatosis. Am J Roentgenol 127: 344
1277. Pras M, Itzchaki M, Prelli F et al. (1985) Amyloid arthropathy; characteristics of the amyloid protein. Clin Exp Rheumatol 3: 327
1278. Pratt PW, Estren S, Kochwa S (1968) Immunoglobulin abnormalities in Gaucher's disease; report of 16 cases. Blood 31: 633
1279. Prelli F, Tummolo D, Solomon A et al. (1986) Novel human light chain V segment: serologic and structural analyses of the III-like Bence-Jones protein. J Immunol 136: H169
1280. Presacco D, Pellegrini A, DiMaggio C (1987) L'ingrandimento radiologico delle mani. Radiol Med (Torino) 73: 159
1281. Prince DS, Luna RF, Cohn MH et al. (1975) Osteophyte induced dysphagia occurrence in ankylosing hyperostosis. JAMA 234: 77
1282. Pritchard MH, Jessop JD (1977) Chondrocalcinosis in primary hyperparathyroidism. Ann Rheum Dis 36: 146

1283. Proell F (1949) Neuere Erkenntnismöglichkeiten und wissenschaftliche Deutungsversuche der Herdinfektionslehre. Dtsch Med Wochenschr 74: 1167
1284. Puhl W (1974) Die Mikromorphologie gesunder Gelenkknorpeloberflächen. Z Orthop 112: 6
1285. Puhl W (1976) Synovektomie bei entzündlichem Rheumatismus. Diagnostik 9: 621
1286. Puhl W, Dustmann HO (1973) Die Reaktionen des Gelenkknorpels auf Verletzungen. Z Orthop 111: 494
1287. Puhl W, Scharf HP (1985) Pathophysiology of the hemophilic arthritis. In: Doehring S, Schulitz KP (eds) Orthopaedic problems in hemophilia. Zuckschwerdt, München
1288. Punzi L (1986) Esame de liquido sinoviale: attualita e prospettive. Reumatismo 38: 221
1289. Punzi L, Todesco S, Toffano G et al. (1986) Phospholipids in inflammatory synovial effusions. Rheumatol Int 6: 7
1290. Putti VP (1920) Arthroplasty of the knee joint. J Orthop Surg 2: 530

1291. Queneau R (1952) A propos de la correction des formes graves du genu flexum paralyticum. Rev Chir Orthop 38: 42

1292. Rabl DRH (1923) Kalkmetastase (Kalkgicht). Gefäßverkalkung und Nierenfunktion. Klin Wochenschr 2: 202
1293. Radin EL (1976) Etiology of osteoarthrosis. Clin Rheum Dis 2: 509
1294. Radin EL (1984) Chondromalacia of the patella. Bull Rheum Dis 34: 1
1295. Radin EL, Paul IL (1972) A consolidated concept of joint lubrication. J Bone Joint Surg [Am] 54: 607
1296. Radin EL, Paul IL, Rose RM (1972) Role of mechanical factors in pathogenesis of primary osteoarthritis. Lancet 1: 519
1297. Rafii M, Firooznia H, Golimbu C (1985) Computed tomography of septic joints. CT J Comput Tomogr 9: 57
1298. Raisman V, Courten F (1952) The importance of stretching in the treatment of acute and convalescent poliomyelitis. N Y State J Med 52: 3005
1299. Ralston HI, Miller WR, Kasahara M (1960) Nerve endings in human fasciae, tendons, ligaments, and synovial membrane. Anat Rec 136: 137
1300. Ramadier JO, Lacheretz M (1953) Traitement des ankyloses et des raideurs en extension du genou. Rev Chir Orthop 39: 450
1301. Rampazzo G, Ravenni A, Bolzan M (1980) Studio descrittivo della zona euganea ed indagine sugli esiti della fangoterapia. Med Term Climatol 48: 81
1302. Ranawat CS, Straub RL, Freyberg R et al. (1971) A study of regenerated synovium after synovectomy of the knee in rheumatoid arthritis. Arthritis Rheum 14: 117
1303. Ranawat CS, Ecker ML, Straub RL (1972) Synovectomy and debridement of the knee in rheumatoid arthritis. Arthritis Rheum 15: 571
1304. Ranawat CS, O'Leary P, Pellicci P et al. (1979) Cervical spine fusion in rheumatoid arthritis. J Bone Joint Surg [Am] 61: 1003
1305. Ravid M, Robson M, Hedar I (1977) Prolonged colchicine treatment in four patients with amyloidosis. Ann Intern Med 87: 568
1306. Razemon P, Bizard G (1931) Les tumeurs primitifs des articulations. Rev Chir Orthop 50: 229
1307. Re C, Rivera S (1962) Su un caso di disfagia da spondiloarthrose osteofitosica gigante de C6-C7. Tratamento chirurgico e risultato a distanza. Minerva Ortop 13: 180
1308. Reginato AM, Valenzuela FR, Martinez VC (1970) Polyarticular and familial chondrocalcinosis. Arthritis Rheum 13: 197
1309. Reginato AJ, Schumacher HR, Martinez PA (1973) Ochronotic arthropathy with calcium pyrophosphate crystal deposition. Arthritis Rheum 16: 1705
1310. Reginato AJ, Schumacher HR, Jimenez S et al. (1979) Synovitis in secondary syphilis. Arthritis Rheum 22: 170
1311. Reichert J (1955) Coccidioidomycosis. Ariz Med 12: 1
1312. Reigstad A, Granmark T (1984) Osteoarthritis of the hip treated by intertrochanteric osteotomy: a long term follow-up. J Bone Joint Surg [Am] 66: 1
1313. Reik L, Steere AC, Bartenhagen NH et al (1979) Neurologic abnormalities of Lyme disease. Medicine (Baltimore) 58: 281
1314. Reiman I, Mankin HJ, Trahan C (1977) Quantitative histological analysis of articular cartilage and subchondral bone from osteoarthritic and normal hips. Acta Orthop Scand 48: 63
1315. Reiter H (1916) Über eine bisher unerkannte Spirochaeteninfektion (Spirochaetosis arthritica). Dtsch Med Wochenschr 42: 1535
1316. Renier JC (1958) Arthrites purulentes du genou après hydrocortisone – considérations sur leur traitement. Rev Rhum Mal Osteoartic 25: 677
1317. Resnick D, Oliphant M (1975) Hemophilia-like arthropathy of the knee associated with cutaneous and synovial hemangioma. Radiology 114: 323
1318. Resnick D, Mwayama G, Goergen TG (1977) Comparison of radiographic abnormalities of the sacroiliac joint in degenerative disease and ankylosing spondylitis. Am J Roentgenol 128: 189
1319. Resnick DL (1974) Erosive arthritis of the hand and wrist in hyperparathyroidism. Radiology 110: 263
1320. Revell PA, Mayston V (1982) Histopathology of the synovial membrane of peripheral joints in ankylosing spondylitis. Ann Rheum Dis 41: 579
1321. Rhangos WC, Chick EW (1964) Mycotic infections of bone. South Med J 57: 664
1322. Rice PA, Kasper DL (1982) Characterization of serum resistance of Neisseria gonorrheae that disseminates. Roles of blocking antibody and gonococcal outer membrane proteins. J Clin Invest 70: 157
1323. Richards AJ, Hamilton EBD (1974) Destructive arthropathy in chondrocalcinosis articularis. Ann Rheum Dis 33: 196
1324. Richardson SB, Uttley AHA, Rettingale KW (1977) Acute sacroilitis due to Salmonella okatie. Br Med J 1: 1449
1325. Richter JA, Runge LA, Pinals RS et al (1980) Analysis of treatment with gold and antimalarial compounds. J Rheumatol 7: 153
1326. Riehm W (1953) Der Einfluß des Allergieprinzips und die Pathogenese der fokalen Krankheiten. Münch Med Wochenschr 85: 43
1327. Riese H (1895) Die Reiskörperchen in tuberkulös erkrankten Synovialsäcken. Dtsch Z Chir 42: 1
1328. Rifkind BM, Levy RL (1976) Present status of hyperlipoproteinemia: In: Varco RL, DeLaney JP (eds) Controversy in surgery. Saunders Philadelphia
1329. Rinaldi RZ, Harrison WO, Fan PT (1982) Penicillin resistant gonococcal arthritis. Ann Intern Med 97: 93
1330. Roaf R, Kirkaldy-Willis WH, Cathro AJM (1959) Surgical treatment of bone and joint tuberculosis. Livingstone, Edinburgh
1331. Roberts GD (1976) Laboratory diagnosis of fungal infections. Hum Pathol 7: 161
1332. Roberts J, Burch TA (1966) Osteoarthritis. Prevalence in adults. US Public Health Service publication 1000 series 11, no 15
1333. Roberts MET, Wright V, Hall AGL et al. (1976) Psoriatic arthritis. Follow-up study. Ann Rheum Dis 35: 206
1334. Robinson DR, Dayer JM, Krane SM (1979) Prostaglandins and their regulation in rheumatoid inflammation. Ann N Y Acad Sci 332: 279
1335. Ribitsch V, Rainer F, Robitsch G et al (1981) Biorheolo-

gische Beiträge zum Problem der rheumatischen Gelenkerkrankungen. Z Rheumatol 40: 199
1336. Rodas CU, Ronald AR (1974) Comparison of three serological tests in gonococcal infection. Appl Microbiol 27: 695
1337. Rodnan GP (1985) Neuropathic joint disease (Charcot joint). In: McCarty DJ (ed) Arthritis and allied conditions. Lea and Febiger, Philadelphia
1338. Rooney PJ, Ballantyne D, Buchanan WW (1975) Disorders of the locomotor system associated with abnormalities of lipid metabolism and the lipidosis. Clin Rheum Dis 1: 163
1339. Rooney PJ, Third J, Madkour MM et al. (1978) Transient polyarthritis associated with familial hyperlipoproteinemia. Q J Med 47: 249
1340. Root L, Goss JR, Mendes J (1986) The treatment of the painful hip in cerebral palsy by total hip replacement or hip arthrodesis. J Bone Joint Surg [Am] 68: 590
1341. Ropes MW (1957) Examination of synovial fluid. Bull Rheum Dis 7: S21
1342. Ropes MW, Bauer W (1953) Synovial fluid changes in joint disease. Harvard University Press, Cambridge
1343. Ropes MW, Bennett GA, Cobb S et al. (1958) 1958 revision of diagnostic criteria for rheumatoid arthritis. Bull Rheum Dis 9: 175
1344. Rosales Wynne-Roberts C, Anderson C, Turana AM et al. (1977) Synovial hemangioma of the knee; light and electron microscopic findings. J Pathol 123: 247
1345. Rose HM, Ragan C, Pearce E et al. (1948) Differential agglutination of normal and sensitized sheep erythrocytes by sera of patients with rheumatoid arthritis. Proc Soc Exp Biol Med 68: 1
1346. Rosen RS, Jacobson G (1966) Fungus disease of bone. Semin Roentgenol 1: 370
1347. Rosenbaum JT (1981) Why HLA-B27. An analysis based on two animal models. Ann Intern Med 94: 261
1348. Rosenbaum JT, Theofilopoulos A, McDevitt HP et al. (1981) Presence of circulating immune complexes in Reiter's syndrome and ankylosing spondylitis. Clin Immunol Pathol 18: 291
1349. Rosenberg AM, Petty RE (1982) A syndrome of seronegative enthesopathy arthropathy in children. Arthritis Rheum 25: 1041
1350. Rosenberg L (1970) Physical characteristics of protein polysaccharides prepared by different methods. J Bone Joint Surg [Am] 52: 604
1351. Rosenberg L (1973) Cartilage proteoglycans. Fed Proc 32: 1467
1352. Rosenberg L (1989) Structure and function of proteoglycans. In: McCarty DJ (ed) Arthritis and allied conditions. Lea and Febiger, Philadelphia
1353. Rosenberg L, Choi HU, Fang LH et al. (1985) Isolation of dermatan sulfate proteoglycans from mature bovine articular cartilage. J Biol Chem 250: 6304
1354. Rosenthal L, Olhagen B, Ek S (1980) Aseptic arthritis after gonorrhea. Ann Rheum Dis 39: 141
1355. Rosenthal J, Boll GG, Robinson WD (1980) Acute nongonococcal infectious arthritis. Evaluation of risk factors, therapy and outcome. Arthritis Rheum 23: 889
1356. Rossen RD, Brewer EJ, Person DA et al (1977) Circulating immune complexes and antinuclear antibodies in juvenile rheumatoid arthritis. Arthritis Rheum 20: 1485
1357. Rotes-Querol J (1957) Osteoarticular sites of Brucellosis. Ann Rheum Dis 16: 63
1358. Rotes-Querol J, Granados-Daran J, Ribas-Subiros R et al. (1972) La laxite articulaire comme facteur d'altérations de l'appareil locomoteur. Rhumatologie Aix-le-Bains 3: 179
1359. Roth JA, Enzinger FM, Tannenbaum M (1975) Synovial sarcoma of the neck: a follow up study of 24 cases. Cancer 35: 1243
1360. Rothman RH (1973) The pathophysiology of disc degeneration. Clin Neurosurg 20: 174
1361. Rothstein J, Entel I, Zeviner B (1963) Arthritis associated with ulcerative colitis. Ann Rheum Dis 22: 194
1362. Routson GW, Gingras M (1981) Surgical treatment of tennis elbow. Orthopedics 4: 769
1363. Roux J (1978) La serologie de la Brucellose. Med Hyg 36: 453
1364. Roy S (1967) Ultrastructure of synovial membrane in osteoarthritis. Ann Rheum Dis 26: 517
1365. Roy S, Ghadially FN (1967) Ultrastructure of synovial membrane in human hemarthrosis. J Bone Joint Surg [Am] 49: 1636
1366. Roy SB, Sturgis GP, Massell BF (1956) Application of the antistreptolysin-O titer in the evaluation of joint pain and in the diagnosis of rheumatic fever. N Engl J Med 254: 95
1367. Rubens-Duval A (1972) L'hygroma. Rev Rhum Mal Osteoartic 39: 183
1368. Rubens-Duval A, Kaplan G (1972) Les lésions synoviales de l'arthrose et des arthropathies lytiques. Rev Rheum Mal Osteoartic 39: 691
1369. Rudd P, Fried JF, Epstein WF (1975) Irreversible bone marrow failure with chlorambucil. J Rheumatol 2: 421
1370. Ruddy S (1985) Management of rheumatoid arthritis. In: Kelley WM, Harris ED, Ruddy S, Sledge CB (eds) Textbook of rheumatology. Saunders, Philadelphia
1371. Ruddy S, Britton MC, Schur PH et al. (1969) Complement components in synovial fluid: activation and fixation in seropositive rheumatoid arthritis. Ann N Y Acad Sci 168: 161
1372. Ruddy S, Gigli I, Austen KF (1972) The complement system of man. N Engl J Med 287: 489
1373. Ruddy S, Heck L, Gay RE et al. (1983) Collagen types and breakdown in the rheumatoid arthritis. Arthritis Rheum 26: 831
1374. Rudolph AM, Hoffmann JIE, Axelrod S (1987) Pediatrics. Appleton and Lange, Norwalk
1375. Ruett A, Hackenbroch M (1957) Beiträge zur Arthrosis deformans. Beih Z Orthop 89: 110
1376. Rundles RW, Metz EH, Silberman HG (1966) Allopurinal in the treatment of gout. Ann Intern Med 64: 229
1377. Russek A (1976) Biomechanical and physiological basis for ambulatory treatment of low back pain. Orthop Rev 5: 21
1378. Russel H, Sampson JL, Schmid GP et al. (1984) Enzyme-linked immunosorbent assay and indirect immunofluorescent assay in Lyme disease. J Infect Dis 149: 465
1379. Russell RGG, Bisaz S, Fleisch H et al. (1970) Inorganic pyrophosphate in plasma, urine, and synovial fluid of patients with pyrophosphate arthropathy (chondrocalcinosis or pseudogout). Lancet 2: 899
1380. Russell AS, Edelman J (1983) Lymphocytes. Clin Rheum Dis 9: 117
1381. Russell ML, Gordon DA, Ogryzlo MA et al. (1973) The cauda equina syndrome of ankylosing spondylitis. Ann Intern Med 78: 551
1382. Russell TJ, Lorain MD, Schultz M et al. (1972) Histocompatibility (HL-A) antigen associated with psoriasis. N Engl J Med 287: 738
1383. Ryan LM, McCarty DJ (1985) Calcium pyrophosphate crystal deposition disease; pseudogout; articular chondrocalcinosis. In: McCarty DJ (ed) Arthritis and allied conditions. Lea and Febiger, Philadelphia
1384. Ryan WG (1980) Endocrine disorders. Year Book Medical Publishers, Chicago
1385. Rytel MW (1978) Microbial antigen detection in infectious arthritis. Clin Rheum Dis 4: 83

1386. Sabrazes J, DeGrailly R (1951) Synovialome. C R Soc Biol 108: 1155

1387. Sairanen E, Paronen I, Mahonen H (1969) Reiter's syndrome, a follow-up study. Acta Med Scand 185: 57
1388. Salter N (1955) Methods of measurement of muscle and joint function. J Bone Joint Surg [Br] 37: 474
1389. Salter RB, Gross A, Hall JH (1967) Hydrocortisone arthropathy. An experimental investigation. Can Med Assoc J 97: 374
1390. Salter RB, Simmonds DF, Malcolm BW et al. (1980) The biological effect of continuous passive motion on the healing of full thickness defects in articular cartilage. J Bone Joint Surg [Am] 62: 1232
1391. Samra Y, Hertz M, Shaked Y et al. (1982) Brucellosis of the spine. J Bone Joint Surg [Br] 64: 429
1392. Samuelson KM, Freeman MA, Tuke MA (1982) Development and evolution of the ICLH ankle replacement. Foot Ankle 3: 32
1393. Sandberg R, Balkfors B, Wilson B et al. (1987) Operative versus non-operative treatment of recent injuries of the knee. J Bone Joint Surg [Am] 69: 1120
1394. Sanders LL (1967) Blastomycosis arthritis. Arthritis Rheum 10: 91
1395. Sandy JD, Brown HLG, Lowther DA (1978) Degradation of proteoglycan in articular cartilage. Biochim Biophys Acta 543: 536
1396. Sany JF, Rosenberg R, Bataille H et al. (1977) Chondrocalcinoses secondaires et ossociées. Rev Rhum Mal Osteoartic 44: 565
1397. Saphir O, Langendorf R (1953) Nonspecific myocarditis in acute rheumatic fever. Am Heart J 46: 432
1398. Sapolsky AJ, Altman RD, Woessner JF et al. (1973) The action of cathepsin D on human articular cartilage on polysaccharides. J Clin Invest 52: 624
1398 a. Sauter vanHouten S, Utsinger P (1978) Viral arthritis. Clin Rheum Dis 4: 205
1399. Schaad UB (1980) Arthritis in disease due to Neisseria meningitidis. Rev Infect Dis 2: 880
1400. Schachter J, Marshall GR, Jones JP et al. (1987) Isolation of Bedsonia from joints of patients with Reiter's syndrome. Proc Soc Exp Biol Med 122: 283
1401. Schaller JG (1980) Juvenile rheumatoid arthritis. Pediatrics 2: 163
1402. Schaller JG (1989) Treatment of juvenile rheumatoid arthritis. In: McCarty DJ (ed) Arthritis and allied conditions. Lea and Febiger, Philadelphia
1403. Schaller JG, Wedgewood RJ (1983) Is juvenile rheumatoid arthritis a single disease? A review. Pediatrics 50: 940
1404. Schaller JG, Bitman S, Wedgewood RJ (1989) Ankylosing spondylitis with childhood onset. J Pediatr 74: 505
1405. Scheinberg MA, Mendes NF, Kopersztych S et al. (1976) Clinical application of T-, B- and K-cell determinations in rheumatic diseases: a review. Semin Arthritis Rheum 6: 1
1406. Scheller AD, Mitchell SB, Barber FC (1982) Femoral component fracture in revision hip arthroplasty. In: Turner RH, Scheller AD (eds) Revision total hip arthroplasty. Grune and Stratton, New York
1407. Schiff B, Mizrachi D, Orgad S et al. (1982) Association of HLA-AW31 and HLA-DR1 with adult rheumatoid arthritis. Ann Rheum Dis 41: 403
1408. Schiller AL (1985) Tumors. In: Kelley WN, Harris ED, Ruddy S, Sledge CB (eds) Textbook of rheumatology. Saunders, Philadelphia
1409. Schirmer A, Boeni A (1967) Kritische Stellungnahme zur Diagnostik des Reiter Syndroms. Z Rheumaforsch 26: 142
1410. Schirmer O (1903) Studien zur Physiologie and Pathologie der Tränenabsonderung und Tränenfluß. Arch Ophthalmol 56: 197
1411. Schittenhelm A, Schlecht H (1918) Über Polyarthritis enterica. Arch Klin Med 12: 329
1412. Schlein AP (1976) Semiconstrained total elbow arthroplasty. Clin Orthop 121: 222
1413. Schlesinger A (1926) Über den Hydrops articulorum intermittens und seine familiäre Form. Wien. Klin Wochenschr 39: 68
1414. Schlesinger H (1901) Erkrankungen der Knochen und Gelenke bei Syringomyelie. Mitt Grenzgeb Med Chir 16: 214
1415. Schlesinger H (1925) Die Arthrolues tardiva und ihre Behandlung. Springer, Vienna
1416. Schlosstein LH, Terasaki PI, Bluestone R et al. (1973) High association of an HLA antigen W27 with ankylosing spondylitis. N Engl J Med 288: 704
1417. Schmid FR (1984) Routine drug treatment of septic arthritis. Clin Rheum Dis 19/2: 293
1418. Schmid FR (1985) Bacterial arthritis. In: McCarty DJ (ed) Arthritis and allied conditions. Lea and Febiger, Philadelphia
1419. Schmidt MB (1913) Kalkmetastase und Kalkgicht. Dtsch Med Wochenschr 39: 59
1420. Schmorl G, Junghanns H (1953) Die gesunde und kranke Wirbelsäule in Röntgenbild und Klinik. Thieme, Stuttgart
1421. Schneider R (1974) Hip arthrodesis with cobra head plate and pelvic osteotomy. Reconstr Surg Traumatol 14: 1
1422. Schnitzer TJ (1989) Viral arthritis. In: Kelley WN, Harris ED, Ruddy S, Sledge CB (eds) Textbook of rheumatology. Saunders, Philadelphia
1423. Schoenbaum SC, Coleman WF, Dowdle WR et al (1976) Epidemiology of influenza in the elderly. Evidence of virus recycling. Am J Epidemiol 103: 166
1424. Schoentag RA (1989) Hematology analyzers. In: Lifschitz M, DeCresce R (eds) Clinics in Laboratory Medicine. Saunders, Philadelphia, p. 207
1425. Scholnick GK, Buchanan TM, Holmes KK (1976) Gonococci causing disseminated gonococcal infection are resistant to the bactericidal action of normal human sera. J Clin Invest 58: 1163
1426. Schonholtz GJ (1984) Complications of arthroscopic surgery. In: Shariaree H (ed) O'Connors textbook of arthroscopic surgery. Lippincott, Philadelphia
1427. Schubert M, Hammerman D (1968) A primer on connective tissue histochemistry. Lea and Febiger, Philadelphia
1428. Schulitz KP (1972) Lebensfähigkeit von Knorpelgewebe unter verschiedenen Bedingungen. Z Orthop 110: 699
1429. Schulitz KP (1973) Der Wert der Synovektomie bei der Gonarthrose. Z Orthop 111: 537
1430. Schulitz KP (1976) Die Generation der Synovialis. Z Orthop 114: 161
1431. Schulitz KP (1985) Hemophilic arthritis. In: Doehring S, Schulitz KP (eds) Orthopaedic problems in hemophilia. Zuckschwerdt, München
1432. Schulitz KP, Dustman HO, Puhl W (1973) Die Entwicklung der posttraumatischen Arthrose am Beispiel des Schienbeinkopfes. Arch Orthop Chir 76: 136
1433. Schultz JS, Good AE, Sing CF et al. (1981) HAL profile and Reiter's syndrome. Clin Genet 19: 159
1434. Schulz P (1963) Zur Arthropathie bei Syringomyelie. Zentrabl Chir 88: 209
1435. Schumacher HR, Kulka JP (1972) Needle biopsy of synovial membrane: experience with the Parker-Pearson technique. N Engl J Med 286: 416
1436. Schumacher HR (1975) Synovial membrane and fluid morphologic alterations in early rheumatoid arthritis. Microvascular injury and virus-like particles. Ann N Y Acad Sci 256: 39
1437. Schumacher HR (1975) Pathology of the synovial membrane in gout. Arthritis Rheum 18: 771
1438. Schumacher HR (1978) Joint pathology in infectious arthritis. Clin Rheum Dis 4: 33
1439. Schumacher HR (1989) Synovial fluid analysis. In: Kelley WN, Harris ED, Ruddy S, Sledge CB (eds) Textbook of rheumatology. Saunders, Philadelphia

1440. Schumacher HR (1989) Synovial biopsy and pathology. In: Kelley WN, Harris EJ, Ruddy S, Sledge CB (eds) Textbook of rheumatology. Saunders, Philadelphia
1441. Schumacher JR (1985) Ochronosis, hematochromatosis and Hilbert's disease. In: McCarty DJ (ed) Arthritis and allied conditions. Lea and Febiger, Philadelphia
1442. Schumacher HR, Miller JL, Ludovico C et al. (1981) Erosive arthritis associated with apatite crystal deposition. Arthritis Rheum 24: 31
1443. Schur PH, Sandson J (1963) Immunologic studies of the proteins of human synovial fluid. Arthritis Rheum 6: 115
1444. Schur PH, Austen KF (1971/1972) Complement in the rheumatic disease. Bull Rheum Dis 22: 666
1445. Schurman DJ, Parker JN, Ornstein D (1985) Total condylar knee replacement. J Bone Joint Surg [Am] 67: 1007
1446. Schnitzer TJ, Ansell BM (1977) Amyloidosis in juvenile chronic polyarthritis. Arthritis Rheum 20: 245
1447. Schwarz GS, Berenyi MR, Siegel MW (1969) Atrophic arthropathy and diabetic neuritis. Am J Roentgenol 106: 523
1448. Scott Gray M, Philp T (1963) Syphilitic arthritis. Ann Rheum Dis 22: 19
1449. Scott JT (1983) Uric acid and the interpretation of hyperuricemia. Clin Rheum Dis 9: 241
1450. Scott PM (1968) Bone lesions in pigmented villonodular synovitis. J Bone Joint Surg [Br] 50: 306
1451. Scott WN, Ferriter P, Marino M (1985) Intraarticular transfer of the iliotibial tract. J Bone Joint Surg [Am] 67: 532
1452. Scudese VA, Calabro JJ (1963) Vertebral wedge osteotomy – correction of rheumatoid ankylosing spondylitis. JAMA 186: 627
1453. Seddon H (1975) Surgical disorders of the peripheral nerves. Churchill Livingstone, Edinburgh
1454. Seedhom BB, Wright V (1981) Biomechanics. Clin Rheum Dis 7: 259
1455. Seegmiller JE, Howel RR, Malawista SE (1962) A mechanism of action of colchicine in acute gouty arthritis. J Clin Invest 41: 1399
1456. Seegmiller JE, Rosenblum FM, Kelley WN (1967) Enzyme defect associated with a sex-linked human neurological disorder and excessive purine synthesis. Science 155: 1682
1457. Seemann H (1937) Über das Vorkommen des Oestrins in den Hoden und seine Wirkung auf das Knochenwachstum. Endokrinologie 18: 325
1458. Seemen H (1929) Über die Entstehungsbedingungen metaplastischer Gelenkbildungen. Dtsch Z Chir 217: 60
1459. Seglenicks Z, Moore BW (1974) Epidemic polyarthritis in South Australia. Med J Aust 2: 552
1460. Seidel K (1953) Zum Formenkreis der endokrinen Periarthritis. Z Alternsforsch 7: 140
1461. Sellheim H (1913) Der Einfluß der Kastration auf das Knochenwachstum des geschlechtsreifen Organismus. Z Geburtshilfe Gynäkol 74: 362
1462. Selye H (1946) The general adaptation syndrome and the diseases of adaptation. J Clin Endocrinol 7: 117
1463. Selye H (1949) Further studies concerning the participation of the adrenal cortex in the pathogenesis of arthritis. Br Med J 1: 1129
1464. Sennara H, Garry F (1978) Orthopaedic aspects of sickle cell anemia allied to hemoglobinopathies. Clin Orthop 130: 154
1465. Seradge H, Anderson MG (1978) Alkaptonuria and ochronosis. Historic review and update. Orthop Rev 7: 41
1466. Serre H, Simon L, Barjon NC et al. (1962) Les nouveaux corticoides en injections intraarticulaires. Rev Rhum Mal Osteoartic 29: 195
1467. Serre H, Kalfa G, Brousson C et al. (1981) Manifestations osteoarticulaires de la Brucellose. Rev Rhum Mal Osteoartic 48: 143
1468. Serstock DS, Zinneman HH (1975) Pulmonary and articular sporotrichosis. JAMA 233: 1291
1469. Shariaree H (1984) O'Connor's textbook of arthroscopic surgery. Lippincott, Philadelphia
1470. Sharp J (1957) The differential diagnosis of ankylosing spondylitis. Br Med J 1: 975
1471. Sharp JT (1983) Radiographic evaluation of the course of articular disease. Clin Rheum Dis 9: 541
1472. Sharp JT (1985) Reiter's syndrome. In: McCarty DJ (ed) Arthritis and allied conditions. Lea and Febiger, Philadelphia
1473. Shaw RK, Boggs DR, Silberman HR et al. (1981) A study of prednisone therapy in chronic lymphocytic leukemia. Blood 17: 182
1474. Sherman OH, Fetto JF (1983) Systemic diagnosis of knee disorders by symptom complexes. Orthop Rev 12: 109
1475. Sherman OH, Fox JM, Snyder SJ et al. (1986) Arthroscopy – no problem surgery. J Bone Joint Surg [Am] 68: 256
1475a. Sherman OH, Minkoff J (1990) Arthroscopic surgery. Williams and Wilkins, Baltimore
1476. Shiloni E, Bitran D, Rachmilowitz E et al. (1983) The role of splenectomy in Gaucher's disease. Arch Surg 118: 929
1477. Shiota K, Miki F, Kanagama Y et al. (1981) Suppurative coxitis due to Salmonella typhimurium in systemic lupus erythematosus. Ann Rheum Dis 40: 312
1478. Shiozawa S, Shiozawa K, Fujita T (1983) Morphologic observation in the early phase of the cartilage-pannus junction. Arthritis Rheum 26: 472
1479. Shiozawa S, Ziff M (1983) Immunoelectric demonstration of fibronectin in rheumatoid pannus and at the cartilage-pannus junction. Ann Rheum Dis 42: 254
1480. Shiu MH (1984) Diagnosis and management of synovial sarcoma. N Y State J Med 84: 4
1481. Shiu MH, McCormack PM, Hajdu SI et al. (1979) Surgical treatment of tendosynovial sarcoma. Cancer 43: 889
1482. Shoji H, Sakai L, Granda JL (1974) Chondromalacia patellae. N Y State J Med 74: 507
1483. Short CCL (1947) Arthritis in Mediterranean theater of operations. N Engl J Med 236: 468
1484. Siegal S (1964) Familial paroxysmal polyserositis. Am J Med 36: 893
1485. Siegmeth W, Eberl R (1976) Gelenkfernmanifestation der chronischen Polyarthritis. Wien. Klin Wochenschr 88: 81
1486. Siguier F (1957) Maladies vedettes, maladies d'avenir, maladies quotidiennes, maladies d'exception. Editions Paris, Paris
1487. Silberberg M, Silberberg R (1940) Changes in the skeletal tissue of mice following the administration of thyroxin. Growth 4: 305
1488. Silberberg M, Silberberg R (1943) The effects of parathyroid hormone and calcium gluconate on the skeletal tissues of mice. Am J Pathol 19: 839
1489. Silberberg R, Hasler M (1971) Submicroscopic effects of hormones on articular cartilage in adult mice. Arch Pathol 91: 241
1490. Silberberg R, Silberberg M (1961) Male sex hormones and osteoarthritis in mice. J Bone Joint Surg [Am] 43: 243
1491. Silberberg R, Silberberg M (1965) Aging changes and osteoarthrosis in castrated mice receiving progesterone. J Gerontol 20: 208
1492. Silbermann M (1983) Hormones and cartilage. In: Hall BK (ed) Cartilage. Academic, New York
1493. Silverman SL, Schumacher HR (1981) Antibodies to Epstein-Barr viral antigens in early rheumatoid arthritis. Arthritis Rheum 24: 1465
1494. Silverstein E, Friedland J (1983) Angiotensin converting enzyme in cultured fibroblasts in Gaucher and Niemann-Pick disease. Arch Surg 118: 929

1495. Silverstein MN, Kelley PJ (1963) Leukemia with osteoarticular symptoms and signs. Ann Intern Med 59: 637
1496. Silverstein MN, Kelley PJ (1967) Osteoarticular manifestations of Gaucher's disease. Am J Med Sci 253: 569
1497. Simkin PA, Pizzorno JE (1974) Transynovial exchange of small molecules in normal humal subject. J Appl Physiol 36: 581
1498. Simkin PA, Nilson KL (1981) Transynovial exchange of large and small molecules. Clin Rheum Dis 7: 99
1499. Simon DG (1975) Muscle pain syndromes. Am J Phys Med 54: 289
1499 a. Simon DG (1976) Muscle pain syndromes. Am J Phys Med 55: 15
1500. Simon DG, Kaslow RA, Rosenbaum J et al. (1981) Reiter's syndrome following epidemic Shigellosis. J Rheumatol 8: 969
1501. Simon RD, Ford E (1980) Rheumatoid like arthritis associated with colonic carcinoma. Arch Intern Med 140: 698
1502. Simmons DP, Chrisman OD (1965) Salicylate inhibition of cartilage degeneration. Arthritis Rheum 8: 960
1503. Simons RJ, Kimona DW (1989) Fatal colchicine toxicity. Am J Med 86: 356
1504. Sims RE, Genant HK (1986) Magnetic resonance imaging of joint diseases. In: Richardson ML (ed) Magnetic resonance imaging of the musculoskeletal system. Radiol Clin North Am 24/2: 179
1505. Singer JM, Plotz CM (1956) The latex fixation test: I Application to the serologic diagnosis of rheumatoid arthritis. Am J Med Sci 21: 888
1506. Sjoegren H (1951) Some problems concerning keratoconjunctivitis sicca and the sicca syndrome. Acta Ophthalmol 29: 33
1507. Skolnick MD, Bryan RS, Peterson LFA (1976) Polycentric knee arthroplasty. J Bone Joint Surg [Am] 58: 743
1508. Skrede S, Blamhoff JR, Elgja K et al. (1975) Serum proteins in diseases of the liver. Scand J Clin Lab Invest 35: 399
1509. Slama TG (1987) Treatment of septic arthritis. Diagnostic approach and rational use of antibiotics. Orthop Rev 16: 236
1510. Sledge CB (1973) Growth hormones and articular cartilage. Fed Proc 30: 1503
1511. Sledge CB (1977) Joint replacement surgery in juvenile rheumatoid arthritis. Arthritis Rheum 20: 567
1512. Sledge CB (1978) Surgery in infectious arthritis. Clin Rheum Dis 4: 159
1513. Slocum DB, Larson RL (1968) Rotatory instability of the knee. J Bone Joint Surg [Am] 50: 211
1514. Smillie JS (1957) Treatment of osteochondritis dissecans. J Bone Joint Surg [Br] 39: 248
1515. Smith JW, Utz JP (1972) Progressive disseminated histoplasmosis – a prospective study of 26 patients. Ann Intern Med 76: 557
1516. Smith LW (1927) Synoviomata. Am J Pathol 3: 355
1517. Smith PG, Doll R (1982) Mortality among patients with ankylosing spondylitis after a single treatment course with x-rays. Med J 284: 449
1518. Smith PM, Lestas AN, Miller JPG et al. (1969) The differential ferrioxamine test in the management of idiopathic hemochromatosis. Lancet 2: 402
1519. Smith PH, Benn RT, Sharp J (1972) Natural history of rheumatoid cervical luxations. Ann Rheum Dis 31: 431
1520. Smith TWD, Duckworth T, Borgenholtz A et al. (1975) Role of growth hormone on glycosaminoglycan synthesis by articular cartilage. Nature 253: 269
1521. Shmookler BM, Enzinger FM, Brannon RB (1982) Orofacial synovial sarcome. A clinicopathologic study of 11 new cases and review of the literature. Cancer 50: 269
1522. Smythe HA (1989) Nonarticular rheumatism and psychogenic musculoskeletal syndromes: In: McCarty DJ (ed) Arthritis and allied conditions. Lea and Febiger, Philadelphia
1523. Smythe HA, Moldofsky H (1978) Two contributions to the understanding of the fibrositis syndrome. Bull Rheum Dis 28: 928
1524. Snapper I, Turner LB, Moskowitz HL (1953) Multiple myeloma. Grune and Stratton, New York
1525. Snapper I, Goldberg AF (1957) Gaucher's disease presenting as widespread resorption of bone. J Mt Sinai Hosp 24: 1221
1526. Sneppen O, Beck H, Holsteen V (1978) Synovectomy as a prophylactic measure in recurrent hemophilic hemarthrosis. Acta Paediatr Scand 67: 491
1527. Snyderman R, McCarty GA (1978) The role of macrophages in the rheumatic diseases. Clin Rheum Dis 4: 499
1528. Sohar E, Gafni J, Pras M et al. (1967) Familial Mediterranean fever. A survey of 470 cases and review of the literature. Am J Med 43: 227
1529. Sokoloff L (1892) Beitrag zur Casuistik der Erkrankungen bei Gliomatose des Rückenmarkes (Syringomyelia). Dtsch Z Chir 51: 506
1530. Sokoloff L (1975) Biochemical and physiological aspects of degenerative joint diseases with special references to hemophilic arthropathy. Ann N Y Acad Sci 240: 285
1531. Sokoloff L, Hough AJ (1985) Pathology of rheumatoid arthritis and allied conditions. In: McCarty DJ (ed) Arthritis and allied conditions. Lea and Febiger, Philadelphia
1532. Sokoloff L, Hough AJ (1985) Pathology of osteoarthritis. In: McCarty DJ (ed) Arthritis and allied conditions. Lea and Febiger, Philadelphia
1533. Sommer R (1937) Die Endoskopie des Kniegelenkes. Zentralbl Chir 29: 1962
1534. Sonnenschein A (1956) Zu Begriff, Bild und Behandlung der Infektarthritis. Münch. Med Wochenschr 98: 730
1535. Soren A (1937) Zur Claudenbehandlung der Ganglien und Hygrome. Wien. Med Wochenschr 100: 9
1536. Soren A (1938) Ein Beitrag zur Behandlung der Arthrosis deformans. Z Ärztl Fortbild (Jena) 35: 673
1537. Soren A (1950) Ontogenetische Ausbildung des Kniegelenkes beim Mensch. Z Anat 115: 251
1538. Soren A (1954) Zur Verkalkung des Nucleus pulposus. Fortschr Röntgenstrahlther 81: 362
1539. Soren A (1963) On the etiology of proliferative hypertrophic synovitis. Rheumatism 19: 41
1540. Soren A (1964) Bindegewebsveränderungen bei Lipaemie. Wien. Med Wochenschr 114: 511
1541. Soren A (1965) Treatment of musculoskeletal disorders with ultrasound. J Occup Med 7: 434
1542. Soren A (1973) Transport of salicylates from blood to joint fluid. Arch Intern Med 132: 668
1543. Soren A (1978) Histodiagnosis and clinical correlation of rheumatoid and other synovitis. Thieme, Stuttgart
1544. Soren A (1980) The diagnostic significance of certain histopatholgic changes for rheumatoid arthritis. Z Rheumatol 39: 74
1545. Soren A (1981) Joint inflammations as complications in intestinal inflammations. Z Rheumatol 40: 1
1546. Soren A (1984) Stabilization of the hip joint after resection of caput and collum femoris by osteotomy of the femur. Acta Orthop Belg 50: 449
1547. Soren A, Klein W, Huth F (1976) Microscopic comparison of the synovial changes in rheumatoid arthritis and osteoarthritis. Z Rheumatol 35: 249
1548. Soren A, Klein W, Huth F (1978) The synovial changes in posttraumatic synovitis and osteoarthritis. Rheumatol Rehabil 17: 38
1549. Soren A, Waugh TR (1980) Zuverlässige Einfügung eines Knochenspanes bei Arthrodese. Z Orthop 118: 291
1550. Soren A, Waugh TR (1980) The pathology of ganglion. Zentralbl Allg Pathol 124: 454

1551. Soren A, Waugh TR (1982) Les altérations de la membrane synoviale dans l'arthrite psoriasique. Rev Rhum Mal Osteoartic 49: 671
1552. Soren A, Waugh TR (1982) Surgical treatment of hallux valgus. Orthop Rev 11: 71
1553. Soren A, Cooper NS, Rosenberger JA et al. (1983) The synovial changes in rheumatoid arthritis under corticosteroid treatment. Z Rheumatol 42: 107
1554. Soren A, Waugh TR (1983) The morphologic and pathogenetic bases of heterotopic bone formation in the extremities. Zentralbl Allg Pathol 127: 91
1555. Soren A, Waugh TR (1984) The snapping knee joint. Orthop Rev 13: 661
1556. Soren A, Cooper NS, Waugh TR (1988) The nature and designation of osteoarthritis determined by its histopathology. Clin Exp Rheumatol 6: 41
1557. Sotelo-Ortiz, F (1955) Chronic coccidioidal synovitis of the knee joint. J Bone Joint Surg [Am] 37: 49
1558. Sourek J, Vymola F, Trojanova M et al. (1979) Enterotoxins produced by staphylococcus aureus. J Clin Microbiol 9: 266
1559. Sperling O, Persky-Brosh S, Boer P et al. (1973) Human erythrocyte 5-phosphoribosyl pyrophosphate synthetase activity mutationally altered in regulatory properties. Biochem Med 7: 389
1560. Spilberg I, Meyer GJ (1972) The arthritis of leukemia. Arthritis Rheum 15: 630
1561. Spink WW (1951) What is chronic brucellosis? Ann Intern Med 35: 358
1562. Sprenger TR, Foley CJ (1982) Hip replacement in a Charcot joint. Clin Orthop 165: 191
1563. Stauffer RN (1982) Ten year follow-up study of total hip replacement. J Bone Joint Surg [Am] 64: 983
1564. Stauffer RN (1989) Correction of arthritic deformities of the hip. In: McCarty DJ (ed) Arthritis and allied conditions. Lea and Febiger, Philadelphia
1565. Stecher RM (1955) Heberden's nodes. A clinical description of osteoarthritis of the finger joints. Ann Rheum Dis 14: 1
1566. Stecher RM, Heuser H (1948) Heberden's nodes: roentgenological and clinical appearance of degenerative joint disease of fingers. Am J Roentgenol 59: 328
1567. Stedtfeld G (1956) Beitrag zur Klinik and Histologie der Xanthome. Z Orthop 87. 298
1568. Steere AC, Malawista SE, Hardin JA et al. (1977) Erythema chronicum migrans and Lyme arthritis. The enlarging clinical spectrum. Ann Intern Med 86: 685
1569. Steere AC, Broderick TE, Malawista SG (1978) Erythema chronicum migrans and Lyme arthritis: epidemiologic evidence for a tick vector. Am J Epidemiol 118: 812
1570. Steere AC, Green J, Hutchinson GJ et al. (1984) Curing Lyme arthritis: successful antibiotic therapy of established joint involvement. Arthritis Rheum 27: S26
1571. Steere AC, Malawista SG (1985) Lyme disease. In: McCarty DJ (ed) Arthritis and allied conditions. Lea and Febiger, Philadelphia
1572. Stefanich RJ (1986) Intraarticular corticosteroids in treatment of osteoarthritis. Orthop Rev 15: 65
1573. Steffen C (1978) Grundlagenuntersuchungen über die chronische Polyarthritis als Kollagen – Autoimmunkrankheit. Z Rheumatol 32: 131
1574. Stein H, Duthie RB (1981) The pathogenesis of chronic hemophilic arthropathy. J Bone Joint Surg [Br] 63: 601
1575. Stein HB, Paterson AC, Offer RC et al. (1980) Adverse effects of penicillamine in rheumatoid arthritis. Ann Intern Med 92: 24
1576. Steinberg PL (1956) Syringomyelia with multiple neuropathic joints. Ann Phys Med 3: 103
1577. Steinberg CL, Duthie RB, Piva AE (1962) Charcot-like arthropathy following intraarticular hydrocortisone. JAMA 181: 851
1578. Steinbrocker O, Traeger C, Batterman R (1949) Therapeutic criteria in rheumatoid arthritis. JAMA 140: 659
1579. Stenkvist B, Westermark P, Wibell L (1974) Simple method of diagnostic screening for amyloidosis. Ann Rheum Dis 33: 75
1580. Stewart A, Glass J, Patel A et al. (1982) Lyme arthritis in Hunter Valley. Med J Aust 1: 139
1581. Stewart JG (1975) Causation and symptomatology of multiple neuritis. Br Med J 2: 461
1582. Stewart NJ, Bland WG (1958) Compression in arthrodesis. A comparative study of methods of fusion of the knee in ninety-three cases. J Bone Joint Surg [Am] 40: 585
1583. Stewart SM, Alexander WRM, Duthie JJR (1969) Isolation of diphtheroid bacilli from synovial membrane and fluid in rheumatoid arthritis. Ann Rheum Dis 28: 477
1584. Stewart SR, Gershwin MF (1981) Diagnostic tests and procedures in rheumatic diseases. In: Halsted JA, Halsted CH, (eds) The Laboratory and clinical medicine. Saunders, Philadelphia
1585. Stieda A (1909) Über eine typische Verletzung am unteren Femurende. Arch Klin Chir 85: 815
1586. Still GF (1897) On a form of chronic joint disease in children. Med Chir Trans 82: 47
1587. Stillman JS (1981) Antimalarials in the treatment of JRA arthritis in childhood. In: Moore TD (ed) 80th Ross conference on pediatric research. Ross Laboratories, Columbus
1588. Stillman JS, Barry PE (1977) Juvenile rheumatoid arthritis. Arthritis Rheum 20: 171
1589. Stockwell RA, Meachim G (1979) The chondrocyte. In: Freeman MAR (ed) Adult articular cartilage. Pitman Medical, Kent
1590. Stoeber E (1981) Prognosis in juvenile chronic arthritis. Follow-up of 433 chronic rheumatic children. Eur J Pediatr 135: 225
1591. Stoker DJ, Murray RN (1974) Skeletal changes in hemophilia and other bleeding disorders. Semin Roentgenol 9: 185
1592. Stokes G (1976) An improved Congo red method for amyloid. Med Lab Sci 33: 79
1593. Stollerman GH (1983) Global strategies for the control of rheumatic fever. JAMA 249: 431
1594. Stollerman GH (1989) Rheumatic fever. In: Kelley WN, Harris ED, Ruddy S, Sledge CB (eds) Textbook of rheumatology. Saunders, Philadelphia
1595. Stoltze CA, Hanlon DG, Pease GS et al (1960) Keratoconjunctivitis sicca and Sjoegren's syndrome. Arch Intern Med 106: 513
1596. Storti E, Ascari E (1975) Surgical and chemical synovectomy. Ann N Y Acad Sci 240: 316
1597. Stout AP (1948) Myxoma, the tumor of primitive mesenchyme. Ann Surg 127: 706
1598. Stout AP, Lattes R (1967) Tumors of soft tissues. In: Atlas of tumor pathology, vol I. Armed Forces Institute for Pathology, Washington DC, pp. 67
1599. Strand V, Talal N (1979) Advances in the diagnosis and concept of Sjoegren's syndrome. Bull Rheum Dis 30: 1046
1600. Strandberg B (1964) Intraarticular steroid therapy. Acta Rheumatol Scand 10: 29
1601. Strasser T (1978) Rheumatic fever and rheumatic heart disease in the 1970's. WHO Chron 32: 18
1602. Straub LR, Smith JW, Carpenter GK et al. (1961) The surgery of gout in the upper extremity. J Bone Joint Surg [Am] 43: 731
1603. Suit HD, Proppe KH, Mankin HJ et al. (1981) Preoperative radiation therapy for sarcoma of soft tissue. Cancer 47: 2269

1604. Sunderman FWJr, Sunderman FW (1957) Interstitial calcinosis. Am J Med Sci 234: 287
1605. Sutherland RIL, Matheson D (1975) Inflammatory involvement of vertebrae in ankylosing spondylitis. J Rheumatol 2: 296
1606. Sutker WL, Lankford LL, Thompsett R (1979) Granulomatous synovitis, the role of atypical mycobacteria. Rev Infect Dis 1: 729
1607. Sutton FSJr, Thompson CH, Lipke J et al. (1976) The effect of patellectomy on knee function. J Bone Joint Surg [Am] 58: 537
1608. Svartman M, Potter EV, Poon-King T (1975) Immunoglobulins and complement components in synovial fluid of patients with acute rheumatic fever. J Clin Invest 56: 111
1609. Swann DA (1981) The lubricating activity of synovial fluid glycoproteins. Arthritis Rheum 24: 22
1610. Swann M, Ansell BM (1986) Soft tissue release of the hips in children with juvenile chronic arthritis. J Bone Joint Surg [Br] 68: 404
1611. Swanson AB (1972) Flexible implant arthroplasty for arthritic finger joints. J Bone Joint Surg [Am] 54: 435
1612. Swanson SAV (1979) Friction, wear, and lubrication. In: Freeman MAR (ed) Adult articular cartilage. Pitman Medical, Kent
1613. Sweezey RL, Weiner SR (1989) Rehabilitation medicine and arthritis. In: McCarty DJ (ed) Arthritis and allied conditions. Lea and Febiger, Philadelphia
1614. Swett P (1938) A review of synovectomy. J Bone Joint Surg 20: 68
1615. Swift HF (1949) The etiology of rheumatic fever. Ann Intern Med 31: 715
1616. Swift HF, Boots RH (1923) Arthritis of serum sickness. JAMA 80: 12
1617. Sylven B, Paulson S, Hirsch C et al. (1951) Biophysical and physiologic investigations on cartilage and other mesenchymal tissue. J Bone Joint Surg [Am] 33: 333

1618. Talal N (1989) Sjoegren's syndrome. In: McCarty DJ (ed) Arthritis and allied conditions. Lea and Febiger, Philadelphia
1619. Talal N, Sylvester RA, Daniels TE et al. (1974) T and B lymphocytes in peripheral blood and tissue lesions. J Clin Invest 53: 188
1620. Talbott JH (1967) Gout. Grune and Stratton, New York
1621. Talbott JH, Coombs FS (1965) Metabolic studies on patients with gout. JAMA 110: 1977
1622. Talbott NB (1939) The effect of estrogen on the skeletal age of immature rats. Endocrinology 25: 325
1623. Tandler J (1929) Lehrbuch der systematischen Anatomie. Nervensystem und Sinnesorgane. Vogel, Leipzig
1624. Tannenbaum H, Schur PH (1974) The role of lymphocytes in rheumatic diseases. J Rheumatol 1: 392
1625. Taranta A (1989) Rheumatic fever. In: McCarty DJ (ed) Arthritis and allied condition. Lea and Febiger, Philadelphia
1626. Taranta A, Markowitz M (1981) Rheumatic fever. MTP Press, Boston
1627. Teel HM, Cushing H (1930) Studies in the physiological properties of the growth promoting extracts of the anterior hypophysis. Endocrinology 14: 157
1628. Tenenbaum MJ, Greenspan J, Kerkering TM (1981) Blastomycoses. Crit Rev Microbiol 9: 139
1629. Tesh RB (1982) Arthritides caused by mosquito-borne viruses. Ann Rev Med 33: 31
1630. Testa NN (1979) What's causing your patient's knee pain, and what to do about it. Mod Med (Chicago) 47: 24
1631. Testa NN, Potter LA (1985) Painful feet. In: McCarty JD (ed) Arthritis and allied conditions. Lea and Febiger, Philadelphia
1632. Thabe H (1980) Das Synovialhaemangiom des Kniegelenkes. Z Rheumatol. 39: 95
1633. Thannhauser SJ (1958) Lipidoses. Diseases of the intracellular lipid metabolism. Grune and Stratton, New York
1634. Thiemeyer JL (1954) Monarticular coccidioidal arthritis. J Bone Joint Surg [Am] 36: 387
1635. Thomas G (1966) Die Strecksteife des Kniegelenkes. Arch Orthop 60: 248
1636. Thomas J, Collipp PJ, Sharma RK (1981) Thyroid acropathy. Am J Dis Child 125: 745
1637. Thomas LB, Forkner CE, Frei E et al. (1961) The skeletal lesions of acute leukemia. Cancer 14: 608
1638. Thompson GR, Manshady BM, Weiss JJ (1978) Septic bursitis. JAMA 240: 2280
1639. Thompson RC, Robinson HJ (1981) Articular cartilage matrix metabolism. J Bone Joint Surg [Am] 63: 327
1640. Thornberry DR, Brandt DK, Rosenthal J (1982) Histoplasmosis presenting with joint pain and hilar adenopathy. Arthritis Rheum 25: 1396
1641. Thurner J (1984) Traumatische Gelenkerkrankungen. In: Aufdermaur M, Baur E, Fassbender HG et al. (eds) Pathologie der Gelenke und Weichteiltumoren, vol 1. Springer, Berlin Heidelberg New York, p 559 (Spezielle pathologische Anatomie, vol 18)
1642. Thurner J (1984) Gelenkprothesen. In: Aufdermaur M, Baur E, Fassbender HG et al. (eds) Pathologie der Gelenke und Weichteiltumoren, vol 1. Springer, Berlin Heidelberg New York, p 623 (Spezielle pathologische Anatomie, vol 18)
1643. Thurner J, Binazzi R (1978) Deformierende Insertionstendopathie. Wien. Med Wochenschr 128: 522
1644. Tillman K (1973) Chemische Synovektomie. Orthopädie 2: 10
1645. Tillman K (1983) Die operative Behandlung des polyarthritischen Schultergelenkes. Chir Praxis 30: 485
1646. Tillman K (1985) Dringliche Operations-Indikationen in der Rheumaorthopädie. Z Rheumatol 44: 26
1647. Tight RR, Warner JF (1976) Skeletal involvement in secondary syphilis detected by bone scanning. JAMA 235: 2326
1648. Todd AW (1932) Antigenic streptococcal hemolysin. J Exp Med 55: 267
1649. Todesco S (1981) Retinol-binding protein in rheumatoid arthritides. Arthritis Rheum 24: 105
1650. Todesco S, Punzi L, Montanaro D et al. (1976) Beta-2-microglobulin in synovial fluid of rheumatoid arthritis. Arthritis Rheum 19: 966
1651. Tooms RE (1987) Arthroplasty of ankle and knee. In: Crenshaw AH (ed) Campbell's operative orthopaedics. Mosby, St Louis
1652. Toone EC, Kelly J (1965) Joint and bone disease due to mycotic infection. Trans Am Clin Climatol Assoc 67: 91
1653. Torres J, Rathbun HK, Greenbough WB (1973) Pneumococcal arthritis: report of a case and review of literature. Johns Hopkins Med J 132: 234
1654. Townes AS (1967) Complement levels in disease. Johns Hopkins Med J 120: 337
1655. Townes AS, Sowa JM (1970) Complement in synovial fluid. Johns Hopkins Med J 127: 23
1656. Townley CO (1982) Hemi- and total articular replacement arthroplasty of the hip with the fixed femoral cup. Orthop Clin North Am 13: 869
1657. Townley CO (1983) The anatomic total knee resurfacing arthroplasty. Clin Orthop 192: 82
1658. Traldi A, Melanotte PL, Africano A et al. (1985) Twenty years experience with synovectomy for hemophilic arthropathy. In: Doehring S, Schulitz KP (eds) Orthopaedic problems in hemophilia. Zuckschwerdt, München
1659. Treves A (1957) Synovite syphilitique du genou. Rev Rhum Mal Osteoartic 24: 54
1660. Trumble HC (1937) Fixation of the hip joint by means of an extraarticular bone graft; late results. Br J Surg 24: 728

1661. (1976) Tuberculosis in USA (1976) US Public Health Service Publication CDC 76-8322
1662. (1981) Tuberculosis – United States (1980) MMWR 30: 325
1663. Tuli SM, Kumar K, Sen RC (1977) Penetration of antitubercular drugs in clinical osteoarticular tubercular lesions. Acta Orthop Scand 48: 362
1664. Turner AF, Budin K (1970) Arthrography of the knee: A simplified technique. Radiology 97: 505
1665. Turner JH (1983) Posttraumatic avascular necrosis of the femoral head predicted by preoperative technetium 99 m scan. J Bone Joint Surg [Am] 65: 786
1666. Turner R, Collins R, Nombir AM (1979) Extraarticular manifestations of rheumatoid arthritis. Bull Rheum Dis 29: 986 A
1667. Turner RH, Emmerson RH (1982) Femoral revision total hip arthroplasty. In: Turner RH, Scheller AD (eds) Revision total hip arthroplasty. Grune and Stratton, New York

1668. Umber F (1926) Die endokrine Periarthritis. Dtsch Med Wochenschr 52: 1631
1669. Urowitz MB, Gordon DA, Smythe HA et al. (1973) Azathioprine in rheumatoid arthritis. A double blind cross-over study. Arthritis Rheum 16: 411
1670. US Public Health Service (1969) Manual of tests for syphilis. US Public Health Service publication 411
1671. Utz JP, Garriques JL, Sande MA et al. (1975) Therapy of cryptococcosis with a combination of fluorocytosine and amphotericin B. J Infect Dis 132: 368

1672. Vainio K (1967) Arthroplasty of the elbow and hand in rheumatoid arthritis. In: Chapchal G (ed) Synovectomy and arthroplasty. Thieme, Stuttgart
1673. Valk J, MacLean C, Algra PR (1985) Basic principles of nuclear magnetic resonance imaging. Elsevier, Amsterdam
1674. Van Boxel JA, Paget SA (1975) Predominant T-cell infiltrate in rheumatoid synovial membrane. N Engl J Med 293: 517
1675. VanCreveld S, Hoedemaker PJ, Kingma MJ et al (1971) Degeneration of joints in hemophiliacs under treatment by modern methods. J Bone Surg [Br] 53: 296
1676. VanderLinden S, Valkenburg HA, Cats A (1984) Evaluation of diagnostic criteria for ankylosing spondylitis. Arthritis Rheum 27: 361
1677. VanPatter WN, Bargen JA, Dockerty NB (1954) Regional ileitis. Gastroenterology 26: 347
1678. VanSauter S, Utsinger PD (1978) Viral arthritis. Clin Rheum Dis 4: 225
1679. Vartiainen J, Hurri L (1964) Arthritis due to salmonella typhimurium. Acta Med Scand 175: 771
1680. Vasan N (1980) Proteoglycans in normal and severely osteoarthritic human articular cartilage. Biochem J 187: 781
1681. Vasey FB (1984) Spondyloarthropathies. Orthop Rev 13: 93
1682. Vaughan JH, Bayles TB, Favour CB (1951) Serum complement in rheumatoid arthritis. Am J Med Sci 222: 186
1683. Veil E (1929) Orale Sepsis and rheumatische Infektion. Zahnärztl Rundsch 38: 471
1684. Vendsborg P, Hansen LF, Olesen KH (1968) Decreasing incidence of a history of acute rheumatic heart disease. Cardiologia 33: 332
1685. Verse M (1912) Über Calcinosis universalis. Beitr Pathol Anat 53: 212
1686. Versfeld GA, Solomon A (1982) A diagnostic approach to tuberculosis of bones and joints. J Bone Joint Surg [Br] 64: 446
1687. Veys EM, VanLacre M (1973) Serum IgG, IgM and IgA levels in ankylosing spondylitis. Ann Rheum Dis 32: 493
1688. Victor M (1975) Polyneuropathy due to nutritional deficiency and alcoholism. In: Dyck PJ, Thomas PK, Lambert EH (eds) Peripheral neuropathy. Saunders, Philadelphia
1689. Vignon E, Arlet M (1978) Etude du cartilage arthrosique. Données histologique et histochimique. Rev Rhum Mal Osteoartic 45: 541
1690. Villiaumey J (1983) Les lésions extra-articulaires de la spondylarthrite ankylosante. Med Hyg 41: 1093
1691. Villiaumey J, Larget-Piet B (1973) Les osteo-arthropathies du diabète. Monde Med 83: 289
1692. Villiaumey J, Caron JP, Larget-Piet B et al. (1973) Arthropathie destructive de l'épaule revelatrice d'un syndrome syringomyelique. Rev Rhum Mal Osteoartic 40: 277
1693. Villiaumey J, Jean-Baptiste G (1980) Les lésions de la charnière cervico-occipitale au cours de la polyarthrite rhumatoide. Med Hyg 38: 1173
1694. Villiaumey J, Avouac B (1981) La chondrocalcinose articulaire. Encycl Med Chir Appar Locomotor 1427/A10: 4
1695. Virchow R (1866) Ein Fall von allgemeiner Ochronose der Knorpel und knorpelähnlichen Teile. Arch Pathol Anat 37: 212
1696. Vittorio N, Crissman JD, Hopson CM et al. (1986) Histologic assessment of cathepsin D in osteoarthritic cartilage. Clin Exp Rheumatol 4: 221
1697. Volkmann R (1882) Ganglion, Überbein. In: Pitha V, Billroth J (eds) Handbuch der allgemeinen und speziellen Chirurgie. Enke, Stuttgart
1698. Volpe R (1977) The role of autoimmune in hypoendocrine and hyperendocrine function with special emphasis on autoimmune thyroid disease. Ann Intern Med 87: 86

1699. Waaler E (1940) On occurrence of factor in human serum activating specific agglutination of sheep blood corpuscles. Acta Pathol Microbiol Scand 77: 173
1700. Wagenhäuser SJ (1969) Die Rheumamorbidität. Eine klinisch – epidemiologische Untersuchung. Huber, Bern
1701. Wagner H (1964) Traitement operatoire de l'osteochondrite dissequante, cause de l'arthrite deformante du genou. Rev Chir Orthop 50: 335
1702. Wagner H (1978) Surface replacement arthroplasty of the hip. Clin Orthop 134: 102
1703. Wagner H, Zeiler G, Bauer W (1985) Indikation, Technik und Ergebnisse der supra- und infracondylären Osteotomie bei Kniegelenkarthrose. Orthopädie 14: 172
1704. Wagner LC (1948) Fixed extension of knee due to capsular contraction. N Y State J Med 48: 194
1705. Waine H, Bennett GA, Bauer W (1945) Joint disease associated with acromegaly. Am J Med Sci 209: 671
1706. Waine H, Nevinny D, Rosenthal J et al. (1961) Association of osteoarthritis and diabetes mellitus. Tufts Folia Med 7: 13
1707. Waisman J (1982) Aspiration of thyroid nodules by fine needles. West J Med 136: 428
1708. Walker OR, Hall RA (1954) Coccidioidal tenosynovitis. J Bone Joint Surg [Am] 36 A: 391
1709. Walker RJ, Dymock JW, Ansell IA et al. (1972) Synovial biopsy in hemochromatosis arthropathy. Ann Rheum Dis 31: 98
1710. Wall JJ, Hunt DD (1968) Acute hematogenous pyarthrosis caused by hemophilus influenzae. J Bone Joint Surg [Am] 50: 1657
1711. Wallace SL, Robinson H, Masi AT et al. (1977) Preliminary criteria for the classification of the acute arthritis of primary gout. Arthritis Rheum 20: 895
1712. Ward LE, Cohen AS, Bauer W (1963) The diagnosis and therapy of acute suppurative arthritis. Arthritis Rheum 6: 650
1713. Wardle EN, Patton JT (1969) Bone and joint changes in hemochromatosis. Ann Rheum Dis 28: 15
1714. Warin RP, Evan CD, Hewitt M et al. (1957) Reticulohistiocytosis (lipoid dermatoarthritis). Br Med J 1: 1387
1715. Warr W, Bates JH, Stone A (1968) The spectrum of pulmonary cryptococcosis. Ann Intern Med 69: 1109
1716. Warren CPW (1970) Arthritis associated with Salmonella infections. Ann Rheum Dis 29: 483

1717. Wasserman A, Neisser A, Bruch C (1905) Eine serodiagnostische Reaktion bei Syphilis. Dtsch Med Wochenschr 32: 745
1718. Watanabe M (1979) Arthroscopy: the present state. Orthop Clin North Am 10: 505
1719. Watanabe M, Takeda S, Ikuchi H (1969) Atlas of arthroscopy. Igaku Shoin, Tokyo
1720. Watkins PJ (1982) Diabetic neuropathy. Br Med J 285: 493
1721. Waugh TR (1985) Total knee arthroplasty. Clin Orthop 192: 40
1722. Waugh TR, Smith RC, Orofino CF et al. (1973) Total knee replacement, operative technic and preliminary results. Clin Orthop 94: 179
1723. Waugh TR, Evanski PM, McMaster WC (1976) Ankle arthroplasty. Clin Orthop 114: 180
1724. Waugh TR, Soren A (1984) The ankle. In: Cruess RL, Rennie WRJ (eds) Adult orthopaedics. Livingstone, New York
1725. Weed LA, Dahlin DE, Pugh DG et al. (1952) Brucella in tissues removed at surgery. Am J Clin Pathol 22: 10
1726. Wegelin C (1928) Über falsche und echte Tumoren der Kniegelenkskapsel. Schweiz. Med Wochenschr 9: 722
1727. Weichselbaum A (1877) Die senilen Veränderungen der Gelenke und deren Zusammenhang mit der Arthritis deformans. Sitzungsber Akad Wiss Wien 75: 198
1728. Weichselbaum A (1889) Über seltenere Lokalizationen bei pneumonischen virus (Diplococcus pneumoniae). Wien. Klin Wochenschr 1: 659
1729. Weil MP (1947) Ne confondons pas rheumatisme et arthrite. Presse Med 55: 2
1730. Weinberger HJ (1962) Reiter's syndrome re-evaluated. Arthritis Rheum 5: 202
1731. Weiner AD, Ghormley RK (1956) Periodic benign synovitis. Idiopathic intermittent hydraarthrosis. J Bone Joint Surg [Am] 38: 1039
1732. Weiner MH, Yount WJ (1976) Mannan antigenemia in the diagnosis of invasive Candida infection. J Clin Invest 58: 1045
1733. Weinstein GD, Frost P (1971) Methotrexate for psoriasis. A new therapeutic schedule. Arch Dermatol 103: 33
1734. Weiss AS, Markenson JA, Weiss MS et al. (1978) Toxicity of D-penicillimine in rheumatoid arthritis. Am J Med 64: 114
1735. Weiss C, Mirrow S (1972) An ultrastructural study of osteoarthritic changes in the articular cartilage of human knees. J Bone Joint Surg [Am] 54: 954
1736. Weissman G (1966) Lysosomes and joint disease. Arthritis Rheum Dis 9: 834
1737. Weissman G (1976) Rheumatoid arthritis: how the nonsteroidal antiinflammatory agents work. Med Times 104/9: 64
1738. Weissman G (1984) Pathways of arachidone oxidation to prostaglandins and leukotrienes. Semin Arthritis Rheum 13: 123
1739. Weissman G, Pras M, Rosenberg L (1967) Arthritis induced by filipin in rabbits. Arthritis Rheum 19: 325
1740. Weissman G, Spilberg I (1968) Breakdown of cartilage protein polysaccharide by lysosomes. Arthritis Rheum 11: 162
1741. Weitzman G (1965) Lipoma arborescens of the knee: report of a case. J Bone Joint Surg [Am] 47: 1030
1742. Werblin TP, Rheinstrom SD, Kaufman HE (1981) The use of slow release artificial tears in the longterm management of keratitis sicca. Ophthalmology 88: 78
1743. Wernicke C (1881) Lehrbuch der Gehirnkrankheiten für Ärzte und Studierende. Fischer, Kassel
1744. Woolley DE, Crossley JJ, Evason JM (1977) Collagenase at sites of cartilage erosion in the rheumatoid joint. Arthritis Rheum 20: 1231
1745. Weseloh G (1985) Indications and preoperative considerations for surgical treatment. In: Doehring S, Schulitz KP (eds) Orthopaedic problems in hemophilia. Zuckschwerdt, München
1746. Whaley K, Williamson J, Chisholm MD et al (1973) Sjoegren's syndrome: I. Sera components. Q J Med 42: 279
1747. Whaley K, Webb J, McAvoy B et al. (1973) Sjoegren's Syndrome: II. Clinical associations and immunological phenomena. Q J Med 42: 513
1748. Whaley K, Alspaugh NA (1985) Sjoegren's syndrome. In: Kelley WN, Harris ED, Ruddy S, Sledge CB (eds) Textbook of rheumatology. Saunders, Philadelphia
1749. White TG, Peels JL, Mikitans FK (1977) Rabbit arthritis induced by cell free extract of erysipelothrix. Infect Immun 3: 715
1750. White SH, Newcomer V, Mickey M et al. (1972) Disturbance of HLA-antigen frequency in psoriasis. N Engl J Med 287: 740
1751. Whitnack E, Stollerman GH (1985) Antistreptococcal antibodies in the diagnosis of rheumatic fever. In: Cohen AS (ed) Laboratory diagnostic procedures in the rheumatic diseases. Grune and Stratton, Orlando
1752. Widdowsen JP, Maxsted WR, Notley CM et al. (1974) The antibody responses in man to infection with different serotypes of group A streptococci. J Med Microbiol 7: 483
1753. Wiernik PH (1972) Amyloid joint disease. Medicine (Baltimore) 51: 465
1754. Wilding K, Nade S (1975) Actinomycosis of bone. Aust N Z J Surg 45: 61
1755. Wiles P, Andrews OL, Bremner RA (1960) Chondromalacia of the patella. J Bone Joint Surg [Br] 42: 65
1756. Wiley AM, Older NVJ (1980) Shoulder arthroscopy. Investigations with a fibro-optic instrument. Am J Sports Med 8: 31
1757. Willkens RF, Watson MF, Paxon CS (1980) Low dosemethotrexate therapy in rheumatoid arthritis. J Rheumatol 7: 501
1758. Willkens RF, Arnett FC, Bitter T et al. (1982) Reiter's syndrome. Evaluation of preliminary criteria for definite disease. Bull Rheum Dis 32: 31
1759. Wilkinson MC (1955) The treatment of tuberculosis of the spine by evacuation of paravertebral abscess and curettage of vertebral bodies. J Bone Joint Surg [Br] 37: 382
1760. Wilkinson MC (1969) Tuberculosis of the hip and knee treated by chemotherapy, synovectomy, and debridement. J Bone Joint Surg [Am] 51: 1343
1761. Willems C (1919) Treatment of purulent arthritis by wide arthrotomy followed by immediate active mobilization. Surg Gynecol Obstet 28: 546
1762. Williams JGP (1977) Surgical management of traumatic noninfective tenosynovitis of the wrist. J Bone Joint Surg [Br] 59: 408
1763. Williams DN, Goddes AM (1970) Meningococcal meningitis complicated by pericarditis, panophthalmitis and arthritis. Br Med J 2: 93
1764. Williams PO (1952) The assessment of mobility in joints. Lancet 2: 169
1765. Williams RC, DeBoard JR, Mellbye PJ et al. (1973) Studies of the T and B lymphocytes in patients with connective tissue diseases. J Clin Invest 52: 283
1766. Williams RC, McCarty DJ (1985) Clinical picture of rheumatoid arthritis. In: McCarty DJ (ed) Arthritis and allied conditions. Lea and Febiger, Philadelphia
1767. Williams WJ, Bentler E, Eislev AJ et al. (1990) Hematology. McGraw-Hill, New York
1768. Williamson J, Dvig WM, Forrester JV et al. (1984) Management of the dry eye in Sjoegren's syndrome. Br J Ophthalmol 58: 798
1769. Willis RA (1967) Pathology of tumours Butterworths, London
1770. Wilson FC (1976) Total replacement of the knee in rheumatoid arthritis. Part II of a prospective study. Clin Orthop 120: 39
1771. Wilson MG (1962) Advances in rheumatic fever 1942–1961. Harper and Row, New York

1772. Wilson NIL, DiPaola M (1986) Acute septic arthritis in infancy and childhood. J Bone Joint Surg [Br] 68: 584
1773. Wilson PD, Eyre-Brook AL, Francis JD (1938) A clinical and anatomical study of the semimembranous bursa in relation to popliteal cyst. J Bone Joint Surg 20: 963
1774. Winchester RJ, Agnello V, Kunkel HG (1970) The joint fluid G-globulin complexes and their relations to intraarticular complement diminution. Ann N Y Acad Sci 168: 195
1775. Winter FE, Runyon EH (1965) Prepatellar bursitis caused by mycobacterium marinum. J Bone Joint Surg [Am] 47: 375
1776. Winter WG, Larson RK, Honeggar MM et al. (1975) Coccidioidal arthritis and its treatment. J Bone Joint Surg [Am] 57: 1152
1777. Wintrobe MM, Lee GR, Boggs DR et al. (1984) Clinical hematology. Lea and Febiger, Philadelphia
1778. Woessner JF, Sapolsky AL (1975) Breakdown of protein polysaccharide complexes by cartilage proteases. Ann Rheum Dis 34: S 67
1779. Wolfgang GL (1978) Tuberculosis joint infection. Clin Orthop 136: 257
1780. Wolkow M, Baumann W (1891) Über das Wesen der Alkaptonurie. Z Physiol Chem 15. 288
1781. Woo RYG, Morrey BF (1982) Dislocation after total hip arthroplasty. J Bone Joint Surg [Am] 64: 1295
1782. Woodruff JM, Erlandson RA, Horten BC (1989) Pathology of peripheral nerves and gangliomas. In: Silverberg G (ed) Principles and practice of surgical patholgy. Churchill Livingstone, New York
1783. Woolley DE, Crossley JJ, Evanson JM (1977) Collagenase at sites of cartilage erosion in the rheumatoid joint. Arthritis Rheum 20: 1231
1784. Worrell RV (1975) A comparison of patellectomy and prosthetic replacement of the patella. Clin Orthop 111: 284
1785. Wright PH, Sim FH, Soule EH et al. (1982) Synovial sarcoma. J Bone Joint Surg [Am] 64: 112
1786. Wright-Smith RJ (1945) The pathology of rheumatic carditis. R Melbourne Hosp Clin Rep 16: 13
1787. Wright V (1965) The diagnosis of Reiter's syndrome. Rheumatism 21: 30
1788. Wright V (1979) Conference on measurement of joint movement. Rheumatol Rehabil 18: 261
1789. Wright V (1985) Psoriatic arthritis. In: Kelley WN, Harris ED, Ruddy L, Sledge LB (eds) Textbook of rheumatology. Saunders, Philadelphia
1790. Wright V, Watkinson G (1965) The arthritis of ulcerative colitis. Br Med J 11: 670
1791. Wright V, Dawson D (1976) Lubrication and cartilage. J Anat 121: 187
1792. Wroblewski MV, delSol HJ (1980) Urethral instrumentation and deep sepsis in total hip replacement. Clin Orthop 146: 209
1793. Wustman C (1925) Beitrag zur Frage der xanthomatösen Riesenzellenneubildungen. Dtsch Z Chir 192: 380
1794. Wyke B (1981) The neurology of joints: a review of general principles. Clin Rheum Dis 7: 223
1795. Wyllie JC (1969) The stromal cell reaction of pigmented villonodular synovitis: an electron microscopic study. Arthritis Rheum 12: 205
1796. Wyllie JC (1983) Histopathology of the subchondral bone lesion in rheumatoid arthritis. J Rheumatol 10: S 11–26
1797. Wyngaarden JB (1974) Metabolic defects of primary hyperuricemia and gout. Am J Med 56: 651

1798. Yacobucci GN, Scutilli MD (1981) Sporotrichosis of the knee. Orthopedics 9: 387
1799. Yates DB, Maini RN, Scott JT et al. (1975) Complement activation in Reiter's syndrome. Ann Rheum Dis 34: 468
1800. Yee NM, Katz M, Neu HC (1975) Meningitis, pneumonitis and arthritis caused by Neisseria meningitidis group Y. JAMA 232: 1354
1801. Youmans GP (1975) Histoplasmosis, coccidioidomycosis, blastomycosis. In: Youmans GP, Paterson PJ, Sommers HM (eds) The biological and clinical basis of infectious diseases. Saunders, Philadelphia
1802. Young JM, Houdacek AG (1954) Experimental production of pigmented villonodular synovitis in dogs. Am J Pathol 30: 799
1803. Yu TF (1982) The efficacy of colchicine prophylaxis in articular gout. Semin Arthritis Rheum 12: 256
1804. Yunus M, Calabro JJ, Miller KA et al. (1981) Family studies with HLA typing in Reiter's syndrome. Am J Med 70: 1210
1805. Yunus M, Maso AJ, Calabro JJ et al. (1981) Primary fibromyalgia (fibrositis): clinical study of 50 patients and matched normal controls. Semin Arthritis Rheum 11: 151

1806. Zagala IG, Feinstein AR (1962) The preceding illness of acute rheumatic fever. JAMA 179: 863
1807. Zampa G (1933) Lo stato anafilattico nella genesi de alcune artropathia. Chir Organi Mov 18: 12
1808. Zanasi R (1962) Artrosinovite chroniche aspecifiche asettiche del ginocchio (anatomia patologica). Chir Organi Mov 48: 89
1809. Zenni EJ, Carothers JA (1980) Total knee arthroplasty, current state of the art. Orthop Rev 9: 51
1810. Ziff M (1971) Viruses and the connective tissue diseases. Ann Intern Med 75: 957
1811. Ziff M (1974) Relation of cellular infiltration of rheumatoid synovial membrane to its immune response. Arthritis Rheum 17: 313
1812. Ziff M (1977) Immunological aspects of rheumatoid synovitis – 25 years. Arthritis Rheum 20: S31
1813. Ziff M (1979) General mechanisms of inflammations in rheumatoid arthritis. Bull Schweiz Akad Wiss 35: 275
1814. Ziff M (1983) Factors involved in cartilage injury. J Rheumatol 10 (suppl 11): 13
1815. Zitnan D, Sitaj L (1963) Chondrocalcinosis articularis: I. Clinical and radiological study. Ann Rheum Dis 22: 142
1816. Zizic TM, Marcoux C, Hungerford DS et al. (1983) Radiography, scintigraphy, and hemodynamics. Diagnosis of ischemic necrosis of bone (abstr) Arthritis Rheum 26: S 37
1817. Zizic TM, Hungerford VS (1985) Avascular necrosis of bone. In: Kelley WN, Harris ED, Ruddy S, Sledge CB (eds) Textbook of rheumatology. Saunders, Philadelphia
1818. Zubler RH, Nydegger U, Perrin LH et al. (1976) Circulating and intraarticular immune complexes in patients with rheumatoid arthritis. J Clin Invest 57: 1308
1819. Zucker-Franklin D (1966) The phagosomes in rheumatoid synovial fluid leukocytes. A light, fluorescence and electron microscope study. Arthritis Rheum 9: 24
1820. Zuckner J, Baldassare A, Chang F et al. (1977) High synovial fluid leukocyte count of noninfectious etiology. Arthritis Rheum 20: 270
1821. Zvaifler NJ (1960) Chronic postrheumatic fever (Jacoud's arthritis). N Engl J Med 207: 10
1822. Zvaifler NJ (1973) Immunopathology of joint inflammation in rheumatoid arthritis. Adv Immunol 16: 265
1823. Zvaifler NJ, Martel V (1960) Spondylitis in chronic ulcerative colitis. Arthritis Rheum 3: 76
1824. Zvaifler NJ, Reefe WE, Black RL (1960) Articular manifestations in primary hyperparathyroidism. Arthritis Rheum 5: 237
1825. Zwahlen P (1935) Sur les sarcomes des gaines tendineuses. Bull Assoc Fr Etude Cancer 24: 682

Index